Occupational
Therapy
for Children

Occupational Therapy

for Children

4th edition

Edited by

Jane Case-Smith, EdD, OTR/L, FAOTA

Associate Professor
Occupational Therapy Division
The Ohio State University
Columbus, Ohio

with illustrations by
Jeanne Robertson
Jody Fulks, MS, medical illustrator
Ted Bolte

40 *contributors*
297 *illustrations*

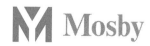 Mosby

A Harcourt Health Sciences Company

St. Louis   London   Philadelphia   Sydney   Toronto

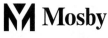
Mosby

A Harcourt Health Sciences Company

Editor in Chief John Schrefer
Editor Kellie White
Associate Developmental Editor Leslie Mosby
Project Manager Linda McKinley
Project Specialist Rich Barber
Cover Design Stephanie Foley
Internal Design Dana Peick
Design Manager Amy Buxton

Mosby, Inc.
A Harcourt Health Sciences Company
11830 Westline Industrial Drive
St. Louis, Missouri 63146

Printed in the United States of America

ISBN 0-323-00764-3

00 01 02 03 04 CL/KPT 9   8   7   6   5   4   3   2   1

contributors

Susan J. Amundson, MS, OTR/L
Executive Director
O.T. Kids, Inc.
Homer, Alaska

Jill Anderson, MS, OTR/L
Supervisor, Occupational Therapy
Step by Step Infant Development Center
Brooklyn, New York
Occupational Therapy Early Intervention
Herbert G. Birch Early Childhood Center
Jamaica, New York
Adjunct Clinical Professor
Occupational Therapy Program
New York University
New York, New York

Beth Ann Ball, MS, OTR/L
Occupational Therapist
Columbus Public Schools
Columbus, Ohio

Margaret J. Barnstorff, MOT, OTR
Occupational Therapist
Poudre School District
Private Practice
Pediatric Therapy Associates
Fort Collins, Colorado

Anne F. Cronin, PhD, OTR, BCP
Assistant Professor
Division of Occupational Therapy
West Virginia University
Morgantown, West Virginia

Debora A. Davidson, MS, OTR
Assistant Professor
Occupational Therapy Program
School of Health Professions
Maryville University
St. Louis, Missouri

Brian J. Dudgeon, MS, OTR
Lecturer
Department of Rehabilitation Medicine
University of Washington
Seattle, Washington

Snaefridur Thora Egilson, MS, OT
Assistant Professor
Occupational Therapy Program
Department of Health Sciences
University of Akureyri
Akureyri, Iceland

Charlotte E. Exner, PhD, OTR/L, BCP, FAOTA
Professor
Occupational Therapy
Acting Dean
College of Health Professions
Towson University
Towson, Maryland

Sharon G. Gartland, MA, OTR/L
Staff Therapist
Chicago Public Schools
Adjunct Instructor
Department of Occupational Therapy
University of Illinois
Chicago, Illinois

Catherine Yanega Gordon, EdD, OTR/L
Associate Professor and Chairperson
Department of Occupational Therapy
Ithaca College
Ithaca, New York

Ruth Humphry, PhD, OTR/L
Associate Professor
Division of Occupational Science
University of North Carolina
Chapel Hill, North Carolina

Jan G. Hunter, MA, OTR
Neonatal Clinical Specialist
Children's Hospital
Assistant Professor
Department of Occupational Therapy
School of Allied Health
University of Texas Medical Branch
Galveston, Texas

Jan Haas Johnson, OTR/L, BS, MS
Occupational Therapist
Patagonia Elementary School
Patagonia, Arizona

Mary Law, PhD, OT(C)
Professor and Co-Director
CanChild Centre for Childhood Disability Research
School of Rehabilitation Science
McMaster University
Hamilton, Ontario, Canada

Zoe Mailloux, MA, OTR, FAOTA
Director of Administration and Practice
Pediatric Therapy Network
Torrance, California

Peggy Metzger, MS, OTR/L
Staff Therapist
Northwestern Illinois Association
Geneva, Illinois

Cheryl Missiuna, PhD, OT(C)
Assistant Professor
School of Rehabilitation Science
Co-Investigator
CanChild Centre for Childhood Disability Research
McMaster University
Hamilton, Ontario, Canada

Christine Doyle Morrison, MS, OTR/L
Pediatric Occupational Therapist
Brookfield, Illinois

Deborah S. Nichols, PhD, PT
Director and Associate Professor
Physical Therapy Division
The Ohio State University
Columbus, Ohio

L. Diane Parham, PhD, OTR, FAOTA
Associate Professor
Department of Occupational Science and Occupational
  Therapy
University of Southern California
Los Angeles, California
Director of Research and Education
Pediatric Therapy Network
Torrance, California

Nancy Pollock, MSc, OT
Associate Clinical Professor
School of Rehabilitation Science
Co-Investigator
CanChild Centre for Childhood Disability Research
McMaster University
Hamilton, Ontario, Canada

Pamela K. Richardson, PhD, OTR
Assistant Professor
Department of Occupational Therapy
San José State University
San José, California

Jan Rogers, MS, OTR/L
Private Practice
Pickerington, Ohio

Sandra L. Rogers, PhD, OTR
Assistant Professor
Occupational Therapy Division
The Ohio State University
Columbus, Ohio

Karen E. Schanzenbacher, MS, OTR/L
Occupational Therapist
Cattaraugus—Allegany Board of Cooperative
  Education Services
Olean, New York

Colleen M. Schneck, ScD, OTR/L, FAOTA
Professor
Department of Occupational Therapy
Eastern Kentucky University
Richmond, Kentucky

Joanne S. Schoelkopf, MBA, OTR/L
Contract Occupational Therapist
Orange County Public Schools
Pediatric Services of America (PSA) Kids Medical Club
Orlando, Florida

Winifred Schultz-Krohn, MA, OTR, BCP, FAOTA
Assistant Professor of Occupational Therapy
Department of Occupational Therapy
San José State University
San José, California

Jayne Shepherd, MS, OTR
Assistant Professor
Department of Occupational Therapy
Virginia Commonwealth University
Richmond, Virginia

Elizabeth Snow-Russel, PhD(c), OTR
Consultant
Burbank, California

Karen C. Spencer, PhD, OTR
Associate Professor
Department of Occupational Therapy
Colorado State University
Fort Collins, Colorado

Linda C. Stephens, MS, OTR/L, FAOTA
Director and Owner
Atlanta Children's Therapy, Inc.
Atlanta, Georgia

Debra Stewart, MSc, OT
Assistant Clinical Professor
School of Rehabilitation Science
Research Coordinator
CanChild Centre for Childhood Disability Research
McMaster University
Hamilton, Ontario, Canada

Katherine B. Stewart, MS, OTR/L, FAOTA
Clinical Associate Professor
School of Occupational Therapy and Physical Therapy
University of Puget Sound
Tacoma, Washington

Yvonne Swinth, PhD, OTR/L
Assistant Professor
School of Occupational Therapy and Physical Therapy
University of Puget Sound
Tacoma, Washington

Susan K. Tauber
Executive Director
Adaptive Learning Center for Infants & Children, Inc.
Atlanta, Georgia

Barbara B. Marin Wavrek, MHS, OTR/L
Lecturer
Occupational Therapy Division
The Ohio State University
Columbus, Ohio

Marsha Weil, MS, OTR/L
Occupational Therapist
Bellevue School District
Bellevue, Washington

Christine Wright-Ott, MPA, OTR
Occupational Therapist
Rehabilitation Technology & Therapy Center
Lucile Packard Health Services at Stanford
Palo Alto, California

foreword

One measure of civilization is the value it places on its children. Jane Case-Smith, EdD, OTR/L, FAOTA, the editor of the fourth edition of *Occupational Therapy for Children,* has combined her expertise with that of colleagues to create a comprehensive introduction to pediatric occupational therapy that reflects this valuing of children. The book, although designed specifically as a pediatric text for entry-level students, is equally useful as a resource for practicing therapists.

The strengths of this text include its comprehensiveness, its overall organization, and the study aids included in each chapter. The book lays the foundation for occupational therapy practice and identifies the broad knowledge base required for this endeavor. Building on this foundation, the book progresses logically from assessment through intervention with specific foci on postural control, hand function, visual perception, psychosocial and emotional development, feeding and oral motor skills, self-care and adaptation for independent living, play, handwriting, augmentative communication and computer access, and mobility. Specific strengths in content that merit emphases are the attention to the psychosocial development and needs of children, the use of technology to increase function, the importance of families and others in the child's system through the continuing process of adaptation, and the legislation that is relevant to children with disabilities and their families.

The book's concluding section on arenas of pediatric occupational therapy practice is addressed from a developmental perspective. This section provides integrative function, facilitating understanding of the therapy process starting in the neonatal intensive care unit, progressing through early intervention and preschool and school programs, and appropriately concluding with the transitioning from school to adult life. For pediatric therapists this longitudinal perspective assists with understanding a child's program within the context of the child's past, present, and future.

Understanding of the needs of students when using a textbook is reflected in the editor's careful inclusion of study aids in each chapter. Key terms, chapter objectives, and study questions are strategically offered to guide learning and provide opportunities to apply and integrate knowledge.

The editor has coordinated the efforts of an impressive group of authors, reflecting a broad range of expertise in pediatric practice. The diverse and rich contributions of these individuals are organized logically and meaningfully so that this knowledge can be used by students and therapists who work daily to facilitate the potential of children to play, to care for themselves, and to work. The fourth edition of *Occupational Therapy for Children* reflects caring, empowering, and respect. It is a treasure for occupational therapists and for children with disabilities and their families.

Jean Deitz, PhD, OTR/L, FAOTA
Professor and Graduate Program Coordinator
Department of Rehabilitation Medicine
University of Washington

preface

Since the first edition of *Occupational Therapy for Children* was published, the practice of occupational therapy has experienced tremendous growth and change. In the first edition of this book, Pratt and Allen described the roles and functions of pediatric occupational therapists, the core knowledge of the profession, and the occupational therapy process as it existed in 1983. Because this comprehensive text was essentially the first to describe occupational therapy with children, many educational programs adopted it.

Approximately 3 years later, Pratt and Allen began a text revision that was published in 1989, adding content specific to the treatment of cerebral palsy, changing the assessments presentation, and adding a section on management.

In the 1990s the field of occupational therapy expanded, and its leaders, scholars, and researchers refined core theories and practices. External forces, including new legislation and federal programs, brought about some of the changes in the profession. Amendments to the Individuals with Disabilities Education Act (IDEA, 1990, 1997) had significant impact on service delivery by increasing services to infants and young children and their families, improving access to assistive technology in schools, and encouraging inclusion. The Americans with Disabilities Act (1990) increased opportunities for occupational therapists to assume roles as consultants, helping organizations and agencies make accommodations for individuals with disabilities. Maternal Child Health Training Grants promoted the development of pediatric occupational therapy throughout the 1980s and 1990s by funding university programs and supporting conferences on pediatric occupational therapy.

In addition to legislative changes and government-supported programs, professional resources and focused research studies that were new at the time supported pediatric occupational therapy practice. Internal forces of the profession included the works of the members of the American Occupational Therapy Association to define best practices and to join with other disciplines to articulate the national issues affecting the care of young children with disabilities and their families.

The third and fourth editions of *Occupational Therapy for Children* reflect many of these changes brought about by the research and legislation of the 1980s and 1990s. These editions also acknowledge our continual refinements of the theories that are core to occupational therapy practice. The cadre of authors represents experts in the specialty areas of pediatric practice; they bring their insights and experience-based knowledge to the reader.

The current edition has four sections with complementary purposes. Section I describes foundational knowledge that forms the basis for pediatric practice. This section uses theories of human development and occupation as a basis for understanding the child's acquisition of functional skills and social roles. Models of practice that evolve from theory are described. These theories and models serve as guideposts for making clinical decisions and for designing occupational therapy programs. Theories and models presented in Section I are exemplified throughout the text.

Additional changes in the first section include expanded and updated information on physical disabilities and neurologic problems. The chapter on families has been revised to reflect the great variation in current family structures and life styles. Family-centered intervention as a philosophy and practice is described and applied to families of diversity. To exemplify this philosophy, Section I concludes with a discussion of strategies for supporting families who struggle with socioeconomic and health issues.

Section II includes three chapters on occupational therapy assessment of children. Evaluation is explained as a process in Chapter 7, focusing on analysis of functional performance within natural contexts. Chapter 8 describes how to administer standardized tests and interpret the findings. Chapter 9 builds on the first two by explaining how evaluation information is synthesized with intervention goals and the development of an intervention plan. Section II explains the critical nature of occupational therapy evaluation to the family's understanding of the child and the team's ability to establish a comprehensive plan.

Performance areas of importance to occupational therapy are described in detail in Section III. These chapters have been updated in the fourth edition to include information on revised models of practice, advocated service delivery models, recently developed intervention methods, and new technology. Research findings are used to define a scientific base for occupational therapy practices, and efficacy study results are presented to lend support to the interventions described. The evolution of our theoretical approaches is documented in this third section. Intervention using sensory integration theory has changed based on recent research using the Sensory Integration and Praxis Tests and new measures of sensory responsivity. Children's sensory processing abilities, which are affected in many developmental disorders, are recognized as an important basis for functional performance. Neurodevelopmental theories have been expanded to include motor learning, motor control, and dynamical systems theories. Our understanding of the use of play in intervention and the variables that relate to playfulness has increased.

Section IV describes arenas of occupational therapy practice. This section was developed in recognition of the importance of the environment to the child's performance. Current practice has shifted from an emphasis on the individual to the individual within his or her social and physical environments. Therefore the performance areas addressed in therapy must always consider the demands and resources of the child's environment. In many cases, the goals of occupational therapy shift from changing the individual to modifying the environment, enabling therapy to support the child's performance and functional independence. This section explains how the selection of intervention approaches and service delivery models relate to the systems in which the occupational therapist practices. Contrasting examples of therapy in medical, community, private practice, residential, and educational environments illustrate the varying roles of occupational therapists. A developmental framework (birth to adulthood) organizes Section IV on the arenas of practice. This life-span perspective helps promote understanding of how occupational therapists manage the functional problems imposed by disabilities at different ages and in different contexts. For example, early intervention services with infants who have neuromotor impairments are essentially different from school-based services. Developmental theories, although critical for young children, are less important as the child enters school and develops compensatory strategies for functioning in the classroom.

The text also emphasizes cultural competence. The case studies exemplify children of different cultures and emphasize cultural sensitivity in evaluation and intervention. Case studies that emphasize the child's social and physical context have greater potential to teach clinical reasoning than those studies that emphasize clinical information.

We have maintained the primary purpose of the book as an undergraduate text; however, we recognize that some of the content is beyond entry level. For example, the chapter on practice in the neonatal intensive care setting reflects advanced knowledge and skill required to work with preterm infants. Chapters on mobility and augmentative communication also contain information relevant to specialized areas of practice. Reference and resource lists provide helpful information to practitioners who may continue to use the text. In the interest of manageable book size, information on low incidence conditions is presented only when illustrating a frame of reference, intervention approach, or practice setting.

I acknowledge with gratitude those who have contributed to this book and have guided its development. Many clinicians, too many to list, helped inspire the authors and me to present information that is helpful in developing professional skills. Clinicians who have guided me and assisted in developing the chapters include Beth Ball, Mary Stover, Debora Davidson, Jan Rogers, Cindy Iski, Lori Schoeppner, Cathy Tela, and Becky Selegue. I also acknowledge the original editors of the book, Pat Pratt and Anne Allen, who established a comprehensive text that described pediatric occupational therapy using theories and philosophies of the profession in combination with examples of clinical practice. Mosby editors have been resourceful and helpful in developing this edition. In particular, I appreciate the expertise and support of Dana Peick and Leslie Mosby. Finally, I acknowledge my family, Greg, David, and Stephen, for their ongoing support and patience. They have donated many "family hours" to the mission of completing this text.

Jane Case-Smith, EdD, OTR/L, FAOTA

contents

Occupational
Therapy
for Children

section **1**

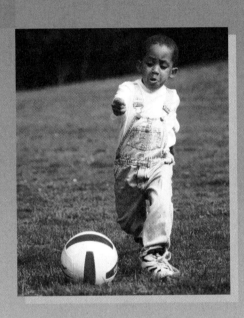

KNOWLEDGE BASE OF OCCUPATIONAL THERAPY IN PEDIATRICS

chapter 1

An Overview of Occupational Therapy for Children

Jane Case-Smith

key terms

Participation
Activity
Impairment
Clinical reasoning
Emerging technology
Natural environments
Evidence-based practice

■ CHAPTER OBJECTIVES

1. Explain how occupational therapists use clinical reasoning in the evaluation process.
2. Apply the International Classifications of Impairment, Activities and Participation in evaluation and intervention planning.
3. Explain a model that defines the aims and strategies of occupational therapy intervention to children and families.
4. Discuss models of service delivery used in a child's natural environment.
5. Explain emerging trends in assistive technology.
6. Discuss evidenced-based practice of occupational therapy with children.

A child's job of growing into adulthood involves continual adaptation to the demands of the environment and assimilation of its opportunities. The dynamic nature of this interaction is created by the child's internal clock of maturation as he or she adapts to a changing environment. Changes in the child's physical and social environment are influenced by his or her developmental needs and by variables external to the child. For example, the caregiver adapts the level of assistance provided during bathing and dressing activities as the child gains independence. Likewise, the caregiver's interactions with the child may change if the caregiver becomes ill or begins new employment. These changes in the child's social environment may prompt unexpected independence in self-care.

Occupational therapy practice is based on an understanding of the interactions among children, their activities, and their environments. Therefore when occupational therapists evaluate a child's performance, they determine whether limitations in performance relate primarily to the child's innate ability or to external factors in the environment. Occupational therapists have yet to unravel the complexity of the interrelationships between environment and person; however, their analyses of these relationships within individual scenarios can foster sound clinical decisions. At the same time that occupational therapists systematically analyze the child's functional performance and impairments, they acknowledge that the spirit of the child determines who he or she is and will become.

This text presents theories, principles, and strategies that are used in occupational therapy with children. Its pages present intervention strategies to help children cope with disability and master activities that have meaning to them. Although this theoretical and technical information is important to occupational therapy practice with children, it is childhood, itself, that creates meaning for the practitioner. Childhood is hopeful, joyful, and ever new. The spirit, the playfulness, and the joy of childhood create the context for occupational therapy with children.

The first section of this chapter describes how occupational therapists use clinical reasoning in evaluation and intervention planning. The process of evaluating participation, activities, and impairments is described. Interventions that (1) establish a higher level of functioning, (2) compensate for activity limitations through adaptation and assistive technology, (3) modify environments, or (4) change systems to increase participation are defined. The second section of this chapter discusses best-practice concepts in pediatric occupational therapy.

■ CLINICAL REASONING IN EVALUATION

Participation and Participation Restrictions

The occupational therapist begins his or her assessment of the child by gaining an understanding of the child's *level of participation in daily activities* with his or her family and in preschool or school activities with other adults and peers (Figure 1-1). Initially, the therapist surveys multiple sources to acquire a "sense" of the child's performance and to form a picture of the child. This initial picture is based on (1) concerns of the parents, (2) concerns of other adults who interact with the child, (3) informal observations of the child in his or her natural environment, (4) administration of a screening instrument, and (5) review of evaluation reports written about the child by other professionals. This background information gives the occupational therapist a direction for

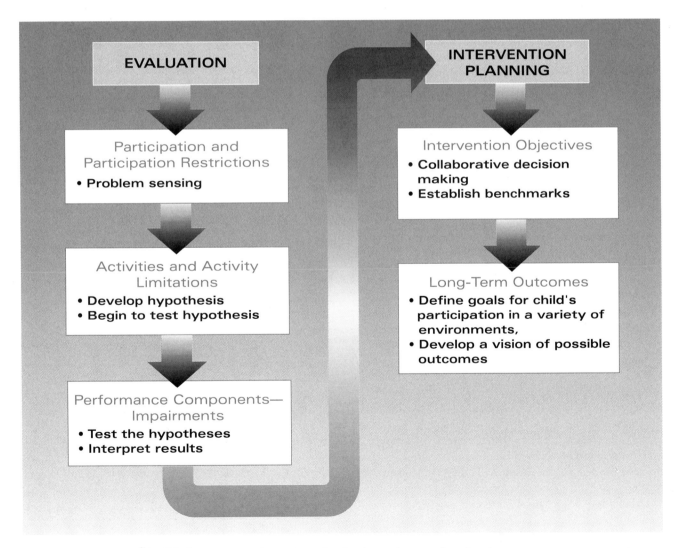

figure**1-1**   Conceptual overview of evaluation to intervention planning process.

additional, more intense evaluation, as it raises awareness of the issues defining the problem.

Underpinning the occupational therapist's evaluation and intervention is clinical reasoning (Table 1-1). Two types of reasoning are emphasized when the therapist first gathers data about a child's social and physical participation. First, *procedural reasoning* is used to gather and organize facts about the child, environment, and activity limitations. This initial process is termed *problem sensing*. Identifying information, which is needed to plan intervention, is a primary objective of surveying the child's ability to participate in multiple environments and in various social roles (Figure 1-2). Initial assessment of the child's participation also involves evaluating the environment to identify problems or potential problems that appear to affect the child's participation.

Narrative reasoning is also used to assess a child's participation in his or her environments. In narrative reasoning, the therapist identifies which story he or she is in with the child. Over time, the story unfolds as the therapist gains understanding of the child, family, and context. Mattingly (1994) explains that prospective stories are useful because they give the therapist a starting point for evaluation; however, the therapist willingly adjusts and adapts the story as new information becomes known. This unique story assists the occupational therapist in identifying what is significant and meaningful to the child (Figure 1-3). The occupational therapist uses the story to

create meaningful experiences that engage the child and are valued by the child and his or her family. For example, the child who loves to go fishing with a grandfather may be highly motivated by a fishing expedition in a "rocking boat" in the preschool's gross motor room. Meaningful

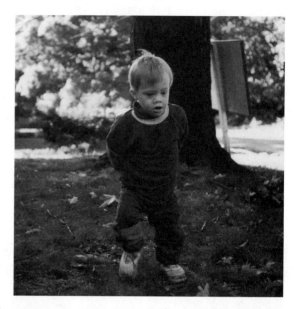

figure**1-2** Assessment in multiple environments familiar to the child gives the therapist a complete picture of the child's function.

	table **1-1**	**Clinical Reasoning Involved in Evaluation and Intervention Planning**
Step	**Phase of Problem Solving**	**Clinical Reasoning**
EVALUATION		
Participation	Problem sensing	Procedural Narrative
Activities; activity limitations	Hypothesis generation Hypothesis testing	Procedural Interactive Narrative
Performance components; impairments	Cue interpretation Hypothesis testing	Procedural Narrative
INTERVENTION PLANNING		
Setting objectives	Collaborative decision making	Conditional Pragmatic
Establishing long-term goals	Visioning	Conditional

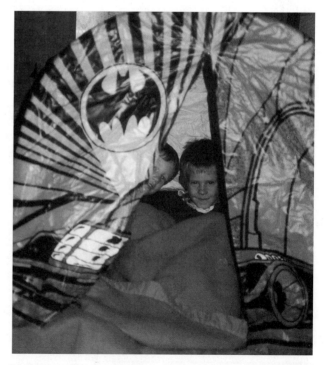

figure**1-3** Special places and favorite play partners have high significance to young children.

and significant experiences between therapist and child are potent intervention outcomes, often equal to achieving the child's established goals and objectives.

Activity and Activity Limitations

With an understanding of the child's participation, the therapist continues the evaluation process to define *specific activities and activity limitations*. Activities according to the International Classification of Impairments Activities and Participation (ICIDH-2) (World Health Organization [WHO], 1997) describe the nature and extent of functioning of a person. In occupational therapy with children, the focus is everyday, common *activities in play, self-care, and school occupations*. Therapists use quantitative and qualitative observational assessments to judge activity limitations. In addition to documenting whether expected activities for the child's age are missing, delayed, or deficient, occupational therapists note whether the activity becomes possible or is performed at a higher level when the child is given assistance. Is the child able to perform the activity with adapted equipment or assistive technology? When the child performs well with adapted equipment or environmental accommodations, the activity is not considered limited and is probably not an appropriate focus of intervention. An activity is limited when the child can perform it in only one environment (e.g., at home) but not in another environment (e.g., at school). For example, a child with physical disabilities and high distractibility is independent in self-feeding at home; however, because of the noise level, physical arrangement, high level of activity, and time restrictions, this child requires assistance to eat in the school cafeteria.

Activity limitations can be measured by duration, quality of performance, degree of assistance required, safety, and developmental level (Holm, Rogers, & James, 1998). Occupational therapists observe children playing or performing in the classroom and home as part of this evaluative process. Careful observation allows the therapist to understand the qualitative aspects of performance, to determine the relative influence of the environment and the innate abilities of the child. Procedural reasoning leads to pattern recognition and *hypothesis generation* (Fleming, 1994). The occupational therapist identifies children with whom she or he has worked who exhibited a similar pattern. When a child fits a known pattern of activity and activity limitations, the occupational therapist contemplates the match between the goals of the child who exhibited similar patterns and the child under observation. This comparison becomes important as the therapist assesses the performance problems and hypothesizes the basis for these problems.

During observation the therapist often provides facilitation or cues to determine how therapeutic methods of assistance influence the child's performance. Assessing the quality of assisted performance helps the

therapist judge how the child may respond to social, sensory, or physical assistance, support, or accommodations. Interpreting the child's response to assistance or adaptation of the activity allows the therapist to test his or her hypotheses about which interventions to apply and what outcomes are realistic. The following example illustrates how the therapist applies intervention strategies to gain a more complete understanding of the child's performance and the potential for improving performance (Box 1-1).

---

box 1-1 *Evaluating potential effects of intervention*

Four-year-old Ryan had been recently diagnosed with autism when he was first evaluated by the occupational therapist. In a telephone conversation with the therapist before the evaluation, Ryan's mother reported that his communication and play with other children was extremely limited. He appeared disengaged from those around him, and his play with toys appeared repetitive and without purpose. Ryan had not yet attended preschool, and most of his time was spent at home [with his] younger brother. When he entered the clini[c he sa]t with the therapist and wa[lked around the ro]om to find a metal bowl si[. . . . Ry]an to spin the bowl, appear[. . . . . sp]inning. After 1 to 2 minut[es the therapi]st sat beside him and made [. . . . . a]ctions, to which Ryan [. . . . .] then remarked, "Let'[s . . . . . bow]l," and dropped a plas[tic . . . makin]g a clanking sound. Rya[n . . . . . fo]r a few seconds. The th[erapist said, "would you] like more fruit?" and p[ut . . . . f]ruit into the bowl. Ryan picked up a near[by ... and] dropped it into the bowl. His response of imitating the therapist was highly encouraging. She verbalized praise of his action. He did not verbally respond, but his face seemed to brighten slightly. Ryan then removed the objects from the bowl and returned to spinning it. In response, the therapist began to arrange the play dishes on the table next to him, as if she were setting the table. Ryan occasionally stopped his spinning to watch her actions. His interest in and his singular response to her actions were encouraging to the occupational therapist. Through this initial observation, the therapist felt that increased engagement and interaction in play with others and purposeful pretend play with objects were realistic outcomes for Ryan.

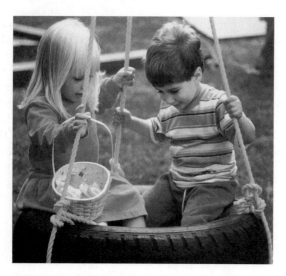

figure**1-4**   The interests of the child are influenced by siblings and his or her physical surroundings.

Interactive reasoning is used at this stage of evaluation to discover what interests and motivates the child (Figure 1-4). The therapist gathers information about the child's temperament and personality that may be helpful in building a relationship with the child. The therapist looks for interactive secrets to build an alliance with the child. Clues from parents and teachers are sought to determine which sensory systems are preferred for learning, which play interests are favored, and how the child's temperament influences his or her actions.

As the occupational therapist analyzes the activity limitations, she or he uses narrative reasoning to continue to refine the child's story. The therapist seeks to uncover those activities that have the greatest meaning to the child, those that relate to the child's perceived self-esteem, and those that seem unimportant to the child or family. Generally, qualitative social or sensory aspects of an activity become most important in developing an intervention plan. *Narrative reasoning* helps the therapist identify what motivates the child: Does the child exert more effort when music is played? Does the child demonstrate greater skill and motivation with peers or adults involved in the activity? Does the child enjoy animals? Would including a pet in therapeutic activities elicit the child's optimal participation? Through narrative reasoning the therapist identifies family's preferences, past experiences, and cultural values that appear to affect the child's performance.

Performance Components and Impairments

With an explicit understanding of activity limitations, the therapist seeks to uncover the impairments associated with these limitations. The ICIDH-2 (WHO, 1997) de-

fines impairment as a loss or an abnormality of body structure or a loss or an abnormality of a physiologic or psychologic function. At this level of evaluation, the therapist identifies performance components that are delayed, deficient, or missing, thus limiting participation. The occupational therapist also identifies performance components that are strengths and those on which the child relies to perform an activity. Because children perform differently in different environments, performance components are always defined within specific contexts. The therapist explores the associations between impairments and activity limitations that may explain the performance problems, and he or she explores the performance components that have the greatest potential to improve the level of participation in age appropriate, desired occupations.

Performance components of greatest interest to occupational therapists are sensory, motor, perceptual, cognitive, and psychosocial. To identify missing or impaired performance components, the therapist can administer a standardized test, such as the Peabody Developmental Motor Test (Folio & Fewell, 2000), Developmental Test of Visual Perception (Hammill, Pearson, & Voress, 1993), or the Evaluation Tool for Children Handwriting (Amundson, 1996). At this point in the evaluation, the therapist has moved *beyond hypothesis generation to cue interpretation and hypothesis testing.* Standardized tests are helpful to confirm or invalidate the hypothesized reasons for activity limitations. The therapist brings specific evidence that identifies which performance components seem to be most associated with activity limitations. The therapist also decides whether the impairment will improve with remediation and whether a method of compensation is needed. An understanding of impairments and intervention possibilities helps the therapist establish realistic goals and outcomes. For example, in over the course of a school year a child with autism who is extremely disengaged may develop interactive skills with play objects, but he or she may not develop interactive play skills with peers. In contrast, a preschool child with Down syndrome who has very few play skills may develop consistent associative and cooperative play with other children. The therapist can predict and facilitate these outcomes by understanding the impairments involved and the performance components associated with the performance delays.

Testing hypothesis involves *procedural* and *narrative reasoning,* as the therapist refines the story by identifying the targeted components and associating these components with environmental factors and activity limitations.

At this point, the therapist has completed the evaluation, confirmed the hypothesis, and identified a pattern that fits the child and his or her story. By moving from evaluation of participation to activities and then to performance components, the therapist has a good understanding of the broad concerns and problems and of the individuals involved (e.g., child, parent or caregiver, family members, teachers). The therapist also understands how to interact with the child to build a trusting and a positive relationship.

■ CLINICAL REASONING IN INTERVENTION PLANNING

Interpreting the information gained from the evaluation for intervention requires that the therapist rethink the child's activity limitations and participation, but from the perspective of a future orientation (see Figure 1-1). Activity limitations are often the basis for establishing short-term goals and objectives, and participation restrictions are the basis for establishing long-term outcomes. Goal statements concerning the activities the child will perform include the environmental conditions, environmental modifications, and activity assistance (e.g., adaptive equipment) to ensure the child's optimal participation. To formulate outcome statements, the occupational therapist, team, and family members envision how the child can participate in new social roles and how he or she can more fully participate in current ones. For example, which interventions will enable the child to play independently on the playground, to participate in a regular education classroom for a full day, or to make new friends? The occupational therapist contributes to the vision because he or she understands the possibilities and has experiences with similar children.

To establish meaningful outcomes with the family, the occupational therapist uses conditional reasoning (see Table 1-1). In conditional reasoning, the therapist assimilates all the information about the child and his or her occupations and environments to create a future picture of the child. Fleming (1994) defined conditional reasoning as forming an image of future life possibilities for the person. The child's impairments are understood, as are the constraints of the environment. The use of adaptive equipment, compensatory techniques, and environmental accommodations are all considered in developing a vision for the child and an outcome of increased participation.

Pragmatic reasoning is also important in intervention planning (Schell, 1998). Potential outcomes may not be feasible, depending on funding, time, and system constraints. Certain outcomes may be more practical, more realistic, or more appropriate when considering these constraints. For example, will the family support the child's use of an augmentative communication device? Will family members be able to handle a power wheelchair weighing 40 pounds? Is the parent interested in and does he or she have the time to implement a therapeutic program at home? Through pragmatic reasoning, the therapist identifies the most practical ways to reach meaningful outcomes.

■ INTERVENTION: PURPOSES AND STRATEGIES

The occupational therapist continues to use clinical reasoning to design and implement therapeutic activities. Almost all intervention activities with children have playful qualities, since play is an occupation of high relevance and importance to a child. The child who is playing is active, goal directed, and intrinsically motivated (Rubin, Fein, & Vandenberg, 1983). During play a child exhibits an internal sense of control (Bundy, 1997). With a play goal established through collaboration of the occupational therapist and child, the child is given choices about the activity to further motivate him or her. Play begins with the child's current skills level, but play evolves into challenging activities. The therapist guides the activity to a point in which it becomes challenging and somewhat stressful. The therapist offers assistance as the child faces a challenge to ensure that he or she succeeds and masters the task. The therapist may need to adapt or modify the stressful activity to make certain the child does not fail or become frustrated.

Intervention focuses on enhancing a child's ability to perform everyday activities and to participate in multiple environments. Interventions include the following aims:
1. Establishing a higher level of functional performance
2. Compensating for activity limitations by adapting task or providing assistive technology
3. Modifying environments
4. Changing the system (Table 1-2)

To achieve these intervention aims, the occupational therapist consistently incorporates the therapeutic use of occupation with the child and educates and consults the child's caregivers and teachers.

Establishing a Higher Level of Functional Performance
Using occupation as means

The focus of most occupational therapy interventions with children is to establish developmentally and functionally higher performance. Childhood is a period of great change, and occupational therapists guide that change in positive directions. Various practice models or frames of reference guide how the occupational therapist approaches intervention to improve functional performance. The authors of this text in (e.g., Chapters 3, 12, and 17) and others (e.g., Kramer & Hinojosa, 1999) explain these practice models. To establish new skills, the therapist uses occupation as means. An activity is selected that has meaning for the child and successfully engages

<table>
<tr><th colspan="2">table 1-2 *Intervention Aims and Strategies*</th></tr>
</table>

Intervention Aims	Strategies
Establishing a higher level of functional performance	Using occupation as means
	Implementing graded activity: the "just right" challenge
	Improving performance components
	Augmented and individualized sensory cueing and feedback
	Therapeutic use of self
	Education and consultation with caregivers and teachers surrounding the child
Compensatory approaches:	Individual-activity environmental fit
	Concurrent developmental and functional goals
	Education and consultation with adults who support use of compensatory methods
Environmental modifications	Improving fit between child and environment
	Consultation and negotiation with adults in environment
Systems change	Working with systems and administrators
	Communication, negotiation, consensus building within the child's community

box 1-2 *Grading an activity: challenging and eliciting full participation*

Aaron, a 10-year-old child with autism, participated in a cooking activity with the occupational therapist and three peers. The children were proceeding in an organized manner—sharing cooking supplies and verbalizing each step of the activity. As they proceeded, Aaron had great difficulty participating in the task; the materials were messy, and the social interaction was frequent and unpredictable. He performed best when the activity was highly structured, the instructions were very clear, and the social interaction was kept at a minimum. To help him participate at a comfortable level, the occupational therapist suggested that his contribution to the activity be to put away supplies and retrieve new ones. The other children were asked to give him specific visual and verbal instructions as to what they needed and what should be replaced in the refrigerator or cupboard. With this new rule in place, the children gave simple and concrete instructions that Aaron could follow. Importantly, this strategy included the support of his peers to elicit an optimal level of participation and could be generalized to other small group activities involving Aaron and his peers.

the child. Such an activity generally has a purpose or goal that is valued by the individual child. The therapist often entices the child into an activity by defining its purpose. "Let's build a castle." "Would you like to make a bracelet?" "Can you swing to the edge of the mat and pick up some dog bones to feed our hungry dog?" The theme must have meaning to the child to enhance and sustain the child's efforts (Trombly, 1995).

Graded activities: the "just right" challenge

Occupational therapists select highly adaptable activities and, as a result, can carefully raise or lower the task's difficulty level on the basis of the child's performance. To promote change in the child, the activity must be challenging and create a degree of stress. The stress is meant to elicit a higher level of response, not to cause failure. It is important to avoid failure. The therapist's interactions with the child are similar to those of a dance, in which the therapist poses a problem or challenge to the child who is motivated by that challenge and responds. The therapist facilitates or supports the child's action so that he or

she successfully responds at a higher level. The therapist then gives feedback regarding the action and presents another problem of greater or lesser difficulty, based on the success of the child's response. By precisely assessing the adequacy of the child's response, the occupational therapist finds the "just right" challenge. Cognitive, sensory, motor, perceptual, or social aspects of the activity may be made easier or more difficult (Box 1-2). At this action-reaction level, the child demonstrates his or her highest level of adaptive response and succeeds in the task presented.

Improving performance components

At times, the therapist focuses on the performance components that are the building blocks of occupations. A focus on performance components is appropriate when specific systems are impaired and appear to be interfering with performance. For example, a child with cerebral palsy may experience tightness in the shoulder girdle. Certain passive techniques may be used to elongate and relax the muscles around the shoulder to improve range of motion and freedom of movement. This increased range allows the child to participate in a reaching or weight-bearing, on-hands activity. The activity must relate to a valued occupation. The biomechanical nature of the activity must be combined with a cognitive goal (e.g., child places magnetic letters on a vertical board to spell words), with a playful goal (e.g., child lines up toy bears on the top shelf as a put-away activity), or with a psychosocial goal (e.g., child participates in a contest to see who can stack blocks highest).

Occupational therapists often focus on sensory systems that appear to interfere with functional performance. Children with hypersensitivity or sensory defensiveness may need calming or help in organizing responses before they can engage in an activity. The therapist may begin a session by applying vestibular or proprioceptive input to calm the child, improve his or her focus and attention, or improve the processing of sensory input. Sensory preparation is a well-accepted therapeutic principle (Koomar & Bundy, 1991; Miller & Heaphy, 1998). The effects of vestibular, tactile, and proprioceptive input related to a child's performance need further scientific investigation, but practitioners testify to the immediate and powerful effects of these proximal senses (Kimball, 1999).

Augmented and individualized sensory cueing and feedback

To promote the individual child's performance during an activity, the therapist uses a variety of techniques. The techniques are selected based on the child's learning style and patterns of performance. The therapist uses the child's preferred sensory systems to support performance that appears deficient. The therapist may use a multisensory approach with more guidance and augmented feedback about his or her performance. For example, the child with visual perceptual problems may benefit from manipulating cutout wooden letters to learn manuscript handwriting. For the child with performance problems and language deficits, visual cueing or modeling are preferred strategies for teaching new skills. The child with autism may require a picture card with a written instruction to move to the next activity. The child with low muscle tone and a poor sense of his or her body's movements in space can use heavy objects or a weighted vest to enhance sensory feedback from movement. Sensory feedback can help the child compensate for limited perception and delayed performance by augmenting the sensory systems that are used to compensate.

Therapeutic use of self

The occupational therapist establishes a relationship with the child that encourages and motivates. The therapist becomes invested in the child's success and makes evident to the child the importance of his or her efforts. The therapist first establishes a relationship of trust. Although the therapist presents challenges and asks the child to take risks, the therapist also supports or facilitates the performance so that the child succeeds or feels "okay" when he or she fails. This trust enables the child to feel safe and willing to take risks. The occupational therapist shows interest in the child, enjoys his or her unique characteristics, and values his or her preferences and goals. The unique traits and behaviors of the child become the basis for designing activities that will engage the child and provide the "just right" challenge. By individualizing activities so that the child feels important and by grading the activity to match the child's abilities, the child achieves mastery and a sense of accomplishment.

Children's self-esteem and self-image are influenced by skill achievement and their success in mastering tasks. Generally, the intrinsic sense of mastery is a stronger reinforcement to the child than external rewards, such as verbal praise or other contingent reward systems. The occupational therapist vigilantly attends to the child's performance during an activity to provide precise levels of support that enable the child to succeed in the activity.

The occupational therapist remains highly sensitive to the child's emerging self-actualization and helps the team and family provide activities and environments that support the child's sense of self as an efficacious person. Self-actualization, as defined by Fidler and Fidler (1978), occurs through successful coping with problems in the everyday environment. It implies more than the ability to respond to others; self-actualization means that the child initiates play activities, investigates problems, and initiates social interactions. A child with a positive sense of self seeks experiences that are challenging, responds to play opportunities, masters developmentally appropriate tasks, and forms and sustains relationships with peers and adults.

Caregiver and teacher education and consultation

Children acquire skills through practice. The high-level responses that a child demonstrates in a therapy session must be practiced and reinforced in the child's natural environments to become part of his or her repertoire. Often the child's performance continues to require some cueing or assistance from an adult (Figure 1-5). It also may require specific materials that offer the "just right" challenge. For example, in an actual occupational therapy session, a child succeeded in stacking magnetic blocks to build a house because the blocks were heavier and stuck together. However, he could not stack the wooden blocks at home. In this example the therapist allowed the parents to borrow the magnetic blocks so that the child could practice building houses at home. She demonstrated three-dimensional designs that he had accomplished and suggested other designs to be tried. The therapist also explained how support of his trunk and proximal arm helped increase the control of his hands in constructing block designs.

In another example, the therapist suggested calming sensory preparation activities to the preschool teachers of

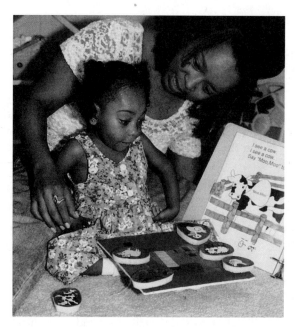

figure**1-5**   Verbal, physical, and visual cueing are used to elicit the child's full participation in the activity.

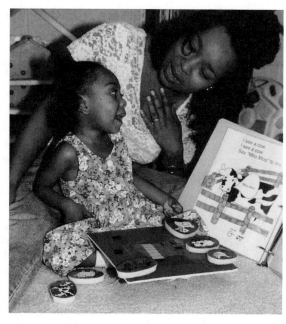

figure**1-6**   Therapists consult with parents to help them offer the "just right" challenge for the child to perform the activity.

a 4-year-old boy. The child was swung while prone in a hammock, and then deep pressure was applied by rolling him up in a blanket. This successful sensory preparation was then implemented on a daily basis to encourage the child to listen at story time. Soon he learned to ask to be rolled up when he felt disorganized, which signified an improved ability to self-regulate according to his sensory needs.

Consultation is an essential part of therapy. The therapist helps develop solutions that fit into the child's natural environment and promote the child's transfer of new skills into a variety of environments. Skills demonstrated in therapy session within the preschool classroom with the support of the therapist do not automatically generalize to other environments. It is important that the child feels safe to try new skills in other environments. Sometimes simply informing caregivers and teachers about an emerging skill or a new activity is sufficient for others to encourage and support practice in other environments. It is most helpful for the therapist to share the level of support or type of facilitation and cueing that the child needs to perform at a higher level (Figure 1-6). As the therapist teaches other adults how to implement activities with the child, the therapist adjusts to the adult's learning style and learning preferences. Pragmatic reasoning is used to judge how much time and effort the teacher or parent will be able to give to an individualized activity with a child.

Pragmatic reasoning is also used to determine when it is appropriate to teach strategies that involve some risk to the child when implemented improperly. If a highly specific, technical activity is needed to elicit a targeted re-

sponse, then teaching others may not be appropriate, and the activity should remain in the direct therapy session. Because children often feel unstable and are easily frightened on a therapy ball, for example, ball activities are most appropriately implemented by occupational therapists and physical therapists. Particularly when children have difficulty maintaining postural alignment, teaching others to implement activities on a therapy ball is not advised. Sometimes extended practice with the therapist is beneficial to ensure success in less supportive environments.

Compensatory Approaches: Adapting Activities or Providing Assistive Technology
Individual fit of environment and activities

Occupational therapists help children compensate for delays or deficits in performance by adapting activities or applying assistive technology (Figure 1-7). Compensatory approaches are particularly appropriate in self-care and school functions. These functional activities are important to the child and family during the toddler years and increase in importance as the child becomes school aged and older. Adapted techniques may be used when the child first learns to dress. For example, in children with poor balance the therapist may suggest that they dress while sitting in the bedroom's corner or lying in bed. A child with hemiparesis is taught to dress his or her affected extremities first. (Chapter 16 offers many examples of adapted techniques to increase a child's independence in self-care.)

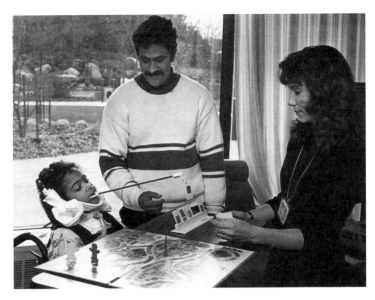

figure**1-7**   The occupational therapist designed a mouth stick and game board setup so that the child can play the game with his father.

Adapted techniques are also used at school to help the child successfully participate in school functions such as managing and manipulating his materials, transitioning between classes, moving within the classroom, and eating independently in the cafeteria. Examples of adapted techniques used to increase function at school are methods to grasp pencils or scissors or one-handed techniques for eating, for handling books and papers, and for writing.

Generally, most compensatory methods incorporate adapted equipment or assistive technology. Technology is pervasive throughout society and has become increasingly versatile so that it is easily adaptable to a child's individualized needs. (Technology solutions are described throughout this text and are the focus of Chapters 16, 19, and 20.) Appropriate use of assistive technology involves thorough assessment of the activity to be performed, the individual's abilities, and the environmental constraints and supports.

Low technology solutions are often applied to enhance self-care performance or to increase a child's independence in self-care. Examples include built-up handles on utensils, weighted cups, elastic shoelaces, and electric toothbrushes. High technology solutions are often used to increase mobility or functional communication. Examples include power wheelchairs, augmentative communication devices, and computers. The use of high technology, which involves computer processing and switch or keyboard access (e.g., augmentative communication devices), requires that adults in the child's daily environment support its use. High assistive technology for children is carefully selected so that it is durable and can grow with the child. For example, the size of the wheelchair is adjustable or the number of

keys on the augmentative communication device can be increased.

Concurrent developmental and functional goals

The role of assistive technology with children is not simply to compensate for a missing or delayed function, but it is also used to promote development in targeted performance areas. It is widely recognized that increased mobility with the use of a power wheelchair increases social and perceptual skills (see Chapter 20). The use of an augmentative communication device can enhance language and social skills and may prevent behavioral problems common in children who have limited means of communicating. Therefore the occupational therapist selects compensatory methods that not only enable the child to participate more fully in functional activities, but they also enhance the development of skills related to a specific functional area. For example, when a child has a physical disability with motor impairments, the therapist may set up a computer game as a play activity. The computer game simulates reading a book to promote preliteracy skills and uses an expanded keyboard to promote computer skills (Figure 1-8).

Educating adults who support the use of compensatory methods

The application of technology usually involves educating parents, care providers, and teachers. This education needs to include how to use the technology, how to adapt or adjust it, and how to troubleshoot when it does not work.

Assistive technology solutions continually change as devices become more advanced and more versatile. Cur-

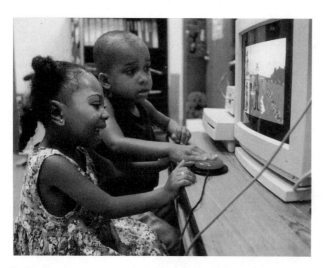

figure 1-8   A switch activates the computer program that simulates a story book.

rent technology offers a wide array of choices in devices with varying levels of complexity. The occupational therapist needs to be sensitive to the learning needs of those who will support the use of this technology. Often, it is important to talk through and model each step in the use of the technology and to remain available and supportive to others when the technology is first implemented. Strategies for integrating the technology into a classroom or home environment (i.e., discussing the ways the device can be used throughout the day) are helpful so that the greatest benefit is derived. The entire team needs to update their skills continuously so that they have a working knowledge of emerging technology. (See the following section of this chapter).

Summary

Compensatory methods promote a child's functional performance and promote developmental skills across domains. The following statements guide the occupational therapist in the use of compensatory approaches.

- Compensatory methods should be selected according to the child's individual abilities (intrinsic variables), expected or desired activities, and environmental constraints (extrinsic variables).
- Techniques and technology should be adaptable and flexible so that devices can be used across environments and over time as the child develops.
- Technology should be selected with a future goal in mind and a vision of how the individual and environment will change.
- The method should be selected in consultation with or input from caregivers, teachers, and other professionals and all adults who support its use.
- Extensive training and follow-up should accompany the use of compensatory methods.

Environmental Modifications
Improving the fit between child and environment

To succeed in a specific setting, a child with disabilities often benefits from adaptations to the environment. Environmental modifications include temporary or permanent adaptations that enhance a child's performance, increase safety or sense of safety, and improve comfort. Children with physical disabilities may require specific environmental adaptations to increase accessibility or safety. For example, although a school's bathroom may be accessible to a child in a wheelchair, the therapist may recommend the installation of a bar beside the toilet so that the child can safely perform a standing pivot transfer. Ramps may need to be installed or desk heights and chairs may need to be adjusted for the child in a wheelchair. Many of the physical accommodations to improve accessibility are in place as schools and community facilities comply with the Americans with Disabilities Act (ADA) (1990).

Often the role of the occupational therapist is to recommend adaptations to the sensory environment that accommodate children with sensory processing problems. Preschool and elementary school classrooms usually have high levels of auditory and visual input. Classrooms with visual clutter may be overwhelmingly disorganizing to a child who does not filter visual input. Young children who need proprioceptive input or quiet times during the day may need a bean bag chair in a pup tent in the corner of the room. The therapist may suggest that a preschool teacher implement a quiet time or turn down the lights for a period (Haack & Haldy, 1998). Sitting on movable surfaces (e.g., liquid-filled cushions) can help a child's posture and improve arousal and attention. The intent of recommendations regarding the classroom environment is often to maintain a child's arousal and level of alertness without overstimulating or distracting him or her.

Consultation and negotiation with adults in the child's environment

Environmental adaptations can only be accomplished through consultation with the adults who manage the environment. High levels of collaboration are needed to create optimal environments for the child to attend and learn at school and at home.

Environmental modifications often affect everyone in the room, so they must meet the needs of and be appropriate for all children in that environment. The therapist articulates the rationale for the modification and negotiates the changes to be made by considering what is most appropriate for all, including the teacher and other students. Through discussion, the occupational therapist and teacher reach agreement as to what the problems are. With consensus regarding the problems and desired outcomes, often the needed environmental modification logically follows. It is essential that the therapist follow through by evaluating the impact of the modification on the targeted child and others. Adaptations to the environment may require adjustments throughout the year, and therefore monitoring the effects of environmental modifications is always required (Hanft & Place, 1996).

System Change
Working with the system and administrators

Therapists may advocate for system change to improve accessibility, modify curriculum materials, develop educational materials, or help improve attitudes toward disabilities. By participating in curriculum revision or course material selection, therapists can help establish a curriculum with sufficient flexibility to meet the needs of children with disabilities. Often a system problem that negatively affects one child is problematic to others as well. The occupational therapist needs to recognize which system problems can be changed and how these changes can be encouraged. For example, if a child has difficulty reading and writing in the morning, he or she may benefit from physical activity before his deskwork. The occupational therapist cannot change the daily schedule and move recess or physical education to the beginning of the day, but she or he may convince the teacher to begin the first period of the day with warm-up activities. If the teacher indicates that time for warm-up cannot be allotted, she or he may allow the student to hold and handle "fidgets" during reading. Sometimes a crunchy snack can increase arousal and alertness. The occupational therapist can work with the teacher to establish a policy that allows children to eat a snack in the morning and then encourage parents to pack a crunchy snack.

To affect system change, the occupational therapist must become part of the system. This has not always occurred in schools; often therapists with a health care background and medical-based education feel like a "visitor" in the classroom. It has been difficult for occupational therapists to become an integral part of the educational system because of their limited understanding of the system. Similarly, teachers and principals do not always understand occupational therapy. To become part of the system, occupational therapists need to make conscious efforts to (1) define their profession and their roles, (2) determine the roles of school personnel, and (3) learn the rules, both overt and unspoken, that govern the system. Importantly, the occupational therapist needs to spend time with teachers and administrators and develop relationships with them. By participating in school routines (e.g., helping at recess, lunch, or assembly time), the occupational therapist demonstrates his or her interest in supporting the work of teachers and the school's overall operation. Participating in school activi-

ties also gives the therapist insight into the child's ability to cope with the routine and to participate in all school functions. The therapist also gains insight as to how to establish working relationships with teachers and how to approach problems that may be primarily an issue of difficult interaction between a child and teacher.

Communication and negotiation in the child's community

To change the system on behalf of all children or children with disabilities requires communication with stakeholders or persons who are invested in the change (Case-Smith, 1998). Strong rationale and negotiation are needed. When a change in the system (e.g., curriculum) is considered, inevitably many points of view are expressed and need to be considered. A system change is most accepted when the benefits appear high and the costs are low. Can all children benefit? Which children are affected?

Building an accessible playground is one example of a system change. Occupational therapists are frequently involved in designing playgrounds that are accessible to all and promote the development of sensory motor skills. Another example is helping school administrators select computers that are accessible to children with disabilities. The occupational therapist can also serve on the school committee that selects computer software for the curriculum and can advocate for software that is easily adaptable for children with physical or sensory disabilities. A third example is helping administrators and teachers select a handwriting curriculum to be used by regular and special education students. The occupational therapist may advocate for a curriculum that emphasizes prewriting skills or one that takes a multisensory approach to teaching handwriting. The occupational therapist may also advocate for adding sensory-motor-perceptual activities to an early childhood curriculum. These examples of system change suggest that the occupational therapists become involved in helping educational systems improve health care and prevent disability among children at risk, as well as compensate for children with specific diagnoses.

■ BEST PRACTICES WITH CHILDREN
Inclusion and Services in Natural Environments

Legal mandates and best practice guidelines require that services to children with disabilities be provided in environments with children who do not have disabilities. The Individuals with Disabilities Education Act (IDEA, 1997) requires that services to infants and toddlers be provided in "natural environments," and that services to preschool and school-aged children be provided in the "least restrictive environment." The young child's natural environment is most often his or her home, but it may include a child care center or preschool setting. The family must define the natural environment. (See further discussion in Chapter 22.) This requirement shifts when the child reaches school age, not in its intent but with recognition that community schools and regular education classrooms are the most natural and least restrictive environments for services to children with disabilities. School-aged children with severe medical or behavioral problems sometimes receive services in the home, but this environment is considered restrictive (see Chapter 30). Inclusion in natural environments or regular education classrooms only succeeds when specific supports and accommodations are provided to children with disabilities. Occupational therapists are often important team members in making inclusion successful for children with disabilities. (This concept is further discussed in Chapter 24.)

A recent focus of educators and related health care service providers, such as occupational therapists, is the inclusion of children with disabilities as not only a physical arrangement but also an opportunity for optimal learning and a method for reaching educational outcomes on par with those expected from all students. Therefore the goal of inclusion of students with disabilities is full participation in the school's curriculum and activities. This goal requires that teachers work closely with related service personnel to design course materials for the child with disabilities and to adapt learning experiences to ensure that he or she can achieve many of the same learning goals as do his or her peers.

Goals and strategies

With the team focused on inclusion, its goals, strategies, and methods lean toward outcomes that make inclusion successful (e.g., children functioning and learning with their peers in regular education classrooms). Inclusion of all children in schools include the following outcomes:

1. Children with disabilities are full participants in school activities, accessing all school environments and participating as independently as possible in school functions.

2. Children with disabilities have friends and relationships with their peers.

3. Children with disabilities learn and achieve with the general educational curriculum to the best of their abilities.

4. All children learn to appreciate individual differences in people.

5. Children with disabilities participate to the fullest extent possible in their communities.

Occupational therapists contribute in meaningful ways to all these outcomes. Often, the primary reason children fall short of reaching their goals is social or be-

havioral problems. Teachers can adapt the curriculum for specific learning issues, but behavioral problems are more difficult to manage because they disrupt the entire class and can negatively affect other children's ability to learn. Children who are extremely active, aggressive, impulsive, loud and boisterous, or oppositional are disruptive to classes and are a great concern of teachers.

Occupational therapists routinely address specific goals that are essential to a child's ability to function in a regular education classroom and promote the teacher and peers' acceptance of the child (Table 1-3). Occupational therapists approach these goals with important insight into the student's ability to respond to sensory input and to self-regulate (e.g., inhibit impulsive reactions). By sharing their understanding of the reasons a

table 1-3 *Occupational Therapy Goals for Promoting Inclusion*

Goals	Examples of Strategies
1. Decrease student's disruptive behaviors	Promote calming Decrease sensory-seeking behaviors by providing appropriate outlet for sensory seeking (e.g., break for jumping on trampoline or for applying deep pressure)
2. Increase student's time management	Give strategies for completing tasks on time Give method for cueing transition to new activities
3. Decrease student's aggressive behaviors	Decrease frustration by simplifying challenging activities Meet sensory needs throughout day
4. Improve student's interpersonal skills	Help child initiate and sustain interaction with peers Increase understanding of social norms
5. Improve student's responsiveness and self-regulation	Facilitate arousal, using appropriate but enhanced sensory input
6. Improve student's attention span and decrease distractibility	Provide materials that enhance visual focus
7. Improve student's ability to organize and manage materials	Teach compensatory methods for locating and assembling correct materials

child responds in certain ways, the occupational therapist may help teachers, parents, aides, and other professionals reframe the problem. Often, reframing the problem is an important step in developing the most appropriate solutions to the student's problems.

Occupational therapists also use behavioral approaches that include comprehensive behavioral programs designed by the team, and they rely on these strategies to help manage the child's behaviors. Behavioral approaches are effective when they are consistently applied across situations and environments. Therefore it is important to gain consensus and support for a behavioral program from all adults working with a child. With his or her understanding of the child's sensory, motor, and cognitive skills, and social function, the occupational therapist can contribute insights as to which behavioral strategies have a high probability for success.

Service delivery models

The goal that children should participate to the fullest extent possible in their natural environment also suggests that occupational therapists adopt certain methods of service delivery. The occupational therapist needs to work within the classroom or other natural environments. To be invited into the classroom or home environment, the occupational therapist must observe appropriate etiquette and have an appreciation for the adults who manage the environment. Becoming acquainted with the adults in the environment is an important first step. Often the best intervention for the child is support of the adults who are with the child on a daily basis (Case-Smith, 1998). The occupational therapist provides teachers and parents ongoing education and is instrumental in solving problems. Strong skills in consultation and collaboration are needed to help children function effectively in their natural environments. Once the occupational therapist becomes part of the system and acknowledges the importance of other roles and the skills of the adults who teach and work with the child, he or she can make recommendations for modifications and accommodations to the environment and curriculum that will be implemented and appreciated.

Consultation is most effective when a collaborative approach is taken. Hanft and Place (1996) described the critical elements of effective consultation as the following: (1) dynamic interaction over time, (2) respectful relationships, and (3) collaborative efforts to reach common ground. With collaborative consultation, the occupational therapist commits to developing and sustaining relationships with parents and other professionals to solve the problems incurred by a student. When the occupational therapist suggests solutions, he or she is sensitive to the needs of these adults and offers practical solutions that recognize time constraints, environmental restrictions, and learning priorities. All suggestions involve follow-up and adaptations to the approach to ensure that the most workable and effective strategy is implemented.

Occupational therapists also attend to the style in which they provide consultation. As much as possible, the therapist should match the learning style and interaction style of those being consulted (e.g., teacher). For example, if the teacher is a visual learner, pictures or handouts of positions and activities to use with a student should be provided. If the teacher is a kinesthetic learner, the occupational therapist may suggest that the teacher practice a movement or handling technique to build confidence before applying it with a child. When the person being consulted has an interaction style reflecting that she or he is an achiever, the occupational therapist must also recognize that recommendations need to produce short-term effects. If the person has an analytic style, details and specificity are important when making recommendations (DeBoer, 1986).

Summary

Occupational therapists support inclusion by (1) focusing on goals that enable the child to be successful in inclusive environments, (2) providing services in the least restrictive environment or in the child's natural environment, and (3) using consultation and education as primary methods of service delivery. Helping students function in inclusive settings implies that occupational therapists integrate their services into these settings, that they become an integral part of the system, and that skills in consultation with adults complement the occupational therapist's skill in working directly with students.

New and Emerging Technologies

New technologies have significantly improved the quality of life for persons with disabilities. Computers, power mobility, augmentative communication devices, and environmental control units have greatly enhanced functional performance, making it possible for children to participate in roles previously closed to them. Similar to the legislation that supports inclusion, IDEA and other laws encourage states to provide assistive technology to children. These laws have increased the momentum for using assistive devices with children; however, the IDEA mandate is not funded, meaning that local school districts and other sources need to provide the funding for assistive technology. In delivering technology services, the occupational therapist functions as consultant and educator. The use of this technology not only requires that the team perform an in-depth evaluation to ensure appropriate recommendations, it also requires that the occupational therapist teach the child and adults around the child how to use the technology.

Often the occupational therapist is part of an assistive technology team that troubleshoots technology failures, determines technology needs, and provides ongoing education to staff and families.

Two trends in the development of technology have broad implications for occupational therapists: universal access and greater availability of new, highly complex systems.

Universal access

The concept of universal access is now widespread, and it refers to the movement to develop devices and design environments that are accessible to everyone. It is now possible for children in power or manual wheelchairs to access all environments, including recreational facilities, sports arenas, swimming pools, playgrounds, and community centers. Schools are now designed to accommodate additional computers in classrooms. Desks are designed for laptop computers, and some desks are accessible to wheelchairs. In addition, current computer programs are easily adaptable; for example, the cursor can be enlarged and most computer application and word processing programs offer multiple methods of augmented visual and auditory feedback. Keyboards are highly adaptable, and often access can be programmed to a single switch (see Chapter 19).

Hammel and Niehaus (1998) outlined the involvement of occupational therapists in general technology to ensure accessibility for students with disabilities. School-based occupational therapists should demonstrate the following competencies:

- Operate major computing systems used in public schools and troubleshoot system problems
- Make major operating systems accessible to persons with disabilities
- Establish networks using telecommunications systems
- Operate general application programs (e.g., word processing, databases, graphics), teacher utility tools, and computer-based instruction

New, highly complex systems

New, complex technologies are becoming more available. Occupational therapists are required to have a high level of expertise to help schools and families make appropriate choices, set up equipment, and train students to use the technology. This expertise is developed through participation in continuing education and hands-on experience (Hammel & Niehaus, 1998). The use of complex technologies requires the support of specialized, advanced services to ensure high-quality, safe application. For example, students can access a computer program using an infrared switch that enables the student to select from a virtual keyboard on the screen. Head and eye gaze systems are available for indirect selection access to word processing and other computer programs. Power wheelchairs now can have integrated controls that enable switches on the chair to function as environmental control units (Cook & Hussey, 1995).

These two trends require that all occupational therapists who work with children in any setting develop skills in assistive technology. However, the prevalence of these new systems also suggests that assistive technology specialists are needed. These occupational therapists may pursue certification by Rehabilitation Engineering Society of North America (RESNA) or attend continuing education classes on assistive technology. Occupational therapists with expertise in assistive technology can join technology teams now present in many school districts or can function as consultants to teachers and related services personnel in the school system. They can also act as team members in assistive technology clinics in hospitals and rehabilitation centers. These clinics typically provide in-depth evaluation, family education regarding new technologies, device and equipment loans for trial use, and assistance in securing funding.

Evidenced-Based Practice

With the goal of providing the best services possible, occupational therapists and other health care professionals are seeking and using practices and approaches that have evidence of effectiveness. The use of databases on evidence-based medicine has become essential to clinical decision making. Outcomes studies, when applicable to the individual child, contribute to procedural and conditional reasoning. Sackett and others (1996) defined evidence-based medicine as "the conscientious, explicit, and judicious use of current best evidence in making decisions about the care of individual patients" (p. 71). Evidence-based practice implies that the occupational therapist must perform the following functions:

1. Research databases to find studies relevant to his or her practice (e.g., similar diagnoses, outcomes, settings).

2. Evaluate the research and assess its applicability to his or her practice (e.g., similar core elements).

3. Apply the research to his or her clients in logical ways. Clinical decisions need to be made regarding which parts of the study are applicable and how the evidence should be considered in clinical problem solving.

Outcomes research can help practitioners establish benchmarks or standards for identifying the levels of performance improvement they can expect. With outcomes research, the occupational therapist can identify the type of client who will likely derive benefit from intervention. To appropriately use outcomes research, the results of efficacy studies must be used carefully, with attention given to differences among subgroups of clients and the levels of change associated with intervention.

Research on the effects of occupational therapy with children has been limited to only a few studies until the past two decades. Although the number of occupational therapy studies continues to lag behind those in other health care professions, the number and quality of occupational therapy outcomes studies have significantly increased in the 1990s. In addition, many studies of efficacy from other disciplines have applicability and utility for occupational therapists. Three areas of occupational therapy with children have been a focus of outcomes studies: sensory integration, neurodevelopmental treatment (NDT), and consultation. Occupation, as an intervention means, has also been the focus of study. Although these studies most frequently use adult subjects, the results are relevant to occupational therapy with children.

Studies of sensory integration with children (discussed in Chapter 12) demonstrate that its effects are positive but small (Varga & Camilli, 1999). Recent studies have found that the effects of intervention using a sensory integration approach are equivalent to the effects of alternative treatment approaches. The original studies that compared sensory integration with no treatment (e.g., Ayres, 1972; Ayres, 1977) demonstrated significant positive effects. Recent studies of children with learning disabilities (e.g., Polatajko, Law, Miller, Schaffer, & Macnab, 1991) have demonstrated no differences in outcomes when sensory integration was compared with other treatments. Sensory integration has been associated with improvement in motor planning but not academic skills (Humphries, Wright, McDougall, & Vertes, 1990; Humphries, Wright, Snider, & McDougall, 1992).

Outcomes of NDT with children who have cerebral palsy or delayed motor function have also been studied. Results of these studies are inconclusive. Two early studies of NDT found significant improvement in the sample receiving intervention using NDT (Carlsen, 1975; Scherzer, Mike, & Ilson, 1976). A more recent study with infants who exhibited delayed or abnormal motor behavior compared intensive with less intensive NDT and found a positive effect in the sample that received intensive NDT (Mayo, 1991). The results of two studies comparing NDT and alternative therapies in children with cerebral palsy or neuromotor disabilities were positive for the alternative therapy (D'Avignon, 1981; Palmer et. al., 1988). Three studies found no differences in the performance of children who received NDT and those who received no treatment or an alternate treatment (Law et. al., 1991; Sommerfeld, Fraser, Hensinger, & Beresford, 1981; Wright & Nicholson, 1973). A recent study by Law and others (1997) found that functional performance in children who received intensive NDT and casting were no different than the performance of children who received regular occupational therapy that emphasized functional activities. Together, the studies of NDT indicate weak support for this interventional method. By clinical report, it is effective for certain children, primarily those with cerebral palsy, in developing specific motor skills. These studies suggest that an NDT approach should be selectively applied to achieve specific outcomes. The inconclusive evidence also suggests that the performance areas targeted when using NDT should be specifically and routinely measured to determine whether progress toward expected outcomes is satisfactory.

The types of service delivery have been the focus of outcome studies. In occupational therapy, the use of consultation has been examined, comparing it with one-on-one models of intervention. These studies have shown that consultation is as effective or more effective than direct services. In a study with preschool children that extended 7 months, direct individual services (n = 8) were compared to group consultation services (n = 8) (Davies & Gavin, 1994). The progress of the children's motor skills was similar in the two samples, indicating that positive outcomes could be achieved when group interventions with consultation were used. In a pilot study of 14 kindergarten children, the levels of achievement of individualized education program (IEP) goals were compared with the achievement levels of children who received direct intervention or consultation. Children achieved nearly three fourths of their IEP goals whether they received consultation or direct services (Dunn, 1990). Teachers expressed feedback that was more positive toward the occupational therapy services when the therapist provided consultation. Kemmis and Dunn (1996) examined the effectiveness of weekly occupational therapy consultation with teachers. During each week of the school year, teachers and occupational therapists dedicated 60 minutes to plan intervention. Students who were the focus of these weekly meetings achieved a success rate of 63% on their intervention goals. Although these studies of consultation used small sample sizes, together, they suggest that consultation facilitates achievement of the child's goals and has positive benefits in developing relationships between occupational therapists and other professionals who are working with the child.

Finally, occupation as a means for improving performance has been well-researched. Occupations that are effectively used as means to intervention outcomes must have purpose and meaning (Trombly, 1995). The purpose is the goal of the intervention activity, and the meaning is the value of the activity. As discussed in the first part of this chapter, through clinical reasoning the therapist learns what the child values and what has meaning. When possible, the goal should be the same as that of the child's, although the goal is often established by external demands (e.g., children are expected to learn keyboarding in fifth-grade curriculum). Perhaps most importantly, the meaning or theme of an activity should reflect the child's values and interests.

Although most studies of the effectiveness of meaningful occupation or purposeful activity use adults as subjects, the results have important implications for occupational therapy with children. These studies support the use of occupation as a means for improving client performance and suggest that occupational therapists continue to refine their occupation-based models of intervention.

Examples of studies of the effects of occupational context on performance are replete in the occupational therapy literature. A few examples are described in this section. Lin, Wu, Tickle-Degnen, and Coster (1997) completed a meta-analysis of studies of occupation as means. They concluded that intervention providing purposeful activity produces better quality client performance (e.g., improved motor function) than a therapist and client focus on movement in isolation. To evaluate the effect of having a concrete goal, Van der Weel, Van der Meer, and Lee (1991) compared children's range of motion in supination when moving a drumstick to moving to an abstract command. The movement range was significantly greater with the concrete task. Sietsema and others (1993) also investigated the difference in shoulder range of motion when participants with brain injury reached to play a computer game versus when they reached for an abstract target. Range of motion was significantly greater when playing the game.

Nelson and colleagues extensively investigated the effect of enhanced context or enhanced meaning on client performance during an activity. In these studies (e.g., Bloch, Smith, & Nelson, 1989; Lang, Nelson, & Bush, 1992; Miller & Nelson, 1987; Riccio, Nelson, & Bush, 1990), the clients were given either a rote exercise or a meaningful activity with enhanced context with a purposeful goal. Their studies and others (e.g., Murphy, Trombly, Tickle-Degnen, & Jacobs, 1999) demonstrated that when the meaning of an activity was enhanced by producing an end-product, playing a game, or providing a specific context, the clients performed longer, with greater effort, and with higher quality (e.g., greater range of motion, smoother, more organized movement). All these outcomes suggest that meaningfulness in intervention activities motivates children to perform at optimal levels. By extension, it is probable that meaningful intervention activities are practiced in and generalized to other contexts, because the child values them. The effectiveness of occupation as an intervention means and consultation as the primary model of service delivery are important concepts in practice with children. The evidence supports the effectiveness of these concepts and validates the model presented in this chapter that included these concepts as essential elements of occupational therapy intervention.

■ SUMMARY

This chapter introduces the text presented in the next chapters by defining basic concepts in occupational therapy evaluation and intervention. It also describes evolving concepts that support best practices with children. It concludes by presenting the commitment of occupational therapists to using evidence-based outcomes research in clinical problem solving. Through this commitment, occupational therapists make decisions on the basis of their knowledge of efficacy and their understanding of individual concerns and priorities.

Occupational therapy practice with children has matured in the last two decades from a profession that relied on basic theory to drive its decisions to one that recognizes the complexities and essential nature of clinical reasoning. The profession is dedicated to refining theory by using efficacy research and to providing best care within the constraints of today's service delivery systems.

STUDY QUESTIONS

1. Describe the characteristics of scales and measures that are used in the first part of evaluation when the occupational therapist assesses the child's participation. What characteristics of scales and measures are used to assess activity limitations and impairments? (See Chapter 8.)

2. Give examples of appropriate scales or tests to use to evaluate (a) participation, (b) activity and activity limitations, and (c) performance components and impairments in a 5-year-old child with severe cerebral palsy. (See Chapters 7 and 8.)

3. Define narrative reasoning. Why is this type of reasoning important to all levels of evaluation? List important sources that the therapist uses to develop the "child's story."

4. How does the least restrictive environment change for a child from the time of infancy to school age? Compare the rules and etiquette when providing services in the home versus services in the classroom.

5. Consider a second-grade student who uses high technology (e.g., power mobility, augmentative communication device, adapted computer) to function in the classroom. Define methods that help integrate his assistive technology into classroom routine. Describe how the occupational therapist can include the teacher, teacher's aide, and student's peers in this goal.

References

Americans with Disabilities Act. (1990). Public Law 101-336, 104.

Amundson, S. (1996). *Evaluation Tool of Children's Handwriting.* Homer, AK: OK Kids.

Ayres, A.J. (1972). Improving academic scores through sensory integration. *Journal of Learning Disabilities, 5,* 339-343.

Ayres, A.J. (1977). Effect of sensory integrative therapy on the coordination of children with choreoathetoid movements. *American Journal of Occupational Therapy, 31,* 291-293.

Bloch, M.W., Smith, D.A., & Nelson, D.L. (1989). Heart rate, activity, duration, and effect in added-purpose versus single-purpose jumping activities. *American Journal of Occupational Therapy, 43,* 25-30.

Bundy, A. (1997). Play and playfulness: What to look for. In D. Parham & L. Fazio, (Eds.) *Play and occupational therapy for children* (pp. 52-66). St. Louis, MO: Mosby.

Carlsen, P.N. (1975). Comparison of two occupational therapy approaches for treating the young cerebral-palsied child. *American Journal of Occupational Therapy, 29,* 267-272.

Case-Smith, J. (1998). Thinking out of the box. In J. Case-Smith (Ed.), *Occupational therapy: Making a difference in school based practice.* Bethesda: AOTA, Inc.

Cook, A., & Hussey, S. (1995). *Assistive technologies: Principles and practice.* St. Louis: Mosby.

Davies, P.L., & Gavin, W.J. (1994). Comparison of individual and group/consultation treatment methods for preschool children with developmental delays. *American Journal of Occupational Therapy, 48,* 155-161.

Deboer, A. (1986). *The art of consulting.* Chicago: Arcturus books.

Dunn, W. (1990). A comparison of service-provision models in school-based occupational therapy services: A pilot study. *Occupational Therapy Journal of Research, 10* (5), 300-320.

Fidler, G.S., & Fidler, J.W. (1978). Doing and becoming: Purposeful action and self-actualization. *American Journal of Occupational Therapy, 32,* 305-310.

Fleming, M. (1994). Procedural reasoning: Addressing functional limitations. In C. Mattingly & M.H. Fleming, *Clinical reasoning: Forms of inquiry in a therapeutic practice* (pp. 137-177). Philadelphia: F.A. Davis.

Folio, R., & Fewell, R. (2000). *Peabody Developmental Motor Scales* (2nd ed.). Pro Ed.

Haack, I., & Haldy, M. (1998). Adaptations and accommodations for sensory processing problems. In J. Case-Smith (Ed.), *Occupational therapy: Making a difference in school system practice.* Bethesda: American Occupational Therapy Association, Inc.

Hammel, J., & Niehues, A. (1998). Integrating general and assistive technology into school-based practice: Process and information resources. In J. Case-Smith (Ed.), *Occupational therapy: Making a difference in school system practice.* Bethesda: American Occupational Therapy Association, Inc.

Hammill, D.D., Pearson, B.N.A., & Voress, J.K. (1993). *Developmental Test of Visual Perception* (2nd ed.). Austin, TX: Pro Ed.

Hanft, B., & Place, P.A. (1996). *The consulting therapist.* San Antonio, TX: Therapy Skill Builders.

Holm, M., Rogers, J.C., & James, A.B. (1998). Treatment of activities of daily living. In M.E. Neistadt & E.B. Crepeau (Eds.), *Willard & Spackman's occupational therapy* (pp. 323-363). Philadelphia: Lippincott.

Humphries, T., Wright, M., McDougall, B., & Vertes, J. (1990). The efficacy of sensory integration therapy for children with learning disability. *Physical and Occupational Therapy in Pediatrics, 10* (3), 1-17.

Humphries, T., Wright, M., Snider, L., & McDougall, B. (1992). A comparison of the effectiveness of sensory integrative therapy and perceptual-motor training in treating children with learning disabilities. *Developmental and Behavioral Pediatrics, 13* (1), 31-40.

Individuals with Disabilities Education Act. Amendments of 1997 (P.L. 105-17). 20 U.S.C. 1400 et seq.

Kemmis, B.L., & Dunn, W. (1996). Collaborative consultation: The efficacy of remedial and compensatory interventions in school contexts. *American Journal of Occupational Therapy, 50,* 709-717.

Kimball, J. (1999). Sensory integration frame of reference: Postulates regarding change and application to practice. In P. Kramer & J. Hinojosa, *Frames of reference of pediatric occupational therapy* (2nd ed.). Philadelphia: Lippincott Williams & Wilkins.

Koomar, J., & Bundy, A. (1991). The art and science of creating direct intervention from theory. A.G. Fisher, E.A. Murray, & A.C. Bundy (Eds.), *Sensory integration: Theory and practice* (pp. 251-313). Philadelphia: F.A. Davis.

Kramer, P., & Hinojosa, J. (1999). *Frames of reference for pediatric occupational therapy.* (2nd ed.). Philadelphia: Lippincott Wilkins & Williams.

Lang, E.M., Nelson, D.L., & Bush, M.A. (1992). Comparison of performance in materials-based occupation, imagery-based occupation, and rote exercise in nursing home residents. *American Journal of Occupational Therapy, 46,* 607-611.

Law, M., Cadman, D., Rosenbaum, P., Walter, S., Russell, D., & DeMatteo, C. (1991). Neurodevelopmental therapy and upper-extremity inhibitive casting for children with cerebral palsy. *Developmental Medicine and Child Neurology, 33,* 379-387.

Law, M., Russell, D., Pollock, N., Rosenbaum, P., Walter, S., & King, G. (1997). A comparison of intensive neurodevelopmental therapy plus casting and a regular occupational therapy program for children with cerebral palsy. *Developmental Medicine and Child Neurology, 39,* 664-670.

Lin, K-C., Wu, C-Y., Tickle-Degnen, L., & Coster, W. (1997). Enhancing occupational performance through occupationally embedded exercise: A meta-analytic review. *Occupational Therapy Journal of Research, 17,* 25-47.

Mattingly, C. (1994). The narrative nature of clinical reasoning. In C. Mattingly & M.H. Fleming, *Clinical reasoning: Forms of inquiry in a therapeutic practice* (pp. 239-269). Philadelphia: F.A. Davis.

Mayo, N.E. (1991). The effects of physical therapy for children with motor delay and cerebral palsy. *American Journal of Physical Medicine and Rehabilitation, 70,* 258-267.

Miller, H., & Heaphy, T. (1998). Sensory processing in preschool children. In J. Case-Smith (Ed.), *Occupational therapy: Making a difference in school system practice,* Bethesda: American Occupational Therapy Association, Inc.

Miller, L., & Nelson, D. (1987). Dual-purpose activity versus single-purpose activity in terms of duration on task, exertion level, and affect. *Occupational Therapy in Mental Health, 7,* 55-67.

Murphy, S., Trombly, C., Tickle-Degnen, L., & Jacobs, K. (1999). The effect of keeping an end-product on intrinsic motivation. *American Journal of Occupational Therapy, 53,* 153-157.

Nelson, D.L., Konosky, D., Fleharry, K., Webb, R., Newere, K., Hazboun, V.P., Fontane, C., & Licht, B.C. (1996). Effects of an occupationally embedded exercise on bilaterally assisted supination in persons with hemiplegia. *American Journal of Occupational Therapy, 50,* 639-646.

Palatajko, H.J., Law, M., Miller, J., Schaffer, R., & Macnab, J. (1991). The effect of a sensory integration program on academic achievement, motor performance, and self-esteem in children identified as learning disabled: Results of a clinical trial. *Occupational Therapy Journal of Research, 11,* 155-176.

Palisano, R. (1989). Comparison of two methods of service delivery for students with learning disabilities. *Physical and Occupational Therapy in Pediatrics, 9* (3), 79-99.

Palmer, F.B., Shapiro, B.K., Wachtel, R.C., Allen, M.C., Hiller, J.E., Harryman, S.E., Mosher, B.S., Meinert, C.L., & Capute, A.J. (1988). The effects of physical therapy on cerebral palsy. *New England Journal of Medicine, 318,* 803-808.

Riccio, C.M., Nelson, D.L., & Bush, M.A. (1990). Adding purpose to the repetitive exercise of elderly women through imagery. *American Journal of Occupational Therapy, 44,* 714-719.

Rubin, K., Fein, G.G., & Vandenberg, B. (1983). Play. In P.H. Mussen (Ed.), *Handbook of child psychology: Vol. 4* (4th ed.). (pp. 693-774). New York: Wiley & Sons.

Sackett, D.L., Rosenberg, W.M.C., Muir Grany, J.A., Haynes, R.B., & Richardson, W.S. (1996). Evidence-based medicine: What it is and what it isn't. *British Medical Journal, 312,* 71-72.

Schell, B. (1998). Clinical reasoning: The basis of practice. In M.E. Neistadt & E.B. Crepeau (Ed.), *Willard & Spackman's occupational therapy,* (pp. 90-102). Philadelphia: Lippincott.

Scherzer, A.L., Mike, V., Ilson, J. (1976). Physical therapy as a determinant of change in the cerebral palsied infant. *Pediatrics, 53,* 47-52.

Sietsema, J.M., Nelson, D.L., Mulder, R.M., Mervau-Scheidel, D., & White, B.E. (1993). The use of a game to promote arm reach in persons with traumatic brain injury. *American Journal of Occupational Therapy, 47,* 19-24.

Sommerfeld, D., Fraser, B.A., Hensinger, R.N., & Bereford, C.V. (1981). Evaluation of physical therapy service for severely mentally impaired students with cerebral palsy. *Physical Therapy, 61,* 338-344.

Tickle-Degnen, L. (1998). Using research evidence in planning treatment for the individual client. *Canadian Journal of Occupational Therapy, 65* (3), 152-159.

Trombly, C.A. (1995). Occupation: Purposefulness and meaningfulness as therapeutic mechanisms. *American Journal of Occupational Therapy, 49,* 960-972.

Varga, S., & Camilli, G. (1999). A meta-analysis of research on sensory integration treatment. *American Journal of Occupational Therapy, 53,* 189-198.

World Health Organization. (1997). *ICIDH-2: International classification of impairments, activities, and participation.* Geneva, Switzerland: WHO.

Wright, T., & Nicholson, J. (1973). Physiotherapy for the spastic child: An evaluation. *Developmental Medicine and Child Neurology, 15,* 146-163.

chapter 2

Teaming

Jane Case-Smith

key terms

Related professionals
Collaboration
Model of team dynamics
Team interaction models
Team process

■ CHAPTER OBJECTIVES

1. Describe professionals in other disciplines who provide services to children with disabilities and to their families.
2. Describe the dynamics of team function.
3. Compare team function in medical, educational, and early intervention systems.
4. Describe the elements of team process, including communication, decision making, consensus building, and conflict resolution.
5. Discuss issues in the team process that affect team effectiveness.

A child with disabilities benefits most from holistic intervention. Therefore the collaborative efforts of a multidisciplinary team of professionals are needed to design and provide the intervention program. In medical, educational, and community-based settings where children are served, individualized plans of intervention are developed and child outcomes become the responsibility of teams of professionals. Often the child's individualized plan calls for the involvement of specialized professionals who then make up the team for the child, that is, certain services become responsible for implementing the plan.

The members of the team are determined by the type and severity of the child's disability, as well as the child's age, support systems, and environments. For example, a child with a high-level spinal cord injury will benefit from the services of an occupational therapist, a physical therapist, a nurse, a social worker, a rehabilitation engineer, and others, depending on the child's situation. A child with Down syndrome often receives services from an occupational therapist, a speech-language pathologist, a physical therapist, a special educator, a nurse, a social worker, an optometrist, and a physician.

The professionals involved with the child and family will change over time, and new professionals will participate in the child's care during medical crises and hospital admissions, during periods of vocational training, and with transitions from early intervention to preschool and from preschool to school. Because a team of professionals from multiple disciplines defines the context for almost all pediatric occupational therapy practice, it is essential that the therapists develop collaborative skills. Effective teaming skills can be as important as the technical and professional skills that define their professions.

This chapter describes the professionals of other disciplines who work with occupational therapists. A model of team dynamics is explained and then exemplified for medical, educational, and early intervention teams. Finally, effective team processes are identified and discussed.

■ SERVICE PROVIDERS WHO WORK WITH OCCUPATIONAL THERAPISTS

Physicians

The primary physician for children is often a pediatrician or family practitioner. Physicians in pediatric specialty areas may also provide medical care (e.g., pediatric neurology, surgery, orthopedics, ophthalmology). Physicians who provide medical care to children have completed internships and residencies in pediatrics and related specialty areas and have successfully completed board certification examinations. Standards of pediatric practice mandate the identification of developmental delays as part of the routine care for the well child. Because most children obtain health care on an ongoing basis from birth, pediatricians and family practitioners are in an ideal position to identify, evaluate, treat, and refer children with developmental delays.

Roles for the pediatrician or family practitioner include identifying children for referral for early intervention and providing families with information about early intervention (Wachtel & Compart, 1996). The family often needs a physician's referral to become eligible for early intervention services and specific prescriptions for physical and occupational therapy services.

In addition to identifying children at risk and making appropriate referrals, the physician manages diagnostic work-up examinations to determine the causes of disability. Often, it is important to research the medical cause of a disability to determine its course and prognosis, and, in the case of a genetic problem, it is essential to identify the likelihood of reoccurrence of the disability within the family. Some conditions (e.g., autism, attention-deficit disorder) benefit from pharmaceutical treatment, which must be initiated and managed by a physician.

Children with disabilities generally have more medical problems than other children. For example, children with spina bifida are vulnerable to orthopedic, respiratory, and circulatory problems. Children with cerebral palsy require ongoing medical management related to orthopedic, neurologic, and respiratory concerns. All children with chronic medical problems require ongoing monitoring by their pediatricians and other medical specialists. The role of the physician on the team varies from consultant to leader, depending on the system in which the team is functioning and the medical stability of the child.

Nurses

Registered nurses (RNs) make up the largest segment of the health care workforce. To become an RN or a pro-

fessional nurse, candidates must graduate from a state-approved school of nursing. The program may be a two-year associate degree program, usually offered at community colleges; a three-year diploma program, usually based at a hospital; or a four-year baccalaureate degree program from a college or university. Generic nursing education includes courses in the biological, behavioral, and social sciences. Basic courses include biology, anatomy and physiology, pharmacology, pathophysiology, nutrition, growth and development, system theory, and interpersonal relationship. Nurses prepared at the bachelor's degree level receive education in community health, including principles of interdisciplinary and interagency service coordination or care management and nursing research (Cox, 1996).

Twenty years ago, most nurses graduated from associate degree programs. Today, most nurses graduate from associate or baccalaureate degree programs, and over 20% of RNs have postgraduate degrees. RNs who specialize as pediatric nurses receive their training through a variety of sources. Some are trained on the job, and others complete graduate degrees in pediatric nursing. These nurses can establish their own practices in a community, but generally they establish a close working relationship with a specific physician or group of physicians.

The *clinical nurse specialist* has an advanced nursing degree that allows him or her to function more independently than a nonspecialist. Therefore the clinical nurse specialist can implement certain procedures traditionally performed by a physician or under the direct supervision of a physician. The roles of the clinical nurse specialist include (1) assessing health status, (2) diagnosing human responses to actual or potential health problems, (3) planning and implementing specific therapeutic intervention, and (4) evaluating client outcomes (American Nurses' Association Council of Clinical Nurse Specialists, 1986).

Nurse practitioners hold an advanced degree in a specialty area of nursing practice. These nurses can practice independently, that is, without direct physician supervision. The major activities of nurse practitioners include screening, completing health histories, performing physical and psychologic examinations, managing care during wellness and illness, teaching, consulting and collaborating, conducting client follow-up examinations and referrals, promoting positive health, and managing personnel and administration (Cox, 1996).

All RNs must pass licensure examinations after completing their accredited generalist educational program. Each state defines the scope of nursing practice and standards for licensure in a Nurse Practice Act. Many states have developed continuing education requirements for nurses as a prerequisite to maintaining licensure (American Nurses' Association, 1990).

In 1992, approximately two thirds of employed RNs worked in hospitals, almost 10% worked in community or public health settings, and 8% worked in ambulatory care settings, most often physicians' offices (American Nurses' Association, 1999). Today, nurses who work with children are employed in diagnostic clinics, child development centers, outpatient and health department clinics, and home health services. Nurses who work in schools provide medical care by administering medicine, implementing routine medical procedures (e.g., asthma treatment or catheterization), and providing health screenings. The role of nurses in early intervention includes (1) diagnosing and treating health problems with children and families; (2) screening and assessing the psychologic, physiologic, and developmental characteristics of the child and family for early identification, referral, and intervention; (3) planning and coordinating with the family and interdisciplinary team; (4) providing intervention to the family to improve child and family's health and developmental status; and (5) evaluating the effectiveness of nursing care provided (American Nurses' Association Consensus Committee—Maternal Child Nursing, 1993).

Nurses often serve as case managers in early intervention (Collins, 1995; Hansen, Holaday, & Miles, 1990). Their case management activities may include locating community activities, helping family members gain understanding of the child's individual education plan, making periodic telephone calls to assess status, providing information about parent groups, and helping parents contact families with similar problems.

Licensed practical nurses (LPNs) complete 12- to 16-month training programs, usually after high school, and complete examinations in the state in which they will practice. LPNs provide bedside care and work under the supervision of RNs. Nurse's aides are trained at the associate degree level in vocational or on-the-job programs in medical facilities. These programs last generally one year and do not necessarily result in a degree.

Physical Therapists

Physical therapists work closely with occupational therapists in a variety of settings. Known together as the rehabilitation therapies (or related services in the schools), occupational therapists and physical therapists share similar or common goals for their clients and offer complementary approaches to intervention. For example, both therapies address activities of daily living (ADLs), but would approach these outcomes using different techniques and theories. They would make complementary recommendations to the family. Physical therapists assess joint motion, muscle strength and endurance, function of heart and lungs, and performance of activities required in daily living, among other responsibilities. Treatment includes therapeutic exercise, cardiovascular endurance training, and training in ADLs (American Physical Therapy Association [APTA], 1999).

The minimum educational requirement to become a physical therapist will be a master's degree after 2002. In 1999, 173 colleges and universities nationwide offered professional educational programs in physical therapy, and 7 university programs offered an entry-level doctoral program. Other universities are developing clinical doctoral programs (APTA, 1999). Physical therapists and educators have proposed that the doctor of physical therapy is the appropriate professional level in the profession, but this opinion has generated discussion and controversy (Soderberg, 1993). At all entry levels of physical therapy education, the graduates must pass a state-administered licensure examination, enabling the candidate to practice in that particular state.

Physical therapy professional educational programs prepare students to be generalists, capable of entering general settings, such as hospitals or rehabilitation centers. The entry-level curriculum provides basic information about working with children and families; however, pediatric content is not a primary emphasis of the course work. Physical therapists provide intervention to children with neuromuscular, musculoskeletal, or cardiopulmonary impairments. Competencies for physical therapy with young children have been developed. These competencies can be achieved through experience, continuing education, and graduate studies (Box 2-1).

Physical therapist assistants work under the supervision of physical therapists. They assist the physical therapist in implementing treatment programs, training children in exercises and ADLs, and conducting treatment, and they report the child's responses to the physical therapist. A physical therapist assistant must complete a 2-year educational program, typically offered through a community or junior college. The program consists of 1 year of general education and 1 year of technical courses on physical therapy procedures and clinical experience.

Speech-Language Pathologists

Occupational therapists work closely with speech-language pathologists, particularly when children have feeding and oral motor problems, augmentative communication needs, or global neuromotor and developmental delays. Occupational therapists share knowledge and philosophy with speech therapists. Speech-language pathologists hold master's or doctoral degrees. To practice they must receive the Certificate of Clinical Competence of the American Speech-Language-Hearing Association (ASHA), and in most states speech-language pathologists can only practice with a license (ASHA, 1999).

According to ASHA (1999), speech pathologists work to prevent speech, voice, language, communication, swallowing, and related disabilities. They screen, identify, assess, diagnose, refer, and provide treatment and intervention, including consultation and follow-up services to children at risk for speech, voice, language, communica-

box **2-1** *Physical therapist working with children and families*

The major roles of physical therapists who work with infants and preschool-aged children and their families include providing the following services:

1. Screening for neuromusculoskeletal, cardiopulmonary, and general developmental dysfunction
2. Assessing neuromusculoskeletal status and motor skills for differential diagnoses
3. Assessing cardiopulmonary status
4. Designing, implementing, and monitoring therapeutic interventions
5. Evaluating intervention effectiveness and modifying programs as needed
6. Identifying family concerns, resources, and priorities
7. Developing family recommendations and monitoring their implementation
8. Participating in interdisciplinary planning
9. Consulting with family members and caregivers
10. Consulting with and referring to other professionals and community agencies
11. Serving as service coordinator
12. Recommending or fabricating adaptive equipment and mobility devices
13. Recommending and implementing environment modifications

Adapted from Cochrane, C.G., Farley, B.G., & Wilhelm, I.J. (1990). Preparation of physical therapist to work with handicapped infants and their families: Current status and training needs. *Physical Therapy, 70,* 372-380.

box **2-2** *The practice of speech-language pathology*

Speech-language pathologists provide the following:

1. Screening, identifying, assessing, diagnosing, treatment intervention, and follow-up services for disorders that affect the following:
   - Speech, articulation, fluency, voice
   - Language, syntax, semantics, pragmatics
   - Oral, pharyngeal, cervical esophageal, and related functions
   - Cognitive aspects of communication
   - Social aspects of communication
2. Consultation, counseling, and referrals
3. Training and support for family members and other communication partners
4. Effective augmentative and alternative communication techniques and strategies
5. Instrumental technology to diagnose and treat disorders of communication and swallowing

Adapted from Scope of Practice in Speech-Language Pathology, American Speech-Language Hearing Association, 1999, (http://www.asha.org).

tion, swallowing, and related disabilities. Speech-language pathologists select, prescribe, dispense, and provide services that support the effective use of augmentative and alternative communication devices and other communication prostheses and assistive devices (Box 2-2).

The practice of speech pathology with young children has shifted its focus from language to the broad area of communication in recognition of the importance of social behaviors and cognition in addition to language (Lorsardo, 1996). Speech therapists or communication specialists also appreciate the relationship between communication and other domains of development (e.g., motor performance, social-emotional function, or adaptive behaviors). Almost 60% of all speech therapists work in schools. Most school-based speech-language pathologists have earned master's degrees. ASHA encourages the inclusion of speech therapy support personnel (e.g., individuals with undergraduate degrees) to expand the services offered in public schools (ASHA Task Force on Support Personnel, 1994).

School Psychologists

A school psychologist is a professional psychologist who has completed a field placement program in school psychology. All psychologists have a master's or doctoral degree and have satisfactorily completed at least 1 year of supervised experience. School psychologists function as independent practitioners. They conduct multifactored psychologic and psychoeducational assessments of children and adolescents (National Association of School Psychologists [NASP], 1999). Their primary role in assessment is to identify an educational diagnosis and assist in determining the level of inclusion that would be most beneficial to the student. Psychologic and psychoeducational assessment includes the following areas:

- Intelligence and cognitive functioning
- Scholastic aptitude
- Adaptive behavior
- Language and communication skills
- Academic knowledge and achievement
- Sensory and perceptual motor function
- Career and vocational development (NASP, 1999)

Although most occupational therapists associate school psychologists with assessment and diagnosis, their roles are more comprehensive. The goals of school psychologic services are to promote mental health and facilitate student learning. To meet these goals, school psychologists consult and collaborate with parents, school, and outside personnel regarding mental health, behavioral, and educational concerns. They design and develop procedures to prevent mental health and learning problems, and they provide educational opportunities related to these goals. School psychologists also provide direct services to individual students and groups to enhance mental health, behavior, social competency, and academic status. These services often entail counseling or family dialogue. Most often, school psychologists intervene for behavioral and mental health issues affecting a student's performance. Using consultation and monitoring models, school psychologists interface with teachers and related service providers who interact with the students on a daily basis.

Social Workers

Professional social workers are the nation's largest group of providers of mental health services. The primary focus of the social work profession is to help people participate in their social environments. Social workers help children and families link to community agencies, obtain financial assistance, and find resources when mental health is at risk. They also provide counseling to clients and coordination of interagency services for clients.

A professional social worker has earned a bachelor's or a master's degree in social work and meets state certification or licensure requirements. Most states that certify clinical social workers require a master's degree in social work, at least 2 years' experience, and an examination. Social workers practice in many settings, including family service and child welfare agencies, community mental health centers, schools, and hospitals. The social worker with a bachelor's degree can work in a variety of settings, primarily performing case management activities. Social work case managers help link clients to community resources and help coordinate services for clients who need comprehensive care (National Association of Social Workers [NASW], 1999, www.socialworkers.org).

Social workers in clinical and school settings provide counseling and consulting services. They are credentialed at four levels (Box 2-3).

Teachers and Special Educators

Teachers in collaboration with special educators provide instruction to students with disabilities. Occupational therapists and certified occupational therapy assistants work closely with teachers, often directly in the classroom. Therapists consult with teachers and provide other support (e.g., teaching, modifying curriculum for students with disabilities, setting up assistive technology for classroom use).

---

box 2-3 *Levels of certification*

- Certified Social Workers
- School Social Work Specialists (SSWS)
- Qualified Clinical Social Workers (QCSW)
- Diplomate in Clinical Social Work (DCSW)

Each credential requires a master's or doctoral degree, supervised clinical experience, and successful completion of an examination (NASW [1999], www.socialworkers.org).

Teachers and special educators are certified or licensed in specialty areas of instruction that define the grades and types of student they are qualified to teach (e.g., early childhood, low incidence). All teachers and early intervention specialists—sometimes called developmental specialists—have at least a bachelor's degree. With a bachelor's or master's degree in special education and successful completion of a teaching internship, the individual earns a teaching certificate in one of the student categories. To maintain their license or certification, most states require teachers to complete graduate courses. Many states require teachers to work toward and achieve a master's degree within specified periods after employment.

Educators work with other team members in child assessment, program planning, and implementation. They administer tests and collect evaluation data on the students. Often, they coordinate comprehensive assessments of students to ensure that all relevant areas are evaluated and the process is completed in a timely manner. The special educator calls together the planning meeting to develop the Individualized Education Program (IEP) or the Individualized Family Service Plan (IFSP) and coordinates the meeting time, participants, and place. With an individualized program in place, the educator selects, adapts, and implements instructional strategies that address the developmental and educational needs of the child. They select, manage, and present the curriculum and learning materials, and they manage the classroom environment, creating surroundings conducive to learning. In the case of home schooling or home-based services, the special educator helps families establish home environments that promote development and learning. Teachers often ask for consultation from related service personnel (e.g., occupational therapists) to help solve problems when specific issues arise or students fail to meet expectations. The standards of practice as published by the Council of Education of Children (CEC) are listed in Box 2-4.

Most classrooms have teaching assistants or aides who are trained to assist the professional teacher in the classroom. Aides help with the logistics of student function, (e.g., getting dressed for recess, monitoring hallways, assisting in feeding, setting up learning areas). Aides often work directly with children with disabilities, assisting them in classroom activities. A teaching assistant usually has an associate of arts degree and a certificate as a teach-

ing associate. Teaching assistants have a minimum of a high school diploma, and aides do not have any minimal degree requirement.

Summary

A number of trends in education, certification, and qualifications can be observed in the related professions that work with occupational therapists and certified occupational therapy assistants. Most of these related professions require a master's degree to practice with children and families, and most are licensed or certified according to state law. Therefore these professionals have legal definitions and scopes of practice. Most professionals who work with children have multiple levels of education and credentialing that define levels of authority and independence in practice. With support personnel to assist in teaching and implementing intervention, collaborative teams of supervisors and associates (e.g., occupational therapists and certified occupational therapy assistants) work together to provide comprehensive and cost-effective services.

The national organizations for the professions discussed in this section have established standards of practice that define the roles and values of each profession. The national organizations publish ethical statements

---

box 2-4 Standards for special education personnel

1. Identify and use instructional methods and curricula that effectively meet individual needs of persons with exceptionalities
2. Participate in the selection and use of appropriate instructional materials, equipment, supplies, and other resources
3. Create safe and effective learning environments that contribute to fulfillment of needs, stimulation of learning, and self-concept
4. Maintain class size and case loads that are conducive to meeting the individual instructional needs of persons with exceptionalities

Adapted from CEC Code of Ethics and Standards of Practice, 1999, (www.cec.sped.org).

---

table 2-1 Disciplines Listed in the Individuals with Disability Education Act

Part B: School Programs	Part C: Early Intervention

FAPE offers services that meet state standards; they are provided under public supervision by qualified personnel.
FAPE includes the following:
• Special education (specially designed instruction) that meets unique educational needs of the child, including classroom, physical education, home, hospital, and institution instruction, and vocational education if specially designed
• Related services needed by the child to benefit from special education are the following:
  1. Speech and hearing therapy
  2. Psychologic sessions
  3. Physical and occupational therapy
  4. Recreation
  5. Social work
  6. Counseling
  7. Medical diagnosis and evaluation
  8. Parent training and counseling
  9. Assistive technology devices and instruction
  10. Rehabilitation counseling
  11. School health program
	Early intervention is designed to
	• Meet developmental needs of the child and family relative to the child's development; and
	• Meet state standards, providing services under public supervision by qualified personnel.
	Early intervention includes the following services:
	• Family training, counseling, home visits
	• Special instruction
	• Speech therapy
	• Hearing therapy
	• Occupational therapy
	• Physical therapy
	• Psychologic sessions
	• Service coordination
	• Medical diagnosis or evaluation
	• Early identification, screening, and assessment
	• Health program
	• Social work
	• Vision
	• Nursing
	• Nutrition
	• Assistive technology devices and instructions
	• Transportation and financial counseling

FAPE, Free appropriate public education.

with their standards of practice that confirm the profession's ethical values and assure the public that its professionals are fair, truthful, competent, and respectful of the consumers' confidentiality and individual rights.

This section describes only a few of the professionals who work with occupational therapists and certified occupational therapy assistants. (See the list of services under IDEA in Table 2-1). Each profession has its own scope of practice and makes unique contributions to the medical, school-based, or early intervention team. Learning about the educational background and scope of practice of other professionals on the team is the first step in collaborative teamwork. With this knowledge, appropriate referrals can be made and each professional's expertise can be used in team decisions. An understanding of discipline-specific roles of each member promotes team communication and process as described in the next sections.

Model of Team Dynamics

The team of professionals who provide services to children tends to be fluid and dynamic with roles and membership shifting in response to client needs and system changes. Team interaction is one of the most rewarding and potentially challenging aspects of pediatric occupational therapy. To become an effective team member requires a unique set of competencies. Skills in interpersonal communication, conflict resolution, decision making, consultation, and leadership are among the skills that are essential for the effective team member. This section describes a model of team dynamics based on interacting components that determine a team's effectiveness and productivity (Figure 2-1). The model's components are the team's (1) mission and purpose, (2) composition and structure, and (3) interaction model. These team elements determine how the team functions and are nested in a system or practice context. The primary contexts for children's services are hospitals or medical systems, schools, and community early intervention programs.

The context or organizational system often determines the team's mission, structure, and interaction model, which can vary, even within one system (e.g., teams in the public school system may use multidisciplinary or interdisciplinary models). This section applies the model of team dynamics to medical, educational, and early intervention systems.

■ MEDICAL SYSTEMS

Team Mission

Children's hospitals and hospitals with pediatric units provide medical, surgical, and psychiatric testing and treatment for children who are ill or have been injured or are newborns with medical problems. The aim of a hospital-based team is to restore or promote health (Figure 2-2). Related to the individual's health, medical systems also promote function, generally defined in medical settings as independence in ADLs. Various health care professionals provide care under the direction of a physician. From the first day of admission, the desired outcome for the child is discharge from the hospital as medically stable or healthy. Therefore the goal on entrance into the system is that the child will leave the system as quickly and medically well as possible. A secondary goal of the hospital team is placement in appropriate services that meet the child's developmental, functional, and educational needs.

When the child has a specific diagnosis or health problem, care plans and critical pathways are developed to guide the medical intervention. A critical pathway is a standard protocol used to guide a child's treatment and judge whether the most efficacious treatments are being used. Critical pathways also provide a method for evaluating outcomes. (Ideally, the client follows the pathway). Care plans determine when specific services are initiated and then provide broad guidelines for what should be provided. They are one tool that helps hospital personnel

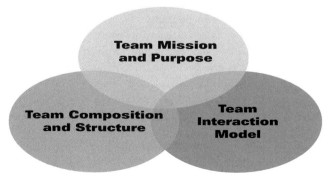

SYSTEM-PRACTICE CONTEXT

figure2-1   Model of team dynamics.

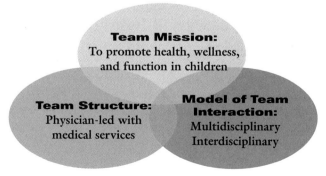

MEDICAL SYSTEM:
Hospitals and Rehabilitation Centers

figure2-2   Example of team dynamics in the medical system.

make efficient use of resources, reduce length of hospital stay, and lower readmission rates. They reflect the expanding focus of hospitals toward cost-effective measures, examination of outcomes, and management of resources.

Team Composition and Structure

Hospitals have traditionally used a physician-led team model. A child is admitted to the physician's care, and the physician determines the tests, procedures, and treatments that the child receives. The physician refers the child to other health professionals when another professional's scope of practice matches the treatment interventions that the child needs. Sometimes the team is made up of a physician and nurse. Other clients require the services of nurse, social worker, occupational therapist, physical therapist, and speech-language pathologist. The child's medical problem determines the composition of the team and the unit on which he or she is admitted. Teams may form quickly and temporarily around a single case (e.g., the physical therapist or occupational therapist who can take a new referral is on the team). Hospitals also have long-standing core teams with stable membership (e.g., a multidisciplinary feeding team, a developmental neonatal intensive care unit [NICU] team, or a myelomeningocele team).

The roles of the medical team members are usually inequitable, and the physician is designated as the leader. The physician-led team is essential to the operation of intensive care, surgical, or acute care units. The leadership position of the physician is not as established in rehabilitation or chronic care teams. When care is long term and less medically critical, a nurse or rehabilitation therapist may share in the leadership roles. A hierarchy of power and linear relationships among team members may not be as apparent. On these chronic care or rehabilitation teams, the physician may function as a consultant and members may have more equality. In other clinical practices managed by health management organizations (HMOs), nurse practitioners may provide numerous medical services and are considered leaders of the medical team.

Team Interaction Model: Multidisciplinary and Interdisciplinary

Although the lines of authority may vary in certain medical teams, most use multidisciplinary team models. This model evolves when the membership of the team frequently changes, generally in response to the child's medical problem. In multidisciplinary teams, members function relatively autonomously. Each is respected for his or her expertise in a defined practice area. Members have a good understanding of other professionals' scopes of practice and rely on these team members to fulfill their

roles. For example, in a NICU, all team members acknowledge that the dietitian provides new mothers with information on infant feeding formulas before discharge. This team also relies on the physical therapist to provide positioning recommendations to parents at the time of the newborn's discharge. Teams that are more established and are assigned to units with children who have comprehensive rehabilitation needs may use interdisciplinary models. (This model and the multidisciplinary model are described in this section.)

In a multidisciplinary model, professionals complete separate assessments and make individual treatment plans. Intervention is generally carried out in separate one-on-one sessions. Communication is informal (e.g., a quick call from the nurse to the occupational therapist to inform him or her that an infant appears alert and ready for an oral feeding). The medical chart is a primary form of communication. Communication tends to focus on essential elements of the child's care and tasks that need to be accomplished to restore health or meet the functional goals that will lead to discharge. Communication often results in actions and leads to other immediate communications, reflecting the rapid pace of the medical system. The medical goals are held as priorities and usually supercede social and behavioral goals.

A multidisciplinary, hospital-based team functions well when membership is stable and when team members perceive that they have equal status with one another. Teams are most likely to achieve equality of member status when goals for the client expand beyond the child's medical needs to social, developmental, and functional needs. Hospitals and medical systems have long-standing teams on special units (e.g., NICU, rehabilitation units) or in specialty clinics (e.g., cerebral palsy clinic). These teams establish developmental and functional goals for the client in addition to health goals. On these teams, interdisciplinary models are used.

In contrast to the multidisciplinary team, the interdisciplinary team requires group synthesis (Box 2-5). The professionals have substantial knowledge of the other disciplines, and this awareness enables each professional to speak and understand the language of the others. Roles on an interdisciplinary team are more flexible and more equitable. Inpatient rehabilitation programs (see Chapter 28) generally have interdisciplinary teams. A well-defined program often prescribes the team roles. The Commission for Accreditation of Rehabilitation Facilities (CARF) requires that programs define admission and discharge criteria, services, and protocols for certain conditions, as well as methods for program evaluation.

On rehabilitation units, comprehensive plans involving multiple services are developed for individual children. The team members work together on mutually agreed on functional outcomes. Co-treatments are common; therapists meet with the child's family to address problem issues such as selection of mobility devices, selection of augmentative communication devices, or strategies for managing posttraumatic brain injury aggression. Although assessment may be carried out in one-on-one sessions, members participate together in program and discharge planning. A case manager, who is usually a nurse or sometimes a social worker, coordinates the individualized care plan. The case manager is not only knowledgeable about the rehabilitation unit's services and the team's therapists, but he or she is also familiar with the services the child and family will need as they transition into the community.

Parents' roles on the hospital team are usually limited and prescribed. Family members defer to the physician and other health care personnel because of their expertise and professional prestige (Gilkerson, 1990). Although parents are the experts about their child, they admit that they are not the authority on health conditions. In particular, parents of a child with a newly diagnosed illness or disability may find it difficult to understand or accept their child's condition. Therefore they are not prepared to participate as members of a hospital-based team. Parents' participation is also affected by the stress induced by the child's illness and hospitalization, external demands of their lives that continue in spite of the trauma (e.g., other children in the family), and the simple logistics of scheduling team and parent meetings. Often parents form individual relationships with the professionals of the team and recognize that limited participation on the team may be adequate, particularly when their individual communication is shared with other team members.

■ EDUCATIONAL SYSTEM

Team Mission

The mission of a school-based team is to prepare children with the knowledge and skills to live productive lives in society (Figure 2-3). Public schools are primarily (i.e., approximately 80%) funded by their local communities and are therefore responsible to those communities. As knowledge expands and the complexity of tech-

---

box 2-5 *Hospital-based interdisciplinary team*

After suffering severe head trauma, Phil was a patient for 2 months at Children's Hospital on its rehabilitation unit. An interdisciplinary team, which included a nurse, social worker, occupational therapist, certified occupational therapy assistant, physical therapist, and speech-language pathologist, cared for Phil during his stay. A school psychologist, dietician, and clinical psychologist also consulted with the team. In the first weeks the team evaluated and monitored Phil as he transitioned from a comatose state to a conscious condition. The certified occupational therapy assistant implemented a sensory stimulation program, and the physical therapist initiated upright posture and performed passive range-of-motion exercises.

Phil became alert and responsive 2 weeks after his injury. At that time, both therapists completed a separate evaluation related to each professional domain of concern. At the beginning of the third week, all team members met with the family to review their assessment results and recommendations. After an hour's discussion the team developed a plan that reflected the parents' concerns and priorities, the medical concerns, and the therapists' recommendations.

Initially, the emphasis was placed on mobility and ADLs, and the physical and occupational therapists took leadership roles in determining his daily regimen of activities. By the fourth week the team met and decided to prioritize speech goals for the following 2 weeks and to evaluate and order assistive technology, including a wheelchair and laptop computer. Both would be needed for his return to school. Phil's ADLs remained an emphasis with these expanded goals.

At the end of the sixth week the hospital team met with the school-based team to determine revised priorities, based on the expectations of his school environment. Written and oral communication and school functions were emphasized.

In the last 2 weeks of his admission, team members frequently met to discuss his technology needs for the home and school and to plan a home program. They discussed which scenarios were optimum for follow-up, and it was determined that the school therapists could carry out most of his program with limited outpatient follow-up by the hospital team.

This example of an interdisciplinary medical team demonstrates how its members function individually to provide treatment. It illustrates the need for frequent meetings at critical points to make program changes, to address technology needs, to develop recommendations, and to complete discharge planning. Although the roles are delineated, members understand the benefit of frequent communication, and the goals reflect the input of several members, including the family. Flexible models of intervention are used, including co-treatments, consultations with other professionals, and transference of leadership among various team members.

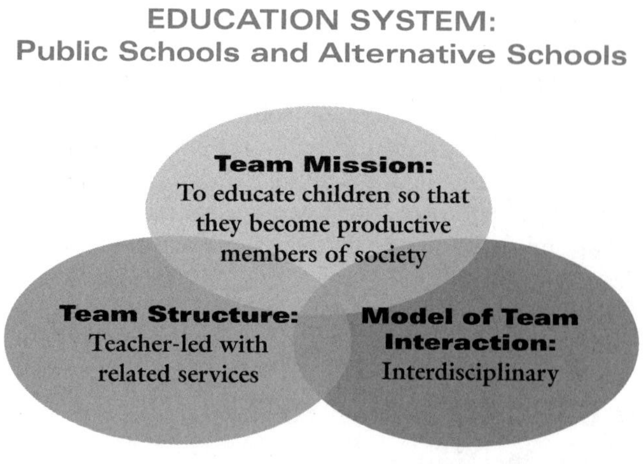

EDUCATION SYSTEM:
Public Schools and Alternative Schools

Team Mission:
To educate children so that they become productive members of society

Team Structure:
Teacher-led with related services

Model of Team Interaction:
Interdisciplinary

figure 2-3 Example of team dynamics in the educational system.

nology increases, public schools must reflect on both. As stated by Fullan, "Education has a moral purpose to make a difference in the lives of students regardless of background and to help produce citizens who can live and work productively in increasing dynamically complex societies" (1993, p. 4). He reasoned that educators must continually improve and reinvent the school's curriculum to prepare students to succeed in this ever-changing world.

Team Composition and Structure

The members of the school-based team are defined by and related services are listed in IDEA (see Table 2-1). In addition to the services of the regular and special educators, a student is entitled to related services that enable him or her to benefit from special education (IDEA, 1997). Although some educational teams (e.g., diagnostic teams) have stable membership, more often the membership of an educational team fluctuates according to the needs of the student.

A child's IEP defines which service providers will participate in a child's educational program, and it determines the level of service to be provided. Therefore an IEP defines how a team organizes and structures levels of participation around an individual child. When services are defined as "consultation," interaction and communication between therapists (the consultants) and teacher (the consultee) become the predominant method of service delivery. When the team decides that occupational therapy direct services are needed, a combination of service delivery models is implemented. These service delivery models may include (1) one-on-one intervention inside or outside the classroom, (2) consultation with the teacher and other related service providers, and (3) group sessions. Therefore team structure is governed by decisions made at the beginning of the year, and they

reflect parent priorities, assessment results, educational priorities, and educational outcomes as defined by the school system.

The teacher or special educator is often the leader of the team, coordinating the related services listed on the IEP and ensuring that certain educational priorities are achieved. The teacher's role as leader is a natural one, because he or she spends the most time with the students in the classroom. The teacher is most knowledgeable of the grade's curriculum and expected learning outcomes and often has greater access to the parents for ongoing communication. Because team members have equal status, roles and responsibilities are shared, all members contribute to problem solving, and decisions about a student's program are made collaboratively.

When therapy services are contracted from other agencies, school teams are considered interagency; therefore the related service personnel are not actual employees of the school system. This structure can be challenging for the team, particularly when the contract therapist is considered an outsider or is consistently unavailable for team meetings. When members are not full participants, the fractured team may result in duplication of services or missed opportunities for the student. Intra-agency teams create challenges for the team leader, and extra steps must be taken to maintain the flow of communication among all members.

Although the occupational therapist has the guidance of IDEA in determining the discipline-specific role in the school, Giangreco identified issues in team roles of related services. His studies (Giangreco, Edelman, & Dennis, 1991; Giangreco, Dennis, Edelman, & Cloninger, 1994) found that many professionals continue to assess, plan, make service provision decisions, implement, and evaluate in relative isolation, in spite of their belief that collaborative teamwork is ideal. Often professionals come to the IEP meeting with goals and recommendations already formulated. In many schools it is not uncommon for the person from each related service discipline to generate a separate set of goals that reflect outcomes valued by his or her respective discipline. In spite of this research, which reports that therapists act from the perspectives their own disciplines, IDEA clearly sets forth a process for interdisciplinary collaboration through the law's description of assessment and planning (i.e., writing the IEP).

Team Interaction Model: Interdisciplinary

As described under medical system teams, members of school-based interdisciplinary models value the contribution of each discipline and work to ensure regular and systematic communication. Team members recognize that their knowledge, skills, roles, and responsibilities overlap and therefore routinely meet to discuss and clarify their roles regarding a specific student. Essential to the success of an interdisciplinary educational team is the support of the school's administration. The research confirms the need for this support, as well as an organizational structure that recognizes the importance of team collaboration (Giangreco, 1995).

Six components contribute to the success of a school-based interdisciplinary team:

- Goal development through consensus
- Collaborative strategies
- Proximity
- Formal and informal meetings
- Flexibility
- Decision making through consensus

Goal development through consensus

The members of an interdisciplinary team develop the student's goals through a consensus process. In this process, discussion and disagreement are welcomed as part of determining optimal goals for the student.

Collaborative strategies

Members identify appropriate strategies. An emphasis is placed on collaborative strategies that teachers and therapists design together or implement together. For example, the preschool teacher and occupational therapist may decide to implement a sensory-motor activity with 5-year-olds before their writing and spelling lesson. Each child takes turns on the balls, scooter boards, trampoline, and swings in games led by the teacher and occupational therapists. These activities emphasize various themes including body scheme, numbers and counting, seasons, and holidays.

Proximity

Members work in proximity to each other. Working in a classroom, rather than in a separate clinic or area, helps promote interdisciplinary teaming. When in the classroom, the therapists are allowed to model for the teacher, to learn from the teacher, and to best address educational outcomes that relate to the classroom curriculum. Informal communication while in the classroom contributes to each other's understanding.

Block scheduling, a method particularly suited to preschool classrooms, refers to a block of time in the morning or afternoon during which a therapist is in one classroom. In some settings, the blocked time is shared with other therapists (e.g., both speech and occupational therapists are in the kindergarten room on Wednesday afternoons). During this time, the therapist may work with several different children, lead one or two small group activities, and participate in general classroom instruction. Often, most of the children in the room receive direct input from the therapist during the block of time. Block scheduling allows (1) support activities to be scheduled at the same time, (2) time for teachers and practitioners to work intensively with small groups of students, (3) minimal disruption of instruction, and (4) time for teachers and therapists to hold team meetings (Snell, Lowman, & Canady, 1996).

Formal and informal meetings

The school administration must recognize the importance of formal and informal meetings and allow time for both when scheduling and staffing. Administrators who do not recognize the value of team meetings may write contracts for occupational therapy services that cover only the treatment times specified on the IEP. As result, therapists are not paid and cannot afford to schedule time for meetings or for communications. This lack of administrative support is detrimental to the team.

Flexibility

Interdisciplinary teams must be flexible. Team leadership is shared by all team members and shifts from member to member, depending on the issue or task. The leadership qualities of team members are recognized and promoted. Flexibility regarding discipline roles is necessary (Box 2-6).

Decision making through consensus

Consensus in decision making is important to the function of interdisciplinary teams. When members agree, goals and plans can be supported and implemented. When team members do not achieve consensus, relationships tend to erode and conflicts develop. Conflicts can be destructive to the implementation of a child's program. Conflict resolution involves objectively examining the issues and then reexamining the child's goals. Generally, focusing on the child's goals helps resolve conflict concerning discipline-specific strategies. (Consensus building and conflict resolution are discussed in the final section of this chapter.)

Summary

When interdisciplinary teams in the school succeed, it is always the student who benefits. The challenge comes in learning how to support the teacher. The occupational therapist may have to sacrifice scheduled time with a student to listen to a teacher's concerns, or express an interest in what the class is learning, or solve a problem that has become a troubling issue to the teacher. Support of the teacher and his or her role and responsibilities is essential to develop a climate in which the team can flourish. This collaboration is often returned in the form of support for the goals that are the occupational therapist's responsibility. Time with the teacher supports the communication that is critical to understanding the student's progress in the curriculum and his or her needs that interfere with that progress.

box 2-6   *Flexible discipline roles*

Patricia is a 9-year-old student with spastic hemiparesis and severe communication delays. The team developed an IEP that identified mobility, keyboarding, and communication goals. Initially, emphasis was placed on ambulation using a hemiwalker, and the physical therapist had precedence in the child's schedule. The occupational therapist and teacher helped emphasize this primary goal.

Half way through the year, the family and team decided that powered mobility was optimum during the school day, and a powered wheelchair was obtained. The team met to revise Patricia's IEP. Independent ambulation became a secondary goal, and concerns about her difficulty with oral and written communication were given priority in the team's discussion. With new goals in speech and written communication, the level of direct services provided by the speech-language pathologist and occupational therapist increased. Keyboarding and

use of an augmentative communication device became the emphasis of the occupational therapy intervention. The occupational and speech-language therapists scheduled in-class time together to help Patricia learn to use her new device in her classroom. They used in-class time to determine how, when, and where Patricia could best use the device.

By the end of the year, Patricia's homeroom teacher supported the use of her device in the classroom. The occupational therapist switched to working with Patricia during her computer laboratory time using "Intellitool" programs, and the speech-language therapist assumed a leadership role in developing an appropriate vocabulary that related to the curriculum of her classroom on her augmentative communication device.

This example emphasizes the level of flexibility needed by team members to accommodate the evolving needs of the student.

In summary, team relationships require nurturing. Time together, positive interactions, trust, and respect are essential foundations to building team collaboration. Trust and respect develop when a therapist contributes to the classroom routine and supports the teacher and other team members through listening and acting on promises. To enhance the student's functional performance, the therapist asks for the opinions of team members and welcomes feedback regarding recommendations she or he has made.

■ EARLY INTERVENTION SYSTEM

Team Mission

The early intervention system is designed to provide multidisciplinary, interagency services to infants and toddlers with disabilities and their families (Figure 2-4). A major role of early intervention systems is the identification of infants who are at risk for disability and those who will benefit from these services. Once an infant enters the early intervention system, optimizing his or her developmental function becomes the focus. Professionals recognize the importance of intervention during this early period of neuroplasticity and rapid development of function. In addition, professions embrace the concept that the family is the constant in the infant's life, and services must include support of the family's ability to promote the child's development. An emphasis on family involvement has become a universal characteristic of early intervention programs. In family-centered services, pro-

EARLY INTERVENTION SYSTEM: Community agencies, homes, childcare centers

Team Mission: To provide family-centered services that promote the development of infants and toddlers with disabilities

Team Structure: Fluid, interagency, one primary service provider

Model of Team Interaction: Transdisciplinary Interdisciplinary

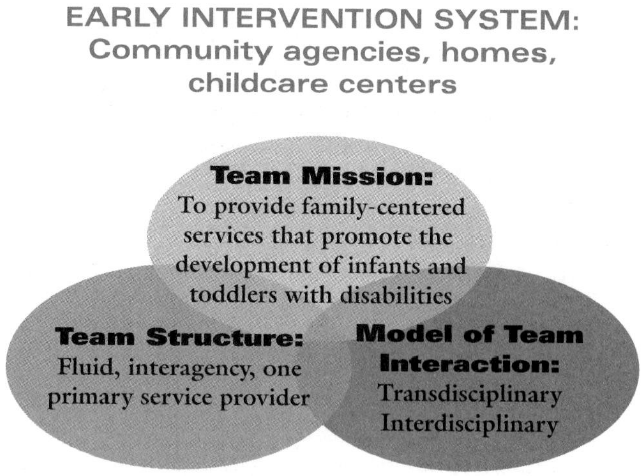

figure **2-4**   Example of team dynamics in early intervention systems.

fessionals form partnerships with parents to develop a mutually agreed-upon program for the infant. This program may include direct services to the infant or direct services to the parents or both. Parents participate in early intervention services to the extent that they are willing and comfortable. At times, parents may be the leader of the team; in other instances, parents may primarily be the recipients of services.

Several aspects of early intervention systems are different from medical or educational systems. First, early intervention systems were built on a range of services established for families and children that existed in each state before the implementation of early intervention legislation. Today, as a result, multiple agencies participate in providing services and interagency agreements characterize every intervention system. Teams in this system are not only multidisciplinary in nature, but they are also interagency in structure. Because members of the team are employed in different agencies, the need to coordinate the services is great. The role of service coordinator is highlighted in the early intervention legislation and plays an important role in early intervention teams. This individual coordinates the IFSP process to ensure that it is consistent and comprehensive and that it helps link the family with other community agencies.

Second, with the family as the center of the team, members acknowledge the need to assume roles with flexibility. When supported by other team members, professionals act in roles that are outside their discipline's scope of practice; they also teach parts of their roles to other members of the team. According to IDEA, services must be provided in the child's natural environment, which is often the home or childcare center. The IFSP is viewed as a dynamic or fluid document, and families can add goals or revise goals as intervention progresses without reconvening a full team meeting.

Team Composition and Structure

The early intervention services that are available to families as defined by IDEA are listed in Table 2-1. In addition to this list of professionals, the law clearly places the parents in an essential role as members on the early intervention team. The IFSP lists both infant and family goals, as well as the needed supports related to the concerns and priorities the family has for the infant. The structure of the early intervention team is circular with members sharing equal status. Leadership roles are shared, and service delivery is flexible so that services accommodate family priorities. Community based teams tend to have stable and enduring membership, which can strengthen the team's cohesiveness. Because a high level of flexibility is required and the family is the center of services, transdisciplinary models of teamwork are developed.

Team Interaction Model: Transdisciplinary and Interdisciplinary

A transdisciplinary approach is based on the assumption that coherence is promoted when the family primarily interacts with one professional (McGonigel & Garland, 1988). Team members work together to evaluate the infant and to design a program that is implemented by one team member. The family's entrance into therapy and intervention programs becomes easier because the family primarily relates to only one individual. This individual consults with other professionals on the team to answer the family's questions and design appropriate intervention strategies. Role release is inherent in this model, and the occupational therapist frequently provides consultation or becomes the recipient of consultation. The transdisciplinary approach is particularly appropriate for the infant who is medically fragile and does not tolerate multiple sources of stimulation.

In this model, assessment is planned, implemented, and summarized by the team as a whole. All team members assess the child, often in an arena assessment (see Chapter 22). In the arena model, one team member interacts with the child while other members observe the child and interact with the parents; asking them to help interpret the child's behaviors. Throughout the process, team members explain the assessment model to the parents and encourage them to ask questions. After observing the child, the team assembles to interpret their observations.

All team members (including the parents) come together with assessment results and their interpretations to develop the IFSP. Planning begins by asking the family to communicate their concerns and priorities. The team helps the family members articulate what they would like the early intervention team to address in the form of outcomes. Each outcome has prescribed services (e.g., occupational therapy, nutrition, social work) that will take responsibility for achieving it. The service delivery setting (e.g., home, clinic) is also defined, based on family preferences. Services in the infant's natural environment are emphasized. The natural environment includes home and community settings in which children without disabilities participate.

In the transdisciplinary model, all team members commit to teaching, learning, and working across disciplinary boundaries (Bruder & Bologna, 1993). Team members share information from their disciplinary skills that meet the child's needs. After the IFSP meeting, one or two members assume responsibility for carrying out the recommendations and strategies. The primary interventionist and the parents learn to recognize when the expertise of the occupational therapist or another therapist is needed. Because responsibility for the plan rests primarily with one individual, team members must be well versed in the skills and resources of the other professionals on the team. This model, sometimes termed role release, works only when team members frequently call on their colleagues to solve problems and for consultation. Role release is inappropriate when the occupational therapist has recently learned an intervention technique and is not yet comfortable with applying it. In addition, role release is not appropriate when the team member responsible for its implementation does not appear to have it mastered. Highly specialized techniques should not be transferred to other professionals, particularly when incorrect application could be detrimental to the infant (Garland, 1994).

The advantage of a transdisciplinary model is that unnecessary duplication and fragmentation are avoided. The team adopts the family goals; as a result, these integrated, goals are functional and holistic and in the context of the child's natural environment. The transdisciplinary model enables professionals to learn from each other and expand their professional knowledge into related disciplines. "At its best, the transdisciplinary approach can limit the intrusiveness in and disruption of family lives that occurs when teams require families to work separately with each discipline" (Garland, 1994, p. 99).

Using a transdisciplinary approach requires that professionals willingly share discipline-related information. Teaching someone else one's discipline-specific skills may be initially perceived as a threat. The occupational therapist needs to determine or ask about a fellow team member's preferred learning style. The style used to teach occupational therapy techniques can then be tailored to that learning style. Judgment is needed to decide what is critical knowledge for the successful implementation of a strategy with an infant and what is "bonus" information—specifics that are not necessary and perhaps not appreciated. Decisions must be made to determine whether a therapy technique is appropriate for someone who does not have knowledge of the discipline to implement the strategy. When strategies have the potential to be unsafe, it is the therapist's responsibility to recommend whether the strategy should be applied and, if so, how.

Summary

Early intervention teams create equality of roles across disciplines and agencies. Nontraditional team members may be involved because of the expanded focus of child and family. Team members share roles that sometimes fall outside the scopes of practice for their disciplines. Transdisciplinary teams can provide consistent, holistic services to young families when team members achieve a high level of collaboration and communication.

■ TEAM PROCESS

Team Communication

The goal of team communication is that professionals and family members develop *shared meaning* about their concerns and priorities for the child and about the system (Case-Smith & Wavrek, 1997). Because the language used by health care professionals is often technical and medically related, families can easily misunderstand its meaning. Occupational therapists and other team members must make a concerted effort to use layperson terminology to describe function, rather than neurophysiologic components, and to work with families to develop shared meaning about the child and the system. Descriptive *everyday language* adds to the comfort level and understanding of fellow team members. Even when professionals use simple and direct language, the message can be misunderstood. Parents are often preoccupied with their home and work lives, making it difficult to listen with understanding. The family's ability to assimilate information may also be limited in times of stress, for example, when the child is in the hospital. Therefore professionals should use simple messages and repeat information when it is essential that parents understand.

Parents and professionals develop *different understandings* of intervention services because they speak different languages (i.e., everyday language versus medical or discipline-specific terminology). When parents and professionals meet to discuss the child's diagnosis or to identify specific problems of a child as revealed in the medical or educational assessment, the parents may feel vulnerable and threatened. These meetings, as well as those that involve planning a year's program (e.g., IEP meeting), weigh heavily on parents who worry about the outcomes. In such meetings, professionals typically communicate at two different levels (McClellan, 1991). When professionals speak to professionals, the language is often technical, discipline-specific, and medical; when professionals speak with parents, layperson terms are often used. Using both levels of terminology to communicate the same or similar concepts can be confusing to parents. The use of specific medical terminology, although helpful to the physician or other professionals, can be baffling to the parent. Clear translation of technical terms for the parents should be offered without intimidating them or losing the intent of the specific communication.

Parents will usually reinforce intervention goals when team members explain recommendations in sufficient depth, reinforce each other's suggestions, welcome parental feedback, and incorporate parents' ideas into a suggested activity. Such collaboration requires time and willingness to develop a shared meaning of what is best for the child.

In teams whose members have developed effective communication systems, collaboration and integrated service delivery becomes possible. Teams use three methods for reaching decisions: problem solving, decision making by consensus, and conflict resolution. Each method is based on open lines of communication, a willingness and initiative to share information, and a commitment to team collaboration.

Team Problem Solving

In the first step of team problem solving, it is often important to identify who needs to be involved in discussing the problem. Not all team members must participate, but access to those with relevant expertise is critical to the process. In team problem solving, the members use a five-step process to ensure all solutions are considered and to encourage all members to contribute. The steps of the model as defined by Johnson and Johnson (1987) are presented in Figure 2-5. Team problem solving offers the following advantages:

1. More diverse knowledge and perspectives are brought to bear on the problem.
2. Great interest in the problem is stimulated because of the attention of numerous individuals.

3. The resulting solution is greater than the sum of the individual contributions.
4. Inappropriate solutions are rejected.

An educational team, in particular, engages in a problem-solving process when the student's performance does not match the expectations of the curriculum or when anticipated progress is not achieved. In problem-solving meetings in the schools, teams search for the least intrusive solutions that can be implemented in the regular classroom and those that are consistent with the IEP in place. School teams work to develop creative solutions that use in-place resources, because resources are often limited.

Step 1: Define the problem

Team members need to reach consensus about the definition of the problem. A clear definition of the problem enables the team members to agree on what the problem is. Therefore the first problem-solving step is to get valid, reliable, and correct information about the child and the environmental issues affecting the child's performance. Commitment to solving the problem rests with agreement as to the existence of the discrepancy between current and desired circumstances and an understanding of its importance.

Step 2: Diagnose the problem

The second step is to diagnose the dimension and determine the variables that are causing the problem. What barriers need to be overcome? What forces and factors are in place that may help solve the problem?

Step 3: Formulate alternative strategies

The third step is to formulate strategies and alternative ways to solve the problem. Creativeness, divergent thinking, opposition among ideas, and inventiveness are essential for this phase. Alternative solutions should address strengthening the child's current skills, improving his or her functional level, and removing barriers of the environment that interfere with functional performance. In specifying alternative strategies for change, the team members should think of as many ways as possible to solve the problem and promote the child's function. Outside consultation may be benefi-

Step 3: Formulate alternative strategies—cont'd

cial to increase the range of possible solutions. This step essentially involves brainstorming, and divergent thinking should be encouraged with no right or wrong answers at this time.

Step 4: Decide on and implement a strategy

Once all the possible strategies have been identified and formulated in specific terms, the team selects a solution. First, the team members engage in decision making by discussing the benefits for each alterative strategy, identifying resources needed to implement each alternative, and evaluating the probability of success if the alternative is implemented. Once a decision has been made, a plan is developed for implementing the solution. This may involve assigning specific team members the responsibility for carrying out parts of the plan and developing a time line for complete implementation. A detailed plan is desirable for accountability. The plan should be evaluated for its fit with the overall intervention plan for the child. Adjustments need to be made to the intervention plan or the newly formulated solu-

Step 5: Evaluate the success of the strategy

The decision if evaluated by determining (1) whether the strategies were successfully implemented, and (2) what the effects of the strategies were. To evaluate the strategy effectively, criteria are needed.

figure 2-5 Steps in team problem solving.

Decisions by Consensus

Decisions in medical, educational, and early intervention systems are rarely or never made unilaterally. Although each professional may assess the child, these interpretations and recommendations must always be given to the team so that the recommendations can be prioritized and integrated with other similar interpretations of team members. Decision making is therefore never reductionistic; the team and family make all important decisions. Although this process requires time and resources, it eliminates duplication and the team is able to focus on the most important goals and services for the child and family.

Therefore innovative and effective plans that the team and family can commit to implementing require the "buy in" of all members. When all members agree to implement an intervention plan, the participation of each member will increase and the plan will more likely succeed. To reach team consensus, members must actively participate and negotiate, with the voice of each member equally important. Decisions by consensus take more time and require more adaptability and flexibility by team members than other decision-making models. However, consensus building around individual children is summative and, over time, enhances team cohesiveness.

In team planning meetings that include parents (e.g., an IFSP or IEP meeting), the parent has the deciding voice. To assume the role of decision maker, a parent must be informed about how the team operates, how he or she can participate in the process, and how an intervention plan is developed. Given clear and specific information about the team's assessment and planning process and the type of intervention the program offers, the parents can take leadership roles in building consensus for their important concerns regarding their child. Bailey (1991) made the following suggestions for practices that can increase the family's role in reaching team consensus.

1. At the beginning of the meeting, the team leader states the purpose of the meeting and its desired outcome. All participants describe their roles as they relate to the child.

2. Members explain to the parents the format, that is, what they can expect to happen during the meeting.

3. Families are invited to speak first. They should be asked to share their perspectives and describe their observations of the child.

4. Any medical, technical, or discipline-specific terms are immediately explained in layperson's language.

5. Members readily admit when they do not know the answer to a question. Honesty is most important. Misinformation can have severely negative effects on relationships and trust building.

6. Families should never be placed in the middle of a professional disagreement. When professionals disagree, they should be open about their opinions but make every attempt not to confuse the family or break their trust in the team.

7. Consensus on goals for the child and intervention strategies results when professionals communicate openly and clearly and when they consider child and family needs above their professional identities and personal interests. (Additional discussion of communication strategies for consensus building is found in Chapter 5.)

Conflict Resolution

When disagreement arises regarding the intervention plan or service implementation, negotiation strategies should be employed to resolve the conflict in a positive and constructive way. Negotiation is a process by which people, who want to come to an agreement but disagree about the nature of the agreement, establish a plan accepted by all. Negotiation requires clear communication of the options and possible solutions. Team members should present clear rationales for the goals or solutions that they propose. The goals proposed should relate directly to the entire team's concerns and priorities and particularly to those of the family.

The first step in negotiation among team members is to identify the overall goal. When the team members disagree on specific objectives or activities, a global goal (e.g., promotion of the child's optimal health and development) on which all members agree becomes the starting point for compromise. Common interests related to the general goal can be established by first reconfirming the common purpose. With overall goals in mind, compatible intervention strategies can be identified. Conflicting interests need to be made explicit (Brandt, 1993).

Successful negotiation and problem resolution are more likely to be attained when (1) members are separated from the problem, (2) mutual interests and gains are accentuated, and (3) objective criteria are used to evaluate the solutions generated (Fisher & Ury, 1981). Therefore the problem needs to be depersonalized or viewed as separate from the individuals involved and their interpersonal interactions. All common interests and concerns should be identified, and they should relate to the child or to the concerns of family members. The solutions generated should be specific and concrete. They may need to be prioritized so that the team has an initial emphasis. Finally, criteria should be established to evaluate progress toward resolution of the conflict. Short-term objectives with explicit criteria allow the family and team to measure immediate progress and adjust to the plan to avoid negative feelings and conflict. These problem-solving strategies help the team reach agreement on intervention goals and to support each other and the family in reaching the goals.

■ SUMMARY

An occupational therapist's teaming skills are as important to effective intervention as discipline-specific techniques. Contributing to a team, collaborating with its members, and negotiating opinions are competencies that require effort and team experience to develop. Garland (1994) summarized how professionals can become contributing, collaborative team members:

1. Strive for consistency among one's discipline-specific goals and philosophy and those of the team's.
2. Ask for clarification regarding one's role and the roles of other team members.
3. Promote openness and clarity of communication.
4. Offer one's knowledge and skills, and express a willingness to use the resources of the other team members.
5. Develop decision-making and problem-solving skills.
6. Communicate a willingness to accept responsibility for the work of the team.
7. Develop skills in managing and using conflict productively.
8. Seek and use performance feedback from team colleagues.

As described in the model of team dynamics, the environment must be conducive to the growth and development of a collaborative team. Administrative and organizational supports are essential to team function, and these supports influence the type of team interaction that evolves.

STUDY QUESTIONS

1. Describe the role of the physician and nurse in the hospital, school, and early intervention systems. What are the implications for the team when the roles of medical professionals shift from team leaders to consultants?

2. What is the role of the teacher in the hospital? Given a child with head trauma who has spent two months on a rehabilitation unit, describe how the hospital-based teacher may optimally function during the child's transition from hospital to his former classroom.

3. Compare the advantages and disadvantages of primary communication with other professionals on your team through (a) written reports, (b) files and charts, (c) electronic mail, (d) telephone contact, (e) face-to-face meetings, and (f) informal conversations in the lunchroom.

4. Identify the variables that promote the effectiveness of a team, including system and individual characteristics important to the development of a cohesive team.

References

American Nurses' Association. (1999). *Nursing facts: Today's registered nurse—Numbers and demographics.* www.nursingworld.org

American Nurses' Association. (1990). *Standards of clinical nursing practice.* Washington, DC: ANA.

American Nurses' Association Council of Clinical Nurse Specialists. (1986). *The role of the clinical nurse specialist.* Kansas City, MO: Author.

American Nurses' Association Early Intervention Consensus committee. (1993). *National standards of nursing practice for early intervention services.* Lexington: University of Kentucky College of Nursing.

American Physical Therapy Association. (1999). APTA Background Sheet 1999, www.apta.org

American Speech-Language-Hearing Association (ASHA). (1999). Scope of practice in Speech-Language pathology, www.asha.org

Bailey, D.B. (1991). Building positive relationships between professionals and families. In M.J. McGonigel, R.K. Kaufmann, & B.H. Johnson. (Eds.), *Guidelines and recommended practices for the Individualized Family Services Plan* (pp. 29-38). Bethesda, MD: Association for the Care of Children's Health.

Brandt, P. (1993). Negotiation and problem-solving strategies: Collaboration between families and professionals. *Infants and Young Children, 5* (4), 787-884.

Bruder, M.B., & Bologna, T. (1993). Collaboration and service coordination for effective early intervention. In W. Brown, S.K. Thurman, & L.F. Pearl. (Eds.), *Family-centered early intervention with infants and toddlers: Innovative cross-disciplinary approaches* (pp. 103-127). Baltimore: Brookes Publishing.

Case-Smith, J., & Wavrek, B. (1997). Models of service delivery and team interaction. In J. Case-Smith (Ed.), *Pediatric occupational therapy and early intervention* (pp. 83-109). Boston: Butterworth Heineman.

Cochrane, C.G., Farley, B.G., & Wilhelm, I.J. (1990). Preparation of physical therapist to work with handicapped infants and their families: Current status and training needs. *Physical Therapy, 70,* 372-380.

Collins, R.M. (1995). Nurses in early intervention. *Pediatric Nursing, 21* (6), 529-531.

Council for Exceptional Children. (1999). *CEC Code of Ethics and Standards of Practice.* www.cec.sped.org

Cox, A.W. (1996). Preparing nurses. In D. Bricker & A. Widerstrom, (Eds.), *Preparing personnel to work with infants and young children and their families: A team approach* (pp. 161-180). Baltimore: Brookes Publishing.

Fisher, R., & Ury, W. (1981). *Getting to yes: Negotiation agreement without giving in.* New York: Viking Publishers.

Fullan, M. (1993). *Change forces: Probing the depths of educational reform.* New York: The Falmer Press.

Garland, C.W. (1994). World of practice: Early intervention programs. In H. Garner & F. Orelove, (Eds.), *Teamwork in human services: Models and applications across the life span* (pp. 89-116). Boston: Butterworth Heinemann.

Giangreco, M.F. (1995). Related services decision making: A foundational component of effective education for students with disabilities. In *Occupational and physical therapy in educational environments* (pp. 47-68). New York: Haworth Press.

Giangreco, M.F., Dennis, R., Edelman, S., & Cloninger, C. (1994). Dressing your IEPs for the educational climate: Analysis of IEP goals and objectives for students with multiple disabilities. *Remedial and Special Education, 15* (5), 288-296.

Giangreco, M.F., Edelman, S., & Dennis, R. (1991). Common professional practices that interfere with the integrated delivery of related services. *Remedial and Special Education, 12* (2), 16-24.

Gilkerson, L. (1990). Understanding institutional functioning style: A resource for hospital and early intervention collaboration. *Infants and Young Children, 2,* 22-30.

Hansen, S., Holaday, B., & Miles, M.S. (1990). The role of pediatric nurses in a federal program for infants and young children with handicaps. *Journal of Pediatric Nursing, 5* (4), 246-251.

Individuals with Disabilities Education Act (IDEA) Amendments of 1997 (P.L. 105-17). U.S.C. 1400 (et seq.)

Johnson, D.W., & Johnson, F.P. (1987). *Joining together: Group theory and group skills,* Englewood Cliffs, NJ: Prentice-Hall.

Lorsardo, A. (1996). Preparing communication specialists. In D. Bricker & A. Widerstrom, (Eds.), *Preparing personnel to work with infants and young children and their families: A team approach* (pp. 91-114). Baltimore: Brookes Publishing.

McClellan, M. (1991). *The discourse of interdisciplinary health care assessment: Toward a biosocial model,* Unpublished doctoral dissertation, Ohio State University, Columbus.

McGonigel, M.T., & Garland, C.W. (1988). The individualized family service plan and the early intervention team: Team and family issues and recommended practices. *Infants and Young Children, 1,* 10-21.

National Association of School Psychologists. (1999). *Standards for the provision of school psychological services.* www.naspweb.org

National Association of Social Workers (1999). *Credential and social work.* www.socialworkers.org

Snell, M.E., Lowman, D.K., & Canady, R.L. (1996). Parallel block scheduling: Accommodating students' diverse needs in elementary schools. *Journal of Early Intervention, 20* (3), 265-278.

Soderberg, G.L. (1993). The twenty-seventh Mary McMillan lecture: On passing from ignorance to knowledge. *Physical Therapy, 73,* 797-808.

Wachtel, R.C., & Compart, P.J. (1996). Preparing pediatricians. In D. Bricker & A. Widerstrom (Eds.), *Preparing personnel to work with infants and young children and their families: A team approach* (pp. 181-198). Baltimore: Brookes Publishing.

chapter **3**

Foundations for Occupational Therapy Practice with Children

Mary Law
Cheryl Missiuna
Nancy Pollock
Debra Stewart

key terms

Theories of occupation
Foundational theories
Risk and resilience
Family-centered service
World Health Organization International Classification
Developmental theories
Integrative theories
Occupation-based models of practice
Neuromaturation-based models of practice

■ CHAPTER OBJECTIVES

1. Explain the history and evolution of developmental theories.
2. Define the term *occupation*, and describe the study of occupation with emphasis placed on the occupations of children.
3. Explain what is meant by person-environment congruence.
4. Articulate the concepts and principles that define family-centered services.
5. Explain the developmental and learning theories of the early and middle 1900s, which provided the foundation for occupational therapy theories.
6. Explain and apply cognitive models of practice.
7. Use a dynamical systems approach to explain how children develop motor skills.
8. Explain how the person-environment-occupation model is used with other specific models of practice in occupational therapy intervention with children.
9. Describe and apply acquisitional theories and approaches.
10. Define and explain the appropriate use of neurodevelopmental and sensory integration therapy approaches.
11. Describe strategies that exemplify each practice model using client examples provided.
12. Compare and contrast intervention activities derived from different theoretical approaches and practice models.

■ INTRODUCTION

Chapter 3 discusses the current conceptual and theoretical foundations of occupational therapy practice with children. This chapter is organized in four sections, beginning with a brief overview of the historical and current perspectives of the theories that underlie current service provision: development, occupation, and environment. Section 2 focuses on foundational theories for occupational therapy practice. In Section 3 the overall framework for occupational therapy practice with children is discussed, based on a person-environment-occupation (PEO) perspective. This discussion is followed by overviews of current models of practice, ranging from a neuromaturation-based approach to an occupation-based approach. Section 4 of this chapter illustrates the application of these models of practice to specific practice scenarios, demonstrating the connection of theories, models of practice and assessment, and intervention strategies.

Occupational therapists have developed and used theory as the basis for professional practice for many years. Early developers of occupational therapy focused on the theories of occupation and the use of time (Meyer, 1922; Slagle, 1922), and theories of development and their influence on occupation began to be used in the 1920s and 1930s. However, theories and models of practice related to neurointegrative and environmental approaches were not developed until the 1940s (McColl, Law, & Stewart, 1993). In the past three decades, there has been a reemergence of the theories of occupation, and several models of practice have been developed using these concepts.

---

section 1
OCCUPATIONAL THERAPY PRACTICE WITH CHILDREN

When recalling childhood, summer is remembered as a time when friends spent the entire day playing outside. Children moved from activity to activity as a group, enjoying each another and participating in a variety of play activities. Most adults have fond memories of these days. At the time, however, the children did not think about the reasons they engaged in play activities or why particular activities were enjoyable. It was just fun! Occupational therapists, however, have a different perspective on play.

Play is considered one of the primary occupations of childhood. Occupational therapists understand that play is essential for development, and they study the concepts and assumptions that underlie the theories of play. Occupational therapists realize that multiple interrelated factors influence a child's ability to engage in play. All therapists, either implicitly or explicitly, base their practice on a theoretical rationale: play is the primary occupation of childhood. Through the use of theory, assessment, and clinical reasoning, occupational therapists hypothesize and then develop interventions to improve the occupational performance of children.

Theory is defined as a set of facts, concepts, and assumptions that together are used to describe, explain, or predict phenomena. Theories help organize selected aspects of the world in a systematic manner. Using theory, occupational therapists organize knowledge, understand observations, and explain or predict occupational function and dysfunction. Theories therefore provide a guide or rationale for occupational therapy intervention. Theories form the foundation for models of practice, or frames of reference, that guide the day-to-day delivery of occupational therapy services. A model of practice is the practical expression of theory and provides therapists with specific methods and guidelines for occupational therapy intervention. Models of practice draw from one or more theories and use concepts and assumptions to delineate the specific details of an occupational therapy practice, including who receives intervention, what intervention strategies are used, and when and where intervention is provided. The expected results from the delivery of an occupational therapy service is also based on the model of practice and the results that are expected in each practice situation.

■ CONCEPTS INFLUENCING OCCUPATIONAL THERAPY PRACTICE WITH CHILDREN

Development

Perspectives on development and occupation have changed over the past century as the knowledge about children, factors affecting their development, and basic needs for engagement in purposeful tasks and activities have changed. Developmental theories focus on explaining the processes by which infants mature and gain skills to become fully functioning adults. At the core of developmental theories is an explanation of the relationship between human biologic capacity and maturation and the influence of the environment on the behavioral experiences of the individual. In fact, developmental theories tend to be distinguished from each other by the specific weighing of these two factors, nature or nurture, or by the emphasis on a particular aspect of human biologic function or environment. For example, behavioral theories focus more on the influence of the environment on human development as compared with psychoanalytic theories that focus on biologic determinants of behavior. Although the emphases can differ, developmental theorists generally agree that human development is both the process and the product of biologic maturation and environmental experiences. Development may be defined as the sequential changes in the function that occurs with maturation of the individual or species. These sequential changes should be differentiated from the concept of growth, which refers to maturational changes that are physically measurable. In the past, different dimensions of development have been emphasized. For example, longitudinal development focuses on the stages of development, whereas hierarchical development focuses on the prerequisite skills needed for higher-level skills. Evolving views and theories of development place less emphasis on the stages and components of development and more on the person as a whole and his or her development in relation to environment, roles, and occupations. The emerging theories of person-environment relations and complex systems have influenced these changes.

Occupation

Theories of occupation have changed since the early 1900s. The ideals of moral treatment were prominent in the early part of the twentieth century, particularly the concept that daily routines and occupations improve a person's health. Although the profession of occupational therapy had not yet developed, physicians and others in health care began to focus on the use of a "work cure." The following excerpt from the *Journal of the American Medical Association* is an excellent example of the value placed on occupation at the time.

"How does occupation affect a cure? One thing is certain, that the coated tongue, the obstinate constipation, the diminished secretions, the sallow complexion and the other symptoms of ill health that very stubbornly resist other methods of treatment gradually disappear when patients are engaged in suitable occupation, and we can nearly always look forward with confidence for a marked improvement in mental condition" (Moher, 1907, p. 1666).

The decade after this article was published saw the beginning of a new profession called occupational therapy. Throughout the 1920s and into the 1930s, the focus of occupational therapy was the development of the idea of occupation as cure and it defined the occupations that were best used for specific medical problems. Occupational therapists used the principles of graded, purposeful activity and a balance of work, rest, and play as the basis for treatment methods (McColl, Law, & Stewart, 1993; Slagle, 1922).

In the 1940s, changes in the medical arena, particularly with the discovery of antibiotics and the advancement of specific medical and surgical techniques, had a tremendous influence on the way in which occupational therapists used occupation in treatment. There was an increase in the development of specific techniques and more focus on programs of activities of daily living. Occupational therapy treatment focused on the prescription of activities with specific aims (Hyatt, 1946). For example, the flexion, extension, pronation, supination (FEPS) loom was developed to ensure that targeted ranges of movement were achieved. The result of these changes was that treatment was "medicalized." In other words, the focus of occupational therapy was a series of technical activities rather than purposeful occupation. The influence of the medical model on the profession dominated for 3 decades, and it remains a predominant influence today.

As the 1960s ended, occupational therapists were increasingly uncomfortable with the technical focus of their profession. There was a call for more emphasis on the development of theory and a renewed interest in the roots of the profession—occupation (Yerxa, 1967). During this time, Reilly (1966; 1974b) described a theory of occupational behavior in which the individual strives to develop skills and competencies directed toward mastery and achievement. Work and play were viewed as the contexts in which these developments occur. Fidler and Fidler (1978) focused on the importance of purposeful activity,

or "doing," as necessary for the development of self and the prevention of dysfunction. Kielhofner and Burke (1980), building on Reilly's work, described a model of human occupation that incorporated a systems theoretical view of the nature of occupation. This model expanded the understanding of life roles and the powerful influence they have on experience and health. In the last 15 years a specific academic discipline named occupational science became the basis of occupational therapy (Yerxa et. al., 1989). This study of the human as an occupational being is essential to understand the complexity of engagement in occupation and the relationship between occupation and human health. Wilcock (1993) described the human need to use time in a purposeful way. "This need is innate and related to health and survival because it enables individuals to utilize their biologic capacities and potential and thereby flourish" (p. 23).

As the study of occupation has developed, occupational therapy scholars have proposed definitions of occupation. Clark and others (1991) defined occupations as "chunks of daily activity that can be named in the lexicon of the culture" (p. 301). Christiansen, Clark, Kielhofner, and Rogers (1995) defined occupation as the "ordinary and familiar things that people do every day" (p. 1015). The definition adopted by the Canadian Association of Occupational Therapists (CAOT) (1997) states that "occupation refers to a group of activities and tasks of everyday life, named, organized, and given value and meaning by individuals and a culture" (p. 34).

Each definition refers to daily activities or "chunks" of activity. Because of this daily activity concept, occupation is often thought of as simple; daily activities that people perform everyday to look after themselves, to be productive, and to enjoy life. The definition of occupation becomes more complex with the inclusion of its meaning or purpose. The meaning of an occupation for an individual or the value of an occupation determined by a culture begins to show the many layers of occupation and the central relationship of occupation to the human experience. Occupation is a basic human need (CAOT, 1997). Dunton (1919) expressed his belief that occupation is as necessary to life as food and drink. Occupation is an important determinant of health. Health can be strongly influenced by a person's engagement in meaningful occupations, and, conversely, the absence of meaningful occupation can have dire health consequences (Wilcock, 1998). Occupation serves as a means of organizing time, space, and materials. Patterns, habits, and roles evolve through the organization of occupation (Kielhofner, 1992). Occupations change over the life span (as do patterns of time used), representing occupational development.

Play is a key area of occupational focus in practice with children. Play is often described as a primary occupation of childhood (Knox, 1997). Most of the focus in the occupational therapy literature has been on play as a therapeutic medium and play as a reflection of development (Stewart et. al., 1996). Parham (1996) referred to this description as the functional view of play, that is, play serves other functions such as the development of motor or cognitive skills. A recent survey confirms that pediatric occupational therapists most often use play in therapy as a medium to develop skills underlying function (e.g., understanding of cause-effect relationships, exploring an object by manipulating it) and understanding rules that guide behavior (e.g., taking turns) (Couch, Deitz, & Kanny, 1998). Occupational therapists often observe children's play and play with them when trying to determine their level of development in performance areas and performance components (Linder, 1994). Less often, but probably more importantly, therapists view play as the outcome of interest or the ends rather than the means. Parham (1996) suggested that therapists will need to understand that "play is important for its own sake, not only because it subserves other important functions" (p. 78).

Occupation plays a dual role in the profession as both the focus of intervention and the media through which occupational therapists often intervene. For example, a child may be struggling at school in successfully fulfilling his or her role as a student because of an attention-deficit disorder. The student's academic occupations are negatively affected, as are his or her social occupation of maintaining positive peer relationships. The occupational therapist analyzes the daily occupations in which the child is expected to participate, determines the personal and environmental factors that are influencing the child's performance, and uses some of these occupations (e.g., entering a play group, independently completing desk work) to facilitate the child's performance. Occupational analysis is frequently used to understand the roles, tasks, activities, and skills required by the individual to perform meaningful occupations successfully in specific contexts (Watson, 1997). The recent development of occupation-focused assessment tools, such as the School Function Assessment (Coster, Deeny, Haltwanger, & Haley, 1998), indicate that the profession is moving forward in applying increased theoretical knowledge about occupation to practice.

When occupational therapists employ an occupation-based model of practice, the desired outcome is the achievement of optimal occupational performance for a child. What do the professionals know about the occupational performance of children with special needs? According to the 1992 to 1994 National Health Interview Survey, 6.5% of children with disabilities are limited to some degree in their participation in daily activities (Newacheck & Halfon, 1998). Children with physical disabilities are "2 to 3 times more likely to be unable to perform their usual activities than children with other conditions" (e.g., asthma) (Newacheck & Halfon, 1998, p. 612). Children with special needs experience lower rates of participation in ordinary daily activities (Brown & Gordon, 1987; Pless, Cripps, Davies, & Wadsworth, 1989). This pattern of restricted occupation appears to start in early childhood and is ingrained by the adolescent years. Children with special needs also experience social isolation (Anderson & Clarke, 1982; Blum, Resnick, Nelson, & St. Germaine, 1991; Cadman et. al., 1987; LaGreca, 1990; Law & Dunn, 1993). Clearly, encouraging participation in the typical activities of childhood needs to be the major focus for pediatric occupational therapy.

Environment

Human ecology is the study of human beings and their relationships with their environments. Environments are those contexts and situations that occur outside individuals and elicit responses from them, including personal, social, institutional, and physical factors. Environmental factors can facilitate or limit engagement in occupation (Law, 1991). A concept prevalent in the environmental literature and more recently in health care is person-environment congruence or "environmental fit," which is described as the congruence between individuals and their environments.

How has environment been historically viewed in occupational therapy? Early in the development of occupational therapy, little was written about the influence of the environment. The few references to the environment in early occupational therapy literature focused on how the physical environment influenced the recovery of the client (McColl et. al., 1993). In the 1930s, environmental theories had not yet been developed, but the literature introduced general ideas about how occupational therapy could provide an environment that was conducive to both recovery and the development of skills. Modification of the environment to influence client behaviors was first suggested in the 1940s. During the 1950s and 1960s, the literature continued to describe the role of the environment in occupational therapy as an influence on behavior and how enrichment of the environment or the creation of "prosthetic environments" could minimize disability.

During the past two decades, occupational therapists have stressed the importance of the interaction between individual and environment. Specific models of practice have been developed with a focus on environment (Dunn, Brown & McGuigan, 1994; Law et. al., 1996). Systems theory, emphasizing the interdependent relationship between individual and environment, formed the basis for concepts that define occupational therapy and models of practice. Primary models of practice address the environment in terms of its cultural, social, institutional, and physical dimensions and the transactional relationship between people and the environments in which they live, work, and play (Yerxa et. al., 1989).

Two theories from environment-behavior studies and theories related to risk and resilience are presented in these pages, because these theories are most applicable to occupational therapy practice in pediatrics. (The reader is directed to Law and others [1996; 1997] for information on other environment-behavior theories and models.)

Bronfenbrenner (1977) came from a background in developmental psychology and focused his study on the *social* development of the individual. He believed that there was an interdependent relationship between a person and social settings. A person is viewed as a social agent who interacts with all levels of the environment to develop and bring meaning to his or her life. The environment is described in terms of the social and cultural settings around a person. Changes at any level of the environment influence a person's behavior. A person, throughout his or her life, constantly adapts to changes in the environment.

Bronfenbrenner's emphasis on the social development of a person is important, because occupational therapists are part of a person's social environment. Bronfenbrenner's concepts help the therapist understand life span changes of clients within the context of their social settings. The interdependence between a person and the social environment assists therapists in pediatrics to expand intervention strategies to include families and communities.

E. Gibson (1988) and J. Gibson (1977, 1979), ecologic psychologists, considered the interdependence of a person with his or her environment as an explanation of *perceptual* development. Gibson (1988) described the motivation of a person to perform meaningful tasks and to learn about the various aspects of the environment that enable the individual to reach his or her goals. Gibson (1977, 1979) described the importance of the environment as constraining or enhancing the performance of tasks, and he termed this relationship "affordance." A person's successful adaptation to the environment occurs when a person matches his or her activities to the affordances of the environment, or the person modifies the environment to allow these activities to take place appropriately.

Gibson and Gibson's theories emphasize the importance of understanding a child's development in the context of daily surroundings and activities. Occupational therapists are encouraged to provide opportunities in which a child can explore and learn about the environment in a manner suitable to achieving his or her goals.

Risk and Resilience

Several theories and research programs have been developed to explain how the environment influences the developmental outcomes of children and adolescents. Most of this work focuses on the participation of children and youth in everyday activities and on factors that either place children and adolescents at risk for poor outcomes or help them achieve optimal outcomes. For example, psychologist Emi Werner had studied the people of Kawaii for over 40 years. Her research indicated that participation in extracurricular activities plays an important role in the lives of resilient adolescents, especially when they participate in activities that are cooperative in nature (Werner, 1989).

The *risk and resilience* literature attempts to explain why some children have better outcomes than others who were raised in similar circumstances. Researchers such as Rutter (1990) and Garmezy (1985) have identified protective factors related to the child, the family milieu, and the social environment. For example, attributes of the child that influence positive outcomes include positive self-esteem and communication skills (Garmezy, 1985; Werner, 1989, 1994). Attributes of the family that influence positive outcomes include family cohesion and harmony (Garmezy, 1985). Attributes of the social environment that promote resilience include extended social support and availability of external resources (Garmezy, 1985). Environmental factors such as family-centered service delivery, accepting community attitudes, supportive home environments, and mentoring relationships with adults have been shown to have a positive influence on child development (Richmond & Beardslee, 1988; Wallander & Varni, 1989; Werner, 1994).

Family-centered service

During the past 20 years, families of children with disabilities have increased their role in determining and implementing services for their children. Families have been leaders in promoting family-centered service, a philosophy of service provision that places emphasis on the central role of families in making decisions about the care their children receive. Although client-centered and family-centered practice first originated in the 1940s after Carl Rogers published a book on the clinical intervention of the problem child (Rogers, 1939), only recently has implementation of the principles of family-centered service become a standard of practice. Challenged by the changes in the health services field and an increased demand by consumers for involvement in the services they receive, health care providers have made great strides in implementing family-centered service.

Family-centered service, a philosophy of service provision, is a term that arose from early intervention programs. Three important concepts that define family-centered service are (1) parents know their children best and want the best for their children; (2) families are different and unique; and (3) optimal child functioning occurs within a supportive family and community context. The child is affected by the stress and coping of other family members (Rosenbaum, King, Law, King, & Evans, 1998).

In family-centered service, the family's right to make autonomous decisions is honored. The relationship between the family and professionals is a partnership in which the family defines the priorities for intervention and, with the service provider, helps direct the intervention process (Dunst, Trivette, & Deal, 1988). In working with families, service providers emphasize education to enable parents to make informed choices about the therapeutic needs of their child (Bazyk, 1989). Intervention is based on the family's visions and values. Service providers recognize their own values and do not impose them on the family. Family roles, interests, environments in which the members live, and culture make up the context for service provision (Law, 1991). Individualization of both the assessment and the intervention processes are essential to family centeredness. Intervention is viewed as a dynamic process in which clients and parents work together as partners to define the therapeutic needs of the child with a disability. Services are designed to fit the needs of the family, rather than the family fitting the needs of the services or intervention philosophies already in place.

There is increasing evidence in the literature that interdisciplinary, family-centered service for children with disabilities leads to increased family satisfaction and may lead to greater functional improvement in children with disabilities. Research has demonstrated that parents have greater control when service providers are positive and proactive and promote parental participation and competency. In contrast, a lack of control is associated with behaviors that are unresponsive to the family's needs, paternalistic, and fail to recognize or accept family decisions (Dunst, Trivette, Davis, & Cornwall, 1988). Moxley-Haegert and Serbin (1983) found that teaching parents to recognize developmental gains in their delayed infants increases parents' participation and enhances developmental gains for the child. Stein and Jessop (1984, 1991), in a randomized controlled trial with 219 families, demonstrated that an integrated, community-based program that focused on the whole family and its needs led to greater parental satisfaction with care and better psychologic adjustment of the child. Occupational therapists who work with children enhance the effectiveness of their services when they practice from a family-centered perspective.

World Health Organization International Classification of Impairment, Activity, and Participation

It is useful for occupational therapists to have knowledge of the *World Health Organization* (WHO) *International Classification* system that is used in the broad rehabilitation and disability arena. The International Classification of Impairments, Disabilities, and Handicaps (ICIDH) was first developed and published in 1980 (WHO, 1980). This system classifies the effects of health conditions on functioning into three levels: the body (impairment), the person (disability), and the roles and society (handicap). The development of software that

categorizes and selects outcome measures (Law et. al., 1999) is an example of how occupational therapists have used this classification. The ICIDH revised classification system is currently titled the International Classification of Impairments, Activities, and Participation (WHO, 1998). This revised classification (ICIDH-2) also includes the domain of environmental factors, because it is recognized that environmental factors have significant influence on a person's activities and participation in activities. Terminology used in occupational therapy parallels that included in the ICIDH-2. Performance components are comparable to "impairments," and "involvement in activities" and "participation" reflect occupational performance.

section 2
FOUNDATIONAL THEORIES

Foundational theories are used to form the basis of occupational therapy intervention approaches. These theories come from many fields of study—from biologic sciences to social sciences to humanities. Occupational therapists draw from a wide range of foundational theories to explain occupational performance. Most theories used by occupational therapists who work in pediatrics are concerned with change. Such theoretical perspectives complement the therapist's view of human development as sequential changes in the function of an individual or a species. Considering the complex nature of the PEO perspective and the transactions that are involved in occupational performance, multiple foundational theories have relevancy. This section reviews the theories that are most commonly used by occupational therapists who work with children and adolescents with disabilities.

■ DEVELOPMENTAL THEORIES

Developmental theories explain and describe different components of a person as they relate to occupational performance. Different theorists have focused on particular components of the individual in an effort to explain developmental function and dysfunction. The most common theories used by occupational therapists are presented.

Freud and Psychosexual Development

Discussion of Sigmund Freud's theory focuses on personality development. Freud (1856-1939) proposed that personality arises from the biologic, instinctual energy of the individual, and that this energy is differentiated through typical environmental experiences at different ages. He believed all behavior is causal in nature.

Freud's model of personality includes three main concepts: id, ego, and superego. The id is the initial, motivating part of a person's personality and is present at birth. It represents the psychic energy, the impetus for all behavior. The id contains both the life and death instincts of the individual. Life instincts, which include hunger, thirst, and sex drive, ensure the survival of the individual and the species. The source of energy for these drives is called libido. Opposing drives are death instincts, which manifest themselves throughout life in the form of destructive energies and aggressive behavior.

Freud is best known for his systematic study and organization of concepts related to the unconscious. Although only parts of the ego and superego exist at the unconscious level, the entire id is located in the unconscious mind. The ego acts as a gatekeeper to the unconscious, channeling the needs of the id that can be met in socially acceptable ways. The superego functions as the moral component of personality, reflecting the learned values of the culture. Libidinal urges that are in conflict with society (and its mirror, the superego) are held back or sidetracked through defense mechanisms (Nye, 1978).

Freud postulated that the impetus for development at different stages of life is centered on obtaining pleasur-

able sensation in the erogenous zones. Each stage of psychosexual development is named for the erogenous zone that presumably provides the greatest source of pleasure and contact between the child and environment at each stage (Table 3-1).

Freud's concepts of the unconscious and psychosexual aspects of personality development have contributed significantly to our understanding of human nature. Many developmental frames of reference and models, including those in occupational therapy, incorporate some of Freud's concepts.

Erikson and Psychosocial Development

Eric Erikson (1963) was a student of Freud's, and his theory of development reflects that affiliation. Erikson is viewed as the father of ego psychology. His work demonstrates a more optimistic view of human nature and focuses on the functions of the ego in response to the environment. He believed that personality is based on more than instinct, and he gave priority to the adaptive response of the ego in the development of the individual.

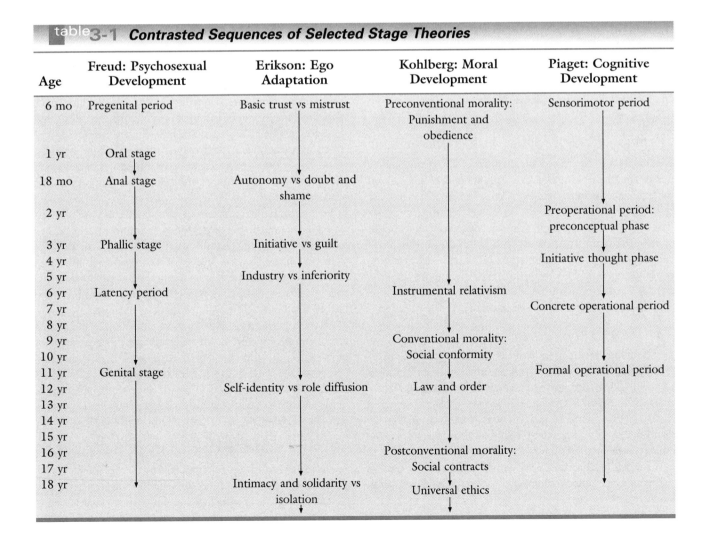

table 3-1   Contrasted Sequences of Selected Stage Theories

Age	Freud: Psychosexual Development	Erikson: Ego Adaptation	Kohlberg: Moral Development	Piaget: Cognitive Development
6 mo	Pregenital period	Basic trust vs mistrust	Preconventional morality: Punishment and obedience	Sensorimotor period
1 yr	Oral stage			
18 mo	Anal stage	Autonomy vs doubt and shame		
2 yr				Preoperational period: preconceptual phase
3 yr	Phallic stage	Initiative vs guilt		
4 yr				Initiative thought phase
5 yr		Industry vs inferiority		
6 yr	Latency period		Instrumental relativism	Concrete operational period
7 yr				
8 yr				
9 yr			Conventional morality: Social conformity	
10 yr				
11 yr	Genital stage			Formal operational period
12 yr		Self-identity vs role diffusion	Law and order	
13 yr				
14 yr				
15 yr				
16 yr			Postconventional morality: Social contracts	
17 yr				
18 yr		Intimacy and solidarity vs isolation	Universal ethics	

Erikson conducted extensive studies of children, including cross-cultural comparisons. He believed that play afforded the best opportunity for observations of adaptive and maladaptive responses of the ego. His theories emphasize environmental influences and are applicable across cultures, which make them especially useful for occupational therapists.

Erikson divided the life span into eight stages of psychosocial development. Each stage is represented by a personal-social crisis that gives impetus to ego growth. His model begins with exploration and leads to mastery. The concepts of mastery and achievement characterize development throughout childhood and adolescence (see Table 3-1). Each stage results in the acquisition of an abstract personality quality, such as hope or wisdom (Hall & Lindzey, 1978). This text briefly describes the first five stages through adolescence.

Basic trust versus mistrust

The infant, from birth to about 18 months, develops psychologic trust, the eagerness to approach new experiences without fear. Trust develops through the caregiving attentions of the parents. The initial sense of trust comes from the infant's realization that survival needs will be met and that he or she can exist in a state of comfort. The most difficult task for the infant is to maintain this trust in the absence of his or her parents. Erikson believed that parents must provide gradual opportunities for separation, yet ones that do not provoke excessive anxiety. Infants who successfully resolve this stage acquire *hope*.

Autonomy versus doubt and shame

The 2- to 4-year-old toddler experiences autonomy rather than doubt and shame. This stage is characterized by holding on and letting go and is exemplified by the crisis that occurs through the toilet-training process. Erikson specified the relationship of autonomy to the child's increasing control over his or her body. This stage brings independent movement away from the parents, enabling the child to explore the environment. Parents must provide opportunities for the child to make choices and develop a sense of self-controlled *will*.

Initiative versus guilt

The newly autonomous preschool-age child has mastered basic motor skills and must now build a repertoire of social skills to deal with the outer world. Central to this development is the achievement of gender role identity. Children primarily learn gender roles through imitation of parents and possibly teachers. Through imitation, children learn to assume responsibility for themselves in familiar and comfortable environments. Evident in their complex play scenarios and newly achieved self-care skills is a sense of *purpose*.

Industry versus inferiority

The elementary school child experiences a period of slow, steady growth. The need for security is transferred from the family to the peer group, as the child attempts to master the activities appropriate for his or her age. The peer group is used as a standard of performance against which the child can measure his or her own skills. Through sports, games, and school achievements the child gains a sense of *competence*.

Self-identity versus role diffusion

Erikson studied the period of adolescence in detail. The masterful school-aged child is suddenly shaken by the physiologic changes of puberty and must struggle to regain control over body, identity, and future. During adolescence, prolonged childhood ends and society asks the adolescent to make choices concerning adult roles. The adolescent experiments with patterns of identity until a sense of continuity and control over the ego is regained and a perspective of the future is acquired. In spite of the often-turbulent conflicts among adolescents and their elders, Erikson believed the actions of both are directed to the same end of helping adolescents clarify their roles as members of society. Through resolution of the identity crisis, the individual gains continuity of the past with the future—a sense of *fidelity*.

Kohlberg and Moral Development

Lawrence Kohlberg (1978) was interested in the relationship between the concepts of cognitive development and the acquisition of moral value schemes. He designed a series of fascinating experiments that presented moral dilemmas to children and young adults of different ages. Like Piaget, whose theories are described in the next section, he did not judge the correctness of children's choices; instead, he collected data about the concepts used by the children to make moral decisions. He found these concepts to be patterned, sequential, and somewhat linked to age. His model of moral development describes three discrete levels: preconventional morality, conventional morality, and postconventional morality. Each of these levels has two complementary stages (see Table 3-1).

It is interesting to note that Kohlberg's stages are chronologically behind those of Piaget, indicating that levels of cognition must be mature before an individual can use the higher-level operative methods to examine abstract issues of morality. The development of morality ends with adults using moral thinking in dealing with everyday situations.

Maslow and the Hierarchy of Basic Needs

Abraham Maslow is generally considered the father of humanistic psychology in the United States (Hall & Lindzey, 1978). He outlined a hierarchy of basic human needs that is believed to follow a longitudinal sequence (Maslow, 1968; 1970; 1971). At the base of his hierarchy are physiologic needs, such as food, water, rest, air, and warmth, which are necessary to basic survival. The next level is characterized by the need for safety, broadly defined as the need for both physical and physiologic security. The need for love and belonging promotes the individual's search for affection, emotional support, and group affiliation. The need for a sense of self-esteem, which is defined as the ability to regard the self as competent and of value to society, is evidenced as an individual grows. The need for self-actualization, which represents the highest level, is attained through achievement of personal goals.

Maslow proposed that each of these needs serves as a motivator to achieve a higher level of human potential. There is a progression of development that begins with the satisfaction of biologic and egocentric needs. It proceeds through the needs for social group affiliation and culminates in the use of intellectual capacities to affect the broader community of the individual. If the lower-level needs are not met, the individual is not able to direct his or her energies toward higher levels. For example, when a child comes to school hungry, it is difficult to concentrate on the classroom learning activities. Recognition of a child's needs and the hierarchy of development of these basic needs are important for occupational therapists who strive to assist children to achieve personal goals.

Rogers and Development of Self

Carl Rogers (1969) believed that people have an inborn need for self-actualization. Central to Rogers' theory is the individual's inner experiencing, that is, how the individual perceives him or herself and his or her relationships and environment. Rogers acknowledged the instrumental influence of the environment in the development of self, but he believed that the individual has the capacity to choose responses to the environment that allow him or her to maintain a sense of personal control.

Rogers is best known for his formulation of client-centered therapy. Like Erikson, Rogers believed that each individual has, and must find within himself or herself, the resources for growth, adaptation, and self-actualization. Client-centered therapy is designed to elicit these resources, and the therapist takes a nondirective role that encourages the client to express his or her own desires and interests and to act on these. Occupational therapists have embraced a client-centered approach to practice for many years, because it fits with the philosophy of the client being actively engaged in the therapy process.

■ INTEGRATIVE THEORIES

Most important to occupational therapy are *integrative theories,* which are theories that integrate concepts about persons, their environments, and their occupations. A discussion of these learning and systems theories follows.

Learning Theories

Development has been defined as an "evolution of predictable sequences of interactions between a child and the objects in his or her environment" (Lyons, 1984, p. 446). Developmental theories, which provide stages or markers of progress against which a child can be compared, are emphasized in the previous section in this chapter. Traditional views of development emphasize the dominant role of the maturation of the central nervous system (CNS). More recently, occupational therapists have begun to understand that cognitive and motor progress is possible through a dynamic process in which the CNS develops as the child attempts to solve cognitive and movement problems. This process is termed learning, that is, the acquisition of knowledge through experience in a way that leads to a permanent change in behavior. In occupational therapy theory, it is helpful to examine theories of motor learning, cognitive progress, and motivation for change. In all three domains, learning occurs when children find solutions to problems and thereby acquire functional skills.

Before examining how children learn, it is important to review the different dimensions along which tasks may vary since each of these is relevant to the way in which they are learned.

1. *Simple-complex.* Simple tasks, such as reaching for an object, require a decision followed by a sequenced response. Complex tasks, such as handwriting, require the integration of information from a variety of sources and the application of underlying rules that guide performance (Colley & Beech, 1989).
2. *Open loop–closed loop.* In an open-loop task a motor program is put into place before the action begins and is not modified during the performance of a task. An example of an open-loop task is throwing a ball. In a closed-loop task the child continues to monitor and respond to feedback that he or she receives intrinsically from the body and extrinsically from the environment. An example of a closed-loop task is cutting out a shape using scissors (Adams, 1971).
3. *Environment changing–environment stationary.* The difficulty of learning a task is tremendously influenced by the extent to which the task is predictable. When the environment is changeable or variable, the child has to learn the movement and learn to monitor the environment to adapt to change. Running on rough terrain or playing soccer are examples of tasks in which the environment is constantly changing. This concept is not to be confused with the open- and closed-loop features of the task previously described. Brushing the teeth and playing the piano

are tasks in which the child must monitor sensory feedback during the performance of the tasks (closed loop), but the environment remains stationary (Sugden & Sugden, 1990).

4. *Novel-acquired.* During the first performances of a task, the child combines what he or she knows about the task with information from the environment. The child then makes a workable procedure that is controlled, slow, and full of effort. With repeat performances of the task, however, multiple procedures are collapsed and run more automatically. With practice, the speed of performance increases and the effort decreases (Anderson, 1982).

5. *Task modality.* The ease or difficulty of learning a task depends on the match between the way the task is presented and the preferred learning style of the child. Some children learn best through auditory or visual methods; others prefer movement and touch. The modality of the task (e.g., visual, oral, physical, figural) is another factor that influences learning.

Skinner and behaviorism

The past 50 years have witnessed tremendous progress in the field of learning theories. Early learning theorists, such as Thorndike, emphasized the association between a behavior and the resulting reward or punishment as a simple explanation of behavioral change. Skinner (1953) described perhaps the best-known learning theory from this era. Skinner believed that the environment shapes all human behaviors and that behaviors may be randomly emitted in response to an environmental stimulus. In other words, a person tries a behavior that worked in a previous situation, or an involuntary, reflexive response is elicited by an environmental stimulus. The behavior is then reinforced by the environmental consequences that follow. This sequence—stimulus situation, behavioral response, and environmental consequence—constitutes a "contingency of behavior," the mechanism through which the environment shapes behavior.

Skinner (1976) stated that through natural occurrences in the environment, the child's adaptive behaviors are reinforced, and those behaviors that are not adaptive are ignored or punished. The child usually associates positive reinforcement (reward) with a pleasant experience. Behavior is strengthened and maintained as long as it is generally effective in obtaining positive reinforcement. If reinforcement is absent, that is, not given and therefore negative, positive behavior may be extinguished.

Skinner believed that all behavior is a result of the environmental control of the individual, culture, and species. He specified that humans, species, and culture are all part of the environment, and therefore they control as much as they are controlled. Problems arise when an environment changes and becomes inconsistent with prior contingency patterns. For example, children use one set of behaviors with their families and another set with friends. Behaviors that are reinforced by friends may bring complaints or be ignored by parents.

Extensive research has confirmed that when particular behaviors result in specific, consistent consequences, these behaviors can be modified. Skinner (1953) believed that a process called shaping creates new behaviors. Shaping involves breaking down a complex behavior into subcomponents and reinforcing each behavior individually and systematically until it approximates the desired behavior. Critics of this theory site its failure to explain personality traits (e.g., motivation) and cognitive abilities (e.g., imagination and creativity) and its tendency to generalize across age and gender spectrums with no recognition of developmental differences.

Piaget and cognitive development

Jean Piaget (1971) was concerned with the developmental adaptation of the individual in response to ongoing environmental experiences. He defined adaptation as the child's ability to adjust to change to fit into his or her environment, and he examined adaptation through the child's relationships with human and nonhuman objects and through time and space. Piaget (1952) introduced the idea that children are intrinsically motivated to learn from their surroundings and that they act on, rather than simply react to, their environment (Krantz, 1994). Piaget used the term cognitive structures, or schema, to describe the way in which children represent objects, events, and relationships in their minds. Piaget viewed every interaction as an opportunity to either assimilate new knowledge into existing structures or to adapt existing structures to accommodate new information. Accommodation is new learning and believed to be the way in which cognitive progress is made. Piaget's developmental stages have been the focus of research and critique; however, his descriptions of the gradual accumulation of knowledge in specific content areas remain valid concepts in child development.

Piaget believed the child organizes his experiences into mental schemes (concepts) through mental operations. Operations may be defined as the cognitive methods used by the child to organize his or her schemes and experiences to direct his or her actions. The totality of operational schemes available to the child at any given time constitutes the adapted intelligence, or cognitive competence, of the child.

Piaget believed there was an invariant, hierarchical development of cognition that proceeded from the simple to the complex, from the concrete to the abstract, and from personal to worldly concerns. He specified four maturational levels or periods of cognitive function: sensorimotor, preoperational, concrete operational, and formal operational (see Table 3-1) (Flavell, 1985). He believed that this sequence of development leads to the cognitive maturity of adulthood. The culmination of these levels is a person with values, goals, plans, and an understanding of his or her purpose in society.

Knowledge of Piaget's theory is important to occupational therapists who plan programs for children. Regardless of the therapeutic approach used in treatment, the therapist interacts with a thinking child. The selection and structure of an activity is essential, in accordance with the operational skills and concepts of the child.

The primary focus of Piaget's concept is explaining cognitive learning, but Schmidt (1988) developed the idea further in the area of motor learning. He proposed that motor schemas are formed as combinations of (1) the initial conditions of the movement, (2) the specific parameters used to create it, (3) the knowledge of the results in the environment, and (4) the sensory consequences of the movement. Through repeated experiences, the child abstracts relationships among these four features (Schmidt, 1988) and is considered to have learned a new movement.

Social cognitive theories

The initial acquisition of highly complex and abstract behaviors was difficult for learning theorists to explain until the advent of Bandura's (1977, 1982, 1989) social cognitive theory. This theory introduced the idea that children can learn by observing the behavior of others. Bandura's theory has two important concepts: *acquisition* and *performance*. During acquisition, a child observes the behavior of others and determines the consequences, and these observations are stored in memory for later use. Performance refers to the idea that the child may decide to perform the behavior, depending upon the child's perception of the situation and the consequences. Bandura believed that critical factors in the child influence the learning process, including the child's perception of his or her competencies, a topic that is addressed later in this section. Bandura's introduction of the importance of the social context to the child's ability to learn and his recognition that a child's thoughts and beliefs also influence his or her learning ability are important to occupational therapists.

Vygotsky (1978) also recognized that learning is developed in a social context, and he believed that cognitive development occurs through the gradual internalization of concepts and relationships that are encountered through social interactions. Although he agreed with Piaget that children develop as a result of engagement in activity, he believed that learning also requires interaction with others who were more cognitively competent. He suggested that children first experience activities (e.g., problem solving) in situations in which there is a child, an activity, and a significant other. The adult initially does most of the cognitive work; however, gradually the adult's speech is internalized by the child and, with experience and application, becomes part of the child's cognitive repertoire (Missiuna, Malloy-Miller, & Mandich, 1998).

Vygotsky introduced the critical concept of a zone of proximal development, which he conceptualized as follows:

> The distance between the actual developmental level as determined by independent problem-solving and the level of potential development as determined through problem-solving under adult guidance or in collaboration with more capable peers (Vygotsky, 1962, p. 86).

Vygotsky believed that the zone of proximal development is reflective of the learning potential of the child at a moment in time. When an adult and a child experience an activity together, they interpret the objects and events differently. Vygotsky suggested that the adult uses language to help the child redefine the situation so that both adult and child will have a shared definition. When a learning opportunity is created that provides an optimal balance between the child's existing skills and the challenge of the task, the adult can model language and behavior that will help the child progress. Vygotsky's emphasis on the interaction between children's learning, their environment, the type of instruction provided, and their culture was a precursor to many of the dynamical systems models that influence learning theory today.

Information processing

The computer has served as a source of inspiration for learning theories that study the manner in which children learn, attend, remember, and solve problems. These theories are called *information processing* theories, and they all focus on the system through which children extract information from the environment, interpret the information, and organize a behavioral response. The theories of many widely recognized theorists (e.g., Case, 1985; Shiffrin & Atkinson, 1969; Siegler, 1983) stem from this framework. Although each learning theory differs slightly, there are similarities in the basic beliefs about learning. Information processing theories are usually portrayed as flowcharts that represent the source of the sensory *input,* the method of accessing memories and solving problems (called *throughput* or elaboration), and the *output* that is the result or solution. Some theorists also add a feedback loop to explain the acquisition of knowledge and the use of the results of actions (e.g., Sternberg, 1984). Like social cognitive theory, information processing theory emphasizes change as a continuous process of learning and explains age differences as improvement in children's problem-solving abilities with experience (Krantz, 1994). Information processing theories have been applied and developed in both the cognitive and motor domains.

Summary

One cannot complete a discussion of learning theories without briefly considering the factors in the child that are believed to influence learning; these factors include motivation, attitude, and self-perception. The relationship between learning and other affective components is complex. It is widely accepted that children's motivation to perform occupations is influenced by their perceptions of their efficacy, whether or not these perceptions are correct (Bandura, 1993). If children experience success in learning situations, it is assumed that they increase their perceived competence and internal control, gain support from significant others, and show pleasure at mastering the task. The assumption is made that children are more likely to seek out optimal challenges if they have experienced success. The corollary of this theory is that children who experience repeated failure begin to avoid challenges and are less likely to seek out new learning situations (Harter, 1978). Therapists need to be aware of the importance of providing successful learning opportunities and optimal challenge situations. It is also important to note, however, that when children are young, they may not have the metacognitive awareness required to compare their own performance accurately with that of others. This lack of awareness may actually have an adaptive purpose in childhood. The fact that young children do not evaluate their own performance increases the likelihood that they will put energy and effort into practicing skills in a wide variety of environments with little concern about their actual competency (Bjorklund & Green, 1992).

A final consideration for the occupational therapist relates to what happens to the learning once the skill is acquired. Children do not always automatically transfer the skills that they have learned; they often require instruction and guidance to transfer the knowledge and skills from one task to another and to generalize these skills to different environments. Some researchers propose that generalization receive as much attention and emphasis as is given to initial skill acquisition (Gresham, 1981). As the research on how children learn is reviewed, the ability of theory to explain learning and performance in a functional context and in a variety of settings needs reflection.

Systems Theory

Emerging theoretical ideas from systems theory influence today's thinking about both learning and motor development in children, and these ideas are beginning to lead to the creation of alternative models of practice for therapy intervention. In contrast to a hierarchical model of neural organization, systems theory (also called dynamical systems theory) proposes a flexible model of neural organization in which the functions of control and coordination are distributed among many elements of the system rather than vested in a single hierarchical level

(Van-Sant, 1991). Work that led to the development of dynamical systems theory includes research by Bernstein (1967), who used concepts from physics related to movement and applied these ideas to motor development. Bernstein proposed that the CNS controls groups of muscles (not individual muscles) and that these groups can change motor behavior on their own without CNS control. These ideas challenge the traditional view that the brain controls all motor behavior.

Systems theorists do not believe in the formation of schema, patterns, or representations of learning but, instead, suggest that the parameters of the actual situation influence the learning that takes place at that point in time (Eliasmith, 1998). Systems theory has its roots in geometric concepts, and at the most basic level, a dynamical system is simply something that changes over time. Dynamical systems theorists emphasize that learning does not just occur in the brain "since the nervous system, the body, and environment are all constantly changing and simultaneously influencing each other" (Van Gelder, 1995, p. 373). In this approach, the therapist looks for periods of stability in learning and watches for signs that a child is ready to shift to a qualitatively different type of behavior. Identifying the system variables that will drive the transition from one level to another facilitates learning (Burton & Miller, 1998). These variables can be related to the child, task, or environment. Thelen (1995) suggested variables such as physical growth and biomechanics may be more important for learning in infancy, whereas factors such as experience, practice, and motivation may be more influential when the child is older.

In this theoretical approach, instead of viewing behavior (e.g., motor skills) as predetermined in the CNS, systems theory views motor behavior as emerging from the dynamic cooperation of the many subsystems in a task-specific context. The CNS is seen as only one of the components underlying movement changes. Other elements include the infant's biomechanical, psychologic, and social environments, as well as the task itself (Heriza, 1991).

The dynamical systems approach is developed from a functional rather than a structural framework. It implies that all factors contributing to the motor behavior are important and exert an influence on the outcome. It represents an ecologic approach in that a child's functional performance is dependent on the interactions of the child's inherent and emerging skills, the characteristics of the desired task or activity, and the environment in which the activity is performed. Dynamical systems theory shares many similarities with the emerging occupational therapy theories that focus on PEO relationships.

Dynamical systems theory explains how new motor skills are learned. To learn new movements or ways of completing an activity, previously stable movements break down or become unstable. New movements and skills emerge when there is a critical change in any of the components that contribute to motor behavior. These periods of change are called *transitions*. Motor change in young children is envisioned as a series of events during which destabilizing and stabilizing of movement take place before the transitional phase movement becomes stable and functional (Piper & Darrah, 1994).

The period of instability that occurs within a transitional phase is seen as the optimal time to affect changes in movement behavior. There are three characteristics of the transitional stage:

1. Variability in motor performance increases.
2. When changes in movement occur, it takes longer to return to a stable pattern.
3. Children display more interest in trying a new motor task. For example, when changing to a walk from a crawl, children interrupt the normal efficient crawl by standing up from time to time. They start to take steps when holding onto someone's hand. Children like to be upright and begin to spend less time in crawling. Ultimately they take their first independent steps.

In children with impairments such as cerebral palsy, constraints hinder the emergence of motor functions. Constraints in the child are limitations imposed on motor behaviors by the physical, social, cognitive, and neurologic characteristics of the child. The constraint that has traditionally received most attention is the integrity of the CNS; less frequently, other biomechanical constraints such as biomechanical forces, muscle strength, or disproportionate trunk-to-limb ratios are considered. Environmental constraints include physical, social, and cultural factors not related to a specific task. One example of a physical constraint is gravity, whereas a social constraint could be a parent's lack of reinforcement of the acquisition of motor behaviors. Task constraints refer to restrictions on motor behavior imposed by the nature of the task. Established motor behaviors may be altered by specific task requirements. For example, infants, when faced with the task of crawling on rough terrain, may alter motor behavior by extending their knees and "bearwalking." The size of a ball also serves to shape the approach and grasp that a child will use when handling it. The unique features of these tasks have shaped the child's motor behavior.

section 3
MODELS OF PRACTICE USED BY OCCUPATIONAL THERAPISTS

This section of the chapter focuses on models of practice developed specifically for occupational therapy assessment and intervention with children. Section 3 begins by providing an example of a theoretical framework that focuses on occupation and occupational performance. It is the assertion of the authors of this text that occupational therapy assessment and intervention should always reflect an occupation-based theoretical perspective. Discussion of this overall framework is followed by overviews of specific models of practice used with children and youth. These models of practice are used in conjunction with an overall focus on occupation and occupational performance.

As discussed earlier in this chapter, several theoretical frameworks primarily address the concepts of occupation and occupational performance. These theoretical frameworks provide a means for occupational therapists to understand the PEO relationship and its reflection in clinical practice. Examples of current and emerging frameworks that provide this perspective include the following:

- Person-environment-performance (Christiansen & Baum, 1991, 1997)
- Ecology of human performance (Dunn et. al., 1994)
- Model of human occupation (Kielhofner, 1995)
- Person-environment-occupation model (Law et. al., 1996)
- Occupational adaptation (Schkade & Schultz, 1992)

To illustrate the use of a theoretical framework to ensure that occupational performance is the focus of clinical practice, the PEO model is described in detail.

The PEO model was developed using theoretical foundations from the *Canadian Guidelines for Occupational Therapy*, environmental-behavioral theory, and work by Csikszentmihalyi on the theory of optimal experience. The PEO model outlines concepts of person, environment, and occupation as follows:

Person: A unique being who across time and space participates in a variety of roles important to him or her.

Environment: Cultural, socioeconomic, institutional, physical, and social factors outside a person that affect his or her experiences.

Occupation: Groups of self-directed, functional tasks and activities in which a person engages over the life span (Law et. al., 1996).

The PEO model suggests that occupational performance is the result the dynamic, transactive relationship between person, environment, and occupation as depicted in Figure 3-1. Across the lifespan and in different environments, the three major components—person, environment, and occupation—interact continually to determine occupational performance. Increased congruence or fit between these components represents more optimal occupational performance (Figure 3-2).

The PEO model is used as an analytic tool to identify factors in the person, environment, or occupation that facilitate or hinder the performance of occupations chosen by the person. Occupational therapy intervention can then focus on facilitating change in any of these three dimensions to improve occupational performance. Specific

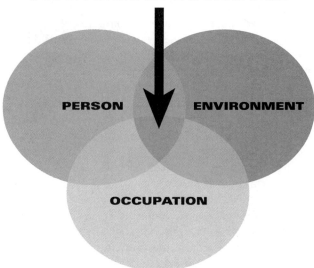

figure**3-1**   Person-environment-occupation model. *(From Law, M., Cooper, B., Strong, S., Stewart, D., Rigby, P. & Letts, L. [1996]. The person-environment-occupation model: A transactive approach to occupational performance.* Canadian Journal of Occupational Therapy, 63 *[1], 9-23. Reprinted with permission.)*

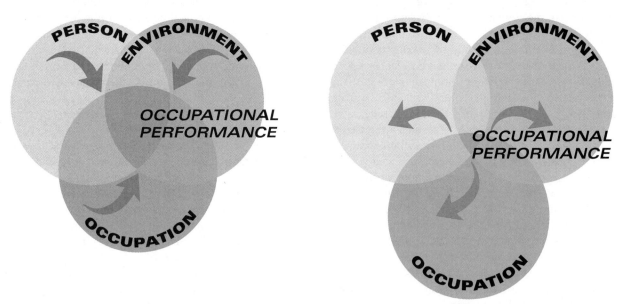

figure**3-2**   Person-environment-occupation analysis. *(From Law, M., Cooper, B., Strong, S., Stewart, D., Rigby, P. & Letts, L. [1996]. The person-environment-occupation model: A transactive approach to occupational performance.* Canadian Journal of Occupational Therapy, 63 *[1], 9-23. Reprinted with permission.)*

models of practice as outlined in the next section of this chapter can be used in conjunction with the PEO model to address specific performance components or environmental conditions that impede occupational performance.

■ SPECIFIC MODELS OF PRACTICE

The models of practice or frames of reference currently used in occupational therapy with children and youth can be classified into two types: occupation-based model and neuromaturation-based model. *Occupation-based models of practice* have been developed more recently, are based on a systems theoretical approach, and emphasize optimal occupational performance as the desired outcome of intervention. *Neuromaturation models of practice,* in contrast, have been used in practice longer, are based on a hierarchical approach to development, and emphasize both performance components and aspects of occupational performance as desired outcomes.

Occupation-Based Models of Practice
Cognitive approaches

Cognitive approaches are "top-down" or occupation-based approaches because the emphasis in therapy is on assisting the child to identify, develop, and use cognitive strategies to perform daily occupations effectively. The following distinct approaches are classified as cognitive models of practice:

- Cognitive behavior modification (Meichenbaum, 1977; Kendall, 1993)
- Cognitive strategy training (McCormick, Miller, & Pressley, 1989)
- Verbal self guidance (Martini & Polatajko, 1998)
- Cognitive orientation to occupational performance

All cognitive approaches emphasize increasing a child's repertoire of cognitive strategies and improving the child's ability to select, monitor, and evaluate their usage during the performance of a task. There is an inherent assumption that improved performance results from the dynamic interaction of the child's movement skills with the parameters of the task in the context in which it needs to be performed. Therefore cognitive strategies are discovered, applied, and evaluated during task performance in the child's typical environments.

The cognitive model of practice requires that the therapist identifies and uses a global problem-solving strategy, which provides a consistent framework within which the child discovers specific strategies that are applicable to tasks that the child either needs or wants to perform. This global strategy is based on the five-stage problem-solving structure that Luria (1961) first outlined. Using occupational therapy terminology, these steps include (1) task analysis, (2) anticipation of the child's difficulties, (3) exploration and selection of task-specific strategies, (4) application of a strategy to the task, and (5) evaluation of its effectiveness (Missiuna, Malloy-Miller, & Mandich, 1998). The task-specific strategies that a child discovers are unique to him or her. However, they may help the child become more aware of his or her personal biomechanics (e.g., "You need to reach out with both hands to catch a big ball."); motor learning (e.g., "Watch someone else first, then try it."); or implicit sensory feedback (e.g., "You need to hold the pen more firmly."); as well as the aspects of the task (e.g., "The cookie dough is easier to knead than stir."). The

strategies that the therapist helps the child discover may initially seem to be compensatory, but once they are internalized, the child's cognitive skills develop and he or she becomes able to approach, learn, and perform tasks more effectively. The atmosphere in the therapy session is one of acceptance and support for taking risks. Although the child guides the selection of activities, the therapist is always aware of the generalization and task-specific strategies that the child needs to learn and creates opportunities for the discovery of these to occur.

Since the selection of tasks is critical to the approach, a client-centered tool must be used that allows the child to identify goals for intervention. An appropriate goal-setting instrument for use with children older than 8 years of age is the Canadian Occupational Performance Measure (COPM) (Law et. al., 1998); for children 5 to 8 years of age, the perceived efficacy and goal setting system can be used (Missiuna & Pollock, submitted). The cognitive approach is probably not a suitable model of practice for children under 5 years of age because of its emphasis on the development of metacognitive skill and knowledge.

One of the key features of a cognitive model of practice is the way in which the therapist helps the child explore strategies, make decisions, apply strategies, and evaluate their usage. The therapist does not give instruction. Rather, he or she uses questions to help children (1) discover the relevant aspects of the task, (2) examine how they are currently performing the task, (3) identify where they are getting "stuck," (4) creatively think about alternative solutions, and (5) try out these solutions and evaluate them in a supportive environment. Once a strategy is found to be helpful, the therapist uses questions to help the child "bridge" or generalize the strategy, eliciting from the child other times and situations in which that strategy may apply (Missiuna, et. al., 1998).

In summary, occupational therapists who use a cognitive model of practice (1) focus on the occupations that a child wishes to perform, rather than on foundational skill building; (2) use a general problem-solving framework that will guide the child to discover, select, apply, and evaluate the use of specific cognitive strategies; (3) use process questions to increase the child's awareness of the use of strategy during the performance of daily tasks; and (4) plan for transfer and generalization of the strategies that the child has learned (Missiuna, et. al., 1998).

Compensatory and environmental approaches

Occupational performance is successful when the demands of the task, the skills of the child, and the features of the environment are congruent. When the skills of the person do not meet the demands of the task in the environment, occupational performance decreases. Most of the models of practice in occupational therapy, particularly with children who are still developing, focus on increasing the child's skills. The compensatory model of practice operates from the assumption that the emphasis should be on adapting the demands of the task or modifying the environment in such a way that will "compensate" for the limitations of the person. Performance of the occupation increases because of the compensation; however, the task is often performed in a manner that is not described as typical. Teaching clients to use compensatory techniques has an immediate and direct link to improved performance on everyday occupations.

The compensatory approach has two major concepts: *compensation,* which involves making children aware of their difficulties and teaching them strategies for coping with these problems; and *adaptation,* which involves changing the task or the environment to accommodate the difficulties (Kielhofner, 1992). In compensatory strategy, the child is trained to compensate for motor patterns or cognitive functions that are ineffective by using intact behaviors or abilities that can be substituted for behaviors that are impaired (Neistadt, 1990). In the motor domain, the child with limited use of intrinsic hand muscles can learn to manipulate objects on a table rather than in the hand. In the cognitive domain, therapists may teach children to use "cognitive prostheses," such as memory notebooks or lists of the sequence of steps in an activity with the expectation that, over time, the child may internalize the content that is supported by these external cues. When skills are still insufficient to enable performance, then task adaptation is used to modify the demands of a task to bring it to the competence level of the child. Task demands are analyzed, functional limitations are identified, and then difficulties are creatively circumvented. For example, a child with a learning disability may be able to complete a page of arithmetic problems when the font is enlarged and the paper has a color tint. With children, the compensatory approach often complements other approaches that focus on skill building. Methods for adapting tasks are selected not only so that the child succeeds at a particular task, but also to promote skills in similar tasks and in other environments. For example, a boy with poor drawing skills can create a picture using peel-off stickers of animals. Although this adaptation allows the boy to create a picture more easily than drawing with markers, pealing off and placing the stickers provide practice of fine motor skills, specifically, bilateral coordination, isolated finger movements, spatial relations, and use of force. Practicing these skills may generalize to other art activities, and

the easy success the child achieves when using colorful animal stickers may encourage him to attempt other art activities.

Psychosocial approaches

Occupational therapists use a variety of psychosocial approaches when they work with children and adolescents who are experiencing problems in occupational performance because of social, emotional, or behavioral issues or difficulties with relationships. Several of these approaches, such as a cognitive approach or the compensatory and environmental approach, are discussed elsewhere in this chapter. These approaches are grounded in theories that focus on the development of self, on family and peer relationships, and on the aspects of the social and cultural environment that influence each of these. Although the number of occupational therapists who work with children with chronic mental health issues is relatively small, all occupational therapists who work in pediatrics use the concepts of psychologic and social development implicitly, since developing the ability to maintain relationships with peers and significant others is an essential part of the occupational performance of childhood and adolescence.

Models of practice that focus on social behavior and the development of self place fairly equal emphasis on the person and the social environment. Personal attributes, such as temperament, self-esteem and self-efficacy, solving problems, and social skills, are considered to be important determinants of healthy functioning. Environmental influences on behavior and social development suggest the need to consider the expectations and social elements of home, school, and community environments and to recognize the importance of friends in a young person's life. For the occupational therapist, the critical consideration is the impact of the person's attributes and environmental influences on the child's ability to participate in daily occupations.

Given the complex nature of behavior and social relationships, occupational therapists often draw on a number of intervention approaches in this model of practice. The therapist's knowledge of normal behavior, vulnerabilities associated with particular disabilities, attachment, coping skills, and compatibility of temperaments may guide intervention with a parent-child dyad. Cognitive behavioral strategies may be used by occupational therapists to assist young people who are depressed or socially withdrawn to develop strategies that encourage participation in social situations.

Coping model. The coping model (Williamson & Szczepanski, 1999; Zeitlin & Williamson, 1994) addresses psychosocial function, uses cognitive behavioral strategies, and is congruent with the PEO model. Therapists applying this model emphasize the use of coping resources that enable the child to meet challenges posed by environment. The goal is to improve the child's ability to cope with stress in personal, social, and other occupational performance areas. When children are successful in coping with their own personal needs and the demands of the environment, they feel good about themselves and their place in the world. Coping strategies are learned, and they build on previous successful experiences in coping with environmental expectations (Zietlin & Williamson, 1994).

All children experience stress when faced with physical, cognitive, and emotional challenges. When these challenges are successfully met by the child's inner resources and caregiving supports, the result is a sense of motivation, learning, and mastery. Stress can evoke negative feelings when the child's resources are poorly matched to the environment's demands (i.e., the child is negatively stressed when picked up quickly from the floor because he or she cannot tolerate the intensity of the stimulation, and parent holding and protection are not available). Both internal and external resources assist in the process of coping. Internal coping resources include coping style, beliefs and values, physical and affective states, and developmental skills. External coping resources include human supports and materials and environmental supports.

Coping style. Children have unique patterns of sensorimotor organization, reactivity, and self-initiation (Zeitlin, Williamson, & Szczepanski, 1988). Children exhibit unique patterns of response to sensory input. Levels of sensory reactivity determine arousal and activity levels and are basic to all interactions. Coping style includes how the child reacts to social interactions and how he or she responds to environmental events. Intrinsically motivated and self-initiated behaviors are part of a child's coping style. Examples of these behaviors are the child's exploration of objects and space, initiation of interaction, and persistence in activities. Self-initiated behaviors are particularly important to occupational therapists, because many children with disabilities exhibit limited spontaneous behaviors when exploring the environment, initiating play, and persisting in activity.

Beliefs and values. Beliefs and values describe how the child views self and the world. Beliefs are reflected in the child's self-esteem and can be inferred from behavior. Values reflect a child's desires and preferences and are demonstrated in activity preferences and task mastery. A child's beliefs and values are strongly influenced by the family's beliefs and cultural background.

Physical and affective states. Physical and affective states influence the child's ability to cope with environmental stress. Energy, endurance, moods, and emotions define the child's ability to respond to, engage in, and persist in activity. Chronic illness, emotional instability,

and depression influence the child's ability to handle the demands of the environment effectively.

Developmental skills and competence. Developmental skills and competence are the internal resources that a child brings to a task. As a child matures, he or she is able to handle increasingly complex demands. Often a child with disabilities is placed in situations that match his or her chronologic age (e.g., a preschooler play group) but not necessarily developmental age. When expected behaviors do not match developmental skills (e.g., to sit quietly and attend), children experience stress and generally seek external coping supports.

Human supports. Human supports are people in the child's environment who support the child's coping efforts. Parents and other primary caregivers are the most significant external resources for coping in the child's early years (Williamson & Szczpanski, 1999). Parents buffer the child's exposure to stress, make demands, model coping behaviors, encourage and assist the child in coping efforts, and give contingent feedback.

Material and environmental supports. The family provides material supports and resources, including food, clothing, shelter, and medical services, as well as toys and activities. Environmental supports are the spaces and materials available to the child. Coping skills are influenced by the organization of materials, light intensity, noise level, and temperature. Environment resources may include adapted equipment and technology associated with comfort and functional support.

Effective coping. The child successfully copes with new challenges when (1) he or she has underlying resources that enable a successful response to an environmental demand or new situation; (2) human supports are provided to facilitate his or her performance (e.g., the therapist gives the child a visual or verbal cue); and (3) environmental supports are provided that enable the child to feel safe and comfortable, be attentive and engaged, and feel calm and organized (e.g., a classroom that is quiet and well-organized with comfortable lighting and temperature). The therapist continually evaluates whether the child's skills (internal resources) and environmental supports (external resources) are adequate to meet the demands of the activity. When the child exhibits ineffective coping strategies, the therapist adjusts the task demands and provides more human or environmental support to enable the child to succeed in his or her coping efforts. The child's failure in an activity is not always avoided because feedback from inadequate performance can help the child learn to evaluate his or her coping efforts and adapt or modify his or her response.

To facilitate effective coping, Williamson and Szczepanski (1999) defined three postulates.

1. The occupational therapist can grade the environmental demands to ensure they are congruent with the

child's adaptive capabilities. For example, the environment of a child with attention-deficit hyperactivity disorder (ADHD) can be adapted by reorganizing materials to reduce visual demands and enhance visual attention. To enhance social skills of children with behavioral disorders, a shortage of materials for an art activity can be placed on the table to encourage sharing among the children.

2. The therapist can design intervention activities to enhance the child's internal and external coping resources. Intervention focuses on the child's resources, including coping style, beliefs and values, physical and affective states, developmental skills, human supports, and material and environmental supports. Coping is supported when beliefs and values contribute to a positive sense of self. The therapist can foster a positive sense of self and can involve the child in activities that promote self-efficacy. For older children, the therapist can facilitate group discussions of personal goals and plans for reaching these goals. Personal social skills may be emphasized by practice of social skills in the context of games with peers. Activities that emphasize group skills, such as problems solving, sharing, and communication, can help older children develop improved personal social skills that can be generalized to school and extracurricular activities.

3. The therapist can provide appropriate, contingent responses to the child's coping efforts. Timely, positive, and explicit feedback to the child's coping efforts helps the child experience a sense of mastery. Feedback that effectively enhances coping efforts emphasizes self-directed, purposeful behaviors. Therefore the therapist supports child-initiated activity and provides feedback that encourages the extension and elaboration of emerging skills (Williamson & Sczcepanski, 1999). Because research suggests that children with disabilities tend to assume passive, dependent roles, highly structured and therapist-directed activities should be replaced with child-initiated activities that are specifically and appropriately reinforced and then generalized to other situations.

Social skills development. Intervention that develops positive coping strategies in children and adolescents with psychosocial dysfunctions can be essential to promote the ability to participate in meaningful daily activities and relationships. Occupational therapists working with older children and adolescents with mental health problems often use social skills groups to promote coping effectiveness and occupational performance. A group milieu allows young people to master developing skills in a safe and supportive environment.

Current intervention approaches may also target the broader environment as the focus of intervention through the following:
- Family education and counseling
- Consultation to caregivers and service providers in schools and community programs

- Peer support and activity groups
- Development of strong social networks

Social networks have been shown to help a person establish positive attitudes and role behavior, maintain and improve self-esteem, and develop moral and social values (Hansen, Watson-Perszel, & Christopher, 1989; Christopher, Nangle, & Hansen, 1993). Other studies have identified the interactive, protective factors in the child, the family, and the social environment that enable a child to be resilient to the effects of disability (Garmezy, 1985; Rutter, 1990).

Research. Research on psychosocial approaches is difficult to review because of its scope and variety of types of practice and their implementation across different disciplines. Evidence in the literature supports the use of specific approaches is minimal. Reinecke, Ryan, and DuBois (1998) completed a meta-analysis of cognitive behavioral approaches for adolescents with depressive symptoms. Six clinical trials were reviewed, and the approach was shown to be effective in alleviating depression with a moderate maintenance of the effect over time. Studies on the effectiveness of social skills training have been conducted with adolescents with conduct disorders (Tisdelle & St. Lawrence, 1988), with depression (Fine, Forth, Gilbert, & Haley, 1991; Pilenis et. al., 1987; Reed, 1994), with schizophrenia (Hayes, Halford, & Varghese, 1991), and with autism (Pilenis et. al., 1987). Although there are methodologic limitations with many of these studies, the results seem to offer support for social skills interventions in improving self-esteem, positive affect, and problem-solving and social behaviors.

Systems approaches

Systems theory concepts are applied in occupational therapy intervention in areas of motor development and play. The application of these concepts is challenging because using this approach broadens the focus of intervention to include all factors (environmental, family, child, occupation) that influence the performance of a specific task. From the literature that discusses the application of systems theory to occupational therapy intervention, the following principles emerge:
- Assessment and intervention strategies must recognize the inherent complexity of task performance. The most useful assessment strategy is to develop a "picture" or "profile" of how performance components and environmental and task factors affect performance of the tasks the child wants to accomplish. Assessment of only one or a few components (e.g., balance, mood, tone) is not likely to lead to the most effective identification of constraints (Hay, 1997).
- The focus of assessment and intervention is on the interaction of the person, environment, and occupation. Therapy begins and ends with a focus on the occupa-

tional performance issues that a child or youth wants to, needs to, or is expected to perform. When a child exhibits readiness and motivation to attempt a task or activity, the focus of intervention on that particular activity can affect changes in his or her performance (Law et. al., 1998).

■ The therapy process focuses on identification and change of child, task, or environmental constraints that prevent the achievement of the desired activity. Some of these factors may be manipulated to enhance the functional motor task or goal; others may be managed by providing the missing component during the execution of the task. Parts of activities can be changed (e.g., different toy sizes). Activities should be practiced in a variety of environments that can facilitate completion of the task and promote the flexibility of movement patterns. Activities incorporated in the daily routine of the child provide increased opportunities to find solutions for functional motor challenges.

■ Intervention using the systems approach will have an equal or a greater focus on changing environments and occupations than on changing the inherent skills of the child or adolescent. Intervention is best accomplished in natural, realistic environments. The accomplishment of whole occupations, not parts of them, is emphasized. The goal in therapy is to enable a child to accomplish an identified activity, rather than promote change in a developmental sequence or improve the quality of the movement.

■ Children must practice a newly found skill. Practice and repetition of activities are also the rule for children without disabilities who are developing any new skill.

Law and colleagues (1998) used the systems theory to develop a family-centered, functional approach to intervention. In their approach the focus of assessment is the child's ability to achieve functional tasks and the identification of factors in the child, task, or environment that enable or constrain performance. The COPM, an individualized, family-centerd measure, has been used with parents to enable them to identify tasks and activities that their child is beginning to do, trying to do differently, or showing an interest in doing (Law et. al., 1998). The actual behavior of the child is the most important determinant of these activities. Therapists and parents then work together to observe these activities to ensure that the child is attempting and remains interested in a new task. Once it has been determined that a child is trying to accomplish a new task or trying to accomplish an already achieved task in a new way, the therapist and parents together identify the constraints (child, environmental, task) that are preventing successful completion of the task.

Intervention focuses on changing constraining factors to facilitate performance. Intervention is only provided when it has been identified that a child is ready to ac-

complish a task and when constraints have been identified for which intervention or compensation can be provided. Intervention emphasizes practice of tasks in context and does not focus on the achievement of performance within a hierarchical developmental framework or on the achievement of improved quality of movement. Intervention focuses on changing a broad range of constraints in the child, task, and environment to facilitate performance.

Reilly and other occupational therapists have focused on play behavior using a systems approach. Mary Reilly (1962, 1974a) originally developed a theory of occupational behavior to conceptualize the roles of being a child, a student, a worker, and an adult. She focused on the importance of play in the development of occupational behavior. She saw play as the occupation of the child, having an organizational effect on behavior. She believed that play forms the basis for adult competence and that play gives meaning to the daily life of a child.

Reilly described two major theoretical orientations: (1) an appreciative system of learning and (2) play progression. The appreciative system of learning states that learning takes place as the individual tries to relate external facts to internal values. The learning process is based on personal values, and through these values a person derives meaning from the external world. The individual's imagination is critical to learning. Play progresses through three hierarchical levels of play: (1) exploration, (2) competence, and (3) achievement. Through play the child learns different rules, which can then be used in future interactions. Play serves as the foundation for adult competency.

Play competence is complex, as it involves the child interacting with different environments (physical, social, cultural) and includes both action and attitude (Ferland, 1997). A child's attitude toward play is termed playfulness. These concepts form the basis of new approaches to occupational therapy assessment and intervention in the area of play (Bundy, 1991; 1993; Ferland, 1997; Parham & Primeau, 1997).

Motor learning

Motor learning as a model of practice focuses on helping the child achieve goal-directed functional actions. It may initially appear to be a skill-building approach because the focus is on the acquisition of skills involved in movement and balance. However, it is actually an occupation-based approach in that motor learning is directed toward searching for a motor solution that emerges from an interaction of the child with the task and the environment.

When a child is learning a new functional task, a general movement structure is brought into place that takes into consideration the relationship between the child's movement capabilities, the environmental conditions, and the action goal. When the task is performed repeatedly, these correspondences become more refined and the goal is achieved more successfully. Specific processes, such as muscle contraction patterns, stabilization and positioning of joints, response to gravity, and other forces, are only crudely organized at first. However, with continued practice these become more organized and finely tuned (Gentile, 1998). These patterns are called movement synergies, or coordinative structures, and they represent the child's preferred strategy to solve a task in the most energy-efficient way (Thelen, 1995). Children with motor programming and motor control deficits often have difficulty establishing the timing and sequencing of synergies of movement. When using a motor learning model of practice, the therapist evaluates and then facilitates the development of the postural control and movement synergies that are necessary for achievement of a functional goal (Blanche, 1998). In addition to knowledge about movement, the major concepts that therapists need to understand include the importance of feedback, both intrinsic and extrinsic, and of the variables that affect practice of a specific task.

Different types of feedback contribute to the motor learning process. Feedback is *intrinsic* when it is produced by the child's sensory systems and is inherent in a task. An example of intrinsic feedback includes information that is available to the child through vision, proprioception, sensation, and kinesthesia. Extrinsic feedback is that which is provided to the child by an external source, such as the therapist, or by observing the results of one's actions (Nicholson, 1996). *Knowledge of results* is a type of extrinsic feedback in which the therapist provides information to the child about the relationship between the actions and the goal—after the fact. For example, a child who is throwing a basketball toward the net may be told that the ball is not going high enough so it is missing the net. *Knowledge of performance* is the type of feedback that emphasizes the pattern of movement and its relationship to achievement of the task. In the same example, the child may be told that his arms are not extending far enough before releasing the ball. In both cases, the therapist's feedback focuses on the outcome of the action, not on the effort of the child.

Research on the scheduling, frequency, and amount of feedback that best promotes learning has been published (e.g., reviewed in Lee, Swinnen, & Serrien, 1994). Studies have shown that immediate extrinsic feedback may keep the learner from paying attention to the intrinsic sources of feedback that are always available, such as vision and proprioception. This lack of attention to intrinsic feedback may make the learner dependent on information from the person providing instruction (Schmidt, 1988). Very little research has focused on the

effect of different types of feedback on task performance with children who are experiencing occupational performance difficulties. Research investigating motor learning principles with children with movement difficulties has suggested, however, that these children may not solve movement problems in a typical way. The research suggests that extrinsic sources of feedback that focus a child's attention on specific aspects of the task and on important sensory cues may be important (Lefebvre & Reid, 1998).

Another important concept in motor learning is the influence of different types of practice on learning and performance. There is no question that practice of a task is beneficial to learning. The difficulty confronting most therapists, though, is the dilemma of whether to practice the *whole* task or to practice only *parts* or components of the task. Study results indicate that the benefits of whole or parts of task practice depend on the inherent goals of the task (Shumway-Cook & Woollacott, 1995). If the task is one in which the coordination or timing of the parts is important to the task, then whole task practice is more effective for learning. Examples of these continuous types of tasks include walking, swinging at a ball, and bicycling. If a task contains distinct parts that can be performed in a serial manner, then they can be practiced as parts of the task. A child learning soccer can be taught how to kick the ball as a discrete task. Most occupations involving movement are actually a combination of continuous and discrete tasks. Consequently, the application of the whole task must follow teaching the parts. Learning to ride a tricycle, for example, does not have the same requirement for integrating balance as bicycling. Therefore the child can focus on learning to pedal separately from steering, but he or she must then combine them.

Another important consideration in planning practice sessions is the use of random versus blocked practice. During random practice, the environmental conditions vary slightly each time, whereas blocked practice involves drilling the task over and over in the same way. Random practice produces better learning because the variable practice allows the child to solve a slightly different movement "problem" every time (Lee, Swinnen, & Serrien, 1994). In this way the child defines more quickly the parameters that are relevant to that particular plan of action (Gentile, 1998).

Some of the key techniques that therapists use within this model of practice include giving verbal instructions and demonstrating movement strategies. Verbal instructions focus on the relationship between the child and the objects in the environment and emphasize key movement features that are directly related to achievement of the functional goal (Gentile, 1998). The extent to which a therapist should use physical handling to guide or demonstrate movement has been a subject of some debate (Nicholson, 1996). Some suggest that providing manual guidance can be helpful during the initial teaching of a movement because it may clarify the goal, guide selective attention, and help the child organize and plan the movement. Others stress that guidance or facilitation of movement should not be used or should be removed as soon as possible, arguing that the therapist rapidly becomes part of the environment, which alters the performance context and the intrinsic feedback that is available to the child (Gentile, 1998).

To summarize, a therapist using a motor learning model of practice takes the following steps:

1. Analyzes the movement synergies that the child is using to achieve the functional action goal
2. Considers the child's stage of learning; determines how to best facilitate the provision of both extrinsic and intrinsic feedback to improve the efficiency of the movement
3. Provides opportunities for optimal practice of the goal
4. Promotes independent performance and decision making as soon as possible

Acquisitional approach

An acquisitional approach to practice relates to the theories of learning and behavior, focusing on how behavior is learned or acquired. Occupational therapists and other professionals use this approach to promote learning and development in areas of function that involve complex motor skills. It is similar to the "teaching-learning approach" described in occupational therapy literature. In occupational therapy, self-care and handwriting are examples of areas of occupational performance that are compatible with the use of an acquisitional approach.

The underlying assumptions and concepts of an acquisitional approach originate from the field of behavior studies and have evolved with our increased understanding of learning theory. They include the following assumptions and concepts:

1. Acquisitional skills can be improved through practice, repetition, feedback, and reinforcement.
2. The focus of intervention is on the skill itself (e.g., handwriting) and not on the specific components (e.g., fine motor control, in-hand manipulation, grasp). Intervention involves direct training of the skill.
3. Brief, frequent (e.g., daily) treatment sessions are considered most effective for learning a skill.
4. The skill may be divided into subskills (i.e., performance components) and taught at the performance component level. However, as each new subskill or component is acquired, the new learning is com-

bined with the components already mastered to reinforce learning. It is understood that remediation of performance components alone will not necessarily affect change in higher-level skills.

5. The intervention should be matched to the individual needs of the child and should be meaningful to the child for learning to occur.

Although few studies of the effectiveness of the acquisitional approach to handwriting have been published, many remedial handwriting programs are commercially available. A few published studies have demonstrated that the use of acquisitional principles by therapists and educators in a positive, interesting, and dynamic learning environment promotes the development of handwriting (Barchers, 1994; Milone & Waslyk, 1981). Some handwriting studies provide therapists and educators with strategies for remediation (Bergman & McLaughlin, 1988; Graham & Miller, 1980) that use some of the concepts previously listed. Further research is needed to determine the effectiveness of this approach with different populations of children across a broad range of skills.

Sensory processing approach

Sensory processing is an emerging occupational therapy approach that has developed from one particular aspect of sensory integration theory (see the next section). The focus of this approach is on the modulation of sensory input by the nervous system and how it affects task performance. It is hypothesized that some children are either underresponsive to sensory input or overresponsive or a combination of both. This inability to modulate sensory input results in problems such as hypersensitivity or gravitational insecurity and is hypothesized to affect sensorimotor and cognitive development, behavior, social interactions, and daily occupational performance. Children with a sensory processing disorder may show poor registration of sensation, be hyper-sensitive to stimuli, avoid certain sensations, or seek particular inputs (Dunn, 1997). These disorders may be present in children with a variety of developmental disorders, and are often described in children with pervasive developmental disorders or autism (Yack, Sutton, & Aquilla, 1998). Dunn and colleagues (Dunn, 1994; Dunn & Brown, 1997; Ermer & Dunn, 1997) have developed evaluation tools for identifying sensory processing problems. A number of authors have proposed treatment programs to address sensory processing disorders (Reisman & Hanschu, 1992; Wilbarger, 1995; Williams & Shellenberger, 1994). Currently, however, the literature lacks any controlled trials that evaluate the efficacy of these treatment approaches. Although there is significant intuitive appeal for sensory processing disorders as explanatory models for children's observed behaviors, more research is required to validate these theories.

Neuromaturation Approaches

Neuromaturation approaches in occupational therapy refer to approaches that are based primarily on a hierarchical, staged development of the nervous system, and they focus largely on changing performance components during therapy intervention. They are supported primarily by developmental theories.

Neurodevelopmental therapy

Historically, the primary concept underpinning a neurodevelopmental therapy approach to practice is that normal postural reactions are necessary for normal movement and that these postural reactions are for the most part automatic (Bobath, 1980). In therapy the therapist facilitates normal movement patterns and postural reactions through handling techniques while abnormal movement patterns and reflex activity are inhibited. The therapist adjusts the amount of handling and challenges the child to attain more normal postures and function as postural control increases.

Treatment using this approach is based on a neuromaturational theory of motor development that proposes a reflex and hierarchical model of motor control, with subcortical-controlled postural activity underlying cortical-controlled volitional movement. It assumes that a lack of higher-level control over movements and a release of primitive and abnormal reflexes at lower levels are the results of CNS lesions. According to Bobath, the lesion in the CNS of the patient with cerebral palsy results in a lack of inhibition of primitive total patterns and in insufficiently developed postural reflex mechanisms.

Because this treatment is based on a hierarchical model, intervention is directed primarily toward the inhibition of abnormal movement, facilitation of automatic responses, and encouragement of voluntary movements. Because of the belief that the CNS can learn both abnormal and normal movement patterns, children may be encouraged to delay the beginning of functional activities, such as walking, for fear that abnormal, compensatory patterns may become ingrained (Horak, 1991). The ultimate goal is to provide children with more "normal" patterns of posture and movement. Hence, there is an inherent emphasis on "quality" of movement.

Clinical evaluation studies of the neurodevelopmental therapy approach have also raised questions about its efficacy. Nine comparison studies of this approach for children with cerebral palsy have been conducted over the past 20 years. In these studies this approach has been compared with no therapy (Wright & Nicholson, 1973), functional therapy (Carlsen, 1975; Scherzer, Mike, & Ilson, 1976; Sommerfeld, Fraser, Hensinger, & Bereford, 1981), infant stimulation (Palmer et. al., 1988), Vojta

therapy (D'Avignon, 1981) and differing intensities of therapy (Law et. al., 1991; 1996; Mayo, 1991). The results of these trials are mixed with four demonstrating no difference (Law et. al., 1991, 1996; Sommerfeld et. al., 1981; Wright & Nicholson, 1973), three supporting neurodevelopmental therapy (Carlsen, 1975; Mayo, 1991; Scherzer et. al., 1976), and two supporting alternate treatments (Palmer et. al., 1988; D'Avignon, 1981). The more rigorous randomized clinical trials have generally produced results that do not support the efficacy of the neurodevelopmental approach (Ottenbacher, 1986; Piper, 1990).

During the past decade, motor learning and other therapy approaches have been used as parts of a neurodevelopmental approach. The use of these methods together has not been evaluated. Because of the tendency to combine approaches, it is rare to see a "pure" neurodevelopmental approach to therapy in current practice. The use of the name, neurodevelopmental therapy, persists, but what it refers to often varies in different regions of the country.

Sensory integration

The theory of sensory integration, together with the treatment approach derived from the theory, grew from the work of Jean Ayres (1969, 1972a, 1972b). Ayres developed her theory in an effort to explain behaviors observed in children with learning difficulties based on neural functioning. Specifically, she hypothesized that some children with learning difficulties experience problems in "organizing sensory information for use" (Ayres, 1972a). She named this neural process sensory integration. Since Ayres' original work, she and many others have conducted research aimed at evaluating the process of sensory integration, defining subtypes of sensory integrative dysfunction and determining the efficacy of sensory integration therapy (SIT).

SIT is based on assumptions drawn from neuromaturation theory and systems theory (Fisher & Murray, 1991). Neuromaturation concepts, such as hierarchical organization of cortical and subcortical areas, developmental sequence of learning and skill acquisition, and neural plasticity, are key to the understanding of the mechanisms of sensory integration. Systems theory also underlies sensory integration, since the focus is on the child seeking sensory input and using adaptive behavior as an organizer of the input. Based on these assumptions, the SIT approach seeks to provide the child with enhanced opportunities for controlled sensory input, with a particular emphasis on vestibular, proprioceptive, and tactile input in the context of meaningful activity. In intervention the therapists facilitates an adaptive response, which requires the child to integrate the sensory information. Through this process, sensory integration is hypothesized to improve.

Much of Ayres' work, and that of her colleagues, was devoted to the development of evaluation tools, which could clearly identify individuals with sensory integrative dysfunction. The Southern California Sensory Integration Tests (Ayres, 1972c, 1980), the Southern California Postrotary Nystagmus Test (Ayres, 1975), and the more recent Sensory Integration and Praxis Tests (Ayres, 1989) are the result of this work. Included in this area of identification and evaluation are a number of studies aimed at describing different subtypes of sensory integrative dysfunction (Ayres, 1965; 1972d; 1977; 1989; Ayres, Mailloux, & Wendler, 1987). These identified dysfunction subtypes include somatodyspraxia, bilateral integration and sequencing, postural ocular movements, and sensory modulation. Some of these results have been called into question based on the validity of the methods used to determine the subtypes (Cummings, 1991).

Another area of intense research effort has focused on evaluating the efficacy of SIT for children with learning problems. Early work by Ayres (1972b; 1978) and others (Ottenbacher, Short, & Watson, 1979; Ayres & Mailloux, 1981) reported positive changes resulting from SIT in such outcomes as motor, academic, and language performance. Reviews of these more recent studies have cited the substantial methodologic flaws in the research methods used and called these results into question (Hoehn & Baumeister, 1994). Studies in the late 1980s and 1990s evaluated the efficacy of SIT using methods that are more rigorous including randomized controlled trials. In a systematic review of these studies, Polatajko, Kaplan, and Wilson (1992) concluded that "the review has failed to find any statistical evidence that SIT improves the academic performance of learning disabled children more than a placebo. With respect to sensory or motor performance, the results are not consistent, but do suggest that, statistically, overall SIT may be similar to perceptual motor training" (p. 337). Using meta-analysis techniques, Vargas and Camilli (1999) concurred with these conclusions. They found that early efficacy studies of sensory integration produced large positive effects, but studies conducted after 1982 did not yield significant positive effects. The more recent studies of SIT demonstrated equal effects to alternative treatments in the participants' psychoeducational and motor performance areas with no improvement noted in sensory perceptual areas (Vargas & Camilli, 1999).

In spite of the negative findings related to sensory integration research, SIT is widely practiced in the field of occupational therapy and remains a powerful force in clinical reasoning in the field of pediatrics. Kaplan, Polatajko, Wilson, and Faris (1993) suggest the following possible explanations for this continued support:

1. An intense bond is formed between the child and therapist during SIT that has multiple the positive influences

2. The child is perceived to improve even though SIT may not be the cause of the improvement

3. Sensory integration theory is useful in reframing the thinking about what underlies a child's behavior, leading to a more positive view of the child

Ayres' work has had a potent impact on occupational therapy practice with children and, because of its controversial nature, has led to an increased sophistication and rigor in the scholarly work accomplished within the field of occupational therapy.

Developmental approaches

Occupational therapists have developed approaches for their work with children that are based on earlier developmental theories from other disciplines. These theories attempt to explain the functioning and growth of children and adolescents from an occupational therapy perspective and are often referred to as developmental frames of reference for occupational therapy practice.

Lela Llorens (1969; 1976; 1991) identified a developmental frame of reference that focuses on the physical, social, and psychologic aspects of life tasks and relationships. Her theoretical base draws from several developmental theorists including Erikson (1963), Havighurst (1972), Piaget (1971), and Freud (1966).

The major premise of her theoretical framework is that the child is viewed from two perspectives: the specific period of life, which Llorens refers to as horizontal development, and the course of time, which is longitudinal development. Both perspectives are viewed as continua that occur simultaneously. The integration of these two aspects of life is critical to normal development. Llorens viewed the role of the occupational therapist as facilitating development and assisting in the mastery of life tasks and the ability to cope with life expectations.

A spatiotemporal adaptation model of practice that views development as a spiraling process, moving from simple to complex, was proposed by Gilfoyle, Grady, and Moore (1990). Adaptation is viewed as a continuous process of interaction between the individual and time and space. Many of the concepts are drawn from an understanding of the CNS and theoretical material from Piaget (1971) and other developmental theorists.

The adaptation process involves four components: assimilation, accommodation, association, and differentiation. *Assimilation* is the reception of sensory stimuli from internal and external environments. *Accommodation* is the motoric response to these stimuli. *Association* is the organized process of relating current sensory information with the current motor response and then relating this relationship to past responses. *Differentiation* is the process of identifying the specific elements in a child's situation that are useful and relevant to another situation to refine the responsive pattern. Based on prior experience, the child develops a sense of what is useful and what is not useful to motor activity in the current situation. In this view of development, the child is continually modifying older, more primitive behaviors for effective motor responses, rather than continually acquiring new skills.

section 4
CLINICAL APPLICATION EXAMPLES

In this section, three case examples are discussed as a means of outlining the different assessment and intervention strategies and expected outcomes that are used when implementing the models of practice discussed in

Section 3. The examples include a young child with CP, a school-age child with developmental coordination disorder, and an adolescent with sensory modulation and behavioral problems. For each example, the most commonly used approaches are selected for the clinical situation. These choices do not mean that other approaches cannot be used, but they are applied less often.

Stacey is a 3-year-old girl who has CP with moderate involvement of all four limbs. She is able to walk short distances using a walker. Her parents have set current goals for Stacey that include household mobility, participation in dressing tasks, and improving participation with peers in play in her preschool setting. In this example, this discussion focuses on the goal of participation in play with peers (Table 3-2).

table 3-2   *Case Study 1: Stacey*

	Assessment Strategy	Clinical Reasoning Used to Explain Client Problem	Clinical Reasoning Used to Guide Intervention and Predict Outcome	Expected Outcomes
Dynamic systems	Using COPM, the parents identify the tasks that Stacey is trying to accomplish but having difficulty doing so. The therapist and parents work together to identify factors in the child, environment, and task that enable or hinder task achievement.	Stacey tries to accomplish the task of playing with her peers, but environmental, child, or task constraints hinder her ability to accomplish the task. Intervention is provided only when Stacey is ready to accomplish a task and when constraints have been identified for which intervention or compensation can be provided.	Intervention focuses on changing identified constraints to enable improved performance. The constraints that are easiest to change are initially targeted (e.g., changes to play environment). Intervention emphasizes practice of tasks in context. Intervention is provided only for a short period, after which reassessment occurs. The effects of intervention are evaluated in the context of achievement of the identified task. If constraints cannot be changed, then intervention focuses on compensation for the constraint.	Stacey performs the identified task functionally, efficiently, and environmentally appropriate, without particular concern for the quality of movement.

COPM, Canadian Occupational Performance Measure; *ROM,* range of motion.

Brian is a 9-year-old child with developmental coordination disorder. He is isolated from his peers at school, is clumsy, has difficulty performing any tasks requiring handwriting, is poorly organized, and has trouble staying on task (Table 3-3). A COPM was completed with Brian, and he identified the following occupational performance issues:

1. Messy desk
2. Disorganized written work; illegible handwriting
3. Difficulty getting out for recess on time

Chris is a 15-year-old high school student who is currently struggling to complete grade 10. He has dropped one subject in the current year and has been labeled an "underachiever." He has difficulty taking notes in class and reorganizing his work. He has been referred to a community psychiatric service because of problems with low mood, lack of motivation in his academic and social life, poor social adjustment, and disturbed family relations.

His parents complain that Chris regularly lies to them about petty thefts from the home and that he requires hours of confrontation and badgering from them to get the truth. They report various other instances of misbehavior. Chris has had trials of medication for ADHD and depression with limited success, and on one occasion he took a dangerous overdose of medication.

He presents himself as a somewhat disheveled youth who denies any knowledge or insight into his difficulties. His parents are firm in their conviction that he requires intensive intervention (Table 3-4).

table 3-2 Case Study 1: Stacey—cont'd

	Assessment Strategy	Clinical Reasoning Used to Explain Client Problem	Clinical Reasoning Used to Guide Intervention and Predict Outcome	Expected Outcomes
Motor learning	Motor requirements of various play situations are observed in the preschool environment. Stacey's current ability to walk to the play area, to sit in a stable position, and to use both hands in play are observed.	Stacey participates in play situations more easily when she is able to move to and from the play areas and to use her hands for play while in a seated position.	Therapist identifies movement positions or transitions necessary for play and sets up the environment to facilitate practice of these activities. During practice, the therapist uses oral instruction or physical guidance to improve performance.	Through varied practice in situations that motivate Stacey, she learns to use intrinsic and extrinsic feedback more effectively to guide movement. Over time, the movement positions or transitions become more functional, and she is able to engage in play situations more easily.
Neuro-development	Stacey's movements in the environment, her movement transitions in particular, are observed. Physical assessment of tone, ROM, strength, reflex development, righting reactions, and equilibrium responses are performed. The Gross Motor Function Measure is used to assess gross motor skills.	Atypical tone and movement patterns inhibit the development of more normal patterns and limits Stacey's mobility.	Therapy is provided to decrease influence of tone and promote development of normal movement patterns. The sensory motor experience of normal movement will reinforce new movement strategies. Handling and facilitation techniques are used to accomplish these goals.	Stacey demonstrates a reduced influence of abnormal tone on movement and an increase of normal movement patterns; increased functional movement, allowing engagement in play with peers; and decreased risk for contractures and deformities.

table 3-3 *Case Study 2: Brian*

	Assessment Strategy	Clinical Reasoning Used to Explain Client Problems	Clinical Reasoning Used to Guide Intervention and Predict Outcome	Expected Outcomes
Cognitive	Brian is observed performing each of the tasks identified by COPM. The specific strategies that he does or does not use are identified, and the points at which he appears to get "stuck" are noted.	Brian does not know the strategies that he needs to complete each task effectively and efficiently nor is he able to select appropriate strategies to achieve his goal.	Using guided discovery and mediation, it is possible to teach Brian strategies that will help him organize his desk, his written work, and the sequence in which he dons his outdoor clothing for recess.	Brian will be able to implement task-specific and global strategies that will help him to organize any task that has multiple parts or requires a sequence of actions. Brian will be able to generalize these strategies to other settings and transfer them to other tasks.
Compensatory/adapt task	Classroom materials and procedures that are in place for each task are observed. The options for making each task easier for Brian are discussed with the teacher.	Brian currently does not have the skills needed to cope with the demands of the tasks. Each task needs to be adapted to ensure Brian's success in the classroom.	Brian will be provided with modified materials that will help him organize his desk (e.g., color-coded notebooks to match textbooks, colored schedule on the wall), his written output (e.g., raised-lined paper), and his locker (e.g., sequence of instructions posted on locker door).	With modifications in place, Brian will become more successful at performing these tasks. Brian will ultimately improve his ability to complete tasks efficiently and to participate with his peers. Over time, other interventions can be used to improve his skills.

CNS, Central nervous system; *COMPS,* Clinical Observation of Motor and Postural Skills; *COPM,* Canadian Occupational Performance Measure; *ETCH,* Evaluation Tool of Children's Handwriting; *ROM,* range of motion; *SIPT,* Sensory Integration and Praxis Tests.

table 3-3 *Case Study 2: Brian—cont'd*				
	Assessment Strategy	**Clinical Reasoning Used to Explain Client Problems**	**Clinical Reasoning Used to Guide Intervention and Predict Outcome**	**Expected Outcomes**
Sensory integration	With tools such as the SIPT, COMPS, and ETCH, as well as observing Brian in the classroom, playground, and home, Brian's performance is assessed. Brian, his teacher, and his parents are interviewed.

Using observations, interviews, and checklists (e.g., Sensory Profile) to examine Brian's behavior and history in different environments, patterns of behavior that potentially indicate underlying difficulties in processing or modulating sensory input are examined. | Brian is not integrating sensory input from different sensory systems effectively, which is leading to maladaptive responses, limiting the development of new skills and the ability to respond effectively to environmental demands.

Brian's behavior and functioning is a reflection of sensory processing and modulation abilities. He is seeking to modulate input to the CNS through various sensory systems. | Controlled sensory input, in particular tactile, vestibular, and proprioceptive input, is provided to Brian with a demand for an adaptive response through goal-directed, meaningful play activities. This input facilitates sensory integration.

Task and environmental factors are modified to alter sensory experience for Brian, working toward the goal of Brian taking responsibility for adapting tasks and the environment to meet his own needs. Some therapists use specific sensory input (e.g., deep pressure to change the child's CNS state) to increase Brian's awareness of what he needs. They help him identify ways to enhance sensory input through functional activities and in a socially acceptable manner. | Brian will interact more effectively in his environment and generalize his reactions to all environments as he progresses. A closer relationship between environmental expectations and Brian's performance or response will be achieved.

Improved modulation of sensory input will prepare Brian for learning and will help him benefit from classroom instruction and participation in school activities. |

table 3-4 *Case Study 3: Chris*

	Assessment Strategy	Clinical Reasoning Used to Explain Client Problem	Clinical Reasoning Used to Guide Intervention and Predict Outcomes	Expected Outcomes
Acquisitional models	School-based "skills" (areas of occupational performance) are assessed, including handwriting and organizational skills.	Chris' acquisitional skills (handwriting, organization) appear to have significant gaps that would benefit from a behavior or learning approach.	Chris' handwriting and organizational skills could improve with an intensive, repetitive program that focuses on the acquisition of these skills.	If Chris identifies a need to improve his handwriting and organizational skills and he is motivated to work on acquiring these abilities, a regular program can be successful in improving his occupational performance in these two areas.
Sensory processing	Chris' ability to process sensory information (e.g., tactile, vestibular, visual, auditory, proprioceptive) is assessed.	Chris has difficulty modulating sensory stimuli when there is input from more than one source (e.g., visual and auditory combined). Poor proprioceptive feedback and low tone in the upper extremities affect handwriting skills.	A multisensory handwriting program may improve his speed and legibility.	Chris and his teachers will develop strategies to modulate sensory stimuli at school, which will enable Chris to focus more on the tasks of schoolwork. Handwriting speed and legibility may improve somewhat, enabling Chris to keep up with the written demands at school.
Compensatory/ adapt environment	Chris' current environment and the fit of environmental demands are assessed with Chris' skill level.	Demands of the school environment are not matched to Chris' skills, resulting in anxiety and behavioral problems. Family is concerned but confused about Chris' behavior.	If Chris and his teachers develop an awareness of his sensory processing challenges, he will be able to develop cognitive strategies to cope with multiple sensory input. If Chris becomes more aware of his difficulties in the school environment, he can use compensatory strategies to cope with the demands. Environmental adaptation of difficult tasks and people's expectations are needed to create a more supportive environment for Chris.	With the development of compensatory strategies and environmental adaptations, the person-environment fit will improve, and Chris will experience increased satisfaction with his school performance. Family and teacher education will help his parents understand his difficulties and will increase supportive strategies.

STUDY QUESTIONS

1. As the occupational therapist, you recently initiated services with a 10-year-old girl with spina bifida. Her lesion is T1 and she uses a motorized wheelchair. She has difficulty with lower extremity dressing and the dressing involved in catheterization. Using the dynamical systems model, identify variables that would likely affect dressing goals.

2. You work with a 4-year-old boy with autism who has severe communication problems, stereotypic movement, and hypersensitivities. This boy has particular problems in making transitions from the classroom to the playground, cafeteria, and bus. Describe two strategies using a compensatory approach that you might use to help him make transitions without causing a temper tantrum. Describe one strategy using a sensory processing approach that should be considered to help him make transitions out of the classroom.

3. In therapy with a child with dyspraxia, you are working on cutting with scissors. At present the child alternates hands, holds the scissors with forearm pronated and wrist flexed, and makes only snips when attempting to cut paper. Use a motor learning approach to design an intervention activity to promote scissors cutting. Explain the types of feedback that you would give him or her to reinforce learning.

4. An 8-year-old girl with sensory processing problems is referred to the school-based occupational therapist. She appears to be sensory seeking and is very active in the classroom. She hits and bites other children and does not seem aware that these behaviors are socially inappropriate. She focuses most effectively when given deep pressure, but her attention span remains limited to 10 minutes. Apply the coping model to design three intervention strategies that will help her cope and develop peer relations in the second grade classroom.

References

Adams, J.A. (1971). A closed-loop theory of motor learning. *Journal of Motor Behavior, 3,* 111-149.

Anderson, E.M., & Clarke, L. (Eds.). (1982). *Disability and adolescence.* New York: Methuen.

Anderson, J.R. (1982). Acquisition of cognitive skill. *Psychological Review, 89,* 369-406.

Ayres, A.J. (1965). Patterns of perceptual motor dysfunction in children. A factor analytic study. *Perceptual and Motor Skills, 20,* 335-368.

Ayres, A.J. (1969). Deficits in sensory integration in educationally handicapped children. *Journal of Learning Disabilities, 2,* 160-168.

Ayres, A.J. (1972a). *Sensory integration and learning disorders.* Los Angeles: Western Psychological Services.

Ayres, A.J. (1972b). Improving academic scores through sensory integration. *Journal of Learning Disabilities, 5,* 338-343.

Ayres, A.J. (1972c). *Southern California sensory integration tests manual.* Los Angeles: Western Psychological Services.

Ayres, A.J. (1972d). Types of sensory integrative dysfunction among disabled learners. *American Journal of Occupational Therapy, 26,* 13-18.

Ayres, A.J. (1975). *Southern California postrotary nystagmus test manual.* Los Angeles: Western Psychological Services.

Ayres, A.J. (1977). Cluster analyses of measures of sensory integration. *American Journal of Occupational Therapy, 31,* 362-366.

Ayres, A.J. (1978). Learning disabilities and the vestibular system. *Journal of Learning Disabilities, 11,* 18-29.

Ayres, A.J. (1980). *Southern California sensory integration tests manual: Revised.* Los Angeles: Western Psychological Services.

Ayres, A.J. (1989). *Sensory integration and praxis tests.* Los Angeles: Western Psychological Services.

Ayres, A.J., & Mailloux, Z.K. (1981). Influence of sensory integrative procedures on language development. *American Journal of Occupational Therapy, 35,* 383-390.

Ayres, A.J., Mailloux, Z.K., & Wendler, C.L.W. (1987). Developmental dyspraxia: Is it a unitary function? *Occupational Therapy Journal of Research, 7,* 93-110.

Bandura, A. (1989). Human agency in social cognitive theory. *American Psychologist, 44,* 1175-1184.

Bandura, A. (1993). Perceived self-efficacy in cognitive development and functioning. *Educational Psychologist, 28,* 117-148.

Bandura, A. (1982). Self-efficacy mechanism in human agency. *American Psychologist, 37,* 122-147.

Bandura, A. (1977). Self-efficacy: toward a unifying theory of behavior change. *Psychological Review, 84,* 191-215.

Barchers, S.I. (1994). *Teaching language arts: An integrated approach.* Minneapolis: West Publishing.

Bazyk. S. (1989). Changes in attitudes and beliefs regarding parent participation and home programs: An update. *American Journal of Occupational Therapy, 43,* 723-728.

Bergman, K.E., & McLaughlin, T.F. (1988). Remediating handwriting difficulties with learning disabled students: A review. *Journal of Special Education, 12,* 101-120.

Bernstein N. (1967). *Coordination and regulation of movements.* New York: Wiley.

Bjorklund, D.F., & Green, B.L. (1992). The adaptive nature of cognitive immaturity. *American Psychologist, 47,* 46-54.

Blanche, E.I. (1998). Intervention for motor control and movement organization disorders. In J. Case-Smith (Ed.), *Pediatric occupational therapy and early intervention* (2nd ed.). (pp. 255-276). Boston, MA: Butterworth-Heinemann.

Blum, R.W., Resnick, M.D., Nelson, R., & St. Germaine, A. (1991). Family and peer issues among adolescents with spina bifida and cerebral palsy. *Pediatrics, 88* (22), 280-285.

Bobath, K. (1980). *A neurophysiological basis for the treatment of cerebral palsy.* London: Heinemann Books.

Bronfenbrenner, U. (1977). Toward an experimental ecology of human development. *American Psychologist, 32,* 513-531.

Brown, M., & Gordon, W. (1987). Impact of impairment on activity patterns of children. *Archives of Physical Medicine and Rehabilitation, 68,* 828-832.

Bundy, A.C. (1991). Play theory and sensory integration. In A.G. Fisher, E.A. Murray, & A.C. Bundy (Eds.), *Sensory integration. Theory and practice* (pp. 46-68). Philadelphia: F.A. Davis.

Bundy, A.C. (1993). Assessment of play and leisure: Delineation of the problem. *American Journal of Occupational Therapy, 47,* 217-222.

Burton, A.W., & Miller, D.E. (1998). *Movement skill assessment.* Champaign, IL: Human Kinetics.

Cadman, D., Boyle, M., Szatmari, P., & Offord, D.R. (1987). Chronic illness, disability, and mental and social well-being: Findings of the Ontario child health study. *Pediatrics, 79,* 805-813.

Canadian Association of Occupational Therapists. (1997). *Enabling occupation: An occupational therapy perspective.* Ottawa, ON: CAOT.

Carlsen, P.N. (1975). Comparison of two occupational therapy approaches for treating the young cerebral-palsied child. *American Journal of Occupational Therapy, 29,* 267-272.

Case, R. (1985). *Intellectual development: Birth to adulthood.* Orlando, FL: Academic Press.

Christiansen, C., & Baum, C. (1991). *Occupational therapy: Overcoming human performance deficits.* Thorofare, NJ: Slack.

Christiansen, C., & Baum, C. (1997). *Occupational therapy: Enabling function and well-being.* Thorofare, NJ: Slack.

Christiansen, C.H., Clark, F., Kielhofner, G., & Rogers, J. (1995). Position Paper: Occupation. *American Journal of Occupational Therapy, 49,* 1015-1018.

Christopher, J.S., Nangle, D.W., & Hansen, D.J. (1993). Social skills interventions with adolescents. *Behavior Modification, 17,* 314-338.

Clark, F.A., Parham, D., Carlson, M.E., Frank, G., Jackson, J., Pierce, D., Wolfe, R.J., & Zemke, R. (1991). Occupational science: Academic innovation in the service of occupational therapy's future. *American Journal of Occupational Therapy, 45,* 300-310.

Colley, A.M., & Beech, J.R. (1989). *Acquisition and performance of cognitive skills.* New York: John Wiley and Sons.

Coster, W. (1998). *School Function Assessment.* San Antonio: Psychological Corporation.

Couch, K.J., Deitz, J.C., & Kanny, E.M. (1998). The role of play in pediatric occupational therapy. *American Journal of Occupational Therapy, 52,* 111-117.

Cummings, R.A. (1991). Sensory integration and learning disabilities: Ayres' factor analysis reappraised. *Journal of Learning Disabilities, 24,* 160-168.

D'Avignon M. (1981). Early physiotherapy ad modum vojta or bobath in infants with suspected neuromotor disturbance. *Neuropediatrics, 12,* 232-241.

DCD Research Group. (1995). CO-OP: *Cognitive orientation to daily occupational performance.* Unpublished manuscript. London, ON: University of Western Ontario.

Dunn, W. (1994). Performance of typical children on the sensory profile: an item analysis. *American Journal of Occupational Therapy, 48,* 967-974.

Dunn, W. (1997). The impact of sensory processing abilities on the daily lives of young children and their families: A conceptual model. *Infants and Young Children, 9,* 23-35.

Dunn, W., & Brown, C. (1997). Factor analysis on the sensory profile from a national sample of children without disabilities. *American Journal of Occupational Therapy, 51,* 490-495.

Dunn, W., Brown, C., & McGuigan, A. (1994). The ecology of human performance: A framework for considering the effect of context. *American Journal of Occupational Therapy, 48,* 595-607.

Dunst, C., Trivette, C., & Deal, A. (1988). *Enabling and empowering families—principles and guidelines for practice.* Cambridge, MA: Brookline Books, Inc.

Dunst, C.J., Trivette, C.M., Davis, M., & Cornwall, J. (1988). Enabling and empowering families of children with health impairments. *Child Health Care, 17,* 71-81.

Dunton, W.R. (1919). *Reconstruction therapy.* Philadelphia, PA: Saunders.

Eliasmith, C. (1998). The third contender: A critical examination of the dynamicist theory of cognition. In P. Thagard (Ed.), *Mind readings: Introductory selections on cognitive science* (pp. 303-333). Cambridge, MA: MIT Press.

Erikson, E.H. (1964). *Childhood and society* (2nd ed.). New York: W.W. Norton.

Ermer, J., & Dunn, W. (1997). The sensory profile: A discriminant analysis of children with and without disabilities. *American Journal of Occupational Therapy, 51,* 283-290.

Ferland, F. (1997). *Play, children with physical disabilities and occupational therapy: The Ludic model.* Ottawa, ON: University of Ottawa Press.

Fidler, G.S., & Fidler, J.W. (1978). Doing and becoming: purposeful action and self-actualization. *American Journal of Occupational Therapy, 32,* 305-310.

Fine, S. , Forth, A., Gilbert, M., & Haley, G. (1991). Group therapy for adolescent depressive disorder: A comparison of social skills and therapeutic support. *Journal of the American Academy of Child and Adolescent Psychiatry, 30,* 79-85.

Fisher, A.G., & Murray, E.A. (1991). Introduction to sensory integration theory. In A.G. Fisher, E.A. Murray, & A.C. Bundy (Eds.), *Sensory integration: Theory and practice* (pp. 3-26). Philadelphia: F.A. Davis.

Flavell, J. (1985). *Cognitive development.* Englewood Cliffs, NJ: Prentice-Hall.

Freud, S. (1966). *Standard edition of the complete psychological works of Sigmund Freud.* London: Hogarth.

Garmezy, N. (1985). Stress-resistant children: The search for protective factors. In J.E. Stevenson (Ed.), Recent research in developmental psychopathology. *Journal of Child Psychology and Psychiatry Book,* (Suppl. No. 4, pp. 213-233). Oxford: Pergamon Press.

Gentile, A.M. (1998). Implicit and explicit processes during acquisition of functional skills. *Scandinavian Journal of Occupational Therapy, 5,* 7-16.

Gibson, E. (1988). Exploratory behavior in the development of perceiving, acting and acquiring of knowledge. *Annual Review of Psychology, 39,* 1-41.

Gibson, J. (1977). The theory of affordances. In R. Shaw, & J. Bransford (Eds.), *Perceiving, acting and knowing* (pp. 67-82). Hillsdale, NJ: Erlbaum.

Gibson, J. (1979). *The ecological approach to visual perception.* Boston: Houghton-Mifflin.

Gilfoyle, E.M., Grady, A.P., & Moore, J.C. (1990). *Children adapt* (2nd ed.). Thorofare, NJ: Slack.

Graham, S., & Miller, L. (1980). Handwriting research and practice: a unified approach. *Focus of Exceptional Children, 13,* 1-16.

Gresham, F. (1981). Social skills training with handicapped children: A review. *Reviews in Educational Research, 51,* 139-176.

Hall, C.S., & Lindzey, G. (1978). *Theories of personality* (3rd ed.). New York: John Wiley.

Hansen, D.J., Watson-Perczel, M., & Christopher, J.S. (1989). Clinical issues in social skills training with adolescents. *Clinical Psychology Review, 9,* 365-391.

Harter, S. (1978). Effectance motivation reconsidered: Toward a developmental model. *Human Development, 21,* 34-64.

Hayes, R.L., Halford, W.K., & Varghese, F.N. (1991). Generalization of the effects of activity therapy and social skills training on the social behavior of low functioning schizophrenic patients. *Occupational Therapy in Mental Health, 11,* 3-20.

Havighurst, R.J. (1972). *Developmental tasks and education.* New York: David McKay.

Heriza, C.B. (1991). Motor development: traditional and contemporary theories. In M. Lister, (Ed.), *Contemporary management of motor control problems: Proceedings of the II-step conference.* Alexandria, VA: Foundation for Physical Therapy.

Hoehn, T.P., & Baumeister, A.A. (1994). A critique of the application of sensory integration therapy for children with learning disabilities. *Journal of Learning Disabilities, 27,* 338-350.

Horak, F.B. (1991). Assumptions underlying motor control for neurologic rehabilitation. In M. Lister, (Ed), *Contemporary management of motor control problems: Proceedings of the II-step conference.* Alexandria, VA: Foundation for Physical Therapy.

Hyatt, G.B. (1946). Occupational therapy: Can doses be exact? *Occupational Therapy and Rehabilitation, 25,* 57-61.

Kaplan, B.J., Polatajko, H.J., Wilson, B.N., & Faris, P.D. (1993). Re-examination of sensory integration treatment: A combination of two efficacy studies. *Journal of Learning Disabilities, 26,* 342-347.

Kendall, P.C. (1993). Cognitive-behavioral therapist with youth: Guiding theory, current status and emerging developments. *Journal of Consulting and Clinical Psychology, 61,* 235-247.

Kielhofner, G. (1992). *Conceptual foundations of occupational therapy.* Philadelphia: F.A. Davis.

Kielhofner, G. (1995). *A model of human occupation: Theory and application* (2nd ed.). Baltimore: Williams and Wilkins.

Kielhofner, G., & Burke, J. (1980). A model of human occupation. Part 1. Conceptual framework and content. *American Journal of Occupational Therapy, 34,* 572-581.

Knox, S. (1997). Development and current use of the Knox Preschool Play Scale. In L.D. Parham, & L.S. Fazio (Eds.), *Play in occupational therapy for children.* St. Louis: Mosby.

Kohlberg, L. (1978). Revisions in the theory and practice of moral development. *New Directions in Child Development, 2,* 83-87.

Krantz, M. (1994). *Child development: Risk and opportunity.* Belmont, CA: Wadsworth.

LaGreca, A.M. (1990). Social consequences of pediatric conditions: Fertile area for future investigation and intervention? *Journal of Pediatric Psychology, 15,* 285-307.

Law, M. (1991). The environment: A focus for occupational therapy. *Canadian Journal of Occupational Therapy, 58,* 171-179.

Law, M., Baptiste, S., Carswell, A., McColl, M., Polatajko, H., & Pollock, N. (1998). *Canadian Occupational Performance Measure* (3rd ed.). Ottawa, ON: CAOT Publications.

Law, M., Cadman, D., Rosenbaum, P., DeMatteo, C., Walter, S., & Russell, D. (1991). Neurodevelopmental therapy and upper extremity casting: Results of a clinical trial. *Developmental Medicine and Child Neurology, 33,* 334-340.

Law, M., Cooper, B., Strong, S., Stewart, D., Rigby, P., & Letts, L. (1996). The person-environment-occupation model: A transactive approach to occupational performance. *Canadian Journal of Occupational Therapy, 63* (1), 9-23.

Law, M., Cooper, B., Strong, S., Stewart, D., Rigby, P., & Letts, L. (1997). Theoretical contexts for the practice of occupational therapy. In C. Christiansen & C. Baum (Eds.), *Occupational therapy. Enabling function and well-being.* Thorofare, NJ: Slack.

Law, M., & Dunn, W. (1993). Perspectives on understanding and changing the environments of children with disabilities. *Physical and Occupational Therapy in Pediatrics, 13* (3), 1-17.

Law, M., King, G., MacKinnon, E., Russell, D., Murphy, C., & Hurley, P. (1999). *All about outcomes.* (CD-ROM). Thorofare, NJ: Slack.

Lee, T.D., Swinnen, S.P., & Serrien, D.J. (1994). Cognitive effort and motor learning. *Quest, 46,* 328-344.

Lefebvre, C., & Reid, G. (1998). Prediction in ball catching by children with and without a developmental coordination disorder. *Adapted Physical Activity Quarterly, 15,* 299-315.

Linder, T.W. (1994). *Transdisciplinary play-based assessment.* Baltimore: Paul H. Brookes.

Llorens, L.A. (1969). Facilitating growth and development: The promise of occupational therapy. *American Journal of Occupational Therapy, 24,* 93-101.

Llorens, L.A. (1976). *Application of developmental theory for health and rehabilitation.* Rockville, MD: American Occupational Therapy Association.

Llorens, L.A. (1991). Performance tasks and roles throughout the life span. In C. Christiansen & C. Baum (Eds.). *Occupational therapy: Overcoming human performance deficits* (pp. 45-68). Thorofare, NJ: Slack.

Luria, A. (1961). *The role of speech in the regulation of normal and abnormal behaviors.* New York: Liveright.

Lyons, B.G. (1984). Defining a child's zone of proximal development: Evaluation process for treatment planning. *American Journal of Occupational Therapy, 38,* 446-451.

Martini, R., & Polatajko, H. (1998). Verbal self-guidance as a treatment approach for children with developmental coordination disorder: A systematic replication study. *Occupational Therapy Journal of Research, 18,* 157-181.

Maslow, A.H. (1968). *Toward a psychology of being.* Princeton: Van Nostrand.

Maslow, A.H. (1970). *Motivation and personality.* New York: Harper and Row.

Maslow, A.H. (1971). *The farther reaches of human nature.* New York: Viking.

Mayo, N.E. (1991). The effect of physical therapy for children with motor delay and cerebral palsy. *American Journal of Physical Medicine and Rehabilitation, 70,* 258-267.

McColl, M., Law, M., & Stewart, D. (1993). *Theoretical Basis of Occupational Therapy: An annotated bibliography of applied theory in the professional literature.* Thorofare, NJ: Slack.

McCormick, C.B., Miller, G., & Pressley, M. (1989). *Cognitive strategy research: From basic research to educational applications.* New York: Springer-Verlag.

Meichenbaum, D. (1977). *Cognitive-behavior modification: An integrative approach.* New York: Plenum Press.

Meyer, A. (1922). The philosophy of occupational therapy. *Archives of Occupational Therapy, 1,* 1-10.

Milone, M.N. Jr., & Waslyk, T.M. (1981). Handwriting in special education. *Teaching Exceptional Children, 14,* 58-61.

Missiuna, C., Malloy-Miller, T., & Mandich, A. (1998). Mediational techniques: Origins and application to occupational therapy in pediatrics. *Canadian Journal of Occupational Therapy, 65,* 202-209.

Missiuna, C., & Pollock, N. (submitted). Goal setting and perceived competence in young children. Submitted to *Canadian Journal of Occupational Therapy.*

Moher, T.J. (1907). Occupation in the treatment of the insane. *Journal of the American Medical Association, 158,* 1664-1666.

Moxley-Haegert, L., & Serbin, L.A. (1983). Developmental education for parents of delayed infants: Effects on parental motivation and children's development. *Child Development, 54,* 1324-1331.

Neistadt, M.E. (1990). A critical analysis of occupational therapy approaches for perceptual deficits in adults with brain injury. *American Journal of Occupational Therapy, 44,* 299-304.

Newacheck, P., & Halfon, N. (1998). Prevalence and impact of disabling chronic conditions in childhood. *American Journal of Public Health, 88* (4), p.610-617.

Nicholson, D.E. (1996). Motor learning. In C.M. Fredericks, & L.K. Saladin (Eds.), *Pathophysiology of the motor systems: Principles and clinical presentations* (pp. 238-254). Philadelphia, PA: F.A. Davis.

Nye, R.D. (1978). *Three psychologies: perspectives from Freud, Skinner and Rogers.* (2nd ed.). Monterey, CA: Brooks/Cole.

Ottenbacher, K., Short, M.A., & Watson, P.J. (1979). Nystagmus duration changes in learning disabled children during sensory integrative therapy. *Perceptual and Motor Skills, 48,* 1159-1164.

Palmer, F.B., Shapiro, B.K., Wachtal, R.C., Allen, M.C., Hiller, J.E., Harryman, S.E., Mosher, B.S., Meinert, C.L., & Capute, A.J. (1988). The effects of physical therapy on cerebral palsy: A controlled trial in infants with spastic diplegia. *The New England Journal of Medicine, 318,* 903-908.

Parham, L.D (1996). Perspectives on play. In: R. Zemke & F. Clark (Eds.) *Occupational science: The evolving discipline.* Philadelphia: F.A. Davis Company.

Parham, L.D., & Primeau, L. (1997). Play and occupational therapy. In L.D. Parham, & L. S. Fazio (Eds.). *Play in occupational therapy for children.* St. Louis, MO: Mosby.

Pelinis, A.J., Hansen, D.J., Ford, F., Smith, S., Stark, L., & Kelly, J. (1987). Behavioral small group training to improve the social skills of emotionally-disordered adolescents. *Behavior Therapy, 18,* 17-32.

Piaget, J. (1952). *The origins of intelligence in children.* New York: International Universities.

Piaget, J. (1971). *Psychology and epistemology: towards a theory of knowledge.* New York, NY: The Viking Press.

Piper, M.C. (1990) Efficacy of physical therapy: Rate of motor development in children with cerebral palsy. *Pediatric Physical Therapy, 2,* 126-130.

Piper, M.C., & Darrah, J. (1994). Motor assessment of the developing infant. Philadelphia: W.B. Saunders.

Pless, I.B., Cripps, H.A., Davies, J.M.C., & Wadsworth, M.E.J. (1989). Chronic physical illness in childhood: Psychological and social effects in adolescence and adult life. *Developmental Medicine and Child Neurology, 31,* 746-755.

Polatajko, H.P., Kaplan, B.J., Wilson, B.N. (1992). Sensory integration treatment for children with learning disabilities: Its status 20 years later. *Occupational Therapy Journal of Research, 12,* 323-341.

Reed, M.K. (1994). Social skills training to reduce depression in adolescents. *Adolescence, 29,* 293-302.

Reilly, M. (1962). Occupational therapy can be one of the great ideas of 20th century medicine. *American Journal of Occupational Therapy, 16,* 87-105.

Reilly, M. (1966). A psychiatric occupational therapy program as a teaching model. *American Journal of Occupational Therapy, 20,* 61-67.

Reilly, M. (1974a). *Play as exploratory behavior.* Beverly Hills, CA: Sage.

Reilly, M. (1974b). Occupational behavior: A perspective on work and play. *American Journal of Occupational Therapy, 25,* 291-296.

Reinecke, M.A., Ryan, N.E., & DuBois, D.L. (1998). Cognitive-behavioral treatment of depression and depressive symptoms during adolescence: A review and meta-analysis. *Journal of the American Academy of Child and Adolescent Psychiatry, 37,* 26-34.

Reisman, J., & Hanschu, B. (1992). *Sensory integration inventory—Revised for individuals with developmental disabilities.* Hugo, MN: PDP Press.

Richmond, J.B., & Beardslee, W.R. (1988). Resiliency: Research and practical implications for pediatricians. *Journal of Developmental and Behavioral Pediatrics, 9,* 157-163.

Rogers, C.R. (1939). *The clinical treatment of the problem child.* Boston MA: Houghton-Mifflin.

Rogers, C.R. (1969). *Freedom to learn.* Columbus, OH: Merrill.

Rosenbaum, P., King, S., Law, M., King, G., & Evans, J. (1998). Family-centred service: A conceptual framework and research review. *Physical & Occupational Therapy in Pediatrics, 18,* (1), 1-20.

Rutter, M. (1990). Psychosocial resilience and protective mechanisms. In J. Rolf, A.S. Masten, D. Cicchetti, K. Nuechterlein, & S. Weintraub (Eds.), *Risk and protective factors in the development of psychopathology* (pp. 181-214). Cambridge: Cambridge Press.

Scherzer, A.L., Mike V, & Ilson J. (1976). Physical therapy as a determinant of change in the cerebral palsied infant. *Pediatrics, 53,* 47-52.

Schkade, J.K., & Schultz, S. (1992). Occupational adaptation: Toward a holistic approach for contemporary practice, Part 1. *American Journal of Occupational Therapy, 46,* 829-837.

Schmidt, R.A. (1988). *Motor control and learning: A behavioral emphasis.* Champaign, IL: Human Kinetics.

Shiffrin, R.M., & Atkinson, R.C. (1969). Storage and retrieval processes in long-term memory. *Psychological Review, 76,* 179-193.

Shumway-Cook, A., & Woollacott, M.H. (1995). *Motor control: Theory and practical applications.* Baltimore, MD: Williams & Wilkins.

Siegler, R.S. (1983). Five generalizations about cognitive development. *American Psychologist, 38,* 263-277.

Skinner, B.F. (1953). *Science and human behavior.* New York: Free Press.

Skinner, B.F. (1976). *Walden two.* New York, NY: Macmillan.

Slagle, E.C. (1922). Training aides for mental patients. *Archives of Occupational Therapy, 1,* 11-17.

Sommerfeld, D., Fraser, B.A., Hensinger, R.N., & Beresford, C.V. (1981). Evaluation of physical therapy service for severely mentally impaired students with cerebral palsy. *Physical Therapy, 61,* 338-344.

Stein, R.E.K., & Jessop, D.J. (1984) Does pediatric home care make a difference for children with chronic illness? Findings from the pediatric ambulatory care treatment study. *Pediatrics 73,* 845-853.

Stein, R.E.K., Jessop, D. (1991). Long-term mental health effects of a pediatric home care program. *Pediatrics 88,* 490-496.

Sternberg, R.J. (1984). Mechanisms of cognitive development. *American Psychologist, 38,* 263-277.

Stewart, D., Pollock, N., Law, M., Ferland, F., Rigby, P., Toal, C., Sahagian, S., & Harvey, S. (1996). Occupational therapy and children's play. Practice paper. *Canadian Journal of Occupational Therapy, 63,* insert.

Sugden, D.A., & Sugden, L. (1990). *The assessment and management of movement skill problems.* Leeds: School of Education.

Thelen, E., & Fisher, D.M. (1982). Newborn stepping: An explanation for a "disappearing reflex." *Developmental Psychology, 18,* 760-775.

Tisdelle, D.A., & St. Lawrence, J.S. (1988). Adolescent interpersonal problem-solving skill training: Social validation and generalization. *Behavior Therapy, 19,* 171-182.

Van Gelder, T. (1995). What might cognition be, if not computation? *Journal of Philosophy, 91,* 345-381.

Van-Sant, A.F. (1991). Neurodevelopmental treatment and pediatric physical therapy: A commentary. *Pediatric Physical Therapy, 3,* 137-141.

Vargas, S., & Camilli, G. (1999). A meta-analysis of research on sensory integration treatment. *American Journal of Occupational Therapy, 53,* 180-198.

Vygotsky, L.S. (1962). *Thought and language.* Cambridge, MA: MIT Press (first published in Russian in 1934).

Vygotsky, L.S. (1978). Mind in society: The development of higher mental processes. In M. Cole, V. John-Streiner, S. Scribner, & E. Souberman (Eds.), *Mind in society.* Cambridge, MA: Harvard University Press.

Wallander, J., & Varni, J. (1989). Social support and adjustment in chronically ill and handicapped children. *American Journal of Community Psychology, 17,* (2), 185-201.

Watson, D.E. (1997). *Task analysis: An occupational performance approach.* Bethesda, MD: AOTA, Inc.

Werner, E.E. (1989). High-risk children in young adulthood: A longitudinal study from birth to 32 years. *American Journal of Orthopsychiatry, 59,* 72-81.

Werner, E.E. (1994). Overcoming the odds. *Developmental and Behavioral Pediatrics, 15,* 131-136.

Wilbarger, P. (1995). The sensory diet: Activity programs based on sensory processing theory. *Sensory Integration Special Interest Section Newsletter, 18,* 1-4.

Wilcock, A. (1993). A theory of human need for occupation. *Occupational science: Australia, 1,* 17-24.

Wilcock, A. (1998). Reflections on doing, being, becoming. *Canadian Journal of Occupational Therapy, 65,* 248-256.

Williams, M.S., & Shellenberger, S. (1994). *How does your engine run? A leader's guide to the alert program for self-regulation.* Albuquerque, NM: Therapy works.

Williamson, G., & Sczcepanski, M. (1999). Coping frame of reference. In P. Kramer, & J. Hinojosa (Eds.), Frames of reference in Pediatric Occupational Therapy. Baltimore: Williams and Wilkins.

World Health Organization. (1980). *International classification of impairments, disability and handicap.* Geneva: World Health Organization.

World Health Organization. (1998). *International classification of impairments, activities and participation: ICIDH-2 Beta Draft.* Geneva: World Health Organization.

Wright, T., & Nicholson, J. (1973) Physiotherapy for the spastic child: An evaluation. *Developmental Medicine and Child Neurology, 15,* 146-163.

Yack, E., Sutton, S., & Aquilla, P. (1998). *Building bridges through sensory integration.* Weston, ON: Authors.

Yerxa, E.J. (1967). Authentic occupational therapy. *American Journal of Occupational Therapy, 21,* 1-9.

Yerxa , E.J., Clark, F., Frank, G., Jackson, J., Parham, D., Pierce, D., Stein, F., & Zemke, R. (1989). Occupational science: The foundation for new models of practice. *Occupational Therapy in Health Care, 6,* 1-17.

Zeitlin, S., & Williamson, G.G. (1994). *Coping in young children: Early intervention practices to enhance adaptive behavior and resilience.* Baltimore: Brookes.

chapter 4

Development of Childhood Occupations

Jane Case-Smith

■ CHAPTER OBJECTIVES

1. Describe historic and current theories of child development.
2. Explain the development of functional performance using dynamical systems theory.
3. Apply the person-environment-occupation model to child development.
4. Explain how individual systems and the environment contribute to a child's occupational performance in the first 10 years of life.
5. Describe the development of play in children.

Understanding child development is the foundation of knowledge for pediatric occupational therapists. Researchers from multiple disciplines, including medicine, psychology, education, sociology, and occupational therapy, have contributed to the literature on human development. The different perspectives they provide in this literature bring important insights to the understanding of how children become adults.

Occupational therapists want to know *what* developmental changes occur in children and *how* they take place. The answers to these questions provide essential knowledge for evaluating children and interpreting what are appropriate materials, activities, and environments to promote their skill development.

This chapter describes child development theories, with emphasis on concepts that have emerged in the past 2 decades. The first section describes emerging concepts that explain how children develop. In the second part of the chapter, a model for the development of childhood occupations is presented and then applied to children's development of play in the first 10 years of life.

■ DEVELOPMENTAL THEORIES AND CONCEPTS

Researchers of the 1930s and 1940s were concerned with identifying the sequence of skill maturation that defined normal development. Gesell (1945; Gesell & Amatruda, 1947; Gesell et al., 1940) and McGraw (1945) assumed that normal development is revealed through a specific sequence skills that reflected maturation of the central nervous system (CNS). They believed that the sequence of motor, cognitive, social-emotional, and language-skill development was relatively unaffected by the infant's experiences. The work of these neuromaturational theorists in documenting this developmental sequence has been well-respected and used in developmental assessment. The sequence of normal development has been particularly important in identifying children with disabilities. Gesell believed that variations in the normal sequence of development indicate CNS dysfunction. Identification of children with developmental deficits or significant delays remains an important function of physicians, nurses, occupational therapists, and others who provide early intervention services.

Based on neuromaturational theory, we acknowledge that brain stem structures develop first, as evidenced by the reflexive responses of the newborn (e.g., automatic grasp, asymmetric tonic neck reflex) that are controlled by neural pathways originating in the brain stem. Cortical structures appear to develop later, as evidenced by the coordinated and planned actions of the child. The infant's increasing control of action and movement indicates not only development and myelination of the midbrain and cortical structures, but this control also indicates simultaneous inhibition of brain stem control of movement. Three principles form the foundation of neuromaturational theory:

1. Movement progresses from primitive reflex patterns to voluntary, controlled movement. Motor reflexes of the newborn and young infant provide the first methods of interaction with the environment (e.g., reflexive grasp) and are essential to life (e.g., sucking and swallowing reflex). Because early reflexive movements serve functional needs, the newborn appears surprisingly competent. These reflex patterns subside as balance, postural reactions, and voluntary motor control emerge (i.e., when the infant learns to roll, sit, creep, stand, and walk).

2. The sequence and rate of development are consistent among infants and children. The developmental scales of Gesell and Amatruda (1947), Illingworth (1966; 1984), Bayley (1993), and others are based on a typical rate and sequence of development. By assuming that the sequence of milestones (i.e., major motor accomplishments) is constant and predictable, the normative developmental sequence can be used to diagnose neurologic impairment and disability.

3. Low-level skills are prerequisite foundations to certain high-level skills. For example, cephalocaudal development is evidenced when the infant develops head control, then trunk control sufficient for independent sitting, and finally pelvic control sufficient for standing and walking.

In assuming a hierarchy of CNS function, the neuromaturational theory limited the thinking about how a child learns to act in the environment. Using current research models (e.g., Thelen, 1995), it has become apparent that multiple variables at different levels influence the child's development. The child learns occupations through interaction with his or her environment rather than through the emergence of a predetermined scenario reflecting neuromaturational principles.

Piaget expanded our understanding of child maturation by emphasizing that development is interplay between the environment and the child's innate abilities (see Chapter 3). Piaget emphasized the maturation of cognitive structures that enable the child to understand the environment, language, and social action. The impact of environment on the child's development changes as the child becomes increasingly able to assimilate the complexities of physical and social events. Piaget documented the child's acquisition of symbolic thought and formal cognitive operations, because these reflect genetic endowment and are reinforced by experiences in an environment that responds in predictable ways.

Another early developmental theorist, Vygotsky (1978), believed that children learn in social interactions. He demonstrated that children learn through scaffolding, or support, provided by caregivers and teachers. A "just right" challenge in the child's zone of proximal development enables the child to take the next step in skill development. Parents and other family members intuitively provide environmental challenges that encourage the infant to exhibit a higher skill level and then support the infant's efforts to reach that level. Parents and siblings naturally promote the infant's development by modeling actions, assisting the infant's first attempts to perform an action and reinforcing his or her efforts with praise and expressions of delight.

The early developmental theorists were concerned with the similarities of children at different ages, and they developed age-related descriptions of skill development. Using cross-sectional studies of children at each age milestone, average skills for each age group were identified. These average, or expected, skills for age groups continue to be used today in assessments (e.g., the Bayley Scales of Infant Development [Bayley, 1993]) and curricula (e.g., the Hawaii Early Learning Profile [Furuno et. al., 1984]).

Since the time of Gesell, researchers of child development have documented differences in the rate of development in socioeconomic groups, regions, and individuals. For example, rates of development appear different in rural versus urban areas (Touwen, 1979; Von Hofsten, 1993). There is also evidence that the rate of development differs between cultural groups and generations, in part because of differences in nutrition and childcare practices.

When individuals are compared, some children develop quickly at certain ages and slowly at others. These variations may relate to differences in physical growth and to the effects of body size and extremity length on a child's ability to perform an action. Often during growth, a child's actions become more awkward as he or she adjusts motor plans for actions previously learned.

Other research has shown that cognitive structures develop at earlier ages than Piaget assumed. Infants as young as 1 month demonstrate abilities to associate learning from one sensory system to another. For example, they recognize objects with their eyes that they previously felt in their mouths (Mandler, 1990). In addition, infants at 9 months can remember an event 1 week after it happened (Metzoff & Moore, 1992).

At the present, emphasis is placed on how human development transpires through a dynamic interplay between the child and the environment. In human development research, current emphasis is on the variations expressed by individual infants and on what human systems and environmental constraints contribute to these variations. For example, when first learning to creep across the carpet, a child must overcome biomechanical problems related to how much strength it requires to lift and hold the body over hands and knees, as well as how much forward momentum is needed to move on the carpeted surface.

Studies that analyze the uniqueness of individual performance use longitudinal approaches in which the same child is studied over a period. Because these longitudinal studies document the patterns of development over time, they uncover how individual systems are constructed and assembled. Longitudinal approaches make it possible to relate transitions of subsystems to each other and to other dynamic growth parameters (Von Hofsten, 1993). Understanding *how* children acquire qualitative differences in functional performance and *how* they become unique individuals can begin by focusing on the uniqueness of each child's developmental course.

▪ DYNAMICAL SYSTEMS THEORY

This section describes current theories of development that offer explanation as to how interplay and interdependence between the environment and child influence the child's acquisition of function. Dynamical systems theory refers to performance or action patterns that emerge from the interaction and cooperation of many systems. In the context of child development, performance patterns emerge from the interaction of an individual's systems and performance contexts as the child strives to achieve a functional goal (Mathiowetz & Haugen, 1994, 1995). The body and brain, as well as the environment in which a child lives, influence his or her functional performance.

In this model a child's behaviors and actions are initially highly variable with many degrees of freedom. The first actions of the infants have been described as random and uncontrolled. Development of skill proceeds by constraining these degrees of freedom as the child gains control of his or her actions. Therefore behavior is not pre-

scribed by a hierarchical arrangement of the CNS, but it emerges from external and internal constraints. These constraints provide information to the brain and body systems that set the boundaries or limits for the child's behavior (Clark, 1997).

Constraints to behavior come from three sources: (1) the child, (2) the environment, and (3) the task (Newell, 1986). The organism constraints are those constraints embodied in the individual (e.g., motor, sensory, perceptual, skeletal, and psychologic). Environmental constraints refer to the physical and sociocultural environments surrounding the individual. Tasks are the activities that define occupations; they are the steps or pieces to occupational performance.

Humans are complex biological systems composed of many subsystems. These subsystems are in constant flux, interacting according to the task at hand and conditions in the environment. The child's actions during the performance of a task, then, are the result of the subsystems interacting with each other and with the environment. These individual systems come together and self-organize in a coordinated way to achieve the child's goal. For example, initially a child is interested in exploring the sensory characteristics of a toy. As he or she reaches for the toy, grasps it, brings it to midline in hand-to-hand play, and finally to the mouth, the child's attention and cognitive focus are not on planning each of these actions. Instead, they are on assimilating the toy's actions and perceptual features.

Longitudinal studies reveal that children demonstrate unique trajectories of development and that variations in functional performance among children persist into adulthood. Thelen and her colleagues demonstrated the uniqueness of motor development in a study of reaching in 4- and 5-month-old infants (Thelen et. al., 1993). Each 5-month-old infant was able to reach toward an object, but the patterns demonstrated were quite unique. Certain infants demonstrated a slow, cautious first approach to the object, whereas others make ballistic arm movements in an attempt to reach it. Although all first reaches tended to be circuitous, the amount of correction made to obtain the object, the speed at which the attempt was made, and the angle at which arms were held toward the object were different.

In a similar way, between 8 and 10 months most infants acquire the motivation to be independently mobile. The need to self-initiate movement from place to place emerges as an important task, or goal, to accomplish. This goal reflects the infant's curiosity about the environment, a desire to explore space, and a determination to reach a specific play object. Although mobility becomes a common goal of an infant toward the end of the first year, the method used to achieve that mobility varies greatly. Some infants roll to another space in the room, whereas others scoot on their buttocks in a sitting position. Some infants push backwards while lying in a prone position, and others creep forward to explore their environment. How the infant achieves mobility is influenced by many contributing body systems (e.g., strength, coordination, and sense of balance and movement). Conditions in the environment also influence infant mobility (e.g., the surfaces on which the child plays, the encouragement provided by the caregivers, and the way in which the task is presented).

Perceptual Action Reciprocity

Perception and action are interdependent and inextricably linked. An individual's perception of the environment informs action, and the individual's actions provide feedback about movement, performance, and consequences in the environment. Initially, many of the child's actions are exploratory in nature; that is, the child moves fingers over the surfaces of objects to learn their shape, texture, and consistency. The child waves an object in the air to hear the sounds that it makes and to feel its weight. These actions help the child perceive sensory and perceptual features (affordances) of objects. Affordance refers to the fit between the child and his or her environment (Gibson, 1979, 1997). The environment and objects in it offer the child opportunities to explore and act. This action is based on what the environment affords, as well as the child's perceptual capability to recognize affordances in that environment. For example, colorful, noise-making toys afford manipulation because they have movable parts, rounded surfaces, and easily fit into an infant's hand. Individual finger movements, thumb opposition, hand-to-hand transfer, and eye-hand coordination are facilitated by the characteristics of the toy.

Manipulation is guided by visual, tactile, and kinesthetic input (Rochat, 1989; Ruff, 1989). The sensory information helps the infant adjust and modify finger movement and force, so that precise grasp and manipulation are possible. Through object manipulation, the child develops haptic sense (i.e., an understanding of shape, texture, and mass). When manipulating objects, sensory information enters the CNS as a unit and is integrated at all levels, affecting neuronal centers for motor, perceptual, and cognitive behaviors. Therefore a child learns to perform and refines performance from integrated sensory input. Impairment in sensory responsiveness or processing will limit refinement of movement patterns, because the child receives imprecise feedback.

Functional Performance: Flexible Synergies

As mentioned, the infant begins life with few constraints on performance, permitting the greatest variability within the system for the generation of spontaneous movements. This variability permits flexibility for explo-

ration of the environment and rapid perceptual and cognitive learning. The infant quickly selects functional synergistic movement patterns. For example, from birth the infant demonstrates a pattern of hand-to-mouth movement (e.g., to calm him or herself by sucking on a fist). This synergistic pattern (shoulder rotation and horizontal adduction, elbow flexion and forearm pronation, followed by supination and neutral wrist position) makes only minimal adaptive changes as the child learns to feed him or herself with various utensils.

Synergies that enable tool use are softly assembled around the goal of the task at hand; therefore they are stable but flexible units. Synergies have specific consistent characteristics, such as the sequence of movements and the ratio of joint movement, which can be adjusted to accommodate each new situation. This *adaptable stability* is a hallmark of normal movement (Cioni et al., 1997).

The functional synergies that characterize a child's development of occupations are highly adaptable and highly reliable. The child self-organizes these synergies around goals, and his or her first goals are embedded in and organized around play (as described in the second part of this chapter).

New Tasks and Occupations

How does a child learn new tasks? How does competent occupational performance develop during childhood? Children generally transition through three stages of learning to acquire a new skill (Gibson, 1997; Piper & Darrah, 1994). The first stage involves exploratory activity. Exploration occurs naturally in all human beings. Through exploration, a child learns about self and the environment. In this stage the child experiments with objects and tasks using different systems, new combinations of perception and movement, and new sequences of action.

In the second phase of learning the child begins to use the feedback and reinforcement received from his or her exploration. At this time, variability of action patterns decrease, and the child shows greater consistency in the movement patterns exhibited. The second phase can be characterized as a phase of perceptual learning, and certain actions that were initially tried are discarded as ineffective. Interest in the activity remains high as perceptual learning continues and is inherently motivating and meaningful to the child.

In the third phase the child selects the action pattern that works best to achieve a goal. The pattern selected is comfortable and efficient for the child. Selection of a single pattern indicates both perceptual learning and increased self-organization. During this end stage of learning, the child demonstrates flexible consistency in performance. The child uses the same pattern and approach to the task, but easily adapts the pattern according to task requirements. High adaptability is always characteristic of a well-learned task. Other attributes of learned performance are that the action patterns used are orderly and economical. Children continue to practice performance when given opportunities in the environment. The third phase of learning, skill achievement, leads to exploration of new and different tasks. Therefore a child's learning continues into new performance arenas, expanding his or her occupations.

■ DEVELOPMENT OF HUMAN OCCUPATION

The activities or tasks performed in occupations, the individual, and the environment contribute to a child's development (Figure 4-1). Occupational performance reflects the complexity of the activity; the inherent facility of the individual, including genetic endowment; and the supports and constraints within the environment. Although the relative importance of each component to the child's performance shifts, a child's performance can only be understood by assessing the interaction of occupation, individual, and environment.

Occupations and Activities

Occupations include combinations of tasks that have meaning (i.e., are purposeful) for the child and reflect the expectations, constraints, and supports of the environment. Occupations define a child's role in home, school, and community environments. Individual ability, presenting tasks and activities, and environmental accommodations and supports determine the level of participation in play, self-care, social roles, and school activities.

Occupations are organized into functional sequences of tasks. Tasks and activities are specific to occupations at particular ages in specific environments. Each task or activity defines a goal for the child or an end state that organizes the child's actions. The activity's goal may require a simple action (e.g., reaching for a toy), or it may require a series of actions (e.g., moving into a parent's lap, eating a bowl of cereal, or climbing a jungle gym). Children tend to accomplish certain occupations and their corresponding tasks at similar ages. However, how children accomplish these tasks is unique for each child. Variations in how the child plays (e.g., waves and mouths a rattle, builds a fence of wooden blocks, uses scissors to cut out a circle) provide clues as to how a child learns.

Individual Systems

How a child learns new occupations relates to the facility that the individual brings to the task. Motor, cognitive, sensory or perceptual, communicative, and social-emotional systems contribute to occupational performance. Strengths and constraints of each system determine the quality and developmental level of performance. These systems are interdependent: they work together, such that strengths in one system (e.g., visual) can support limitations in others (e.g., kinesthetic). Which systems are recruited for the task varies according to the novelty of the activity and the degree to which the task has become automatic. For example, research has shown that handwriting involves visual, perceptual, kinesthetic, visual-motor, cognitive, and language systems (Cornhill & Case-Smith, 1996; Tseng & Murray, 1994). Initially, handwriting is guided by the visual system, but after it is practiced and learned, handwriting is primarily guided by the kinesthetic system. Occupations such as feeding may involve somatosensory systems more than visual systems. Feeding behaviors are reflexive at birth and continue to involve primarily automatic responses as the infant becomes a child.

Environments

The child's social and physical environments change through the course of development and tend to expand as the child matures. However, this expansion depends on the family's composition, structure, social status, and cultural values. The environment surrounds and supports the child's action; it forces the child to adapt and assists, or accommodates, that adaptation. As a child perceives the affordances of the environment, the child learns to act on those affordances, expanding a repertoire of actions. At the same time, an understanding of how the world responds to his or her actions increases. In spite of a belief in the strong influence of the environment on the child's development and the importance of play objects to enhance the child's development, studies of play (playful) environments and their direct influence on a child's performance are few. Although it is intuitively believed that the materials and spaces available to a child to explore highly relate to the course of development a child follows, more research is needed to better understand this relationship.

OCCUPATIONAL PERFORMANCE

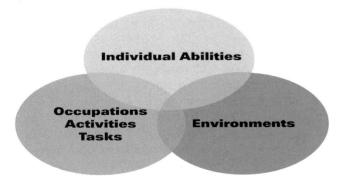

figure 4-1   Model of the development of child occupations.

---

table 4-1 *Development of Play Occupations: Infants 0 to 6 Months*

PLAY OCCUPATIONS	Cognitive
Exploratory play	Repeats actions for pleasurable experiences
Sensorimotor play predominates	Integrates information from multiple sensory systems
Social play	*Psychosocial*
Focused on attachment and bonding	Coos, then squeals
	Smiles, laughs out loud
INDIVIDUAL ABILITIES	Expresses discomfort by crying
Fine motor/manipulative	Communicates simple emotions through facial expressions
Develops accurate reach to object	
Uses variety of palmar grasping patterns	**ENVIRONMENTS**
Secures object with hand and brings to mouth	Home is primary; may also experience childcare center
Transfers objects hand to hand	Floor and carpet
Examines objects carefully with eyes	Infant seat
Plays with hands at midline	Infant swing
Posture/gross motor/mobility	Parents' laps
Lifts head (3-4 mo) raises trunk when prone (4-6 mo)	Caregivers' arms
Sits propping on hands	Highchair
Plays (bounces) when standing with support from parents	Crib
Rolls from place to place	

Application of the Person-Environment-Occupation Model

In the following section the person-environment-occupation (PEO) model is applied to the development of play occupations. For three age groups—infancy, early childhood, and middle childhood—typical play occupations and activities are described. The individual abilities and environments that contribute to the development of play occupations are then identified. Although children's occupations are similar at various age levels, the environments, individual abilities, and activities in play occupations are varied and diverse, resulting in a unique occupational performance for each child. The uniqueness of a child's development and how these components relate in individuals are the keys to analyzing the development of occupational performance.

This chapter describes the development of play occupations, acknowledging that it includes both physical and social activities. Although the child learns occupations other than play (e.g., those related to school function), occupational therapists most often use play activities to engage the child in the therapeutic process. Play activities serve as the means to improve performance, because they are self-motivating and offer goals around which the child can self-organize (Parham & Primeau, 1997). Children place effort and energy into play activities, because they are inherently interesting and fun. (Further description of play as a goal and modality of therapy is found in Chapter 17.) Description of a child's development of feeding, self-care, and school function is presented in other chapters (Chapters 15, 16, 18, and 23). The contribution of communication abilities is also important to the development of play and other childhood occupations, but it is not described in this chapter because language and communication are not primary concerns for occupational therapists.

■ INFANTS: BIRTH TO 2 YEARS

Play Occupations

The play occupations of infants in the first 12 months are exploratory and social; that is, they are related to bonding with caregivers (Tables 4-1 and 4-2). As in every stage, these occupations overlap (i.e., bonding occurs during exploratory play with the parent's hair and face, and the parent's holding supports the infant's play with objects). Much of the infant's awake and alert time is spent in exploratory play, often play that occurs in the caregiver's arms or with the caregiver nearby.

Exploratory play is also termed *sensorimotor play*. Rubin (1984) defined exploratory play as an activity that is performed simply for the enjoyment of the physical sensation it creates. It includes repetitive movements to create actions in toys for the sensory experiences of hearing, seeing, and feeling. The infant places toys in his or her mouth, waves them in the air, and explores their surfaces with his or her hands. These actions allow for intense perceptual learning and bring delight to the infant (without any more complex purpose).

table 4-2 *Development of Play Occupations: Infants 6 to 12 Months*

PLAY OCCUPATIONS

Exploratory play

 Sensorimotor play evolves into functional play

Functional play

 Begins to use toys according to their functional purpose

Social play

 Attachment, relating to parents or caregivers

INDIVIDUAL ABILITIES

Fine motor/manipulation

 Mouths toys

 Uses accurate and direct reach for toys

 Plays with toys at midline; transfers hand to hand

 Banging objects together to make sounds

 Waves toys in the air

 Releases toys into container

 Rolls ball to adult

 Grasps small objects in finger tips

 Points to toys with index finger, using index finger to
  explore toys

 Crudely uses tool

Posture/gross motor

 Sits independently

 Rolls from place to place

 Independently gets into sitting

 Pivots in sitting position

 Stands, holding on for support

 Plays in standing when leaning on support

 Crawls initially, then creeps on all fours (10 mo)

 Walks with hand held (12 mo)

Cognitive

 Responds to own name

 Recognizes words and family members' names

 Responds with appropriate gestures

 Listens selectively

 Imitates simple gestures

 Looks at picture book

 Begins to generalize from past experiences

 Acts with intention on toys

Psychosocial

 Shows special dependence on mother

 Plays contently when parents are in room

 Interacts briefly with other infants

 Plays give and take

ENVIRONMENTS

Home and childcare center

Floors with variety of surfaces and textures

Parents may use gates to protect, given infant's new mobility

Highchair and other sitting devices (e.g., car seat)

Yards and outside environments (e.g., grass or sandbox)

Small swimming pool

In the second year of life, the infant engages in functional, or relational, play; that is, an object's function is understood, and that function determines the action (Tables 4-3 and 4-4). Initially, children use objects on themselves (e.g., pretending to drink from a cup or pretending to comb hair). These self-directed actions signal the beginning of pretend play (Piaget, 1952). The child knows cause and effect and repeatedly makes the toy telephone ring or the battery-powered doll squeal to enjoy the effect of the initial action.

By the end of the second year, play has expanded in two important ways. First, the child begins to combine actions into play sequences (e.g., he or she relates objects to each other by stacking one on the other or by lining up toys beside each other). These combined actions show a play purpose that matches the function of the toy. Second, 2-year-old children now direct actions away from themselves. The objects used in play generally resemble real-life objects (Linder, 1993). The child places the doll in a toy bed and then covers it. The child pretends to feed a stuffed animal or drives toy cars through a toy garage. At 2 years of age, play remains a very central occupation of the child, who now has an increased attention span and the ability to combine multiple actions in play. The emergence of

symbolic or imaginary play with toys and objects offer first opportunities for the child to practice the skills of living.

The child also engages in gross motor play throughout the day. As the child becomes mobile, exploration of space, surfaces, and large action toys becomes a primary occupation. Movement is also enjoyed simply as movement; the child delights in swinging and running or attempting to run and moving in water or sand. Deep proprioceptive pressure and touch are craved and requested. As in exploratory object play, the child's exploration of space involves simple, repeated actions in which the goal appears to be sensation. Often extremes in sensation seem to be enjoyed and are frequently requested. Repetition of these full-body kinesthetic, vestibular, and tactile experiences appears to be organizing to the CNS. In addition, this repetition is important to the child's development of balance, coordination, and motor planning. Hence, the occupational goal of movement and exploration becomes the means for development of multiple performance areas.

In the first year the goal of an infant's *social play* is attachment, or bonding, to the parent. As described by Greenspan (1990), this is a period in which the infant falls in love with his or her parents and learns to trust the en-

table 4-3   *Development of Play Occupations: Infants 12 to 18 Months*

PLAY OCCUPATIONS

Relational and functional play

Simple pretend play directed toward self (pretend eating, sleeping)

Links 2-3 schemes in simple combinations

Imitative play from an immediate model

Gross motor play

Explores all spaces in room

Rolls and crawls in play close to ground

Social play

Begins peer interactions

Parallel play

INDIVIDUAL ABILITIES

Fine motor/manipulation

Holds crayon and makes marks; scribbles

Holds two toys in hand and toys in both hands

Releases toys inside containers, even small containers

Stacks blocks and fits toys into form space (places pieces in board)

Attempts puzzles

Opens and shuts toy boxes or containers

Points to pictures with index finger

Uses two hands in play, one to hold or stabilize and one to manipulate

Gross motor/mobility

Sits in small chair

Plays in standing

Walks well, squats, picks up toys from the floor

Climbs into adult chair

Flings ball

Pulls toys when walking

Begins to run

Walks upstairs with one hand held

Pushes and pulls large toys or boxes on floor

Cognition

Acts on object using variety of schema

Imitates model

Understands how objects work

Understands function of objects

Uses trial-and-error in problem solving

Recognizes names of various body parts

Psychosocial

Moves away from parent

Shares toys with parent

Responds to facial expressions of others

ENVIRONMENTS

Home and childcare center

Floors; all surfaces

Gates used for safety

Climbs onto furniture

Highchair

Small chairs at table

Increased outdoor play

Toddler gym set

Sand box; small pool

---

vironment because of the care and attention provided by the parents or caregivers. These occupations are critical foundations to later occupations that involve social relating and demonstration of emotions. At 1 year of age, infants play social games with parents and others to elicit responses. Although infants at this age engage readily with individuals other than family, they require their parents' presence as an emotional base and return to them for occasional emotional refueling before returning to play.

By the second year, children exhibit social play in which they imitate adults and peers. Imitation of others is a first way to interact and socially relate (Papalia & Olds, 1995). Both immediate and deferred imitation of others is important to social play as children enter preschool environments and begin to relate to their peers.

Individual Systems
Sensorimotor

The newborn's motor responses contribute to perceptual development and organization. Gross motor activity begins prenatally in response to vestibular and tactile input inside the womb. The first movements of newborns appear reflexive, however, on closer examination they reveal the ability to process and integrate sensory information. The newborn demonstrates orientation and attention to visual, auditory, and tactile stimuli. Importantly, the newborn also exhibits habituation, or the ability to extinguish incoming sensory information (e.g., ability to sleep by blocking out sound in a noisy nursery).

In the first month of life, the infant moves the head side to side when in a prone position and rights the head when sitting. By 4 months, the prone infant lifts the head to visualize activities in the room. This ability to lift and sustain an erect-head position appears to relate to the infant's interest in watching the activities of others, as well as improved trunk strength and stability. As the infant reaches 6 months, he or she demonstrates increased ability to maintain upright posture when in a prone position. The infant can also move side to side on forearms, then hands, and lift an arm to grasp a toy. In the following 6 months, this dynamic, postural stability prepares the infant to become mobile.

table 4-4 *Development of Play Occupations: Toddlers 18 to 24 Months*

PLAY OCCUPATIONS

Functional play
- Multischeme combinations
- Performs multiple-related actions together

Pretend or symbolic play
- Makes inanimate objects perform actions (dolls dancing, eating, hugging)
- Pretends that objects are real or symbolize another objects

Social play
- Participates in parallel play
- Imitates parents and peers in play
- Participates in groups of children
- Watches other children
- Beginning to take turns

Gross motor play
- Enjoys sensory input of gross motor play

INDIVIDUAL ABILITIES

Fine motor/manipulation
- Completes 4- to 5-piece puzzle
- Builds towers (e.g., 4 blocks)
- Holds crayon in finger tips and draws simple figures (straight stroke or circular stroke)
- Strings beads
- Begins to use simple tools (e.g., play hammer)
- Participates in multipart tasks
- Turns pages of book

Gross motor/mobility
- Runs; squats; climbs on furniture

- Climbs on jungle gym and slides
- Moves on ride-on toy without pedals (kiddy car)
- Kicks ball forward
- Throws ball at large target
- Jumps with both feet (in place)
- Walks up and down stairs

Cognitive
- Links multiple steps together
- Has inanimate object perform action
- Begins to use nonrealistic objects in pretend play
- Continues to use objects according to functional purpose
- Object permanance is completely developed

Psychosocial
- Expresses affection
- Shows wide variety of emotions: fear, anger, sympathy, joy
- Can feel frustrated
- Enjoys solitary play, such as coloring, building
- Laughs when someone does something silly

ENVIRONMENTS

Home, childcare center, outside settings, homes of extended family and family friends
Moves over all surfaces, including sidewalks and gravel
Uses small chairs and adult chairs
Stairs and areas around stairs
Play grounds
Jungle gyms
Stays in yard or fenced-in area
Parents may no longer use gates in home

Rolling is usually the infant's first method of becoming mobile and exploring the environment. Initially, rolling is an automatic reaction of body righting; usually the infant first rolls from the stomach to the side and then from the stomach to the back. By 6 months the infant rolls sequentially to progress across the room. Heavy or large babies may initiate rolling several months later, and infants with hypersensitivity of the vestibular system (i.e., overreactivity to rotary movement) may avoid rolling entirely.

Most infants enjoy supported sitting at a very early age. As their vision improves in the first 4 months, they become more eager to be supported in a sitting position. The newborn sits with a rounded back and a head that is erect only momentarily. Head control emerges quickly. By 4 months, the infant can hold the head upright with control for long periods, moving it side to side with ease. The 6-month-old infant sits alone by propping forward on arms using a wide base of support with legs flexed. However, this position is precarious, and the infant easily topples when tilted. Many 7-month-old infants sit independently. Often their hands are freed for play with toys, but they struggle to reach beyond arm's length.

If not sitting independently, most infants play while comfortably sitting with back support provided by a chair or a pillow. By 8 to 9 months the infant sits erect and unsupported for several minutes. At that time, or within the next couple months, the infant may rise from a prone posture by rotating (from a side-lying position) into a sitting position. This important skill gives the infant the ability to progress by creeping to a toy; and then, after arriving at the toy, to sit and play. By 12 months, the infant can rise to sitting from a supine position, rotate and pivot when sitting, and easily move in between positions of sitting and creeping.

After experimenting with pivoting and backward crawling in a prone position, the 7-month-old infant crawls forward. The infant may first attempt crawling using both sides of the body together. However, reciprocal arm and leg movements quickly emerge as the most successful method of forward progression. Creeping in a hands-and-knees posture requires more strength and coordination than crawling. The two sides of the body move reciprocally. In addition, shoulder and pelvic stability are needed for the infant to hold body weight over

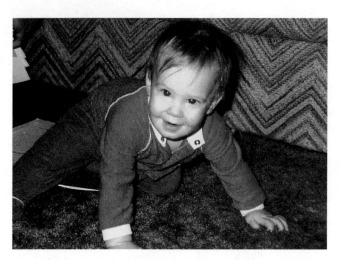

figure**4-2**   Creeping allows the child to develop trunk rotation and transitional movements.

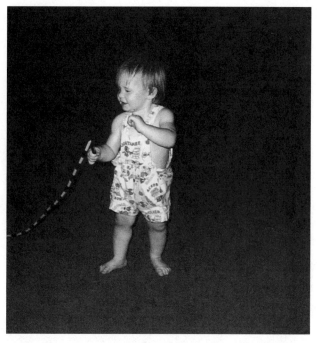

figure**4-3**   Infant's first stance is characterized by a wide base and high guard arm position.

hands and knees. Mature, reciprocal creeping also requires slight trunk rotation (Figure 4-2). Through the practice of creeping in the second 6 months of life, the child develops trunk flexibility and rotation. Most 10- to 12-month-old infants creep rapidly across the room, over various surfaces, and even up and down inclines.

Infants at 5 and 6 months delight in standing, and they gleefully bounce up and down while supported by their parents' arms. The strong vestibular input and practice of patterns of hip and knee flexion and extension are important to the development of full upright posture after 1 year. The young infant also prepares for a full upright posture by standing against furniture or the parent's lap. A 10-month-old infant practices rising and lowering in upright postures while holding onto the furniture. At this time the infant becomes interested in objects that are unavailable or have been denied. This interest stimulates an even stronger desire to stand when objects are moved out of reach. At 12 months the infant learns to shift body weight onto one leg and step to the side with the other leg. The infant soon takes small steps forward while holding onto furniture or the parent's finger.

The infant's first efforts toward unsupported forward movement through walking are often seen in short erratic steps, use of a wide-based gait, and arms held in high guard (Figure 4-3). All of these postural and mobility skills contribute to the infant's ability to explore space and obtain desired play objects. By 18 months, the infant prefers walking to other forms of mobility, but balance remains immature and falling is frequent. The infant continues to exhibit a wide-based gait and has difficulty with stopping and turning. However, walking brings new avenues of exploration and a sense of autonomy, and the parent must now protect the infant from objects that could not previously be reached and from spaces that could not previously be explored.

The newborn moves his or her arms in wide ranges, mostly to the side of the body. In the first 3 months, the infant contacts objects with the eyes more than with the hands. However, the infant soon learns to swipe at objects placed at his or her side. This first pattern of reaching is inaccurate, but by 5 months the accuracy of reaching toward objects greatly increases. The infant struggles to combine grasp with reach and may make several efforts to grasp an object held at a distance. As postural stability increases, the infant also learns to control arm and hand movements as a means for exploring objects and materials in the environment. By 6 months a direct unilateral reach is observed, and the infant is able to extend his or her arm smoothly toward a desired object (Von Hofsten, 1993).

Grasp changes dramatically in the first 6 months (Figure 4-4). Initially, grasping occurs automatically (when anything is placed in the hand) and involves mass flexion of the fingers as a unit. The object is held in the palm rather than distally in the fingers or fingertips. Therefore 3- to 4-month-old infants squeeze objects within their hands, and the thumb does not appear to be involved in this grasp. At 4 to 5 months the infant exhibits a palmar grasp in which flexed fingers and an adducted thumb press the object against the palm. At 6 months the infant uses a radial palmar grasping pattern in which the first two fingers hold the object against the thumb. The infant secures small objects using a raking motion of the fingers, with the forearm stabilized on the surface.

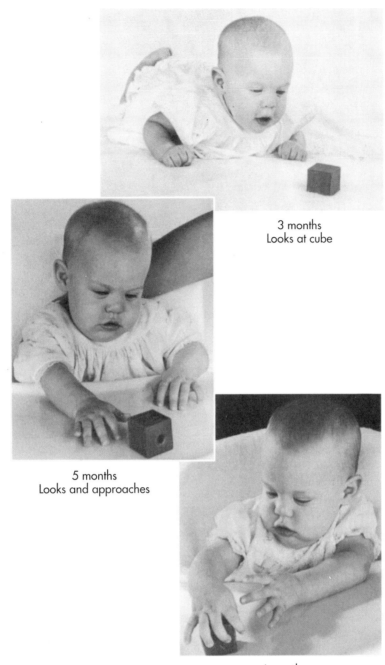

3 months
Looks at cube

5 months
Looks and approaches

6 months
Looks and crudely grasps with whole hand

figure4-4   Development progression of prehensile behavior. *(From Ingalls, A.J., & Salerno, M.C. [1983]. Maternal and child health nursing [3rd ed.]. St. Louis: Mosby.)*

Continued

Grasp continues to change rapidly between 7 and 12 months (Corbetta & Mounoud, 1990). A radial digital grasp emerges in which the thumb opposes the index and middle finger pads. At approximately 9 months, wrist stability in extension increases, and the infant is bet- ter able to use fingertips in grasping (e.g., the infant can use fingertips to grasp a small object, such as a cube or cracker). A pincer grasp, with which the infant holds small objects between the thumb and finger pads, devel- ops by 10 to 11 months. The 12-month-old infant uses

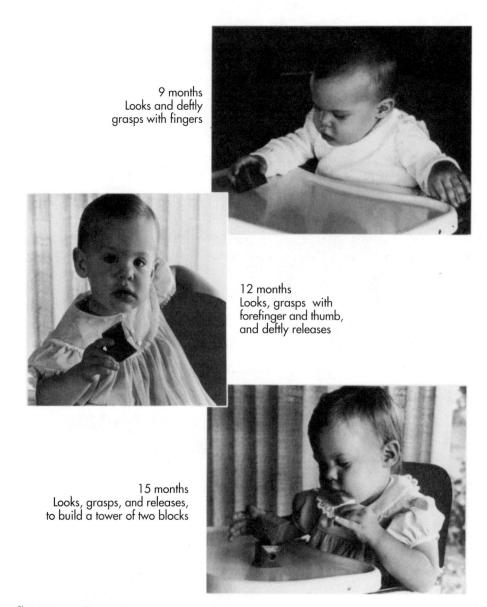

9 months
Looks and deftly
grasps with fingers

12 months
Looks, grasps with
forefinger and thumb,
and deftly releases

15 months
Looks, grasps, and releases,
to build a tower of two blocks

figure **4-4, cont'd** Development progression of prehensile behavior. *(From Ingalls, A.J., & Salerno, M.C. [1983]. Maternal and child health nursing [3rd ed.]. St. Louis: Mosby.)*

a variety of grasping patterns, often holding an object in the radial fingers and thumb. The infant may also grasp a raisin or piece of cereal with a mature pincer grasp (i.e., one in which the thumb opposes the index finger).

In the second year of life, grasping patterns continue to be refined. The child holds objects distally in the fingers, where holding is more dynamic. By the end of the second year, a tripod grasp on utensils and other tools may be observed. Other grasping patterns may also be used, depending on the size, shape, and weight of the object held. For example, tools are first held in the hand using a palmar grasp and then a digital grasp. Blended grasping patterns develop toward the end of the second year, which enable the child to securely hold a tool in the ulnar digits while the radial digits guide its use.

Voluntary release of objects develops at about 8 months. The first release is awkward and is characterized by full extension of all fingers. The infant becomes interested in dropping objects and practices release by flinging them from the high chair. By 10 months objects are purposefully released into a container, one of the first ways the infant relates separate objects. As the infant combines objects in play, release becomes important for stacking and accurate placement. For example, the play of 1-year-old children includes placing objects into containers, dumping them out, and then beginning the activity again.

Between 15 and 18 months, the infant demonstrates release of a raisin into a small bottle and the ability to stack two cubes. Stacking blocks is part of play, since the infant now has the needed control of arm in space, precision grasp without support, controlled release, spatial relations, and depth perception. The infant can also place large, simple puzzle pieces and pegs in the proper areas. At the same time the infant acquires the ability to discriminate simple forms and shapes. Perceptual skills are supported by increasing manipulative abilities, and increased perceptual discrimination promotes the practice of manipulation (Pehoski, 1995).

The complementary use of both hands to perform a desired task develops between 12 months and 2 years. During this time one hand is used to hold the object while the other hand manipulates or moves the object. In general, the 1-year-old child switches which hand is the "doing" hand and which is the "holding" hand. It is not until the third year that children consistently demonstrate use of two hands, in simultaneous coordinated actions (e.g., using both hands to string beads or button a shirt) (Fagaard, 1990).

Cognitive

In the first 6 months the infant learns about the body and the effects of its actions. Interests are focused on the actions of objects and the sensory input that these actions provide. The infant's learning is through the primary senses: looking, tasting, touching, smelling, hearing, and moving. The infant enjoys repeating actions for their own sake, and play is focused on the action that can be performed with an object (e.g., mouthing, banging, shaking), rather than the object itself (Linder, 1993).

By 12 months the understanding of the functional purpose of objects increases. Play behaviors are increasingly determined by the purpose of the toy, and toys are used according to their function. The infant also demonstrates more goal-directed behaviors, performing a particular action with the intent of obtaining a specific result or goal. Tools become important at this time, as the infant uses play tools (e.g., hammers, spoons, shovels) to gain further understanding about how objects work.

In the second year, the child can put together a sequence of several actions. For example, placing small people in a toy bus and pushing it across the floor. The sequencing of actions indicates increasing memory and attention span. Some of the first sequential behaviors il-

lustrate the child's imitation of adult or sibling actions. Therefore increased ability to imitate and increased play sequences appear to develop concurrently (Figures 4-5 and 4-6).

Psychosocial

The infant's emotional transition from the protective, warm womb is dramatically changed at the moment of birth. The primary concern of the newborn is to maintain body functions (i.e., cardiovascular, respiratory, gastrointestinal systems). However, as the infant matures the focus moves to increasing competence in interacting with the environment. The sense of basic trust or mistrust becomes a main theme in the infant's affective development and is highly dependent on the relationship with the primary caregivers. According to Erikson (1963), the first demonstration of an infant's social trust is observed in the ease with which he or she feeds and sleeps.

The basic trust relationship has varying degrees of involvement. Parent-infant bonding is not endowed but is developed from experiences shared between parent and child over time. These feelings are seen in the progression of physical contact between the parent and infant. Klaus and Kennell (1976) discussed the importance of the face-to-face position and eye-to-eye contact between parents and infant as part of the attachment process.

Temperament is an important attribute in the child's social interaction. According to Thomas and Chess (1977), temperament refers to the child's behavioral style, and it is believed to be innate and learned. Nine areas of temperament have been identified: (1) activity level, (2) approach or withdrawal, (3) distractibility, (4) intensity of response, (5) attention span and persistence, (6) quality of mood, (7) rhythmicity, (8) threshold of response, and (9) adaptability. Each of these areas contributes uniquely to the child's ability to form social relationships and to respond to the social environment (Thomas & Chess, 1977).

Each of these areas of temperament forms a continuum: extreme temperament levels are associated with problematic behaviors, and moderate levels are related to easy and appropriate behaviors. Children who exhibit extreme temperament characteristics (e.g., those who are highly active, moody, irritable) have been identified as *difficult*. Others with happy moods and moderate intensity of response are considered *easy*. Temperament certainly influences the types of play in which the child engages. In addition, temperament influences the intensity of play and the child's persistence in play. It is also critical to attachment; a match of parent and infant temperament can facilitate strong attachment, just as a mismatch can create difficulties in attachment. (Temperament is further explained in Chapter 13.)

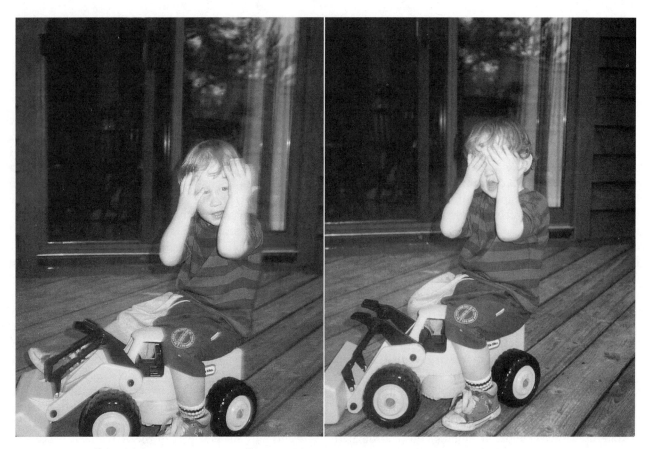

figure**4-5 and 4-6**   This 2-year-old boy engages in social play, imitating an adult, sequencing action, taking turns, and demonstrating understanding of object permanence on self (e.g., hiding his eyes).

In the second year of life, the parents (or caregivers) remain the most important persons in the child's life. Toddlers practice their autonomy around parents, but they have no intention of giving up reliance on them and may become upset or frightened when parents leave. Two-year-old children are interested in other children, but they tend to watch them rather than verbally or physically interact with them. In a room of open spaces, it is likely that these children will play next to each other. Their side-by-side play often involves imitation with few oral acknowledgments of each other.

Environments

Although many infants have a supplemental play area in a childcare center, the home provides the infant's true play environment. The crib is often a play environment, providing a place for comforting toys (e.g., music boxes, and colorful mobiles). Other early play spaces include the playpen, infant seat, or swing. The infant also spends time playing on the floor's carpeted surface or on a blanket. Because the infant is not yet mobile, safety is not as much of a concern as it will be in the next 2 years of life. Early play also occurs in the parent or caregiver's arms. Exploratory play and attachment occupations are pursued on the parents' laps, and the infant is fascinated by the parents' faces and clothing. At the same time the infant feels safe and comforted by the parent's presence.

In the second 6 months the infant requires less support to play and a major role of the parent becomes one of protector from harm. As the infant becomes more mobile, spaces are closed and objects now within reach are removed. Exploration of all accessible spaces becomes an infant's primary goal.

In the second year of life, the child's environment may expand to the yard, to the neighbors' homes and yards, and to previously unexplored spaces in the home. Most children have opportunities for play in their home's yard or in the fenced-in areas of their childcare centers. Although the child's increasing interest in visiting outdoor spaces provides important opportunities for sensory exploration, it also creates certain safety concerns. Therefore parents invest in gates and other methods for restricting the child's mobility to safe areas.

table 4-5 *Development of Play Occupations: Preschoolers 24 to 36 Months*

PLAY OCCUPATIONS

Symbolic play

Links multiple scheme combinations into meaningful
    sequences of pretend play

Uses objects for multiple pretend ideas

Uses toys to represent animals or people

Plays out drama with stuffed animals or imaginary friends

Constructive play

Participates in drawing and puzzles

Imitates adults using toys

Gross motor play

Likes jumping, rough-and-tumble play

Makes messes

Social play

Associative, parallel play predominates

INDIVIDUAL ABILITIES

Fine motor/manipulation

Snips with scissors

Traces form such as cross

Colors in large forms

Draws circles accurately

Builds towers and lines up objects

Holds crayon with dexterity

Completes puzzles of 4 to 5 pieces

Plays with toys with moving parts

Gross motor/mobility

Rides tricycle

Catches large ball against chest

Jumps from step or small height

Begins to hop on one foot

Cognitive

Combines actions into entire play scenario (e.g., feeding
    doll, then dressing in nightwear, then putting to bed)

Interested in wearing costumes; entire scripts of imagina-
    tive play

Psychosocial

Cooperative play, takes turns at times

Interest in peers, enjoys having companions

Begins cooperative play and play in small groups

Shy with strangers, especially adults

Engages in dialogue of few words

ENVIRONMENTS

Home; has access to all rooms; goes up and down stairs
    without supervision

May have pets; interacts with pets

Stays inside yard with fence

Multiple community environments

Often attends preschool or childcare center with indoor and
    outdoor play areas

Climbing equipment

Enters new environments without fear

Tries playground equipment using new actions

■ EARLY CHILDHOOD: AGES 2 TO 5 YEARS

Play Occupations

The three types of play that predominate in early
childhood are (1) dramatic, or symbolic play; (2) constructive play; and (3) rough-and-tumble, or physical
play (Tables 4-5, 4-6, 4-7, and 4-8). Similar changes are
observed in each type of play. First, the child's play becomes more elaborate; that is, the child now combines
multiple steps and multiple schema. Short play sequences
become long scripts involving several characters or actors
in a story (Knox, 1997; Linder, 1993). Second, play becomes more social. The preschool-age child orients play
toward peers, involving one to two peers in the story and
taking turns playing various roles. When playing with
peers, the interaction appears to be as important as the
activity's goal. As the child approaches 5 years, all play
becomes increasingly social, generally involving a small
group of peers (Papalia & Olds, 1995).

Beginning at 2 years of age and continuing through
the early childhood years, the child's play is *symbolic and
imaginative*. The child pretends that dolls, figurines, and
stuffed animals are real. The child may also imitate the
actions of parents, teachers, and peers. At ages 3 and 4,
pretend play becomes more abstract, and objects, such as
a block, can be used to represent something else. Pretend
play now involves many steps that relate to each other.
Children develop scripts as a basis for their play (e.g., one
child is the father and one is the mother). They base these
scripts on real-life events and play their roles with enthusiasm and imagination, creating their own stories and enjoying the power of their imaginary roles. Their dramatic
play is quite complex at this time. However, when in
small groups, their interaction with their peers seems to
be more important than the play goal, and they can easily
turn to new activities suggested by one of the group. By
5 years of age, this imaginary play is predominantly social, as small groups of two and three join in cooperative
play. About one third of the time, a 5-year-old child engages in pretend play (Rubin, Maioni, & Hornung,
1976). However, this pretend play is based on imitation
of real life and dressing up to play certain roles (e.g., fireman, policeman, ballerina). Although children of this age

---

table 4-6 *Development of Play Occupations: Preschoolers 3 to 4 Years*

PLAY OCCUPATIONS

Complex imaginary play
  Creates script for play where pretend objects have actions that reflect roles in real or imaginary life

Construction play
  Creates art product with adult assistance
  Puzzles and blocks

Rough and tumble play
  Enjoys physical play, swinging, sliding at playground, jumping, running

Social play
  Participates in circle time, games, drawing and art time at preschool
  Singing and dancing in groups
  Associative play: play with other children, sharing and talking about play goal

INDIVIDUAL ABILITIES

Fine motor/manipulation
  Uses precision (tripod) grasp on pencil or crayon
  Colors within lines
  Copies simple shapes; begins to copy letters
  Uses scissors to cut; cuts simple shapes
  Constructs three-dimensional design
  Draws face

Gross motor/mobility
  Demonstrates skills in jumping, climbing, and running
  Begins to skip and to hop

Cognitive
  Uses imaginary objects in play
  Dolls and little men carry out roles and interact with other toys
  Categorizes and sorts objects

Psychosocial
  Attempts challenging activities
  Prefers play with other children; group play replaces parallel play
  Follows turn-taking in discourse and is aware of social aspects of conversation
  Interested in being a friend
  Prefers same sex playmates

ENVIRONMENTS

Home and yard
Homes of peers
Neighbor's yard and home with supervision
Multiple community environments
Preschool:
  Environment with high levels of sensory stimulation
  Frequent interaction with peers and adults
  Playgrounds; gross motor play areas; centers for art, fine motor activities, and manipulation; reading; circle time

---

demonstrate some understanding of adult roles, they erroneously assume that roles are one dimension (e.g., a fireman has one role, that of putting out fires). Through pretending, children develop creativity, problem solving, and understanding of another person's point of view (Singer & Singer, 1990).

Play that involves building and *construction* also teaches the child a variety of skills during early childhood. At first these skills are demonstrated in completion of puzzles and toys with fit-together pieces. However, with mastery of simple pegs and puzzles, the child becomes more creative in construction. For example, the 4-year-old child can develop a plan to build a structure with blocks and then carry out the steps to complete the project. With instructions and a model, the 5-year-old child can make a simple art project or create a three-dimensional design. A 5-year-old child can also put together a 10-piece puzzle. The final product has become more important, and the child is motivated to complete it and show others the final result. The planning and designing involved in building-and-construction play helps

the child to acquire an understanding of spatial perception and object relations. This activity also appears to be foundational to academic performance in school.

Children from 2 to 5 years of age are extremely active and almost always readily engage in *rough-and-tumble play*. They continue to delight in movement experiences that provide strong sensory input. Activities such as running, hopping, skipping, and tumbling are performed as play without any particular goal. Although rough-and-tumble play generally involves other children, it is generally noncompetitive and rarely organized. Children enjoy this activity for the simple, simultaneous enjoyment of movement that it brings them as they play together.

In associative physical play, children are generally more interested in being with other children than with the goal of the activity. However, it is important to note that some children enjoy primarily social play, whereas others enjoy solitary play. These differences do not relate to ability as much as they relate to preferences and temperament (Papalia & Olds, 1995).

table 4-7 *Development of Play Occupations: Preschoolers 4 to 5 Years*

PLAY OCCUPATIONS

Games with rules
  Begins group games with simple rules
  Organized play with prescribed roles
  Participates in an organized gross motor game such as kick
    ball, "duck, duck, goose"

Construction play
  Takes pride in products
  Interested in the goal of the art activity
  Constructs complex structures

Social play; dramatic play
  Participates in role play with other children
  Participates in dress up
  Tells stories
  Continues with pretend play that involves scripts with
    imaginary characters

INDIVIDUAL ABILITIES

Fine motor/manipulative
  Draws with dexterity, using a dynamic tripod grasp
  Copies simple shapes
  Completes puzzles of up to 10 pieces
  Uses scissors to cut out squares and other simple shapes
  Colors within the lines
  Uses two hands together well, one stabilizing paper or
    object and other manipulating object
  Draws stick figure, or may begin to draw trunk and arms
  Copies own name

Gross motor/mobility
  Highly mobile on all surfaces
  Jumps down from high step; jumps forward
  Throws ball
  Hops for long sequences
  Climbs on playground equipment, swinging from arms or
    legs
  Throws ball and hits target
  Skips for a long distance

Cognitive
  Understands rules to a game
  Remembers rules with a few reminders
  Makes up stories that involve role playing with other
    children
  Participates in cooperative play with 2 to 3 other children
    that is goal-oriented (treasure hunt)
  Participates in planning a play activity
  Beginning of abstract problem solving

Psychosocial
  Enjoys clowning
  Sings whole songs
  Role playing is based on parents' roles

ENVIRONMENTS

Home and neighborhood
Preschool: playground, gross motor room, art center, circle,
  fine-motor center
Community centers, library, churches, and temples

table 4-8 *Development of Play Occupation: Kindergarten 5 to 6 Years*

PLAY OCCUPATIONS

Games with rules
  Board games
  Computer games with rules
  Competitive and cooperative games

Dramatic play
  Elaborate imaginary play
  Role-play stories and themes related to seasons or
    occupations
  Emphasis is on reality
  Reconstructs real world in play

Sports
  Participates in ball play

Social play
  Participates in group activities
  Organized play in groups
  Goal of play (winning) may compete with social interaction
    at times

INDIVIDUAL ABILITIES

Fine motor
  Cuts with scissors
  Prints name from copy
  Constructs a complex building
  Completes puzzles of up to 20 pieces
  Copies printed letters

  Manipulates tiny objects in finger tips without dropping
  Uses two hands together in complementary movements

Gross motor
  Hops well for long distances
  Skips with good balance
  Kicks with accuracy

Cognitive
  Reasons through simple problems
  Play is based more on real life than imaginary world
  Organized games
  Complex scripts are used in play
  Deferred imitation

Psychosocial
  Groups of 2 to 4 play in organized, complex games
  Has friends (same sex)
  Enjoys singing and dancing; reflects meaning of words and
    music
  Demonstrates understanding of others' feelings

ENVIRONMENT

Spends at least ½ day in school
Defined areas of school for gross motor play, eating, fine
  motor play, and storytime
Community environment becomes more important and child
  accesses recreation centers, ball fields, camps

Individual Systems

Sensorimotor

Young children are amazingly competent individuals, whose repertoire of motor function leaps forward during the preschool years. By age 2, the child walks with an increased length of stride and an efficient, well-coordinated, and well-balanced gait. Children do not exhibit true running (characterized by trunk rotation and arm swing) until 3 and 4 years of age, because running requires greater strength and balance than walking. The 4-year-old child demonstrates a walking pattern similar to that of an adult. By 5 to 6 years of age the mature running pattern develops, and children test their speed by challenging each other to races.

As mobility develops, children access spaces that were previously unavailable to them. By 2 years of age, a child climbs stairs without holding onto a parent's hand, and when 2½ years old the child climbs downstairs without support. The 3½-year-old child walks up and down stairs, alternating feet and without needing to hold onto a rail.

Running and stair climbing become possible, in part, because the child's balance increases. Emerging balance can be observed as the 2-year-old child briefly stands on one foot. By 5 years of age the child can balance on one foot for several seconds and walk on a curb without falling (Folio & Fewell, 2000). Between 3 and 5 years, the child may successfully attempt to use skates or roller blades (Figure 4-7).

Jumping is first observed in the 2-year-old child. This skill requires strength, coordination, and balance. By

3 years of age the child can jump easily from a step. Hopping requires greater strength and balance than jumping and is first observed at 3½ years. Skipping is the most difficult gross motor pattern, because it involves sequencing a rhythmic pattern that includes a step and a hop. A coordinated skipping pattern is not observed until 5 years of age (Knobloch & Pasamanick, 1974).

Two-year-old children begin to pedal tricycles and move small riding toys. By 3 years of age they can pedal a tricycle but may run into objects. However, the 4-year-old child can steer and maneuver the tricycle around obstacles.

By 2½ years most children can catch a 10-inch ball. This pattern of maturity enables the 4-year-old child to catch a much smaller ball successfully, such as a tennis ball (Folio & Fewell, 2000). The first pattern of throwing involves a pushing motion, with the elbow providing the force for the throw. The 4-year-old child demonstrates more forward weight shift with throwing, therefore increasing the force of the ball and the distance thrown. Kicking emerges in the 2- to 3-year-old child, with accurate kicking to a target exhibited by 6 years of age. Ball skills become increasingly important as the child begins participating in organized sports during the primary grades.

Early childhood is a time of rapid improvement in fine-motor and manipulation performance. By 4 years of age, children learn to move small objects efficiently within one hand (i.e., in-hand manipulation). By 4 years of age a child can hold several small objects in the palm of the hand while moving individual pieces with the radial fingers (Pehoski, 1995). In-hand manipulation indicates that isolated finger movement is well-controlled and that the thumb easily moves into opposition for pad-to-pad prehension. These skills also indicate that the child can modulate force and that he or she has an accurate perception of the gentle force that is needed to handle small objects with the fingertips (Pehoski, 1995; Case-Smith & Berry, 1998).

With efficient in-hand manipulation, the preschool child also learns functional use of drawing and cutting tools. The preschool child grasps a pencil using a tripod or quadripod grasp (i.e., with the pencil resting between the thumb and first two fingers or between the thumb and first three fingers). At first the child holds a pencil with a static tripod grasp and uses forearm and wrist movement to draw. However, the 5-year-old child develops a mature, dynamic tripod. In this grasp pattern the pencil is held in the tips of the radial fingers and is moved using finger movement. By controlling the pencil using individual finger movements, the child can make letters and small forms.

Drawing skill progresses from drawing circles, to lines that intersect and cross in a diagonal (e.g., an "**X**"). The 5-year-old child can draw a person with multiple and recognizable parts. Drawing is often a strong interest at this

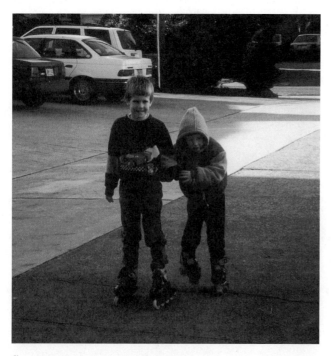

figure **4-7** Preschool children demonstrate sufficient equilibrium for roller skating.

age and therefore contributes to the child's imaginative play. He or she can also draw detailed figures created in the imagination (i.e., monsters, fairies, and other fanciful creatures).

The development of scissors skills follows the development of controlled pencil use. The first cutting skill, observed at 3 years, is snipping with alternating full-finger extension and flexion. Between 4 and 6 years, bilateral hand coordination, dexterity, and eye-hand coordination improve, enabling the child to cut out simple shapes. Mature use of scissors is not achieved until 5 to 6 years, because it requires isolated finger movements, simultaneous hand control, and well-developed eye-hand coordination for cutting accuracy (Folio & Fewell, 2000).

Other fine-motor skills acquired during the preschool years are important to the child's constructive and dramatic play. Activities such as putting puzzles together, building towers, stringing small beads, using keys, and cutting out complex designs usually require dexterity, bilateral coordination, and motor planning.

Cognitive

Preschool age children create symbolic representations of real-life objects and events during play. In addition, they begin to plan pretend scenarios in advance, organizing who and what are needed to complete the activity. Play becomes an elaborate sequence of events that is remembered, acted out, and later described for others. For example, the child may act out the role of an adult, imitating action remembered from an earlier experience. This form of role play demonstrates the child's understanding of how roles relate to actions and how actions relate to each other (e.g., the child may role play a grocery store clerk, displaying items for sale, take money from the customer, and place it in a toy cash register).

Abstract thinking begins in the preschool years as the child pretends that an object is something else. For example, the child may pretend a block is a doll bed; later the same block may become a telephone receiver or a train car.

The motor skills noted in early childhood also reflect cognitive skills. To construct a three-dimensional building, the child needs to have the ability to discriminate size and shape. Building in three dimensions also requires spatial understanding and problem-solving skills. When building from a set of blocks, the child usually must first categorize and organize them. Next, the child must solve the problem of how to fit them together to replicate a model or create the imagined structure.

In a similar way the emergence of drawing skills reflects cognitive abilities, as well as fine motor skills. The 3-year-old child makes crude attempts to represent people and objects in drawings. By 4 years of age a child can draw a recognizable person, demonstrating the ability to select salient features and represent them on a two-dimensional surface. The 4-year-old child not only identifies the parts of a person but also relates them correctly, although the size of the parts is rarely proportional to real life. At 5 years, the child's drawing is more refined, more realistic, and better proportioned. By this age, pictures begin to tell stories and reflect the emotions of the child (Linder, 1993).

Psychosocial

In early childhood, interaction and play with peers take on increasing importance. Children become social beings and identify themselves as individuals (i.e., separate from parents). Erikson (1963) defined the first psychosocial phase of early childhood as *autonomy versus shame and doubt*. Autonomy dominates the psychosocial development from 2 to 4 years. The child is adamant about making personal decisions. The development of trust in the environment and improvements in language bring forth control over self, strengthening the child's autonomous nature.

The discovery of the body and how to control it promotes independence in self-care. The success in acting independently instills a sense of confidence and self-control. However, the negative side of autonomy is a sense of shame or doubt. This feeling comes when the child acts independently and is told that he or she has done something wrong, (i.e., misbehaved). The child needs to learn which independent actions meet the approval of adults.

Erikson described the latter part of early childhood as a period of *initiative versus guilt*. Children need to achieve a balance between initiative to independently act and the responsibility they feel for their own actions. Children, aged 4 and 5, explore beyond the environment, discovering new activities. They seek new experiences for the pleasure of learning about the environment and for the opportunities it offers for exploration. If the child's learning experiences are successful and effective and his or her actions meet the parental approval, a sense of initiative is developed. Through these activities the child learns to question, reason, and find solutions to problems.

Adult-child relationships and early home experiences also influence later peer relations. According to research, children whose attachments to their mothers are rated as secure tend to be more responsive to other children in childcare settings. They are also more curious and competent (Jacobson & Wille, 1986; Youngblade & Belsky, 1992). Peer play becomes an important avenue for the child's development of social and cognitive abilities.

The development of autonomy provides a foundation for the child's imagination. Now the young child explores the world not only through the use of his or her senses but also by thinking and reasoning. Although play can be reality based, it usually includes fantasy, wishes, and role play. Words, rhymes, and songs also complement this type of play (Figure 4-8).

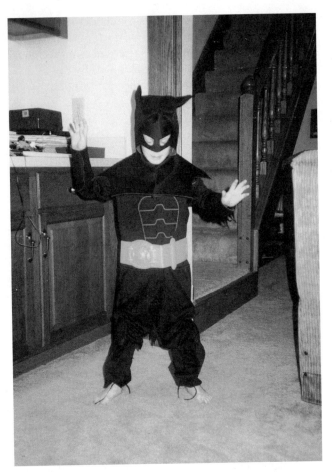

figure**4-8** Children, ages 3 and 4 years, love dressing in costumes and spending hours in the character suggested by those costumes.

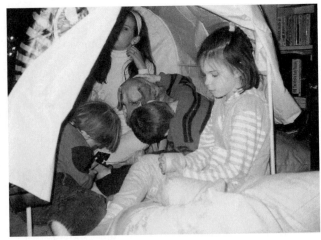

figure**4-9** Pup tents become a haven for quiet play.

Environments

By the age of 5, a child's outdoor environment has expanded beyond the areas around the home and childcare center. A variety of outdoor environments offer spaces for rough-and-tumble play, and expanded social and physical environments give the child new opportunities for learning (and generalizing) the skills he or she has achieved. Although adult supervision remains essential, the entire neighborhood may become the child's playground.

The availability of new indoor environments is also to be expected. Preschool classrooms usually have centers for different types of activities (e.g., creating art, listening to stories, playing games). In addition, community groups often sponsor a variety of indoor activities (e.g., preschool gymnastics, organized play programs) in which the child can take part.

Expanded environments offer children the opportunity to adapt play skills learned at home to the constraints of new spaces. For example, the child who climbs and slides down the stairs at home learns to climb a 6-foot ladder and slide down the slide in the neighborhood park. Parks and playgrounds also provide the child with new surfaces that challenge balance and equipment that offers intense vestibular experiences.

Preschool-age children also enjoy spending time in quiet spaces. Children, especially those who demonstrate overreactivity to sensory input, may feel drawn to quiet, enclosed spaces (e.g., a space behind the couch, the safe haven of their bedrooms, a small tent in the corner of the playroom) (Figure 4-9). Quiet spaces can be organizing and calming after a day in a childcare center. Other children who may have underreacting sensory systems may seek stimulating environments that are full of activity, or they may create their own high activity in an otherwise quiet space.

When placed in new environments, children often respond by instinctively exploring the new spaces (e.g., hallways, cupboards, corners, furniture). Exploring the features of an environment can help orient children to the spaces that surround them, can promote perceptual learning, and can provide an understanding of the play possibilities in that environment.

▪ MIDDLE CHILDHOOD: AGES 6 TO 10 YEARS

Play Occupations

Although 6-year-old children continue to enjoy imaginative play, they begin to increasingly structure and organize their play. By 7 and 8 years of age, structured games and organized play predominate (Table 4-9). *Games with rules* are the primary mode for physical and social play. Groups of children organize themselves, assign roles, and explain (or create) rules to guide the game they plan to play. The goal of the game now competes

table 4-9   *Development of Play Occupations: Middle Childhood 6 to 10 Years*

PLAY OCCUPATIONS

Games with rules
   Computer games, card games that require problems
      solving and abstract thinking
Crafts and hobbies
   Has collections
   May have hobbies
Organized sports
   Cooperative and competitive play in groups/teams of
      children
   Winning and skills are emphasized
Social play
   Play includes talking and joking
   Peer play predominates at school and home

INDIVIDUAL ABILITIES

Fine Motor/manipulative
   Good dexterity for crafts and construction with small
      objects
   Bilateral coordination for building complex structure
   Precision and motor planning evident in drawing
   Motor planning evident in completion of complex puzzles
Gross motor
   Runs with speed and endurance

Jumps, hops, skips
Throws ball well at long distances
Catches ball with accuracy
Cognitive
   Abstract reasoning
   Performs mental operations without need to physically try
   Demonstrates flexible problem solving
   Solves complex problems
Psychosocial
   Cooperative: less egocentric
   Tries to please others
   Has best friend
   Is part of cliques
   Less impulsive, able to regulate behavior
   Has competitive relationships

ENVIRONMENTS

School is now primary environment
Lunchroom and playground are important play environments
Multiple community environments with adults and peers
Forms various relationships with adults (e.g., coach, teacher)
Community programs for sports, scouts, dance, and choral
   groups

---

with the reward of interacting with peers, and children become fascinated with the rules that govern the games they play.

At 7 and 8 years of age, children do not understand that rules apply equally to everyone involved in the game, and they are often unable to place the rules of the game above the personal need to win (Florey & Greene, 1997). However, breaking the rules may reap the criticism of peers, who also acknowledge the importance of rules at this time. By 9 and 10 years of age, children are more conscientious about obeying rules.

By 8 and 9 years, children become interested in sports, and parents are generally supportive of sport activities. Although a form of play, organized sports can assume a serious nature (i.e., intrinsic motivation and internal sense of control are overridden by the external demands of practice and serious competition with peers).

There is a continuing interest in creating craft and art projects in middle childhood. During this time, the child shows increased abilities to organize, to solve problems, and to create from abstract materials. However, the completion of craft and art projects continues to require the support of adults to organize materials and identify steps. The final product, which is relatively unimportant to younger children, is now valued.

In middle childhood, children play in cooperative groups and value interaction with their peers. When friends come together, almost all activity is play and fun. Simply talking and joking become playful and entertaining. Children spend over 40% of their waking hours with peers (Cole & Cole, 1989). In these peer groups, children learn to cooperate but also to compete (Florey & Greene, 1997). They are now interested in *achievement* through play; they recognize and accept an outside standard for success or failure and criteria for winning or losing. With competition in play comes risk-taking and strategic thinking. Children who compete in sports and other activities exhibit courage to perform against an outside standard (Reilly, 1974).

Individual Systems
Sensorimotor

During the elementary school years, sensorimotor development continues to focus on refining previously acquired skills. With this refinement, hours of repetition of activities to attain mastery of common interests are observed. Children ride bicycles, scale fences, swim, skate, and jump rope (Knobloch & Pasamanick, 1974; Stone & Church, 1973) (Figure 4-10). Although motor capabili-

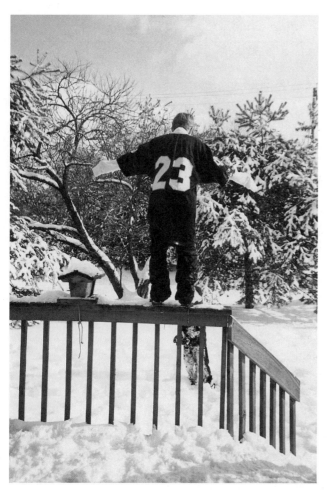

figure**4-10**   Balance is excellent in 9- and 10-year-old children, who skillfully conquer icy railings.

Cognitive

In middle childhood, concepts and relationships in the physical world are understood and applied. The child relates past events to future plans and comprehends how situations change over time. Thinking has become more flexible and abstract. The child has become a reasoning individual, who can solve problems by understanding variables and weighing pertinent factors before making decisions.

In the past, children could only apply one solution, and they were often stuck when the solution of choice did not work. However, by 8 and 9 years of age, they recognize that different solutions can be tried, and they arrive at answers through abstract reasoning rather than through concrete trial and error. At this age, children can also pay attention to more than one physical characteristic at a time and can systematically put elements together (Papalia & Olds, 1995).

In play, children order objects by size or shape, demonstrating the ability to discriminate perceptual aspects of objects and to order them accurately. They also understand the relationship of whole to parts, and they imagine pieces as parts of a whole. Children at 9 and 10 years of age can give instructions to others and tell stories in detail.

By middle childhood, children learn to combine tasks and routines into complex games and competitive sports. Because multiple rules are needed to play sports, such as baseball or hockey, the child understands the need to combine the rules into a complete game. To participate in the activity successfully, he or she also understands when rules apply and how they relate to each other.

Psychosocial

Children in this age group focus on meeting challenges in themselves and challenges presented by others. Children appreciate the recognition that comes with successfully completing assignments or projects. Comparison with peers is increasingly important during this time. If a child's schoolwork is compared with the work of a more successful student, a negative evaluation can decrease his or her sense of mastery and may produce feelings of inferiority.

School-age children seek independence of identity. They are not as egocentric as young children and demonstrate a more objective view of themselves. Children at this age have a definite subculture, or clique, that includes only certain friends (Papalia & Olds, 1995). At this age, children are quick to criticize those who do not conform to the group esthetic. Therefore rejection by the child's peers may result from a lack of conformity in dressing or physical appearance. Children who are rarely praised by their peers, who have difficulty communicating, or who do not know how to initiate relationships are less likely to have close friendships.

ties are highly varied for this age group, balance and co-ordination improve throughout the middle childhood years, providing children with the agility to dance and play sports with proficiency. Research indicates that children who master physical skills tend to exhibit high self-esteem (Short-DeGraff, 1988). Not only does self-esteem improve as children master physical skills, but peer acceptance improves as well.

Performance of fine motor skills in middle childhood includes efficient tool use (e.g., scissors, tweezers) and precise drawing skills. Children handle and manipulate (fold, sort, adhere, cut) materials with competency. The drawing skills of 8- and 9-year-old children demonstrate appropriate proportions and accuracy, and handwriting skills improve in speed and accuracy as children learn manuscript and then cursive writing. These improvements provide evidence of increased dexterity and coordination. Construction skills, manipulation, and abilities to use tools continue to generalize across performance areas with increases in speed, strength, and precision.

During middle childhood, children become disinterested in adults, including their parents. Values from peers become significantly more important than those of adults. Data indicate that children between 7 and 10 years of age are highly compliant to their peers and easily shift in the direction of their peers (Costanzo & Shaw, 1966).

The child's progression from games with some structure and flexible rules to highly competitive games demonstrates progression in moral development. Early in the child's thinking (before 7 years of age), rules are viewed as absolute, sacred, and unchangeable. Children 7 to 10 years old recognize that rules come from someone in authority, and they accept what this authority says. However, late in the elementary school years, children cast aside their beliefs in the absolute infallibility of rules, because they have gained the knowledge that people are the creators of rules. Questioning the rules and the authority who makes them begins at this age (Florey & Greene, 1997).

Environment

The child's play environment is now large and complex; more activities take place in the neighborhood and at school. The school's playground supports both social and physical play of small groups (or pairs) of children. Play occurs in ball fields, community centers, amusement parks, and sports arenas. Organized activities often take place in churches or YMCAs. By middle childhood, children have the mobility skills to maneuver through all environments (e.g., rough terrain, busy city streets). The society of school-age children dominates neighborhood streets and backyards, with bicycle races and spontaneous street hockey games. They explore the woods and go on adventures in nearby parks to find areas unexplored by others. Although supervision by adults is still needed at times, intermittent supervision usually suffices.

■ SUMMARY

A child's development of occupational performance is influenced by multiple systems and variables in the individual and the environment. The individual patterns observed in children provide insight as to how and why a child follows a certain developmental trajectory. Biomechanical, sensorimotor, cognitive, and psychosocial characteristics are related to the child's performance in play occupations, as are variables such as temperament, social supports, and physical constraints.

As an essential occupation of childhood, play provides a window through which development can be understood and appreciated. A child's play reveals the complexities of individual, activity, and environmental interaction. To identify how individual systems and the environment constrain or facilitate a child's performance, occupational therapists often analyze occupational performance by considering the role of the child as a player. This analysis becomes the basis for using play as a means and an end of occupational therapy.

STUDY QUESTIONS

1. Describe three toys that would likely engage optimal-play performance in a 12-month-old boy, in a 2-year-old girl, and in a 3-year-old boy.

2. Describe the development of social play of a child from age 2 to 6 years. Explain how an occupational therapist would use this information when designing an intervention plan. Define ideal group size at 2 years and at 6 years.

3. Compare the sensorimotor play of a 2-year-old to that of a 5-year-old child.

4. Two 4-year-old children are playing house together; one is the father and one is the mother. They have decided to have a play dinner that they will make in their play kitchen. At this time, they are setting the table using play silverware and plates from the small kitchen's cupboard. Analyze this play activity by identifying the motor, sensory, perceptual, cognitive, and psychosocial abilities needed to set the table for a play dinner. List two environmental variables that would constrain or limit this task and two that would facilitate completion of dinner.

References

Bayley, N. (1993). *Bayley Scales of Infant Development* (Rev. ed.). San Antonio, TX: Psychological Corporation.

Case-Smith, J., & Berry, J. (1998). Preschool hand skills. In J. Case-Smith (Ed.), *Making a difference in school based practice* (pp. 1-45). Bethesda, MD: AOTA, Inc.

Cioni, G., Ferrari, F., Einspieler, C., Paolicelli, P., Barbiani, T., & Prechtl, H.F. (1997). Comparison between the observation of spontaneous movements and neurologic examination in preterm infants. *Journal of Pediatrics, 130,* 704-711.

Clark, J. (1997). A dynamical systems perspective on the development of complex adaptive skill. In C. Dent-Read & P. Zukow-Goldring (Eds.), *Evolving explanations of development: Ecological approaches to organisms-environment systems.* Washington, DC: American Psychological Association.

Cole, M., & Cole, S. (1989). *The development of children.* New York: Scientific American Books.

Corbetta, D., & Mounoud, P. (1990). Early development of grasping and manipulation. In C. Bard, M. Fleury, & L. Hay (Eds.), *Development of eye-hand coordination across the life span.* Columbia, SC: University of South Carolina Press.

Cornhill, H., & Case-Smith, J. (1996). Factors that relate to good and poor handwriting. *American Journal of Occupational Therapy, 50,* 732-739.

Costanzo, P.R., & Shaw, M.E. (1966). Conformity as a function of age level. *Child Development, 37,* 967-975.

Erikson, E.H. (1963). *Childhood and society* (2nd ed.). New York: W.W. Norton.

Fagaard, J. (1990). The development of bimanual coordination. In C. Bard, M. Fleury, & L. Hay (Eds.), *Development of eye-hand coordination across the life span.* Charleston, SC: University of South Carolina Press.

Florey, L.L., & Greene, S. (1997). Play in middle childhood: A focus on children with behavior and emotional disorders. In L.D. Parham & L. Primeau (Eds.), *Play in occupational therapy for children* (pp. 26-143). St. Louis: Mosby.

Folio, M.R., & Fewell, R.R. (2000). *Peabody Developmental Motor Scales* (Rev. ed.). Austin, TX: Pro-Ed.

Furono, S., O-Reilly, K.A., Hosaka, C.M., Inatsuka, T.T., Zeisloft-Falbey, B., & Allman, T. (1984). *Hawaii Early Learning Profile.* Palo Alto, CA: VORT.

Gesell, A. (1945). *The embryology of behavior: The beginnings of the human mind.* New York: Harper and Brothers.

Gesell, A., & Amatruda, G. (1947). *Developmental diagnosis* (2nd ed.). New York: Harper & Row.

Gesell, A., Halverson, H.M., Thompson, H., Ilg, F.L., Castner, B.M., Ames, L.B., & Amatruda, C.S. (1940) *The first five years of life.* New York: Harper & Row.

Gibson, E.J. (1997). An ecological psychologist's prolegomena for perceptual development: A functional approach. In C. Dent-Read & P. Zukow-Goldring (Eds.), *Evolving explanations of development: Ecological approaches to organisms-environment systems.* Washington, DC: American Psychological Association.

Gibson, J.J. (1979). *The ecological approach to visual perception.* Boston: Houghton-Mifflin.

Gilfolye, E., Grady, A., & Moore, J. (1990). *Children adapt.* (2nd ed.). Thorofare, NJ: Slack.

Goldfield, E.C., Kay, B.A., & Warren, W.H. (1993). Infant bouncing: The assembly and tuning of action systems. *Child Development, 64,* 1128-1142.

Greenspan, G. (1990). *Infancy and early childhood: The practice of clinical assessment and intervention with emotional and developmental challenges.* Madison, WI: International Universities Press.

Illingworth, R.S. (1966). The diagnosis of cerebral palsy in the first year of life. *Developmental Medicine and Child Neurology, 8,* 178-194.

Illingworth, R.S. (1984). *The development of the infant and young child.* Edinburgh: Churchill Livingstone.

Jacobson, S.L., & Wille, D.E. (1986). The influence of attachment pattern on developmental changes in peer interaction from the child to the preschool period. *Child Development, 57,* 338-347.

Klaus, M.H., & Kennell, J.H. (1976). *Maternal-infant bonding.* St. Louis: Mosby.

Knobloch, H., & Pasamanick, B. (1974). *Gesell & Amatruda's developmental diagnosis* (3rd ed.). New York: Harper & Row.

Knox, S. (1997). Development and current use of the Knox Preschool Play Scale. In L.D. Parham & L. Primeau (Eds.), *Play in occupational therapy for children* (pp. 35-51). St. Louis: Mosby.

Linder, T. (1993). *Transdisciplinary play-based assessment* (Rev. ed.). Baltimore: Paul Brookes Publishers.

Mandler, J.M. (1990). A new perspective on cognitive development in infancy. *American Scientist, 78,* 236-243.

Mathiowetz, V., & Haugen, J. (1994). Motor behavior research: Implications for therapeutic approaches to central nervous system dysfunction. *American Journal of Occupational Therapy, 48,* 733-745.

Mathiowetz, V., & Haugen, J. (1995). Evaluation of motor behavior: Traditional and contemporary views. In C.A. Trombly (Ed.), *Occupational therapy for physical dysfunction* (4th ed.) (pp. 157-186). Baltimore: Williams & Wilkins.

McGraw, M. (1945). *The neuromuscular maturation of the human infant.* New York: Maxmillan.

Metzoff, A.N., & Moore, M.K. (1992). Early imitation within a functional framework: The importance of person identity, movement, and development. *Infant Behavior and Development, 15,* 470-505.

Newell, K.M. (1986). Constraints on development of coordination. In M.G. Wade & H.T.A. Whiting (Eds.), *Motor development in children: Aspects of coordination and control* (pp. 341-360). Dordrecht, Netherlands: Martinus Nijhoff.

Papalia, D.E., & Olds, S.W. (1995). *Human development* (6th ed.). New York: McGraw-Hill, Inc.

Parham, L.D., & Primeau, L. (1997). Play and occupational therapy. In L.D. Parham & L. Fazio (Eds.), *Play in occupational therapy for children* (pp. 2-22). St. Louis: Mosby.

Pehoski, C. (1995). Object manipulation in infants and children. In A. Henderson & C. Pehoski (Eds.), *Hand function in the child* (pp. 136-153). St. Louis: Mosby.

Piaget, J. (1952). *The origins of intelligence in children* (M. Cook, Trans.) New York: International Universities Press.

Piper, M.C., & Darrah, J. (1994). *Motor assessment of the developing infant.* Philadelphia: W.B. Saunders.

Reilly, M. (Ed.). (1974). *Play as exploratory learning.* Beverly Hills, CA: Sage Publications.

Rochat, P. (1989). Object manipulation and exploration in 2- to 5-month-old infants. *Developmental Psychology, 25,* 871-884.

Rubin, K. (1984). *The play observation scale.* Ontario, Canada: University of Waterloo.

Rubin, K.H., Fein, G.G., & Vandenberg, B. (1983). Play. In E.M. Hetherington (Ed.), *Handbook of child psychology: Socialization, personality and social development* (pp. 693-774). New York: John Wiley & Sons.

Rubin, K., Maioni, T.L., & Hornung, M. (1976). Free play behaviors in middle-class and lower-class children: Parten and Piaget revisited. *Child Development, 47,* 414-419.

Ruff, H.A. (1989). The infant's use of visual and haptic information in the perception and recognition of objects. *Canadian Journal of Psychology, 43,* 302-319.

Short-DeGraff, M. (1988). *Human development for occupational and physical therapists.* Baltimore: Williams & Wilkins.

Singer, D.G., & Singer, J.L. (1990). *The house of make-believe: Play and the developing imagination.* Cambridge, MA: Harvard University Press.

Stone, J.L., & Church. J. (1973). *Childhood and adolescence: A psychology of the growing person* (3rd ed.). New York: Random House.

Thelen, E. (1995). Motor development: A new synthesis. *American Psychologist, 50,* 79-95.

Thelen, E., Corbetta, D., Kamm, K., Spencer, J., Schneider, K., & Zernicke, R. (1993). The transition to reaching: Mapping intention and intrinsic dynamics. *Child Development, 64,* 1058-1098.

Thomas, A., & Chess, S. (1977). *Temperament and development.* New York: Brunner/Mazel.

Touwen, B.C.L. (1979). *Examination of the child with minor neurological dysfunction. Clinics in Development Medicine 71.* London: Heinemann.

Tseng, M., & Murray, E. (1994). Differences in perceptual-motor measures in children with good and poor handwriting. *Occupational Therapy Journal of Research, 14,* (1), 19-36.

von Hofsten, C. (1982). Eye-hand coordination in the newborn. *Developmental Psychology, 18,* (3), 450-461.

von Hofsten, C. (1993). Studying the development of goal-directed behaviour. In A.F. Kalverboer, B. Hopkins, & R. Geuze (Eds.), *Motor development in early and later childhood: Longitudinal approaches.* New York: Cambridge Press.

Vygotsky, L.S. (1978). *Mind in society: The development of higher psychological processes.* Cambridge, MA: Harvard University Press.

Youngblade, L.M., & Belsky, J. (1992). Parent-child antecedents of 5-year-olds' close friendships: A longitudinal analysis. *Development Psychology, 28* (4), 700-713.

chapter 5

Working with Families

Ruth Humphry
Jane Case-Smith

key terms

Family systems and subsystems
Structure, boundaries
Family traditions and rituals
Sources of family diversity
Family functions
Family life cycle
Family resources and strengths
Coping and adaptation of families

Parent-professional partnerships
Communication strategies
Vulnerability and resilience
Families facing multiple challenges

■ CHAPTER OBJECTIVES

1. Use the terms about families to describe family situations.
2. Discuss the sources of diversity in family structure.
3. Depict forces within the family that promote a child's resilience.
4. Analyze a family system and discuss implications of a systems perspective for occupational performance of family members.
5. Analyze the implications of a child with special needs on parent-child co-occupations and family function.
6. Synthesize information about family life cycle and transitions to identify times of potential stress for families.
7. Value an ecological and systems perspective of the parenting process.
8. Specify the roles of the occupational therapist in collaborating with families.
9. Understand how to establish and maintain collaborative relationships with a family.
10. Enact alternative methods of communication that promote family-therapist partnerships.
11. Describe ways families may participate in intervention services.

12. Explain strategies for supporting strengths of families facing multiple challenges.

■ WHY WORK WITH FAMILIES?

It has long been recognized that when a medical condition, disease, or disability challenges a child's development, the ultimate outcome is highly influenced by the caregiving environment (Sameroff & Chandler, 1975). Many of the children served by occupational therapists have conditions (e.g., autism, hyperactivity, cerebral palsy [CP], and attention deficit disorder) that produce developmental differences across the life span. However, this does not mean the ultimate outcome and quality of their occupational performance is predetermined.

Researchers and those working with children are developing a richer understanding of what makes a difference in young people's lives (Kirby & Fraser, 1997). Factors that increase the child's vulnerability to negative outcomes are *individual* (e.g., physical impairment, difficult temperament, family history of depression) or *contextual* (e.g., single mother who is working two jobs, living in a violent inner city neighborhood).

Some children appear to overcome factors that look like significant disadvantages and develop to their greatest potential, leading lives composed of socially valued, productive, and enjoyable occupations. Positive forces that produce the resilience necessary to overcome negative pressures contribute to adaptive responses and optimal outcome. These positive factors can be *internal* (e.g., child's outgoing personality) or *external* (e.g., child's positive family situation). Features of families (where and how they function) are factors that contribute to the *vulnerability* and *resilience* of children.

To help an individual with disabilities, it is necessary to look beyond the sequence of development and the characteristics of the child's special needs to see additional sources of vulnerability and resilience. Using an epidemiologic approach, McDermott and others (1996) found that problem behaviors in children with CP are five times more likely than in typically developing children. Children with CP who do not show behavioral problems, such as dependency, hyperactivity, and disruptive actions, may have external support or internal resiliency that prevents these negative outcomes. Occupational therapists work with families because the people that make up a child's family and the experiences they provide contribute to a child's resilience. In addition, certain family characteristics can be risk factors if not addressed. Interventions that enhance or strengthen forces of resilience will help the child develop to the best of his or her potential.

Over the last two decades researchers have used dynamical systems and ecological models to explain the child's development as being inseparable from the family context (Bronfenbrenner, 1986, Fraser, 1997; Thelen & Smith, 1994). The family creates the child's earliest occupational context, and an important part of parenting is managing the pattern of activities and learning opportunities that the child is shown throughout the day (Park, 1995). Parent's choices about toys, available playmates, and opportunities to explore enable the young child to acquire new movement and communication skills. The family's socioeconomic status influences the types and quality of experiences in childcare centers, schools, neighborhoods, clubs, and after-school jobs. The role of the family in influencing development and promoting resilience has particular importance when the child has special needs.

In addition to organizing and enabling daily occupations, the family represents the most enduring set of relationships throughout childhood and early adulthood. During the course of a lifetime, an individual with a disability interacts with and relates to a multitude of professionals. These may be short-term relationships, or they may endure for several years. However, relationships always change as the child moves into new life stages and service systems. The young person's family represents a source of continuity. Family members with their unique emotional involvement and everyday contact have gathered insight into the child's needs, abilities, and occupational interests. The occupational therapist recognizes the family's position as the expert on the young person. They strive for a collaborative relationship that follows the family's lead and supports its efforts to promote the health and optimal development of its members (Lawlor & Mattingly, 1998).

The critical perspective families bring to services for children with special needs and their power in promoting development are reflected in federal legislation. Requiring their input and permission on any assessment, intervention plan, and placement decision reinforces the role of the child's parent or guardian. The importance of the family in the early part of the child's life (birth to 3 years old) is reflected by the emphasis on family-centered services in Part C of the Individuals with Disabilities Education Act (IDEA) (IDEA, 1990). The Individualized Family Service Plan (IFSP) is developed through dialogue with the parents regarding what resources the family needs to help promote the child's development. (The IFSP and early-intervention legislation are further described in Chapter 22.)

After 3 years of age the child's program may become more focused on the child and his or her education. However, input from parents on the Individualized Educational Program (IEP) is an important part of the process. Although a specific parental role in IEP development is defined in IDEA, the parent's involvement does not stop with planning the child's educational program. The expectation of development is that the young person will leave home and live in the community. Acquisition of independent living and prevocational skills enables the student with special needs to move from school to community participation. In services for young adolescents with special needs, IDEA recognizes the importance of family in forming transition plans. The law confirms that parents are in the best position to guide the adolescent's transition planning process.

■ WHAT IS A FAMILY?

Given the powerful role families play in their children's health, development, and education, it is important that the occupational therapist understand how families work. Contemporary families defy a single definition of who is part of a child's family. An outsider, such as a service provider, cannot decide what people or relationships constitute a family (Levin & Trost, 1992). Families do have specific *boundaries* that determine whether an individual is part of the unit, and membership in the family may change with life events. For example, a person may be added to the family unit by birth, by adoption, or by marriage. Although heterosexual relationships have traditionally been assumed to be the basis for the formation of a family with children, this is no longer the case as more lesbian couples choose to use artificial insemination to become parents (Park, 1998). Families also lose members because of divorce, death, limited contact, or decreased emotional commitment. Asking a client to *"describe the family"* is one way an occupational therapist can avoid suggesting any preconceived ideas about family membership.

A family can also be seen as the interdependent relationship of two or more people who share an enduring emotional commitment to each family member's well being. Regardless of membership or cultural background, all families address particular issues to ensure members' well being. *Family functions* include (1) fostering affection, (2) providing emotional support, (3) socializing members for participation in occupations outside the family, (4) ensuring opportunities for recreation, (5) promoting health and independence in self-care, and (6) fostering readiness for education and development of potential productivity.

To accomplish these functions, family members engage in a variety of different occupations such as home management, caregiving, and leisure activities. Some family members engage in productive occupations to acquire and maintain physical resources such as shelter, food, and clothing. Energy and time are intangible resources that one or more of the family members need to succeed in their occupations. Physical, financial, and emotional resources have to be shared among the members. As a result, a family must set priorities and allocate resources. Frequently, families are organized in a hierarchy so one or two members have more power to determine how the family resources are allocated.

■ FAMILY AS A SYSTEM

To understand how families fulfill their functions, occupational therapists have learned from social scientists in anthropology, developmental psychology, sociology, and occupational science. A common theoretic approach is to view the family as a dynamic, interacting system (Box 5-1) (Minuchin, 1985). Each aspect, or principle, of a family system is discussed in terms of the implications the principles have on occupations that take place in a family context.

Through a systems model, the family can be seen as a *group of individuals with interrelated occupations*. Therefore changes in one family member's occupational performance potentially affects all other members. For example, when a child starts to walk, the new form of functional mobility and potential for exploratory play affects other members of the family. The parent experiences occupational change when caregiving behaviors become more disciplinary in nature (e.g., setting limits

---

box 5-1 *Key concepts of a family system model*

1. A family system is composed of individuals that are interdependent with reciprocal influences.
2. Within the family, subsystems are defined with their own patterns of interaction and recurrent behaviors.
3. A family must be understood as a whole, and it is more than the sum of the abilities of each member.
4. The family system works to achieve homeostasis on a day-to-day basis and to be part of a larger community.
5. Change and evolution are inherent in a family.
6. A family, as an open system, is influenced by its environment.

---

on the child's exploration of the home). The older sister's occupational context changes because the younger sibling can explore her room and toys. The child's grandmother, who provides childcare during the day, also experiences a change in her occupations as she feels more fatigue and has less energy to pursue leisure interests in the evenings.

The occupational therapist that recognizes that the pattern and performance of each family member's occupations are interdependent is able to see the complexity that results when the performance of one member changes. In addition to the *direct effect* of the child's new form of an occupation, there are *indirect consequences* among family members. For example, the grandmother's increased vigilance in watching the child, who moves rapidly from one room to the next, makes it less likely that she will have time to help her granddaughter with homework. Therefore an indirect effect of the child's new mobility is a change in his sister's occupational performance at school.

Family members come together and form *interactive subsystems* with their own boundaries and shared or co-occupations. The caregiving process frequently means that the parent and child subsystems are engaged in co-occupations such as dressing or feeding (Zemke & Clark, 1996). A couple planning the family vacation reflects the parent subsystem, whereas two sisters playing "house" is an example of a co-occupation of the sibling subsystem. In co-occupations the performance of one family member is part of the social context of the other family member's experience in the shared occupation. As a result, co-occupations set in place a reciprocal process, influencing the performance of each member of the subsystem. In co-occupations the less-skilled member of the subsystem (usually the younger child) is enabled to participate at a more sophisticated performance level than when engaged in the occupation alone. In pediatric practice the occupational therapist may primarily interact with the parent and child subsystems (Lawlor & Mattingly, 1998). At the same time the clinician recognizes that not all family functions are accomplished by the mother-child subsystem. For example, a session that involves a sibling may effectively enhance occupational performance in play because play opportunities occur most frequently in the sibling subsystem.

How a family works cannot be completely understood by separately gathering information about occupational performance of each individual. The family's functions are a product of an *interacting unit that must be viewed as a whole.* Just as occupational performance cannot be understood by knowing the developmental status of individual components, the family needs to be considered as a whole. For example, knowing that all the siblings are old enough to get dressed for school independently does not mean the therapist can assume that mornings run smoothly; nor can the therapist assume that the parent can give the child with special needs extra attention to promote self-care in the mornings. The occupational therapist cannot directly observe all aspects of family life and shared occupations that may affect the child with special needs. However, interviewing the primary care providers and collaborating with the family in program development increases the probability that any intervention ideas consider the interactive operatives of the whole family.

A family system works to *achieve a degree of homeostasis.* Creating family routines and rituals can maximize resources (e.g., time and energy) and meet family functions (e.g., nurturing, emotional well being, sense of continuity among family members). Families can operate in a variety of ways to accomplish the same outcome. The great variety of patterns reflected in different cultures illustrates the degree of freedom with which families fulfill their functions. Families who report that they have established rituals that are important to them tend to demonstrate higher levels of family cohesiveness and work effectively together (Fiese, Hooker, Kotary, & Schwagler, 1993). These routines and rituals appear in daily occupations, family traditions, and special celebrations.

In the context of daily, shared lives, *interactive routines in occupations and co-occupations* help define who does what, when, and how (Fiese et. al., 1993). For example, a variety of occupations ensure physical hygiene (e.g., children can wash in the sink, shower, or tub). This can be done alone or with another family member at different times during the day or night. To be efficient, the family must determine how and when the occupations are accomplished by establishing guidelines and rules. Maintaining homeostasis is essential to family function

and disruption to homeostasis usually becomes a high priority and the focus of the family's energy.

In addition to helping the family operate effectively and anticipate members' behaviors, routines take on symbolic and emotional meaning. Frequently, co-occupations such as sharing meals, getting ready for bed, or leaving each other to go to work or school are ways families express affection, thereby fulfilling a powerful family function.

When a therapist asks how something is done at home, he or she may hear about the observable form the occupation takes, not about the meaning it holds. For example, a parent and daughter with severe motor impairments routinely bathe together (the mother sits in the bathtub and supports the daughter). The occupational therapist hears about the routine and orders a bath chair. However, because the form of the co-occupation held special meaning, the bath chair remains unused. In a family-centered approach, the occupational therapist would ask the mother if the bath-time routine was comfortable and pleasurable and if there was any interest in changing the routine. If an interactive routine in the co-occupation is valued, the family members may not wish to change or adapt it, in spite of the time and effort required.

In addition to routines and rituals for daily occupations, families also establish occupations for special events. *Family traditions,* such as cooking special food for birthday celebrations or sharing leisure activities on Sunday afternoons, help families develop a sense of group cohesion and make each family feel unique. These traditions are another way family members maintain a predictable pattern in their lives over time. Families may decide to maintain its tradition, rather than address an individual member's needs. For example, a family that traditionally visits the grandparents for several weeks in the summer may experience conflict with the occupational therapist if the therapist assumes they will cancel a vacation to attend weekly treatment sessions. When the occupational therapist asks the family to set priorities, the members consider all their traditions and determine how they want occupational therapy to fit into their lives.

Celebrations are family rituals that are shared with the community. These religious or community celebrations also guide family conduct and contribute to homeostasis. The forms occupations take in family celebrations are common with other families who share the same background, and celebrations give the family a sense of belonging to a larger group. Participation of the child with special needs in celebrations is one way a family confirms that their child is like other children (Figure 5-1).

To maintain homeostasis, families may resist changing shared occupations that are part of routines, rituals, traditions, and celebrations. However, over time family systems experience *metamorphosis and adaptation* related to family occupations. Although families develop and grow

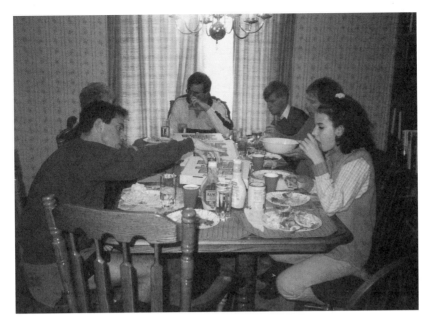

figure 5-1   Family meals on the holidays are often an important part of family celebrations.

(even when there are no children in the family), most models of family development are linked to the ages of children. At the different stages of family development, there are common developmental pressures the family must address. (These stages are described in a later section on *family life cycles.*) With each new stage of a child's development, the forms of occupations and co-occupations change. In addition, unanticipated events can require the family to adapt routine occupations. The extent to which family members share, adapt to, or change responsibilities in occupations that support family functions and alter interactive routines in occupations varies. During times of transition to a new stage of family development, a flexible family may experience shifts with slight confusion and no interruption in meeting family functions. The more fixed the family routines, the more disruption the family will experience when developmental changes or unexpected events interrupt the way things are done. For example, the husband who believes paid employment and yard care are his contributions to family function may not assume responsibility for childcare while his wife recovers from an illness. Therefore the family may not fulfill all its functions during this time, and therapy sessions may be missed.

Families are *open systems* and are influenced by their environments. Forces beyond the family boundaries determine influences that encourage and constrain family members' occupations. Because each family is seen as part of a greater set of systems, the *ecological model* is critical to appreciating how families influence the development of children (Bronfenbrenner, 1986). An ecological perspective of families enables the occupational thera-

pist to understand how the family's operations are supported (creating optimal resilience) or limited (increasing risk factors) by their context and the time in which the family exists.

■ ECOLOGY OF FAMILIES

Resources that support family function, such as socialization and recreation, are available to most families in the neighborhood and local community. Proximity to local churches, stores, and friends are part of the family's ecology. At a slightly more removed level, family resources are created by a community commitment to children, (e.g., the health department that runs an immunization clinic, the volunteer group that helps parents make good choices about childcare centers). The advantage of an ecological perspective is that it calls attention to how factors removed from the family and beyond its control can influence the child (Garbarino & Kostelney, 1995). Forces that change the family ecology can be even more distant from the child and family. For example, a large corporation that decides to cut its workforce causes job loss in the neighborhood and forces people to leave the area to find employment. Suddenly the parents no longer have a baby-sitter, and the local grocery store closes. On an even more distant level, social attitudes and public policies influence families. For example, a decision to reform welfare reflects a societal attitude about welfare recipients and has the potential to affect many families with children (Seccombe, James, & Walters, 1998).

When working with children with special needs, it is especially important that the occupational therapist take an ecological perspective of how their families operate. The therapist should also realize that each community varies in its support for families who provide care for special children. In addition to funding early intervention programs and related services in the schools, some civil organizations provide additional support. For example, a community group that raises funds to modify a park to accommodate a special-needs child expands the family's ability to engage in recreational activities.

■ SOURCES OF DIVERSITY IN FAMILIES

Families with children who need occupational therapy services come in many different forms, and therapists working with children have the rewarding opportunity to learn about a variety of families. It is the therapist's challenge to help the members of each family feel accepted and respected for whomever they are. A frequently recommended step for increasing sensitivity to diversity is to become familiar with one's own culture and values. With self-knowledge, the therapist is better prepared to appreciate individual differences in families and how background influences attitudes, values, and behaviors. Because differences create variations in the occupational contexts of children, occupational therapy services are adjusted to be consistent with the backgrounds of its families.

Families vary according to their structure, lifestyle, ethnic background, and socioeconomic status. When a family has a child with special needs and does not conform to the image of what constitutes a family as expressed in the dominant culture, the family may feel especially alienated from mainstream services (Lynch & Hanson, 1998).

Much of the diversity among families is translated into *variation in occupational form*. Family diversity is also translated into variation in the meaning of interactive routines and rituals, family traditions, and parenting styles. An individual family has a unique pattern of characteristics (e.g., family structure, adult lifestyle, parental background) and has a unique cultural background (e.g., social, ethnic, religious). Therefore generalizations about diverse family groups are rarely accurate, and sensitivity to the unique cultural differences of each family is always needed.

Family Structure

Family structure is determined by relationships among family members and by the designation of certain members to fulfill key occupations. An important consideration in understanding family structure is to determine who is the head of the household. This person (or subsystem of adults) determines how family resources are committed and can actively support or hinder changes in interactive routines in co-occupations. This may or may not be the same family member who is responsible for the acquisition of financial and or physical resources.

With children and two parents present, the family structure can be described as a *nuclear family*. Single-parent households can be considered a modified form of the nuclear family. In 1996 the U.S. Bureau of Census estimated that more than 26% of all children lived with a single parent: 21% lived with their mother and 5% lived with their father. In a study of adults who became single parents, several family strengths and weaknesses were identified (Richards & Schmiege, 1993). The family strengths included better communication between parent and child, increased personal growth, and enhanced family-management skills. Without another adult to share the parenting role, children in single-parent families may be given more household chores, which may possibly enhance the child's sense of responsibility. The problem most frequently identified by single mothers and fathers was feeling too much responsibility, such as being the only source of family income. Concerns over money occur most often when the single parent is a woman; 80% of the women who became single parents identified this issue (Acock & Kiecolt, 1989). Men who were single fathers were more likely to experience continuing problems with the former spouse, who may share custody of the children (Richards & Schmiege, 1993).

Although many children experience being a member of a single-parent family sometime in their lives, this is not always a permanent state. *Blended families* occur when adults become partners, forming a family structure in which one of the adults is biologically related to the child and the other acts as a stepparent. The *extended family* is made up of additional relatives who may or may not live in the same house. Depending on the culture and family circumstances, a family member other than the parent may be the head of the household. An *augmented family* includes individuals who are not relatives but are considered members of the family because of the close relationships they have formed with family members. In general, an extended or augmented family is likely to have more resources to help promote the child's development (Slaughter-Defoe, 1993). The *skipped-generation family* is a growing, diverse family structure in which the child (or children) is in the care of a grandparent or great grandparent. In this family structure the parent is not living with the family or is not engaged in caregiving (Goldberg-Glen, Sands, Cole, & Cristofalo, 1998).

Adult Lifestyle

Another variation of family structure is created by the lifestyle of the adult. Children can be born or adopted into families headed by homosexual partners (Park,

1998), or the child, who is a product of a parent's heterosexual relationship, can become a member of a blended family when that parent takes a new partner of the same sex. The number of children living with gay or lesbian parents is difficult to estimate because many parents with same-sex partners fear that they will lose custody of their children (Patterson, 1995). Much of the literature concerning children of gay or lesbian parents has been generated to explore the impact of the parent's lifestyle on the child's development. Park (1998) emphasized that the sexual orientation of the parent has not been associated with negative outcomes. Even so, many families with same-sex partners continue to experience social prejudice.

A strength of families with same-sex parents is the high egalitarian approach they take toward occupations associated with caregiving and home maintenance (Park, 1998). Without the influence of gender stereotyping, these families can be more flexible in role behaviors, and it may be easier for them to adjust to new circumstances. Another ecological advantage of this family structure is that the gay and lesbian community can act as a support system by forming support groups for parents and play groups for children with the same family structure (Patterson, 1995).

Homosexual partners express many of the same needs and stresses as heterosexual couples with children. They also experience some unique issues (Hare, 1994). A primary concern is whether they will be accepted as a family if they "come out" to people who work with the child. For example, when registering her child for kindergarten, a mother is asked the name, phone number, and relationship of another adult to contact in case of emergency at the school. Questions such as these create a dilemma for a mother with a same-sex partner, because she must decide whether she should deny her partner's co-parenting status or inform the school clerk of her sexual orientation. Occupational therapists working with children parented by gay or lesbian couples can communicate that they recognize the partners as co-parents by naming both parents in invitations to IFSP or IEP meetings. If the team extends an open invitation to bring significant others who share responsibility for the child, the option is left to the parent.

Ethnic Background

Ethnic variations can contribute to cultural differences between families (Lynch & Hanson, 1998) and differences between roles of fathers and mothers within families (Julian, McKenry, & McKelvey, 1994). Julian and colleagues (1994) compared responses of parents with black, white, Asian, and Hispanic backgrounds. They concluded that parents of all ethnic groups use similar techniques for socializing their children (e.g., modeling, reinforcement, and identification of desired behaviors),

but they place different emphasis on the child's independence, performance in school, and ability to control temper. How the family values independence versus interdependence is of particular importance to the occupational therapist. For example, if the parents of a child with Down syndrome do not place a high priority on independence, the therapist's suggestion to work on the child's community travel skills may be rejected.

In a qualitative study of American mothers who had emigrated from Asian countries, a Korean mother expressed how cultural differences affected her experiences with her son who had suffered a traumatic brain injury.

> You know that oriental men are not used to doing household chores. My social worker would tell my husband about all the work that I have to do and ask him what work he would be willing to take over to give me relief. She laid the foundation for my husband to begin to help me, but it is hard for him to know what to do. In Asian culture, men do not ask for help since their role is that of a provider. When we were told about getting monetary help for my son from SSI and Medicaid, we were very reluctant since we wanted to provide for him (Raghavan, 1998, p. 62).

Parents who are members of minority groups are faced with the double task of socializing children to their own culture and helping them to interact with members of the dominant culture. The values and experiences of each culture influence what the parent selects to pass on to the children. For example, black mothers who place a high priority on the children's independence and ability to control their temper may do so to prepare children to deal with the negative impact of racism on their lives (Julian et. al., 1994). To understand a family's cultural background, therapists should consider the interrelationship between an ethnic group's culture of origin, history of economic concerns, and experience with racism.

Socioeconomic Background and Family Resources

The occupational therapist's recognition of the power of the family's socioeconomic status (SES) on members' health and occupations is of critical importance (Sussenberger, 1998). Information about a child's SES is gained through details that the family presents about the structure, educational background, income level, and prestige and nature of work performed by employed family members (Entwise & Astone, 1994). Families of low SES have limited resources and restricted opportunities to participate in a wide range of occupations (Sussenberger, 1998). The family's SES can be viewed as a complex indicator of resources the family has to support the child's development and ability to participate in the community. Understanding the nature of SES helps occupational therapists appreciate how to adapt recommendations effectively to be consistent with family resources and background. In addition, factors contributing to higher parental SES can act as a protective force for certain children, eliminating risk factors (e.g., poor nutrition) that would make them more vulnerable to poor developmental outcome (McCormick, McCarton, Brooks-Gunn, Belt, & Gross, 1998). If the therapist appreciates the forces that contribute to positive resources for family functioning, he or she can identify family strengths.

Entwisle and Astone (1994) used three critical elements to describe the social and economic environments of families: (1) financial capital, (2) human capital, and (3) social capital.

Financial capital

Financial capital, or household income, is needed to provide shelter and purchase physical goods and services for family members. Children thrive in a wide variety of physical settings, but substandard housing and a limited diet are obvious risk factors to a child's health. Monetary resources determine some of the occupations and experiences that families share at home and in the community. For example, children of a financially limited family may be expected to contribute more to home-management activities, such as doing the laundry or mowing the lawn. Helping with household duties enable children to contribute to the well-being of their families and may be the foundation for practicing prevocational skills. For other families with more financial resources, hired help, such as a gardener or baby-sitter, allows children and adults to engage in alternative occupations, such as taking special classes to pursue a musical interest or spending more time at the office to follow career goals. The family's financial status may determine whether a child is covered by insurance or whether a parent can afford to take time away from work to bring the child to therapy or to attend an IEP meeting scheduled during regular business hours.

Human capital

Human capital is also an important part of the family's SES environment (Coleman, 1988; Entwisle & Astone, 1994). Typically recorded as the number of years of education and type of employed work performed by adults, human capital reflects the intellectual environment of the household. Educational background and work setting are frequently interdependent variables and suggest something about a parent's fund of knowledge, exposure to new ideas, and potential ability to access and synthesize information used to solve problems.

Families face a variety of challenges in meeting the needs of their children, and human capital is an important resource that may be available to them, even when financial capital is limited. For example, the availability of human capital is important in the case of two 21-year-old mothers who each receive welfare and raise a 1-year-old son alone. Even though both women have the same income, the atmosphere in the families is different because of human capital. Although the first woman dropped out of her junior year in college when she found she was pregnant, the second woman dropped out of high school and worked in a textile mill packing nylons until she found she was pregnant. Both women decide to continue their education but need additional assistance to pay for childcare. Their differences in human capital are reflected in reading ability, knowledge of how systems work, and comfort talking to welfare workers, all of whom have college degrees. These differences are exemplified in what the mother does in the waiting room of a social services office. The first mother reads a brochure about a welfare-to-work program and realizes she has to prove she qualifies. She brings her son's birth certificate and negotiates the application process in one visit. The second woman does not understand the welfare-to-work brochure and does not realize that she has to prove her relationship to her son to qualify for the program. Therefore two trips to the social services office are required to complete the application, and she misses the starting date for the Graduate Equivalency Degree program that semester.

Human capital is expressed in the occupations in which a parent becomes involved with the child. Higher education can translate into giving more help with homework, having conversations that are more complex, or prioritizing more time for incidental learning (e.g., reading bedtime stories, making museum trips). In visits to pediatricians, parents with more education and financial resources are more likely to recall details about prescription medication correctly. They are also more likely to call the clinic to clarify instructions given to them by the physician (Heffer et. al., 1997). Similarly, a parent with greater human capital is more likely to understand how to access the Internet to learn about a child's condition and explore treatment options, interact with professionals on the team, and select developmentally appropriate intervention goals for the child.

Social capital

Social capital is another resource that benefits a child (Coleman, 1988). Social capital includes the time, energy, and interpersonal connections that ensure informal assistance and access to information. Social capital through family members (especially the adults) connects a child with positive opportunities in the community and concerned individuals who can offer the family support. For example, a friend of a parent with an autistic child may offer to hire the child for a supported work situation. Similarly, a parent's membership in a religious group may provide connections with adults who volunteer to care for a child with chronic health problems occasionally.

Social capital can be increased or decreased over time. Families that move out of state can lose social capital because they lack connections in the new community. A family where the demands of several young children exceed an adult's energy may be low in social capital because the mother focuses all of her energy on caring for the children. Low levels of social support can contribute to increased vulnerability to poor developmental outcome. For example, a mother who is depressed and overwhelmed by her child's disability may be unresponsive and withdraw from contacts outside of the family. These responses to the problem reduce her social capital and therefore the child's exposure to other adults and to learning opportunities through an early intervention program. However, if the same mother and child were members of a blended or extended family, they would have greater social resources because of the increased number of adults involved with the child. Alternative family members that assume the parenting role provide a support if a parent is not always able to meet the child's needs. For example, if the depressed mother lives with her sister, the child's aunt can provide needed caregiving and ensure that the therapist's recommendations for a stimulating environment are implemented.

Parenting Style

The characteristics and individual style of the adults providing childcare is a key factor in understanding the diversity of families. One or more adults parent every child. Therefore all people are exposed to some form of parenting. Through socialization during childhood, adults have formulated some ideas about *what is* or *is not* appropriate parenting style. The phrase, *"Parenting is something that is caught, not taught,"* reflects the influence that past childhood experiences have on parenting behaviors. It also suggests that occupational therapists bring their own ideas about parenting to their interactions with caregivers.

Dialogue between parents and therapists (about what the child needs to be able to do or how to organize occupations to compensate for an impairment) do not always work smoothly, and the collaborative nature of the relationship is sometimes lost. If the parent and therapist hold different ideas about parenting style, tensions may arise because the therapist disapproves of the parent's priorities or prefers that the parent emphasize specific child behaviors. Parents receiving services express the concern that they are being judged as a *"good,"* not a *"bad,"* parent (Lawlor & Mattingly, 1998). Collaborative problem solving is limited when the therapist expects parent compliance, or follow through, on therapist-generated recommendations. The professional cannot assume greater

knowledge about what the child needs or the parenting style that best accommodates those needs. In appreciating variations in parenting style, it is helpful to reflect on the occupation of parenting.

Ideas about how to be a good parent have always been of common interest. Advice columns, magazine articles, and books about raising children are numerous and easily available to the public. Word of mouth is also a great resource for parents seeking advice. Neighbors and friends constantly share stories about problems their children present and the techniques they use to solve problems. However, caregiving styles seem to be the product of a process influenced by a complex interaction of the adult's personality and own history of being parented (Vondra & Belsky, 1993). The occupations associated with parenting are not always guided by advice on specific techniques. In writing about his experiences in parenting, Krieger (1996) pointed out that formal advice on parenting is most effective in helping the adult relax. When confronted with a child signaling a need for food, comfort, or entertainment, the parent is "in the moment." What the parent acquired through books and lectures (even by well-intended occupational therapists) is only background information. Parenting, then, is not something that rests just with the adult; it is co-constructed between the parent and child (Hinde, 1995). Parenting is a process, and adult and child work out solutions while engaged in their co-occupations.

What is it about parenting style that is so powerful in shaping the occupations of children? Primeau (1998), in her qualitative study of parents' play with their children, found that parents use different strategies in balancing the many occupations involved in play, caregiving, and home maintenance. In this study some parents described a conflict between household work and children's play, and they reported that they took a break from housework to play with their children. By segregating the activities, they felt able to get things done around the home and give children their full attention at other times. Other parents solved the problem by embedding playful experiences in household work. For example, they might have asked the child to help sort silverware or plan a trip to the store. In sharing the occupation, the parent made the task fun for the child and organized it to match the child's developmental level.

Two broad dimensions of parenting style are the *extent the adult works to nurture or support the child* and the *degree of control the parent exerts over the child* (Peterson & Leigh, 1990). Although parents most often feel warm and committed to their children, they may hold different ideas regarding which traits are important. Ecology of the family, as determined by the employed work experiences of one or more parents, can overflow and influence parenting behaviors. Parents come to understand what it takes to "make it" at work, and they want to enhance these characteristics in their children (Luster, Rhodes, & Haas, 1989). Parents with less education and less-skilled jobs are thought to value traits that will help their children follow directions and work cooperatively with a team. For these parents, obedience and good manners in their children are important. For parents with white-collar jobs, career success requires more problem-solving and independent work. As a result these parents tend to have goals that encourage self-direction and curiosity, and they select play experiences accordingly.

■ WHAT DOES IT MEAN TO HAVE A CHILD WITH A DISABILITY?

As explained in the discussion of the family as a system, any significant family event that influences the occupational performance of one member affects all family members. It is important to acknowledge that a child's disability does not imply a deficit in the family. However, differences in the child elicit family members' accommodations.

In review of a longitudinal study of families who were raising children with special needs, Bernheimer and Keogh (1995) concluded: "The majority of our families are doing quite well. Like the children in our study, they share common characteristics but are strikingly unique in many ways. They are adapting and adjusting within their physical and cultural environments, and are making decisions about the organization of their lives and about their children, consistent with their values and beliefs and with what they think is important" (p. 429).

As a place to gain insight into some of the issues and choices that families make, this section first discusses family subsystems; then considers family functions.

Parent-Child Subsystem

The impact of a child with special needs on a family will vary according to (1) the age and abilities of the child, (2) the meaning that the particular impairment or disability has to the family, (3) the adult's motivation and skill in dealing with the child's disability, (4) the meaning the adult brings to occupations associated with parenting.

In describing optimal parenting, scholars have examined parent-child interactions and identified *involvement* and *responsivity* as important features (Mahoney, Boyce, Fewell, Spiker, & Wheeden, 1998). In addition to interacting with the child, the parent is extremely important in managing the organization of the child's occupations during the day (Park, 1995). For the parent of a child with special needs, managing occupa-

tions may assume additional dimensions (e.g., accessing educational programs, maintaining health, promoting developmentally enriching experiences).

Studies have found that additional time in caregiving co-occupations is required in *mother-child* subsystems in which the child has a disability (Brotherson & Goldstein, 1992; Crowe, 1993). The type of disability the child has and its severity determines the amount of time required. Disabilities that seem to create more stress and time for the family include autism, severe and multiple disabilities, behavior disorders, and medical problems that require frequent hospitalization and in-home medical care. Considering the demands, it is not surprising that mothers of children with special needs sometimes report less sense of parental satisfaction and competence (Hombeck et. al., 1997).

The mother, who is typically the primary parent working with the intervention team, faces greater demands on time and communication skills (Lawlor & Mattingly, 1998). She often becomes the conduit for communication, trying to transfer information and expectations between clinic and family. Therefore mothers must be sensitive to the perspectives of both the professionals and family members.

Regardless of whether the father lives in or out of the home, the *father-child* subsystem warrants consideration. Scholars have come to recognize the multidimensional process influencing what fathers do and why they do it (Park, 1995). They also have noted that fathers are more sensitive than mothers to the influence of the ecology of the family and the attitude of others. Systematic barriers to greater paternal responsivity include the fact that, if a marriage ends, women are granted custody more often than men. In addition, in a nuclear family, time at work is often greater for men than women. Young and Roopnarine (1994) found that fathers spend about one third the time caring for the children when compared with mothers. Father-child occupations and co-occupations also vary.

May (1990) and Sparling, Berger, and Biller (1992) identified typical differences in the roles of mothers and fathers:

1. A father may be more concerned with the child's relationship to the external world and the social stigma that may result from a disability.

2. A father may be more concerned with physical appearance.

3. A father may have fewer ways to interact with a child whose physical or mental delays limit ability to participate in recreational activities, such as sports. Interaction may be most limited when the child is a boy and has a physical disability.

4. A mother may have additional demands on her role as caregiver for a child who continues to require assistance in feeding, bathing, and dressing.

5. A mother may feel needed and competent and gain more satisfaction from her role as caregiver.

6. A father's employment may support his adaptation. Employment offers the father a chance to "get away" and to distance himself from the strain of childcare.

These statements do not apply to all families. Mothers have described the positive roles that they perceive their husbands to have: "I always think that [my child] likes [his father] more than he likes me because I have to do all the things that he doesn't like . . . make him take a bath . . . and when [his father] comes home his savior has arrived. Dad takes over in the evening and allows me to cook dinner and take care of the house" (Nastro, 1992, p. 43).

The occupational therapist who recognizes the power of social capital wants to support involvement of all adults. In general, fathers appear not to be always included in intervention programs. One father reported a recurring situation when his son's teachers and therapists telephoned his home: "Whenever they call about Tim, they immediately ask for my wife. Why don't the therapists want to talk with me? Do they feel I will not understand the information? Will I not answer their questions? Do they think that I don't care to learn about what is happening at school? I used to feel hurt and hand the phone to my wife, but now I reply that if they have information or a question about Tim they can talk with

me" (Ballard, 1991, personal communication, August 12, 1991).

Ninio and Rinott (1988) recommended a number of strategies for encouraging the father's participation. Programs that seem to best support the father's involvement include the following components:

1. Involve the father in program planning.
2. Offer convenient scheduling (e.g., evenings, Saturdays).
3. Focus on providing information about the disability and community resources.
4. Provide opportunities for the father to enjoy activities with his child.

Meyer developed a model for father support groups (Meyer, Vadasy, & Fewell, 1986). The programs were based on the support, education, and involvement of fathers. Support was generated from their peers, other men in similar situations. Discussion revolved around common joys and concerns, the impact of the disability on the family, and the changing role of the father in society. The educational components included information about the nature of the child's disability, resources and materials available, and medical and educational systems. Fathers also learned positive ways to interact with their children and effective strategies for advocating for their children (Figures 5-2 and 5-3).

Sparling and others (1992) explained the importance of involving the father if he is the family's primary decision maker and will decide how the family's resources are spent. For the father to support ongoing therapy, new equipment, and other resources for the child, he must thoroughly understand all the benefits and advantages of treatment. Fathers need ongoing information to understand the course of intervention and to participate in decision making. When many options for fathers' involvement are presented, their ongoing involvement is more likely.

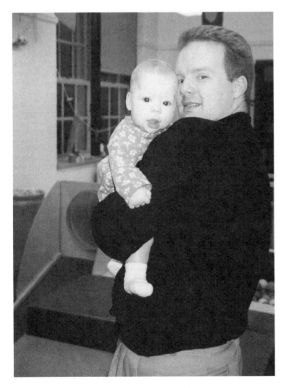

figure5-2   Father enjoys holding his child when his family attends an early intervention program in the evening.

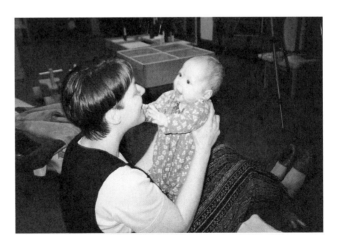

figure5-3   Mother and infant enjoy face-to-face play. Sound play and touches add to their delight.

Parent Subsystem

Regardless of the type of family structure (e.g., traditional, nontraditional, blended, or extended), adults sharing parental duties need to coordinate childcare efforts. These adults form the *parent subsystem* of the family, which can be a positive force and contribute to the child's ability to face developmental challenges. In original research on family systems, marital dysfunction was assumed to be a consequence of having a child with a disability. Today researchers find a number of different solutions in how parents distribute childcare, realizing that the different forms may all be adaptive if they enable the system to operate and meet family functions (Hombeck et. al., 1997; Weiss, Marvin, & Pianta, 1997). Similar levels of marital satisfaction are found in traditional families in which the mother stays home and provides all the care, families where the parents act as a team and evenly distribute tasks, and other families where extended family members are actively involved in care.

Sibling Subsystem

Living with a child with special needs affects siblings in different ways. The factors that contribute to the *sibling subsystem* include the severity of the disability, the ages and birth order of the children, and the family's attitude toward the disability. When interviewing families of children with behavioral disorders, Turnbull and Ruef (1997) found that sibling relationships were frequently negative and worrisome to the parents. Parents revealed that siblings expressed frustration about having property destroyed, embarrassment about problem behaviors in public, and resentment about the amount of time and attention required for the sibling with problem behaviors. In comparison, a comprehensive study of college-age siblings indicated that more than one half believed they had benefited from having a brother or sister with special needs. Grossman (1972) and Meyer (1993) reported that benefits perceived by siblings included (1) increased understanding of others, (2) heightened tolerance and compassion, and (3) greater appreciation of health and ability.

Comments made by siblings show the importance of growing up with a brother or sister who has a disability:

"Stacy [my sister] has taught me to never judge people without understanding them first. A hasty judgment of Stacy does not reveal her acute perceptiveness. . . . As a result I hesitate to classify other people too quickly" (Levitt, 1988, p. 5).

"My experience with my sister has been one of the most important in my life . . . it has definitely shaped my life and channeled my interests" (Itzkowitz, 1990, p. 4).

Parents have indicated that siblings, particularly older siblings, are of great help in managing childcare and the extra needs of the child with a disability. Siblings usually take on the extra responsibility willingly. Older sisters are most often expected to take responsibility for the sibling with special needs (Cleveland & Miller, 1977). Siblings are often willing to help with caregiving or teaching while living with their family of origin, but they express concern and anxiety about future responsibilities they may have for their disabled brother or sister.

The needs and importance of siblings can be addressed in intervention programs. Many centers and some schools run sibling workshops. These vary in format from educational, informational workshops to sibling support groups (Meyer, 1993). The workshops are typically designed to help siblings learn more about the disabilities, how to handle situations that may occur with their siblings, and ways to be helpful to their siblings. In peer support groups, siblings meet in a relaxed and recreational atmosphere. These groups generally have open-ended discussions about what it means to have siblings with disabilities. When possible, siblings should be involved in occupational therapy sessions. They are likely to be the best playmates and can often elicit maximum effort from their brother or sister. In addition, sibling involvement gives the therapeutic activity additional meaning (play), and siblings can act as models to teach new skills and provide needed support in a natural context (e.g., help the special-needs child with a puzzle or game).

Extended Family

In the extended family the meaning and experience of having a child with special needs depends on the meaning family members bring to their relationship with the child. For some *grandparents,* grandchildren represent a link to the future and opportunity for vicarious achievement. Researchers find that when children have disabilities, grandparents express both positive and negative feelings and go through a series of adjustments similar to those of the parents (Schimoeller & Baranowski, 1998). Many of the negative feelings, such as anger and confusion, appear to decrease with time. However, some never completely disappear. Positive feelings, such as acceptance and a sense of usefulness, increase over time. A grandparent's educational level and sense of closeness to the child are positively associated with greater involvement with the child. Factors, such as the grandparent's age, the grandparent's health, and how far away the grandparent lives from the child, do not appear to influence involvement. Grandparents learn information about their grandchild's condition primarily through the child's parents. However, some seek information from other sources, such as support groups for grandparents of special-needs children. As part of the extended family, grandparents can provide significant social capital and should be welcomed to therapy sessions.

Patterson, Garwick, Bennett, and Blum (1997) interviewed parents of children with chronic conditions about the behavior of extended family members. Family members, such as grandparents, uncles, and aunts of the child, were especially important to fathers and mothers for emotional and practical assistance. When extended family members were not supportive, parents expressed frustration and hurt by their lack of contact. In addition, parents recalled examples of when family members made insensitive comments about the child, ignored the child, or did not want to talk about the child's disability. Parents of children with behavioral problems reported that extended family members tended to blame the child's actions on the parents' inability to discipline correctly (Turnbull & Ruef, 1997).

Because members of the extended family can provide important social support, it is important to include them in the intervention process. With the consent of the parents, occupational therapists can encourage extended family members to become more involved by offering to share information with them and inviting them to intervention sessions.

■ INFLUENCE OF A CHILD WITH SPECIAL NEEDS ON FAMILY FUNCTIONS

Understanding how families operate to fulfill their functions is critical, because families of special-needs children have much in common with families of typically developing children. Patching and Watson (1993) pointed out that at some time, most families can benefit from support, and families with children who have special needs are no different. However, families who have a child with a disability must also assume extra tasks and responsibilities, such as finding and accessing medical and educational services.

With increased and varied responsibilities, the family's functions shift to meet the child's specific developmental needs. Priorities shift and solutions to everyday problems may differ from typical families. For example, the logistics of a trip to the grocery store becomes more complicated when a child with autism or a child that requires a wheelchair or a ventilator accompanies the parent.

With finite social and financial capital, a family's emphasis on one function can take resources from other functions. In certain cases, the family's resources of time, money, and physical and emotional energy may be directed primarily to the needs of the child with a chronic condition. For example, a mother who has a full-time job to help pay bills (economic and productive functions) and spends 4 hours a day feeding her severely disabled child (socialization and health functions) has limited time remaining to plan special family recreation. Children who need 2 hours of extra help each night on their homework (education function) have families with less time committed for socialization. Brotherson and Goldstein (1992) discussed how, in families with disabled children, choices about family resources committed to daily function appear to be controlled externally by people, institutions, and events that impose expectations and requirements on the family. Therefore it is not just the needs of the child that may have a special influence on family functions; it is also the implied demands from external sources.

Economic Acquisition and Allocation Function

The child with special needs usually has a direct impact on family economics. First, expenditures can increase because the child requires additional medical care, therapy, and equipment. Second, one parent may choose to stay home to provide extra caregiving, thereby reducing income. Mothers may decide they cannot manage full-time employment and have time for therapy visits, pediatrician appointments, and educational programming (Gallimore, Weisner, Bernheimer, Guthrie, & Nihira, 1993).

Parents with children with disabilities also have many hidden and ongoing expenses (Patterson, 1993). In a study of how parents spend their time, mothers of children with Down syndrome worked significantly fewer paid hours than mothers of children without disabilities. As a result, the mothers of children with Down syndrome had reduced earning capacity (Barnett & Boyce, 1995). When children are hospitalized, many expenses (e.g., childcare for siblings, transportation, meals, motel rooms) are incurred in addition to costs not covered by insurance. Children who require extensive medical treatment can bring economic devastation to a family, especially when their insurance coverage is inadequate (Kirk, 1998).

Although financial problems create added stress, therapists are often reluctant to discuss finances, especially costs associated with their own services. In a sample of mothers of children with CP, Nastro (1992) found that insurance coverage was inadequate to meet their needs. One mother reported her experiences: ". . . each piece of equipment has a big price tag. Even the smallest piece has a couple hundred dollar price tag . . . most insurance companies do not cover it. Medicaid does not cover everything" (p. 52).

Another mother explained how her family managed: "The insurance covers 15 OT [occupational therapy] visits, 15 PT [physical therapy] visits, and 15 speech each year, so we pay for Martin's therapy ourselves. We took out a home equity loan to pay for it . . . There isn't anything free if you have a middle income status. Insurance would not pay for Pedisure, which is $35 a case . . . We did access respite services" (p. 52).

Another mother reported that therapy cost $11,000 for her twins with CP in the first year. This mother also explained that she and her husband took vacation time and leave without pay during periods that their children were in the hospital for surgical procedures and illnesses (Nastro, 1992).

Developing Independence in Self-Care and Health-Maintenance Function

Children with disabilities often are dependent on caregivers longer than typically developing children and can have extra daily care needs that extend for many years. The amount of time spent in co-occupations around caregiving can be wearing and frustrating, and it can reduce the family's time for recreation and social gatherings. The mother who spends hours feeding a child with severe oral-motor problems has less time to spend with her other children, less energy to give to her husband, and may experience less satisfaction with the productivity of her occupation as the child changes slowly to acquire self-feeding independence. When a child needs range of motion, which is included in bathing routines, an enjoyable task may assume a more worklike meaning. In a study of over 200 families of children with Down syndrome, mothers spent three times as much time in childcare than the mothers of typically developing children. In addition, the fathers of children with Down syndrome spent twice as much time in childcare as fathers of typically developing children (Barnett & Boyce, 1995). When parents spend most of their day caring for their children's needs, they sometimes overlook their own needs.

Occupational therapists who understand the nature of co-occupations can help parents manage and adapt daily living tasks with their children. The therapist asks first about daily routines and tasks that seem the most difficult. Then the therapist asks the parent where help is needed. After observing the parent feeding or dressing the child, the occupational therapist engages the parent in a discussion of alternatives that help the child perform daily living activities with greater skill and independence (Figure 5-4). With knowledge of the biomechanics of lifting and moving, the therapist considers whether the task is performed in a way that conserves energy and avoids injury. This consideration is especially important when a physical impairment significantly limits mobility. Strategies to help a 5-year-old bathe, dress, and use the toilet may no longer be safe for the parent's back when the child becomes an adolescent.

Routines that lead to more independence in self-care provide opportunities to enrich the child's learning. During dressing, the child can improve strength by pulling up pants and increase language by naming colors found on the clothing. Therapists can suggest how to turn tasks

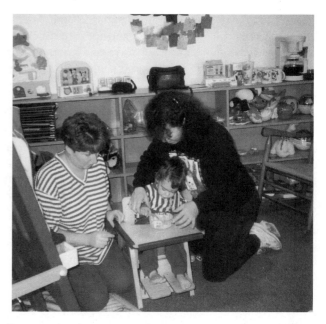

figure **5-4** Therapist gives the mother recommendations to increase the child's skills in self-feeding. Supportive-positioning equipment and adapted-feeding utensils make the task easier for the child and the mother.

into learning situations. As with all suggestions, the parent weighs the costs and benefits. Often, the occupational therapist hears, "That just won't work for us." When this happens, a number of different strategies are needed to reach the same goal.

Becoming independent in self-care occupations frequently requires repeated practice until performance becomes a habit. Occupational therapists who understand principles of behavior management can help parents reinforce a child's efforts at independence. Continuity in frequently repeated self-care occupations, such as using the toilet and eating with utensils, is increased through communication between the occupational therapist, teacher, parents, and others. A notebook that the child carries between school and home may serve this purpose.

Any extra time that the therapist asks the parent to spend teaching new steps in self-care should be in response to a parent's identified need. In addition, the effort should be justified by evidence that the altered routine has a good chance of bringing an immediate change. Alternative suggestions should be quickly made when an adapted technique does not work. The goal of occupational therapy recommendations should be to benefit the entire family by increasing the child's independence at minimal cost in time and energy to the parent. As stated by Bernheimer and Keogh (1995): "successful interventions are the ones that can be woven back into the daily routine; they are the threads that provide professionals with the means to reinforce, rather than fray, the fabric of everyday life" (p. 430).

Family Recreation and Leisure Function

Healthy families are able to relax and enjoy recreational activities together and create leisure opportunities that meet personal agenda. Shared recreational occupations form the basis for many family traditions, leading to a sense of family unity and identity. Through group recreation, a family also fulfills the function of socialization. Individual's play and leisure may not have the priority of other areas of function, such as development of members' potential for education and productivity skills. Therefore time for leisure activities is replaced by educational or therapeutic tasks. Diamond (1981) explained this need when he related the experiences he had as a young child:

> Something happens in a parent when relating to his disabled child: [she] forgets [he] is a kid first. I used to think about that a lot when I was a kid. I would be off in a euphoric state, drawing or coloring or cutting out paper dolls, and as often as not the activity would be turned into an occupational therapy session. "You're not holding the scissors right," or "sit up straight so your curvature doesn't get worse." The era was ended when I finally let loose a long and exhaustive tirade. "I'm just a kid! You can't therapize me all the time! I get enough therapy in school everyday! I don't think about my handicap all the time like you do" (p. 30).

Occupational therapists can communicate that they respect the value of recreation and leisure by including it in assessment and intervention plans. Therapists can suggest adapted equipment the child can use to make recreational activities possible. With the passage of the Americans with Disabilities Act (1990), more recreational opportunities are available to individuals with disabilities. Information about community recreational activities is often available in local newsletters. Therapists can note which activities are accessible and appropriate for children with disabilities. Scheduling therapy and education programs to enable families to engage in recreational activities can also support family function.

Socialization and Participation in Social Activities

Experiences in occupations within families are the foundation for socialization, which is a vital aspect of each family member's life. Socialization is not only needed for health, it is an important mechanism to prepare family members to enter their cultural group and participate in community activities. Frequently, parents organize the children's daily routines to encourage social interactions with peers, and they feel concern over whether the child will have friends. Although inclusive educational programs have increased children's social opportunities, peer relations can remain problematic. Children with disabilities engage in fewer social interactions and have less mature social behaviors than their peers without disabilities (Odom, McConnell, & McEvoy, 1992). Delayed social skills may relate to language or cognitive delays or to the negative attitudes of peers. Children with disabilities may be in more adult-directed situations, and they may lack social interaction skills when dealing with peers or siblings.

The presence of a disability in the child may also create barriers to the parents' opportunities to socialize. Families of special-needs children often feel that they have less time to spend participating in social activities. Because childcare is typically difficult to arrange and must be set up in advance, involvement in spontaneous social opportunities is rarely possible (Patterson & Blum, 1996). Children who act out or demonstrate disruptive behaviors may be particularly difficult to take into social situations. Patterson and others (1997) found that members of the parent's social network frequently did not know how to respond when they learned the parent's child had a chronic disability. Families reported that the attitudes and behaviors of people in the community were often a greater source of stress for the family than having a child with a chronic condition. Parents who experienced hurtful interactions with others eliminated those people from their social network. Unfortunately, a reduced social network also diminished the potential for social support from neighbors or friends. One parent described the changes she experienced in her circle of friends.

> Before Peter, we had many good friends in our neighborhood. I used to walk Peter in his stroller, however, each time we ran into neighbors they would ask how he was doing and ask if he was walking yet. I would always reply that he was doing well and that he wasn't walking yet. Then they were silent, like they did not know what to say next. I don't seem to have anything in common with my old friends now that I have Peter (NY, personal communication, April 11, 1992).

Parents should be encouraged to participate in social situations because they often develop new friendships with other parents who are experiencing similar circumstances. Vincent (1988) described the importance of an informal social support system:

> Parents are most likely to rely upon family members, friends, neighbors, or co-workers for support when confronting problems in raising their children. Social integration with the community and the informal supports of friends and neighbors are critical to the family's ability to cope. Only as a last resort do they consult professionals. The implication of this finding for us is that we need to focus more of our attention in helping families develop and strengthen their own support networks. We need to emphasize to families that they are the ones best able to solve their own problems (p. 4).

In summary, family members' connections with others are important to the child's development. Social-skill development is usually delayed in children with disabilities. Therefore opportunities to observe and to imitate family members socializing can be critical to acquiring and enhancing social interaction skills.

Affection and Emotional Support Functions

The family is the first place where a child experiences affection. Affection is the bond that creates and sustains the family (Figure 5-5). A child with a disability can have a positive or a negative effect on the family's expression of affection for each other. Often the child has a positive influence and draws the family members closer together.

The sister of Billy, who had Down syndrome, described her appreciation of her brother:

> Billy has a deep concern for the feelings of other people. He has a kind nature, and I cannot remember ever hearing a malicious word leave his mouth. When anyone in the family travels, Billy calls to be sure we arrived safely. And when someone has a problem, is ill, or has died, Billy's sincere sympathy is heartwarming (Schulz, 1993, p. 38).

Lori expressed her family's affection for her son with Apert's syndrome:

> I think Sean has enriched our family . . . even my extended family. He is a hero to them because of all the things he's had to deal with. And he has a sunny personality. He's sort of an example to the rest of us when we complain about little things. We've had fun watching him grow up . . . He's a gift. He seems larger than life (Riley, 1998, page 81).

Like other areas of function, expressing affection may become an issue when the child with a disability becomes an adolescent and is not able to understand or properly express sexual desires. When affection for peers of the opposite sex is not reciprocated or is not understood, self-esteem can be affected. The issues of expressing sexuality and affection among adolescents can be a difficult and challenging situation for the family. Once again, information on making this transition is needed. The therapist may suggest positive ways to express affection to peers.

Closely linked to shared affection is each member's sense of identity and self-esteem (Figure 5-6). In particular, siblings need to be helped to understand that they are *related to* but *separate from* their sibling with a disability. Siblings who assist in caring for the child with special needs may gain feelings of self-esteem from their role as a helper. When other children make unkind comments about the disability, the sibling should be given positive strategies for managing the situation. Turnbull and Turnbull (1990) suggested that all family members should develop self-identity (in areas other than the child's disability) by pursuing their own interests, hobbies, and personal goals. Patterson and Blum (1996) explained that when internal family boundaries are clear, all relationships benefit. One parent's intense involvement with a child can detract from the marital relationship. It can also harm the self-esteem and self-identity of the siblings.

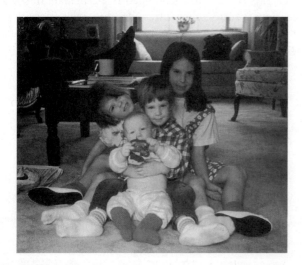

figure**5-5** Affection between siblings is an important family function.

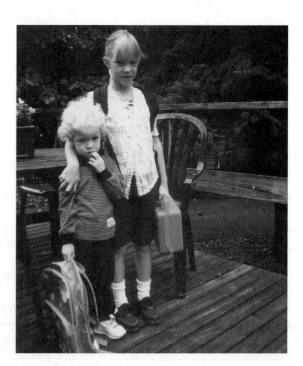

figure**5-6** Sister's first day of school.

Fostering Readiness to be a Student and Developing Vocational Potential

As part of its function to support development, family life must be sufficiently organized around enabling the child to move into educational and training opportunities in the community. When a child has a disability, educational and vocational activities (including occupational therapy as it relates to the educational program) can require more time and receive greater emphasis. Although parents and family members of children with disabilities express appreciation for the educational system, they also report being overwhelmed by the demands of the educational program (Brotherson & Goldstein, 1992). In addition to communicating with the regular teacher and working on supplemental school activities, parents of children receiving related services are asked to attend IEP meetings and communicate with teachers and therapists. The parent may believe that providing extra help and attention helps the child maintain the same pace of learning as classmates. The amount of homework and therapy performed in the evening can increase by small increments; then, suddenly, the parents realize that every evening is spent in therapy or working on school-related tasks.

Both parents and therapists need to strive toward balancing educational activities with other family functions. Parents should always be given choices regarding their level of participation (Gartner, Lipsky, & Turnbull, 1990; McBride, Brotherson, Joanning, Whiddon, & Dermitt, 1993). A balance of activities (e.g., recreational, social, educational, daily care) helps the family maintain their equilibrium and should remain a priority of the intervention team (Turnbull & Winton, 1984).

As children with disabilities reach preadolescence, the number of accommodations made by their families increase. However, most parents report no increase in the stress and effort of adapting their lives and the environment. Apparently, making accommodations has become integrated into their lifestyle (Gallimore, Coots, Weisner, Garnier, & Guthrie, 1996). However, the educational system can put up roadblocks, and the family may still have to push for inclusion and advocate for services.

■ FAMILY LIFE CYCLE

As discussed earlier, family systems undergo metamorphosis and adapt as family members change. Some transitions can be anticipated with developing children and seem to be tied to age more than ability. For example, *normative events* in children that require adjustments in families include the birth of a child, starting kindergarten, transitions between schools, leaving high school, and living outside the home. Other changes in the family are not anticipated. *Non-normative events* may include a grandparent coming to live with the family or a parent accepting a different job in another city. Families that are cohesive and adaptable adjust interactive routines, reorganize occupational patterns, and return to homeostasis. If interactive routines and role designation are too rigidly set, the family may not be able to operate effectively through periods of transition. This is especially true if the family experiences unanticipated, threatening events, such as a job loss or a medical crisis. All families use coping strategies to accommodate periods of transition. (Some of these coping strategies are described in the next section.)

The normative family life stages have particular meaning for families who have children with disabilities. Parents have told their stories of experiences throughout the life cycle (Turnbull & Turnbull, 1985; Turnbull & Turnbull, 1990). An understanding of the entire family life cycle helps a therapist recognize that the family's roles will change across all developmental stages. For many parents of children with disabilities, the role of caregiving will continue through adulthood. Lawlor and Mattingly (1998) found that families express frustration that therapists do not engage them in anticipatory planning. Parents want to understand that they have reason to expect their disabled child will have a place in society and an opportunity to engage in socially valued occupations throughout adulthood.

Another advantage in understanding the family life cycle is recognizing that families can experience greater challenges during the transitions between stages than during any one stage where homeostasis of family routines occurs. When the child begins a new program or undergoes a rapid physiologic change (e.g., puberty), demands on the family's adaptations increase. The family's time and energy are needed to refocus and move through these transitions.

Occupational therapists must also understand that all families are unique. Although life-cycle models consist of predictable events, the individuality of each family is acknowledged. The characteristics and issues at each life stage are highly variable, and each family moves through the stages at different rates. For example, a family may experience and resolve their feelings when they first learn about their child's diagnosis. However, the family will also experience cycles of sadness and acceptance later, within and between life stages. Issues that the family seemed to resolve when the child was an infant may occur again when the child reaches school age and an "educational diagnosis" is made or a learning problem is identified. Other stage-related events, such as the child's ability to develop friendships when first entering grade school, may become an issue again when the child enters high school.

Finally, the nature of the family structure can result in different members of the family being at different stages at the same time. Therefore characteristics of the family members and the child's phase of development must be considered. For example, in a skipped-generation family, grandparents frequently have to deal with changes associated with old age at the same time they are parenting their grandchildren. In other families, parents may be taking care of their elderly parents in addition to caring for a child with special needs. Similarly, a young couple may have more energy and resources to cope with the birth of a child with special needs than an older couple with four other children participating in school activities; consequently, regular attendance in an early intervention program is problematic for the older couple.

Turnbull and Turnbull (1990) described the tasks that families undertake at key stages of the life cycle. Although each stage emphasizes different activities, precise distinctions between stages cannot be made because developmental events occur at different times. Families from different cultures may experience different life cycles that may include longer periods of dependency and may not consider allowing the child to live apart from the family of origin. Therefore the following brief descriptions of developmental stages are general and not proven, but they give occupational therapists a framework for exploring where and how family members view the life cycle.

Early Childhood

After a child is born, the first task of any family is loving and nurturing the child (Figure 5-7). The new child generally brings great joy and results in pulling family members together around their new responsibility (Figure 5-8). Many times families of infants are not immediately aware that the child has special needs (Rolland, 1987). Frequently, families can recall a period of uncertainty when they were aware something was different, but they could not identify the problem. After receiving a diagnosis and seeking a period of stability, the family may not immediately seek early intervention services (Calhoun, Calhoun, & Rose, 1989). Instead, the family may pull together to be with the infant and support each other (Rolland, 1987). Once they feel stable, the family is usually ready to find help for its newest member.

When a child's impairment or disability is identified, families usually begin gathering information about the diagnosis. Gathering information about the child's disability helps them take control of the situation and learn how to help their child develop (Gowen, Christy, & Sparling, 1993). Sometimes their search for more information leads the parents to pursue further testing and to visit numerous "experts" and specialists. These parents often have minimal prior knowledge of early intervention programs and their alternatives. To negotiate early childhood systems successfully, parents must learn about legal

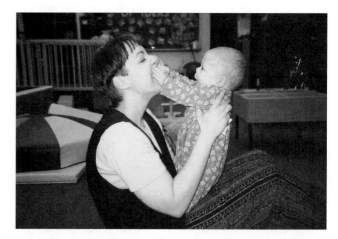

figure**5-7** Mother-infant affection.

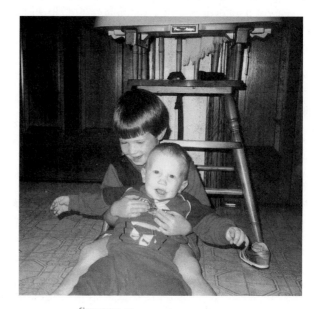

figure**5-8** Brotherly affection.

issues, parental rights, local programs, community resources, and therapy and educational services.

When parents participate in early childhood programs, they can assume new roles (e.g., coordinating services, helping with therapy and education, advocating the rights of special-needs children). Research has found that mothers of young children with disabilities can be directive and controlling when interacting with their children, often focused on teaching discrete skills (Hanzlik, 1990; Mahoney, Finger, & Powell, 1985). By helping parents prioritize natural play interactions over structured teaching sessions, occupational therapists can allow parents to relax and enjoy their young children.

Parents often seek as much information as possible about the disease and what they can expect for the child's future. Sometimes parents of young children ask questions such as: "Do you think he can go into a regular class-room?" "Do you think he will be able to live on his own some day?" Thoughtful responses to these questions recognize the parents' need for optimism and hope. However, they must be honest and realistic. Even therapists with years of experience and extensive knowledge about disability and development cannot make definitive statements about the future. Long-range predictions about when the child will achieve a certain milestone or level of independence are always speculative. However, parents experience frustration when told that the future cannot be predicted. Therapists can help parents understand the range of possibilities by telling them about the continuum of services for older children and young adults in the community. Talking with parents of older children with a similar condition or hearing the therapist's story of a child with the same characteristics provides some insight into the future. Even without knowing the child's developmental course, parents start to develop an understanding that services are in place, and they begin to create new stories about their child's future.

Sometimes the parents' questions about the future reflect their desire to express and discuss their anxiety. The occupational therapist may ask the parents about concerns, dreams, and hopes for the future, emphasizing the importance of sharing this information. Parents should also be encouraged to share their vision with other professionals who work with the child. As one parent expressed, "The greatest anxiety for parents of handicapped children is uncertainty of the future. The services established for [our children] have only been stopgaps. With the exception of rare, lifelong institutional placements, we don't have plans for the future" (Schulz, 1985, p. 17).

Armed with information about the system, their rights, and the resources available to them in their communities, parents can solve problems and independently access needed services. The caregiving routines of parents whose young child has a disability are not particularly different from those of all parents of young children. At this time in the child's life, the parent's work consists of managing the child's play environment and introducing new, developmentally appropriate objects and materials. The parent ensures safety and may adjust or arrange the play environment so that the infant can access objects of interest. Feeding, diapering, bathing, and daily care are also natural parenting activities at this time. Only when infants and young children have serious medical conditions or behavioral problems are daily occupations significantly altered.

When children are medically unstable but still at home, a family may have home-based nursing for extended periods (i.e., months to several years). Murphy (1997) described the stress when nurses and professional care providers are constantly present in the home. Role ambiguity often results when parents feel that they must take on unpaid nursing work and nurses take on parenting roles. Parents also report stress from a lack of privacy and the continual feeling that they are "on duty." Parents of medically fragile children must make tremendous accommodations and should elicit high levels of sensitivity and responsiveness from professionals. For example, when parents have a medically unstable infant and around-the-clock, in-home nursing care, services such as respite become a priority.

School Age

When the child enters school, the typical family is excited about the new opportunities for learning and the child's new demonstration of independence. However, school entry is not always a positive event for families of children with disabilities. Families who experienced early intervention services may be disappointed to find fewer family services and less family support offered by the school. Typically, parents are not encouraged to attend classes or school-based therapy sessions. Many parents view the transition to school as an opportunity to be less involved and a sign of their child's maturation. To ease the transition from home to school, the parents of special-needs children should learn about the school's programs, schedules, rules, and policies.

For children with mild learning disabilities, entry into school may be the first time that the gap between the child's abilities and expected occupational performance is identified. Therefore this may also be the first time parents with children who have not previously been identified as having special needs receive that information. When this is the case, parents will experience the same reactions and issues that the parents of children who were already identified as having special needs faced earlier in their children's lives.

To the school-age child, making friends and maintaining friendships become critically important. Some parents report concern if their children appear lonely, isolated, and friendless. Turnbull and Ruef (1997) found that children with behavioral problems have no friends, leaving the parents with the additional responsibility of creating and supervising play opportunities with other children. Teachers and therapists can use different strategies to promote friendships in inclusive environments. Typically developing peers can take turns being the child's "specially buddy," and they can offer assistance with projects or tutoring. In situations where social stigma is an issue, peer relations can be promoted by explaining the disability to the other children and by designing classroom activities that promote cooperation and positive interaction.

Inclusive models of education seem to have successfully increased social opportunities for children with disabilities and, by extension, their ability to enjoy friendships (Odom & Brown, 1993; Odom & McEvoy, 1988).

Increased accessibility to playgrounds, theaters, and children's recreation areas promotes more opportunities for friends to participate in community activities. However, this is not always true if the child lives outside of an urban area. "Because we live in a rural area, there are few social activities designed for handicapped people. . . . As a result, Billy has learned to enjoy his own company and the solitude of his home" (Schulz, 1985, p. 17).

Adolescence

Adolescence is a challenging and potentially stressful time for all families. Several issues emerge in the lives of children with disabilities when they reach adolescence. Parents may need to prepare the young person to handle his or her growing sexual needs. In certain cases parents face decisions about their child's use of birth control and protection from sexually transmitted diseases. With adolescence, new concerns about a son or daughter's vulnerability increase.

Although the child usually is well-accepted by family members, the social stigma with peers and others may increase during adolescence. As one mother expressed, "The community accepts our children much more easily when they are small and cute. Babyish mannerisms are no longer acceptable. . . . [Our son] has had real problems with his social relationships. He simply does not know how to initiate a friendship. He has difficulty maintaining a sensible conversation with his peers. He doesn't handle teasing well, so he is teased unmercifully" (Anderson, 1983, p. 90).

The cute child with unusual behaviors may become a not-so-cute adolescent with socially unacceptable behaviors. As one parent explains why her son was not invited to a Christmas party, "Everyone in the family was invited except Billy. I thought it must be an oversight, but the friend later explained apologetically, 'I thought Billy's presence might make the other guests uncomfortable.' This kind of attitude is difficult to accept, particularly when he had been included very successfully in a similar party. I find myself crying at the unfairness" (Schulz, 1985, p. 16).

Others have expressed difficulty in caring for their child's growing physical needs. As the child reaches adulthood, parents who are reaching middle age may feel their strength and energy decline.

> The sapping of energy occurs gradually. The isolation it imposes does too. As I work professionally with young mothers, I see them coping energetically with the demands of everyday life. They are good parents, caring ones, doing everything possible to help their retarded child reach full potential, sometimes doing more than they have to; and if they have other children, they are doing the same for them. Most of these mothers even get out, see friends, attend meetings, volunteer in the community, and do all the things their friends and families

expect them to do. All this is at least possible when one's child is little, though it demands enormous energy. But to look at the mothers of children who have turned into teenagers is to see the beginnings of the ravages. Their lifestyle is changing. They go out less, see fewer people, do less for their children. They are stripping their living to the essentials (Morton, 1985, p. 144).

The parents of a young person with a severe disability may face the possibility of institutionalization of their child for the first time, as they begin to wonder whether they can continue to provide the necessary care for their adolescent. Schulz (1993) wrote:

> There are serious issues in the future. There is the age-old question of who will care for him if something happens to me. We have planned the best we can; we have provided for Billy financially; he has skills that with supervision, should enable him to continue his contented life. But who will supervise him? Who will provide his transportation? What if he loses his job? Who will be his aggressive, persistent advocate? I find myself thinking, as many parents of persons with disabilities have thought before me, that it would be easier if I outlive him. These are issues that we can't laugh about, or shrug off (pp. 38-39).

■ FAMILY ADAPTATION AND COPING

An important philosophic shift has occurred in the last decades in how families of children with special needs are viewed by professionals. The original assumption that the presence of a disabled member led to family dysfunction and a life of recurring sorrow has been replaced with more neutral descriptions of the adjustment process (Helff & Glidden, 1998). Parents of children with special needs explained that their children bring growth-producing challenges, a sense of pride, fulfillment, and joy to their families (Stallings & Cook, 1997; Turnbull, et. al., 1988). The strength and resilience of many families to meet life events and achieve a level of happiness and life satisfaction can be a source of inspiration to occupational therapists.

The fact that most families successfully adjust to children's disabilities should not lead occupational therapists to ignore the initial and ongoing challenges that families face. Times of coping and adaptation vary according to whether one discusses adjustment to an acute traumatic event leading to a disability or one develops a gradual, unfolding understanding of the child's developmental differences. After the diagnostic period, when the child's problems are identified, the family goes about the process of living. During this period there are varying demands for adaptation and coping. When viewing the family as a dynamic system within its unique sociocultural niche, it is not a surprise that one model does not completely explain how the family of a child with special needs adapts to normative and non-normative events. In the following sections, two models with different perspectives are examined.

Stages-of-Adjustment Model

A model of family adjustment serves as a guide to understand how adults respond, especially when confronted with an unanticipated illness or accident that threatens a child. In this approach, the responses of families' are described as "stages" of adjustment (Rape, Bush, & Slavin, 1992). Typically, there are four stages: (1) initial shock, (2) relief and denial, (3) working through it, and (4) getting on with the business of living.

Initial shock

When family members first learn that their child has a problem, they may experience *initial shock*. In the case of injury or sudden illness, this stage may have a sudden onset in which the child's life is threatened and the family feels immediate confusion, anger, and concern. In other cases, children's developmental disabilities are frequently not identified at birth, and there may be a prediagnostic period where, over months or years, the parents grow concerned that something is wrong. The diagnostic period (and sense of shock and uncertainty) may last months, while a variety of tests are completed. Families may be told that a final diagnosis may take many months of waiting and watching to understand how the symptoms unfold. When conflicting information is given about the diagnosis, the family's anger and disorganization heighten.

Relief and denial

The second stage includes a sense of *relief* that the uncertainty is over and *denial* that the family member is as disabled as professionals have suggested. For children with acquired injury or disabling illness, the family may anticipate things will return to normal. Families may hope that therapy will help their child "catch-up," and they may make a concentrated effort to focus family resources on developing educational readiness. During this period of adjustment, family members may surprise professionals with what appears to be unrealistic expectations for the child's future. For example, after a severe, closed head injury to a child, the parent may talk about a time in the future when the son learns to drive or when he leaves for college. Therapists realize a family's expression of highly optimistic expectations does not mean that the parents do not accept the diagnosis: the high expectations reflect the family's need for hope. An image of a different future for their child gradually crystallizes as the family moves into the next phase and acknowledges that the child has health problems or developmental challenges. When a young child has problems but no visible sign of a disability, parents may anticipate a life like every other child, with entry into regular educational programs

(Kraus-Mars & Lachman, 1994). In this case, families may find excuses (e.g., "He is just lazy," or "His teacher does not explain things the right way,") to explain why the child does not do well.

Working through it

The next stage of adjustment is described as one of *"working through it."* This is a process of giving up the image of the child as healthy and like all other children and developing a new image of the child's future abilities. It is not clear that all families experience the sorrow and mourning process (Rape et. al., 1992). The lack of a mourning period may be especially true when the child has been born with the disability, so the parents know very early that their child will be different. Parents of children with congenital conditions (e.g., mental retardation [MR]) appear less likely than parents of children with unexpected physical injuries (e.g., closed head injuries) to express regret about the child's condition (Batten & Cutler, 1990).

Getting on with the business of living

The final phase of adjustment is one of acceptance and *"getting on with the business of living"* (Rape et. al., 1992; Rolland, 1987). All families experience a process of reorganization when a new member joins the family. Therefore when a child has been born with a disabling condition, the reorganization may be integrated with the typically occurring developmental transition of the family. Actual restructuring of the family may occur only when the child's disabilities are caused by an accident or illness experienced after infancy. A family focused on the process of raising a special-needs child often comes to realize that the child is not that different from other children in the neighborhood.

Describing family adjustment as having stages has several limitations. First, many of the stages are based on clinical observation and become shared theories among professionals. However, the stages have not been confirmed through research (Rape et. al., 1992). A second limitation is that not all families go through all the stages, and some families adapt better than others. A third limitation concerns the fact that the stages cannot be thought of as a set developmental process, because anticipated and unanticipated events may cause a family to return to previous stages. For example, anticipated events, such as a child's birthday or entrance into school, may cause the parent to experience feelings of grief from an earlier stage. Parents may also experience grief and adjustment at unexpected times for reasons not apparent to the professional. For example, when the neighbor's child first walks or learns to ride a bike. A fourth limitation is that individual family members may be at different stages at the same time. For example, when both parents attend a support group, one parent may refuse to participate in discussions about the child, while the other actively participates in group discussions.

Family Coping and Adaptation Model

When a child has special needs, it can be more effective to frame the ongoing accommodations required in light of the family's strengths, resources, and coping strategies (Bernheimer & Keogh, 1995; Judge, 1998). Over time, all families have to adjust to life events and will experience varying degrees of stress. Although stressful events (e.g., the birth of a second child, a family member starting a first job) occur in many households, other events may be unique to families with special-needs children (e.g., placing the child in a special school, planning guardianship of a young adult).

The stresses and demands that families experience can be very wearing over time. Singer and Yovanoff (as cited in Patterson & Blum, 1996) reported that parents of children with disabilities are twice as likely to report depression; compared with parents of children without disabilities. Although some families show increased risk for psychosocial problems, other families adapt to the added demands of the child's disability without apparent effect on family function. Certain families seem to become stronger and increase their ability to function as a family. The differences in family adaptation seem to be primarily related to coping style and coping effectiveness.

Coping strategies are essential to every family's ability to deal with stress, trauma, and change. A variety of coping strategies have been identified in the literature, including active problem solving, seeking social supports, positive reframing, turning to religion, and denial. Parents effectively use problem-solving strategies by (1) actively seeking information; (2) energetically working to solve problems; (3) communicating their feelings; and (4) balancing personal, family, and illness needs.

Other parents express the need for emotional support in addition to, or more than, these problem-solving strategies. These parents actively seek support from friends and extended family, or they may turn to their faith or religion. Parents have voiced that emotional support is as important as instrumental and informational support, and therapists and professionals should openly acknowledge its value. Denial may also be viewed as a coping strategy that many parents use from time to time. As expressed in the parent's story at the end of this chapter, denial can provide a valuable temporary reprieve, during which parents gain the energy that they need to fight the battles that they will face (e.g., finding educational services most appropriate for their child).

Hill (1958) proposed a model that has become a classic way of framing the family coping and adaptation process. He recognized that the extent to which an event disrupts a family and creates a crisis depends on several interacting elements. Using the Hill model, the occupational therapist recognizes sources of individual differences in a family's unique sociocultural niche and resources it will use to enact different coping strategies. Table 5-1 applies the ABC = X Family Crisis Model to a family dealing with the potential crisis of losing services when an adolescent with special needs graduates from high school.

A family attempts to adjust to the demands of the event while maintaining homeostasis. The family works to restore homeostasis by doing one or more of the following: (1) getting more resources and learning new skills, (2) reducing the number of demands, or (3) redefining the situation problem or making emotional adjustments (Lazarrus & Folkman, 1984; Patterson, 1988). The occupational therapist supports the family in their adaptation process (see Table 5-1). The therapist may

table 5-1	Interactive Elements: How a Family Adjusts to a Critical Event (X) in Their Child's Life
ELEMENT OF THE MODEL	**EXAMPLE**
Stress event (A)	Son will graduate from high school next month but has not yet achieved the skills needed for employment and community travel.
	Family is notified that their son will not be eligible for services through the schools.
Family's resources for meeting the crisis (B)	Formal resources for meeting the crisis may be the school's team, which has identified the skills the adolescent needs to learn, and an appropriate job in the community.
	Informal resources for meeting the crisis may include friends who have had a daughter graduate from the high school's special education program 2 years earlier.
	Family resources include time and role flexibility, so all members of the family work together to practice community living.
Meaning the family makes of the event (C)	Family worries that their son is not ready to graduate. They recognize that additional resources are needed to prepare him. They identify that their son has perseverance and has taken risks in the past.
Family adapts to the stressful event (X)	Family contacts a social services agency to obtain a part-time coach for their son.

first address resources by providing additional information or may offer social support by identifying some of the skills to be addressed, making the process less overwhelming to the family. Finally, the therapist helps the family develop a positive, confident attitude about their future.

Because the resources, the demands of the disability, and the parents' coping styles contribute dynamically to the family's adaptation, families respond differently to similar events. The family's unique cluster of financial, human, and social capital, which provides the resources and strategies that help family members frame and cope with stress, will also help the family determine their ability to meet demands (Patterson, 1988). With an open definition of sources of problems (not just the child's needs), therapists recognize that stress can accumulate and deplete resources. For example, an event such as having the child catch a new bus in the morning may require adjustments in the family routine. Although most families can organize their lives to get the child to the bus on time, this demand may appear insurmountable to a family dealing with unemployment and neighbors that keep them awake at night. By using this model, the therapist recognizes that additional resources are needed before the family can adjust their schedule to get the child up and ready for the bus.

■ DEFINING FAMILY-CENTERED SERVICES

There is increasing evidence that formal and informal social support is a powerful resource for families who are raising children with chronic illnesses or developmental differences (Dunst, Trivette, & Jodry, 1997). Judge (1998) found an association between actively seeking social support as a coping mechanism and positive family functioning. Professionals working with children and young people with special needs are part of the formal social support system and are in a position to encourage the family's efforts to network among friends, family members, and parent groups. Although parents' needs change as the child grows, a number of themes consistently occur when parents are surveyed or asked about the services they value. First, the professional should communicate with the parent in a way that does no harm. The therapist must also be sure to provide comprehensive and sensitive services (Patterson et. al., 1997). A family-centered approach is demonstrated when the therapist appreciates that the child with special needs is part of an interactive family system and enables the parent to become an equal team member (Brown, Humphry, & Taylor, 1995). The components of a family-centered approach are best defined by the families who receive these services. Therefore most of the following descriptions are based on the voices of parents

(Mahoney & Bella, 1998; Mahoney & Filer, 1996; Summers et. al., 1990; Turnbull & Ruef, 1997).

Establishing a Partnership

The first interactions of the therapist with a family open the door to establishing a partnership. In a family-centered approach, the therapist demonstrates a family orientation that establishes trust and builds rapport. The practitioner conveys to the family "a willingness to orient services to the whole family, rather than just the child." (McWilliam, Tocci, & Harbin, 1998). The therapist's initial interview reflects an interest not only in the child's behaviors but also in the family's concerns with managing these behaviors. These first interactions demonstrate that an equal partnership is desired and encourage a give-and-take of information. At the same time, parents begin to understand that professionals are there to help them and to provide information and resources that support the child's development.

Trust building is not easily defined, and it is associated with nonverbal language and words. Thinking the best of families is important to developing this partnership. This may not always be easy, particularly when the family's lifestyle contradicts that of the professional. Being positive and maintaining a nonjudgmental position with a family can be very difficult, but it is essential to establish trust and build on a trusting relationship.

In a parent-therapist partnership, the family and therapist collaborate using agreed upon roles to obtain agreed upon goals for the child (Dunst, 1991). Therapists and parents develop partnerships to promote the child's functional skills. Partnerships imply a solid working relationship with open communication that is built on mutual respect. Parent-therapist partnerships may seem easy to accomplish, but a number of barriers have traditionally prevented strong collaborative models of service delivery. Often when obtaining services, parents have reported feeling "intimidated, unheard, or dismissed by the professionals who are trying to help them" (Singer & Irvin, 1989).

Both the parent and therapist bring certain perspectives and have certain responsibilities in the partnership. Dunst (1991) indicated that the therapist must assume greater responsibility for ensuring the success of the family-professional relationship.

It is incumbent upon them to share all information openly and honestly right from the start and to treat families with respect and dignity. Families, however, may choose to withhold information, understanding, and support until such time as they feel a trusting relationship has been established (p. 69).

The goal is not for parents to become quasiprofessionals. Parents and therapists have different relationships with the child. A parent's relationship with the child is individual, intimate, lifelong, and subjective. The professional's involvement with the child is time limited and objective. As with most partnerships, a successful relationship emerges when persons with differing skills and expertise are brought together (Gartner et. al., 1990). The importance of partnerships suggests that long-term therapist-parent relationships are beneficial. Parents report that "starting over" with new therapists is stressful and disruptive to the intervention process (Case-Smith & Nastro, 1993).

Healy, Keesee, and Smith (1989) provided guidelines for establishing partnerships with parents. Their wisdom included the following key points:

1. Although parents with at-risk and disabled children may at times be parents in crisis, they are not disabled parents. They have capacities for creative problem solving and coping that professionals need to respect, promote, and encourage.

2. Parents and involved professionals may have widely differing perspectives, experiences, and goals for a particular at-risk or disabled child. The difficult process of sharing and learning to understand these differing perspectives is an important part of care for the child.

3. Finding the professional balance between promoting competence and independence in families and providing needed expertise and emotional support is part of a developmental process. A particular kind of support at one time may promote inappropriate dependence later.

4. The professional needs to share large amounts of information, often of a technical nature, with the parents of special-needs children. This process can be aided by appropriate translation of technical language, the provision of relevant written materials, open acknowledgment of unknowns, and direction to other service providers.

Providing Helpful Information

Parents of young children with disabilities report that they desire information first and that information should cover the following concerns in order of priority: (1) the child's disability, (2) the services available for the child, (3) the future, (4) the services for the parents, (5) general child development, and (6) the services for the siblings (Summers et. al., 1990). Suggested formats range from written materials to videotapes and oral explanations. Parents want informational materials not only for themselves but to help explain the child's needs to their other children and extended family members. Participants agree that early intervention programs should be prepared to repeat information in several formats, if necessary, as family members' changing emotional states allow them to attend to the information.

Although the primary type of information that intervention programs provide relates to the child, programs also provide resources and information of direct help to the family. In a study of family-centered early intervention programs, mothers reported the frequency of specific family services. The services provided, in order of frequency, were (1) child information, (2) educational activities, (3) systems engagement, (4) personal-family services, and (5) resource assistance (Mahoney & Bella, 1998). The information that therapists provide to families about the intervention system prepares the families to work with existing systems, to use resources available, and to understand their rights as consumers. This information also enables the family members to become informed decision makers and to choose their level of participation in the intervention program.

The child-related information that may be of benefit to parents includes information about the child's development, the disability, the child's health, and test results. Although parents express that child and diagnostic information is desired, it must be given in a supportive manner. Service providers who focused on the negative aspects of the child's condition or compared the child to typically developing peers were viewed as not supportive (Patterson et. al., 1997). Once a deficit is identified and the child qualifies for services, hearing the child's developing abilities expressed as delays or deficits can be hurtful. Describing what the child has accomplished using a criterion-referenced instrument, such as using the Pediatric Evaluation of Disability Inventory (Haley, Coster, Ludlow, Haltiwanger, & Andrellos, 1992), helps parents remain positive and encouraged. Using an occupation-centered approach, the therapist asks what self-care activities the child is attempting or what play skills are emerging. Articulating a therapeutic goal linked to an emerging skill that the parents have identified reduces professional jargon and helps parents understand how the intervention plan relates to their child. Typically, parents hope to receive recommendations for activities that help the child play, for toys that match the child's abilities, or for strategies that lead to independence in self-care. They also look to the therapist for help in managing motor impairments or differences in sensory processing that limit occupational performance.

Respecting and Accepting Family Diversity

Respecting and accepting family diversity is demonstrated when professionals acknowledge that all families have strengths and resources. The positive aspects of families are recognized and used as the foundation for the intervention program. This principle becomes particularly relevant when families are of different racial, ethnic, cultural, and socioeconomic status.

Families from different cultures often have different perspectives on child rearing, health care, and disabilities.

Table 5-2 lists cultural characteristics, examples, and the possible consequences for intervention programs.

The occupational therapist needs to recognize the balance of family roles and responsibilities and how much emphasis is placed on nurturing the child versus promoting the child's independence. The family may appear to be overprotective of the child when they are, in reality, behaving according to their cultural norm. In some families, autonomy is valued; in others the child is expected to obey rules and not question authority.

Therapists need to be sensitive to the implications of these subtle differences in child rearing. For example, in one family all of the children slept in the parents' bed for their first 12 years. This tradition made it difficult to increase the independence and self-sufficiency of a 10-year-old boy with myelomeningocele. Although the therapist was concerned about the child's dependence in bedtime routines, the parents were not. If the therapist gave the family recommendations for increasing independence that included having the child sleep in his own bed, the parents' responses may have been negative. Choosing to change a family routine is entirely a parental decision. The parents may indicate that they prefer that the occupational therapist focus on activities other than those that challenge the family's values.

Seligman and Darling (1989) proposed five principles for establishing rapport with families who are culturally diverse (Box 5-2). One important way to understand a family's culture is to visit their home, because family members are often most comfortable there. In addition, viewing the home environment gives the occupational therapist an opportunity to better understand cultural traditions and family values. With this understanding, the therapist can adjust expectations and strategies to fit into the family's routines. For example, if the home is very simple and sparsely furnished, recommending state-of-the-art electronic equipment may not be well received. With a home visit, the therapist can learn more about family rituals and celebrations that need to be considered in the therapy schedule and program.

Flexible, Accessible, and Responsive Services

Because each family is different and has individualized needs, services must be flexible and adaptable. The occupational therapist should continually adapt the intervention activities as the family's interests and priorities change. Responsiveness entails "doing whatever needs to be done" and may, at times, require that a practitioner holds back and does not push his or her agenda (McWilliam et. al., 1998). Although therapists are often flexible and responsive to the child's immediate needs and the parent's concerns, the range of

---

box 5-2 Suggestions for trust building with culturally diverse families

1. Invite an interpreter or bilingual family member to meetings or therapy.
2. Provide written materials in the family's native language.
3. Use community representatives and peers to develop initial relationships.
4. Be sensitive to logistical constraints and be flexible in working with the family to find viable solutions that are comfortable for them.
5. Encourage families to share their view of their situation. Listening to the family's story and perspective can reinforce your genuine interest and concern.
6. To the greatest extent possible, take the "shoes test" and try to assume the family's point of view.

Modified from Seligman, M., & Darling, R.B. (1989). *Ordinary families, special children: A systems approach to childhood disability.* New York: The Guilford Press.

---

possible services is sometimes limited by the structure of the system. When a parent desires additional services, a change in location (e.g., home-based versus center-based care), or services to be held at a different time, the therapist may or may not be able to accommodate the parent because of the therapist's tight schedule. Often the agency or school system enforces policies regarding the therapists' caseloads and scope of services. Practitioners are caught in the middle, between the system's structure and individualized family needs. A ready solution does not always exist for the therapist who is constrained by time limitations and the demands of a large caseload.

Much of the time the therapist recognizes that he or she cannot change the structure of the system and must work as efficiently as possible within the system. At the same time the therapist should inform the family regarding the program's rules and policies so that they are aware of the constraints of the system. The therapist may recommend additional services through other agencies or similar activities that can complement the effect of therapy (e.g., swimming lessons, gymnastics, horseback riding). The occupational therapist can also take the initiative to work toward change in the system that allows more flexibility in meeting family needs. When a therapist has a caseload of 40 children each week, can he or she provide services that are responsive to family priority concerns for each of these children? Large caseloads and tight schedules limit the degree to which services can be flexible in meeting family needs.

table 5-2 *Suggestions for Cultural Considerations*

Cultural Considerations	Examples	May Determine
Meaning of the disability	Disability within a family may be viewed as shameful and disgraceful or as a positive contribution to the family.	Level of acceptance of the disability and the need for services
Attitudes about professionals	Professionals may be viewed as persons of authority or as equals	Level of family members' participation; may be only minimal in the partnership out of respect and fear
Attitudes about children	Children may be highly valued	Willingness of the family to make many sacrifices on behalf of the child
Attitudes about seeking and receiving help	Problems within the family may be viewed as being strictly a family affair or may be easily shared with others	Level of denial; may work against acknowledging and talking about the problem
Family roles	Roles may be sex specific and traditional or flexible. Age and sex hierarchies of authority may exist	Family preferences; may exist for the family member who takes the leadership role in the family-professional partnership
Family interactions	Boundaries between family subsystems may be strong and inflexible or relaxed and fluid	Level of problem sharing/solving in families; family members may keep to themselves and deal with problems in isolation, or they may problem solve as a unit
Time orientation	Family may be present or future oriented	Family's willingness to consider future goals and future planning
Role of the extended family	Extended family members may be close or far, physically and emotionally	Who is involved in the family-professional partnership
Support networks	Family may rely solely on nuclear family members, on extended family members, or on unrelated persons. Importance of godparents	Who can be called on in time of need
Attitude toward achievement	Family may have a relaxed attitude or high expectations for achievement	Goals and expectations of the family for the family member with the disability
Religion	Religion and the religious community may be a strong or neutral factor in some aspects of family life	Family's values, beliefs, and traditions as sources of comfort
Language	Family may be non-English speaking, bilingual, or English speaking	Need for translators
Number of generations removed from country of origin	Family may have just emigrated or be several generations removed from the country of origin	Strength and importance of the cultural ties
Reasons for leaving country of origin	Family may be emigrants from countries at war	Family's readiness for involvement with external world

From Turnbull, A.P., & Turnbull, H.R. (1990). *Families, professionals and exceptionality: A special partnership* (pp. 156-157). Columbus, OH: Merrill.

Parents have offered advice on providing flexible and responsive services (Turnbull & Turnbull, 1990):
1. Listen with empathy to understand family concerns and needs.
2. Verbally acknowledge family priorities.
3. Make adaptations to services based on parents' input.
4. Explain the constraints of the system when the parents' requests cannot be met.
5. Suggest alternative resources to parents when their requests cannot be met within the system.
6. Discuss parents' suggestions and requests with administrators to increase the possibilities that policies and agency structure can change to benefit families.

Family Roles in Decision Making

Parents should be the primary decision makers in intervention for their child. Although professionals tend to acknowledge readily the role of the parents as decision makers, they do not always give parents choices or explain options in ways that enable parents to make good decisions. Too often, plans that should be family-centered are written in professional jargon and do not always address family concerns (Boone, McBride, Swann, Moore, & Drew, 1998). Parents are involved in decision making about their child in the following ways:

1. They can defer decision making to the therapist. Deferring to the therapist may reflect confidence in the therapist's judgment and may be an easy way for parents to make a decision about an issue that they do not completely understand.

2. Parents have veto power. It is important that parents know that they have the power to veto any decision made or goal chosen by the team. Awareness of the legitimacy of this role gives parents assurance that they have an important voice on the team and can make changes, should they desire them. This role appears to be quite satisfying to parents (McBride et. al., 1993).

3. Parents share in decision making. As described in the previous section, when parent-professional partnerships have been established, the parents fully participate in team discussions that lead to decisions about the intervention plan. Service options and alternatives are made clear, and parents have the information needed to make final decisions. Requests of parents are honored (within the limitations of the program).

In a qualitative study in which families were interviewed, McBride and others (1993) found that although family members assumed limited roles in decision making and were provided few meaningful choices, most families reported satisfaction with these practices. Families cannot always be given a wide range of choices about who will provide services and when and where these services will be provided. However, their role in decision making should still be emphasized. Families who are empowered to make decisions early in the intervention process will be better prepared for that role throughout the course of the child's development. In most cases, assessment of choices and good decision making will be a skill that parents promote in their children as they approach adulthood.

■ COMMUNICATION STRATEGIES

As previously discussed, a priority of parents is to receive information regarding typical child development, diagnosis of disability, therapeutic activities to enhance the child's skills development, and methods to cope with the disability within the family's routine. Therapists have tremendous amounts of information to impart to parents. Effective helping is most likely to occur when the information given is requested or sought by the parent (Dunst, Trivette, & Deal, 1994). Effective communication is built on trust and respect; it means honesty and sensitivity to what the parent needs to know at the moment.

Occupational therapists communicate with parents using a variety of methods: formal and informal, written, verbal, and nonverbal. The following section describes communication strategies consistent with the principles described earlier. The strategies are based primarily on feedback from parents regarding what they have found to be effective help from occupational therapists (Hinojosa, 1990; Case-Smith & Nastro, 1993).

Formal Team Meetings with Families

Sometimes the therapist's first meeting with a family is a formal team meeting to develop the IFSP or IEP. To increase the parents' participation and comfort level in such a meeting, it is important to provide them with specific information about the purpose, structure, and logistics of the meeting. They should be provided with specific information about their role and questions the team members may ask. Parents should receive assessment results before the IFSP or IEP meeting. Therapists may contact the parents by phone to express their concerns and to suggest possible goals. As a result, parents have an opportunity to think about the assessment and goals and to be prepared to discuss them in the team meeting. A telephone call before the meeting also gives the therapist an opportunity to ask about the parents' concerns and to prepare options for meeting those concerns in the child's educational program or intervention plan.

Turnbull and Turnbull (1990) use the work of Stephens and Wolfe (1980) to describe the components of a parent-professional conference. They suggested that each conference have four components: (1) building a rapport, (2) obtaining information, (3) sharing information, and (4) summarizing and following up.

Building a rapport

Family members need to feel comfortable and connected to the other team members. All members should be introduced, and the purpose of the meeting should be reviewed. Parents should be encouraged to ask questions, express opinions, or take notes.

Obtaining information

Family members should be encouraged to share information, using open-ended questions. For example, the therapist might begin, "What are your primary concerns about Jim and school right now?" All team members should respectfully attend to what the parents say, ask for clarification when needed, and indicate understanding by paraphrasing or summarizing the information. Summers and others (1990) found that families appreciated an "unhurried atmosphere [that conveyed] the sense that family concerns and needs are important to practitioners" (p. 85).

Sharing information

Jargon-free language should be used, avoiding technical terms. When technical terms are used, they should be explained in ways that everyone understands. Professionals should begin with positive points and then explain problems and deficits. In describing the problems, anecdotes or real examples of the child's performance should be given. When giving information, the occupational therapist should be sensitive to the parent's response and provide opportunities for questions. Information should be provided in writing so that parents have an opportunity to read it later without the presence of a group of professionals.

Summarizing and following up

After plans and decisions about goals are made, they should be summarized. Plans should be specific and include dates, tasks, and names of those who are responsible for the plans. The meeting should end on a positive note, with plans made for another meeting or the next mode of communication. Again, verbalized plans should be given to the parents in writing as soon as possible.

Informal Meetings

Many parents prefer informal, individual meetings with the occupational therapist rather than structured, more formal meetings. When parents are interested in a one-on-one conference, they should be given a list of times that the therapist is available. Meetings during or after the child's therapy, although convenient, are not always ideal. The therapist needs to be organized and prepared for parent encounters. Often the answer to a casual question such as, "How is Sherry doing in occupational therapy?" holds great importance to the parent. Casual or general responses are not adequate. The therapist should either describe specific examples of recent performance or state when reevaluation will occur and how those results will be reported.

When unplanned meetings occur, the therapist needs to listen to and acknowledge the parent's concerns. When the parent asks for specific information about intervention or intervention goals, the therapist should indicate that he or she prefers to respond after reviewing daily notes and charts on the child. The therapists can later make a telephone call to the parent with the child's chart in hand to avoid giving the parent erroneous or misleading information.

Written Communication

In many intervention settings, particularly in the schools, parents are not physically present, and regular communication with family members relies on written strategies. Because written communication does not require the sender and recipient to be in the same place at the same time, it is a practical and important way to maintain communication with parents.

Notebooks

Notebooks shared between therapists and parents seem to be a highly valued and successful way for parents to keep important information and to have a regular, reliable method for expressing concerns. In the notebook team members may describe a new skill the child demonstrated that day, an action by the child that delighted the class, an upcoming school event, or materials requested from the parent. It may also include snack information or the current strategy for working on self-feeding. The parents can share their perception of the child's feelings, new accomplishments at home, or new concerns. Regardless of whether the therapist and parent have face-to-face contact, notebooks are important. Home-based therapists may initiate a notebook for the parent to record significant child behaviors and for the therapist to make weekly suggestions for activities. In the neonatal intensive care unit, notebooks are sometimes kept at the infant's bedside. These notebooks provide a method for the parents and therapists to communicate with the nursing staff on successful strategies for feeding and handling the infant.

Handouts

When judiciously used and appropriate to the child, handouts can be helpful and valued by the parents. Handouts should be individualized and applicable to the family's daily routine. Handouts copied from books and manuals are appropriate if they are individualized. Many parents prefer pictures and diagrams. One mother expressed her appreciation of handouts: "The home-based therapist who came out would not only show me and do things, she would watch me handle Martin and correct me if I did it wrong. She brought me pictures and diagrams and explained what each meant. . . . I still go back to them at times" (Nastro, 1992, p. 70).

Other mothers have expressed that photographs are helpful. In the hospital, occupational therapists often take photographs of the child in a good position for feeding or other caregiving tasks to serve as a reminder to parents and staff of how to improve postural alignment.

Electronic mail and other methods of communication

Electronic mail has become an easy way to stay in touch with parents. As an end-of-the-day activity, it can offer the therapist a method for noting any particular daily occurrences that would be of interest to parents. Whether or not the family has access to electronic communication, a regular progress report is important to parents. A simple report covering a few areas of performance may be more meaningful to the parents than a lengthy, complicated report. Child quotes and reports of specific performance send the message that the child is receiving individualized attention.

Many options are available for communication between parents and therapists. Telephone calls and simple notes sent home are good ways to maintain communication regarding issues in which both parties have common understanding. However, informal communication methods are not appropriate when the therapist has concerns or issues about the child. If the therapist expects a lengthy discussion, the telephone is not the method of choice, although a call may be used to set up a meeting.

Some therapists use videotapes to convey information about handling, feeding, and positioning methods. When selecting videotaping as a method of conveying information, it should be recognized that parents must invest time in watching the tape; short clips of direct relevance to current goals are most efficient.

■ HOME PROGRAMS

Throughout this text, recommendations have been given for ways to implement therapeutic activities into the daily lives of children, with the clear recognition that learning occurs best in the child's natural environment. Skills demonstrated in therapy translate into meaningful functional change only when the child can generalize the skill to other settings and demonstrate the skill in his or her daily routine. Therapists often recommend home activities for parents to implement with their child, so he or she can apply new skills at home. A number of studies have supported the importance of suggestions for the home and have helped define what types of home programs are most beneficial to parents.

Rainforth and Salisbury (1988) described an approach for developing home programs that fit into the family's daily routine. Before making specific recommendations for home activities, the parents are asked about daily routines or asked to chart the typical flow of family activities during the week. Together the therapist and parents discuss co-occupations during the day and whether therapeutic goals can be addressed at these times. The parents can be empowered to identify naturally occurring opportunities to teach the child new skills by understanding what needs to occur and deciding when it will work for them. The result of this close examination of the typical week enables the therapist and parent to embed goals and activities into interactive routines where the therapeutic process does not diminish the value and pleasure with the ritual in these co-occupations.

Hinojosa (1990) and Case-Smith and Nastro (1993) examined how mothers use home programs and the characteristics of home programs that parents value and implement. Hinojosa completed a qualitative study in which eight mothers of preschool children with CP were interviewed. Most of the mothers did not carry out the prescribed home programs. Mothers reported that they did not have the time, energy, or confidence to follow the programs effectively. Hinojosa (1990) suggested that it is inappropriate to expect mothers to follow a strict home program. Instead, therapists should assist mothers in adaptive ways to meet their children's needs with minimal disruption to their lives. He described the resultant home intervention as "mother directed," meaning that the mother made the decision as to how therapy might be implemented at home.

Case-Smith and Nastro (1993) replicated Hinojosa's study using a sampling of mothers from Ohio who had young children with CP. Each had accessed private and public-funded therapies. Initially, when their children were infants, these mothers had participated extensively in home programs. They indicated that these efforts were self-motivated and did not feel that the specific home programs were "an imposed expectation" on the part of the therapists. As the children reached preschool age, the mothers no longer implemented home programs with their children. Reasons for discontinuing home programs included lack of time and increased resistance on the part of their children. Lyon (1989) expressed a mother's perspective on implementing therapy at home:

> I've come to terms with being "only human." If I could ensure that Zak could go through the day always moving in appropriate ways, flexing when he should flex, straightening when he should straighten, and play and learn and experience and appreciate . . . I would; but, that is not possible. I do have a responsibility to help Zachary develop his motor skills, but I also have a responsibility to help him learn about life. So on those days when we have so much fun together or are so busy that bedtime comes before therapy time, I finally feel comfortable that I have given him something just as vital to his development, a real mom (p. 4).

Although mothers tend not to implement specific prescribed strategies, they report appreciating the therapists' suggestions and ideas about home activities that promote child development or make caregiving easier. Case-Smith and Nastro (1993) found that the mothers in their sample frequently used the handouts with specific activities and recommendations long after they had been given to them. Summers and others (1990) explained that parents found written materials and videotapes helpful because they were "not always ready to hear, understand, or accept some information, but that it could be available for later use" (p. 91). At the same time it is important to realize that written material may be a less-effective form of communication for families where reading is not an already established way to learn about child development.

Summary

Positive relationships with families seem to develop when open and honest communication is established, and parents are encouraged to participate in their child's program to the extent that they desire. When asked to give advice to therapists, parents stated that they appreciated (1) specific objective information, (2) flexibility in service delivery, (3) sensitivity and responsivity to their concerns, and (4) positive, optimistic attitudes (Case-Smith & Nastro, 1993). One mother expressed that hope and optimism are always best. "Given a choice, I would want my therapist to be an optimist and perhaps to strive for goals that might be a bit too optimistic, keeping in mind that we might not come to that" (Nastro, 1992, p. 64).

■ WORKING WITH FAMILIES FACING MULTIPLE CHALLENGES

Features that contribute to diversity in families are characteristics that occupational therapists welcome and accommodate in providing individualized services. The principles presented in this text remain critically important, but they are more difficult to implement when working with families confronted with multiple challenges. Challenges to a family's ability to fulfill its functions (e.g., living in poverty, acute onset of a disability in the parent) increase the vulnerability of children with special needs and add unique challenges to family operations. By identifying protective factors supporting the child's resilience, the therapist can approach issues from a positive perspective to support strengths, capitalize on family assets, and work to make maximum use of community resources.

The occupational therapist grounded in family systems theory and committed to empowering families can work effectively with a whole family system in a family-centered manner, regardless of the type of disability of one or more family members (Brown et. al., 1997). Understanding how the family system orchestrates members' occupations to fulfill family function and the value of co-occupations in promoting development prepares the occupational therapist to take a holistic view of the family's needs and priorities. Although parents advocate a positive view, it is important to recognize when an unusual parental behavior reflects family dysfunction (e.g., child abuse, child neglect). When family dysfunction is pervasive, most occupational therapists need input from colleagues with expertise in counseling and family systems. Services for the child with special needs continue, but the therapist considers ecological and family systems factors in collaborating with the team to set priorities and provide services.

Families in Chronic Poverty

Chronic poverty has a pervasive effect on family and child experiences. The majority of families receiving public assistance are children and mothers with poor educational backgrounds, inconsistent work history, and low-wage jobs. Welfare recipients are often stereotyped as lazy, unmotivated, and having children just to make money off the system (Seccombe, James, & Walters, 1998). The process of having to "qualify" for services can be frustrating, depersonalizing, and degrading. Once qualified, resources are not always enough for the family to make ends meet. In interviews with hundreds of single mothers living on welfare or working in low-paying jobs, Edin and Lein (1996) found both groups had to engage in a variety of survival strategies to access enough resources to meet their families' needs. Both groups reported sharing apartments and working on the side or having a second job. In addition, both groups relied on financial assistance from their social network, such as the child's father or family and friends.

Seccombe and colleagues (1998) conducted an ethnographic study of women receiving welfare and asked about their reasons for needing assistance. Although the participants realized that the United States culture tended to emphasize individual responsibility for rising above poverty, many of the women believed that luck was a primary reason their families needed assistance. Single parents are particularly vulnerable (Edin & Lein, 1996); without family members to help, these mothers lacked control over the events in their lives. Unexpected events, such as a car breaking down or special meetings at school about a child, can cause the parent to miss hours at a job and increase financial strain. Some of the women in Seccombe's study reported that they returned to welfare and Medicaid "for the child." Poverty represents a multidimensional issue, and therapists cannot make assumptions about the reasons a family lives in poverty.

Poverty is a burden born by a disproportionate number of children who are members of ethnic minority groups. In 1995 it was estimated that 20% of all children lived in poverty, and 41.5% of the children who were black and 39% of the children who were Hispanic lived in poverty (U.S. Bureau of Census, 1997). Because children in families with poor housing and low access to basic services are more likely to experience health problems, occupational therapists frequently have to incorporate issues related to poverty in making their interventions appropriate to family SES. Recognizing that poverty creates a unique cultural worldview will enable therapists to consider what it means to provide family-centered services (Humphry, 1995). For example, a different worldview of time, with the emphasis on the here and now, makes it harder to schedule or keep appointments. Families of low SES are rarely able to follow through with their plans.

Therefore, planning for the future has little meaning, and participating in setting annual goals at IFSP or IEP meetings may not be considered important.

Further, increasing the vulnerability of children with special needs who live in poverty are the multiple challenges that make their parents at greater risk for poor parenting. Almost one half (45%) of the mothers in one study struggled with depression, and less than one half reported they had a family member who could help baby-sit (Schteingart, Molnar, Klein, Lowe; Hartmann, 1995). Even with incentives such as diapers, toys, and food, low-income mothers got their children to an early intervention program only 40% to 50% of the time, compared with the 75% of the time for middle-income mothers (Brinker, 1992). Low income influences the parents' psychologic health, their sense of well-being, and the quality of their interactions within the parenting subsystem (Brody et. al., 1994). Therapists who are aware that poverty creates special conditions strive to individualize intervention plans and consider how formal support can replicate the positive effects of social support to promote better parenting (Brinker, 1992; Dunst et. al., 1997). The following case study describes intervention that reinforces family strengths and addresses important environmental issues that influence this child's development.

Case Study

Jason and his mother, Ms. Thorp, lived in a government subsidized one-bedroom apartment, and they received food stamps and welfare. Because it was a dangerous neighborhood, Ms. Thorp tried to keep Jason inside as much as possible. At his 4-year-old annual physical, the physician noticed that Jason was not completely toilet trained. His mother stated that he did not use a spoon, and he demonstrated limited expressive vocabulary. An interdisciplinary assessment at the Developmental Evaluation Center revealed a short attention span, below average self-care standard score on the Pediatric Evaluation of Disabilities Inventory, and 20% delay in expressive language. The occupational therapist also noted that Jason demonstrated poor fine motor skills (i.e., he did not complete puzzles, color with a crayon, or cut along a line). On the fine motor scales of the Peabody Developmental Motor Scales, Jason was below the 10th percentile. Because Jason had not been exposed to a varied learning environment, the team recommended that he enroll in a childcare program with children his own age. They also recommended that the speech language pathologist and occupational therapist consult with his teacher.

In developing an IEP, his mother, with input from the social worker, had selected a childcare program. It was near her home, so she could walk Jason to school, saving him an hour-long van ride to the Head Start program on the other side of town. The teachers welcomed him and thought that they could work on toilet training, but they insisted that Jason needed to be able to feed himself lunch before he entered the program.

The therapist discussed Jason's use of a spoon with Ms. Thorp, but she remained vague about whether she could force Jason to use utensils. The therapist recalled hearing that children living in poverty were less likely to have meals in a particular location or at regular times, and she realized strategies at different levels would be needed to achieve spoon feeding.

The therapist decided she could be supportive and effective in changing mealtime routines by providing services in the home, rather than at the clinic. Therefore she visited Jason's home later that week. At the beginning of the home visit, the therapist realized that the family had no kitchen table. In talking about their daily schedule, Ms. Thorp reported that they did not awaken at any specific time. However, Jason was usually up by 11:30 AM to watch his favorite television show. She reported that watching television together was an activity she enjoyed with her son.

Ms. Thorp gave Jason a cheese sandwich sometime in the late morning. She selected cheese sandwiches because the nutritionist said they were good and Jason did not make a mess when he walked around with them. Ms. Thorp reported that she was not a "morning person," so she frequently did not have breakfast or lunch. Instead, she snacked during the day. For dinner, she frequently made chicken or hamburgers, which she and Jason ate in the living room. The plate was placed on the coffee table, and Jason stood near it and finger fed himself. If she made something like pinto beans, Ms. Thorp fed Jason so he would not make a mess. She explained, "When we moved in, there were bugs everywhere. I fought hard to kill them because I know they are dirty. I know if he makes a mess with food the bugs will be right back!"

The therapist brought a cup of pudding as a treat for Jason, and she asked him to spoon it himself. They sat Jason in the corner of the sofa. When he was handed the spoon, he dipped it into the pudding, inverted the spoon as he brought it to his mouth, and sucked the pudding from the spoon. Ms. Thorp became upset when pudding dropped from his spoon onto his shirt. She took the spoon away and fed him the rest of the pudding.

The therapist wanted to understand Jason's weekly routine. She learned that Jason spent every Tuesday night with his father, who would take him out for an ice cream cone. His maternal grandmother occasionally watched Jason on weekends when Ms. Thorp supplemented their income by filling in as a cook's assistant in a coffee shop. The therapist interpreted the family's strengths as:

1. Ms. Thorp is a devoted mother who wants her son to be healthy and wants a clean apartment.

2. Ms. Thorp listens to and follows the advice of the nutritionist.
3. The Thorps share an interactive routine around a television show in the morning, which helps create temporal organization.
4. Jason's family includes extended family, who see him regularly.

Her concerns about Jason learning to spoon feed include:

1. Jason does not have a place for meals, and he rarely sees another person using a spoon.
2. Meals are typically foods that can be eaten with fingers.
3. Jason does not use tools well, and Ms. Thorp does not want him to be messy.
4. Ms. Thorp is easily overwhelmed by details, and she does not seem to solve problems easily.

The next time she visited, the therapist brought a stool from the physical therapy equipment library. They adjusted the height so that it could be pulled up to a coffee table, creating a place for Jason to sit and eat. She also purchased two place mats with his favorite cartoon hero on them. The therapist brought a can of macaroni and cheese for Jason to eat. Jason loved his "chair" and table. When given the spoon to eat macaroni from a bowl he scooped but inverted the spoon on the way to his mouth. He looked surprised and finger fed himself the noodles. Together they planned that Jason would have "noodles" as lunch, and they agreed that lunch would occur immediately before Jason's favorite TV show.

On her third home visit, the therapist arranged to come in the evening when Jason's father came to take him for ice cream. When she arrived, Ms. Thorp returned the stool because her mother had a stool he could use. The therapist explained to Jason's father that his son needed more practice using a spoon. He agreed to get cups of ice cream instead of ice cream cones and eat with Jason.

Within 4 weeks of the therapist's third visit, Ms. Thorp reported that Jason was successfully using a spoon. The team arranged for Jason to begin preschool the next week.

Parents with Special Needs

Parents themselves may have special needs that require an emphasis on supportive services. Parents who face physical or sensory challenges may need help in solving problems, such as monitoring the activity of an active child or being alerted to the cry of an infant (Meadow-Orlans, 1995). Occupational therapists, who work from the perspective that parenting reflects a process of co-occupation, can assist the parent in the modification of tasks. For example, adapting the location of routines, such as diaper changing and infant bathing, can enable parents with physical limitations to participate in caregiving and simple routines that build affection between the parent and child. Therapists can explore the use of adaptive equipment, such as motion detectors or sound activated alarm systems, to compensate for the parents' sensory deficits and ensure responsivity to their child's cues. Most parents who have had long-term experiences with a physical limitation independently develop creative solutions to provide care for their children, and they only occasionally seek a therapist's assistance in determining how to perform specific caregiving tasks.

Parents who struggle with drug addiction or mental illness (MI) often require counseling, mental health services, and opportunities to participate in support groups. When parents have special needs that strongly influence their caregiving ability, often their needs become the first emphasis of intervention.

Parents with MR, MI, or drug addiction are at risk for having children with developmental disabilities. Professionals have questioned the competency of parents with MR. However, with support systems in place, these parents can be surprisingly successful. Parents at risk because of MR or MI appear to be most successful in caring for young children when they are married, have few children, have adequate financial support, and have multiple sources of support (Tymchuk, Andron, & Unger, 1987).

In providing support to parents with MR, Espe-Sherwindt and Kerlin (1990) recommended that professionals focus on the parents' internal and external control, self-esteem, social skills, and problem-solving skills. Therapists can help empower parents to make their own decisions; increasing their sense of self-control. Often individuals with MR or drug addiction have low self-esteem and lack confidence in their ability to make decisions. Because self-esteem is important in interactions with children, this aspect of interaction should be considered.

Professionals should also focus on helping parents with MR and MI build problem-solving skills. Everyday care for children requires constant problem solving. Many times professionals give advice or recommendations without encouraging the parents to solve the problem or independently to try their own actions first. When others direct parents, they become more dependent. However, when parents successfully solve a problem, they become empowered to act independently in daily decision making. Problem solving can be taught and modeled. Espe-Sherwindt and Kerlin (1990) suggested that teaching problem-solving skills in daily caregiving could be critical to parents' development of caregiving competence.

When occupational therapists work with parents with MR or MI, it becomes essential to know their learning styles and abilities. Many times instructions need to be repeated and reinforced. Therapists must use good judgment in what techniques are taught to these parents, with emphasis on safe and simple methods. The occupational therapist should also recognize the need for additional supports to help parents with MR access those supports. Regular visits in the home by aides, nurses, or teaching assistants can meet the level of support needed. If the occupational therapist communicates his or her goals and strategies to the visiting aide, therapy activities are more likely to be implemented by the parents and other professionals working with the family.

Working with parents who are MR or have MI can be frustrating when appointments are missed or requests are not followed. Therefore an understanding of the parents' needs is essential. Development of simple, repetitive routines and systems that the parents can learn and follow enables them to become competent caregivers. With support, they can offer a child a positive and loving environment that fosters both health and development.

Professionals use a variety of strategies to deal with challenging families. When families have continual stress and problems, it is important for therapists to begin to slowly build trust, to share observations and concerns, and to accept parents' choices (DeGangi, Wietlisbach, Poisson, Stein, & Royeen, 1994). When parents do not seem to understand the intervention process, professionals can attempt to establish rapport by using concrete, simple terms; providing both written and oral information; and providing ideas that would immediately help the child. Professionals also report that parents can better articulate their concerns when services were home based; when lay terminology is used; and when services are presented in a slow, nonjudgmental way (DeGangi et. al., 1994). Focusing on the child's strengths and developing trust and responsiveness are also believed to be important when parents have difficulty articulating concerns.

■ SUMMARY

Working with families is one of the most challenging and rewarding aspects of pediatric occupational therapy. The family's participation in intervention is of critical importance in determining how much the child can benefit. Therapy goals and activities that reflect the family's priorities often result in meaningful outcomes.

This chapter described families as systems with unique structures and interaction patterns. The potential effects of a child with a disability on family function were related to implications for the occupational therapist's role. Issues that arise during different stages of the family's life cycle were described. In the final section, principles and strategies for working with families were discussed. The strategies included communication methods to inform and involve parents in the intervention program. Of critical importance is the occupational therapist's sensitivity

to the family's values and interests, respect for these interests, provision of information, and consistent support of family members.

STUDY QUESTIONS

1. Take random selection of 10 friends (include at least 5 people of different ages). Ask them to write down the names of everyone in their family and to include anyone they want. Write a definition of "the family" that would include all the characteristics of the families described by your subjects. (Idea adapted from Levin and Trost, 1992.)

2. Use Table 5-2 to identify your own cultural characteristics. Of which characteristics would you want an occupational therapist to be aware if he or she were giving services to your family?

3. The priorities of parents change over the life cycle. Describe two priorities of the parents of a low-functioning infant with severe and multiple disabilities. Describe priorities of the same parents during the child's early school years and adolescence. Describe the role of the occupational therapist in meeting each priority need.

4. List three strategies that the occupational therapist might use in working with a family of low SES in which the father is of normal intelligence and the mother has moderate MR. Neither parent works outside the home, and they have a 2-year-old daughter with moderate delays in language and fine-motor skills.

References

Acock, A.C., & Kiecolt, K.J. (1989). Is it family structure or socioeconomic status? Family structure during adolescence and adult adjustment. *Social Forces, 68,* 553-571.

American with Disabilities Act of 1990, 42, U.S.C.A . § 12134 *et. seq.* (Publisher and Year).

Anderson, D. (1983). He's not "cute" anymore. In T. Dougan, L. Isbell, & P. Vyas (Eds.), *We have been there* (pp. 90-91). Nashville, TN: Abington Press.

Barnett, S., & Boyce, G.C. (1995). Effects of children with Down syndrome on parents' activities. *American Journal of Mental Retardation, 100,* (2), 115-127.

Batten, B., & Cutler, P. (1990). *A comparison of coping strategies used by families with children with special needs based upon the time of onset of the disability.* Unpublished manuscript, University of North Carolina at Chapel Hill, Chapel Hill, N.C.

Bernheimer, L.P., & Keogh, B.K. (1995). Weaving interventions into the fabric of everyday life: An approach to family assessment. *Topics in Early Childhood Special Education, 15,* 415-433.

Boone, H.A., McBride, S.L., Swann, D., Moore, S., & Drew, B.S. (1998). IFSP practices in two states: Implications for practice. *Infants and Young Children, 10,* (4), 36-45.

Brinker, R.P. (1992). Family involvement in early intervention: Accepting the unchangeable, changing the changeable, and knowing the difference. *Topics in Early Childhood Special Education, 12,* (3), 307-332.

Brody, G.H., Stoneman, Z., Flor, D., McCrary C., Hastings, L., & Conyers, O. (1994). Financial resources, parent psychological functioning, parent co-caregiving, and early adolescent competence in rural two-parent African American families. *Child Development, 65,* 590-605.

Bronfenbrenner, U. (1986). Ecology of the family as a context to human development. Research perspectives. *Developmental Psychology, 22,* 723-745.

Brotherson, M.J., & Goldstein, B.L. (1992). Time as a resource and constraint for parents of young children with disabilities: Implications for early intervention services. *Topics in Early Childhood Special Education, 12,* (4), 508-527.

Brown, S.M., Humphry, R., & Taylor, E. (1997). A model of the nature of family-therapist relationships: Implications for education. *American Journal of Occupational Therapy, 51,* 597-603.

Calhoun, M.L., Calhoun, L.G., & Rose, T.L. (1989). Parents of babies with severe handicaps: Concerns about early intervention. *Journal of Early Intervention, 13,* 146-152.

Case-Smith, J. (1998). Defining the early intervention process. In J. Case-Smith (Ed.), *Pediatric occupational therapy and early intervention* (pp. 27-48). Boston, MA: Butterworth-Heinemann.

Case-Smith, J., & Nastro, M. (1993). The effect of occupational therapy intervention on mothers of children with cerebral palsy. *American Journal of Occupational Therapy, 46,* 811-817.

Cleveland, D.W., & Miller, N. (1977). Attitudes and life commitments of older siblings of mentally retarded adults: An exploratory study. *Mental Retardation, 15,* (2), 38-41.

Coleman, J.S. (1988). Social capital in the creation of human capital. *American Journal of Sociology* (Suppl. 94), S95-S120.

Crowe, T.K. (1993). Time use of mothers with young children: The impact of a child's disability. *Developmental Medicine and Child Neurology, 35,* 612-630.

DeGangi, G.A., Wielisback, S., Poisson, S., Stein, E., & Royeen, C. (1994). The impact of culture and socioeconomic status on family-professional collaboration: Challenges and solutions. *Topics in Early Childhood Special Education, 14,* (4), 503-520.

Diamond, S. (1981). Growing up with parents of a handicapped child: A handicapped person's perspective. In J.L. Paul (Ed.), *Understanding and working with parents of children with special needs* (pp. 23-59). New York: Holt, Rinehart & Winston.

Dunst, C.J. (1985). Rethinking early intervention. *Analysis and Intervention in Developmental Disabilities, 5,* 165-201.

Dunst, C.J. (1991). Implementation of the individualized family service plan. In M.J. McGonigel, R.K. Kaufmann, B.H. Johnson (Eds.), *Guidelines and recommended practices for the individualized family service plan.* Bethesda, MD: Association for the Care of Children's Health.

Dunst C.J., Trivette, C.M. & Deal, A. (1994). *Supporting and strengthening families: Methods, strategies and practices.* Cambridge, MA: Brookline Books.

Dunst, C.J., Trivette, C.M., & Jodry, W. (1997). Influences of social support on children with disabilities and their families. In M.J. Guralnick (Ed.), *The effectiveness of early intervention* (pp. 499-522). Baltimore: Paul H. Brookes.

Edin, K., & Lein, L. (1996). Work, welfare, and single mothers' economic survival strategies. *American Sociological Review, 61,* 253-266.

Entwisle, D.R., & Astone, H.M. (1994). Some practical guidelines for measuring youth's race/ethnicity and socioeconomic status. *Child Development, 45,* 1521-1540.

Espe-Sherwindt, M., & Kerlin, S.L. (1990). Early intervention with parents with mental retardation: Do we empower or impair? *Infants and Young Children, 2,* (4), 21-28.

Fiese, B.H., Hooker, K.A., Kotary, L., & Schwagler, J. (1993). Family rituals in the early stages of parenthood. *Journal of Marriage and the Family, 55,* 633-642.

Fraser, M.W. (1997). The ecology of childhood: A multisystem perspective. In M.W. Fraser (Ed.), *Risk and resilience in childhood: An ecological perspective* (pp. 1-9). Washington, DC: National Association of Social Workers.

Gallimore, R., Coots, J., Weisner, T., Garnier, H., & Guthrie, D. (1996). Family responses to children with early developmental delays II: Accommodation intensity and activity in early and middle childhood. *American Journal on Mental Retardation, 101,* (3), 215-232.

Gallimore, R., Weisner, T.S., Bernheimer, L.P., Gurthrie, D., & Nihira, K. (1993). Family responses to young children with developmental delays: Accommodation activity in ecological and cultural context. *American Journal on Mental Retardation, 98,* 185-206.

Garbarino, J., & Kostelney, K. (1995). Parenting and public policy. In M.H. Bornstein (Ed.), *Handbook of parenting, Vol. 3.* (pp. 419-436). Mahway, NJ: Lawrence Erlbaum.

Gartner, A., Lipsky, D.K., & Turnbull, A.P. (1990). *Supporting families with a child with a disability: An international outlook.* Baltimore: Brookes.

Goldberg-Glen, R., Sands, R.G., Cole, R.D., & Cristofalo, C. (1998). Multigenerational patterns and internal structures in families in which grandparents raise grandchildren. *Families in Society, 79,* 477-489.

Gowen, J.W., Christy, D.S., & Sparling, J. (1993). Informational needs of parents of young children with special needs. *Journal of Early Intervention, 17,* 194-210.

Grossman, F.K. (1972). *Brothers and sisters of retarded children: An exploratory study.* Syracuse, NY: Syracuse University Press.

Haley, S.M., Coster, W.J., Ludlow, L.H., Haltiwanger, J.T., & Andrellos, P.J., (1992). *Pediatric Evaluation of Disability Inventory.* San Antonio: Psychological Corporation.

Hanzlik, J. (1990). Nonverbal interaction patterns of mothers and their infants with cerebral palsy. *Education and Training In Mental Retardation, 25,* 333-343.

Hare, J. (1994). Concerns and issues faced by families headed by a lesbian couple. Families in society. *The Journal of Contemporary Human Services, 75,* 27-35.

Healy, A., Keesee, P.D., & Smith, B.S. (1989). *Early services for children with special needs: Transactions for family support* (2nd ed.). Baltimore: Brookes.

Heffer, R.W., Worchel-Prevatt, F., Rae, W.A., Lopez, M.A., Young-Saleme, T., Orr, K., Aikman, G., Krause, M., & Weir, M. (1997). The effects of oral versus written instructions on parents' recall and satisfaction after pediatric appointments. *Developmental and Behavioral Pediatrics, 18,* 377-382.

Helfer, C.M., & Glidden, L.M. (1998). More positive or less negative? Trends in research on adjustment of families rearing children with developmental disabilities. *Mental Retardation, 36,* 457-464.

Hill, R. (1958). Generic features of families under stress. *Social Casework, 49,* 139-150.

Hinde, R.A. (1995). In M.H. Bornstein (Ed.), *Handbook of parenting, Vol. 1* (pp. xi-xii). Mahwah, NJ: Lawrence Erlbaum.

Hinojosa, J. (1990). How mothers of preschool children with cerebral palsy perceive occupational and physical therapists and their influence on family life. *Occupational Therapy Journal of Research, 10,* (3), 144-162.

Hombeck, G.N., Gorey-Ferguson, L., Hudson, T., Seefeldt,T., Shapera, W., Turner, & Uhler, J. (1997). Maternal, paternal, and marital functioning in families of preadolescents with spina bifida. *Journal of Pediatric Psychology, 22,* 167-181.

Humphry, R. (1995). Families living in poverty: Meeting the challenge of family-centered services. *American Journal of Occupational Therapy, 49,* 687-693.

Individuals with Disabilities Education Act of 1990, 20 U.S.C.A. § 1400 *et. seq.* (Publisher and Year).

Itzkowitz, J. (1990). Siblings' perceptions of their needs for programs, services and support: A national study. *Sibling Information Network Newsletter, 7,* (1), 1-4.

Judge, S.L. (1998). Parental coping strategies and strengths in families of young children with disabilities. *Family Relations, 47,* 263-268.

Julian, T.W., McKenry, P.C., & McKelvey, M.W. (1994). Cultural variations in parenting: Perceptions of Caucasian, African-American, Hispanic, and Asian-American parents. *Family Relations, 43,* 30-37.

Kirby, L.D., & Fraser, M.W. (1997). Risk and resilience in childhood. In M.W. Fraser (Ed.), *Risk and resilience in childhood: An ecological perspective* (pp. 10-33). Washington, DC: National Association of Social Workers.

Kirk, S. (1998). Families' experiences of caring at home for a technology-dependent child: A review of the literature. *Child: Care, health and development, 24,* (2), 101-114.

Kraus-Mars, A.H., & Lachman, P. (1994). Breaking bad news to parents with disabled children: A cross-cultural study. *Child: Care, Health and Development, 20,* 101-113.

Krieger, M.H. (1996). A phenomenology of motherhood. In R. Zemke, & F. Clark (Eds.), *Occupational science: The evolving discipline* (pp. 243-246). Philadelphia: F.A, Davis.

Lawlor, M.C., & Mattingly, C.F. (1998). The complexities embedded in family-centered care. *American Journal of Occupational Therapy, 52,* 259-267.

Lazarus, R.S., & Folkman, S. (1984). *Stress, appraisal, and coping.* New York: Springer.

Levin, I., & Trost, J. (1992). Understanding the concept of family. *Family Relations, 41,* 348-351.

Levitt, M. (1988). Away from home for the first time. *The Exceptional Parent, 18,* (5), 55.

Luster, T., Rhoades, K., & Haas, B. (1989). The relationship between parental values and parenting behavior: A test of the Kohn hypothesis. *Journal of Marriage and the Family, 51,* 139-147.

Lynch, E.Q., & Hanson, M.J. (1998). *Developing cross-cultural competence: A guide for working with young children and their families.* Baltimore: Brookes.

Lyon, J. (1989). I want to be Zak's mom, not his therapist. *Developmental Disabilities Special Interest Section Newsletter, 12,* (1), 4.

Mahoney, G., & Bella, J. (1998). An examination of the effects of family-centered early intervention on child and family outcomes. *Topics in Early Childhood and Special Education, 18,* (2), 83-94.

Mahoney, G., Boyce, G., Fewell, R.R., Spiker, D., Wheeden, C.A., (1998). The relationship of parent-child interaction to the effectiveness of early intervention services for at-risk children and children with disabilities. *Topics in Early Childhood Special Education, 18,* 5-17.

Mahoney, G., & Filer, J. (1996). How responsive is early intervention to the priorities and needs of families? *Topics in Early Childhood Special Education, 16,* 437-457.

Mahoney, G., Finger, J., & Powell, A. (1985). The relationship of maternal behavior style to the developmental status of mentally retarded infants. *American Journal of Mental Deficiency, 90,* 296-302.

May, J. (1990). *Fathers of children with special needs: New horizons.* Bethesda, MD: Association for the Care of Children's Health.

McBride, S.L., Brotherson, M.J., Joanning, H., Whiddon, D., & Dermitt, A. (1993). Implementation of family-centered services: Perceptions of families and professionals. *Journal of Early Intervention, 17,* 414-430.

McCormick, M.C., McCarton, C., Brooks-Gunn, J., Belt, P., & Gross, R.T. (1998). The infant health and development program: Interim summary. *Developmental and Behavioral Pediatrics, 19,* 359-370.

McDermott, S., Coker, A.L., Mani, S., Krishnaswami, S., Nagle, R.J., Barnett-Queen, L.L., & Wuori, D.F. (1996). A population-based analysis of behavior problems in children with cerebral palsy. *Journal of Pediatric Psychology, 21,* 447-463.

McWilliam, R.A., Tocci, L., & Harbin, G.L. (1998). Family-centered services: Service providers' discourse and behavior. *Topics in Early Childhood and Special Education, 18,* (4), 206-221.

Meadow-Orlans, K.P. (1995). Parenting with a sensory or physical disability. In M.H. Bornstein (Ed.), *Handbook of parenting, Vol. 4.* (pp. 57-84). Mahwah, NJ: Lawrence Erlbaum.

Meyer, D.J. (1993). Lessons learned: Cognitive coping strategies of overlooked family members. In A.P. Turnbull, J.M. Patterson, S.K. Behr, D.L. Murphy, J.G. Marquis, M.J. Blue-Banning. (Eds.), *Cognitive coping, families, and disability* (pp. 81-94). Baltimore: Brookes.

Meyer, D.J., Vadasy, P.F., & Fewell, R.R. (1986). *Sibshops: A handbook for implementing workshops for siblings of children with special needs.* Seattle: University of Washington Press.

Minuchin, P. (1985). Families and individual development: Provocations from the field of family therapy. *Child Development, 56,* 289-302.

Morton, K. (1985). Identifying the enemy: A parent's complaint. In H.R. Turnbull, & A. Turnbull (Eds.). *Parents speak out: Now and then* (pp. 143-148). Columbus, OH: Merrill.

Murphy, K.E. (1997). Parenting a technology assisted infant: Coping with occupational stress. *Social Work in Health Care, 24* (3/4), 113-126.

Nastro, M. (1992). *An ethnographic study of mothers of children with cerebral palsy and the effect of occupational therapy intervention on their lives.* Unpublished master's thesis, Ohio State University, Columbus.

Ninio, A., & Rinott, N. (1988). Fathers' involvement in the care of their infants, and their attributions of cognitive competence to infants. *Child Development, 59,* 652-663.

Odom, S.L., & Brown, W.H. (1993). Social interaction skills interventions for young children with disabilities in integrated settings. In C.A. Peck, S.L. Odom, & D.D. Bricker (Eds.), *Integrating young children with disabilities into community programs.* Baltimore: Brookes.

Odom, S.L., McConnell, S.R., & McEvoy, M.A. (1992). Peer-related social competence and its significance for young children with disabilities. In S.L. Odom, S.R. McConnell, & M.A. McEvoy (Eds.), *Social competence of young children with disabilities: Nature, development and intervention* (pp. 3-35). Baltimore: Brookes.

Odom, S.L., & McEvoy, M.A. (1988). Social integration of young children with handicaps and normally developing children. In S.L. Odom, & M.B. Karnes (Eds.), *Early intervention for infants and children with handicaps: An empirical base* (pp. 241-268). Baltimore: Brookes.

Park, C.A., (1998). Lesbian parenthood: A review of the literature. *American Journal of Orthopsychiatry, 68,* 376-389.

Park, R.D. (1995). Fathers and families. In M.H. Bornstein (Ed.), *Handbook of parenting Vol. 3.* Mahwah, NJ: Lawrence Erlbaum.

Patching, B., & Watson, B. (1993). Living with children with an intellectual disability: Parents construct their reality. *International Journal of disability, development and education, 40,* 115-131.

Patterson, C.J. (1995). Lesbian and gay parenthood. In M.H. Bornstein (Ed.), *Handbook of parenting, Vol. 3* (pp. 255-273). Mahwah, NJ: Lawrence Erlbaum.

Patterson, J.M. (1988). Families experiencing stress. *Family Systems Medicine, 6,* 202-237.

Patterson, J.M. (1993). The role of family meanings in adaptation to chronic illness and disability. In A.P. Turnbull, J.M. Patterson, S.K. Behr, D.L. Murphy, J.G. Marquis, M.J. Blue-Banning (Eds.), *Cognitive coping, families, and disability* (pp. 221-238). Baltimore: Brookes.

Patterson, J., & Blum, R.W. (1996). Risk and resilience among children and youth with disabilities. *Archives Pediatric Adolescent Medicine, 150,* 692-698.

Patterson, J.M., Garwick, A.W., Bennett, F.C., & Blum, R.W. (1997). Social support in families of children with chronic conditions: Supportive and nonsupportive behaviors. *Developmental and Behavioral Pediatrics, 18,* 383-391.

Peterson, G.W., & Leigh, G.K. (1990). The family and social competence in adolescence. In T.P. Gullotta, G.R. Adams, & R. Montemayer (Eds.), *Developing social competency in adolescence* (pp. 97-138). Newbury Park, CA: Sage.

Primeau, L.A. (1998). Orchestration of work and play within families. *American Journal of Occupational Therapy, 52,* 188-195.

Raghavan, B. (1998). *An ethnographic study of Asian mothers of children with disabilities: Implications of cultural influences for health care professionals.* Unpublished master's thesis, Ohio State University, Columbus.

Rainforth, B., & Salisbury, C. (1988). Functional home programs: A model for therapists. *Topics in Early Childhood Special Education, 7,* (4), 33-45.

Rape, R.N., Bush, J.P., & Slavin, L.A. (1992). Toward a conceptualization of the family's adaptation to a member's head injury: A critique of developmental stage models. *Rehabilitation Psychology, 37,* 3-22.

Richards, L.N., & Schmiege, C.J. (1993). Problems and strengths of single-parent families: Implications for practice and policy. *Family Relations, 42,* 277-285.

Riley, K. (1998). *The experiences of mothers having children born with Apert syndrome: A qualitative study.* Unpublished master's thesis, Ohio State University, Columbus.

Rolland, J.S. (1987). Chronic illness and the life cycle: A conceptual framework. *Family Process, 26,* 203-221.

Sameroff, A.J., & Chandler, M.J. (1975). Reproductive risk and the continuum of caretaking causality. In F. Horowitz (Ed.), *Review of child development research (Vol. 4).* Chicago: University of Chicago Press.

Schimoeller, G.L., & Baranowski, M.D. (1998). Intergenerational support in families with disabilities: Grandparents' perspective. *Families in Society: The Journal of Contemporary Human Services, 79,* 465-476.

Schteingart, J.S., Molnar, J., Klein, T.P., Lowe, C.B., & Hartmann, A.H. (1995). Homelessness and child functioning in the context of risk and protective factors moderating child outcomes. *Journal of Clinical Child Psychology, 24,* 320-331.

Schulz, J.B. (1985). The parent-professional conflict. In H.R. Turnbull & A.P. Turnbull (Eds.), *Parents speak out: Then and now* (2nd ed.) (pp. 3-22). Columbus, OH: Merrill.

Schulz, J.B. (1993). Heroes in disguise. In A.P. Turnbull, J.M. Patterson, S.K. Behr, D.L. Murphy, J.G. Marquis, & M.J. Blue-Banning (Eds.), *Cognitive coping, families, and disability* (pp. 31-42). Baltimore: Brookes.

Seccombe, K., James, D., & Walters, K.B. (1998). "They think you ain't much of nothing:" The social construction of the welfare mother. *Journal of Marriage and the Family, 60,* 849-865.

Seligman, M., & Darling, R.B. (1989). *Ordinary families, special children: A systems approach to childhood disability.* New York: The Guilford Press.

Singer, G.H.S., & Irvin, L.K. (1989). Family caregiving, stress, and support. In G.H.S. Singer & L.K. Irvin (Eds.), *Support for caregiving families: Enabling positive adaptation to disabilities* (pp. 3-26). Baltimore: Brookes.

Slaughter-Defoe, D.T. (1993). Home visiting with families in poverty: Introducing the concept of culture. *The future of children: Home visiting* (pp. 173-183). Los Altos, CA: Center for the Future of Children.

Sparling, J.W., Berger, R.G., & Biller, M.E. (1992). Fathers: Myth, reality, and public law 99-457. *Infants and Young Children, 4*(3), 9-19.

Stallings, G., & Cook, S. (1997). *Another season: A coach's story of raising an exceptional son.* Boston: Little, Brown.

Stephens, T.M., & Wolf, J.S. (1980). *Effective skills in parent/teacher conferencing.* Columbus: Ohio State University, National Center for Educational Material and Media for the Handicapped.

Summers, J.A., Dell'Oliver, C., Turnbull, A.P., Benson, H., Santelli, E., Campbell, M., & Siegel-Causey, E. (1990). Examining the individualized family service plan process: What are family and practitioner preferences? *Topics in Early Childhood Special Education, 10,* (1), 78-99.

Sussenberger, B.B. (1998). Socioeconomic factors and their influences on occupational performance. In M.E. Neistadt & E.B. Crepeau (Eds.), *Willard & Spackman's occupational therapy* (9th ed.), (pp. 67-78). Philadelphia: Lippincott.

Thelen, E., & Smith, L.B. (1994). *A dynamic systems approach to the development of cognition and action.* Cambridge, MA: MIT Press.

Turnbull, A. P., & Ruef, M. (1997). Family perspectives on inclusive lifestyle issues for people with problem behavior. *Exceptional Children, 63,* (2), 211-227.

Turnbull, A.P., & Turnbull, H.R. (1990). *Families, professionals and exceptionality: A special partnership* (2nd ed.). Columbus, OH: Merrill.

Turnbull, A.P., & Winton, P.J. (1984). Parent involvement policy and practice: Current research and implications for families of young severely handicapped children. In J. Balcher (Ed.), *Severely handicapped children and their families: Research in review* (pp. 377-397). New York: Academic Press.

Turnbull, H.R., Guess, D., & Turnbull, A.P. (1988). Vox Pouli and Baby Doe. *Mental Retardation, 26,* 127-132.

Turnbull, H.R., & Turnbull, A.P. (1985). *Parents speak out: Then and now* (2nd ed.). Columbus, OH: Merrill.

Tymchuk, A.J., Andron, L., & Unger, O. (1987). Parents with mental handicaps and adequate child care: A review. *Mental Handicap, 15,* 49-54.

United States Bureau of the Census (1997). *Statistical abstract of the United States: 1997* (117th ed.). Washington, DC: U.S. Government Printing Office.

Vadasy, R.F., Fewell, R.R., & Meyer, D.J. (1986). Grandparents of children with special needs: Insights into their experiences and concerns. *Journal of the Division of Early Childhood, 10,* (1), 36-44.

Vincent, L.J. (1988, Fall). What we have learned from families. *Family Support Bulletin,* 3.

Vondra, J., & Belsky, J. (1993). Developmental origins of parenting: Personality and relationship factors. In T. Luster & L. Kodak (Eds.), *Parenting: An ecological perspective* (pp. 1-34). Hillsdale, NJ: Lawrence Erlbaum & Associates.

Weiss, K.L., Marvin, R.S., & Pianta, R.C. (1997). Ethnographic detection and description of family strategies for child care: Application to the study of cerebral palsy. *Journal of Pediatric Psychology, 22,* 263-278.

Werner, E. (1990). Protective factors and individual resilience. In S.J. Meisels & J.P. Shonkoff (Eds.), *Handbook of early childhood intervention* (pp. 97-116). Cambridge, MA: Cambridge University Press.

Werner, E., & Smith, R.S. (1989). *Vulnerable but invincible: A longitudinal study of resilient children and youth.* New York: Adams Bannister Cox.

Wolin, S.J., & Bennett, L.A. (1984). Family rituals. *Family Process, 23,* 401-420.

Young, D.M., & Roopnarine, J.L. (1994). Fathers' childcare involvement with children with and without disabilities. *Topics in Early Childhood Special Education, 14,* (4), 488-502.

Zemke, R., & Clark, F. (1996). Co-occupations of mothers and children, Introduction. In R. Zemke & F. Clark (Ed.), *Occupational science: The evolving discipline.* Philadelphia: F.A. Davis.

Ziskin, L. (1985). The story of Jennie. In H.R. Turnbull & A.P. Turnbull (Eds.), *Parents speak out: Then and now* (2nd ed.) (pp. 65-80). Columbus, OH: Merrill.

A Parent's Perspective

When I was first asked to contribute to this chapter, I reflected on the myriad of experiences and feelings that have emerged as a result of having children with disabilities. This seemed too vast a topic to be captured in a few typed pages. The following is a brief glimpse into my thoughts and feelings about life with my three disabled children. There is much more than facts or history about our lives. There is, of course, emotion—deep and undeniable—and there is poetry. There is the first shed tear of realization that my child will have a life that is more difficult than most. There is the happy smile of childhood shared with supportive therapists and teachers. There is the frustrated panic of adolescence, when social situations are hard and troublesome and when the phone does not ring on Saturday night.

Initial Response

Learning about the disabilities of each of my children came at different times in their lives. The impact varied, because of the timing of the news and the disability of each child. Benjamin was born on a warm June day in 1971. On the delivery table, the nurse turned the mirror away, and I didn't understand why I couldn't see the baby. Everything seemed to happen in slow motion. The physician held him up and announced that he was a boy, but there was a small problem. His right arm tapered from the elbow to a thumblike digit for a right hand, and his left arm ended in a modified claw hand, having a center cleft halfway into his palm and syndactyl webbing between the outside fingers.

The nurse placed him on my tummy and he peed a fountain all over the sterile drapes. She said, "That works," which was comforting, but scary, because I had not considered that other things could be wrong.

It was not until that night when I had him all to myself in the privacy of my own room, that I felt the bifid femur of his right leg; the block at his knee that refused to let it extend; the very thin lower leg, which turned out to be missing the tibia; and the clubfoot. I discovered all of these problems one at a time. The sick feeling in my stomach was guilt. There must have been something that I had done wrong that had caused this.

Even though I had followed all the doctor's instructions, I must have missed something. What would everyone think? I must not be good enough to have a child.

Mick, my husband, and I were lucky to have a wonderful pediatrician whose first advice was exactly what we needed to hear. He told us not to withdraw from our family and friends (alluding to the feelings of shame and guilt that we had not overtly expressed). He told us to allow them to give us support; that they would only want to help. The unspoken message that they would not judge us was very important.

And so we started on our journey of new experiences with orthopedic surgeons, prosthetists, genetic counselors, neurologists, urologists, internists, and pediatricians. Later came occupational therapists, physical therapists, ENT (ear, nose, and throat) specialists, vision therapists, special education teachers, and psychologists. We searched for answers to, "Why?" We searched for options to deal with the issues of discrepancies in leg length and hand function. We searched for resolution to our own feelings. But we were fortunate because, as husband and wife, we never blamed each other.

Mick and I started the journey together, and we have always turned to each other for support. Sometimes it was an "us against the world attitude" and a fierce, protective response that got us through the hard times. When joyous times came, they did so with the realization that it had taken all our efforts to get there. The reason that we have been able to deal with the problems and come out on top is that we have a commitment to each other and deep faith in God. This statement is much too simplistic for the deep feelings of need, grace, and oneness that we have. This oneness has allowed us to go forward to meet challenges as they have come.

Another reason we have been able to go forward is that we see each of our children as a gift. They are grace without gracefulness. They are charm without all the social skills. They are fun with a sometimes struggling sense of humor. They are individuals who have enriched our lives and given us humility, wonder, and awe at their commitment to living, loving and succeeding.

Accessing Services and Resources

Gaining services and resources for our children has not come without pain, questioning, depression, and anger. It has been a constant struggle. We faced the first barrier when we attempted to find the money to cover the costs of prosthetics and medical care for our son. When we were told that it would be better to amputate Benj's leg above the knee than try to keep it and work through the lack of joints and musculature, we were also told about the costs of prosthetics. One of the first things that our orthopedic surgeon told us was that we needed to find a source of funding, because prosthetics would cost more than a small house by the time Benj was 16.

I will not go into all the details, but I will give you a few insights into what parents must face when they do not know where to turn to find funds. The doctors have a few ideas, but they are not the source of information in this area. Agencies and hospitals may have more information, but getting connected to the right person to gain the information is not an easy task. A major stumbling block to searching and finding help is a set of feelings that include shame for "begging" and not being good enough to support the needs of the child yourself.

In the search for money to cover the costs of prosthetics, we approached a well-known agency because we knew that they worked with individuals who had physical disabilities. They had fundraising campaigns that were earmarked for this purpose. After being told that providing prosthetics was not among their services, and because this was the third or fourth rejection that we had encountered, Mick broke down and joined me with some tears. We were then informed that we had better "pull ourselves together." This was our child and our responsibility, and we had better "face it." Shame turned to anger as we left. I felt judged, and included in the anger was the fear that we would not be able to provide for Benj. How could this man judge us? Why didn't this administrator of an agency that provides services to children with disabilities and parents have more empathy for our situation? If he didn't help, then to whom could we turn?

This experience made us more leery of asking for assistance. Luckily, the Shriners accepted our application, and they provided most of the funds for Benj's prosthetics until he turned 18. I do not want to think of what might have happened if we had not had their help. Dealing with financial issues created a new level of trauma (from outside of the family) that was added to our earlier pain.

However, what we discovered from this process were the necessary, and valuable, aspects of networking. It was through work, friends, and family that we made contact with the Shriners. It was through people at school that we were put in touch with the local Special Education Regional Resource Center and became a part of the Parent Advisory Council. It was through many of the parents that we met in these places that we learned about

The Ohio Coalition for the Education of Children with Disabilities. It has always been invaluable to us to be able to share with other parents who have similar feelings, frustrations, and breakthroughs. If it had not been for these people and these agencies, we would not have received valuable personal, educational, and emotional support that we needed.

Whose Grief, Whose Struggle?

Many people have tried to describe the feelings that occur when a child with a disability comes into a family. The "grief cycle" (the same cycle that we go through when a loved one dies) is sometimes used to explain how families deal with the news that their child is disabled. When my children were small, the path of feelings about their disabilities could be set aside for the new dream of having the brightest, cutest, most-wonderful child with special needs. I dreamed of the well-spoken poster child. These dreams might have also been called denial and led others to believe that I was unaware of the true impact of my children's problems. In truth, that may have been so.

The feelings do not come from the big picture of the disability. They come from all the little incidents. For example, when Benj was 12 or 13 months old, I took him out of a nice warm tub of sudsy water and stood his chubby, slippery, little nude body next to the tub so he could hold on while I toweled him dry. He stood straight and tall on his left leg, but as I watched, he tried to bear weight on his useless, dangling right leg. He bent his left leg so that his right toes touched the floor, and then he leaned forward to see why he could not reach the floor with his right foot. It was a moment of revelation for me. Until that moment, I think that all the focus had been on me: my inadequacy, my problem, my pain. This was harder; it was too deep even for tears. This was Benj's life, his surgeries, his pain, and his inability to run swiftly through life. My role was to help and support him. Of course, every now and then I have my own private pity party. However, it is not my pain that is the issue; it is theirs. Somehow, for me, there is a deeper pain in watching someone I love struggle than the pain I feel when struggling myself.

In our minds, Jessica, our second child, had no disabilities through her first 5 years of life. She did have four eye surgeries by age 5 (due to crossed eyes and rotary nystagmus). During her preschool years, she attended a church-related preschool. At parent conference times, when the teacher would indicate problems or ask pointed questions about behaviors at home, I would justify Jessica's performance by telling myself, or Mick, that every surgery sets a child back about 3 months.

When Jessica was old enough to go to kindergarten, we were called into a special conference where they carefully told us that she was not ready to do so. I did not hear anything else that day. The impact of that statement and the carefully worded explanation was like an icy shower. It was almost as if I had awakened from a dream with a clear vision of how disabled and delayed my daughter really was. I felt guilty and ashamed. I am an occupational therapist, and I know developmental milestones. I had let my doctor and others calm my fears about delays in walking, ataxia, and fine-motor challenges because I did not want to believe that this second child of mine could have more than visual impairments. I was in denial for 5 years, helped by well-meaning people who did not want to hurt me. Jessica's diagnoses from her new physicians included: mild CP, amblyopia, monocular vision, strabismus, and minimal peripheral vision.

It's Okay to be this Way

One night after Jessica's conference, I received an answer to my prayer of "Where do I go from here?" I attended a presentation by Ken Moses, a psychologist and counselor who writes and speaks about parenting children with disabilities. I then experienced a new step on my journey. He spoke about the grief cycle and how we are grieving, not for a lost child, but for a lost dream. His discussion supported what I had been feeling and experiencing. The most important factor to me was the "permission" that he gave me to feel the way I did. He emphasized how important denial is in helping us to deal with life-affecting decisions. He pointed out that denial buys us the time to gather our resources so that we can deal head on with problems.

Ken Moses also spoke about the importance of recognizing that anger gives us the energy to take action. Many times our children's disabilities required so many appointments, surgeries, exercises, prescriptions, individual education plan (IEP) meetings, and other details, that I was left with only enough energy to put one foot in front of the other. I ignored, or put on hold, things or decisions that I should have taken care of immediately. Often, it was anger that got me off my duff and sparked my determination to get things done. I learned that unless anger is turned inward or unleashed on others, it can actually help. I came away from this talk with a sense of relief. To have these feelings was normal, and I was not a bad person, mom, or therapist. It continues to bother me when professionals criticize parents for being in denial. My position is that these parents don't yet have the resources that they need to deal with their child's disability. So give them some!

Where Do We Go From Here?

Decisions are forced on parents. There are medical decisions, therapy decisions, educational decisions, second-opinion decisions, as well as decisions made in the middle of the night and in the emergency room. There are some decisions that are avoided until the last possible moment. Decision making starts immediately with a diagnosis or

with the search for a diagnosis. What doctor should we use? What hospital? What about insurance? How much intervention do we need? How much do we want? What will they think if we say no to this "thing" that they think is important for our family? Is it important?

When Jessica was in elementary school, we would wait for the bus together. Each morning while sitting on our staircase landing, Jessica and I spent 20 minutes practicing "eye exercises." Some days it was easy; other days Jessica would complain, resist, and attempt to divert my attention from the task. One day, when she was 7 or 8 years old, we were doing her exercises and discussing her braces, her eye surgery, and her occupational therapy session scheduled for that afternoon. She wanted to know for the thousandth time why we had to do these things. I explained that we were trying to fix things so she would have an easier time of it. She suddenly looked up at me and asked, "Is there anything about me that you don't have to fix?" I quickly named all of her gifts and attributes that I treasured. Later, as Jessica's bus turned the corner, I was left sitting on the steps with feelings of emptiness and guilt. I also had a new insight into the impact of countless therapy sessions, surgeries, and home programs.

This incident also made me face another aspect of denial. There is an unavoidable fact that there are some aspects of disabilities that cannot be fixed. I became an occupational therapist so that I could help people and make things better for them. I truly believed (and believe) that I could help eliminate some problems, that I could help heal hurts, and that I could provide training so that people could be more independent. Once I "saw" Jessica's problems, I was off and running. I wanted to make up for lost time. Fear drove me to leave no stone unturned if I thought that it would help Jessica "get better."

There have been several types of denial that I have experienced: I denied that there was a problem. I denied my feelings about the problem. I denied that the problem may still exist, even after a lot of intervention. In the school setting, I denied that there were some areas that did not need to be addressed, and I pushed for intervention where it sometimes was not needed. Recently, I have recognized another form of denial: that helping our children with their schoolwork might create a dependency on others for that help. Mick and I always helped our children with their homework and school projects. I rationalized that their success with their schoolwork would help them achieve in life. Their work ethic for school was high. Unfortunately, because we provided continual support in completing their homework, they never had the opportunity to fail. It is now very clear to me that children have to learn responsibility for themselves, and that failure is a vital part of the learning process. I wanted to cushion my children's self-esteem by having them be successful in school. However, with the complex pattern of learning and growth, there is no clear path for children who have more challenges than most. Children with disabilities do need more help with schoolwork, but how much is too much? Lessons learned later are just as valuable, but they are more challenging because there is more at stake.

School

Other than their child's medical issues, qualifying for special education is one of the greatest traumas that a parent of a special-needs child will encounter. It is obvious that Benj has an orthopedic handicap. However, to qualify for special education we had to go through an intake process. Benj had to be tested, and we waited with baited breath. He did qualify, and Benj attended kindergarten through third grade in a school that had an orthopedic handicap program. He was in a self-contained classroom for disabled children until third grade.

When attention turned to education instead of surgeries and therapies, we found that physical disabilities are more apparent than learning disabilities. Soon our priorities switched to cognition and classroom skill building. During that time Benj was retained in first grade because the teachers had decided that he had a "learning disability." This evaluation provided another chance for the ever-present grief cycle to jump up and bite us. "Accepting" the physical part of the disability was almost in place. However, this new evaluation crushed my new dream of having the brightest, most socially adept, disabled child. I went through an equally (if not more so) bitter period of blame and self-pity. Once again, I also feared for his success.

When Jessica was tested, we requested the testing because the preschool had prepared us for the possibility that she would have trouble learning. The school said that it was too early to find a discrepancy, but we pursued it and one was found. She qualified for the learning-disabled program. For each of the next 5 years, Jessica's resource room moved from one school to another. This meant that each year she had to adjust to a new building, new teachers, and new classmates. When Jessica was in fourth grade, we were told to take her to counseling because she was withdrawn and had no friends on the playground. Guess why? When she was in the sixth grade, we moved to another district because it had neighborhood schools with special-education resources in each building. There, too, the resource room for her particular grade level was not in the neighborhood school. We couldn't win!

When Benj was in third grade, Mick and I decided that he would benefit from being in the regular classroom for most of his instruction. We were a little ahead of the curve regarding inclusion, and our request received quite a response! In 1980, Benj was a pioneer. That year was difficult for us because we decided to change priorities to allow the learning-disabled program to meet his needs. One of the most intimidating places in the world is a room full of educators, including heads of programs, psychologists, teachers, occupational therapists, and physical therapists. The only ones that believe that you are doing the right thing for the child seem to be you and your husband. Allowing the school's program to meet our son's needs turned out to be the right decision, but I still get stomach cramps when it is time for an IEP meeting (even an IEP meeting in which I am the occupational therapist).

When we find ourselves making judgments about families, a red flag needs to go up. As was pointed out earlier in this chapter, each family has a different structure and different values. Decision making in each family is complicated and sacred. I know many people thought we were crazy when we decided to have a third child. Some were even brave enough to tell us so to our faces. Service providers held their breath, and educators looked for another Ball child in their classrooms. Having another child was a decision about which Mick and I prayed. This time in our lives was like a pause in a heartbeat, filled with hope and fear, but also with the knowledge that we were in it together.

Alexander was born on a cold day in February of 1981. He had no physical problems, but he was just as colicky as the other two children. He walked at 9 months and never stopped after that. He was very busy. In preschool meetings, I was the one to point out discrepancies in Alexander's progress. The teacher complimented me on being accepting, and I carefully informed her that I had been through this twice before and had not been as accepting then. I told her that that was okay, too. My children had not fallen off the face of the earth because it took time for me to face their delays. They were doing just fine, and parents need to be allowed to feel the way they do. However, that did not mean that professionals should not be honest with them!

Receiving sympathetic and respectful honesty is the only way to know that I know I have all the facts before I make a decision. Honesty is a gift that you give parents. It does not mean that parents will hear you, that they will follow your suggestions, or even that you are always right. But your honesty gives parents a piece of the picture and the truth that they need to help their child succeed. It helps if you take the time to listen to parents' dreams, or if you help them put words to those dreams. Many times I could not even express my dreams because they were caught under the lump of fear deep in my soul. There were, and still are, weeks that I cannot deal with the long term. I can only take it one crisis at a time. There are days that I do not even know that I have a dream for my children. But there are other days when I clearly see the life that my children may achieve, and that is where I like to be.

Alexander has turned out to be borderline gifted and learning disabled, with attention deficit disorder and dyslexia. His disabilities were identified between kindergarten and first grade, again at our insistence. Alexander continues to reverse letters as he reads and writes. He often reads the end of words first. He once wrote out, in bold letters on a T-shirt, a commitment to avoid drugs: "Lust say on." Classic notes left for me on the kitchen counter often tell me that his "homework is bone" or the "bog has ben out."

Alexander's disability has also been difficult on me and my husband. The feelings of loss and sadness that accompanied identification and the knowledge that we had somehow failed resurfaced. Again I had to fight for services. I also had to watch him struggle through years of extra tutoring, vision therapy, and occupational therapy just to begin to decode words. Alexander has born the burden of being the articulate, social child. He has struggled with feelings of guilt that his disabilities are not as great as those of his siblings. He has received counseling to help him deal with these feelings as well as feelings of his own inadequacy.

However, part of Alexander's disability has been a gift for me. He always needed books read to him for school. When he could not get a particular book on tape, or he needed to complete one in a hurry, I have spent time reading with him. We have shared insights on comparisons of religions, how Native Americans smoke peace pipes, and how to save yourself if you become lost in the middle of a forest. It has been cherished time that would not have occurred if he had the ability to read on his own.

Gifts and Dreams

Recently, I heard that old saying, "I'm playing the hand I've been dealt." I think that applies to all of us. It seems to me that everyone has many sources of grief in their lives. We, as the parents of children with disabilities, can focus on the delays and the fears. We should be allowed to feel the feelings that are associated with this situation. However, I think that you'll find that most of us are proud of our children's accomplishments: learning to put on a prosthesis alone, learning to turn a somersault by herself, or hitting the right key on the keyboard to match the screen.

There are some things that our children will never be able to do; activities they choose not to attempt. Jessica has chosen not to pursue bike riding. Benj has chosen not to alternate his feet on the stairs. Alexander has chosen not to read piano music. All of these things would be next to impossible for them to do, but I never told them

that they couldn't do them. Parents are always in the position of encouraging the impossible. Because they are more objective, help givers and professionals think that parents are denying reality. However, the reality is that it is the child who will ultimately determine what he or she can or cannot do. We have made, and will make, many mistakes parenting our children with disabilities, but we refuse to let their disabilities limit the possibilities.

I remember crying over *The Velveteen Rabbit* when I read it to the kids. It seemed that the problems of my children kept them from being "real" too. But I knew that all the love that I was showering on them could not change their physical make up. However, I also knew that the love that I was showering on them might help them cope with their "realness." Benj has told me that he will run in heaven, and I believe that. I also know that they "run" in their hearts everyday here, and that others seeing them are challenged to be more themselves.

Benj is now 28 and has married a young lady with spina bifida. They are working towards independence in all areas of their lives. Jessica is working at a childcare center and just got courage enough to ask for a raise. Alexander just graduated and is planning to major in Recreation and Wildlife Management in college. As parents of children with disabilities, we continue to be very involved in our children's lives beyond the usual time. My dreams for them remain the same as when they were small: that they will be happy, that they will be as independent as they can be, and that they will always have someone who loves them. As the kids have grown into adults, we have had to practice involvement and support without control. We have also had to deal with our emotions, because the disabilities our children have are for life.

In all stages and all ages, families of people with disabilities value support and resources. If you take the time to hear a parent's dream, you may hear the sound of laughter and tears. You may hear the strong heartbeat of anger or the resistance to a life that is less than it can be. You are a gift to parents whose lives you touch. You have a solution to some of their frustration. You have the opportunity to be as honest as you can be and provide them with the information they need to make decisions. You are the answer to some parent's question. Thank you.

Editor's note: Beth Ball is the mother of three children with disabilities. She is also an occupational therapist and has worked in the school system a number of years.

chapter 6 Common Diagnosis in Pediatric Occupational Therapy Practice

Sandra L. Rogers
Catherine Yanega Gordon
Karen E. Schanzenbacher
Jane Case-Smith

key terms

Cardiopulmonary dysfunctions
Musculoskeletal disorders
Neuromuscular disorders
Traumatic brain injuries
Developmental disabilities
Pervasive developmental disorders
Toxic agents
Infectious conditions
Neoplastic disorders
Burn injury

■ CHAPTER OBJECTIVES

1. Describe the incidence, signs and symptoms, causes, and pathologic conditions of common medical diagnoses in children.
2. Describe the primary medical conditions associated with major developmental disabilities.
3. Explain how functional performance is affected by various medical and pathologic conditions.
4. Explain precautions and special considerations for working with children who have specific medical conditions.

This chapter is intended to familiarize the occupational therapist with some of the major medical conditions and diseases found in pediatric occupational therapy practice. Pediatric conditions can be differentiated in several ways: congenital or acquired, occurs at different stages of development, acute or chronic, stable or aggressive, discrete or pervasive, or body systems affected. None of these alone is totally satisfactory; however, the body systems approach is the simplest and most useful for educational and reference purposes.

This chapter is therefore organized in a body systems format and includes sections on traumatic brain injury, burn injury, and pervasive developmental disorders. The chapter provides information on the incidence and prevalence, signs and symptoms, causes, pathologic abnormalities, general medical treatment, and prognosis of the conditions described. Functional performance and treatment issues are also introduced. Pediatric psychiatric conditions are reviewed in Chapter 14, and neonatal medical conditions are described in Chapter 21. No single chapter can provide complete information about all conditions that may affect children. Many of the other chapters detail appropriate occupational therapy evaluation, planning, treatment, and follow-up guidelines. A list of more comprehensive medical texts is provided at the end of the chapter.

■ CARDIOPULMONARY DYSFUNCTIONS

This section addresses *cardiopulmonary dysfunctions,* which are conditions that affect the cardiac and respiratory systems of the infant and child. Included are congenital and acquired conditions that affect the child's health and ability to participate fully in life's occupations and roles.

Congenital Cardiac Defects

Most cardiac problems in children are congenital in nature or secondary to other conditions. When they occur, they are serious, frightening, and sometimes life threatening. This section discusses several of the major anomalies found in the heart and major vessels.

Congenital heart disease is the major cause of death in the first year (other than prematurity) and occurs in approximately 4 to 10 children per 1000 births (Wong, 1997). According to the Centers for Disease Control and Prevention (CDC), an average of 4423 babies are born in the United States each year with heart malformations (CDC, 1997).

Three major cardiovascular changes must take place at birth. The foramen ovale, the hole between the right and left atria, must close. In addition, the ductus arteriosus and ductus venosus must close to allow blood to flow to the lungs and to the liver, respectively. Many complications can arise when these changes do not occur. One of the most common conditions found in premature newborns is *patent ductus arteriosus* (PDA). In this condition the ductus arteriosus does not constrict, which can lead to heart failure and inadequate oxygenation of the brain. Treatment includes the administration of the drug indomethacin, which often triggers closure of the arterial wall. Surgery follows if the drug is not an effective treatment (Brook, 1998; Clark, 1997).

Another cardiovascular complication that may occur during the perinatal period is *intracranial hemorrhage.* This condition may occur prenatally, during the birth process, or postnatally. The site and the extent of the bleeding affect the prognosis. For example, extracranial bleeding, or cephalhematoma, is considered minor and usually does not cause permanent damage. Conversely, subdural, subarachnoid, and intraventricular hemorrhages are more serious and, depending on the extent of damage, may cause seizures, brain damage, cerebral palsy, and death.

The other major congenital malformities are *atrial septal defects* (ASDs), *ventricular septal defects* (VSDs), *tetralogy of Fallot* (TOF), and *transposition of the great vessels* (TGV). An ASD is an opening in the septum between the right and left atrial chambers (Figure 6-1). This opening may be any size and can occur anywhere along the septum. As a result, when the left atrium contracts, blood is sent into the right atrium. This is called a *left-to-right shunt* and causes more blood than normal to be sent to the lungs, resulting in "wet lungs," a condition that makes the lungs more susceptible to upper respiratory infections. Left-to-right shunt also causes the right atrium, and especially the right ventricle, to work much harder, and it can eventually cause heart failure in the older child. Symptoms include poor exercise tolerance and small size for age. Information for diagnosis is gathered from listening to the characteristic heart murmur, evaluating chest x-ray

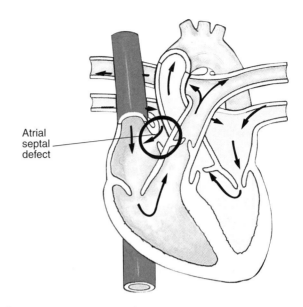

Atrial
septal
defect

figure 6-1   Atrial septal defect. *(From Wong, D.L. [1999].* Whaley and Wong's nursing care of infants and children *[6th ed.]. St. Louis: Mosby.)*

films and electrocardiograms, and performing echocardiograms or heart catheterization.

Surgical procedures are implemented if the child is in distress. The surgery may be performed early, or it may be postponed until the child is 4 or 5 years of age. Until that time the child is closely watched for complications, especially for signs of heart failure (Brook, 1998; Clark, 1997). VSDs are the most common type of congenital cardiac malformation and are often more serious than ASDs. The VSD consists of a hole or opening in the muscular or membranous portions of the ventricular septum (Figure 6-2).

In a VSD the blood flows from the left ventricle to the right ventricle (a left-to-right shunt), and as in an ASD, an increased amount of blood is pumped to the lungs. The defect is considered less serious if the opening is in the membranous section of the septum and more serious if there are multiple muscular holes (Brook, 1998).

Symptoms associated with VSDs include feeding problems, shortness of breath, increased perspiration, fatigue during physical activity, increased incidences of respiratory infections, and delayed growth. Causative factors are often idiopathic, but congenital infections, various teratogenic agents, and genetic predisposition may contribute to the cause (Clark, 1997; Monnett & Moynihan, 1991).

As in ASDs, the diagnosis of VSDs is based on the murmur, chest x-ray film results, electrocardiograms, echocardiograms, and heart catheterization. Improvement often occurs after 6 months of age, and more than 50% of the cases correct themselves by 5 years of age (Clark, 1997). However, if the extent of damage is great or if the hole

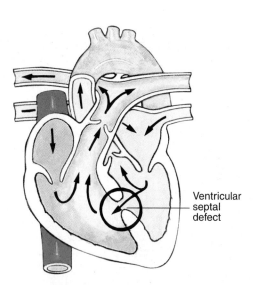

figure 6-2 Ventricular septal defect. *(From Wong, D.L. [1999]. Whaley and Wong's nursing care of infants and children [6th ed.]. St. Louis: Mosby.)*

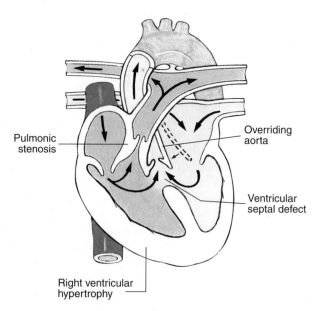

figure 6-3 Tetralogy of Fallot. *(From Wong, D.L. [1999]. Whaley and Wong's nursing care of infants and children [6th ed.]. St. Louis: Mosby.)*

does not repair itself, surgical procedures to close the defect may need to be performed early in the child's life.

Careful monitoring of children with VSDs must occur to prevent the life-threatening situation known as *Eisenmenger's complex,* in which pulmonary vascular obstruction has occurred as a result of prolonged exposure to increased blood flow and high pressure. Eventually the heart is no longer capable of pumping against the increased pulmonary pressure, the child goes into congestive heart failure, and blood pools in the right ventricle. This development is a medical emergency that requires immediate surgical intervention.

The prognosis for infants with VSDs continues to improve as surgical techniques and management of heart failure progress. These children are at risk for several serious complications, including cardiovascular accident (CVA), embolism, brain abscess, growth retardation, seizures, and death (Brook, 1998).

As its name implies, TOF is associated with four different problems: (1) pulmonary valve or artery stenosis with (2) VSD present prenatally, causing (3) a right ventricular hypertrophy and (4) an overriding of the ventricular septum by the aorta (Figure 6-3). Physiologically the unoxygenated blood that is returning from the body cannot easily exit to the lungs because of the pulmonary stenosis. Instead, it takes two paths of least resistance: the defect, creating a right-to-left shunt, and the aorta (Clark, 1997; Monnett & Moynihan, 1991).

Symptoms of TOF include central cyanosis, coagulation defects, clubbing of fingers and toes, feeding difficulties, failure to thrive, and dyspnea (Wong, 1997). The cause of TOF is probably similar to that of VSD. It

is believed that the insult to the developing fetus occurs in the early weeks of fetal development when the right ventricle is at a critical stage (De La Cruz, Gomez, & Cayre, 1991).

Diagnosis of TOF is usually based on cyanosis, analysis of the heart murmur, right ventricular hypertrophy and right axis deviation demonstrated on the electrocardiogram, a chest x-ray film showing the characteristic "boot-shaped heart," and echocardiography demonstrating the overriding aorta (Clark, 1997; Wong, 1997).

Initial management consists of medication, and surgery is delayed as long as possible. In severe cases a temporary shunt may be put in to bypass the stenosis. Usually the Blalock-Taussig surgical procedure is used until "total corrective surgery" can be performed, in which the pulmonary outflow obstruction is removed, the VSD is closed, and the aorta may be enlarged.

As with VSD, prognosis is improving as techniques and maintenance improve. The operative mortality rate has been reduced to 5% to 10%, but surgery is still a dangerous and complicated procedure (Brook, 1998; Wong, 1997).

TGV involves the anatomic transfer of the great arteries. Severity depends on the amount of circulatory mixing between the two sides. This can be accomplished by coexisting congenital cardiac defects, such as a VSD or a pulmonary stenosis, or congenital transposition of the ventricles, called *corrected transposition* (Brook, 1998). The severity of the symptoms varies, but cyanosis, congestive heart failure, and respiratory distress are common.

Diagnosis may be helped by the use of echocardiography, which can help identify the transposition, and by heart catheterization. Surgical treatment techniques include enlarging the foramen ovale by inserting a catheter with a balloon tip through the foramen ovale and into the left atrium. Next, the catheter is pulled back through the foramen ovale to enlarge it, thus increasing the flow of oxygenated blood to the right atrium (Brook, 1998). Another procedure involves excising the atrial septum and inserting a patch that redirects the blood flow. A third, more recently developed technique involves severing the great vessels at their bases and reattaching them to the proper ventricles. The operative mortality rate for TGV is 5% to 10%, regardless of the surgical procedure used. In later life these children have been known to develop arrhythmias and ventricular dysfunctions.

The child with congenital cardiac defects that have not yet been repaired can be expected to have reduced endurance for exertion but may be normal in other ways. This child will want to participate in a range of self-care and play activities. Pacing and selecting appropriate activities may be essential to the child's health and ability to participate in family and peer activities.

The involvement of the occupational therapist in congenital cardiac defects may be direct or indirect. For example, congenital heart defects are often found as secondary diagnoses in children with genetic syndromes. Children with Down syndrome or other types of mental retardation (MR) may have histories of congenital heart problems. In these cases, occupational therapists must be aware of the associated signs, symptoms, treatment procedures, complications of medications, and the effect of these conditions on the child's functioning.

Dysrhythmias

Irregular cardiac rhythms, or *dysrhythmias,* are not as common in children as in adults. However, the incidence of these problems is increasing, possibly because more children with congenital heart defects are surviving surgery, which may leave them with a residual dysrhythmia. Three classes of dysrhythmia exist: bradydysrhythmia, tachydysrhythmia, and conduction disturbances. Diagnosis is primarily based on standard and 24-hour electrocardiographic monitoring (Brook, 1998).

Bradydysrhythmia is marked by an abnormally slow heart rate. The most common is a complete heart block, or atrioventricular (AV) block. This condition is common after surgery or myocardial infarction and may occasionally require a pacemaker. Sinus bradycardia can be caused by anoxia or autonomic nervous system disorder. In this condition the child's heart rate may be reduced to less than 60 beats per minute and may have extra beats and slow nodal rhythms (Clark, 1997).

Tachydysrhythmia is an abnormally fast heart rate. Sinus tachycardia may be a symptom of several other conditions, including fever, anxiety, anemia, and pain. Supraventricular tachycardia (SVT) involves a rapid heart beat of 200 to 300 beats per minute and is among the most common disturbances in children. SVT is a serious condition that can lead to congestive heart failure. The child with SVT is irritable, eats poorly, and is pale. In some cases a vagal maneuver, such as the Valsalva maneuver, can reverse the SVT, but in others the child may require hospitalization, esophageal overdrive pacing, or synchronized cardioversion (Wong, 1997).

Conduction disturbances are common after surgery and may be temporary. Premature contractions may be atrial, ventricular, or junctional. These can sometimes be handled with interim or permanent pacing, depending on the nature and severity of the disturbance (Wong, 1997).

Neonatal Respiratory Problems

Respiratory problems are common in newborns and can be dangerous. Some of these problems are acute, and others are considered chronic lung diseases. Respiratory distress problems may be caused by prematurity, aspiration of amniotic fluid or meconium, malformations or tumors of the respiratory organs, neurologic diseases, central nervous system (CNS) damage, use of drugs, air trapped in the chest or pericardium (the sac surrounding the chest), and pulmonary hemorrhages (see Chapter 21) (Kliegman, 1998).

One of the acute respiratory problems often found in any newborn, especially preterm infants, is *respiratory distress syndrome.* This disease is caused by a deficiency of surfactant, the chemical that prevents the alveoli from collapsing during expiration. Because surfactant is not produced until about the 34th to the 36th week of gestation, many premature infants are born with this deficiency. As the air sacs collapse, oxygen absorption and carbon dioxide elimination are hindered. Treatment includes administration of surfactant and supplemental oxygen. Ventilator support may be needed. After 3 to 4 days of treatment, most infants begin to recover as surfactant begins to be produced by the infant's body. Some newborns develop chronic lung problems after respiratory distress syndrome (Kliegman, 1998).

Chronic lung disease implies a long-term need for supplemental oxygen. The chronic lung disease often seen in neonatal centers is *bronchopulmonary dysplasia* (BPD). Initially, these newborns would have had some type of acute respiratory problem that precipitated the prolonged use of mechanical ventilation and other types of necessary, but perhaps traumatic, interventions. In BPD, airways thicken, excess mucous forms, and alveolar growth is retarded. As a result, these children are often susceptible to respiratory infections and other respiratory problems. Problems such as BPD that are associated with the techniques used to save newborns' lives are called *iatrogenic disorders.*

The artificial respirators that are currently used are sophisticated and allow careful control of the oxygen mixtures. They are designed to maintain a constant pressure on the alveoli, thus keeping them open in the absence of surfactant. This is known as *positive end-expiratory pressure* (PEEP), which has significantly lowered the rate of fetal death and overall risk of severe developmental delays (Kliegman, 1998). At present, many newborns with respiratory distress are administered surfactant at birth, allowing them to breathe independently in spite of lung immaturity. Early administration of surfactant has greatly reduced the incidence of BPD and has improved mortality rates in very premature infants.

Asthma

Asthma is an obstructive disorder characterized by bronchial, smooth muscle hyperreactivity that causes airway constriction in the lower respiratory tract, difficulty in breathing, and bouts of wheezing. It is one of the most common long-term respiratory disorders of childhood. Most children who contract asthma have their first symptoms in early childhood, before 5 years of age (Boguniewicz & Leung, 1999). Asthma appears to be an inherited trait and is often associated with familial patterns of allergy.

Allergen exposure, smoking, cold air, exercise, inhalant irritants, or viral infection may trigger asthma attacks (Boguniewicz & Leung, 1999; Wong, 1997). Smooth muscle spasm of the bronchi and bronchioles and inflammation and edema of the mucous membranes with accumulations of mucous secretions characterize asthma attacks. The child has difficulty breathing, particularly in expiration. The forceful expiration through the narrowed bronchial lumen creates the characteristic wheezing. The child also has a hacking, nonproductive cough. This experience can be frightening for the child, and the symptoms may become more severe in response to this panic. The effort of breathing may also result in sore ribs and exhaustion. Status asthmaticus is a serious asthmatic condition in which medications typically prescribed do not improve the condition and emergency medical intervention is needed.

Treatment for asthma may include environmental control measures, skin testing, immunotherapy for allergies, emotional support, and a combination of pharmacologic agents, usually beta-adrenergic agonists and methylxanthine (Boguniewicz & Leung, 1999; Wong, 1997). These drugs may be related to school performance problems and in some cases can cause dependencies. Monitoring the child's schoolwork and teaching him or her the use and abuse of the medications should minimize difficulties in this area.

Children with asthma may be fearful of overexertion and may be concerned about contact with triggering allergens. This may result in a self-limited lifestyle. Assisting the child to manage the condition, respond calmly to stress, and pace activities can be essential to maintaining a normal childhood pattern. Structured peer group activities can also be useful in preventing social isolation. Breathing exercises, stretching, and controlled breathing can assist in managing the attacks.

Cystic Fibrosis

The most common serious pulmonary and gastrointestinal problem of childhood is *cystic fibrosis* (CF). This inherited disorder is related to a gene located on chromosome 7. CF is found in 1 in 1600 births among white children and 1 in 17,000 births among black children in the United States (Boat, 1996; Wong, 1997). CF is a multisystem disease that appears to be related to an impermeability of epithelial cells to chloride, causing the exocrine, or mucus-producing glands, to malfunction and their secretions to be thick, viscous, and lacking in water (Boat, 1996). These thick secretions block the pancreatic ducts, bronchial tree, and digestive tract.

One of the earliest signs of CF, *meconium ileus,* occurs in the newborn. A thickened, puttylike substance that cannot be eliminated blocks the small intestine (Wong, 1997). The abdomen becomes extended, and the child is unable to pass stools, with vomiting and dehydration occurring in the absence of treatment (Boat, 1996).

Chronic pulmonary disease is the most serious complication of CF. A chronic cough, wheezing, lower respiratory infections, abscesses and cysts, hemoptysis, and recurrent pneumothorax are examples of the serious pulmonary complications that develop in CF. Other complications often result from hypoxemia, nasal polyps, and enlargement of the right side of the heart (right ventricular hypertrophy), which may eventually cause heart failure (Wong, 1997).

Additionally, clients with CF typically have sodium absorption–inhibiting factor affected, which causes excessive amounts of sodium chloride to be secreted from the sweat glands onto the skin. Mothers may detect that their children taste salty when they kiss them. This alerts the physician, who will perform the simple diagnostic test known as the "sweat test." In this test an electrode is placed on the skin, causing the child to sweat at the contact site, and a sample of the sweat is taken. If excessive levels of sodium chloride are detected, the diagnosis is made.

Pancreatic insufficiency causes characteristic foul-smelling and greasy stools. Associated problems include malabsorption; clinical diabetes; deficiencies of vitamins A, E, and K; and gastrointestinal obstruction. In the liver, bile ducts also become blocked, resulting in destruction of cells behind the blocked ducts. Although this is a serious problem, a positive point is that children's livers are often capable of regeneration.

Medical management of CF consists of vigorous antibiotic, enzyme, and vitamin therapy and sound nutritional counseling. In an effort to keep the lungs as free as possible, the following physical or respiratory therapy techniques may be employed: mist tent therapy, intermittent positive pressure breathing, aerosol therapy, and postural drainage techniques (Tizzano & Buchwald, 1992).

The child with CF frequently spends time in and out of hospitals with various complications and for various treatments. These children may have a series of crises alternating with periods of comparative health, although there is a general degeneration that occurs. Children whose primary symptoms are gastric inflammation have a better prognosis than those whose initial problems are related to respiratory functioning. All require a careful balance of nutrition, fluid intake, and exercise. Boys generally have a longer life span than girls, but degeneration of body functions and death occur for many in their teens and early twenties (Wong, 1997). Early detection and treatment has been shown to prolong life. The child and family may need assistance in dealing with grief and impending death.

Medical, nursing, dietary, and respiratory therapy staff is central to the treatment of the child with CF. Respiratory therapists may have a key role in providing postural drainage, clapping, and chest expansion exercises. The occupational therapist may be concerned with energy conservation (activities that promote efficient breathing) and prevocational, recreational, and psychosocial support groups. Social, psychologic, and pastoral staff may provide essential family supports.

■ HEMATOLOGIC DISORDERS

Several hematologic disorders affect child development and function. This section addresses some of those most commonly seen by occupational therapists as primary or secondary diagnoses.

Sickle Cell Anemia

More correctly called *homozygous sickle cell disease,* *sickle cell anemia* (SCA) is a hereditary, chronic form of anemia in which abnormal sickle, or crescent-shaped, erythrocytes are present that contain an abnormal type of hemoglobin called *hemoglobin S* (Milne, 1990). In the United States most cases occur in black infants; the incidence is about 8% among black infants. SCA is rare in white infants but can be found in people of Hispanic, Middle Eastern, and Mediterranean ancestry (Wong, 1997). It is now possible to determine when this condition is present in the newborn. A few states require sickle cell screening for all newborns, and more states are considering this course of action.

The clinical course for children with SCA is interspersed with episodes of severe worsening called *sickle cell crises,* which can be grouped into four types (Evans & Rogers, 1990). Aplastic and hyperhemolytic crises are characterized by imbalances in the production and premature destruction of red blood cells. This may cause the hemoglobin to decrease by 50%, necessitating immediate transfusions. Sequestration crises consist of the sudden and rapid enlargement of the spleen. This type of SCA traps much of the blood volume and can cause shock or death. Painful, or vasoocclusive, crises are characterized by pain in the hands, feet, toes, and abdomen.

SCA affects other organs as well. Lungs may become infected, and hypoxemia is common; liver and kidney involvement causes urine problems and hematuria; CVAs may occur; the legs develop ulcers; and spleen damage can leave the child defenseless against major infections (Evans & Rogers, 1990). Additionally, children with SCA also experience chronic anemia, delayed growth, increased risk of septic infection, and delayed sexual maturation (Figure 6-4).

Sickle cell symptoms do not usually appear until the fourth month of life. However, screening can be done on the newborn with a blood test, the *Sickledex.* This test is followed by hemoglobin electrophoresis, which can provide a definitive diagnosis and allows for early identification and treatment (Wong, 1997). There is no cure for sickle cell disease. Treatment focuses on reducing the sickling phenomenon and treating the medical emergencies and their sequelae. Medical management includes bed rest, hydration and electrolyte replacement, oxygen therapy, analgesics, antibiotics, periodic exchange transfusions, and sometimes splenectomy (Wong, 1997). Bone marrow transplantation is being used in some cases and holds promise for a cure, but it is a painful and high-risk procedure.

Even with medical treatment, children with SCA may experience anoxia, CVAs, seizures, and cardiac failure. Disability and death are common (Milne, 1990). Rehabilitation and school-based professionals may provide treatment for the functional deficits created by these serious complications. Supportive counseling, activity adaptation, family support, and monitoring of the child's day-to-day functions are also important roles for occupational therapists.

Hemophilia

The *hemophilias* are a group of conditions characterized by prolonged clotting (coagulation) times and abnormal and excessive bleeding. This bleeding occurs any place in the body, after serious or minor traumas or spontaneously. There are two major types of hemophilia. Hemophilia A, or classic hemophilia, is caused by a deficiency of a factor in plasma necessary for blood coagulation. This factor has been called *factor VIII, antihemophilic globulin,* and *antihemophilic factor.* Hemophilia B (Christmas disease) results from a deficiency of clotting factor IX. The hemophilias are sex-linked hereditary disorders and occur almost exclusively in boys (Wong, 1997).

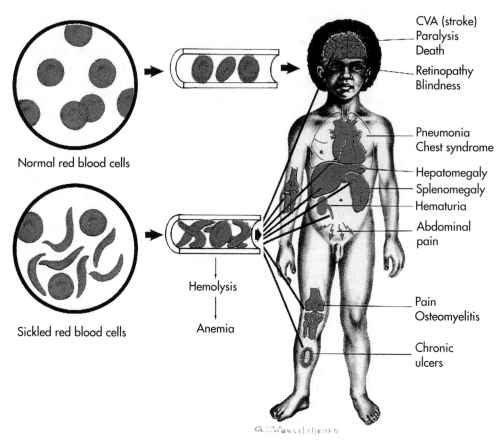

figure **6-4** Differences between normal and sickled blood cells. *(From Wong, D.L. [1999]. Whaley and Wong's nursing care of infants and children [6th ed.]. St. Louis: Mosby.)*

Symptoms are not usually noticeable or bothersome until near the end of the first year of life, when soft tissue hemorrhages begin to occur. Soft tissue hemorrhages and hemarthroses are treated at home by replacing the missing factor to a level that will again control the bleeding. This is called *replacement therapy*, and most children can be trained to administer their own infusions.

Bleeding into joints (hemarthrosis) can cause severe musculoskeletal problems that can lead to joint deterioration if untreated. Consequently, the child may have increasing difficulty with ambulation and functional activities. The following procedures can be used to protect the joints: blood can be drained from a joint, chemical agents can be injected into the joint, and specific preventive range-of-motion (ROM) activities can be initiated. Surgical procedures, such as joint replacements or synovectomies, contain some element of risk for hemophiliac clients (Radel, 1997). Recreational activities must be carefully chosen to avoid trauma, which can be frustrating and limit social interaction. Children with hemarthrosis may frequently miss school during crisis periods.

Prognosis for children with hemophilia depends on the management of the condition and on the avoidance of "bleeds" in critical organs. Intracranial hemorrhage is one of the most dreaded and serious complications of hemophilia. For older hemophiliac clients, acquired immunodeficiency syndrome (AIDS) is also a significant risk. It is estimated that 60% of the hemophiliac clients transfused before the 1980s, when HIV-screening programs were initiated, will acquire AIDS. As they reach the age when they become sexually active, client education related to safe sex is essential. With this exception the treatment of hemophilia has improved sufficiently over the last 20 years to make a normal life expectancy possible (Radel, 1997; Wong, 1997).

■ MUSCULOSKELETAL DISORDERS

Bone tissue is one of the few body tissues that actively regenerates itself. The skeletal system is malleable; it deposits or resorbs bone based on the stresses it receives. Elements of the skeletal system include the bones, joints, cartilage, and ligaments. The muscular system includes the muscle fibers and their covering of fascia; it is activated by the nerves and moves the bones to create functional motion. Tendons connect the muscular and skeletal systems at the origins and insertions of the muscles (Morrissy & Weinstein, 1996).

Bone is mesenchymal tissue. As the child develops, the bone is first laid down as either membranous or cartilaginous and gradually becomes ossified through a calcium deposition process. The bones are formed, initially, early in fetal development. The growth and ossification processes generally occur at the epiphyseal plates, which are located at the ends of the bones. This process continues until 25 years of age, at which time the epiphyses fuse (Morrissy & Weinstein, 1996).

The musculoskeletal system can be affected by genetic and congenital disorders, trauma, infection, and metabolic, endocrine, circulatory, and neurologic disorders (Morrissy & Weinstein, 1996). This section addresses some of the major *musculoskeletal disorders*.

Congenital Anomalies and Disorders

A relatively large number of conditions affecting the musculoskeletal system have a genetic or congenital cause. These conditions often affect the child throughout life, causing disability, deformity, and sometimes death.

Osteogenesis imperfecta (OI), also termed *brittle bones*, is a disorder characterized by decreased bone deposition probably because of the inability to form collagen. It is believed that an autosomal dominant gene transmits OI in most cases. However, the most severe fetal type appears to have an autosomal recessive inheritance pattern (Morrissy & Weinstein, 1996; Wong, 1997). This condition can run several different courses, from mild to severe, with most individuals having a milder form of the disease.

In all cases, however, the bones are unusually fragile, causing the child to fracture bones during minor traumas. The severity of the disorder varies greatly, depending on the time of onset (Table 6-1). Multiple fractures or repeated fractures to the same bone may cause a limb to become misshapen and eventually muscularly underdeveloped because of the long periods of immobilization and disuse. Prevention must be attempted at least with padded arm and leg protectors and orthoses. To provide internal support and to correct deformities that may develop, surgical procedures using metal rods and segmental osteotomies may be helpful. Unfortunately, as the child grows, the rods must be replaced to accommodate the growth.

Over time, children with OI can be expected to develop progressive deformities. Additionally, their activity patterns are affected by caution and time spent in casts. In the fetal and infantile types of this disorder, maternal education on handling and positioning is essential to prevent fractures during childcare activities. Children with OI need to be involved in movement activity, however, so that muscle strength and the postural effects of weight bearing and exercise can be achieved. Children with less severe forms of OI may participate in many normal activities, including some sports.

table 6-1	*Effect of Onset of Osteogenesis Imperfecta*	
Type	Severity	Effect
Fetal	Most severe	Fractures occur in utero and during birth. Mortality is high.
Infantile	Moderately severe	Many fractures occur in early childhood. Severe limb deformities and growth disturbances occur also.
Juvenile	Least severe	Fractures begin in late childhood. By puberty, bones often begin to harden and fewer fractures occur. Dental problems may be present.

Marfan's syndrome, or arachnodactyly, is attributed to an autosomal dominant trait and produces excessive growth at the epiphyseal plates, as well as skull asymmetry and changes in the joints, eyes, heart, and aorta. Joints are lax and hypermobile, and striated muscles are poorly developed. Visual problems are often present because of the dislocation of the lens (Morrissy & Weinstein, 1996). Symptoms include increased height and decreased weight for age, excessively long extremities, scoliosis, coxa vara, depressed sternum, stooped shoulders, elastic skin, and fragility of the blood vessels. A child with Marfan's syndrome may begin walking later than usual because of decreased postural stability, but the child need not have developmental delays. Treatment is symptomatic, addressing any skeletal deformities, such as scoliosis, that interfere with function.

Achondroplasia, or chondrodystrophia, is the most common cause of dwarfism. It is caused by stunted epiphyseal plate growth and cartilage formation. It is an autosomal dominant trait; frequent spontaneous mutations are known to occur. The limb bones continue to grow to appropriate widths but are abnormally short. It is rare for persons with achondroplasia to grow to more than 4 feet in height. Although skull size is normal, face size may be small, with a prominent forehead and jaw and a small nose. Trunk growth is near normal. Skeletal abnormalities include lumbar lordosis, coxa vara, and cubitus varus. There is no known cure for achondroplasia. Adults may experience back pain and, occasionally, paralysis caused by spinal stenosis. Surgical treatment may occasionally be necessary to relieve neurologic complications, improve functional movement, or correct extreme deformities (Morrissy & Weinstein, 1996; Salter, 1983).

Arthrogryposis multiplex congenita is characterized by incomplete fibrous ankylosis of many or all of the child's joints. Its cause is unknown, and it is probably not hereditary. The child has stiff, spindly, and deformed joints and may also have clubfoot, hip dislocation, or characteristic posturing. Knee and elbow joints may appear thickened. Muscles may be absent or incompletely formed. The anterior horn cells of the spinal cord may be absent, in which case the child may also experience paralysis. Treatment focuses on maintaining and increasing functional ROM and strength. Splints, casts, surgery, and daily stretching may be included in this regimen (Morrissy & Weinstein, 1996). Adapted equipment and training for activities of daily living (ADLs), school, play, and work performance may assist the child with arthrogryposis multiplex congenita.

A common abnormality of the foot is *congenital clubfoot*, or *talipes equinovarus*. The incidence of congenital clubfoot is high (1 to 2 per 1000) and much higher in cases where a sibling has clubfoot (1 in 35). In 1997 over 3200 infants were born with clubfoot and boys were affected twice as frequently as girls (CDC, 1997; Morrissy & Weinstein, 1996). The condition may be unilateral or bilateral, with the major clinical features consisting of forefoot adduction and supination, heel varus, equinus of the ankle, and medial deviation of the foot (Figure 6-5). Some of the bones involved may be malformed, and the muscles of the lower leg are often underdeveloped. In a small number of cases paralysis and permanent deformity may be present.

In some cases clubfoot is associated with other congenital problems and conditions, but the exact cause or causes of clubfoot are unclear. During fetal development, something adversely affects the development of the muscles on the medial and posterior aspects of the legs, causing them to be shorter than normal (Morrissy & Weinstein, 1996). These contractions, in turn, lead to the bone and joint problems. The clubfoot deformity can be corrected either through serial casting or with orthopedic surgery. The soft tissue surgeries may be combined with bony operations such as arthrodesis of joints, osteotomies, and the insertion of a bone wedge on the medial side of the calcaneus to correct the line of weight bearing (Morrissy & Weinstein, 1996). This treatment reduces foot mobility but increases function

and stability. Prognosis is good for children who are treated early.

The analogous condition in the upper extremity, *congenital clubhand*, is far less common and is associated with partial or full absence of the radius and bowing of the ulnar shaft. Radial musculature, nerves, and arteries may be absent or underdeveloped as well. Often the hand remains functional. Treatment includes progressive casting and ROM, static or dynamic splinting, or surgery; however, these procedures provide more cosmetic than functional benefit. The child with congenital clubhand may occasionally require some training or adaptations for school or ADLs.

Congenital dislocation of the hip is almost as common as clubfoot, occurring in 1.5 per 1000 live births (Salter, 1983). It is often bilateral and occurs five times more commonly in girls than in boys (Morrissy & Weinstein, 1996). The causes of congenital hip dislocation (head out of socket) and subluxations (head partially out of socket) are both genetic and environmental. Hip laxity may be genetically inherited or may be a result of a hormonal secretion of the uterus. Environmental factors related to hip dislocation include birth complications from uterine pressure and poor presenting positions. In addition, dislocation or subluxation of the unstable hip may be caused by sudden, passive extension or by positioning that keeps the legs extended and adducted.

Early diagnosis of congenital dislocation of the hip is critical because delay can cause serious and permanent disabilities. Three clinical observations that may be used in diagnosing this condition in infants are Ortolani's sign, Galeazzi's sign, and Barlow's test. Ortolani's sign is identified by flexing the infant's knees and hips, alternately adducting and pressing the femur downward, and then abducting and lifting the femur. If the hip is unstable, it will dislocate when it is adducted but can reduce back into the socket as it is abducted. The evaluator feels and often hears a "click" as this happens. Galeazzi's sign consists of one knee being lower than the other when the child is placed in the supine position on a table with knees flexed to 90 degrees. This results from the dislocated femur lying posteriorly to the acetabulum. A positive Barlow's test oc-

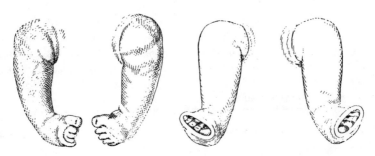

figure **6-5** Bilateral congenital talipes equinovarus. **A,** Before correction. **B,** Undergoing correction in plaster casts. *(From Brashear, H.R., & Raney, R.B. [1986]. Handbook of orthopedic surgery [10th ed.]. [p. 39]. St. Louis: Mosby.)*

curs when the unstable hip clicks out of the acetabulum when the leg is abducted and pressure is placed on the medial thigh (Morrissy & Weinstein, 1996).

In the older child with congenital hip dislocation, a Trendelenburg's sign is seen. Trendelenburg's sign consists of the hip dropping to the opposite side of the dislocation and the trunk shifting toward the dislocated hip when the child is asked to stand on the foot of the affected side.

If treatment is begun within the first few weeks of life, normal development of the hip can nearly always be ensured. The longer the dislocation goes unresolved, the poorer the prognosis. Specific treatment techniques vary according to the age of the client when treatment is initiated, but generally the techniques, ranging from those used on the younger child to those used on the older child, include stabilizing the hip in an abducted and flexed position to facilitate femoral and acetabular development. This stabilization may be accomplished with the use of splints, traction, the hip spica plaster cast, or the pillow splint (Morrissy & Weinstein, 1996). If these methods do not correct the problem, several surgical procedures may be used to correct bony and soft tissue problems. In severe cases, arthrodesis or total replacement arthroplasty may be performed. Again, every infant should be examined for this deformity in the first weeks of life to prevent the complications that this defect can cause.

Hypoplasias or aplasias are relatively rare but do occur in the fibula, tibia, and femur (limiting gait and stability) or in the clavicles and the radius. Other congenital defects occasionally seen are *Sprengel's deformity* (congenital high scapula), recurvatum of the knee, and alignment deformities.

Limb Deficiencies

Limb deficiencies in children are most commonly attributable to congenital malformations. A small number occur also because of accidents or electively to prevent the spread of cancer, such as Ewing's sarcoma. Congenital limb deficiencies occur more frequently in the upper extremities. Limb deficiencies and malformations may be familial, or they may result from early fetal insult or, rarely, from congenital constricting bands. In the latter case the soft tissue and overlying skin on a small body part fail to grow in circumference. If this is severe enough, the band stops distal limb circulation, causing gangrene and intrauterine amputation (Morrissy & Weinstein, 1996; Salter, 1983). Traumatic amputations are becoming less common because of better emergency care and the improved ability of surgeons to reattach a traumatically removed body part. Congenital malformations of the hands or feet occur in 1 of every 600 live births, usually in the fingers and toes (Morrissy & Weinstein, 1996). The CDC (1997) reported that over 3200 babies are born with polydactyly, syndactyly, or adactyly each year.

Polydactyly is an excess of fingers or toes. This is relatively common and may consist of one or more extra complete digits or duplication of only part of a digit. There may be bony changes or just extra soft tissue. In most cases surgical amputation or reconstruction are completed early in childhood, particularly if the hand is involved. *Syndactyly,* or webbing between the fingers or toes, occurs frequently. It is most common in the upper extremity and in boys. It sometimes coexists with polydactyly, which makes repair more complicated. In simple cases the fingers are surgically separated in early childhood (Morrissy & Weinstein, 1996; Salter, 1983). Extensive hand therapy is usually unnecessary, although splinting and scar reduction may be helpful in some cases. *Bradydactyly* and *microdactyly* are overly large or small digits, respectively. Plastic surgical techniques may be used if the digits involved are unsightly or impair function.

Congenital limb deficiencies include amelia, phocomelia, paraxial deficiency, and transverse hemimelia (Figure 6-6). *Amelia* is the absence of a limb or the distal segments of a limb. In *phocomelia* the child may have a full or partially formed distal extremity but is missing one

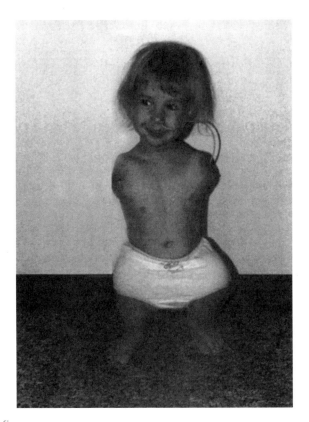

figure 6-6 Child with multiple congenital limb deficiencies, including bilateral transverse upper arm deficiency and bilateral proximal femoral focal deficiency. *(From Stanger, M. [1994]. Limb deficiencies and amputations. In S. Campbell [Ed.], Physical therapy for children. New York: W.B. Saunders.)*

or more proximal segments of the limb. In *paraxial deficiencies* the proximal part of the limb is correctly developed, but either the medial or lateral side of the rest of the limb may be missing. *Transverse hemimelia* is the amputation of a limb segment across the central area. It is common for a child with malformation of one body part to have bilateral or hemilateral problems.

Children with congenital limb deficiencies may require surgery for removal of skin flaps or "nuisance" parts if they interfere with function. It is common for children to have some shoulder, trunk, and rib asymmetries as well. These children are fitted with prostheses as early as 2 months but usually by 6 months of age. This allows the child to incorporate the prosthesis into his or her body image; it promotes balance, prevents scoliosis, facilitates bilateral function, and reduces dependence on the residual limb for tactile input. A multidisciplinary prosthetic team often follows the child's development into adolescence and his or her family.

Initial prostheses often have fixed knees or elbows to simplify prosthetic operation. Young infants with upper extremity amputations are often given a passive mitt, or a terminal device (TD) without cabling. This allows the child to hold objects that are placed in the hand and to develop early eye-hand skills. As the child grows and matures, new prostheses are fabricated that reflect the child's increased size and skills. Active TD use is instituted between 15 and 24 months of age; elbow operation, if necessary, is not introduced until the child is developmentally able to operate the mechanism. As expected, this process is more complex for upper extremity amputees than for lower extremity amputees and for children with multiple amputations.

Acquired limb deficiencies are treated much like those of adults, except that tasks must be developmentally structured and sequenced. Bimanual activities for play, school, and self-care are emphasized. Independent donning, doffing, and care of the prosthesis are also part of the treatment process for school-age children. The child needs to be taught ADL skills, with and without the prosthesis, and may require assistance and adaptations for some school, work, and play tasks. Occasionally, children experience overgrowth of the long bones, causing pain and, if severe enough, skin penetration and infection. Conservative skin stretching and surgical revision may be necessary (Morrissy & Weinstein, 1996). Psychosocial, self-concept, and social play experiences may assist these children, particularly as they approach puberty.

Juvenile Rheumatoid Arthritis

Rheumatoid arthritis is a systemic disease that affects every aspect of an individual's life. It is characterized primarily by inflammatory changes and destruction to the synovial joints (Figure 6-7). Largely a disease of adults, rheumatoid arthritis can also affect children (Melvin,

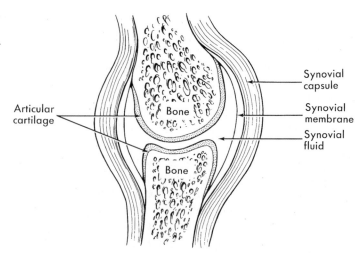

figure 6-7   Components of a typical synovial joint.

1989). *Juvenile rheumatoid arthritis* (JRA) is a major cause of physical disability in children younger than 16 years of age. Approximately 250,000 children in the United States suffer from some form of this disease (Morrissy & Weinstein, 1996). JRA usually begins between 2 and 4 years of age and is more common in girls (Salter, 1983; Wallace & Levinson, 1991).

The exact cause of JRA is unknown, but the following factors are believed to play undefined roles in its cause: genetics, emotional trauma, histocompatibility antigens, viruses, and antigen-antibody immune complexes (Morrissy & Weinstein, 1996).

JRA is usually described as taking three different forms: (1) pauciarticular, (2) polyarticular, and (3) systemic, or Still's disease. The pauciarticular form usually affects only a few joints. Involvement is often asymmetric, and there are few or no systemic manifestations. The joints most often affected are the knee, hip, ankle, and elbow. Overgrowth in the long bones surrounding the inflamed joint often causes gait problems and flexion contractures. Many children suffering from pauciarticular JRA develop iridocyclitis, an inflamed condition of the iris and ciliary body of the eye that can lead to blindness if not treated.

In polyarticular JRA, onset is often abrupt and painful, with symmetric involvement of the wrist, hands, feet, knees, ankles, and sometimes the cervical area of the spine. Other symptoms include a low-grade fever, malaise, anorexia, listlessness, and irritability.

Systemic JRA, or Still's disease, consists of polyarticular symptoms plus involvement in other organs, such as the spleen, and in the lymph nodes (Morrissy & Weinstein, 1996). Signs and symptoms include high fever, rash, anorexia, enlargement of the liver and spleen, and an elevated white blood cell count. Epiphyseal plates adjacent to an affected joint may initially show an acceleration of growth but later may be destroyed, causing local growth delay.

Medical management primarily centers on the use of the following therapeutic drugs (in order of preference): salicylates; nonsteroidal antiinflammatory analgesic drugs; gold salt injections; and adrenocorticosteroids (Rennebohm & Correll, 1984; Salter, 1983). Surgical repair and reconstruction are seldom recommended for children. Other forms of treatment may include splinting, active and passive ROM, and monitoring of joint motions to maintain maximal function and prevent deformity.

The prognosis for JRA varies, depending on a number of factors, but it is important to remember that the largest percentage of children (with the pauciarticular type of JRA) recover completely within 1 to 2 years. Only about 15% of all children with the JRA will have permanent disabilities (Wallace & Levinson, 1991).

Children with JRA may have pain at times, may show signs of fatigue, and may have reduced ROM in one or more joints. As a result they may have difficulty performing ADLs and certain school tasks. Adaptive equipment such as pen and pencil grips, dressing aids, and built-up handles on utensils or other adaptations to feeding equipment often improve functioning and reduce fatigue and stress on joints. Seating needs must be monitored to help reduce fatigue and prevent harmful pressure on joints.

Play and recreational activities may be adapted to allow full participation and to maintain strength and ROM. Children with severe deficits may require prevocational evaluation and treatment. Child and parent education in joint protection and energy conservation techniques is essential for children with JRA at all ages and stages.

Soft Tissue Injury

Children, being active and busy, are frequently subject to traumatic injury, particularly soft tissue injury. *Contusions* include damage and tears to the soft tissue, skin, muscles, and subcutaneous tissue. When they occur, an inflammatory response results and the child experiences pain, swelling, and hemorrhagic responses. Contusions are usually not serious in the normal child but can be difficult for children with disordered response to trauma, such as hemophilia. *Crush injuries* are common in children (e.g., fingers caught in doors), can also involve bone and nails, and may swell and be painful.

A *dislocation* occurs when forces on the joint pull or push the joint out of its socket. This injury creates obvious problems in alignment, deformity, and immobility. Dislocations should be reduced as soon as possible so that inflammation does not increase the pain and difficulty of this procedure. After reduction the child's extremity is usually immobilized for some time to allow healing. If the forces exerted on the ligaments are strong enough to tear them, the injury is called a *sprain*. These

forces also may damage muscles, nerves, tendons, and blood vessels in the area. There are several "special" tests for joint laxity that are used for sprain evaluation. Pain may or may not be severe, but swelling and favoring the extremity usually occur. Sprains must be positioned and immobilized for an extended period and, in severe cases, may be casted or splinted for 3 to 6 weeks.

Fractures

Fractures are extremely common in children. Fractures can occur prenatally and perinatally in children with other pathologic conditions but are uncommon in normal infants. As the child grows older, however, and as independence and activity levels increase, children may be injured in automobile, skateboard, and bicycle accidents; in falls; and while participating in sports. Childhood fractures can also be caused by child abuse. Any child with an unusually high number of fractures may trigger an investigation into the possibility that abuse has occurred.

Fractures may be classified in many ways. An *open,* or compound, fracture refers to an open wound or penetration caused by an object outside the body or caused by the bone penetrating from within the body. A *closed* fracture indicates that no penetration has occurred. Open fractures present added complications because the wound must be closed in addition to treating the fracture. The risks of infection and soft tissue and nerve damage are higher with the open fracture, and complications are more common (Morrissy & Weinstein, 1996).

The fact that bones are displaced and malaligned often complicates traumatic fractures. Figure 6-8 shows some of the most common types of malalignment caused by serious fractures.

Children's fracture patterns are not identical to those of adults. Their bones may buckle or bend rather than break because their bones are thinner and less solid. *Greenstick* fractures occur when the bone is not completely separated on one side, much as a twig breaks when bent. Sometimes the bone breaks completely, but the periosteal covering remains intact, holding the fragments together. This *periosteal hinge* may assist or complicate fracture reduction. *Comminuted* fractures occur when multiple fragments are created by the injury (Morrissy & Weinstein, 1996).

Children's ligaments are often stronger than their epiphyseal plates. Therefore when stress is applied, it is more common to find a fracture than a dislocation or sprain. Fractures involving the epiphyseal growth plate, which account for 15% of childhood fractures, are of particular concern because they may affect the growth and alignment of the bone and the integrity of the joint in later life. The type of problem and its severity depend on the location and extent of the injury in relation to the growth plate. Figure 6-9 illustrates the Salter-Harris classification system (Salter, 1983). Under this system the

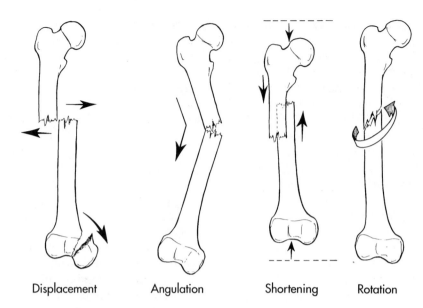

Displacement   Angulation   Shortening   Rotation

figure **6-8**   Types of malalignment caused by fractures.

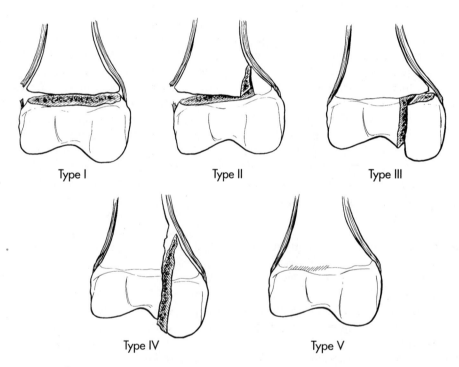

Type I   Type II   Type III

Type IV   Type V

figure **6-9**   Salter-Harris classifications of epiphyseal plate injuries.

more severe injuries are given higher numbers. Injuries that cross the joint surface are generally the most serious because they may result in uneven growth on the joint surface and therefore impair the normal slide, glide, and alignment of the joint in adolescence and adulthood.

Treatment of fractures requires open or closed reduction, or realignment, of the bony fragments and immobilization until the bone heals. Open surgical reduction is rare in children but may be performed for injuries to the

growth plate and serious compound or comminuted fractures (Salter, 1983). Fractures in children heal more quickly than those in adults. Young children and infants may heal in 2 to 4 weeks and school-age children in 6 weeks. Adolescents require immobilization for the same 8 to 10 weeks required by adults with similar injuries (Morrissy & Weinstein, 1996; Wong, 1997).

Immobilization is usually by means of a cast, although in severe cases, pins, traction, and external fixation may be used. The advent of synthetic, fiberglass, and polyurethane resin casting materials are an advantage for children because these materials are waterproof and come in bright colors. Casted children should be checked to ensure that circulation and skin integrity are maintained under the cast and that the cast is not breaking down from active use. The child in traction may need adapted devices and activities to maintain independence while he or she is immobilized. Prevention of skin breakdown is also a concern for any individual for whom bed rest is prescribed.

Torsion Deformities

Particularly in children, prolonged twisting forces may cause changes in epiphyseal plate growth, causing the long bones to twist in the direction of the abnormal force. These are known as *internal, external,* or *combinational torsional deformities.* For example, "toeing out" is common in young children. This deformity is characterized by externally rotated feet and knees and by limited internal rotation of the femur. It is often seen in infants who habitually sleep in the prone position with their legs externally rotated, causing external femoral torsion. Conversely, children who spend a great deal of time sitting on the floor with knees in front, feet out to the side, and femors internally rotated (the "television position," or "W-sitting"), may begin to "toe in," resulting from the internal femoral tension.

Bowlegs, or genu varum, is an example of a deformity caused by combinational torsional forces (i.e., prolonged internal torsion to the tibia and external torsion to the femur). This deformity is often present at birth because of prenatal posturing, but it usually corrects itself unless compounded by specific neuromuscular problems or unusual sleeping and sitting postures that continue to apply the abnormal torsions.

Curvature of the Spine

Lordosis, kyphosis, and *scoliosis* are the terms used to describe the three major deformities of the spine. These conditions may occur functionally, posturally, and structurally; they may be secondary to muscle imbalance, bony deformities, or other pathologic conditions such as cerebral palsy; or they may occur idiopathically. They may be congenital or acquired. In most cases the cause of these disorders is unknown; however, some familial patterns exist.

Lordosis is an anteroposterior curvature in which the concavity is directed posteriorly. Also called *hollow back,* this condition is often secondary to other spinal deformities or anterior pelvic tilt. It is usually predominantly in the lumbar area of the back and is occasionally painful. It can also be secondary to extreme obesity, hip flexion contractures, or conditions such as muscular dystrophy. Lordosis also may occur during the adolescent growth spurt experienced by many girls. Treatment focuses on correcting the underlying conditions, stretching tight hip flexors, and strengthening abdominal musculature. Postural training and occasionally, in severe cases, back bracing is included.

The opposite anteroposterior curvature, with the convexity posterior, is called *kyphosis.* Also called *round back,* and in adolescents *Scheuermann's disease,* the curvature is usually primarily in the upper back. This deformity is common in children and adolescents and is usually secondary to faulty posture. This is particularly true as the teenage girl's skeletal growth outpaces her muscular growth. The deformity can occur in children with spina bifida cystica or arthritis. Treatment depends on the cause and severity of the problem. In mild cases, postural training and strengthening activities such as weight training, swimming, and dance are often useful. In severe cases, Harrington rods may be used to guide and support the spine (Morrissy & Weinstein, 1996).

Scoliosis is the most common and serious of the spinal curvature disorders. Treatment is considered when a lateral curvature of more than 10 degrees is present. Lateral curvature of the spine is often accompanied by rotation of the vertebral bodies. Functional scoliosis is flexible and can be caused by poor posture, leg length discrepancy, poor postural tone, hip contractures, or pain. Congenital scoliosis is usually structural in nature, caused by abnormal spinal or spinal cord structure. Diseases of the nervous system or spine also may create a scoliosis. However, most scoliosis has no known cause.

Scoliosis is rarely painful. About 85% of the cases occur in girls. Diagnosis is based on careful examination and history. If preliminary evaluation and palpation suggest the condition, radiographic analysis is also performed. Structural scoliosis often progresses over time; the vertebral bodies may become wedge shaped and rotate toward the convex part of the curve, and the intervertebral disk may shift and deform (Morrissy & Weinstein, 1996). Curves of less than 20 degrees are considered mild. Those of more than 40 degrees may result in permanent deformity, and those of 65 to 80 degrees may result in reduced cardiopulmonary function. Skin breakdown between the ribs and pelvis may also develop in some cases.

Treatment is usually started early and focuses on postural exercises, maintaining ROM, and strengthening abdominal and spinal musculature. However, these treatments have been found to be of limited value in most cases. If the condition continues unchanged or worsens, surgery and internal fixation of the spine are the usual course of treatment. Common fixation systems are Harrington rods, Luque rods, or Dwyer cable, or a combination of these. Postoperative physical therapy and adapted ADLs are sometimes needed; in general, children and adolescents progress well after surgery and maintain a normal lifestyle into adulthood.

■ NEUROMUSCULAR DISORDERS

Children with *neuromuscular disorders* constitute a large percentage of the clients of occupational therapy practice. Several conditions exist in which the neurologic system is impaired, interfering with the child's ability to interact effectively with the environment. The site of damage may be the brain, spinal cord, peripheral nerves, neuromotor junction, or the muscle itself. It may interfere with the reception and processing of sensory input, the ability to act effectively on the environment, or a combination of these. Neuromuscular deficits may occur before, at, or after birth. This section addresses several of the major conditions in this category.

Cerebral Palsy

Cerebral palsy (CP) is characterized by nonprogressive abnormalities in the developing brain that create a cascade of neurologic, motor, and postural deficits in the developing child. Although a pattern of motor and postural deficits is a defining feature of CP, many secondary disorders typically coexist with this diagnosis. Cognitive, sensory, and psychosocial deficits often compound motor impairments and subsequent functioning (Pellegrino, 1997). Although CP is usually the result of injury or disease at or before birth (congenital CP), children injured in early childhood display similar symptoms and are sometimes classified as having CP (acquired CP). CP is expressed through variable impairments in motor and postural control, coordination of muscle action, and sensation that are typically classified according to the type and distribution of motor impairment (Miller & Clark, 1998).

CP is estimated to occur in 1. 4 to 2. 4 of 1000 live births, and although this has remained constant over a 30-year period, the causes have changed. Because of a rise in the survival rate of very premature infants in both very low birth-weight and extremely low birth-weight categories, a rise in the incidence of CP has been noted for spastic diplegia, often associated with prematurity and low birth weight. On the other hand, athetotoid CP, often attributed to fetal anoxia and hyperbilirubinemia, has decreased in developed countries (Pellegrino, 1997). It is estimated that 5000 infants and 1200 to 1500 preschool children are diagnosed with CP each year.

The various causes of congenital CP can be grouped according to premature birth or term birth. Prematurity now accounts for the majority of known causes for CP because of a preexisting brain abnormality. This increased rate may be associated with the CNS's vulnerability to insult (i.e., increased sensitivity to bleeding near the lateral ventricles, which has a cascading effect on further CNS development) during gestational weeks 26 to 32.

CVA, developmental brain abnormalities, placental abruption, fetomaternal hemorrhage, placental infarction, and maternal exposure to environmental toxins have also been associated with CP. In addition, maternal infections such as cytomegalovirus, syphilis, varicella virus, and toxoplasmosis can be secondary causes of CP. Causes of acquired CP include trauma, intracranial hemorrhage, CNS infections, near drowning, hypoxia, and metabolic disorders.

Early diagnosis of CP is important to elicit the services that the child and family may need to optimize the child's potential for development and to prevent secondary disabilities. To develop a definitive diagnosis, a team of developmental specialists conducts thorough physical and developmental evaluations. These evaluations usually take place over a period of months in early development. The team may include a pediatrician, an occupational and a physical therapist, a developmental nurse, and a speech and language pathologist. Retention of primitive reflexes and automatic reactions, variable tone, hyperresponsive tendon reflexes, asymmetry in the use of extremities, clonus, poor sucking or tongue control, and involuntary movements may indicate the presence of CP. Additionally, motor delays coupled with delays in other developmental areas or with a discrepancy in cognitive development are strong indicators. Infants who weigh less than 1500 grams at birth are particularly vulnerable and need to be monitored closely (Pelligrino, 1997). Each child with CP has a unique set of problems. Comprehensive ongoing medical assessment is necessary in children diagnosed with CP to treat proactively medical sequellae associated with CP.

Characteristically, the child with CP shows impaired ability to maintain normal postures because of a lack of muscle coactivation and the development of abnormal movement compensations. These compensatory patterns develop in certain muscle groups to maintain upright postures and move against gravity. For example, the child's poor head control, resulting from poor coactivation of cervical flexors and extensors, causes the center of gravity to move anteriorly; this results in compensatory reactions in the thoracic and lumbar spine as the child attempts to stay upright. Likewise, hyperreactive responses to tactile, visual, or auditory stimuli may result in fluctuations of muscle tone that often adversely affect postural control and further diminish coordinated responses in everyday activities.

Classification of cerebral palsy

The locale of the lesion affects the development and quality of movement patterns present in the child with CP. For example, CP with spasticity indicates a lesion in the motor cortex. Lesions in the basal ganglia typically cause fluctuations in muscle tone that are described as diakinesis, dystonia, or athetosis. Cerebellar damage tends to produce the unstable movements characteristic of the ataxic child.

The variability of the movement and postural disorder may be classified according to which limbs are affected.

Involvement of one extremity is commonly referred to as *monoplegia,* upper and lower extremities on one side as *hemiplegia,* both lower extremities as *paraplegia,* and all limbs as *tetraplegia* or *quadriplegia.* Diplegia results when the child demonstrates quadriplegia with mild upper extremity involvement and significant impairment of function in lower extremities.

Several classifications of CP have been developed according to quality of tone, disorder distribution, and locale of brain lesions. A combination of these classifications is featured in Table 6-2. Characteristics are described according to quality and distribution of muscle tone, ROM, quality of movement, presence of reflexes and reactions, oral motor problems, associated problems, and personality characteristics.

Although CP is considered nonprogressive, abnormal movement patterns, muscle tone, and sensory function, combined with the effects of gravity and normal growth, may cause the child to develop contractures and deformities over time. Function may become more limited as the child grows to adulthood. Furthermore, the effects of normal aging may result in decreased function, physical discomfort, and arthritic responses over time (Russman & Romness, 1998).

Language and intellectual deficits often coexist with CP. Delays in cognitive development with below-average intelligence have been seen in 50% to 75% of children with CP. This impairment may range from mild to profound (Pellegrino, 1997). Speech disturbances occur in approximately 30% of this population. Articulation problems may be associated with impairment of tongue and lip movements. Speech and language problems may be receptive or expressive, relating to central processing impairment. Limitations in communication tend to isolate the child, may create stress and frustration for the child and parent, and can negatively affect the development of psychosocial skills. Use of augmentative communication equipment can prevent some of these consequences of speech impairment and is critically important for increasing the communication abilities of children with severe CP.

Seizure disorders occur in approximately 50% of children with CP. The incidence appears to be higher among children with spastic disorders (Brown, 1997). In children with severe seizures, some degeneration may continue after birth. Anticonvulsant drugs are commonly used to control seizure activity. These drugs must be carefully monitored and may affect the state of the child's digestion and gums, requiring feeding adjustments and good dental care.

Feeding problems are associated with the abnormal oral movements, tone, and sensation. The child may be hypersensitive or hyposensitive to touch around and in the mouth; sucking, chewing, and swallowing may be difficult to initiate or control (Pellegrino, 1997; Wong, 1997). Diet may need to be adjusted, and special feeding

techniques may be required. These children also may require medication to maintain regularity of elimination. Positioning helps improve postural stability for feeding and toileting.

Several sensory deficits may be present. Problems with the visual system may include impaired vision, blindness, limitations in eye movements and eye tracking, squinting, strabismus, eye muscle weaknesses, and eye incoordination. In addition, children with CP may have visual perception problems that can interfere with school progress. It is estimated that 40% to 50% of children with CP have visual defects of some type (Pellegrino, 1997) and often require glasses, low vision, or visual perceptual training. Auditory disturbances include hearing (acuity) problems that can range from slight hearing loss to total deafness. Auditory perceptual problems and agnosia are also common. An estimated 25% of children with CP have some type of auditory disturbance and may require hearing aides.

Children with CP must be monitored for signs of behavioral problems and psychosocial delays that can become serious problems if not found and corrected early. Evaluation of these areas, emotional support, normalizing social experiences, and behavior management programs should be integral parts of the total assessment and treatment regimen for these special children.

Antispasticity medications can improve motor patterns and range of motion. Muscle relaxants can reduce spasticity or rigidity and improve comfort in older children for short periods. These medications work on the neurotransmitter acetylcholine (ACh) and are fast acting. Significant side effects occur with many children, including drowsiness, excessive drooling, and physical dependency, all of which tend to outweigh the potential benefit of the medication.

Implanted medication pumps are being used with children who have severe spasticity. The pump is inserted into the skin of the abdomen, and the catheter is routed to the lumbar spine where it is placed into the intrathecal space. This placement allows delivery of antispasticity medication (primarily baclofen) into the spinal cord where it can directly inhibit motor nerve conduction. The major advantages to the pump include lower and more controlled doses of the medication and decreased spasticity (Miller & Clark, 1998; Pelligrino, 1997). Mechanical failures, infections, and the need for intensive medical intervention may rule out some children as candidates for this treatment. Additionally, the long-term effects of such treatment for children remain unclear (Miller & Clark, 1998).

In cases where spasticity is severe, neural blocks may be done to disrupt the reflex arc (Pellegrino, 1997). Recently, injectable botulinum toxin has been used to block the nerve-muscle junction effectively. Although botulinum toxin is deadly in the general circulation when in-table 6-2 **Cerebral Palsy Classifications**

	Severe Spasticity	Moderate Spasticity	Mild Spasticity	Pure Athetosis
Quality of tone	Severely increased tone; flexor and extensor cocontraction are constant; tone is high at rest, asleep, or awake; tone pattern is more proximal than distal	Moderately increased tone; near normal at rest but increases with excitement, movement attempts, effort, emotion, speech, sudden stretch; agonists and distal muscles more spastic	Mildly increased or normal tone at rest; increases with effort or attempts to move or attempts at quicker movements	Fluctuation of tone from low to normal; no or little spasticity; no coactivation of flexors and extensors
Distribution of tone	Quadriplegia, but can also be diplegia or paraplegia	Same as severe spasticity	Same as severe spasticity, but more diplegia and hemiplegia	Quadriplegia with occasional hemiplegia
Range of motion	Abnormal patterns can lead to scoliosis, kyphosis, hip/knee/finger deformity; forearm pronation contracture, hip subluxation, heel cord subluxation with equinovarus or equinovalgus; decreased trunk, shoulder, and pelvic girdle mobility; limited midrange control where cocontraction is least balanced	More available movement and more flexor/extensor imbalance can lead to kyphosis, lordosis, hip subluxations or dislocations, hip and knee flexion contractures; tight hip internal rotators and adductors; heel cord shortening and foot rotation	Limitations more distally than proximal; minimal deformities	Transient subluxation of joints such as shoulders and fingers; may have valgus on feet or knees; rarely any deformities
Quality of movement	Decreased midrange, voluntary and involuntary movements; slow and labored stereotypical movements	May be able to walk; stereotypical, asymmetrical, more associated reactions, total movement synergies	Often able to walk; seems driven to move; has increased variety of other movements, some stereotypical	Writhing involuntary movements, more distal than proximal; no change with intention to move; many fixation attempts caused by decreased ability to stabilize
Reflexes and reactions	Obligatory primitive reflexes (positive support, ATNR, STNR, neck righting); protective, righting, and equilibrium reactions are often absent	Strong primitive reflexes—Moro, startle, TNR, TLR, positive support prominent; decreased neck righting; associated reactions strong; righting may be present, but equilibrium reaction develops to sitting and kneeling	Primitive reflexes used for functional purposes and not obligatory; righting, protective, and equilibrium reactions delayed, but not established; may not get higher-level reactions	Primitive reflexes not usually obligatory or evoked; protective and equilibrium reactions usually present but involuntary movements affect grading

Modified from Bobath, B. (1978). *Classification of types of cerebral palsy based on the quality of postural tone.* London: The Bobath Centre.

ATNR, Asymmetric tonic neck reflex; *STNR,* symmetric tonic neck reflex; *TNR,* tonic neck reflex; *TLR,* tonic labyrinthine; *MR,* mental retardation, *URTI,* upper respiratory tract infection.

Athetosis with Spasticity	Athetosis with Tonic Spasms	Choreoathetosis	Flaccid	Ataxia
Fluctuates from normal to high; some ability to stabilize proximally; moderate proximal spasticity and distal athetosis	Unpredictable tone changes from low to very high; either all flexion or extension of extremities	Constant fluctuations from low to high with no cocontraction; jerky involuntary movements more proximal than distal	Fluctuating, markedly low muscle tone; seen at birth or toddler initially as flaccid; later classified as spastic, athetoid, or ataxic	Ranges from near normal to normal; when increased tone is present, usually involves lower extremity flexion
Same as athetosis	Quadriplegia, hemiplegia, or monoplegia	Quadriplegia	Quadriplegia	Quadriplegia
Incidence of scoliosis; some flexion deformities at hips, elbows, and knees; usually full range of motion proximally/hypermobile distally	More pronounced scoliosis; more dislocation of arm because of flailing spasm; possible kyphoscoliosis, hip dislocation on skull side, flexion contracture on hips/knees, subluxation of hips, fingers, or lower jaw	Many involuntary movements with extreme ranges but no control at midrange; deformities rare, but tendency for shoulder and finger subluxation	Hypermobile joints tend to sublux; flat chest; later range limitations due to limited movement	Range is usually not a problem; when present, decreased range is in flexion
Decreased ability to grade movements; decreased midline control and selective movement; proximal stability and distal choreoathetosis; varies with case	Extreme tonic spasm without voluntary control; some involuntary movement, distal more than proximal	Wide movement ranges with no gradation; jerky movements more proximal than distal; no selective movement or fixation of movement; weak hands and fingers	Ungraded movements; slow movements difficult; many static postures as if hanging on to anatomic structures instead of active control	Lack point of stability so coactivation is difficult; use primitive rather than abnormal patterns, hence gross, total patterns; incoordination, thus dysmetria disdiadochokinesia, tremors at rest, symmetric problems
TNR/TLR strong but intermittent and modified by involuntary movements; equilibrium reactions when present are unreliable and may or may not be used	Strong ATNR, STNR, TLR; protective and equilibrium reactions absent during spasm, otherwise present, unreliable, or absent	Intermittent TNR; righting and equilibrium reactions present to some extent, but abnormal coordination. Abnormal upper extremity protective extension but often absent	Usually less reactive because of decreased tone; righting is delayed; delayed protective extension more available than equilibrium reaction	May develop righting reactions but uncoordinated, exaggerated, and poorly used; equilibrium reactions when developed are not coordinated; needs wide base of support because of poor weight shift

Continued

table 6-2   *Cerebral Palsy Classifications—cont'd*

	Severe Spasticity	Moderate Spasticity	Mild Spasticity	Pure Athetosis
Oral motor	Immobile, rigid chest; shallow respiration and forced expiration; lip retraction with decreased lip closure and tongue thrust; communication through forced expiration	Not as involved as severe spasticity	Increased mobility, thus more respiratory function for phonation; shortness of breath limits sentence length; better ability to dissociate mouth parts, but poor lip closure causes drooling	Fluctuations adversely affect gross and fine motor performance; volume of speech may go up or down with breath; feeding may be decreased due to instability and tongue/jaw/swallow incoordination
Associated problems	Seizures; cortical blindness; deafness; mental retardation; prone to URTI; malnutrition	Seizures; MR; perceptual motor problems; imbalance of eye musculature	Seizures; less MR; perceptual problems	Hearing loss; less mental retardation
Personality characteristics	Passive, dependent; resistant and adapts poorly to change; anxious and fearful of being moved; generally less frustrated than athetoid	A lesser picture of severe spasticity	More frustrated and critical about self because of awareness of better performance; more patient than children of same age	Emotional lability; less fearful of movement; more outgoing, but tends to be frustrated

jected intramuscularly in minute quantities, it blocks the neuromuscular junction effectively for 3 to 6 months. This allows the child to use the muscle without interference of spasticity. The long-term benefits of treatment have yet to be well-researched.

Orthopedic surgery has traditionally been used to correct joint deformities, balance uneven muscular action, and reduce contractures that have resulted from abnormal and asymmetric tone. The most frequently performed surgeries include tendon release (permanent lengthening of a muscle) and tendon transfer (moving the point of attachment of a tendon on bone). Both procedures require the use of a cast for 6 to 8 weeks after surgery; and since overall muscle tone is not changed, these procedures may need to be repeated.

Other potential surgeries include correction of hip deformities or dislocations and scoliosis. A new surgical procedure called the *Lucque procedure* is being recommended for the aggressive treatment of scoliosis (Pelligrino, 1997). Orthotic management in support of surgery, or to reduce tone, to prevent contractures, or to stabilize or position, often improves and increases functional activity. Tone-reducing or inhibitive casts made for the lower extremity can gently strengthen and lengthen spastic muscles. Often a series of casts is applied to in-

crease ROM gradually. When ROM within normal limits has been achieved, the cast is worn intermittently to maintain the increased muscle length. Active and passive ROM activities, positioning and handling to enhance postural tone, and orthotics may be used alone or in combination to improve the child's functional independence (Bobath, 1980; Bobath & Bobath, 1972).

Neurosurgical intervention for spasticity has been aimed at the brain, spinal cord, and peripheral nerves. For example, cerebellar or dorsal column stimulators have been implanted but with disappointing results (Chambers, 1997). Currently, selective posterior rhizotomy (SPR) is the most widely used neurosurgical procedure. In SPR 50% of dorsal rootlets at L2-S2 are severed to muscles that are determined to be spastic, as tested by electromyography (EMG) during surgery. Good candidates for SPR include those with a diagnosis of spastic diplegia, normal cognitive status, no fixed deformities, and good underlying muscle strength in the spastic muscles.

The initial studies for SPR provide encouraging data for positive functional changes. Reported changes include improved motor control, gait, upper extremity functioning, sitting balance, and responsiveness to other treatment strategies (Loewen, Steinbok, Holsti, & MacKay, 1998; Steinbok, Reiner, & Kestle, 1997). How-

Athetosis with Spasticity	Athetosis with Tonic Spasms	Choreoathetosis	Flaccid	Ataxia
Difficulty with head control, thus decreased oral motor, strained speech; decreased coordination of suck/swallow, resulting in decreased feeding and speech	Feeding may be difficult because aspiration is unpredictable; severe language and speech impairment caused by decreased control	Facial grimaces; dysarthria; irregular breathing; difficulty in sustaining phonation; poor intraoral and extraoral surfaces	Quiet soft voice because of decreased respiration; delayed speech; increased drooling; often expressionless face	Speech is monotone, very slow; uses teeth to stabilize tongue or hold cup to mouth when drinking; decreased articulation
Same as athetosis	Same as athetosis	Same as athetosis	Obesity; sensory impairment; URTI	Nystagmus; mental retardation; sensory problems; uses vision for righting and as reference point for movement
Same as athetosis	Same as athetosis	Same as athetosis	Visually attentive; cannot move; therefore, is a "good" baby; decreased motivation	Does not like to move

ever, some studies have indicated that serious side effects and long-term complications may exist after SPR is performed, including persistent back pain, neurogenic bowel and bladder, spondylolisthesis, spondylolysis, severe lumbar lordosis, and sensory changes (Miller & Clark, 1997; Steinbok & Schrag, 1998).

Although prognosis varies for each type of CP, children with CP typically live to adulthood, but their life expectancy may be less than that of the normal population. The reason for a shorter life expectancy is not known; it may be related to persistent alterations in physiologic and immunologic functioning, the implications of which are not fully understood (Rogers, Coe, & Karaszewski, 1998). Functional prognosis varies greatly from type to type, with hemiplegia and spastic diplegia having a better prognosis than the more severe, rigid types. Depending on the ability to attain independence or modified independence with assistive devices and technology, children with CP may experience the full range of life events. Children with CP may have limitations in all areas of human occupation to some degree. Functional performance in self-care and independent living, school and work performance, play, and recreation may all need to be addressed at some point in the child's life. Parents may require support and respite, as well as education, to care for the child with CP and to meet the needs of the family as a whole (Scherzer & Tscharnuter, 1990).

Seizure Disorders and Epilepsy

Epilepsy is a group of neuromuscular conditions whose center of dysfunction is in the brain. A *seizure* may be defined as a temporary, involuntary change of consciousness, behavior, motor activity, sensation, or automatic functioning (Menkes, 1995). Individuals are considered to have epilepsy if they have recurring seizures.

A *seizure* starts with an excessive rate and hypersynchrony of discharges from a group of cerebral neurons that spreads to the adjoining cells, called the *epileptogenic focus* (Wong, 1997). Some seizures may be directly attributed to the factor or factors that trigger the seizure. For example, acute factors often described are hypoglycemia, fever, trauma, hemorrhages, tumors, infections, and anoxia. Other seizures may be attributed to previous scarring and structural damage or to hormonal changes. Many seizures, especially in children, have no discernible underlying disease and are therefore idiopathic in nature (Menkes, 1995).

Many authors classify seizures by their clinical characteristics or symptoms and electroencephalographic (EEG) findings. There are two major types of seizures with this form of categorization: (1) generalized seizure, which involves the entire cerebral cortex, and (2) partial seizure, which begins in a single location and remains limited or spreads to become more generalized. Generalized seizures can be further divided into tonic-clonic, absence, atypical absence, myoclonic, and atonic forms. Partial seizures can be either simple or complex and are the most common type of seizure disorder found in childhood; approximately 60% of cases are partial seizures. An individual may experience both generalized and partial seizures, which is called a *mixed seizure disorder* (Brown, 1997; Wong, 1997).

Of the generalized seizures, tonic-clonic occurs most frequently. A child having a *tonic-clonic seizure* may have an aura, or sensation, that the seizure is about to begin. This nonspecific seizure can occur at any age and involves excessive neuronal firing from both hemispheres in a symmetric pattern. This is usually followed by a loss of consciousness during which the body becomes rigid or tonic, and then rhythmic clonic contractions of all the extremities occur. Incontinence is frequent. The seizure may last for 5 minutes, followed by a postical period that may last from 1 to 2 hours in which the child is drowsy or in a deep sleep (Brown, 1997).

A second type of generalized seizures or *absence seizures* are characterized by a momentary loss of awareness and no motor activity except eye blinking or rolling. There is no aura, the seizures usually last only 5 to 10 seconds, and there is no postical period. Onset of seizures occurs in the first decade of life. Abrupt interruption of an activity, glazed look, stares, and unawareness of surroundings characterize a child having an absence seizure. These may be mistaken for daydreaming. Absence seizures are uncommon in children and early adolescents, accounting for only 5% of all seizures (Brown, 1997).

Two other mild forms of generalized seizures are (1) myoclonic seizures that consist of contractions by single or small groups of muscles and (2) akinetic seizures in which the primary problem is a loss of muscle tone. Children rarely have serious seizures for an extended period (30 minutes or more). This condition is called *status epilepticus* and requires medical management to maintain body functions and hydration. Intravenous anticonvulsant medication is also indicated to treat this condition.

In *complex partial seizures,* which usually originate in the temporal lobe, children may show automatic reactions such as lip smacking, chewing, and buttoning and unbuttoning of clothing. These seizures are focal and similar to the characteristics of absence seizures. In addition the individual may appear to be confused and disorganized and may have sensory experiences, such as smelling and tasting items not in the environment and hearing sounds of various types.

Simple partial seizures usually involve the motor cortex and result in clonic activity of the face or extremities.

Psychic symptoms include visual hallucinations, illusions, auditory hallucinations, or olfactory sensations. The typical seizure includes nighttime awakenings and twitching of facial muscles, which spreads to the hands and interferes with speech (Brown, 1997).

Infantile spasms pose a serious threat to development. They typically begin at 6 months and disappear by 24 months. During this time, development appears to stop and skills may be lost. Early treatment with adrenocorticotropic hormone can inhibit the seizure activity; however, the effects on development are almost inevitable. More than 90% of children with known causes for their seizures have MR (Brown, 1997).

The incidence and prevalence of seizures are difficult to estimate. Generalized seizures, including tonic-clonic, absence, and myoclonic seizures, have been reported in approximately 2.5 in 1000 children. Partial seizures have been reported in between 1.7 and 3.6 in 1000 children, with unclassified and mixed seizures accounting for another 2 in 1000 (Menkes, 1995). In young children the most common seizure is associated with the presence of illness or fever. Many of these may occur infrequently and cease as the child matures.

A child who has a seizure must undergo a thorough evaluation to determine the factors causing the seizure. A family history, medical history, and developmental history must be completed, as well as an EEG to help determine the type of seizure.

Anticonvulsive medications are administered in an attempt to control the seizures. In theory these medications increase the intensity required to trigger the seizure or eliminate the recruitment of surrounding cells. Brown (1997) has described some of the common side effects from these anticonvulsive medications: cataracts, weight gain, high blood pressure, pathologic fractures, drowsiness, hair loss or gain, nausea, liver damage, vomiting, gum enlargement, hyperactivity, anorexia, and lymphoma-like syndrome. Commonly prescribed medications include valproic acid (Depakene, Abbott, North Chicago, Ill.), phenytoin (Dilantin, Parke-Davis, Morris Plains, NJ), phenobarbital, ethosuximide (Zarontin, Parke-Davis), and carbamazepine (Tegretol, Geigy, Ardsley, NY).

Balancing the dosage of anticonvulsant medications can be a difficult process and is often repeated at various times as the child grows and matures. Antiepileptic medication is often withdrawn or reduced if the child has been seizure free with a normal EEG for at least 2 years. Withdrawal is done slowly and with caution, and health care workers are often asked to monitor the child closely during this period (Dodson, 1989).

Even with optimal care, only about 50% to 75% of children can be controlled completely on medication. Having a seizure can be frightening to the child and those around him or her. When a child has a seizure, staff must remain calm, move spectators away, and protect the child. Box 6-1 outlines the emergency treatment procedures of seizures.

Muscular Dystrophies

The muscular dystrophies are the most common muscle diseases of childhood. They cause changes in the biochemistry and structure of the surface and internal membranes of the muscle cells and result in progressive degeneration and weakness of various muscle groups, disability, deformity, and sometimes death. For most of the neuromuscular disorders, which all have a genetic basis, the chromosomal location is known and the causal gene has been identified (Chance, Ashizawa, Hoffman, & Crawford, 1998).

Types of muscular dystrophy include *limb-girdle, facioscapulohumeral, congenital,* and *Duchenne's (pseudohypertrophic) muscular dystrophy.* Figure 6-10 graphically demonstrates the differential distribution of paralysis with these dystrophies.

In *limb-girdle* muscular dystrophy the initial muscles affected are the proximal muscles of the pelvis and shoulder girdles. Onset may begin anywhere from the first to the third decades of life, with progression usually slow but sometimes moderately rapid. Its hereditary pattern is autosomal recessive like the congenital form.

Facioscapulohumeral muscular dystrophy is autosomal dominant, and onset usually occurs in early adolescence. Although severity varies greatly among clients, involvement is primarily in the face, upper arms, and scapular re-

box **6-1** *Emergency treatment*

Seizure
Time seizure episode.
Approach calmly.
Protect child during seizure:
  Do not attempt to restrain child or use force.
  If child is standing or sitting in wheelchair at beginning of attack, ease child down so that he or she will not fall; when possible, place cushion or blanket under child.
Do not put anything in child's mouth.
Loosen restrictive clothing.
Prevent child from hitting hard on sharp objects that might cause injury during uncontrolled movements.
  Remove objects.
  Pad objects.
  Move furniture out of way.
Allow seizure to end without interference.
When seizure has stopped, check for breathing; if not present, use mouth-to-mouth resuscitation.
Check around mouth for evidence of burns or suspicious substances that might indicate poisoning.
Remain with child.
When child is able to move, seek help.

From Wong, D.L. (1997). *Whaley and Wong's essentials of pediatric nursing* (5th ed.). (p. 1023). St. Louis: Mosby.

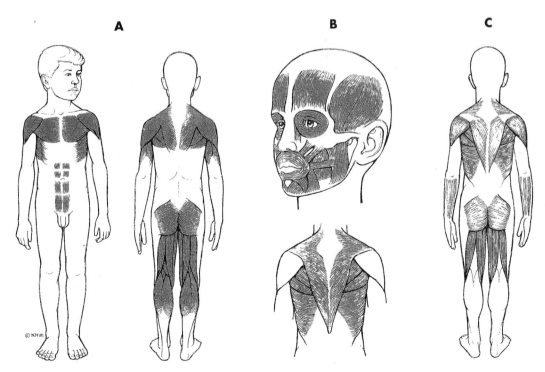

figure **6-10** Initial muscle groups involved in muscular dystrophies. **A,** Pseudohypertrophic. **B,** Facioscapulohumeral. **C,** Limb-girdle. *(From Wong, D.L. [1997].* Whaley and Wong's essentials of pediatric nursing. *[5th ed.]. St. Louis: Mosby.)*

gion, as the name implies. Clinical manifestations include a slope to the shoulders, decreased ability to raise arms above shoulder height, and decreased mobility in the facial muscles that gives a "masked" appearance.

The most common and the most severe form of muscular dystrophy is called *Duchenne's muscular dystrophy*. It is inherited in a sex-linked recessive manner, affects boys, and has an incidence of 1 per 3500 live male births (Wong, 1997).

Symptoms usually begin between the second and sixth years of life. Parents describe their child as having increasing difficulty climbing stairs and rising from a sitting or lying position. The child stumbles and falls excessively and tires easily. A distinctive characteristic of this form is the enlargement of calf muscles and sometimes of forearm and thigh muscles, giving the appearance of strong, healthy muscles. However, this enlargement is caused by extensive fibrosis and proliferation of adipose tissue, which when combined with the other pathologic changes in the muscle tissue actually causes muscle weakness. This phenomenon is referred to as *pseudohypertrophy* of muscles.

Involvement begins in the proximal musculature of the pelvic girdle, proceeds to the shoulder girdle, and finally affects all muscle groups. As leg and pelvic muscles weaken, the child often uses his or her arms to "crawl" up the thighs into a standing position from a kneeling position. This is known as *Gower's sign* and is diagnostically significant (Figure 6-11). Independent ambulation is one of the first functions to be lost, and wheelchair dependence is common by 9 years of age. Gradually the simplest ADLs become difficult and then impossible. In the advanced stages of the disease, lordosis and kyphosis are common, as are contractures at various joints. Death, usually as a result of infection, respiratory problems, or cardiovascular complications, often occurs before the early twenties (Carroll, 1985).

Currently there is no treatment that arrests or reverses the dystrophic process, but antibiotic therapy and other advances in dealing with pulmonary complications have helped extend life expectancy. Steroids can help, but their use remains controversial because of their side effects. Myoblast transfer is used on a trial basis. Although gene therapy is still in the preclinical trial phase, it is a promising option for treatment of Duchenne's and Becker's muscular dystrophies. Two types of treatments are being explored: the use of adenovirus-mediated dystrophin gene transfer and upregulation of a natural dystrophin analogue (Karpati, Gilbert, Petrof, & Nalbantoglu, 1997).

Congenital muscular dystrophies (CMDs) make up a heterogeneous group of muscle disorders with onset in utero or during the first year of life. Several forms of CMD show brain involvement in addition to the neuromuscular disorder (Voit, 1998). CMD is marked by hy-

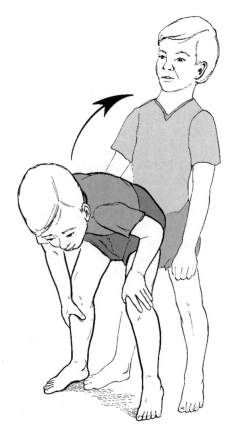

figure 6-11   Child with Gower's sign.

potonia, generalized muscle weakness, and multiple contractures. Four categories have been identified: classic CMD I without severe impairment of intellectual functioning; CMD II with muscle and brain abnormalities; and the less severe types CMD III and IV with muscle, eye, and brain abnormalities (Leyten, Gabreels, Renier, & ter Laak, 1996). Associated problems include clubfoot, torticollis, diaphragmatic involvement, congenital heart defects, and spinal defects. Often little to no progression of the disease is seen after childhood, and some functional improvement may be seen around this time (Thomas & Dubowitz, 1989). Diagnosis is made from the presence of high serum levels of the muscle enzyme creatine kinase, by EMG analysis, and by examination of muscle tissue taken during biopsy. Clinical examination often reveals a "floppy" child with muscle weakness in the face, neck, trunk, and limbs; decreased muscle mass; and absent deep tendon reflexes (Thomas & Dubowitz, 1989).

The use of orthopedic devices and adaptive equipment and activity can increase mobility, minimize contractures, delay spinal curvatures, and maximize independence in ADLs and thus in role functioning. Maintaining the child's independent mobility for as long as possible is a major goal. Children with CMDs appear to degenerate more rapidly once in a wheelchair. Because these children are generally aware of their situation, the therapist working with this child should also be prepared to work with the issues of death and dying. Genetic counseling for parents and female siblings and family support programs are also of value.

All other disorders of muscles are usually called *myopathies*. Congenital myopathies are rare in infants; however, when they occur they are usually caused by autosomal dominant patterns of inheritance but may also be caused by prolonged treatment with certain drugs such as steroids. Symptoms are similar to those of the dystrophies, with proximal muscle weakness of the face, neck, and limbs. Congenital dislocation of the hip, scoliosis, seizures, and reduced cognitive skills may also be present. Diagnosis is made by muscle biopsy. Unlike the dystrophies, this condition progresses slowly or not at all, making the prognosis better (Menkes, 1995).

Neural Tube Defects and Spina Bifida

Neural tube defects refer to malformations early in utero development of the CNS. The three major forms of neural tube deficits are encephalocele, anencephaly, and spina bifida. Encephalocele is a result of the brain protrusion in the occipital region of the brain. These children typically have severe deficits, including MR, hydrocephalus, motor impairments, and seizures (Liptak, 1997). Anencephaly indicates a lack of neural development above the level of the brain stem; these children do not survive infancy.

Spina bifida is the term most commonly used to describe a congenital defect of the vertebral arches and the spinal column. This defect may be mild, with the laminae of only 1 or 2 vertebrae affected and no malformation of the spinal cord, or it may involve an extensive spinal opening with an exposed pouch made up of cerebrospinal fluid (CSF) and the meninges *(meningocele)* or CSF, meninges, and nerve roots *(myelomeningocele)*. These latter conditions are also called *spina bifida cystica*, as opposed to *spina bifida occulta*, where no pouch is evident (Menkes, 1995; Morrissy & Weinstein, 1996) (Figure 6-12). This deficit appears to occur in the fourth week of prenatal development and can be identified by amniocentesis. Hereditary, intrauterine, and environmental factors have been associated with these conditions (Morrissy & Weinstein, 1996). Recently the research suggests that a combination of heredity and a folic acid deficiency may account for up to 50% of cases (Liptak, 1997). Spina bifida cystica is believed to occur from 0.2 to 4.2 times per 1000 live births. The CDC (1997) reported an annual rate of 900 babies born with spina bifida or meningocele in the United States.

The degree of impairment depends on the level and degree of spinal cord involvement. This continuum of impairment can include no functional impairment, mild muscle imbalances and sensory losses, paraplegia, or even death in severe cases.

Many times in spina bifida occulta there are no external manifestations visible, or the skin overlying the defect may be dimpled, pigmented, or covered with hair. Internally the spinal cord may be divided by a bony spur or congenital neoplasm, or there may be a slight bony malformation of one or more vertebrae (Liptak, 1997). Occasionally this area is slightly unstable, and some degree of neuromuscular impairment may occur, including mild gait deficits and bowel or bladder problems.

Spina bifida cystica is more serious and complex. A sac, or meningocele, that is visible above the bony defect characterizes spina bifida with meningocele. This sac is covered with skin and subcutaneous tissue, contains CSF, and although the meninges extend into the sac, the spinal cord remains confined to the spinal canal. In the neonatal period, great care must be taken not to rupture the sac and to prevent infection. Surgical skin closure is usually done soon after birth to protect the cyst. In some cases part or the entire sac is removed.

Spina bifida with myelomeningocele is the most severe form of spina bifida. In this form the sac may be covered with only a thin layer of skin, or the meninges and the spinal cord or nerve roots protrude into the meningocele.

Complications with these forms of spina bifida include meningitis and hydrocephalus. Infection is easily contracted because of environmental exposure of the meninges and spinal cord. Hydrocephalus is a common secondary complication that may be caused by either a developmental defect in the brain, such as aqueduct stenosis, or by the lower portion of the brain (and part of the cerebellum) slipping through the foramen magnum, a condition known as *Arnold-Chiari syndrome* (Liptak, 1997; Menkes, 1995).

Children with myelomeningocele usually display sensory and motor disturbances below the level of the lesion. Most lesions are in the thoracic or lumbar spine, resulting in lower extremity paralysis. Sensory dysfunction is variable. Some children also demonstrate hip, spinal, or foot deformities. Bowel and bladder incontinence is often a problem. Medication, bowel training, and intermittent catheterization may assist significantly in this area (Liptak, 1997).

Children with hydrocephalus or significant motor deficits may demonstrate sensory processing and perceptual problems. Often they exhibit fine motor delays in association with visual perceptual impairment or dyspraxia. Medical management of these children includes surgery for repair of deformities or for shunt implantation and urologic management. Orthotic interventions include lightweight bracing, casting, orthopedic shoes, and assistive devices for ambulation. Family education in skin care, urology, and diet enhances the child's independence. With problems in sensory, neuromotor, and perceptual performance areas, therapists often emphasize self-care, instrumental ADLs, and functional mobility skills.

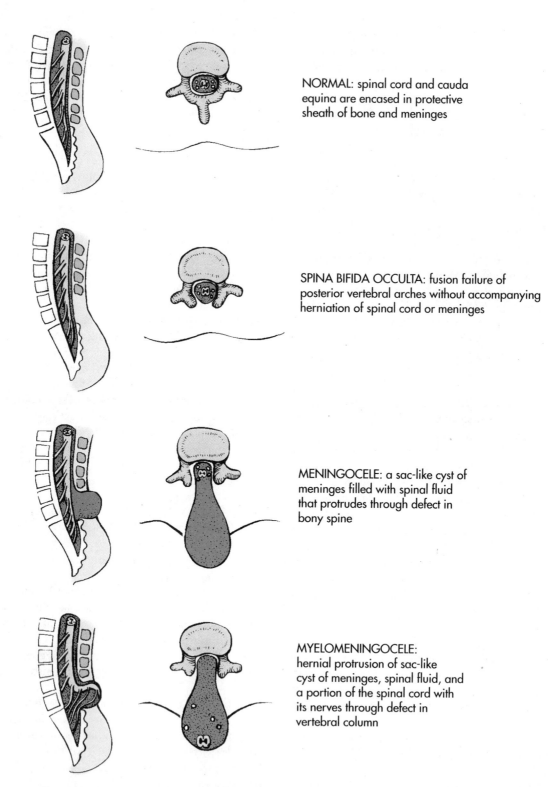

figure 6-12   Three forms of spina bifida. *(From Wong, D.L. [1997]. Whaley and Wong's essentials of pediatric nursing. [5th ed.]. St. Louis: Mosby.)*

NORMAL: spinal cord and cauda equina are encased in protective sheath of bone and meninges

SPINA BIFIDA OCCULTA: fusion failure of posterior vertebral arches without accompanying herniation of spinal cord or meninges

MENINGOCELE: a sac-like cyst of meninges filled with spinal fluid that protrudes through defect in bony spine

MYELOMENINGOCELE: hernial protrusion of sac-like cyst of meninges, spinal fluid, and a portion of the spinal cord with its nerves through defect in vertebral column

Hydrocephalus

Hydrocephalus occurs when CSF builds up in the ventricles of the brain. This occurs when there is an imbalance between the amount of CSF produced and the amount absorbed. Noncommunicating ventricles that obstruct the outflow of CSF from the ventricles, an Arnold-Chiari malformation, or occasionally a tumor may produce this phenomenon.

In infants an early sign of the condition is enlarged head size. In older children, where the head cannot grow, intracranial pressure is increased. Definitive diagnosis may be made by sonography, computed tomography (CT), or magnetic resonance imaging (MRI) scans (Brown, 1997; Liptak, 1997).

Clinical signs of hydrocephalus in infants include abnormal head growth with bulging fontanels, dilated scalp veins, and separated sutures; eyes that appear to deviate downward, producing a "sunsetting" appearance of the iris and visible sclera; and after time, lethargy, irritability, and problems with reflexes, feeding, and tone. In older children, headache, irritability, development of strabismus or nystagmus, and cognitive changes may occur (Johnson, 1997).

The pressure produced by the hydrocephalus can result in visual and perceptual deficits, MR, seizures, and death. If the hydrocephalus is caused by an obstruction, its removal may alleviate the condition. The usual medical treatment for idiopathic hydrocephalus is the placement of a ventriculoperitoneal (VP) shunt. Shown in Figure 6-13, this procedure reduces the CSF pressure by means of a catheter that runs under the skin from one of the ventricles to the abdominal cavity, where the fluid can be safely absorbed. These shunts are usually effective but must be monitored regularly for signs of infection, clogging, kinking, or migration of the tube. Even with shunting, however, many of these children have cognitive, perceptual, visual, or other functional problems (Wong, 1997).

Guillain-Barré Syndrome

Guillain-Barré syndrome is an acute polyneuropathy caused by a virus that attacks the nerve roots. The body then interprets the infected roots as foreign bodies and destroys them with an autoimmune response. The result is a progressive, flaccid muscle paralysis similar to that seen in poliomyelitis. This condition is most often idiopathic in origin (Menkes, 1995). Children are affected by this condition less often than adults. Among children it is most common in middle childhood.

Illness typically begins with an upper respiratory infection and progresses through a period with muscle tenderness, symmetric muscle weakness, and occasionally paresthesias. Paralysis usually begins peripherally and in the lower extremities, ascending to the upper extremities, diaphragm, and occasionally facial area. Respiration and

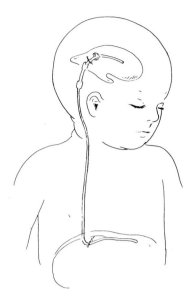

figure**6-13** Ventriculoperitoneal shunt. Catheter is threaded subcutaneously from small incisions at the sites of ventricular and peritoneal insertions. *(From Wong, D.L. [1997]. Whaley and Wong's essentials of pediatric nursing. [5th ed.]. [p. 1027]. St. Louis: Mosby.)*

feeding may be compromised, and the child may require technologic support (Eisen & Humphreys, 1974). The child may experience discomfort and some sensory loss, and incontinence is common (Ropper, 1992).

Muscle function begins to return a few days to a few months after onset. During the early stages of Guillain-Barré syndrome, adaptive devices and palliative care may be provided. In most cases a full recovery can be attained, particularly with physical rehabilitation. Physical and occupational therapy services to initially maintain ROM, regain strength and coordination, and reacquire independent living skills are essential components of the rehabilitation program.

Peripheral Nerve Injuries
Birth injuries

Infants and children occasionally suffer traumatic injuries, perinatally and postnatally, that temporarily or permanently cause peripheral nerve impairment. For example, breech deliveries with after-coming arms can cause *brachial plexus lesions*. These infants may demonstrate weakness or wasting of the small muscles of the hands and sensory diminution in the area of the hand and arm served by this plexus (Menkes, 1995).

This condition, called *Erb-Duchenne palsy*, is usually unilateral and related to the upper brachial plexus only. It is usually a result of stretching the shoulder in extreme shoulder flexion (with the hand over the head). Paralysis of the arm results and is often more pronounced in the shoulder musculature than in the hand. The child often holds his or her arm in a characteristic posture, with shoulder adducted and internally rotated, elbow extended, forearm pronated, and wrist flexed. Prognosis depends on the extent of the damage to the nerves but can be good with early intervention. In *Klumpke's palsy*, or lower brachial plexus paralysis, the stretching injury is generally more severe. Klumpke's palsy results in paralysis of the hand and wrist muscles. A brachial palsy injury can be so severe that the entire arm is paralyzed.

Occupational therapy often involves fabrication of a sling that fits proximally around the humerus and passive and active-assistive exercises. Later in infancy, resistive exercises may be recommended for development of optimal strength in the affected arm.

Traumatic injury of peripheral nerves

In older children, injury to a peripheral nerve is usually caused by an accident, either through severing of the nerve or secondary to fractures, dislocations, excessive exercise, or occasionally medical treatments such as injections. Injuries of this type are common to the radial, ulnar, and median nerves and the brachial plexus, lumbar plexus, peroneal nerves, or sciatic nerves.

Diagnosis is made using a combination of techniques, such as family and medical histories, nerve conduction studies, observations of sensory and motor involvement, muscle biopsies, EMGs, and surgical exploration in serious accidents. Specific treatment depends on the extent, progression, location, and especially the cause of the nerve damage. In general, treatment techniques include rest, splinting, nerve and local anesthetic injections, and surgical intervention to relieve nerve compression.

■ TRAUMATIC BRAIN INJURIES

Traumatic brain injuries (TBIs) or *head injuries* (HIs) during childhood constitute a major medical and public health problem. Approximately 4000 children die each year of head injuries in the United States. Approximately 1 child in 500 children is seriously injured and must endure prolonged hospitalizations and lifelong complications of some degree (Adelson & Kochanek, 1998). Additionally, medical practitioners have begun recognizing the importance of diagnosing minor head injuries, which may result in more subtle but persistent cognitive and functional impairments (Beattie, 1997; Satz et. al., 1997). According to the CDC, the most common causes of head injuries in young children, in order of frequency, are falls, motor vehicle accidents, assault or child abuse, and sports and recreation injuries. In older children, most head injuries are caused, in order of frequency, by motor vehicle accidents, sports-related injuries, and falls. As children reach adolescence, motor vehicle accidents remain the major cause of TBI, followed by assault (primarily abuse and gunshot wounds), sports and recreation injuries, and falls.

Head traumas are classified by the nature of the force that causes the injury and the severity of the injury. Forces, which cause head trauma, are referred to as either *impact* or *inertial* forces. Impact forces will most likely result in skull fractures, focal brain lesions, and epidural hematomas and result from the head striking a surface or a moving object striking the head. Inertial forces are typically the result of rapid acceleration and deceleration of the brain inside the skull, causing a shearing or tearing of brain tissue and nerve fibers. Most TBIs are the result of both types of forces. Severity of the HI is rated as a relatively mild concussion to a more serious injury (Michaud, Duhaime, & Lazar, 1997). Damage to nervous system tissue occurs both at the time of impact or penetration and through secondary damage resulting from brain swelling, intracranial pressure, hematomas, emboli, and hypoxic brain conditions. These secondary causes of nervous system damage can be prevented or at least minimized through early medical intervention (Adelson & Kochanek, 1998).

Loss of consciousness is a prime indicator of significant HI. When an incident occurs and the child does not lose consciousness or loses consciousness momentarily, then later he or she develops symptoms of lethargy, confusion, severe headache, irritability, vomiting, or speech or motor impairments, TBI is implicated. If consciousness is lost longer than momentarily, immediate medical attention is indicated (Michaud et. al., 1997).

Once the child's medical condition is stabilized, the severity of brain injury is determined. One scale that is often used is the Glasgow Coma Scale (Jennett & Teasdale, 1981). This scale rates an individual on eye opening (4 = spontaneous to 1 = nil), best motor response (6 = obeys to 1 = nil) and verbal response (5 = oriented to 1 = nil). Consequently, individuals receive between a 3 and the highest score of 15, with a score of 8 or less considered to be a severe HI. Initial diagnostic procedures typically include an MRI, CT scan, EEG, angiography, and radiography to determine the extent and location of fractures (Beattie, 1997). Medical treatment in moderate or severe HIs includes close monitoring and control of cerebral circulation and of intracranial pressure through the use of sophisticated devices and control systems. When intracranial pressure cannot be controlled by the use of traditional means, a large dose of barbiturate, such as phenobarbital, may be administered. If this attempt fails to control the pressure, lowering the body temperature may help. Withdrawal from the latter two forms of treatment is difficult and may cause sleep disturbances, behavioral problems, apnea, and some decreased intellectual functioning (Raphaely et. al., 1980).

Fortunately, most children who sustain an HI will have only a minor (between 13 and 15 on the Glasgow scale) HI. Children with residual minor head injury deficits may require educational support, environmental modifications and psychologic support. In most cases, the prognosis for these children is very good.

Children who have sustained moderate or severe brain injuries typically follow a behavioral pattern of gradual and full return of consciousness. Depending on the severity of damage, an individual will not initially respond to any external stimuli or will respond in a stereotypical manner. Only a small number of children remain in comas. At this first stage of recovery, children exhibit eye opening to external stimuli and generalized responses to noxious stimuli. The next stage of recovery can be the most difficult for family members because the individual is often agitated and combative; however, the child is rarely aware of his or her actions. As this agitation resolves, the child demonstrates increased appropriate responses to commands, ability to attend and concentrate, and recognition of family members. Through this progress, intervention becomes more goal oriented (Michaud et. al., 1997).

An unfortunate perception of many health professionals is that children have better outcomes from severe HI than adults do, but this belief is not substantiated by fact. Children have similar mortality rates (36% with a Glasgow score >8) and guarded recovery as adults (Johnson & Krishnamurthy, 1998). Persistent deficits can vary widely; individuals who sustain moderate brain damage generally have fewer residual deficits. Performance deficits may include sensorimotor impairments, language and communication impairments, feeding disorders, visual-perceptual deficits, cognitive deficits, and impairment of psychosocial skills. Typically, academic achievement is hindered, and the child will require modifications to the educational setting, including assistive technology or related services (Michaud et. al., 1997).

■ DEVELOPMENTAL DISABILITIES

This section addresses those disorders found in childhood that are not specifically associated with one body system and that delay the developmental progress of the child. In general, *developmental disabilities* are characterized by prenatal, perinatal, or early childhood onset. Some of the factors that negatively affect developmental outcomes are maternal in origin, and others are caused by infant complications. Chapter 21 discusses medical factors during and immediately after birth that place the infant at risk for long-term disability. Each of the developmental disabilities described in this section has the potential to affect multiple areas of the child's development and to impair the child's performance and roles.

Mental Retardation

Mental retardation (MR) is the most common of developmental disabilities, affecting between 0.8% and 3% of the population, depending on the definition used (Batshaw & Shapiro, 1997). These definitions have three key factors: significantly impaired intellectual ability, usually measured on standardized psychoeducational tests; onset before 18 years of age; and impairment of the adaptive abilities necessary for independent living.

Formal testing and history are used to make a diagnosis of MR. Testing usually includes intelligence quotient (IQ) testing and tests of adaptive behavior (basic reasoning, environmental knowledge, and developmentally appropriate daily living and self-maintenance skills). Although the use of IQ scores is controversial, significantly subaverage scores remain a good predictor of future cognitive functioning. Fortunately, intelligence is composed of a wider range of skills than is demonstrated on IQ tests. Additionally, as in typically developing children, developmental outcomes of children with MR are significantly influenced by socioeconomic conditions, environmental events, having at least one parent who is highly committed to the child, and the individual's unique resilience (Horowitz & Haritos, 1998). A child is usually considered to have MR if he or she scores more than two standard deviations below the normative range for age. MR is classified in the fourth edition of the *Diagnostic and Statistical Manual of Mental Disorders* (DSM-IV) by the following levels of severity: *mild, moderate, severe,* and *profound* (APA, 1994). Although this classification has changed over the years and is somewhat artificial (i.e., does not always directly equate to function), it is commonly used to describe children with MR (Figure 6-14).

Intensive debate persists in the literature regarding the rate of development experienced by individuals with MR and the ultimate potential that these individuals possess. These issues have significant implications for identifying, educating, and integrating individuals with MR into society. The modes and strategies of how individuals with MR learn and how they differ in their development are critical issues to resolve for education and the most appropriate therapeutic intervention (Burack, Hodapp, & Zigler, 1998). Children with mild MR have an IQ range of approximately 55 to 70. Characteristics include the ability to learn academic skills at the third to seventh grade levels and the usual achievement of social and vocational skills adequate to live in the community with intermittent support. The employment rate for adults with mild MR is 80%, and 80% are married (Batshaw & Shapiro, 1997).

Children with moderate MR have an IQ range of approximately 40 to 55. These individuals require support to function in society. This group is unlikely to progress past the second grade level in academics; they can usually

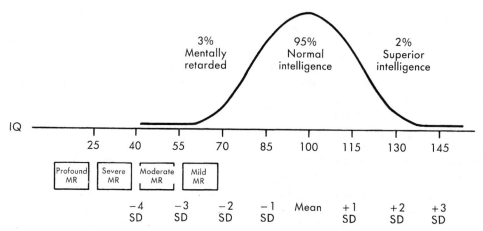

figure 6-14   Criteria for determining the four degrees of severity in mental retardation (MR).

handle routine daily functions and do unskilled or semi-skilled work in sheltered workshop conditions. A group home or supervised housing situation is usually the placement that families choose for these individuals as adults.

Children with severe MR have an IQ range of approximately 25 to 40. These individuals can usually learn to communicate, and they can be trained in basic health habits; however, they require extensive support and supervision to accomplish most tasks.

Children with profound MR have IQs below 25. These children need caregiver assistance for basic survival skills. Usually they have minimal capacity for sensorimotor or self-care functioning. Individuals with profound MR also often have interrelated neuromuscular, orthopedic, or behavioral deficits.

MR is a functional deficit that describes several disabilities. It can occur secondarily to another condition or without apparent cause. It has been estimated that there are more than 300 causes of MR (Batshaw & Shapiro, 1997). These causes are usually categorized into the following headings: problems acquired in childhood (e.g., toxins, trauma, infection); problems of fetal development and birth; chromosomal problems; CNS malformations; congenital anomalies; and neurocutaneous, metabolic, and endocrine disorders.

Approximately 80% of children with MR have additional problems. For example, it is estimated that approximately 50% have speech problems, 50% have ambulation problems, 20% have seizures, 25% have visual problems, and 40% have chronic conditions such as heart disease, diabetes, anemia, obesity, and dental problems (Shapiro & Batshaw, 1993).

Parents, physicians, and allied health professionals who are involved in well-baby care and screening often express concerns about children with MR. Early signs of cognitive impairment include delays in meeting motor and speech milestones, nonresponsiveness to handling and physical contact, reduced alertness or spontaneous play, feeding difficulties, and neurologic soft signs (which include balance, motor symmetry, perceptual motor skills, and fine motor skills). A formal diagnosis of MR is generally made when the child reaches school age because intellectual testing in preschool are limited by test sensitivity. Referrals for psychologic, education, developmental, and speech and hearing evaluation may be made and then interpreted for the parents. Services must be determined, and parents, siblings, and other family members must be given support and advice.

Today, health care professionals, educators, and the general public practice a philosophy of inclusion of persons with MR. Beginning with early intervention, services and programs provide opportunities that enable individuals to reach their maximal level of functioning in the least restrictive environment.

Early programming for children with MR or delays is usually focused on facilitating the attainment of developmental milestones; enriching the environment; developing self-help, language, and motor skills; and educating and supporting the parents. As the child grows, specific deficits may be addressed in special education programs. For the adolescent with MR, the development of vocational interests and skills, social skills and sex education, and community mobility skills are essential (Batshaw & Shapiro, 1997).

Autism and Pervasive Developmental Disorders

Pervasive developmental disorders (PDDs) are a broad class of conditions that reflect a range of deficits, of which *autism* is the most well-documented form. Autism, whose onset is typically before 3 years of age and whose deficits are persistent throughout life, is characterized by severe and complex impairments in social interaction, communication, and behavior (APA, 1994). The most current prevalence rates indicate that autism is seen in 1 to 2 per 1000 persons (NIMH, 1998). These rates are almost twice as high as early epidemiologic reports of autism and may be in part because of an increase in recognition and in the clarification of diagnostic criteria. The National Society for Autistic Children (NSAC, 1996) estimates that approximately four times as many boys as girls are afflicted with autism. Children with autism and PDD are found in families in all racial, ethnic, intellectual, and socioeconomic backgrounds. The other PDD categories include atypical autism, Rett syndrome, other childhood disintegrative disorders, Asperger's syndrome, and pervasive developmental disorder–unspecified (APA, 1994).

PDD and autism are among the most devastating of the chronic developmental disabilities because of the unusual combinations of sensorimotor and behavioral characteristics displayed by these children. Particularly associated with autism are the inability to relate to others and the display of ritualistic, repetitive behaviors. In the almost 40 years since Leo Kanner's elegant description first identified 11 children as having "extreme autistic aloneness," many theories have been proposed for the cause of autism. Today most researchers agree that the cause of PDD and autism is most likely due to a complex combination of familial genetic factors and neurobiologic vulnerability (Cohen & Volkmar, 1997).

Although the location of the exact affected sites in the CNS is not certain, some factors are strongly related to this trilogy of social-behavioral-communication disorders (Mauk, Reber, & Batshaw, 1997; Rapin, 1997). Studies of neurochemical, neurobiologic, and genetic systems have identified leads to the causes of PDD and autism. Overall, neurochemical studies of autism indicate that serotonin levels are elevated and hypothalamic-pituitary-adrenal axis (HPA) dysfunctions and abnormalities in neuroendocrine functioning have been reported (Anderson & Hoshino, 1997).

Currently, autism is accepted to be a disorder of neurologic development. The most current neurobiologic theories suggest impairment in dendritic and synaptic connections, specifically the selective molding and elimination of synaptic connections (Burack et. al., 1998). Initial pathologic anomalies seem to occur at higher-level cognitive processing pathways and involve the cerebral cortex (Mauk et. al., 1997). Genetic influences are also known to be a strong factor in the development of autism; however, the precise mechanisms are not yet known (Rutter, Bailey, Simonoff, & Pickles, 1997).

The behavioral characteristics of PDD and autism are critical to its diagnosis. They can be categorized into the following four subclusters of disturbances (APA, 1994):

1. Disturbances in social interactions
2. Disturbances in communication
3. Disturbances of behaviors
4. Disturbances of sensory and perceptual processing and associated impairments

Disturbances in social interactions affect the child's ability to establish meaningful relationships with people and inanimate objects. Although abnormalities in this area vary with age and degree of severity, they directly involve interactions that require initiative or reciprocal behavior from the child. Specific behaviors that are observed are poor or deviant eye contact, delayed or total lack of a social smile, apparent aversion to physical contact, delayed or absent anticipatory response to being picked up, and an apparent preference for being alone.

Disturbances in communication may be thought of as being on a continuum from severe to mild. At the severe end of the continuum appears a complete lack of speech (mute). At the other end of the continuum, normal language accompanied by only slight articulation or tonal deficits may be observed. Many other communication problems have been described at points along the continuum. For instance, much of the speech of children with autism is repetitive, or echolalic, in nature. Classic echolalia consists of parrotlike repetitions of phrases immediately after the child has been exposed to them, and delayed or deferred echolalia consists of the repetition of phrases at a later time. Echolalic speech occurs out of social context and appears to have little or no communicative value. Other types of speech and language problems include syntax problems, atonal and arrhythmic speech, pronoun reversals, and lack of inflection and emotion during communication (Rutter, 1985).

Disturbances in behavior are seen in the intolerance of deviation from routine, resistance to any type of change, and patterns of behaviors that are best categorized as stereotyped, perseverative, and lacking in representational or pretend play. Additionally, bizarre attachments to unusual objects develop (e.g., intense interest in a vacuum cleaner or a sheet of paper verses stuffed animals or dolls). These patterns of behavior are obsessive rituals where any deviation is not tolerated (Mauk et. al., 1997). Deviations from the routine, however slight, will elicit intense temper tantrums. Additionally, deviant motor patterns may involve the arms, hands, trunk, lower extremities, or entire body. Motor patterns in the upper extremities are common and include wiggling and flicking of fingers, alternating flexion and extension of the fingers, and alternating pronation and supination of the forearm. Other motility patterns often seen include head rolling and banging, body rocking and swaying, lunging and darting movements, toe walking, dystonia of the extremities, involuntary synergies of the head and proximal segments of the limbs, and an inability to perform two motor acts at the same time (Damasio & Maurer, 1978; Howlin & Rutter, 1987).

For almost 30 years, *disturbances of sensory processing and perception* have been reported in children with autism. These include abnormal responses to various visual, vestibular, and auditory stimuli. A. Jean Ayres describes two types of sensory processing problems in children with autistic behaviors. The first deals with the registration of, or orientation to, sensory input. It appears that in these children the neurophysiologic processes that decide that sensory stimuli will be brought to their attention are working correctly at some times but not at others (Ayres & Tickle, 1980). Therefore they react normally to sensory stimuli one minute, and the next minute (hour or day) they may overreact or underreact to the same stimuli.

The second sensory processing disturbance described by Ayres involves the control or modulation of a stimulus once it has entered the system. Again the child with autistic behavior is believed to be capable of exerting control at some times but not at others, resulting in a child who processes tactile information normally at times and who, at other times, appears to be extremely hypersensitive.

Associated impairments in autism include MR, seizure disorders, and discontinuities in developmental rates. The fact that a large percentage of children with autism also suffer from cognitive deficiencies has been a controversial but relatively accepted issue. The cognitive deficiencies exhibited by children with autism are as disabling as those in children with MR, with the same long-term consequences. Seizure disorders occur in high incidence in children with autism. Both tonic-clonic and partial-complex seizures have been reported in this population (Mauk et. al., 1997).

Although most children with autism have normal life expectancies, the functional prognosis is diverse. Some individuals with autism and PDD will live and work independently in the community; some will be fairly independent, needing only minimal support for ADLs and others will continue to depend on support from family and friends. In general, prognosis for children with PDD is closely related to communication skills and intelligence. Higher-functioning individuals may become high-functioning adults with deficits in social interactions. Prognosis of independent functioning through behavioral interventions is encouraging (Bregman & Gerdtz, 1997).

Because no single method of treatment has yet proved to be totally effective in treating autism, an interdisciplinary approach is usually selected. Interventionists generally agree that a combination of behavioral treatment, special education programs, speech-language therapy, pharmacotherapy, and family support constitutes the best management for children with PDD and autism (Mauk et. al., 1997). Various types of therapies have been advocated, including auditory integration training, dietary interventions, discrete trial training, medications, music therapy, sensory integration, speech and language training, and vision therapy. In spite of the wide use and claims of benefits, most of these approaches lack rigorous scientific support. In general, studies to date indicate that individuals with autism respond best to a highly structured, specialized educational program that includes elements of communication therapy, social skill training, and sensory integration therapy (Cohen & Volkmar, 1997). The medications used with these children include sedatives, stimulants, major and minor tranquilizers, antihistamines, antidepressants, and psychotomimetics. It is believed that these medications work best when used in conjunction with an interdisciplinary special education program (Mauk et. al., 1997).

Rett syndrome, exclusively described in girls, is another form of PPD. Although intensively researched, the cause of Rett syndrome has eluded explanation. Heritability studies indicate that maternal lines may contribute to the expression of this disorder. Currently, it is believed that mutation of the X chromosome may cause early abortions of hemizygous male fetuses and a dominant phenotype in heterozygous female fetuses. The male sex is not included in exclusion criteria, but no male infants who meet the strict guidelines for Rett syndrome have been identified. In 1996, 2212 cases of Rett syndrome were identified in the United States (Van Acker, 1997). Worldwide the incidence of Rett syndrome is approximately 1 per 15,000 live female births.

Development appears normal in children with Rett syndrome until about 6 months of age; thereafter the child demonstrates regression in cognition, praxis, and behavior. Microcephaly, spasticity, and seizures develop, and the child develops autistic-like behaviors such as hand mouthing, flapping, or wringing. Functional hand use disappears, and waking hyperventilation is characteristic. Rett syndrome does not appear to be a degenerative disease; rather, it is a disorder of arrested neurodevelopment. Children with Rett syndrome can survive for some time but are usually nonambulatory and nonverbal by late childhood. This is an incurable condition, but carbamazepine may be helpful in reducing symptoms and improving alertness (Menkes, 1995).

Asperger's syndrome is contrasted with autism by no clinically significant delays in language skills. The essential features of Asperger's syndrome include severe and sustained impairments in social interaction and development of restricted, repetitive patterns of behavior, interests, and activities (APA, 1994). The interference with functional daily living skills must be significant. In addition, there are typically no impairments of cognitive development, development of age-appropriate self-help skills, or adaptive behavior aside from social interaction impairments (Klin & Volkmar, 1997). Although language skills are age appropriate, individuals with Asperger's syndrome display idiosyncrasies in verbal communication, characterized by highly circumstantial utterances, long-winded and tangential accounts of events, failure to convey a clear thought, and one-sidedness. Often an obsessive interest in letters and numbers absorbs most of the person's attention and energy. Additionally, these individuals display a lack of nonverbal communication and of empathy, tending to intellectualize feelings and show a poor understanding of others' affect (Klin & Volkmar, 1997).

Asperger's syndrome is more prevalent in boys, but epidemiologic studies have not accurately confirmed this syndrome in the birth rate. Treatment currently consists of supportive and symptomatic intervention. These services include special learning programs, assistance with generalizing adaptive functioning to a wider variety of settings, problem-solving strategies, social skills training, speech and language skills training, and vocational training (Klin & Volkmar, 1997).

Attention-Deficit Hyperactivity Disorder

Regarded as the most common childhood neurobehavioral disorder, *attention-deficit hyperactivity disorder* (ADHD) is a heterogeneous behavioral disorder of uncertain cause that is always evident in childhood but typically persists through adolescence and, for some, into adulthood (Elia, Ambrosini, & Rapoport, 1999). Because of past and recurring difficulties with strict definitions of ADHD, accurate prevalence data are difficult to determine (Barkley, 1998). Using DSM-IV criteria as a standard (APA, 1994), prevalence estimates for ADHD vary between 3% and 5% of the school-age population, or approximately 2 million children. Additionally, it occurs in boys approximately three times as often as in girls.

The prevalence of ADHD subtypes may differ according to the source of referral, with hospital-based clinics, pediatric neurologists, and child psychiatrists treating predominantly a combined subtype and with primary-care practitioners treating a higher rate of inattentive subtype. Data synthesized from the National Ambulatory Medical Care Survey (NAMCS) have documented a 2.8% rise in physician office visits among clients 5 to 18 years of age, resulting in a diagnosis of ADHD from 1990 to 1995, supporting the perception that this diagnosis has dramatically increased in the past decade (Robison, Sclar, Skaer, & Galin, 1999). These increases are thought to be because of better-defined diagnostic criteria and increased sensitivity of physicians to the diagnostic criteria (Greenhill, 1998).

Children with ADHD exhibit inattention, hyperactivity, and impulsivity. Inattention is demonstrated through failure to attend to details, difficulty in sustained attention during play, inability to listen actively to instructions or conversation, difficulty organizing tasks, and avoidance of tasks that require sustained attention. This child is easily distracted and is often forgetful in daily activities. Examples of hyperactivity are frequent fidgeting, inability to sit when remaining seated is expected (e.g., in a classroom), difficulty playing quietly, excessive talking, and being described as "constantly on the go." Impulsivity can be seen in the inability to wait ones turn, frequent and incessant interruptions, and blurting out answers before a question is asked.

The symptoms vary in their degree of impairment, frequency of occurrence, and pervasiveness across settings. The symptoms must occur "often" (to distinguish single symptoms from typical behavior observed in 48% to 52% of children) and across multiple settings (e.g., school, play, home, day-care). Symptoms must persist for at least 6 months to a degree that is maladaptive and subsequently interferes with all occupational activities, including self-care, academic performance, and peer relationships. Three distinct subtypes are identified by DSM-IV (APA, 1994): ADHD combined type, ADHD predominantly inattentive type, and ADHD predominantly hyperactive impulsive type (Barkley, 1998). In the past this disorder has been termed minimal brain dysfunction, hyperactive child syndrome, hyperkinetic reaction of childhood, and attention-deficit disorder with hyperactivity. However, the clinical description for these terms and criteria is now considered sufficiently similar to permit generalizations about cause and treatment (Barkley, 1998).

Over the last decades, researchers have sought to develop and test potential theories of etiology for ADHD. One theory that persists in popular literature is that ADHD is related to food allergies or food additives and the amount of sugar in a child's diet. In 1982, after intensive study, the National Institutes of Health (NIH) (1996) concluded that there is no evidence that diet is responsible for onset of ADHD, and in only 5% of children with ADHD is a restricted diet efficacious in reducing symptoms associated with this disorder. Additionally, a label of minimal brain dysfunction indicated that ADHD was a secondary result of head trauma or birth complications. Although ADHD can result from brain damage, this theory explained only a small number of children with ADHD symptoms.

The current theories, widely supported but still under investigation, include genetic factors, neurologic factors, and neurochemical imbalances. In neural imaging studies, a significant decrease in brain activity in frontal-parietal lobes, which inhibit impulsiveness and control attention, has been demonstrated in adults with ADHD; however, the primary cause of this decreased activity is still unknown (Barkley, 1998; Zametkin & Liotta, 1998). Studies of heritability of this disorder are perhaps the best support that researchers have for linking ADHD with a neurobiologic etiology. It is clear that ADHD runs in families and thus may be one mechanism underlying ADHD symptoms. Neurochemical research into potential causes has failed to identify a single neurotransmitter that is responsible for the clinical deficits in ADHD (Greenhill, 1998). However, medications that influence neurotransmitter functioning are effective in treating some aspects of ADHD, leading researchers to believe that a neurochemical cause remains a viable theory. The selective availability of dopamine and norepinephrine are both candidates for a significant role in this disorder.

The most recent theory to gain acceptance is that of Barkley's (1997), who proposes that the symptoms displayed in ADHD are a result of response inhibition, which then prevents accurate self-regulation to environmental stimuli. He suggests that this response inhibition stems from the underfunctioning of the orbital frontal cortex and its subsequent connections to the limbic system.

Two primary medical treatment intervention strategies include stimulant pharmacotherapy (e.g., amphetamines, methylphenidate) and behavioral interventions. Pharmacotherapy allows 9 out of 10 children to focus and be more successful at school, home, and play (NIMH, 1996). There is no evidence that prolonged use of stimulant drugs is addictive, promotes addictive behavior in adolescence, makes children "high" or jittery, or sedates the child (Barkley, 1998). The realistic side effects of these drugs are weight loss, loss of appetite, interrupted sleep patterns, and in some children slow growth. The results of pharmacologic treatment seem to improve overactivity, attention span, impulsivity and self-control, compliance, physical and oral aggression, social interactions with peers, and academic productivity and accuracy (Zametkin & Ernst, 1999). Rarely, however, are medications alone sufficient to allow a child to function in most settings (Elia et. al., 1999). Deficits that seem to persist are those in reading skills, social skills, learning, academic achievement, and antisocial behavior (Zametkin & Ernst, 1999). Consequently, one or more behavioral interventions are typically needed. The most frequently recommended therapies include cognitive-behavioral therapy, behavior modification, educational interventions, social-skills training, and psychotherapy (Elia et. al., 1999). Although the definitive efficacy of any one strategy is not determined, it is clear that a consistency in responses in all of the child's settings, the environmental adaptations, and counseling to alleviate low self-esteem contribute to improvement in learning and attainment of social skills (Barkley, 1998). Occupational therapists can provide a multitude of successful strategies to the classroom for children with ADHD, including environmental adaptations, social skills training, self-management techniques, and interventions to enhance sensory modulation.

Learning Disabilities

The term *learning disabilities* (LDs) describes a group of problems that affect the ability of a child to master school tasks, process information, and communicate effectively. These disabilities are often not associated with a specific neurologic insult and may be accompanied by MR (Church, Lewis, & Batshaw, 1997). Learning disabilities are often associated with a variety of other neurologic problems (e.g., ADHD). Specific learning disabilities include auditory processing, language disabilities, and perceptual impairments.

Most children with LD have average or above-average intelligence, have adequate sensory acuity (are not blind or deaf), and have been provided with appropriate learning opportunities. In spite of all of these positive features, there is a significant discrepancy between the child's academic potential and the child's educational performance. The term *learning disability* includes conditions such as perceptual disabilities, dyslexia, ADHD, and developmental aphasia. It does not include learning problems that stem from primary sensory deficits, MR, socioeconomic conditions, or psychosocial impairments. The National Joint Committee on Learning Disabilities defines *learning disability* as a generic term that refers to a heterogeneous group of disorders manifested by significant difficulties in the acquisition and use of listening, speaking, reading, writing, reasoning, or mathematic abilities (Hammill, 1990).

Although different studies and agencies report varying incidence figures, the figure most often given is approximately 4% to 5% of the school population, which includes approximately 2 million children. As with autism, more boys than girls are affected; in this instance a 4:1 ratio exists (Church, Lewis, & Batshaw, 1997; Shaywitz & Shaywitz, 1987).

A child with LD may display any number of the behaviors listed under the following eight categories:

1. *Disorders of motor function* include both motor skills and motor activity level. Motor skills dysfunction may range from clumsiness to poor performance in gross or fine motor skills, to problems planning new tasks (dyspraxia), to equilibrium deficits, to sensorimotor problems in a number of areas. Occasionally tics, grimaces, and choreoathetoid movements in the hands may be observed. The child may be described as always being in motion (hyperactive) or being slow and lethargic (hypoactive).
2. *Educational disorders* can occur in one or more academic subjects. Related educational skills that are often limited or delayed are copying from the blackboard, printing and cursive writing, organizing time and materials, understanding written and oral directions, symbolic confusion (reversing letters), cutting, coloring, drawing, and keeping place on the page.
3. *Disorders of attention and concentration* include short attention span and other attention deficits, restlessness, impulsivity, and motor and verbal perseveration.
4. Characteristics included under *disorders of thinking and memory* are poor ability for abstract reasoning,

difficulty with concept formation, and poor short- and long-term memory capabilities.

5. *Problems with speech and communication* may include difficulty shifting topics of conversation; difficulty with "small talk;" difficulty with the sequencing of words, sentences, or sounds; slurred words; and articulation problems.

6. *Auditory difficulties* associated with LD often stem from auditory perceptual and auditory memory problems and not from acuity (hearing) problems. Children with these types of problems are often the ones who cannot remember the oral directions just given to them (auditory memory), cannot sound words out or blend sounds into words (phonemic synthesis), cannot block out background noise (speech-in-noise), and cannot remember the sequencing of sounds, words, or numbers (auditory sequencing). These types of problems often affect school performance and should be explored by an audiologist who is familiar with the specific instruments and programs that are available to assess and treat auditory perceptual (central auditory processing) problems. The high incidence of allergies and ear infections in children with LD places them at risk for auditory perceptual problems.

7. Children with LD often have various *sensory integrative and perceptual disorders.* Many of these children have difficulty with laterality and directionality concepts and tasks that require visual perception skills (Hammill, 1990).

8. Children with LD may have *psychosocial problems.* For example, they may demonstrate temper tantrums or antisocial behavior. Their social competencies may be delayed when compared with chronologic age and mental age. Many of these children are sensitive and decidedly at risk for poor self-esteem and for self-concept problems because they have the intelligence to know when they are being teased and to know the frustration of being good at some things and not at others.

Most children with LD retain some degree of disability as adults; however, most are contributing members of society. As with all disorders, prognosis is affected by the severity of the disability. Therefore individuals with limited impairment should not be limited in their life and career skills, but those with severe LD may need vocational planning, counseling, and adaptations to ensure as high a level of social, emotional, and vocational functioning as possible.

The therapist's role in an intervention program for the child with LD may change as the child develops, depending on the nature and extent of each child's specific disability. With young children, sensory integration, play, and basic socialization and self-help skills may be addressed through early intervention and parent education. As the child progresses into school, sensory integration

intervention may continue, but additional programming to promote social play, perceptual motor integration, and writing skills is indicated. By early adolescence the focus of evaluation and intervention shifts to independent living skills, psychosocial skills, development of compensatory and adaptive techniques, and development of vocational skills, interests, and habits.

Tourette's Syndrome

Tourette's syndrome (TS) is a pervasive disorder affecting neurologic and behavioral function. This condition is believed to be an autosomal dominant trait linked to a gene on chromosome 18. Dopamine dysfunction may be present. Prevalence of the condition varies geographically, but the condition is rare in black children and occurs more frequently in boys than in girls. Symptoms of the condition appear in middle childhood, worsen for about 10 years, and then lessen somewhat. However, they usually continue through the individual's lifetime, although there are periods of remission (Menkes, 1995).

Most characteristic of TS are involuntary vocal and motor tics. Tics are sudden, nonrhythmic, rapid, and recurrent. At some time the child with TS has both vocal and motor tics. The child may also display obsessive behavior and significant dysfunction in social, academic, or occupational skills. Usually tics begin with simple motor movements of the head, including eye movements, grimacing, and shoulder shrugging. Vocal tics may begin with throat clearing, grunting, barking, sneezing, and coughing. As the disease progresses, complex behavioral tics, compulsive echolalia, and cursing may occur. In severe cases, self-mutilation may occur at times. Specific tics tend to appear, recur frequently for a period, and then fade to be replaced by others (Menkes, 1995).

Tics may be suppressed voluntarily at some times, leading to problems in diagnosis and behavioral management; complex tics may be misinterpreted as emotional or behavioral disorders. Children who suppress tics may experience an "explosion" of tics in the later part of the day that may be accompanied by behavioral disturbances. Stress, anxiety, and anticipation of pleasant events can increase the frequency and intensity of tics and behaviors. Many of these children may also demonstrate ADHD, obsessive-compulsive disorders, or LD. These factors combine to impair social, school, and work functions.

Treatment includes clonidine and neuroleptic medication, such as haloperidol. These drugs have significant side effects, however, which also may cause functional deficits. Children who have obsessive-compulsive symptoms may also receive antidepressants. School- and play-based interventions may be necessary to address problems in writing, attention, and perceptual skills. Children may benefit from social skills and stress-reduction programming, as well as understanding from and empathetic interactions with adults and peers. Additional time for testing may also assist school performance.

Genetic and Chromosomal Abnormalities

Human beings normally have 23 pairs of chromosomes in each cell of the body. Smaller or larger numbers of chromosomes can cause significant developmental disabilities. These syndromes may present char acteristic symptom patterns and can often be identified by chromosomal analysis of the child's body tissues. For purposes of prevention, analysis of the amniotic fluid may identify these children before they are born (Batshaw, 1997a).

Genetic diseases are inherited abnormalities caused by abnormal genes that have had a negative effect on development. There are four different patterns of gene inheritance:

1. *Autosomal dominant inheritance* indicates that an abnormal gene is present on one of the non-sex chromosomes. Usually this gene has been directly passed from one of the parents to the child. On rare occasions the gene is not present in either the mother or father, and it is then known as a new, or "fresh," mutation. There is no carrier state; if the gene is present, the baby will have the abnormal characteristics. An example of an autosomal dominant illness is von Recklinghausen's disease (neurofibromatosis).

2. *Autosomal recessive inheritance* indicates that an abnormal gene must be in a paired condition because it is less potent. This condition exists, as with the first pattern, on non-sex chromosomes. Commonly, both parents are carriers but have no symptoms of the illness. Examples of autosomal recessive illnesses are cystic fibrosis, phenylketonuria, and diabetes. Many of the inherited diseases and illnesses have this pattern of inheritance, and in many instances the carrier states can be detected using various diagnostic procedures.

3. In *X-linked inheritance* the abnormal gene sits on the female sex chromosome, the X chromosome. Because this gene is recessive, in girls the normal gene on the second sex chromosome prevents expression of the disease. However, a boy who inherits the abnormal gene on his mother's X chromosome will be affected. Duchenne's muscular dystrophy and hemophilia (factor VIII deficiency) are examples of diseases inherited through this pattern.

4. *Polygenic,* or *multifactorial, inheritance* is a result of the interaction of heredity and the environment. Some congenital heart problems, cleft lip and palate, and meningomyelocele are examples of polygenic inheritance problems.

Excess chromosomal material is evidenced in the trisomy syndromes. The most common trisomy syndrome is *trisomy 21,* or *Down syndrome,* which is characterized by one additional chromosome 21. This syndrome, found in approximately 1 in 660 newborns, causes specific mental and physical problems. Although a range of physical characteristics may be associated with Down syndrome, a few are common to most children. Most of the children have a short and stocky stature with a protruding abdomen. The head is often small and flattened at the back, with upward slanting eyes that have abnormal epicanthal folds. Other common facial features include low-set ears, a flat nose, and often a mouth held slightly open with the tip of the tongue protruding. Extremities are shorter than normal, and fingers and toes are usually broad and short. The palms of the hands usually have a single crease known as the "simian" crease (Roizen, 1997).

Related health problems often include cardiovascular abnormalities, obesity, increased respiratory and other infections caused by immune system inefficiency, thyroid deficiencies, gastrointestinal problems, and an apparent increase in the risk of leukemia (Roizen, 1997). Often visual acuity is poor and requires correction. One problem that is potentially dangerous to the child is the atlanto-axial dislocation, which results in a tendency for dislocation to occur between the first and second cervical vertebrae. If this dislocation is severe, it can result in spinal cord damage. If this dislocation is found through radiographic films, surgery may be performed and precautions may be given to the family about roughhouse play or participation in activities that places stress on this joint.

Life expectancy for children with Down syndrome has improved greatly over the last several years. Those without cardiac anomalies can be expected to live into late adulthood. It is common, however, for these older individuals to develop a syndrome similar to Alzheimer's disease (Pueschel & Pueschel, 1992).

Children with Down syndrome are usually recognized at birth by their facial characteristics. They frequently also have low muscle tone, hypermobile joints, and problems in sucking. Medical examination is performed to ensure that none of the related congenital cardiac and medical problems are present. These problems may extend the hospitalization of the child. As the child grows, developmental delays in all areas of function are noted, although the degree can vary greatly among individual cases. Motor planning skills, language, and cognitive skills develop slowly. Parent support and education, early intervention, and special education assist this child to achieve his or her optimal function.

Other trisomies occur, but most are uncommon and many children who suffer from these problems are stillborn or aborted as fetuses. *Trisomy 18,* or *Edwards' syndrome,* is present in approximately 1 in 3000 births (Menkes, 1995). These children have long, narrow skulls; low-set, malformed ears; prominent occiput; a weak cry and small mouths; syndactyly and webbed neck; congenital heart and kidney malformations; severe MR;

failure to thrive; and early death (Menkes, 1995). The survival rate beyond infancy is only about 10%.

Trisomy 13, or *Patau's syndrome,* occurs in 1 in 5000 births (Menkes, 1995). Children with Patau's syndrome have multiple anomalies, including eye, ear, and nasal anomalies; cleft lip and palate; polydactyly and syndactyly; and microcephaly and neural tube defects (Menkes, 1995). Of the 20% of these children who survive, most are severely retarded and suffer from seizures.

A decrease in the number of chromosomes (45 or less) also causes problems. Many fetuses with this genetic abnormality die early in gestation. One exception to this statement is children born with *Turner's syndrome,* which is found in approximately 1 in 5000 girls (only) and is caused by one missing sex chromosome. These babies may be born with webbing of the neck or congenital edema of the extremities and may have cardiac problems. Small stature, obesity, and underdeveloped ovaries that cause infertility and absence of secondary sexual characteristics are symptoms that must be dealt with in the school-age child and adolescent with Turner's syndrome. Although visual perception problems are common, most of these children do not have MR; therefore their functional prognosis is good.

Other chromosomal abnormalities are caused by a missing portion of an individual chromosome (deletion) or by a portion of a chromosome breaking off and reattaching to another chromosome (translocation). The incidence of these events is more rare than the chromosomal problems described, and because the amount of chromosomal material that is missing or duplicated is variable, the resulting conditions are expressed differently. Problems common in these types of conditions are MR, abnormal brain development, and facial abnormalities.

Cri du chat syndrome is rare (1 in 20,000 live births) and is caused by deletion of part of chromosome 5. This condition is so named because this baby has a weak, mewing cry. These children have a small head and widely spaced, downslanting eyes; cardiac abnormalities; failure to thrive; and profound MR. Additionally, these infants have hypotonia and feeding and respiratory problems (Batshaw, 1997a).

Klinefelter's syndrome is caused by an XXY sex chromosomal pattern. This condition occurs in approximately 1 in 500 live male births and results in a mild disorder that may not be recognized until adulthood. LD and emotional and behavioral problems are characteristic of Klinefelter's syndrome. Those with this syndrome appear tall and slim, have small genitalia, and are infertile. An XYY chromosomal pattern occurs in 4 in 1000 male births, and those with this pattern also appear tall. These individuals may be expected to have mildly depressed IQ scores, tremors, reduced coordination, radioulnar synostosis, and increased incidence of temper tantrums, impulsiveness, and inability to plan or to handle frustration and aggression (Wong, 1997).

Fragile X syndrome represents one third of all X-linked causes of MR. This condition is most evident in boys, who have only one X chromosome. Prevalence studies indicate that it occurs in 0.4 to 0.8 per 1000 boys and in 0.2 to 0.6 per 1000 girls. The genetic transmission of this disorder is more complex, and outcomes can vary when the mother passes on the defective gene. The clinical manifestations become progressively more severe in subsequent generations of expression of fragile X syndrome. This progression is due to the perseveration in the genetic code, which leads to other mutations (Batshaw, 1997b).

In addition to MR, fragile X children have craniofacial deformities, which include elongated faces, prominent jaws and foreheads, large protruding ears, a high arched palate, hyperextensible joints, and flat feet. Other features, including prolapse of the mitral valve and enlarged testicles, become more pronounced with age. Some cognitive features seem to be preserved in male children (e.g., simultaneous processing) even though they are identified as having MR with poor auditory memory and reception. Additionally, participation in daily living skills is preserved, whereas communication and social skills are impaired (Batshaw, 1997b; Wong, 1997). Speech tends to be echolalic, cluttered, and perseverative. Furthermore, these children may be identified as having *pervasive developmental disorders* because of the presence of stereotypic behavior, poor eye contact, unusual sensory stimuli responses, and lack of social skills (Batshaw, 1997b).

Prader-Willi syndrome is associated with a defect in chromosome 15. This condition causes severe obesity, short stature, decreased muscle tone, a long face and slanted eyes, poor thermal regulation, and underdeveloped sex organs. Moderate MR and extreme food-seeking behaviors are classic signs. This condition occurs in 1 in 15,000 live births (Menkes, 1995).

Neurofibromatosis, or von Recklinghausen's disease, has two forms with different genetic patterns. The condition can be called *peripheral neurofibromatosis (type 1),* which is the more common form; or *central neurofibromatosis (type 2).* Incidence is estimated at between 1 in 3000 and 1 in 5000 live births, occurring more commonly in boys, and the condition is associated with a dominant trait (Menkes, 1995). Neurofibromatosis causes multiple tumors, usually neurofibromas, on the central and peripheral nerves, cafe-au-lait spots on the skin, and vascular and visceral lesions. If these tumors occur in critical areas, they may cause death. Mild MR and LD are associated with the condition, as are speech disorders. Hypertension, optic gliomas (type 1), auditory tumors (type 2), skeletal anomalies, and short stature are also associated with the disease. Intervention for the condition may include surgical removal of dangerous or disfiguring lesions, reduction of symptoms, special education, and monitoring for cerebral tumors.

Inborn Errors of Metabolism

Several genetic problems produce errors in metabolism of environmental and internal substances. Untreated, they may cause serious disability and sometimes death. For some, early diagnosis allows treatment or prevention of these consequences, but for others, no known treatment has yet been found. For individuals with errors of metabolism, prenatal diagnosis and genetic counseling may be the only options.

Tay-Sachs disease is a degenerative nervous system disorder caused by the absence of an enzyme, called *hexosaminidase A,* that is usually found in the blood and major organs. This enzyme converts GM2 ganglioside, a product of nerve cell metabolism, into a nontoxic substance. Because this conversion does not take place in individuals with Tay-Sachs disease, the toxic substance builds up in the brain and other body organs and leads to brain damage.

Tay-Sachs disease is common in Jewish individuals whose ancestry can be traced to the Mediterranean region. Today, nearly 1 of every 27 American Jews carries the Tay-Sachs gene (Menkes, 1995). Because Tay-Sachs disease is an autosomal recessive trait, both parents must be carriers of the abnormal gene for the disease to be passed to the child.

Carriers of Tay-Sachs disease can be detected by a simple blood test. In addition, through amniocentesis, the disease can be detected in the fetus by examining the amniotic fluid for the presence of hexosaminidase A. This test, in addition to the relatively small and well-defined population in which the disease is primarily found, makes Tay-Sachs disease hypothetically a preventable condition.

Prevention is particularly important because Tay-Sachs disease is a devastating and fatal condition. Children with Tay-Sachs disease usually appear healthy at birth and develop normally for about 6 to 10 months. The child then becomes listless and regresses cognitively and motorically. A cherry red spot appears in both macular areas. Vision, hearing, loss of voluntary motor control, and seizures appear, leading to death by the age of 3 in most cases. There is no effective treatment for Tay-Sachs disease; medical and therapeutic efforts are essentially palliative and supportive.

Research efforts are focusing on several treatment approaches that may someday offer help for children with Tay-Sachs disease. For example, the search continues for a substance that could substitute for the hexosaminidase A or for a procedure to graft healthy cells into clients with Tay-Sachs disease so that the transplanted cells can produce hexosaminidase A. Research is also progressing on gene transplantation from normal into defective cells. Until an effective treatment is found, the best strategy is prevention through genetic counseling (Menkes, 1995).

Phenylketonuria (PKU) is an inborn error in the metabolism of phenylalanine, an amino acid commonly found in some proteins. This condition affects 1 in 15,000 children but is rare in individuals of Jewish origin and in black children. Untreated, children usually develop blond hair, blue eyes, and severe cognitive and behavioral disabilities, at times mimicking autism. Diagnosis can be made at birth with the Guthrie test. Treatment, which is effective, is dietary and involves withholding foods that have the precursors of phenylalanine. The new food-labeling regulations are helpful.

A similar condition, *galactosemia,* involves the inability of the child to convert galactose, a milk sugar, into glucose. Galactose then builds up in the blood and causes hepatic and splenic dysfunction (Menkes, 1995). Consequences of this condition when untreated include jaundice, vomiting and diarrhea, drowsiness and lethargy, cataracts, systemic infections, and death. Urine testing can detect this condition and is required for newborns in many states. Treatment involves a diet without galactose, including milk, milk products, and breast milk, and is usually effective in compliant children. In poorly controlled cases, some intellectual dulling, perceptual problems, tremors, choreoathetosis, and ataxia may be present (Menkes, 1995).

Lesch-Nyhan syndrome is a progressive neuromuscular disease that is limited to boys and involves the inability to metabolize purines. Children suffering from this condition appear normal for the first year but then experience significant MR, neuromotor degeneration and spasticity, and the compulsive need to bite their lips and fingers and rub their faces. This behavior is involuntary and becomes self-mutilating if unchecked. Vocal tics may also occur. Arthritis, anemia, and renal calculi are also frequent. Treatment usually includes protecting the child from self-mutilation, developmentally focused therapies, and medication to prevent secondary problems and to reduce mutilation. Naltrexone, an opioid antagonist, improves some of the clinical signs of this syndrome (Menkes, 1995).

■ DIABETES

Diabetes mellitus is a metabolic disorder of the pancreas in which the hormone insulin is secreted in insufficient amounts. Increased concentrations of glucose are found in the blood, and several systemic problems occur. The causes of diabetes are unknown, but it has a familial pattern and is now thought to be an autoimmune response to a viral infection in some cases.

There are two major types of diabetes. Type I, or *insulin-dependent diabetes mellitus (IDDM),* usually begins in childhood. This form of the disease tends to be more acute and requires the administration of insulin, carefully balanced with food intake and exercise, to provide adequate metabolic balance. Type II, or *non–insulin-dependent diabetes mellitus (NIDDM),* occurs more frequently in adults older than 40 years of age, is characterized by a resistance to insulin action, and may sometimes be controlled by diet, exercise, or oral medications. Insulin may also be required in some stages of NIDDM.

Virtually all children who develop diabetes are insulin dependent. Onset is usually around age 10 but may occur earlier or later. Early symptoms include polyuria, increased thirst, weight loss, and dehydration. Later symptoms may include acidosis, vomiting, hyperventilation, and coma (Drash, 1989). Overdose of insulin may cause insulin shock or hypoglycemia.

Over the long term, microvascular lesions may result in retinopathy that leads to blindness, nephropathy, and peripheral nerve damage. Sensory loss and increased infection, especially in the extremities, may occur. Individuals with diabetes are at increased risk for heart disease, and diabetic women are at increased risk for complications in pregnancy (Wong, 1997). Because this is a lifelong condition, the child and parents must be taught to administer insulin injections and to adjust and monitor blood glucose and life and dietary patterns. These children must also adjust to being drug dependent. In adolescence this adjustment is often particularly difficult.

The general goals of treatment are to ensure satisfactory growth, ensure emotional development, help the child acquire some degree of normal life, resolve the symptoms, prevent ketoacidosis, and prevent long-term sequelae, such as renal and cardiac damage and eye disease (Drash, 1989). The achievement of these goals is difficult because it depends on maintaining a delicate balance among so many factors: exercise, nutritional intake, hormones, emotions, and many other internal and external influences on blood sugar levels.

■ TOXIC AGENTS

Prenatal Toxins

Several birth defects may be caused by adverse changes within the fetal environment. Substances and factors that negatively affect the developing fetus are called *toxic agents,* or *teratogens.* Drugs, radiation, and chemicals are the most common teratogens known to affect fetal development. Table 6-3 lists some common teratogens and their possible effects on the developing fe-

tus. Several factors determine whether a teratogen will affect the fetus. The dosage, the gestational stage of the infant, and the specific sensitivity of the developing organs at the time of exposure to the teratogen are all factors that contribute to the outcome (Kennard, 1990; Schuster & Ashburn, 1986).

Alcohol-Related Birth Defects and Fetal Alcohol Syndrome

Alcohol-related birth defects (ARBDs), commonly referred to as *fetal alcohol syndrome* (FAS), or *fetal alcohol effects* (FAEs) are the most serious examples of a fetal syndrome caused by maternal exposure to a teratogen. FAS is a specific pattern of altered growth structure and function seen in infants of women who consume high amounts of alcohol during pregnancy (Adams, Victor, & Ropper, 1997). Infants with FAEs, a more mild form of FAS, may lack the distinct facial morphology and growth deficiencies but will share many of the neurobehavioral deficits found in infants with FAS (Abel, 1997).

Conservative estimates indicate that alcohol is the third leading cause of birth defects and the leading cause of MR. ARBD has been reported to occur in 1 to 2 per 1000 live births worldwide for FAS, with at least 1200 children born each year in the United States with this disorder. The estimate for children born with FAE is even higher, with an estimate of between 3 and 5 per 1000 worldwide (Sampson et. al., 1997). However, the risk of FAS or FAE to children born to mild-to-moderate drinkers is currently controversial; some investigators show a high incidence of effects with even small amounts of alcohol and others show few if any effects (Mattson & Riley, 1998). Investigators have demonstrated that the nature and extent of fetal injuries produced by alcohol will depend on several factors, including (1) the amount of alcohol consumed per day, (2) the time during the pregnancy that the alcohol was taken, (3) other stressors experienced by the mother, (4) whether food was eaten near the time of alcohol consumption, (5) whether other substance abuse occurred during the pregnancy, and (6) the general health of the mother (Coles, 1994; Jacobson, 1998).

Alcohol, like other teratogens, causes a spectrum of defects that vary from severe physical and mental problems that are readily detectable at birth to more subtle learning problems that may not be detected until school age (Coles et. al., 1991). The principle features of FAS include prenatal and postnatal growth deficiencies, a pattern of craniofacial malformations, and CNS dysfunction. Newborns are typically small for gestational age (SGA) and continue to show height, weight, and head circumference differences. The pattern of craniofacial malformations seen with FAS includes microcephaly, epicanthal folds, a long philtrum, short palpebral fissures, a flat

table 6-3	*Effects of Common Teratogens on the Developing Fetus and Child*
Substance	**Effect on Fetus or Child**
DRUGS	
Alcohol	Intrauterine growth retardation, mental deficiency, stillbirth. Infants may have complete fetal alcohol syndrome (including facial feature anomalies) or more mild fetal alcohol effects. They may experience withdrawal symptoms, mental retardation, hyperactivity, behavioral disorders, and learning disabilities.
Aspirin	In large amounts may be fatal or cause hemorrhagic manifestations.
Cortisone	Possible relation to cleft palate.
Caffeine	In extremely high levels, may show increased incidence of miscarriage; limb and skeletal malformations. There is no relation to mild intake levels and effects on the fetus.
Dilantin	Fetal hydantoin syndrome (growth and mental deficiency, abnormalities of the face, anomalies of the hands).
Heroin, codeine, morphine	Hyperirritability, shrill cry, vomiting and withdrawal symptoms, decreased alertness and responsiveness to visual and auditory stimuli; can be fatal. In later life, narcotic exposure has been associated with learning disabilities.
Lysergic acid diethylmide (LSD)	Spontaneous abortions, chromosomal changes, suspected anomalies.
Tetracycline	Stains teeth, inhibits bone growth.
Thalidomide	Phocomelia, hearing loss, cardiac anomalies; can be fatal.
Tobacco	Intrauterine growth retardation.
Tranquilizers	All may cause withdrawal symptoms during the neonatal period.
Radiation therapy	Congenital anomalies, growth retardation, chromosomal damages, mental deficiency, stillbirth.
CHEMICALS	
Methylmercury	Congenital abnormalities, growth retardation; can cause abortions.
Pesticides (some types)	Congenital anomalies.
Lead	Spontaneous abortion, intrauterine growth retardation, congenital anomalies, anemia; can be fatal.

Modified from Klaus, M.H., & Farnaroff, A.A. (1979). *Care of the high-risk neonate.* Philadelphia: W.B. Saunders; Schuster, C.S., & Ashburn, S.S. (1986). *The process of human development: A holistic approach* (2nd ed.). Boston: Little, Brown.

midface, and a thin vermilion of the upper lip (Adams et. al., 1997) (Figure 6-15). Musculoskeletal problems include congenital dislocations, foot positional defects, cervical spine abnormalities, specific joint alterations, flexion contractures at the elbows, and tapering of the terminal phalanges. Many of these craniofacial and skeletal defects are secondary to the effect of the alcohol on brain development, and although craniofacial deficits may even recede with growth, microcephaly will not (Batshaw & Conlon, 1997).

Although CNS dysfunction can vary, intellectual capacity is the most frequent disability noted with FAS. It ranges from moderate MR to average intellectual function, with an average IQ of 70 being most recently cited (Mattson & Riley, 1998). Other notable CNS deficits include hyperactivity, attention deficits, vestibular problems, implusivity, poor social skills, learning disabilities, memory deficits, and deficits in visuospatial-perceptual skills and sensory problems, including ocular, auditory,

and possibly vestibular functioning (Church & Abel, 1998).

The prognosis for FAS and FAE children varies with the extent and severity of the various malformations and growth deficiencies. Two important factors to consider are the severity of the maternal alcoholism and the quality and stability of the home environment (Abel, 1997). Studies of the long-term effects of FAS and FAE are just beginning to provide information about the influence of alcohol on the growth and development of the affected child. Size delays appear to continue for some time, with head circumference remaining smaller into middle childhood. The occupational performances of children with FAS or FAE show persistent delays in self-care, school activities, and play. Performance areas, which are typically evaluated, include sensory-motor, psychosocial, and cognitive areas.

Multiple psychosocial issues within the family are present, requiring that the clinician involve the entire

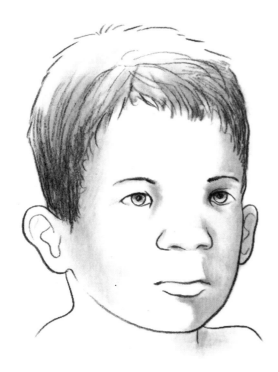

figure 6-15   Typical facial features of a child with FAS.

family in the child's therapy program. In 70% of families the children with FAS are removed from their mothers' care before adolescence (Batshaw & Conlon, 1997). When children remain in their mothers' care, 86% are reported for neglect and 52% for child abuse. In approximately 66% of the cases, the mothers of children with FAS die from alcohol-related causes early in the child's life (Batshaw & Conlon, 1997; Streissguth, Clarren, & Jones, 1985). However, many health care professionals believe that with intensive family intervention (e.g., alcohol recovery programs for the mother and early intervention for the child) and social, medical, and financial support, a better prognosis is possible. Hypothetically, FAS could be completely preventable if the public were educated to the deleterious effects of alcohol on unborn infants and changed its behavior accordingly. The best that can be hoped for is a reduction in the number of newborns with FAS and FAE.

Cocaine and Opiates

The effects of cocaine, crack, and opiates on infants are of increasing concern to developmental specialists. The use of these drugs has increased noticeably in the 1980s and 1990s, particularly the use of cocaine and "crack," a relatively cheap cocaine derivative. Maternal drug use is also complicated by the tendency of abusers to abuse other substances, such as alcohol and tobacco. Additionally, many mothers using these drugs are poorly

nourished and receive less than adequate prenatal care. At this time it is estimated that more than 100,000 infants per year are born to mothers who use drugs during pregnancy, although accurate counts are made difficult by the social and legal implications of reporting drug use (Batshaw & Conlon, 1997; Zuckerman & Frank, 1992).

Cocaine is extremely addictive, causing ecstatic "highs" and significant and prolonged "lows." Addiction to crack is said to be possible after one or two uses (Batshaw & Conlon, 1997). It increases the levels of norepinephrine, serotonin, and dopamine and has strong vasoconstrictive effects. Cocaine crosses the placenta and causes similar effects in the fetus. This vasoconstriction is believed to be damaging to the fetus. Use of opiates, heroin, or methadone by the mother results in an addicted infant who experiences drug withdrawal after birth.

The extent to which abuse of cocaine and other drugs cause developmental problems is still in question (Zuckerman & Frank, 1992). Research in the area continues; however, controlled studies are difficult to accomplish. Several general patterns are emerging. Babies born of addicted mothers are often SGA, with reduced head size and irritability and hypersensitivity to stimuli (Wong, 1997). Cocaine has been associated with congenital anomalies, limb deficiencies, cerebral hemorrhage, increased muscle tone, necrotizing enterocolitis, and rapid shifts of arousal state (Batshaw & Conlon, 1997). Newborns who are exposed to intrauterine narcotics go through active withdrawal, during which time they are irritable, hypertonic, and poor feeders. Often they frantically suck on their hands. Motor coordination is reduced, and activity level may be high. Respiratory distress has also been noted (Wong, 1997). These infants tend to require quiet, low-stimulus environments and may respond positively to swaddling. Parenting these children can be difficult for several months.

Long-term effects are unclear. Some studies have found that by school age these children perform at age-level expectations. However, others have reported performance problems, including hyperactivity and organizational problems, subtle learning and cognitive deficits, and play deficits. Furthermore, the mothers of these children often have few social supports and may be young, homeless, or remain addicted. Children may also be placed in foster care. Early intervention programs and school intervention programs may be necessary to identify, prevent, or minimize the long-term effects of the maternal substance abuse.

Heavy Metals

Heavy metal poisoning is a serious health concern. Because small children often put things in their mouths, they are at particular risk for poisoning by these substances (Menkes, 1995). *Mercury poisoning,* which can cause tremors, memory loss, anorexia, weight loss, diarrhea, and acrodynia (painful extremities), can enter the body through ingestion or inhalation. Liquid mercury evaporates quickly and should be cleaned up immediately to prevent this problem.

Lead poisoning is usually caused by ingestion of environmental lead, such as the lead paint in buildings built and painted before World War II. Lead paint has caused a significant problem in some inner-city communities and in older houses that have been renovated (Menkes, 1995). Lead water piping and some ceramic glazes have also been associated with lead poisoning.

A child may be acutely or chronically affected. Lead affects three body systems in particular: the renal, circulatory, and nervous systems. Renal damage occurs in the proximal tubules of the kidneys, resulting in abnormal excretion of important nutrients and impairment of vitamin D synthesis. Lead severely limits the body's ability to synthesize heme, leading to accumulation of alternate metabolites in the body and, ultimately, anemia (Wong, 1997). The most significant and irreversible effects of lead poisoning on the body occur in the nervous system. Fluid builds up in the brain, and intracranial pressure can reach life-threatening levels (Menkes, 1995). Cortical atrophy and lead encephalitis are usually associated with high levels of blood lead. This can lead to MR, paralysis, blindness, and convulsions. Low-level exposure has been associated with LD, ADHD, hearing impairment, and milder intellectual deficits. Other lead poisoning symptoms include cramping, digestive difficulty, lethargy, headache, and fever (Menkes, 1995).

■ INFECTIOUS CONDITIONS

Maternal Infections

The fetus may be infected by a variety of organisms. Some of these *infectious conditions* are passed from the mother to the fetus during pregnancy (transplacental infections), and others are present in the vagina and are passed to the infant at birth (ascending infections). These infections invade the fetus at a time when it has a limited capacity to ward off disease and, in the case of transplacental infections, at a time when they can have a profound effect on growth and development or the formation of tissues and organs.

The most common maternal infections are the *STORCH infections*, also called *TORCH* or *TORCHS*. Each of these conditions is caused by a specific virus or bacterium and possesses a different set of characteristics. Table 6-4 summarizes these five infections and their effects on the fetus. *Congenital syphilis* can be transmitted in the late stages of pregnancy or during delivery. It is the most virulent form of syphilis and requires isolation of the infected infant. The usual treatment for congenital syphilis is penicillin. Early-stage congenital syphilis is characterized by hepatitis, failure to thrive, neurologic involvement, fever, anemia, restlessness, irritability, and syphilitic rhinitis. Characteristic lesions may be present; hair and nails may be damaged. Osteochondritis at the joints and other bone abnormalities are relatively common. Late-stage congenital syphilis, because of residual damage from the infection, is marked by bony and dental anomalies and visual and auditory deficits (Berhman, Kliegman, & Arvin, 1996).

The mother, through ingestion of raw meat or contact with the feces of newly infected cats, may contract toxoplasmosis, transmitted at any point throughout pregnancy. It is also an increasingly common opportunistic infection in AIDS (McLeod & Remington, 1996; Siegel, 1990a). In the United States the incidence of toxoplasmosis is about 1.3 in 1000 live births (Siegel, 1990a). Stillbirth and death are common. Children born with this condition are often severely mentally handicapped. Hydrocephaly, cerebral calcification, and chorioretinitis are classic symptoms. CP, seizures, cardiac and liver damage, and gastrointestinal problems are also found. Treatment with sulphonomides and py-

---

table 6-4 *Intrauterine Infections (STORCH)*

Name	Cause	Type	Effects on Fetus
Syphilis	Parabacterial infection	A; T	Large liver and spleen; jaundice; anemia; rash; rhinorrhea
Toxoplasmosis	Parasitic infection	T	Deafness; blindness; mental retardation; seizures; pneumonia; large liver and spleen
Rubella	Virus	T	Meningitis; hearing loss; cataracts; cardiac problems; mental retardation; retinal defects
Cytomegalovirus	Virus	T	Hearing loss; in severe form, problems are similar to rubella
Herpes	Virus	A	Localized form: lethargy, rash, respiratory distress, jaundice, enlarged liver and spleen. Generalized form: attacks CNS, causing MR, seizures, and other problems

A, Ascending; *CNS,* central nervous system; *MR,* mental retardation; *T,* transplacental.

rimethamine is usually initiated in infected mothers and children. Once acquired, the neurologic deficits related to the disease can be reduced but not eliminated by maternal treatment (McLeod & Remington, 1996; Siegel, 1990a).

Rubella, a common and fairly mild disease in children, can be devastating when contracted by a pregnant woman, particularly in the first trimester. With the advent of a preventive vaccine, congenital rubella syndrome has declined 99% in the last 25 years; however, the dangers to unvaccinated mothers are significant (Berhman, Kliegman, & Arvin, 1996). Congenital defects, spontaneous abortion, and stillbirth may occur. Central processing hearing loss, MR, microcephaly, and seizures are possible outcomes. Congenital heart defects, including patent ductus arteriosus, are characteristic, as are visual deficits, hepatomegaly, and splenomegaly (Wong, 1997). These children may be SGA and may suffer from numerous respiratory infections in infancy. Late-occurring symptoms include diabetes, encephalitis, hearing loss, and thyroid problems. Functionally, children with congenital rubella symptoms may be expected to have mixed developmental delays and hearing and vestibular deficits. Adjustments to the child's therapy program may be necessary to accommodate cardiorespiratory effects.

Cytomegalovirus, or cytomegalic inclusion disease, has transmission and effects that are similar to rubella. It may be transmitted before, during, or after birth and is a herpes-type viral infection. This infection may also be active or latent in the newborn so that infection-control precautions are appropriate when working with this child. Clinical manifestations include low birth weight, sensorineural hearing loss, microcephaly, hepatomegaly, splenomegaly, and purpuric rash. Jaundice and hepatitis may also be present. Children with cytomegalovirus may be asymptomatic at birth. Symptomatic newborns have a poor prognosis related to neurologic deficits. These children often have learning disabilities and diminished cognitive skills.

The final STORCH infection is *congenital herpes.* The newborn most often contracts this condition during or after delivery by a mother with herpes simplex, often genital herpes (Wong, 1997). The infected child often develops skin, mouth, or eye lesions within 6 to 10 days of contact, but this is not always the case. Some children do not develop overt symptoms. In the disseminated form, a sepsislike picture presents itself and the child may develop internal organ lesions and encephalitis with CNS involvement. Infusion of antiviral agents may reduce the severity of this condition noticeably and has been known to prevent serious brain damage.

Gonorrhea and *chlamydia* are both transmitted to the infant late in fetal development or during delivery. Both may result in eye infections. Gonococcal arthritis, septicemia, and meningitis may also occur. Fortunately, both inflections respond well to antibiotic therapy if discov-

ered early. Other maternal infections known to affect neonatal health include varicella (chicken pox), coxsackie, parvovirus, hepatitis B, listeriosis, Lyme disease, and AIDS.

Acquired Immunodeficiency Syndrome

Acquired Immunodeficiency syndrome (AIDS), caused by HIV, is a major health concern for all, including infants, children, and adolescents. Investigators from the CDC estimate that about 15,000 HIV-infected children were born in the United States from 1978 to 1983. Children with AIDS represent the most serious disease manifestations of HIV. Additionally, the CDC indicates that 7689 cases of AIDS had been reported in children less than 13 years of age by 1996. Of the children with AIDS, 90% were associated with perinatal transmission and 8% were exposed to infected blood or blood products. In 2% of the children infected, the route of transmission was not identified (CDC, 1996). Most perinatal transmission occurs either in utero by transplacental passage of virus, intrapartum through contact with infected maternal blood and cervical secretions, or in the postpartum period through breast-feeding (Hutto & Scott, 1999). Most cases of AIDS in children were reported in minority populations: 58% of the children with AIDS were black, 23% were Hispanic, and 18% were white (Pizzo & Wilfert, 1998).

HIV infection is a disease that infects and damages cells of the immune system, thus making the child vulnerable to life-threatening illnesses that do not affect children with normal immunity. HIV-positive newborns are often asymptomatic at birth. The interval from birth to development of AIDS among perinatally affected infants varies widely. From evaluation of the most current data, there is a subset of perinatally infected children who do not have significant disease for years after their infection and a subset of children who develop the most serious manifestations of infection by 2 years of age (rapid progressors) (CDC, 1996). Onset of serious clinical disease, often before 6 months of age, is a prognostic indicator of survival. Cases of rapid progression of disease are currently under intensive study. Although investigators can identify which factors exist in rapid progressors, they cannot yet offer reasons for this subset of pathogenesis (Pizzo & Wilfert, 1998).

Until the early 1990s, prognosis for children infected with HIV was grim. Although HIV infection is still ultimately fatal, the prognosis has clearly changed, with an increasing proportion of children who are surviving into the second decade of life. The improvement in this prognosis is directly related to potent antiretroviral drugs, better prevention of opportunistic infections, and the use of intravenous drugs to prevent recurrent bacterial infections. Clinical management of HIV-infected children remains intensive with recommendations for clinical evaluations and laboratory assessment to be completed every

3 months. Any viral or bacterial infection is considered a serious breach of immune system integrity and is carefully monitored. Recommendations for HIV-infected children are different, with recommendations for inactivated vaccines for protection and contraindication of live vaccines.

Criteria for a diagnosis of HIV infection include positive results on two separate determinations or the presence of one or more AIDS-defining illnesses. Pediatric classifications for HIV infection are listed in two ways: one set of criteria for immune functioning and a second set of criteria for clinical pathology.

Most HIV specialists indicate that early and aggressive treatment for children with HIV includes combination antiretroviral drug therapy and that intravenous gamma globulin will decrease viral load, which preserves the immune system, provides a longer time to develop the disease, and prolongs survival. As indicated by the diagnostic features, infections are a common occurrence after HIV infection. Children tend to have an increase in minor bacterial infections, including otitis media, urinary tract infections, and pneumonia. Fungal infections include oral candidiasis and candida dermatitis. Children with recurrent infections may benefit from gamma-globulin administered intravenously. *Pneumocystis carinii* pneumonia (PCP) is the most common opportunistic infection seen in children. PCP prevention has become an important focus for care for both HIV and AIDS populations.

Although no cure currently exists for HIV infection or AIDS, antiretroviral drugs can prolong survival. The most commonly used drugs in children are nuceloside analogues that inhibit reverse transcriptase of the virus. These drugs result in a significant slowing of progression of the disease and are associated with prolonged survival times. Initiation of therapy is started immediately after birth, and medical visits include monitoring the HIV infection as well as routine care and immunizations.

As the disease progresses to a severe level, suppression of the immune system, chronic respiratory illness, skin and other infections, and diarrhea often noticeably weaken infected children. These conditions often respond slowly to treatment (Hutto & Scott, 1999). Developmental delays and degeneration may result in delayed or lost motor, speech, and independent living skills. Neurologic deficits, including ataxia, spasticity, rigidity, tremor, and seizures, may be expected as the disease progresses (Hutto & Scott, 1999). Early intervention and rehabilitative and educational services are often indicated (Rutstein, Conlon, & Batshaw, 1997).

Additionally, both the child and family may be socially isolated. Drug-dependent mothers in particular require training in the care and parenting skills needed to work with HIV-infected children. Older children may require opportunities for normal play, social, and prevocational activities. The interactions among children with AIDS, their families, and health care workers need to be positive, accepting, and supportive. The risk of HIV infection from clients to occupational therapists is extremely small. Few health care workers have contracted AIDS from their clients, and nearly all of those who did, did so through prolonged or open skin contact with infected blood products (Lyons & Valentine, 1994). Use of correct universal precautions with all clients should allow any occupational therapist to work safely. Furthermore, the role of preventing HIV infection through client and family education of children with developmental delays and learning and emotional disabilities belongs to all health professionals, including occupational therapists.

Lyme Disease

Caused by a spirochete infection secondary to a bite from a tick of the genus Ixodes, *Lyme disease* has grown to epidemic proportions in recent years (Hollister, 1999; Shapiro, 1996). The disease is often mistaken for JRA in children, and differential diagnosis may be done serologically. Lyme disease may be observed as having three stages, with early treatment often valuable in preventing the disabling effects of the latter stages.

Stage 1 is the actual tick bite, usually from a deer tick. In Stage 2 the individual develops a distinctive, red, target-shaped lesion, often at the site of the tick bite. This lesion usually occurs 3 to 30 days after infection (McIntosh & Lauer, 1999). These lesions may be present for 1 to 3 weeks and may foster secondary lesions in some children (Wong, 1997). The individual may also develop flulike symptoms, including fever, pain, and fatigue. Several weeks or months later, in Stage 3, the child may develop cardiac, neurologic, muscular, or joint disorders. The intensity and duration of the condition may vary considerably. In severe cases, symptoms can be debilitating.

Neurologic involvement includes cranial nerve palsies, meningitis, and radiculoneuropathy, causing pain, nausea, lability, and sensory disturbances. Arthritis-like symptoms are among the most common indications of the syndrome, usually occurring in the large joints. These symptoms are often of sudden onset and affect single joints, although they may be migratory. Attacks may be of short or long duration. Cardiac symptoms are less common and are usually brief. These may include myocarditis or ventricular dysfunctions.

Treatment includes rest and antibiotic therapy, usually penicillin, erythromycin, or in older children, tetracycline (Shapiro, 1996). Intravenous, high-dose penicillin has had some effect. Sequelae of this condition are often treated symptomatically, including pain relief, support, mobilization, and assistance in self-care activities. The child with Lyme disease may also demonstrate reduced endurance, general malaise, and depression if symptoms continue over an extended period.

Encephalitis and Meningitis

Encephalitis and meningitis, infections of the brain and its coverings, are frightening and sometimes dangerous. *Encephalitis* is an inflammation of the brain, which may be caused by bacteria, spirochetes, and other organisms, but usually is caused by a viral infection (Weil & Levin, 1995). The specific cause of encephalitis is often not identified clinically. The condition may be localized or may also include the spinal cord or meninges. Infection of the brain may be direct or secondary to another infection. Mosquitoes spread several of its viral forms; therefore summer onset is common. Herpes simplex has also been associated disproportionately with encephalitis in young children.

The severity of these conditions varies with the cause. Onset may be sudden or gradual, and it is often difficult to distinguish from other infections. Symptoms include fever, headache, dizziness, stiff neck, nausea and vomiting, tremors, and ataxia. In severe cases, stupor, seizures, disorientation, coma, and death may occur. Diagnosis is based on environmental patterns of infection, clinical findings, EEG, and MRI, as well as laboratory examination of blood, brain tissue, or CSF. Treatment may include antibiotics if bacterial infection is suggested but is primarily supportive while the acute disease runs its course (Wong, 1997).

Unfortunately, encephalitis can result in severe-to-mild residual brain damage. The amount of damage depends on the age of the child, type of infection, and care. Young children are at increased risk for neurologic complications. Health care staff must monitor the child's progress and neurologic status after the infection. MR, LDs, behavior disorders, seizures, and neuromotor deficits are common. Neurorehabilitation techniques are applied to limit the disability, and compensatory interventions including assistive technology may assist this child in school, play, and later, prevocational activities (Powell, 1997).

Meningitis is an infection of the meninges, the tissue covering the brain and spinal cord. Meningitis, like encephalitis, may have several causes, including tubercular, fungal, protozoan, viral, and most commonly, bacterial. Clinical manifestations of meningitis vary slightly in newborns, infants, older children, and adolescents, but the clinical picture is not unlike encephalitis. Headache, fever, and rigidity in the neck are classic signs. These may be accompanied by seizures, vomiting, spasticity, behavioral and arousal state changes, and in young children, bulging fontanels. In newborns, jaundice, cyanosis, hypothermia, and respiratory distress may also be present (Weil & Levin, 1995).

Diagnostic evaluation may include lumbar puncture, analysis of CSF, and blood, throat, and nasal cultures. Treatment includes management of the underlying infection with antibiotics, hydration, maintenance of intracranial pressure, and treatment of symptoms and complications. Because many forms of the disease are highly contagious, the acutely ill client may be isolated. The child may be monitored for apnea and cardiac function. As with encephalitis, neuromotor, visual, auditory, seizure, and learning disorders may remain after the acute infection abates. Anticonvulsant and rehabilitative therapy is necessary to manage and remediate these sequelae.

Osteomyelitis

Osteomyelitis is an inflammation of the bone marrow that may be caused by puncture wounds, infection adjacent to the bone, or microorganisms that travel in the blood (Brown, 1997). Initially the organisms settle in the distal end of the metaphysis. As the disease progresses, the infection spreads throughout the bone and outward to the periosteum. Initial symptoms include pain, tenderness, and unwillingness to use or bear weight on the involved limb. Osteomyelitis occurs most commonly in boys between 5 and 14 years of age (Wong, 1997). Fever, soft tissue swelling, and often anorexia follow these symptoms. The child is often ill and experiences pain on movement.

Treatment must be initiated as soon as possible because prolonged infection may cause bone destruction, pathologic fractures, septic arthritis, and eventually growth disturbances (Salter, 1983). Diagnosis is usually made based on clinical signs, and confirmation is made from specimen aspiration test results, blood cell counts, and positive radiographic evidence (Salter, 1983). Initial treatment usually consists of oral or intravenous antibiotic therapy for at least 3 weeks and bed rest and immobility of the affected body part, including splinting. If improvement is not observed, surgery is performed, which includes drilling into the bone to remove the pus and damaged tissue and putting in place drainage tubes and intravenous tubes that are used to infuse the site with a saline and antibiotic solution (Salter, 1983). After these procedures, splinting of the extremity or traction helps prevent the spread of infection, reduces pain, and prevents contractures. Relapses can lead to chronic osteomyelitis that may involve continued discharge of pus from a sinus over the infected area, pain, or the formation of an abscess cavity in the bone itself. Bed rest and antibiotics may clear the problem, or surgical procedures may have to be repeated. Chronic untreated osteomyelitis presents serious medical problems that can be minimized by early detection and prolonged antibiotic therapy.

■ NEOPLASTIC DISORDERS

Cancer is devastating for anyone, but it seems somehow even more insidious when it attacks children. The pain, fear, and life disruption it causes is chronic and affects the child, the child's family, and all of those around the child. The major *neoplastic disorders* that children can acquire are discussed in this section.

Leukemia

Leukemia is a cancer of the blood-forming tissues. It is the most common form of cancer found in children, occurring in 6 to 7 children per 100,000. It occurs in boys more frequently than in girls, almost always in white children, and most frequently in children with Down syndrome. It has a peak incidence between 2 and 5 years of age. Two forms of leukemia recognized in children are acute lymphoid leukemia (ALL) and acute nonlymphoid, or acute myelogenous, leukemia (ANLL or AML) (Wong, 1997). The symptoms of these two forms of cancer are similar, but they react differently to treatment, with ALL having the more favorable response. The causes of leukemia are unknown, but immunologic and chromosomal factors have been associated with the condition.

Leukemia is characterized by the uncontrolled multiplication of immature white blood cells, which prevents the bone marrow from producing normal blood cells (Champlin, 1988). Symptoms include loss of weight, night sweats, chronic fatigue, paleness, a high fever; repeated infections; purpura; and enlarged lymph nodes, spleen, and liver. Examining a specimen of bone marrow for lymphoblasts usually makes diagnosis. Blood counts are also taken.

The goal of medical management is the achievement of complete "cure" by inducing remission, eliminating cells in "sanctuaries" like the CNS, and maintaining the remission. Specifically, treatment is conducted in three phases. The first phase is called *induction therapy* and is designed to rid the bone marrow and the rest of the body of the leukemia cells. The second phase is called *central nervous system prophylaxis* and is aimed at killing cells in the brain and spinal cord. The third phase of treatment is called *maintenance therapy* in which chemotherapy is administered to treat small deposits of cells that remain after remission (Hockenberry & Coody, 1986).

Prognosis for leukemia is much improved over recent years, with the majority of clients with ALL experiencing remission for at least 5 years. Many go long periods with no recurrent signs. Prognosis for children with CNS involvement and ANLL is poorer but still hopeful, particularly with bone marrow transplantation. Furthermore, these children undergo long courses of treatment that can be painful and frightening, and recurrence of the disease and death remain possibilities that must be handled emotionally.

Brain Tumors

Tumors of the brain and spinal cord are the most common tumors of solid tissues in children. Most of these tumors occur in the cerebellum and brainstem, with *medul-*

loblastomas and *astrocytomas* accounting for 30% of all childhood tumors. *Gliomas* and *ependymomas* (ventricular tumors) are also relatively common. The cause of brain tumors is unknown but is believed to be developmental or chromosomal in nature. Tumors may not become evident early in life because they are usually related to increases in intracranial pressure. In the young child the skull is soft enough to provide some accommodation for this phenomenon. Diagnosis is based first on clinical signs and then confirmed with CT scans, MRI images, EEG studies and lumbar puncture.

Symptoms of brain tumors include recurrent and progressive headaches, vomiting (particularly in the morning), loss of coordination or strength, increased reflex activity, changes in behavior, seizures, and vital sign disturbances. Specific symptoms may relate to the location of the tumor. Treatment includes surgical removal of the tumor, radiation therapy, and chemotherapy. Prognosis varies with the type, size, and location of the tumor. The survival rate for astrocytomas (75%) is better than that for medulloblastomas (25% to 35%), which is better than that for glial cell tumors (20% to 30%). Survival with ependymomas varies from 15% to 60%, depending on the study (Maul-Mellott & Adams, 1987). Recurrence of brain tumors is common, and surgery, chemotherapy, and radiation therapy may cause permanent brain damage. Children recovering from these tumors may require a broad spectrum of CNS-based rehabilitation to improve residual sensorimotor and cognitive function.

Hodgkin's Disease

Hodgkin's disease and other *lymphomas* are far less common than leukemia (15 in 1,000,000 people) but are still significant. This condition is commonly a disease of later childhood and adolescence. This cancer of the lymphatic system is marked by painless adenopathy in the cervical region with or without fever. The child may also experience chills and night sweats, anorexia and weight loss, and general malaise. Diagnosis is made by histologic examination of the node. Blood studies may also show characteristic abnormalities. Four stages of the disease have been identified. In stage I, only one node is involved. Stage II demonstrates involvement on only one side of the diaphragm. In stages III and IV, progressively more organs are involved.

Treatment consists of radiation therapy, chemotherapy, or splenectomy. Prognosis is excellent for children in stages I, II and III, but clients with widespread disease have only a 50% survival rate (Maul-Mellott & Adams, 1987).

Non-Hodgkin's lymphomas (NHLs) occur primarily in school-age children. They are more common in boys and are a significant problem for black children. They may also occur as a second malignancy after Hodgkin's disease. Onset is acute, and progression is rapid; most children have disseminated disease at diagnosis. Symptoms include abdominal pain, vomiting, anorexia, diarrhea, ascites, and distention of the abdomen. Fever, a palpable mass, and paraplegia may also be present. Diagnosis is made through physical examination and analysis of laboratory results. Radiation therapy, chemotherapy, and surgery may be initiated to treat these conditions. Prognosis varies with the degree of bone marrow and CNS involvement and with the number and size of tumors present. Between 50% and 80% of those diagnosed survive beyond 3 years (Maul-Mellott & Adams, 1987).

Wilms' Tumor

Wilms' tumor, or nephroblastoma, is a neoplasm of the kidney and is the most common abdominal cancer of children (7.8 in 1,000,000). It is a highly malignant cancer but may be encapsulated for some time and responds well to chemotherapy and surgery. Clinical signs of this tumor include a firm, palpable mass on one side of the body, fatigue and malaise, fever, and occasionally hematuria and hypertension. Wilms' tumor can metastasize to the lung, which may produce respiratory symptoms as well. Surgery is performed as soon as the diagnosis is suggested and includes full or partial nephrectomy, with great care taken to maintain the tumor capsule (Wong, 1997). Survival rates are excellent and improving for most cases, even in some children who experience a recurrence.

Bone Tumors

The two major tumors of the bone, osteosarcoma and Ewing's sarcoma, are relatively uncommon but result in physical disability and, not infrequently, death. Most of these tumors occur in adolescence, more frequently in boys. Survival for both cancers is dependent on early diagnosis before metastatic disease appears. Diagnosis is made by radiologic analysis, with each tumor having a characteristic pattern. Clinical signs include localized pain that may be relieved by change in position, lumps, and reduction in activity level.

Osteosarcoma usually occurs at the end of the long bones, particularly the femur. Large spindle cells and malignant osteoid bone is formed next to the growth plate. A painful mass develops. Frequently a secondary trauma at the site of the tumor brings it to attention. Because osteosarcoma is resistant to radiation therapy, amputation is performed if possible. This is followed by a course of chemotherapy. If metastases occur, they are usually located in the bones or lungs. In their absence the chance of survival is good (up to 50%) but not certain. The child with osteosarcoma also requires prosthetic equipment and training after surgery (Pizzo & Poplack, 1989; Simon, 1988).

Ewing's sarcoma occurs more frequently in the bones of the trunk but also in the long bones and skull. It does not form osteoid tissue but rather small, round groups of cells. This condition spreads its metastases hematologically, particularly to the bones and lungs. Surgery is not performed routinely and often is done only late in treatment. Ewing's sarcoma responds well to radiation therapy and chemotherapy is also routinely prescribed. In the absence of metastases and for distal lesions, survival rates are good (up to 60%). However, if there are metastases, the prognosis is poor (Pizzo & Poplack, 1989).

■ BURNS

Major *burn injury* accounts for a large number of children who must undergo prolonged painful and restrictive hospitalizations. Additionally, countless other children suffer from minor burns. Thermal, electrical, chemical, and radioactive sources can cause burns, but thermal burns are by far the most common. Most burns can be attributed to accidents; however, 10% to 20% of hospital admissions for burns may be attributed to child abuse. Children under 3 years of age account for the majority of thermal burns, and of these, hot water and hot beverage scalds account for 50% to 60% of injuries (Murphy, Purdue, Hunt, & Hicks, 1997). About 30% of burns in older children are related to flame (e.g., match, gasoline, firecracker) or chemical burns. Short periods of high heat or long periods of low heat both can cause significant burns. Chemical burns can cause serious injury, but their effect can often be stopped with prompt emergency treatment. Electrical burns, however, may damage not only the skin, but also underlying bone, muscle, and nerve tissue along the conduction path. Damage can also be caused by smoke inhalation, respiratory failure, shock, and posttraumatic infection (Wong, 1997).

The following criteria determine the prognosis for survival of a child with a burn injury: percentage of body area burned, depth of the burn, location of the burn, age of the child, causative agent, presence of respiratory involvement, length of hospital stay, and presence of other injuries (Baker et. al., 1996).

The percentage of area injured, in children, is assessed according to the total body surface area (TBSA) affected, either by the rule of nines in children older than 10 or by charts specifically designed to accurately estimate the body proportions involved in children of different ages (Murphy et. al., 1997; Wong, 1997). The rule of nines ascribes 9% of TBSA to the head and neck, 9% to each upper extremity, 18% to each lower extremity, 36% to the trunk (18% anterior and 18% posterior), and 1% to the perineum and genitals. In children under 10 years of age, accuracy of TBSA estimations are improved through use of various charts to estimate the modified rule of nines (Figure 6-16). The mortality rates of children under 4 years of age with greater than 30% TBSA are significantly higher than that of older children with the same burn size (46.9% versus 12.5%, respectively) (Morrow et. al., 1996). Inhalation injuries are significantly correlated with

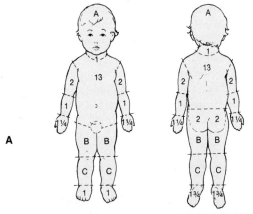

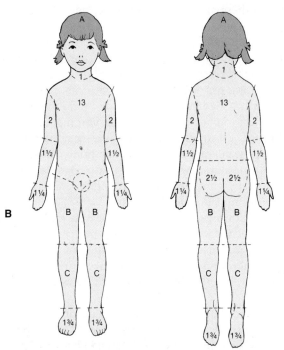

RELATIVE PERCENTAGES OF AREAS AFFECTED BY GROWTH

AREA	BIRTH	AGE 1 YR	AGE 5 YR
A = ½ of head	9½	8½	6½
B = ½ of one thigh	2¾	3¼	4
C = ½ of one leg	2½	2½	2¾

RELATIVE PERCENTAGES OF AREAS AFFECTED BY GROWTH

AREA	AGE 10 YR	AGE 15 YR	ADULT
A = ½ of head	5½	4½	3½
B = ½ of one thigh	4½	4½	4¾
C = ½ of one leg	3	3¼	3½

figure 6-16   Estimation of distribution of burns in children. **A,** Children from birth to 5 years of age. **B,** Older children. *(From Wong, D. [1999]. Whaley and Wong's nursing care of infants and children [6th ed.]. St. Louis: Mosby.)*

death. Additionally, major burns of less than 30% TBSA in children under 4 years of age may result in death in spite of excellent emergency and burn care.

The American Burn Association (1996) also classifies burns as minor, moderate, and severe. In minor burns, less than 10% of the TBSA is covered by a partial-thickness burn; these burns are adequately treated on an outpatient basis. A moderate burn is considered 10% to 20% of the TBSA covered with a partial-thickness burn and requires hospitalization. A major burn is considered any full-thickness burn or greater than 20% of TBSA covered with a partial-thickness burn.

The depth of the burn is assessed according to the number of layers of tissue involved in the injury (Figure 6-17). *Superficial burns,* or first-degree burns, demonstrate minimal tissue damage, although they can be painful. In these burns the skin is red and dry, and healing typically occurs without scaring. *Partial-thickness burns,* or second-degree burns, involve the epidermis and dermis in varying degrees and can be further classified into deep and superficial burns. Superficial partial-thickness burns involve the epidermis and a portion of the dermis, but many of the dermal elements are left intact. Partial-thickness burns appear slightly raised, blistered, reddened, and moist, and they blanch to the touch. These are the most painful of burns and may result in some scarring, although superficial partial-thickness burns may heal spontaneously. In deep partial-thickness burns, both the epidermis and dermis are damaged but the sweat glands and hair follicles of the dermis are left intact. In many cases a deep partial-thickness burn will resemble a full-thickness burn. The appearance of these injuries is dry, soft, and waxy, with no edema or raised appearance. In *full-thickness burns,* or third or fourth degree burns, all layers of the skin are destroyed, as may be some of the underlying subcutaneous tissue (see Figure 6-17). The appearance of full-thickness burns is hard, insensate, leathery, and inflexible eschar. Some systems include a fourth-degree burn classification when the damage extends to underlying muscle, bone, and fascia. These burns may be charred, brown, or red; nerve endings and blood vessels may be damaged; and pain may not be present in the central area. Most third- and fourth-degree burns also have borders of second-degree burns that are painful (Wong, 1997).

When a moderate or major burn occurs, critical care focuses on the maintenance of breathing if there is evidence of respiratory involvement. Additionally, emergency care focuses on immediate replacement of fluids, nutrition, and pain management. The intensive pathophysiologic response to a major burn creates a need to balance the amount of fluid replacement and nutrition carefully to compensate for loss of blood, presence of edema, and critical sodium or potassium changes. Sedation is needed to allow tolerance of treatment and for

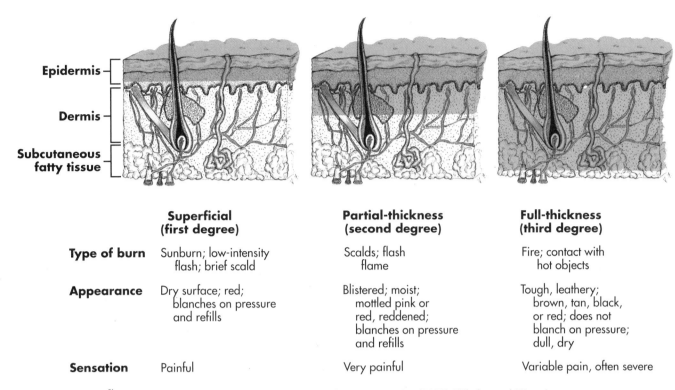

	Superficial (first degree)	Partial-thickness (second degree)	Full-thickness (third degree)
Type of burn	Sunburn; low-intensity flash; brief scald	Scalds; flash flame	Fire; contact with hot objects
Appearance	Dry surface; red; blanches on pressure and refills	Blistered; moist; mottled pink or red, reddened; blanches on pressure and refills	Tough, leathery; brown, tan, black, or red; does not blanch on pressure; dull, dry
Sensation	Painful	Very painful	Variable pain, often severe

figure 6-17   Classification of burn depth. *(From Wong, D. (1997). Whaley and Wong's essentials of pediatric nursing [5th ed.]. St. Louis: Mosby.)*

comfort. Additionally, pain management is ongoing throughout treatment. Morphine, morphine combined with methadone, ketamine, propofol, and nitrous oxide have all demonstrated usefulness in pain management after major burns.

In addition to emergency care, prevention of secondary infection, wound débridement, and wound closure are critical. The application of antimicrobial agents to prevent secondary infection is an ongoing process until the wound is closed. A variety of topical antimicrobial agents are used to help with prevention of infection. Silver nitrate, silver sulfadiazine, mafenide acetate, nystatin, neomycin, povidone-iodine, and bacitracin are the most common (Murphy et. al., 1997; Wong, 1997). However, after a deep partial- or full-thickness burn, primary excision is often required before treatment with topical agents is effective. Additionally, physicians are initiating the use of growth hormone, which has been shown to enhance wound healing and decrease nutritional requirements (Ramirez, Wolf, Barrow, & Herndon, 1998).

Débridement of necrotic tissue is also essential to recovery. Débridement employs use of hydrotherapy to remove debris, cleanse the wound, and allow increased ROM in all body parts. This is typically an extremely painful process undergone twice a day and typically requires the child to be sedated. Tissue is redressed with topical antimicrobial agents and gauze (Murphy et. al.,

1997). Full-thickness, partial-thickness, or meshed skin grafts may be used to cover large burned areas. Wound healing procedures may need to be repeated if the grafts do not "take." Skin-grafting procedures using synthetic and animal skins have significantly improved the prognosis for skin healing. In severe burns, reconstructive surgeries are often needed to limit the long-term effects of burn injuries.

The team approach is essentially universal in burn care units in the United States. The American Burn Association has established guidelines for personnel to be involved in a burn unit team. The team consists of physicians with specialized training in burn care, nurses, occupational therapists, physical therapists, speech therapists, psychologists, and social workers. Occupational therapists are typically involved very early after the burn injury, often within 24 hours (Biggs, de Linde, Banzszewski, & Heinrich, 1998).

The major goals of burn rehabilitation include early skin coverage, correction of cosmetic damage, restoration of function, and integration back into the environment. During the acute period, positioning, hydrotherapy, splinting, active and passive ROM, and ADL modalities are used to prevent contractures and ensure optimal functional and physical outcomes. Many of these procedures are painful, and infection is a continued threat until all burned areas are closed. During this period the child also experiences malaise and may be heavily sedated. Ongoing treatment goals include minimizing problems with scarring, optimizing active ROM, decreasing hypersenstivity, preventing contractures, ensuring good use of hands, and optimizing skills for self-care, home, and school activities (Biggs et. al., 1998; Staley et. al., 1996). These goals include the use of various techniques, including fitting and maintenance of pressure garments, splinting, active and passive ROM, client and family education about stretching and scar formation, emotional support, massage to prevent hypertrophied scaring, and adaptation of ADLs.

Outcome measures used to determine successful burn rehabilitation include resumption of typical daily living skills (e.g., return to school), scar rating, and sensorimotor skills (e.g., ROM, gross and fine motor skills). Numerous rating scales have been developed to characterize or assess a scar. Reliable assessment of the scar surface (e.g., to evaluate healing) includes border height, thickness, and color of a scar (Yeong et. al., 1997). Each of these four characteristics is rated from −1 to 4, with pictorial definitions used for each characterization; a composite score is then generated for the overall scar appearance.

Scar appearance and location are typically believed to influence psychosocial adaptation. Location of the scar on the face or neck is also believed to be correlated with lower self-esteem, less engagement in typical activities, and fewer interpersonal interactions; however, the accuracy of these beliefs is controversial (Kimmo, Jyrki, & Sirpa, 1998; Moore et. al., 1996). Ongoing scar massage techniques have been shown to be effective, if they are initiated before the development of invasive hypertrophied scarring. Splinting continues to be used, primarily after limitations in ROM are noted, except in full-thickness or deep partial-thickness burns where loss of ROM and likelihood of scar contractures are the greatest (Richard, Staley, Miller, & Warden, 1997). The process of scar remodeling, plastic surgery, and revision of skin grafts may be needed for up to 2 years after a major injury.

Possibly more important measures are developmental outcomes and return-to-school outcomes. Developmental outcomes, especially language development and social skills, have been shown to be delayed after burn injury in children, even if physical and functional skills are within normal limits (Gorga et. al., 1999). Adjustment to school after a burn injury is generally successful in spite of the severity of burn, provided that the return-to-school reentry program is comprehensive (i.e., includes peer counseling, encouragement to return promptly to school, early contacts with the school, comprehensive school plan, engaging parents in reentry efforts, social skills training) (Staley et. al., 1999; Wong, 1997). Therapists can be involved in each step of the rehabilitation and return-to-school process, providing ongoing direct services, consultation, and monitoring.

■ SUMMARY

This chapter provides an overview of medical diagnoses in children who often receive occupational therapy services. Knowledge about the child's medical condition is important for developing appropriate intervention plans and for communicating with family and team members. Application of this information should consider that each child's presentation of the diagnosis is unique and that the effect of the disease or disability on the child's function is highly influenced by environmental and developmental variables. The field of medicine continually expands, and the occupational therapist must stay abreast of new developments and current information. Best practice requires thorough research of each diagnosis incurred. To assist in researching the implication of the medical diagnoses discussed in this chapter, key references for each of the diagnoses have been cited and should be accessed to obtain additional information.

STUDY QUESTIONS

1. Describe the classification system for traumatic head injuries. How does this disease affect the child's daily living function?
2. Describe osteogenesis imperfecta. What are precautions in working with a child with this diagnosis?
3. Name two general goals in intervention with children with juvenile rheumatoid arthritis. What is the typical course of this disease?
4. Describe the pathology of two different neuromuscular conditions. Explain how impairment in functional performance results from the conditions.
5. List four functional performance consequences for children with cerebral palsy. Explain the difficulties that may be incurred in self-feeding in the child with (a) upper extremity spasticity and (b) upper extremity athetosis.
6. What are three impairments associated with myelomeningocele? Explain why a child with this diagnosis may have difficulty achieving independence in dressing.
7. Define *autism* and describe the primary problems that affect the child's ability to engage in social play with peers.
8. *Learning disabilities* is used to categorize a multitude of learning problems. Name two types of impairments that are categorized as learning disabilities.
9. The common infections that a mother can transmit to the fetus are called (S)TORCH infections. What are these five infections? Briefly describe each.
10. List three types of cancer common to children. Define the prognosis for each.

References

Abel, E.L. (1997). *Fetal alcohol abuse syndrome revisited*. New York: Plenum Press.

Adams, R.D, Victor, M., & Ropper, A.H. (1997). *Principles of neurology* (6th ed.). New York: McGraw-Hill.

Adelson, P.D., & Kochanek, P.M. (1998). Head injury in children. *Journal of Child Neurology, 13,* 2-15.

American Burn Association. (1996). *Burn severity-rating scale.* New York: Author.

American Psychiatric Association. (1994). *Diagnostic and statistical manual of mental disorders* (4th ed.). Washington, D.C.: Author.

Anderson, G.M., & Hoshino, Y. (1997). Neurochemical studies of autism. In D.J. Cohen & F.R. Volkmar. *Handbook of autism and pervasive developmental disorders* (2nd ed.). (pp. 325-343). New York: Wiley.

Ayres, A.J., & Tickle, L. (1980). Hyperresponsivity to touch and vestibular stimuli as a predictor of positive response to sensory integration procedures in autistic children. *American Journal of Occupational Therapy, 34,* 375-340.

Baker, R.A., Jones, S., Sanders, C., Sandinski, C., Martin-Duffy, K., Berchin, H., & Valentine, S. (1996). Degree of burn, location of burn, and length of hospital stay as predictors of psychosocial status and physical functioning. *Journal of Burn Care and Rehabilitation, 17* (4), 327-333.

Barkley, R.A. (1998). *Attention-deficit hyperactivity disorder: A handbook for diagnosis and treatment* (2nd ed.). New York: Guilford.

Barkley, R.A. (1997). Inhibition, sustained attention, and executive functions: Constructing a unifying theory of ADHD. *Psychological Bulletin, 121,* 65-94.

Batshaw, M.L. (Ed.). (1997a). *Children with disabilities* (4th ed.). Baltimore: Brookes.

Batshaw, M.L. (1997b). Fragile X syndrome. In M.L. Batshaw (Ed.), *Children with disabilities* (4th ed.). (pp. 377-388). Baltimore: Brookes.

Batshaw, M.L., & Conlon, C.J. (1997). Substance abuse: A preventable threat to development. In M.L. Batshaw (Ed.). *Children with disabilities* (4th ed.), (pp. 143-162). Baltimore: Brookes.

Batshaw, M.L., & Shapiro, B.K. (1997). Mental retardation. In M.L. Batshaw (Ed.), *Children with disabilities* (4th ed.). (pp. 335-360). Baltimore: Brookes.

Beattie, T.F. (1997). Minor head injury. *Archives of Disease in Childhood, 77,* 82-85.

Berhman, R.E., Kliegman, R.M., & Arvin, A.M. (Eds.). (1996). *Nelson textbook of pediatrics* (15th ed.). Philadelphia: W.B. Saunders.

Biggs, K.S., de Linde, L., Banaszewski, M., & Heinrich, J.J. (1998). Determining the current roles of physical and occupational therapists in burn care. *Journal of Burn Care and Rehabilitation, 19* (5), 442-449.

Boat, T.F. (1996). Cystic fibrosis. In R.E. Berhman, R.M. Kliegman, & A.M. Arvin (Eds.), *Nelson textbook of pediatrics* (15th ed.). (pp. 1239-1250). Philadelphia: W.B. Saunders.

Bobath, K. (1980). *A neurophysiological basis for the treatment of cerebral palsy.* Philadelphia: J.B. Lippincott.

Bobath, K., & Bobath, B. (1972). Cerebral palsy. In P.H. Pearson & C.E. Williams (Eds.), *Physical therapy services in the developmental disabilities.* Springfield, Ill: Charles C. Thomas.

Boguniewicz, M., & Leung, D.Y.M. (1999) Allergic disorders. In W.W. Hay, A.R. Hayward, M.J. Levin, & J.M. Sondheimer (Eds.), *Current pediatric diagnosis and treatment* (14th ed.). Stamford, Conn: Appleton & Lange.

Bregman, J.D., & Gerdtz, J. (1997). Behavioral interventions. In D.J. Cohen & F.R. Volkmar (Eds.), *Handbook of autism and pervasive developmental disorders* (2nd ed.). (pp. 847-867). New York: Wiley.

Brook, M.M. (1998). The cardiovascular system. In R.E. Berhman & R.M. Kliegman (Eds.), *Nelson essentials of pediatrics* (3rd ed.). (pp. 497-544). Philadelphia: W.B. Saunders.

Brown, L.W. (1997). Seizure disorders. In M.L. Batshaw (Ed.), *Children with disabilities.* (4th ed.). (pp. 553-594). Baltimore: Brookes.

Burack, J.A., Hodapp, R.M., & Zigler, E. (1998). *Handbook of mental retardation and development.* New York: Cambridge University Press.

Carroll, J.E. (1985). Diagnosis and management of Duchenne muscular dystrophy. *Pediatric Review, 6,* 195-200.

Centers for Disease Control and Prevention. (1996). *HIV-AIDS surveillance report* (Vol. 8). (pp. 1-39). Atlanta: Author.

Centers for Disease Control and Prevention. (1997). *National vital statistics reports* (Vol. 47, No. 18). Atlanta: Author.

Chambers, H.G. (1997). The surgical treatment of spasticity. *Muscle and Nerve, 6*(supplement), 121-128.

Champlin, R. (1988). Acute myeleogenous leukemia: Biology and treatment, *Mediguide to Oncology, 8* (4), 1-4, 6, 9.

Chance, P.F., Ashizawa, T., Hoffman, E.P., & Crawford, T.O. (1998). Molecular basis of neuromuscular diseases. *Physical Medicine and Rehabilitation Clinics of North America, 9,* 49-81.

Church, M.W., & Abel, E.L. (1998). Fetal alcohol syndrome. *Obstetrics and Gynecology Clinics of North America, 25* (1), 85, 1998.

Church, R.P., Lewis, M.E.B., & Batshaw, M.L. (1997). Learning disabilities. In M.L. Batshaw (Ed.), *Children with disabilities* (4th ed.). (pp. 471-498). Baltimore: Brookes.

Clark, E.B. (1997). Congenital heart disease. In R.A. Hockelman, S.B. Friedman, N.M. Nelson, & H.M. Seidel (Eds.), *Primary pediatric care* (3rd ed.). (pp. 1253-1259). St. Louis: Mosby.

Cohen, D.J., & Volkmar, F.R. (Eds.), (1997). *Handbook of autism and pervasive developmental disorders* (2nd ed.). New York: Wiley.

Coles, C. (1994). Critical periods for prenatal alcohol exposure. *National Institutes of Health: Alcohol Health and Research World, 18* (1), 112-115.

Coles, C., Brown, B.T., Smith, I.E., Platzman, K.A., Erickson, S., & Falek, A. (1991). Effects of prenatal alcohol exposure at school age. *Neurotoxicology and Teratology, 13,* 357-367.

Damasio, A.R., & Maurer, R.G. (1978). A neurological model for childhood autism. *Archives of Neurology, 35* (12), 777-786.

De La Cruz, M.V., Gomez, C.S., & Cayre, R. (1991). The developmental components of the ventricles: Their significance in congenital heart malformations. *Cardiology with the Young Child, 1* (2), 123-128.

Dodson, W.E. (1989). Medical treatment and pharmacology of antiepileptic drugs. *Pediatric Clinics of North America, 36* (2), 421-433.

Drash, A. (1989). Insulin-dependent diabetis mellitus, *Nursing Clinics of North American, 20,* 191-198.

Eisen, A., & Humphreys, P.(1974). Guillian-Barré syndrome. *Archives of Neurology, 30,* 438.

Elia, J., Ambrosini, P.J., & Rapoport, J.L. (1999). Treatment of attention-deficit-hyperactivity disorder. *New England Journal of Medicine, 340* (10), 780-788.

Evans, J.P.M., & Rogers, D.W. (1980). Sickle cell disease and thalassemia. *Current Opinion in Pediatrics, 2* (1), 121-123.

Gorga, D., Johnson, J., Bentley, A., Siverburg, R., Glassman, M., Madden, M., Yurt, R., & Nagler, W. (1999). The physical, functional, and developmental outcome of pediatric burn survivors from 1-12 months postinjury. *Journal of Burn Care and Rehabilitation, 20* (2), 171-178.

Greenhill, L.L. (1998). Diagnosing attention-deficit/hyperactivity disorder in children. *Journal of Clinical Psychiatry, 59* (supplement 7), 31-41.

Hammill, D.D. (1990). On defining learning disabilities: An emerging consensus. *Journal of Learning Disabilities, 23* (2), 74-84.

Hockenberry, M.J., & Coody, D.K. (1986). *Pediatric oncology and hematology: Perspectives on care,* St. Louis: Mosby.

Hollister, J.R. (1999). Rheumatic diseases. In W.W. Hay, A.R. Hayward, M.J. Levin, & J.M. Sondheimer. *Current pediatric diagnosis and treatment* (14th ed.). (pp. 715-722). Stanford, Conn.: Appleton & Lange.

Horowitz, F.D., & Haritos, C. (1998). The organism and understanding environment. In J.A. Burack, R.M. Hodapp, & E. Zigler. *Handbook of mental retardation and development.* New York: Cambridge University Press.

Howlin, P., & Rutter, M. (1987). *Treatment of autistic children.* New York: John Wiley & Sons.

Hutto, C., & Scott, G.B. (1999). Special considerations in children. In T.C. Merigan, J.G. Bartlett, & D. Bolognesi (Eds.), *Textbook of AIDS medicine* (2nd ed.). (pp. 163-162). Baltimore: Williams & Wilkins.

Jacobson, S.W. (1998). Specificity of neurobehavioral outcomes associated with prenatal alcohol exposure. *Alcoholism: Clinical and Experimental Research, 22* (2), 313-320.

Jennett, B., & Teasdale, G. (1981). *Management of head injuries.* Philadelphia: F.A. Davis.

Johnson, D.L. (1997). Hydrocephalus. In R.A. Hoekelman, B.S.B. Friedman, N.M. Nelson, & H.M. Seidel (Eds.), *Primary pediatric care* (3rd ed.). (pp. 1347-1350). St. Louis: Mosby.

Johnson, D.L., & Krishnamurthy, S. (1998). Severe pediatric head injury: Myth, magic and actual fact. *Pediatric Neurosurgery, 28,* 167-172.

Karpati, G., Gilbert, R., Petrof, B.J., & Nalbantoglu, J. (1998). Gene therapy research for Duchenne and Becker muscular dystrophies. *Current Opinion in Neurology, 10,* 430-435.

Kennard, M.J. (1990). Cocaine use during pregnancy: Fetal and neonatal effects. *Journal of Perinatal and Neonatal Nursing, 3*(4), 53-63.

Kimmo, T., Jyrki, V., & Sirpa, A.S. (1998). Health status after recovery from burn injury. *Burns, 24,* 293-298.

Kliegman, R.M. (1998). Fetal and neonatal medicine. In R.E. Behrman & R.M. Kliegman (Eds.), *Nelson essentials of pediatrics* (3rd ed.). (pp. 167-225). Philadelphia: W.B. Saunders.

Klin, A., & Volkmar, F.R. (1997). Asperger's syndrome. In D.J. Cohen & F.R. Volkmar (Eds.), *Handbook of autism and pervasive developmental disorders* (2nd ed.). (pp. 94-122). New York: Wiley.

Leyten, Q.H., Gabreels, F.J., Renier, W.O., & ter Laak, H.J. (1996). Congenital muscular dystrophy: A review of the literature. *Clinical Neurology and Neurosurgery, 98,* 267-280.

Liptak, G.S. (1997). Neural tube defects. In M.L. Batshaw (Ed.), *Children with disabilities* (4th ed.). (pp. 529-552). Baltimore: Brookes.

Loewen, P., Steinbok, P., Holsti, L., & MacKay, M. (1998). Upper extremity performance and self-care skill changes in children with spastic cerebral palsy following selective posterior rhizotomy. *Pediatric Neurosurgery, 29* (4), 191-198.

Lyons, B.A., & Valentine, P. (1994). Prevention. In R.D. Muma, B.A. Lyons, M.J. Borucki, & E.B. Pollard (Eds.), *HIV: Manual for health care professionals.* Norwalk, Conn.: Appleton & Lange.

Mattson, S.N., & Riley, E.P. (1998). A review of neurobehavioral deficits in children with fetal alcohol syndrome or prenatal exposure to alcohol. *Alcoholism: Clinical and Experimental Research, 22* (2), 279-294.

Mauk, E.J., Reber, M., & Batshaw, M.L. (1997). Autism: And other pervasive developmental disorders. In M.L. Batshaw (Ed.), *Children with disabilities* (4th ed.). (p. 425-448). Baltimore: Brookes.

Maul-Mellott, S.K., & Adams, J.N. (1987). *Childhood cancer: A nursing overview.* Boston: Jones and Bartlett.

McIntosh, K., & Lauer, B.A. (1999). Infections: Bacterial and spirochetal. In W.W. Hay, A.R. Hayward, M.J. Levin, & J.M. Sondheimer (Eds.), *Current pediatric diagnosis and treatment* (14th ed.). Stamford, Conn: Appleton & Lange.

McLeod, R., & Remington, J.S. (1996). Toxoplasmosis. In R.E. Berhman, R.M. Kliegman, & A.M. Arvin (Eds.), *Nelson textbook of pediatrics* (15th ed.). (pp. 831-834). Philadelphia: W.B. Saunders.

Melvin, J.L. (1989). *Rheumatic disease in the child and adult: Occupational therapy and rehabilitation* (3rd ed.). Philadelphia: F.A. Davis.

Menkes, J.H. (1995). *Textbook of child neurology* (5th ed.). Baltimore: Williams & Wilkins.

Michaud, L.J., Duhaime, A.C, & Lazar, M.F. (1997). Traumatic brain injury. In M.L. Batshaw (Ed.), *Children with disabilities* (4th ed.). (pp. 595-620). Baltimore: Brookes.

Miller, G., & Clark, G.D. (1998). *The cerebral palsies: Causes, consequences, and management.* Boston: Butterworth-Heinemann.

Milne, R.I.G. (1990). Assessment of care of children with sickle cell disease: Implications for neonatal screening programs. *British Medical Journal, 300,* 371-374.

Monnett, Z., & Moynihan, P. (1991). Cardiovascular assessment of the neonatal heart. *Journal of Perinatal and Neonatal Nursing, 5* (2), 50-59.

Moore, P., et al. (1996). Competence and physical impairment of pediatric survivors of burns of more than 80% total body surface area. *Journal of Burn Care and Rehabilitation, 17* (6), 547-551.

Morrissy, R.T., & Weinstein, S.L. (Eds.), (1996). *Lovell and Winter's pediatric orthopaedics.* Philadelphia: Lippincott-Raven.

Morrow, S.E., Smith, D.L., Cairns, B.A., Howell, P.D., Nakayama, D.K., & Peterson, H.D. (1996). Etiology and outcome of pediatric burns. *Journal of Pediatric Surgery, 31* (3), 329-333.

Murphy, J.T., Purdue, G.F., Hunt, J.L., & Hicks, B.A. (1997). Burn injury. In D.L. Levin & F.C. Morriss (Eds.), *Essentials of pediatric intensive care* (2nd ed.). (pp. 1010-1021). New York: Churchill Livingstone.

National Institute of Mental Health. (1996). *Attention-deficit-hyperactivity disorder* (NIH Publication No. 96-3572). Washington, DC: Government Printing Office.

National Institute of Mental Health. (1998). *Unraveling autism* (NIH Publication No. 99-4590). Washington, D.C.: U.S. Government Printing Office.

National Society for Autistic Children. (1996). *Autism fact sheet.* Washington, D.C.: Author.

Pellegrino, L. (1997). Cerebral palsy. In M.L. Batshaw (Ed.), *Children with disabilities* (4th ed.). (pp. 499-528). Baltimore: Brookes.

Pizzo, P.A., & Poplack, D.G. (1989). *Principles and practice of pediatric oncology.* Philadelphia: J.B. Lippincott.

Pizzo, P.A., & Wilfert, C. (Eds.). (1998). *Pediatric AIDS: The challenge of HIV infection in infants, children and adolescents* (3rd ed.). Baltimore: Williams & Wilkins.

Powell, K.R. (1997). Meningitis. In R.A. Hoekelman, S.B. Friedman, N.M. Nelson, & H.M. Seidel (Eds.), *Primary pediatric care* (3rd ed.). (pp. 1421-1429). St. Louis: Mosby.

Pueschel, S.M., & Pueschel, J.K. (1992). *Biomedical concerns in persons with Down syndrome.* Baltimore: Brookes.

Radel, E.G. (1997). Hemophilia and other hereditary bleeding disorders. In R.A. Hoekelman, S.B. Friedman, N.M. Nelson, & H.M. Seidel (Eds.), *Primary pediatric care* (3rd ed.). (pp. 1132-1135). St. Louis: Mosby.

Ramirez, R.J., Wolf, S.E., Barrow, R.E., & Herndon, D.N. (1998). Growth hormone treatment in pediatric burns: A safe therapeutic approach. *Annals of Surgery, 228,* 439-448.

Raphaely, R.C., Swedlow, D.B., Downes, J.J., & Bruce, C.A. (1980). Management of severe pediatric head trauma. *Pediatric Clinics of North America, 27,* 715.

Rapin, I. (1997). Classification and causal issues in autism. In D.J. Cohen & F.R. Volkmar (Eds.), *Handbook of autism and pervasive developmental disorders* (2nd ed.). (pp. 847-867). New York: Wiley.

Rennebohm R., & Correll, J.K. (1984). Comprehensive management of juvenile rheumatoid arthritis. *Nursing Clinics of North America, 19,* 647-662.

Richard, R., Staley, M., Miller, S., & Warden, G. (1997). To splint or not to splint. *Journal of Burn Care and Rehabilitation, 18* (1), 64-71.

Robison, L.M., Sclar, D.A., Skaer, T.L., & Galin, R.S. (1999). National trends in the prevalence of attention-deficit/hyperactivity disorder and the prescribing of methylphenidate among school-age children: 1990-1995. *Clinical Pediatrics, 38,* 209-217.

Rogers, S.L., Coe, C.L., & Karaszewski, J.W. (1998). Immune consequences of stroke and cerebral palsy in adults. *Journal of Neuroimmunology, 91* (1-2), 113-120.

Roizen, N.J. (1997). Down syndrome. In M.L. Batshaw (Ed.), *Children with disabilities* (4th ed.). (pp. 361-376). Baltimore: Brookes.

Ropper, A.H. (1992). The Guillain-Barré syndrome. *New England Journal of Medicine, 326* (17), 1130-1136.

Russman, B.S., & Romness, M. (1998). Neurorehabilitation for the child with cerebral palsy. In G. Miller & G.D. Clark (Eds.), *The cerebral palsies.* Boston: Butterworth-Heinemann.

Rutstein, R.M., Conlon, C.J., & Batshaw, M.L. (1997). HIV and AIDS. In M.L. Batshaw (Ed.), *Children with disabilities* (4th ed.). (pp. 163-182). Baltimore: Brookes.

Rutter, M. (1985). The treatment of autistic children. *Journal of Child Psychology and Psychiatry and Allied Disciplines, 26,* 193-214.

Rutter, M., Bailey, A., Simonoff, E., & Pickles, A. (1997). Genetic influences and autism. In D.J. Cohen & F.R. Volkmar (Eds.), *Handbook of autism and pervasive developmental disorders* (2nd ed.). (pp. 344-387). New York: Wiley.

Salter, R.B. (1983). *Textbook of disorders and injuries of the musculoskeletal system* (2nd ed.). Baltimore: Williams & Wilkins.

Sampson, P.D., et. al. (1997). Incidence of fetal alcohol syndrome and prevalence of alcohol related neurodevelopmental disorder. *Teratology, 56,* 317-326.

Satz, P., Zaucha, K., McCleary, C., Light, R., Asarnow, R., & Becker, D. (1997). Mild head injury in children and adolescents: A review of studies. *Psychological Bulletin, 122,* 107-131.

Scherzer, A.L., & Tscharnuter, I. (1990). *Early diagnosis and treatment in cerebral palsy: A primer on infant developmental problems.* New York: Marcel Dekker.

Schuster, C.S., & Ashburn, S.S. (1986). *The process of human development: A holistic approach* (2nd ed.). Boston: Little, Brown.

Shapiro, B.K., & Batshaw, M.L. (1993). Mental retardation. In F.D. Burg (Ed.), *Current pediatric therapy* (14th ed.). Philadelphia: W.B. Saunders.

Shapiro, E.D. (1996). Lyme disease. In R.E. Berhman, R.M. Kliegman, & A.M. Arvin (Eds.), *Nelson textbook of pediatrics* (15th ed.). (pp. 831-834). Philadelphia: W.B. Saunders.

Shaywitz, S.E., & Shaywitz, B.A. (1987). Attention deficit disorder: Current perspectives. *Pediatric Neurology, 3,* 129-135.

Siegel, J.D. (1990a). Toxoplasmosis. In F.A. Oski, C.D. DeAngelis, R.D. Feigin, & J.B. Warshaw (Eds.), *Principles and practice in pediatrics.* Philadelphia: J.B. Lippincott.

Siegel, J.D. (1990b). Rubella. In F.A. Oski, C.D. DeAngelis, R.D. Feigin, & J.B. Warshaw. (Eds.), *Principles and practice in pediatrics.* Philadelphia: J.B. Lippincott.

Simon, M.A. (1988). Limb salvage for osteosarcoma. *Journal of Bone and Joint Surgery, 70A,* 307-310.

Staley, M., Anderson, L., Greenhalgh, D., & Warden, G. (1999). Return to school as an outcome measure after burn injury. *Journal of Burn Care and Rehabilitation, 20* (1), 91-94.

Staley, M., Richard, R., Warden, G.D., Miller, S.F., & Shuster, D.B. (1996). Functional outcomes for the patient with burn injuries. *Journal of Burn Care and Rehabilitation, 17* (4), 362-367.

Steinbok, P., Reiner, A.M., Beauchamp, R., Armstrong, R.W., Cochrane, D.D., & Kestle, J. A Randomized clinical trial to compare selective posterior rhizotomy plus physiotherapy with physiotherapy alone in children with spastic diplegic cerebral palsy. *Developmental Medicine and Child Neurology, 39* (3), 178-184.

Steinbok, P., Reiner, A.M., & Kestle, J.R. (1997). Therapeutic electrical stimulation following selective posterior rhizotomy in children with spastic diplegic cerebral palsy: A randomized clinical trial. *Developmental Medicine and Child Neurology, 39* (8), 515-520.

Steinbok, P., & Schrag, C. (1998). Complications after selective posterior rhizotomy for spasticity in children with cerebral palsy. *Pediatric Neurosurgery, 28* (6), 300-313.

Streissguth, A.P., Clarren, S.K., & Jones, K.L. (1985). Natural history of the fetal alcohol syndrome: A 10 year follow-up of 11 patients. *Lancet, 2,* 89.

Thomas, N.H., & Dubowitz, V. (1989). Muscular dystrophy and other muscle disorders. *Current Opinion in Pediatrics, 1,* 296-300.

Tizzano, E.F., & Buchwald, M. (1992). Cystic fibrosis: Beyond the gene to therapy. *Journal of Pediatrics, 120* (3), 337-349.

Van Acker, R. (1997) Rett's syndrome: A pervasive developmental disorder. In D.J. Cohen & F.R. Volkmar (Eds.), *Handbook of autism and pervasive developmental disorders* (2nd ed.). (pp. 60-93). New York: Wiley.

Voit, T. (1998). Congenital muscular dystrophies: 1997 update. *Brain and Development, 20* (2), 65-74.

Wallace, C.A., & Levinson, J.E. (1991). Juvenile rheumatoid arthritis: Outcome and treatment for the 1990s. *Rheumatic Diseases Clinics of North America, 17,* 891-905.

Weil, M.L., & Levin, M. (1995). Infections of the nervous system. In J.H. Menkes (Ed.), *Textbook of child neurology* (5th ed.). Baltimore, Md: Williams & Wilkins.

Wong, D.L. (1997). *Whaley and Wong's essentials of pediatric nursing* (5th ed.). St. Louis: Mosby.

Yeong, E.K., et al. (1997). Improved burn scar assessment with use of a new scar-rating scale. *Journal of Burn Care and Rehabilitation, 18* (4), 353.

Zametkin, A.J., & Ernst, M. (1999). Problems in the management of attention-deficit-hyperactivity disorder. *New England Journal of Medicine, 340* (1), 40-46.

Zametkin, A.J., & Liotta, W. (1998). The neurobiology of attention-deficit/hyperactivity disorder. *Journal of Clinical Psychiatry, 59* (supplement 7), 17-23.

Zuckerman, B., & Frank, D.A. (1992). Prenatal cocaine and marijuana exposure: Research and clinical implications. In I.S. Zagon & T.A. Slotkin (Eds.), *Maternal substance abuse and the developing nervous system.* San Diego: Academic Press.

Suggested Readings

Batshaw, M.L. (Ed.). (1997). *Children with disabilities* (4th ed.). Baltimore: Brookes.

Berhman, R.E., Kliegman, R.M., & Arvin, A.M. (Eds.). (1996). *Nelson textbook of pediatrics* (15th ed.). Philadelphia: W.B. Saunders.

Menkes, J.H. (1995). *Textbook of child neurology* (5th ed.). Baltimore: Williams & Wilkins

Morrissy, R.T., & Weinstein, S.L. (Eds.). (1996). *Lovell and Winter's pediatric orthopaedics,* Philadelphia: Lippincott-Raven.

Thomas, C.L. (1981). *Taber's cyclopedic medical dictionary.* Philadelphia: F.A. Davis.

Wong, D.L. (1997). *Whaley and Wong's essentials of pediatric nursing* (5th ed.). St. Louis: Mosby.

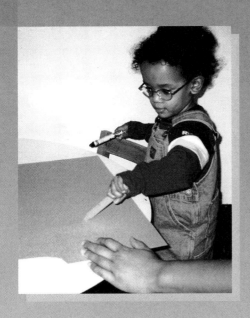

OCCUPATIONAL THERAPY EVALUATION IN PEDIATRICS

chapter 7

Purposes, Processes, and Methods of Evaluation

Katherine B. Stewart

■ CHAPTER OBJECTIVES

1. Identify the dimensions of concern in pediatric occupational therapy evaluation.
2. Define the key terms used in pediatric occupational therapy evaluations.
3. List four primary reasons evaluations are conducted, and discuss the variety of decisions that pediatric occupational therapists make throughout the evaluation process.
4. Describe the specific steps that pediatric occupational therapists follow in the process of evaluating children.
5. Describe the primary evaluation methods commonly used in pediatric occupational therapy.
6. Discuss the major factors that therapists should consider when selecting evaluation methods and measures.
7. Apply the knowledge gained in this chapter to specific case studies of children at risk for or with disabilities.

Those who observe human behavior must be vigilant when examining the details of the behavior and relate those details to each other within the context of that be-havior. Pediatric occupational therapists involved in the evaluation of children face this challenge every day. To fully examine a child's occupational performance, the therapist not only evaluates the child's specific developmental skills, but he or she must analyze how the child's performance is influenced by the physical demands and social expectations of the home, school, and community environments. After identifying the functional activities most important to the child and the child's caregivers, the occupational therapist evaluates the performance components (sensorimotor, cognitive, and psychosocial) of the child's development that are essential for the child's participation in everyday childhood occupations.

The evaluation process is one of the most fundamental, yet complex, aspects of occupational therapy services. The American Occupational Therapy Association (AOTA) defines *evaluation* as the process of obtaining and interpreting data necessary for intervention (Hinojosa & Kramer, 1998). How the occupational therapist views this evaluation process, whether the therapist is open to new ways of understanding the child, which methods and measures the therapist selects to evaluate the child, and how the therapist interprets and documents the evaluation data all contribute to the important decisions regarding the type and degree of occupational therapy intervention that will be provided for the child and family.

This chapter describes the occupational therapy evaluation process with children. The first section of the chapter provides a conceptual framework for evaluating children. The second section outlines the purposes of evaluation and includes specific examples common in pediatric occupational therapy practice. The third section of the chapter describes the evaluation process and provides clinical examples. The fourth section explains the general methods, measures, and principles used in selecting and administering pediatric occupational therapy evaluations.

Four primary concepts are reinforced throughout this chapter:

1. The evaluation of a child is an ongoing, dynamic process that begins with the initial referral for therapy and continues throughout the intervention and discharge phases of occupational therapy services.
2. Evaluations should be ecologically and culturally valid.
3. The views and priorities of the child's primary caregiver and of the child should be held central throughout the evaluation process.
4. The outcome of the evaluation should be an in-depth understanding of the child's participation in childhood occupations meaningful to the child and his or her caregivers.

■ CONCEPTUAL FRAMEWORK FOR EVALUATION

Using a top-down approach to pediatric assessment, the occupational therapist first identifies in the environments and activities in which the child's participation is limited. Occupational centered assessment of children "acknowledges the importance of individual activities that are part of a particular occupation, as well as the context, but is most concerned with the overall process of participation" (Coster, 1998, p. 340). Once limitations in participation are identified, the child's sensorimotor, cognitive, and psychosocial performance and environmental factors that underlie the child's performance in everyday occupations are assessed.

To gain an in-depth understanding of the child's abilities and limitations, the occupational therapist must also assess the features of the environments in which the child performs the tasks. The performance context refers to the physical, temporal, and sociocultural features of the child's environments. Children and their families (Figure 7-1) are embedded in a network of social systems, including extended family, friends, neighbors, daycare,

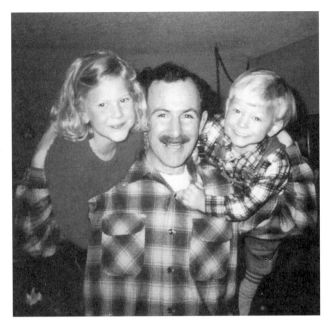

figure 7-1   Family environment: father playing with his two children.

schools, medical and religious institutions, and cultural groups (Bronfenbrenner, Moen, & Garbarino, 1984).

To understand a child and his or her development thoroughly, therapists must view the child within the context of these social environments (Dunn, Brown, & McGuigan, 1994). Although occupational therapists have numerous assessments of performance (e.g., those that examine muscle strength, range of motion, manipulation skills, feeding, and dressing, they have few that measure contextual features such as the physical qualities of an environment, the cultural background of the person, or the effect of friendships on performance (Dunn et. al., 1994).

Coster, Deeney, Haltiwanger, and Haley (1998), the authors of the School Function Assessment (SFA), provide an exemplary model of pediatric assessment. Coster and others recognized the need to develop an assessment tool that measures children's ability to participate in the academic and social aspects of the school environment. The SFA fills an important gap for therapists and educators interested in using a top-down, problem-solving approach, by first considering the student's current level of participation in the educational programs and activities expected of his or her peers, and then identifying the activity settings in which the student's participation is less than expected.

This instrument is based on key concepts from the ICIDH-2: International Classification of Impairments, Activities, and Participation (World Health Organization, 1997). The ICIDH-2 is a classification system that uses abiopsychosocial approach to understand the dimensions of disablement, which is consistent with the basic assumptions of occupational therapy. One purpose of the ICIDH-2 is to promote a more comprehensive and sensitive assessment of problems in the three dimensions of the disablement model: (1) impairments (at the body function level), (2) activities (at the person level), and (3) participation (at the society level). Evaluation using the ICIDH-2 system emphasizes analysis of an individual's level of participation in social and physical environments in addition to analysis of an individual's impairments and activity limitations.

An understanding of the child's participation in a variety of contexts must be gained through observation over time and at different times during the day and week. This type of information is also obtained through interviews with the child's primary caregivers and teachers.

Application

The following case study highlights how specific evaluation measures were selected within the domains and dimensions of concern of occupational therapy for a child with developmental delay.

Kevin is a 6-year-old boy with developmental delay and an attention deficit disorder. Specific deficits that limit Kevin's occupational performance at school and at home include his extreme hyperactivity, fine and gross motor coordination problems, possible visual perceptual deficits, and difficulties in peer interaction.

Kevin attends a special education preschool classroom that consists of 14 children ranging in age from 3 years to 6 years who exhibit mild-to-moderate developmental delays in speech and language, behavior, or motor skills.

Kevin lives with his mother, father, and 3- and 4-year-old younger brothers. The family recently moved to a two-bedroom, one-bath home with a kitchen and living room. Financial resources are limited.

The father, who describes himself as having a learning disability, works part-time as a gardener. The home is situated on a busy urban street in a lower socioeconomic neighborhood. The mother, who does not work outside the home, reported that she attended special education classes throughout her childhood. When asked what they hoped Kevin could accomplish at school in the next year, the parents said they wanted him to become independent in toileting, to print his first name, and to make friends with other children (Figure 7-2).

Given this information, the evaluation measures listed in Table 7-1 would be appropriate options for the occupational therapist to consider. However, assessments of this child would occur over time and would be ongoing with the initiation of occupational therapy services. The section on the process of evaluation provides guidance that is more specific on the sequence of the evaluation process.

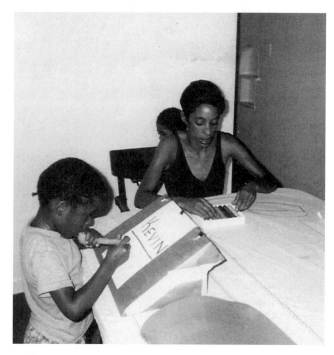

figure**7-2** Kevin learning to print his name at home.

In summary, the occupational therapy evaluation plan should stem from the theoretic base of occupational therapy and include measures of the child's participation in occupations, specific performance of activities, and the performance context in which the child performs daily functional tasks.

■ EVALUATION PURPOSES

Pediatric occupational therapy evaluations are multifaceted, with a focus on obtaining information about the child's developmental and functional status. Evaluation is the process of gathering information for making a clinical decision. This section discusses the decisions that occupational therapists make through various steps of careful screening and comprehensive evaluation of children at risk for or with disabilities.

The six primary purposes for occupational therapy evaluation are as follows:
1. To decide if the child should be further evaluated using assessments that are more comprehensive
2. To decide if the child is eligible for occupational therapy services
3. To assist in the diagnostic process
4. To develop an intervention plan
5. To evaluate the child's progress in therapy and decide if further therapy is warranted
6. To research the efficacy of intervention services and clinical outcomes or to describe patterns of development and functional changes in children with specific diagnoses.

table 7-1   *Appropriate Measures for Kevin's Evaluation*

Evaluation Categories	Evaluation Measures	Rationale
Participation and roles	School Function Assessment	To assess child's performance of functional tasks that support participation in academic and social aspects of school
		To rate child's behavior objectively on specific functional life tasks
Performance of activities and activity limitations	Peabody Developmental Motor Scales	To assess gross and fine motor skills
	Transdisciplinary Play-Based Assessment	To assess development in context of play
	Clinical observations of neuromotor status	To assess child's muscle tone, range of motion, presence of primitive reflexes, automatic reactions, posture, and quality of movement
	Test of Visual Perceptual Skills	To assess child's visual perception
	Informal observations of cognitive and psychosocial skills	To gain insight into child's performance of everyday tasks
	Coping Inventory	To assess child's overall coping style and identify adaptive coping attributes
Performance context	Home Observation for Measurement of the Environment	To assess home characteristics related to child's development
	Interviews with parents, teachers, and other caregivers	To gain insight into perceptions of child's caregivers regarding child's performance on functional tasks

Screening

The primary reason to screen children is to determine whether they warrant a further, more comprehensive evaluation. Pediatric occupational therapists may participate in two levels of screening. The first level (type I) is a basic screening in which the child's general health (e.g., vision and hearing), growth (e.g., weight and height), and development (e.g., physical, social, language, and personal and adaptive skills) are checked. In some settings, such as public school programs, occupational therapists may participate in screening large numbers of children to determine which children should receive further testing.

Public policies, including the Individuals with Disabilities Education Act (IDEA, 1997), Head Start, and Medicaid programs for children, mandate early screening activities to identify those children at risk for disabilities. Some examples of developmental screening tools useful for basic screening of children include the Infant Monitoring System (Bricker & Squires, 1989), the Denver Developmental Screening Test-II (Frankenburg et. al., 1990), and the First STEP (Miller, 1993). The pediatric therapist can refer to several resources for an overview of developmental screening tools (Bailey & Wolery, 1989; Collier, 1991; Gibbs & Teti, 1990; Glascoe, Martin, & Humphrey, 1990).

More frequently, pediatric therapists are involved in the second level of screening children (type II). This type of screening usually occurs after a health or educational professional has identified the child as being at risk for developmental or functional deficits. The child is then referred to the pediatric occupational therapist to obtain a more focused screening of the child's development. At this point in the screening process the therapist, often with other interdisciplinary team members, determines whether the child is a candidate for more comprehensive testing and, if so, what developmental or functional areas need further evaluation. For example, a kindergarten teacher may observe a child's clumsiness in the classroom and refer the child to the occupational therapist or physical therapist to determine if the child needs a comprehensive motor evaluation. In this case the therapist may choose the Quick Neurological Screening Test (Mutti, Sterling, & Spalding, 1978) or the Bruininks-Oseretsky Test of Motor Proficiency—Short Form (Bruininks, 1978) (Figures 7-3 and 7-4).

In addition to administering a standardized screening tool, the therapist gathers pertinent information from the child's parents and teachers, as well as from informal observations of the child's performance in his or her natural environments (e.g., classroom, playground, and home).

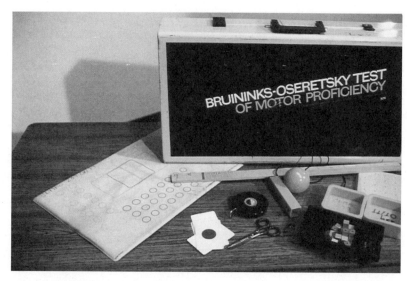

figure**7-3**   Bruininks-Oseretsky Test of Motor Proficiency.

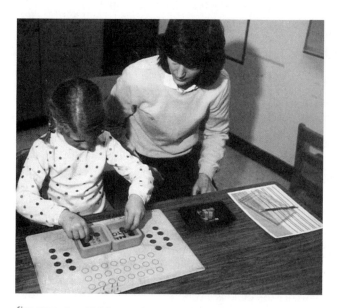

figure**7-4**   Child completing a Bruininks-Oseretsky Test of Motor Proficiency item.

Regardless of the setting and the level of screening (type I or type II), the therapist should consider the following points when screening children to determine whether they warrant further, more comprehensive evaluation:

1. Standardized screening tools should be implemented whenever possible to ensure that results of the screening are reliable and valid. *Standardized tests* require uniform procedures for administration and scoring. Chapter 8 provides more information on using standardized instruments.

2. In addition to standardized screening tools, the therapist should gather relevant information from the child's teacher, parents, or other caregivers.

3. Information gathered during the screening process should include the child's performance across various developmental domains and in different environments to substantiate the need for further evaluation.

4. Screening tools should be carefully evaluated for their cultural validity, and the results should be interpreted cautiously when administered to children from diverse cultural backgrounds. A few instruments, such as the Miller Assessment for Preschoolers (Miller, 1988), have established norms for different ethnic populations.

Comprehensive Evaluations

In pediatric occupational therapy there are several reasons why a *comprehensive evaluation* of the child might be conducted. Five reasons are described in this section. The therapist should keep in mind the purpose of the comprehensive evaluation because, depending on the purpose, different methods and measures may be appropriate for the evaluation. Common assessment tools used by occupational therapists with children are listed in Appendix 7-A.

Eligibility purposes

When evaluating children for the purpose of eligibility or placement, standardized, norm-referenced measures should be used to ensure that the test results are reliable and valid. Many public school systems mandate the use of norm-referenced tests by school personnel, including occupational therapists, when qualifying students for special services. For a specific example, in Washington, children between 3 and 6 years of age must perform at least two standard deviations below the norm on a standardized test in one or more of the specific developmental areas to qualify for related services in the public school setting (Washington Administrative Code, 1990).

Standardized, norm-referenced instruments are helpful in determining how the individual child's performance compares with that of the children in the normative sample. However, caution must be taken when interpreting a child's performance on most standardized developmental instruments. Often these instruments have not been standardized on disabled populations (Farran, 1990). For example, a child with Down syndrome may score more than two standard deviations below the mean for his or her chronologic age, but this rating does not reveal how he or she performs relative to other children with Down syndrome.

The IDEA (1991) mandates that "procedures to assure that testing and evaluation materials and procedures utilized for the purposes of evaluation and placement of children with disabilities will be selected and administered so as not to be racially or culturally discriminatory" (Sec. 1412). Unfortunately, many tools standardized on the U.S. population have limited cultural validity for children who have recently emigrated from other countries or for children from ethnic groups not fully represented in the U.S. norms.

In summary, standardized tools have an important but limited purpose in the occupational therapy evaluation process. Some service systems may require their use for determining eligibility of the child. However, standard scores, when used alone, do not provide complete data on a child and may be misleading, particularly for children with established disabilities. In addition, therapists should carefully interpret standard scores when evaluating children from diverse cultural or ethnic backgrounds.

Diagnostic purposes

Often a child is referred to occupational therapy by another health care provider or educator to gain more information about why the child may be delayed or exhibits performance deficits. This calls for a comprehensive evaluation by the occupational therapist. To assist in the diagnostic process, the therapist should consider a combination of norm-referenced tools and clinical observations. *Clinical observations* (Figure 7-5) are nonstandardized measures that have been developed by therapists to gather data objectively on critical performance components or performance areas. The quality, frequency, and duration of performance are assessed. (The Evaluation Methods section in this chapter] provides information that is more specific regarding the use of skilled ob-

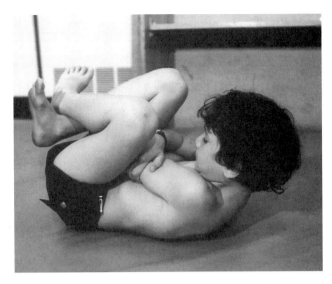

figure **7-5**   Clinical observations of child in supine flexion.

servation.) Box 7-1 provides a sample form for clinical observations of children's neuromotor status. A norm-referenced tool may provide the "anchor" regarding the child's developmental status relative to typically developing children, whereas clinical observations of a child's performance provide rich information on the quality of performance and possible reasons for delayed or deficient performance on quantitative tests. To illustrate how norm-referenced measures are used in combination with nonstandardized clinical observations, the following case example is provided:

> Jason is an 8-year-old boy with mild motor coordination deficits. The therapist administers a norm-referenced tool such as the Sensory Integration and Praxis Tests (Ayres, 1989) to obtain standard scores on his sensory and motor performance. (Figure 7-6 shows the materials provided in the test kit.) In addition, the therapist obtains qualitative data regarding Jason's muscle tone, primitive reflexes, righting and equilibrium reactions, posture, and gait through clinical observations. This information is combined to gain an understanding of Jason's sensory processing and sensory integration and to determine whether direct occupational therapy services are needed.

Intervention planning purposes

Another reason for an occupational therapist to conduct a comprehensive evaluation of a child is to determine the most appropriate intervention plan. When this is the primary reason for evaluation, the therapist should consider evaluation methods that include in-depth observations of the child's performance within his or her natural environments. Interviews with parents and other adults working with the child are another primary

box 7-1 *Clinical observations of neuromotor status*

Checklist for clinical observation of neuromotor status

General instructions: First observe as many of the functional gross and fine motor skills as possible while the child spontaneously plays or moves. Note the child's posture, coordination, and transitional movement patterns during this time. When there is a question or concern regarding the quality of movement or posture during functional gross and fine motor skills, examine the child's muscle tone, primitive reflexes, and automatic reactions through direct testing and physical handling.

Functional gross motor skills
Sit (with or without support?)
Pivot in prone (coordinated use of all four extremities?)
Crawl (on stomach? in quadruped?)
Stand (with or without support?)
Cruise along furniture
Walk (with or without support?)
Ascend and descend stairs (with or without support? alternating feet?)
Jump with both feet (in place? forward?)
Run

Transitional movement patterns
Rolling (prone-to-supine, supine-to-prone) with rotation?
Sit-to-prone with rotation?
Prone-to-sit with rotation?
Supine-to-sit with rotation?
Pull to stand from half-kneel?
Stand to sit with control?

Functional fine motor skills
Reach (bilateral? unilateral? arm preference?)
Prehension patterns (whole hand grasp? partial hand grasp? digital grasp? pincer grasp?)
Release of objects (support of hand on surface? well-controlled?)
Transfer of objects between hands
Manipulation of objects within the hand
Crossing midline of body
Bilateral hand use
Hand preference (hand dominance established?)
Use of scissors (previous experience?)
Use of writing utensil (crayon, marker, and pencil) (Note type and amount of pressure of grasp)
Ability to button and use other fasteners on clothing
Ability to use eating utensils

Posture (Observe symmetry and alignment)
Supine
Prone
Sit
Stand
Prone extension
Supine flexion

Muscle tone
At rest? During movement?
Hypertonia? Hypotonia? Fluctuating tone?
Abnormal tone in extremities? In trunk?
Exaggerated stretch reflex (clonus?)
Asymmetries?

Range of motion
Limitations in upper extremity joints?
Limitations in lower extremity joints?
Limitations from bone or soft tissue contractures?
Asymmetries?

Primitive reflexes
Asymmetric tonic neck reflex
Symmetric tonic neck reflex
Tonic labyrinthine reflex (prone? supine?)
Walking reflex
Neonatal positive support reflex in standing
Grasp reflex
Plantar reflex

Automatic reactions
Equilibrium reactions (head righting? trunk incurvation? extremity counterbalancing?)
Protective arm extension reactions (forward? sideways? backwards?)
Asymmetries?

Ocular-motor skills
Ability to visually focus on object
Ability to visually track a moving object
Esotropia? exotropia? nystagmus?
Peripheral vision

Physical and strength endurance
Physical strength to complete functional tasks
Physical endurance to complete functional tasks

Response to physical handling and movement activities
Response to examiner's or caregiver's touch
Response to activities that require movement through space (e.g., being carried or moved in different positions)

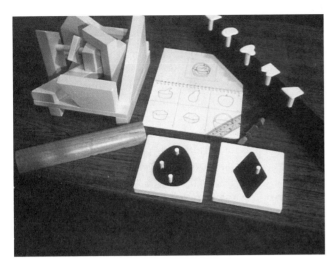

figure7-6   Sensory Integration and Praxis Tests materials.

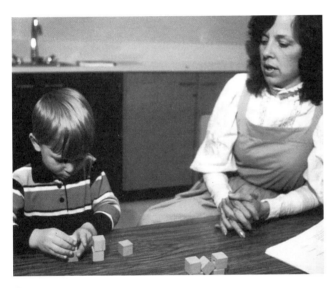

figure7-7   Child completing a fine motor item on the Peabody Developmental Motor Scales.

source of data regarding the child's performance and levels of participation. For intervention planning, norm-referenced instruments may have limited value. Norm-referenced developmental assessments measure skills that are commonly seen in a typically developing population, but they do not necessarily measure what is critical for functional performance in children with disabilities. For example, most 6-year-old children can stand on either foot for at least 10 seconds (Folio & Fewell, 2000). However, is this a critical skill for the child's everyday function? A common mistake of occupational therapists is to design treatment goals and activities directly from items on norm-referenced assessment tools to write a goal regarding stacking blocks (Figure 7-7). Unfortu-

nately this approach not only misses the mark with regard to functional outcomes, but it also invalidates the use of these standardized tests to document the progress of the child and the efficacy of therapy intervention because of the practice effect on the child.

Therapists often use criterion-referenced and curriculum-based measures when the primary evaluation purpose is treatment planning. These measures provide information regarding specific skills important to daily living or school performance. Some examples of criterion-referenced measures used by pediatric occupational therapists include the Hawaii Early Learning Profile (HELP) (Furuno et. al., 1984), the Carolina Curriculum for Infants and Toddlers With Special Needs (Johnson-Martin, Jens, Attermeier, & Hacker, 1991), and the Early Intervention Developmental Profile (Rogers et. al., 1981) (see Appendix 7-A for ordering information).

Reevaluation purposes

The fourth primary reason that an occupational therapist conducts comprehensive evaluations is to reevaluate children's performance so that progress can be measured and the need for continued therapy can be determined. The content and format of the *reevaluation* vary depending on the specific purpose of the reevaluation. If a decision needs to be made regarding whether the child continues to qualify for therapy, the reevaluation will likely include a standardized, norm-referenced measure to ensure reliable results. However, if the primary purpose of reevaluation were to determine whether the child is making progress as a result of therapy, other measures, such as the specific functional goals and objectives written by the therapist during the initial phase of intervention, would be more appropriate and probably more sensitive to developmental and functional changes in the child.

For example, an infant with Down syndrome may show a drop in scores on a standardized test over the course of the intervention year. These standard scores only indicate that the infant with Down syndrome is developing at a slower rate compared with the test's normative group. Measures of progress that are more sensitive to these infants may be the specific goals and objectives written by the early interventionists for each child. These short-term objectives are developed by therapists through task analysis, a process that lists child behaviors that sequentially lead to more advanced behavior in the long-term goals.

It is important to reemphasize that the process of reevaluation of children is an ongoing, dynamic process. Every time a therapist works with a child, the therapist makes clinical judgments regarding the child's response to therapy and functional performance on tasks. The data gathered during each therapy session are analyzed and interpreted by the therapist to determine whether the therapy plan needs to be adjusted.

In summary, although a formal reevaluation is conducted at specific times during therapy intervention, the occupational therapist engages in an ongoing reevaluation of the child and the therapy environment throughout every therapy session.

Clinical research

Instruments used in clinical research are carefully selected to measure the subject's performance and behavior. Although a more complete discussion on standardized tests used for *clinical research* is offered in Chapter 8, a few major points are introduced here.

1. Whether the research design is for a large group or a single subject, the instruments used must be reliable and valid measures of the dependent variable.

2. The measures used depend on the research design and can range from standardized, norm-referenced instruments often used in large-group designs to criterion-referenced instruments or therapy objectives that are operationally defined for single-subject research.

3. One of the most challenging aspects in designing clinical research is finding an appropriate and accurate measure to document change in the subjects. Palisano, Haley, and Brown (1992) describe a research method called *goal attainment scaling (GAS)* as an alternative to norm-referenced scales to document change because of therapy intervention. GAS is an individualized criterion-referenced measure of change that appears to be "advantageous in measuring qualitative change and small, but clinically important, improvement in motor development of children receiving physical therapy" (p. 433).

An important area of research in pediatric occupational therapy is measuring clinical outcomes to document the effectiveness of intervention programs. Law (1999) used a modified ICIDH-2 framework to develop a computerized, self-directed software program designed to assist pediatric therapists in the selection of relevant and appropriate outcome measures for client, service, or program evaluation. With a database of 126 pediatric measures, this software program is an excellent resource for clinicians and researchers in occupational therapy who are conducting clinical outcome studies on children with disabilities.

■ EVALUATION PROCESS

The purpose of this section is to provide a logical sequence of steps that pediatric occupational therapists follow in the process of evaluating children. Kevin's case is a good illustration. After reviewing the numerous tools listed as appropriate for Kevin's occupational therapy evaluation, the occupational therapist may wonder where to begin. All eight assessment tools do not need to be completed before occupational therapy can commence for this child. The process of evaluation in occupational therapy starts with the initial referral and is ongoing throughout the duration of therapy services. The family and the rest of the team, including the occupational therapist, select specific evaluation areas that have priority for completion before developing an intervention plan and initiating therapy. Other areas of evaluation are completed, as the child and family become better known to the therapist. Therefore the therapist must continually consider the new challenges that the child must meet and other priorities that emerge for the family.

To conduct thorough evaluations and provide accurate interpretation and documentation of evaluation results, therapists follow logical steps in the evaluation process. Figure 7-8 illustrates a flow chart of the evaluation sequence.

Referral

Children at risk for or with disabilities are referred to occupational therapists for the evaluation of and intervention for performance deficits. Often the child's diagnosis or deficits in specific developmental areas are listed on the *referral* form. To assist in identification of appropriate referrals, it is critical that the occupational therapist

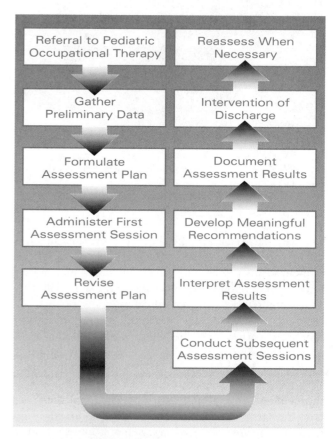

figure 7-8 Flow chart for evaluation process.

be involved in the development of the referral format used in a particular setting.

Evaluation Plan

Once a referral for therapy has been received, the therapist should consult with parents, other caregivers, and professionals from other disciplines to determine which measures to use, the evaluation setting, and the schedule for the occupational therapy evaluation activities. Most therapists find it helpful to formulate a written *evaluation plan* that is based on the child's chronologic age, presenting problems, parent's priorities regarding reasons for referral, availability of evaluation tools, type of service delivery model, and amount of time available for initial evaluation activities. Table 7-2 provides an example of Kevin's initial evaluation plan. The therapist lists the major concerns and the evaluation methods and measures that specifically assess those concerns.

As mentioned previously, the complete evaluation process takes place over time. Given the complexity of problems in children referred to pediatric occupational therapists, it may be difficult to formulate a comprehensive evaluation plan based on the limited referral information. Therefore it is expected that the therapist will revise the initial evaluation plan after the child has been seen at least once by the therapist and more information is gained regarding the caregiver's priorities and the child's developmental status. In the example of Kevin, the therapist learned from the parent interview during the first evaluation session that Kevin's mother is most concerned about his delayed toileting skills. As shown in Table 7-2 Kevin's evaluation plan includes the parents' concern about his delay in developing self-help skills.

Administration of Evaluation Measures

Once the evaluation plan is revised, administration of the various measures selected can proceed. For most entry-level therapists in pediatrics, one of the most challenging aspects of the evaluation process is the management of the child's behavior during the administration of the evaluation measures, particularly when the measures are more formal, structured, and standardized. Testing infants and young children in a structured situation can be enormously demanding on the children, the parents, and the therapist. However, much can be done in the preparation for and during the occupational therapy evaluation to reduce potential behavior problems during testing. Box 7-2 outlines several effective strategies for managing young children's behavior during structured, standardized assessments. Chapter 8 offers a more in-depth discussion on competent administration of standardized tests and outlines some important ethical considerations for therapists when using standardized tests.

The administration of nonstandardized tools, clinical observations, environmental evaluations, and interviews with the child's caregivers should receive the same careful attention and preparation by the occupational therapist as standardized measures require. For some children a combination of standardized tests and nonstandardized measures is appropriate, but for many children who are severely disabled, norm-referenced tests are neither valid nor meaningful. In these cases, data gathered from nonstandardized measures provide the essential information for planning intervention. These evaluation methods, including naturalistic observation, clinical observations, criterion-referenced measures, and interviews with the child's caregivers (e.g., teachers, parents, and day care providers), are more fully described in the Evaluation Methods section.

Interpretation of Results

Once all the initial evaluation information has been gathered on a child's performance the therapist then analyzes these quantitative and qualitative data from standardized test results, clinical observations of the child's performance, caregiver interviews, and environmental

table 7-2	*Initial Evaluation Plan for Kevin*	
Functional Concerns	**Evaluation Methods and Measures**	**Comments**
Difficulty making friends	Coping Inventory Parent interview Teacher interview	Observe Kevin in classroom and at home
Unable to print	Peabody Developmental Motor Scales (PDMS) Test of Visual Perception Skills	May need to adapt standard procedures because of attention deficits
Safety on playground	PDMS Clinical observations of neuromotor status	
Delay in self-help	*Home observation* *Self-help developmental checklist*	*Parent interview*

Note: Information added after initial evaluation visit is printed in italics.

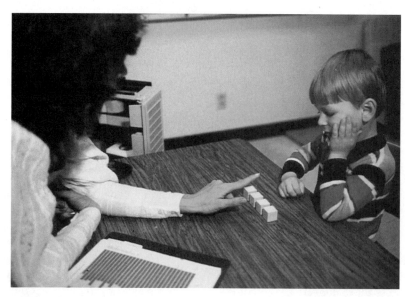

figure**7-9**   Administration of a standardized test (Miller Assessment for Preschoolers).

box**7-2** *Behavior management strategies for testing young children*

1. Be prepared. Know your testing procedures so well that you can focus on the child's behavior and performance, not on the test manual or your paperwork.
2. Be sensitive to the child and parents' physical and emotional needs. Whenever possible, adjust the pace of the examination to match the child's style and acknowledge any concerns that the parents may express.
3. Be purposeful in carrying out the examination. Keep the situation friendly, interesting for the child, and informative for the parent.
4. Be sure that the testing room supports the child's optimal performance. The chair and table should be the appropriate size. Lighting should be sufficient. Remove all auditory and visual distractions. Use test materials that are attractive to children.
5. Build a rapport with the child before physically interacting with or handling the child. Some children may do better when they start with tabletop tasks in which the child sits across from the examiner and observes the situation before being handled physically for motor testing (Figure 7-9). Other children may do better with a spontaneous play situation while the examiner focuses on the parent interview before directly testing the child. Be flexible and follow the child's lead whenever possible.
6. Use positive reinforcement that is meaningful to the child (e.g., praise, stickers, or a fun activity). Be sure to reinforce the child's effort rather than success.
7. Start and end with some easy items (Figure 7-10). This helps the child feel more comfortable at the beginning and leaves a good feeling for both the child and parents at the end.
8. Watch the complexity of your language. Be clear and concise in your instructions to the child. Consider using the parents' level of language complexity as a guide to what the child can understand.
9. Be organized. Keep the test materials arranged neatly in an area that is easily accessible to you but not to the child. It is sometimes helpful to have an attractive toy (not from the test kit) on the table or nearby for the child to play with while you are not directly testing the child.
10. Try to develop reciprocal interactions with the child. When you first show the child a test object, allow him or her to explore it briefly in his or her own way before you give the test instructions. This time provides an excellent opportunity for clinical observations. Then give the child the test instructions and allow him or her to demonstrate his or her skill. If the child continues to be actively engaged with the object when you want to present a new item, it is often effective to present the new test object as you remove the old one.

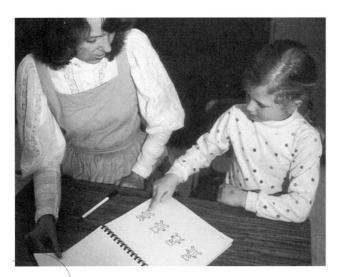

figure 7-10   Administration of the Motor Free Visual Perception Test.

assessments. When a standardized test is used, the therapist must carefully follow procedures outlined in the test manual regarding the interpretation of test results. When nonstandardized measures are used, the therapist must skillfully look for patterns of strength and areas of concern across all measures. Often data obtained from nonstandardized measures can be instrumental in understanding the possible underlying reasons for a child's specific performance on standardized tests. To further illustrate this point, consider the following case study:

> Joey is a 3-year-old boy with motor delays. The quantitative data on the PDMS confirms that he is functioning below age expectations. The qualitative data from the clinical observations of his neuromotor status indicate possible reasons for his motor delay, including low muscle tone and delayed righting and equilibrium reactions.

Accurate and complete interpretation of all accumulated data is one of the most important and demanding tasks of the evaluation process. The occupational therapist must be thorough in examining the details of a child's performance and viewing the child's behaviors within the context of environmental demands and supports. Accurate and complete interpretation of evaluation data allows therapists to make sound clinical decisions, including whether the child is a candidate for occupational therapy and, if so, the frequency, duration, and type of therapeutic intervention that are necessary. Once evaluation data have been analyzed, the therapist then turns to the task of developing recommendations for the child.

Development of Recommendations Based on Results

The first factor the therapist should consider when developing recommendations based on evaluation results is the *functionality of the recommendations.* Functionality refers to the relevance of the recommendation to the child's daily life (Notari & Bricker, 1990). When developing recommendations for a child, the therapist must always ask these questions: "Does this recommendation relate to the child's occupational performance?" "Is this recommendation relevant to the child's everyday function?"

The following examples illustrate how treatment goals can be written in functional terms.

1. *Evaluation finding.* Because of poor fine motor release of objects, Jill was unable to stack 1-inch cubes on the PDMS.
   a. *Inadequate treatment goal.* Jill will stack two 1-inch cubes, three out of four trials, by June 15, 2000.
   b. *Functional goal.* Jill will demonstrate release of small toys into a small container, three out of four trials, by June 15, 2000.
2. *Evaluation finding.* Because of increased muscle tone and poor reciprocal movements in the lower extremities, Ryan was unable to stand from the half-kneel position on either leg, an item on the Gross Motor Function Measure.
   a. Inadequate treatment goal. Ryan will maintain the half-kneel position for 30 seconds, three times over two consecutive therapy sessions, by June 15, 2000.
   b. Functional goal. Ryan will step up on a 6-inch stool to use the classroom toilet without losing his balance, three out of four times, by June 15, 2000.

A second important aspect of meaningful evaluation is that the therapists give priority to the *priorities of the child's caregivers.* Hanft (1994) suggests that every recommendation from an occupational therapist to a parent of a child with special needs should be followed up with the question to the caregiver, "How will this work for you and your child?" For example, during a feeding evaluation in the child's home, a therapist observes a mother and her child with athetoid cerebral palsy and failure to thrive. The therapist notes that the mother has placed the child in an infant walker at mealtime. Because infant walkers have been declared unsafe by the American Academy of Pediatrics, and this particular child would benefit from a more stable seating device that provides trunk and head support needed for optimal oral-motor skills, the therapist might recommend that the infant walker be discontinued and that a special feeding seat be ordered. However, unless the therapist asks the caregiver what the implications of this recommendation may be for the child and the family, the family members may not implement this important recommendation. In this case, additional history taking showed that the child refused to be fed in any position other than in the walker, and the mother was concerned about her child receiving adequate nutrition for growth. Based on the mother's input, the intervention goal became that the child continue to demonstrate oral-motor skills adequate for weight gain and growth. The therapist added a short-term recommendation to provide the parents with information regarding the safety of infant walkers and the importance of proper positioning when eating.

A third consideration of the therapists when developing recommendations from evaluation findings is which *service delivery model* will meet the needs of the child and family. Dunn and Campbell (1991) describe the range of service delivery models in which pediatric occupational therapists work, including direct treatment, monitoring, and consultation. Depending on the service delivery model or combination of models, the therapist's recommendations should be consistent with the primary service delivery model. For example, if the therapist's only role with the child is consultation, recommendations from the initial evaluation would center on how the primary caregiver and other adults working with the child can adapt the child's environment.

A therapist must be able to reconcile these three, sometimes conflicting, factors when developing recommendations. Years of experience can teach a therapist to negotiate through the maze of issues regarding the child, family, team, environments, and service delivery systems. However, entry-level therapists can use several basic strategies to help them become more competent in evaluating children:

1. Find a mentor who is experienced in working with children with various diagnoses and families from diverse backgrounds.
2. Be willing to search continually for new knowledge and resources that are relevant to working with children with special needs.
3. Be open to new ways of viewing children and families.
4. Learn to build effective communication skills and collaboration skills with team members, including the child's primary caregiver.

Documentation of Evaluation Results and Recommendations

The next step in the evaluation process is to provide written and oral reports of the evaluation findings and recommendations. The primary purpose of documenting the results of the pediatric occupational therapy evaluation is to describe to caregivers, physicians, teachers, and other individuals working with the child what the child's current abilities and limitations are on various functional tasks. McClain (1991) suggested the following:

> Effective documentation is telling a true story with a particular style. It calls for the ordinary tasks of day-to-day experience to be succinctly stated in writing. The true story about any child who has a disability is not a simple tale (p. 213).

When providing written documentation the therapist must first consider for whom the reports are intended and then carefully construct reports that are understandable and useful to those individuals. The format and content of evaluation reports may vary significantly, depending on the referral concern, the complexity of the child's problem, and the regulations of the service delivery system in which the child is served (e.g., public school setting, hospital, or home health agency). In some situations, for eligibility purposes, written evaluation reports must also include specific standard scores documenting developmental delay. In all occupational therapy practice settings, documentation stands as a legal record (AOTA, 1986).

Therapists should recognize that their words have great power. Words should be carefully chosen when documenting a child's evaluation results. Hanft (1989) cautions pediatric therapists that "words convey powerful personal images that can be positive and supportive, or negative and destructive". Pediatric occupational therapists should use words that reflect positive attitudes toward children with disabilities. Unfortunately, therapy jargon is filled with technical terms that may not convey the intended message but may confuse or alienate parents. Therapists should always refer to the child first and to the disability as one characteristic of the child (e.g., a child with cerebral palsy, not a cerebral palsied child). Table 7-3 shows how words have either negative or positive attitudes toward children with disabilities.

Box 7-3 provides a written example of how a therapist documented Kevin's evaluation findings and recommen-

table 7-3 Preferred Terms for Documentation

Inaccurate or Negative Terms	Preferred or Positive Terms
Afflicted	Children with disabilities
Defective, deformed	Child with a physical disability
Retarded	Child with developmental delay
Wheelchair-bound	Wheelchair-user
Deaf	Child with hearing impairment
Blind child	Child with visual impairment
Normal child	Nondisabled child

box **7-3** *Initial evaluation summary for Kevin*

University of Puget Sound School of Occupational Therapy Pediatric Clinic

Name:	Kevin	Evaluation Date:	September 18, 1999
School:	Newport Elementary	Date of Birth:	July 15, 1993
Grade:	Kindergarten	Chronologic Age:	6 years 2 months

Occupational therapy initial evaluation
Reason for referral

Kevin was referred to the Occupational Therapy Pediatric Clinic at the University of Puget Sound by his special education teacher, Mrs. Julie White. He has a history of developmental delay and a diagnosis of attention deficit disorder. Approximately 6 months ago Kevin's pediatrician, Dr. Mark Walker, placed him on Ritalin to control his extreme hyperactivity. Primary reasons for referral to occupational therapy include his fine motor delay, possible visual perceptual deficits, poor socialization skills, and gross motor incoordination.

Kevin attends a developmental preschool program five half-days per week. His classroom consists of some non-disabled children and several children who exhibit mild to moderate developmental delays in speech and language, behavior, or motor skills.

Kevin is the firstborn of three children in an African-American family. He lives with both of his parents and his two younger brothers in a small home located in inner city Tacoma.

Formal and informal assessments administered
Peabody Developmental Motor Scales (PDMS)
Clinical observations of neuromotor status
Coping Inventory
Test of Visual Perceptual Skills (TVPS)
Parent interview and home observations
Classroom and playground observations

Behavior during formal (standardized) assessments

Kevin was a friendly child who easily engaged in conversation with the examiner. He had significant difficulty attending to the structured test items, but when provided frequent social reinforcement and tangible rewards (e.g., stickers), he was able to complete most of the items presented. Kevin's hyperactivity and attention deficit limited his performance on some of the items. Therefore his standard scores on the PDMS and the TVPS may underestimate his actual abilities.

Assessment results

The following section describes Kevin's performance on functional tasks within his school and home environments and then provides results of Kevin's performance components on specific measures of motor and visual perception and psychosocial abilities.

Performance areas

Functional areas at school. Based on teacher interview and classroom observation, Kevin is experiencing difficulties in learning to print, making friends, and playing safely on playground equipment. In general, he enjoys school and wants to do well on his classroom activities.

Functional areas at home. Based on parent interview and home observation, Kevin is experiencing difficulties on specific self-help tasks of dressing and toileting. Parents describe him as "difficult to manage" and report he often requires physical punishment. Home observation showed few toys and no space to play outdoors.

Performance components

Fine motor performance. On the Peabody Developmental Fine Motor Scale, Kevin scored solidly through the 30- to 35-month level and successfully completed some items up to the 42-month level. His performance on this scale was more than 2 standard deviations below the mean and was reflective of functional fine motor skills in the approximate 38- to 40-month age range. Kevin preferred his right hand for most tasks that required the skilled use of a tool (e.g., crayons and scissors). He demonstrated hand tremors when attempting various fine motor tasks, but these tremors were not observed at rest. He moved impulsively and, even with verbal cues from the examiner, was unable to slow his movements down.

box 7-3 Initial evaluation summary for Kevin—cont'd

Gross motor performance. On the Peabody Developmental Gross Motor Scale, Kevin scored solidly through the 48- to 52-month level and successfully completed some items up to the 60-month level. His overall performance on this scale was 1.5 standard deviations below the mean and was reflective of functional gross motor skills in the approximate 56- to 58-month age range. Kevin scored within age expectations on tasks requiring speed and agility, but significantly below his age on tasks that required static balance (e.g., standing on one foot) and gross motor tasks that required more precise coordination (e.g., throwing a ball at a target).

Neuromuscular status. Clinical observations showed muscle tone, range of motion, integration of primitive reflexes, and development of automatic reactions (righting and equilibrium responses and protective extension reactions) within the normal range. Posture and gait also appeared normal. His frequent falls and clumsiness on the playground may be more related to his motor impulsivity and his inattentiveness than to delayed balance responses.

Visual perceptual skills. On the TVPS Kevin obtained a percentile rank of 21, indicating an overall performance in the low normal range (−0.8 standard deviation from the mean). His performance on each of the subtests varied significantly, suggesting relative strengths and weaknesses in visual perception. Specific results were as follows:

	Raw Scores	Perceptual Ages	Scaled Scores	Percentile Ranks
Visual discrimination	6	6-9	11	63
Visual memory	2	4-8	6	9
Visual spatial	6	5-2	8	25
Visual form constancy	5	5-11	10	50
Visual sequence memory	1	4-1	5	5
Visual figure-ground	2	4-5	6	9
Visual closure	7	7-6	12	75

Social skills. As measured by the Coping Inventory, Kevin lacked the necessary internal and external resources to meet the demands of his home environment and the unstructured playground environment at school. He demonstrated a minimally effective coping style in these settings, including erratic mood swings and aggressiveness toward others. However, within his classroom environment when the activities were scheduled, structured, and predictable, Kevin could regulate his activity level, and he interacted with peers and adults more successfully.

Summary

Kevin is a 6-year 2-month-old boy with attention deficits and developmental delays. He is currently enrolled in a developmental preschool program. This initial assessment shows that he is functioning almost 2 years below age expectations on the fine motor scale and almost 6 months below on the gross motor scale of the PDMS. Clinical observations of neuromotor status were within normal limits. Kevin's relative strengths and weaknesses in visual perception were substantial, although his overall performance on the TVPS was within the low normal range.

Kevin is a friendly, charming boy, but his extreme hyperactivity and distractibility limit his physical and social performance in both his home and school environments. Kevin's coping effectiveness varied depending on the degree of structure in his environment.

Recommendations

Based on this initial assessment, the following recommendations are suggested:

1. Direct occupational therapy to improve his performance on functional fine motor tasks, particularly learning to print his name.
2. Consult with parents and teachers regarding modifications to his home and school environments to optimize his coping effectiveness.
3. Consult with parents regarding strategies to help teach Kevin self-help skills and behavior management at home.

If there are any questions regarding this report, please contact this therapist at 123-4567.

dations. One important aspect of the report is how the therapist carefully worded it so that the information was helpful to Kevin's parents and to his teacher. The format of the report structures the description of Kevin's occupational performance, including his functional abilities and limitations.

To summarize the major points discussed in the previous sections, occupational therapists should ask themselves the following questions as they evaluate children. Did the evaluation process:

1. Address the caregiver's concerns?

2. Use assessments that measure occupational therapy domains and ICIDH-2 dimensions, including the child's participation in social and physical environments, activities and activity limitations, and body functions and impairments?

3. Use multiple methods of evaluation, including clinical observations, caregiver interview, direct observation of the child in natural environment, and standardized tools?

4. Fully recognize the influence of the child's cultural background on his or her evaluation performance and consider these cultural influences when developing recommendations for the child?

5. Adhere properly to the administration procedures and ethical considerations when using standardized tests?

6. Recognize and acknowledge the child's strengths as well as areas of concern?

7. Result in a summary that contributes meaningful, user-friendly information regarding the child's functional abilities and disabilities?

This section described the evaluation process, including important sequential steps for conducting accurate, thorough evaluations of children and communicating evaluation findings to caregivers and other professionals working with the child. The next, and last, section of this chapter provides the reader with additional detailed information on the methods used in pediatric occupational therapy evaluations.

■ EVALUATION METHODS

Several evaluation methods are available to pediatric occupational therapists. The challenge for therapists is to know which evaluation methods should be selected for a particular child or group of children. The purpose of this section is to describe each of the primary evaluation methods commonly used in pediatric occupational therapy practice and to discuss the major factors that therapists should consider when selecting these methods.

The starting point in the selection process is to identify clearly the purpose of the evaluation and to match appropriate evaluation methods with the identified purpose. Table 7-4 offers a list of the common purposes of

evaluation, described previously in this chapter, and matches evaluation methods appropriate for those purposes. For example, if the only purpose for the evaluation is to determine the child's eligibility for occupational therapy in a public school setting, then the primary evaluation method may be a norm-referenced, standardized test. However, if the primary purpose of the evaluation is to gain information useful for planning an intervention program for the child, the evaluation measures should include skilled observations of the child's functional performance and interviews with the child's caregivers. Often the initial evaluation of a child serves more than one purpose. Therefore therapists frequently use multiple measures and methods when conducting child evaluations. The following sections describe each of the evaluation methods commonly used in pediatric occupational therapy.

Norm-Referenced Tests

Norm-referenced measures are tests that have been developed by administering the test items to a sample of children (in a normative group) who are representative of the population to be tested. The child's score can then be compared with those of the normative group. To evaluate the usefulness of a norm-referenced measure, the pediatric occupational therapist should carefully read in the test manual how the norm-referenced scores were derived and the characteristics of the normative sample. The therapist using norm-referenced tests should also know how to accurately interpret an individual child's scores, including the standard score, and the percentile rank. Chapter 8 provides a more in-depth discussion on the use of standardized tests, including norm-referenced and criterion-referenced measures.

Criterion-Referenced Tests

Criterion-referenced measures are tests that consist of a series of skills in functional or developmental areas, usually grouped by age level. These tests compare the child's performance on each test item with a standard or criterion that must be met if the child is to receive credit for that item. Criterion-referenced tests are made up of items selected because of their importance to the child's school performance or daily living. Because of their importance to everyday function, the items often become intervention targets when the child exhibits difficulty in successfully completing the items.

The primary advantage in using criterion-referenced tests is that the examiner obtains important information regarding the child's strengths and limitations on critical skills. Some examples of criterion-referenced measures used in pediatric occupational therapy include the HELP (Furuno et. al., 1984), the Erhardt Developmental Prehension Assessment (Revised) (Erhardt, 1994), the Assessment and Programming System for

table 7-4 *Selection of Appropriate Evaluation Methods*

Purpose of Assessment	Evaluation Methods				
	Norm Referenced	Criterion Referenced	Skilled Observation	Interview	Checklists
Screening to determine need for further assessment	X		X	X	X
Comprehensive assessment to determine eligibility	X				
Comprehensive assessment to assist in diagnosis	X	X		X	
Comprehensive assessment to determine intervention plan		X	X	X	X
Reevaluation to monitor child's progress and determine need to continue therapy	X	X	X	X	X
Research to investigate clinical populations	X				

Infants and Young Children (Bricker, Bailey, Gumerlock, Buhl, & Slentz, 1986), and the Developmental Programming for Infants and Young Children (Schafer & Moersch, 1981) (see Appendix 7-A). Information gained from criterion-referenced tests is particularly helpful when determining the child's specific skills and when planning appropriate intervention activities to enhance those skills.

Ecologic Assessments

Neisworth and Bagnato (1988) defined *ecologic assessments* as "the examination and recording of the physical, social, and psychological features of a child's developmental context" (p. 39). Consistent with the transactional approach (Sameroff & Chandler, 1975), ecologic assessments are also concerned with the interaction between the individual child and the child's environments (Figure 7-11).

Pediatric occupational therapists are particularly interested in ecologic measures because these tools are a primary mechanism for obtaining data relevant to the child's performance context. Ecologic assessments for children employ techniques that consider the cultural influences, socioeconomic status, and value system of the family or the physical demands and societal expectations of the school setting. Some of these techniques include naturalistic observations, interviews, and rating scales. Ecologic measures familiar to pediatric occupational therapists include the Home Observation for Measurement of the Environment Inventory (Revised) (Caldwell & Bradley, 1984) and the Transdisciplinary Play-Based Assessment (Linder, 1990). The School Function Assessment (Coster et. al., 1998) is another example of an ecologic assessment.

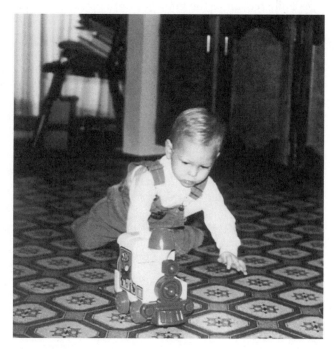

figure **7-11** Observing a child playing in his natural environment.

Skilled Observation

An essential skill of the pediatric occupational therapist is the ability to observe keenly and accurately and record children's behavior in an objective manner. Although formal, standardized assessments are highly valued in pediatric practice, *skilled observation* of a child performing a functional task offers different but equally important information about the child's performance.

Bailey and Wolery (1989) suggest the following:

> Observation of children in familiar settings and routines allows more characteristic views of their abilities and may be actually more reflective of how children can be expected to perform even under the most optimal learning opportunities (p. 256).

For example, skilled observations of a child's performance on functional tasks add important information not gained on standardized motor assessments (Figure 7-12).

Important components of skilled observations include (1) the setting, (2) the behavior of the child, (3) the quality of the behavior, and (4) the frequency and duration of the behavior (Cook, 1991). When skilled observations are used in the evaluation process, therapists must select a systematic, objective recording procedure so that data collected are accurate and reliable. Clark and Miller (1996) proposed a problem-solving approach to functional assessments and databased decision making for occupational therapy practitioners working with children in school settings.

Using direct observations of the child's functional skills at school, the occupational therapist and other team members define the outcome behaviors and identify the relevant dimensions of those behaviors, design a useful data collection system to monitor the progress of the child, and use the data for making decisions about the child's intervention program.

Huber and King-Thomas (1987) proposed that there are at least three different methods, or data collection systems, for recording direct observations. These include (1) recording the rate of behavior (frequency or duration), (2) using a checklist or rating scale, and (3) reporting a specific behavioral event in an anecdotal fashion.

Direct observations within the child's natural environment provide valuable information. Two disadvantages to this method, however, must be noted. First, the examiner loses some control over evaluation conditions. Second, if the examiner is not skilled, he or she may not recognize key behaviors and their meaning when they are viewed within the context of self-care, play, or other daily activities.

Interviews

Another primary method used in pediatric occupational therapy evaluation is the *interview* with the child's primary caregiver, teacher, or other adults working with the child. Caregiver interviews regarding their child's development can serve several functions (Bailey & Wolery, 1989):

1. To collect information about the child's skills from the parents' perspective
2. To validate information collected through direct observations or testing by the professional

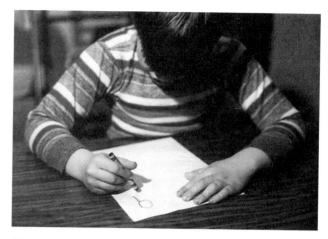

figure 7-12   Skilled observation of child performing a functional task at school.

3. To provide an opportunity for the parents to identify their values and priorities about the skills being evaluated by the therapist

Interviews are best used with other evaluation methods that employ direct observation of the child. An important outcome of the interview is the accurate, meaningful exchange of information between the professional and the parent or other caregiver. Interviews, when done well, can provide an opportunity to build rapport between the therapist and caregivers. They provide a unique opportunity for families to identify and discuss issues that are important to them. Therefore interviews are particularly useful when therapists are interested in family perceptions of children's abilities, the influence of events such as transitions in services on the family, and the family's priorities for services. When interviews are conducted in a flexible, sensitive manner, parents and therapists are able to explore areas of concern as they arise.

Interviews may include closed- or open-ended questions or a combination of both. Specific questions, which are often closed-ended, allow the therapist to gather a predetermined set of information from a caregiver in a relatively short amount of time. Unstructured interviews using open-ended questions allow caregivers to take the lead and set the priorities within the discussion. Open-ended questions invite the caregiver to elaborate on a topic and provide critical information about their child. Conducting an effective interview requires experience and sensitivity.

Several investigators have analyzed and described effective interview skills (Brammer, 1988; Carkhuff & Anthony, 1979; Ivey, 1971) (Box 7-4).

In summary, a skilled therapist conducts interviews with caregivers by carefully selecting questions and sensitively listening to their responses. Interviews offer a unique opportunity for exchange of information between

---

7-4 *Basic strategies for conducting effective caregiver interviews*

1. At the beginning, clarify the purpose of the interview with the caregiver in terms that are meaningful to him or her.
2. Be sensitive to the caregiver's physical and emotional needs throughout the evaluation.
3. Promote interaction by asking open-ended questions, and guide caregivers to where they may sit to participate fully in the conversation.
4. Through careful questioning, attempt to understand what is typical for the family regarding their values and cultural influences in raising their child.
5. Carefully plan when to take notes, preferably after the interview or when the caregiver is busy tending to the child.
6. Remain positive and realistic in your approach with caregivers and in the information you provide.
7. Be flexible throughout the interview, responding sensitively to the caregivers' questions and need for information. If you cannot answer their question, let them know and then figure out a plan with them to begin to find the needed information.
8. Use effective verbal and nonverbal communication skills. Often, nonverbal communication can override verbal information.
9. Avoid the use of therapy and medical jargon. If technical terms are used, be sure they are adequately explained.

---

caregivers and therapists. During the interview, therapists should reciprocate by providing caregivers with accurate, relevant information about the child's functional abilities, the intervention services, and community resources.

Inventories and Scales

A variety of inventories and scales are used to gather data on a child's development, the caregiver-child interactions, or the child's environments. Some published inventories, checklists, and scales are well-developed.

The Pediatric Evaluation of Disability Inventory (PEDI) (Haley, Coster, Ludlow, Haltiwanger, & Andrellos, 1992) is an evaluation of functional capabilities and performance in children 6 months to 7.5 years of age. This assessment is one of the few inventories that has been normed and standardized. The PEDI is administered through structured interview of the parents or by professional judgment of clinicians and educators who are familiar with the child. It measures both capability and performance of functional activities in (1) self-care, (2) mobility, and (3) social function. The inventory consists of 197 functional skills items; the child is scored either 1 (has capability) or 0 (has not yet demonstrated capability, unable) on each item. Twenty additional items rate the amount of caregiver assistance required to complete key functional tasks.

The PEDI was designed for use with young children who have a variety of disabling conditions, although the test authors were primarily concerned with designing an instrument to be used with children who have physical disabilities. The test authors completed a series of reliability and validity studies and developed criterion scores using Rasch Analysis techniques. As a result, the PEDI stands as a well-developed and well-researched assessment tool for evaluating the child's functional performance and capabilities.

Rating scales may provide both quantitative and qualitative data. A rating system usually involves a number scale to rate the quality, degree, or frequency of a behavior. For example, the NCAST Caregiver/Parent-Child Interaction Feeding and Teaching Scales (Sumner & Spietz, 1994) are designed to assess parent-child interactions in the context of feeding and teaching events. Figure 7-13 illustrate the type of data obtained using the feeding scale's rating system.

A parent, teacher, or other caregiver can complete some inventories and rating scales. For example, the Infant Monitoring System (Bricker & Squires, 1989) relies exclusively on parent report. On this scale the items are clearly described, and many are illustrated so that parents can elicit specific behaviors from their children. After each item, parents check the appropriate box: yes, sometimes, or not yet. The Developmental Profile II (DP-II) (Alpern, Boll, & Shearer, 1986) may be given by parent interview exclusively or by direct testing. A classroom teacher or parent can administer the Developmental Checklist for Pre-Dressing Skills (Dunn-Klein, 1983).

Transdisciplinary Arena Assessments

Federal legislation requires that evaluations of infants and young children with disabilities be conducted, when appropriate, by a multidisciplinary team (IDEA, 1991). The form and scope of the multidisciplinary evaluation, however, widely varies depending on the philosophy of the intervention program and the expertise of the professionals. For example, in some settings each professional provides an individual evaluation of the child or family, then meets with the other team members to discuss evaluation findings and recommendations. Sometimes little or

IV. COGNITIVE GROWTH FOSTERING	YES	NO
42. Caregiver provides child with objects, finger foods, toys, and/or utensils.		
43. Caregiver encourages and/or allows the child to explore the breast, bottle, food, cup, bowl, or the caregiver during feeding.		
44. Caregiver talks to the child using two words at least three times during the feeding.		
45. Caregiver verbally describes food or feeding situation to child during feeding.		
46. Caregiver talks to child about things other than food, eating, or things related to feeding.		
47. Caregiver uses statements that describe, ask questions, or explain consequences of behavior, more than commands, in talking to child.		
48. Caregiver verbally responds to child's sound within 5 seconds after child has vocalized.		
49. Caregiver verbally responds to child's movement within 5 seconds of child's movement of arms, legs, hands, head, trunk.		
50. Caregiver avoids using baby talk.		

figure**7-13**   Examples of items from the NCAST Caregiver/Parent-Child Interaction Feeding Scale.

no communication occurs between team members before and during the administration of the evaluation measures. In contrast, a team in another setting may use the transdisciplinary *arena assessment* approach in which one primary team member conducts the evaluation with the child and family and other key team members provide their expertise to the evaluation process through consultation.

One model in transdisciplinary evaluations is the *arena assessment.* An arena assessment allows the child and primary caregiver to interact with one professional throughout the evaluation visit while other professionals observe and, on occasion, directly test the child or interview the caregiver. An excellent example of an arena assessment is Linder's (1990) Transdisciplinary Play-Based Assessment (TPBA). This assessment places a major emphasis on a team approach to the evaluation of young children. The purpose of the TPBA is to obtain developmental information on the child using multidimensional, functional observations of the child during a play session. Parents and professionals together plan, observe, and analyze the child's play session.

Arena assessment of feeding difficulties in children can also be an effective way to gather relevant information without overtesting children or requiring the caregiver to participate in repeated interviews with different professionals. For example, an arena feeding assessment for a child with cerebral palsy and failure to thrive may include an occupational therapist, nurse, and nutritionist. One professional is designated as the lead evaluator, depend-

ing on the primary referral concern. The occupational therapist may take the lead if the child has oral-motor deficits, such as chewing or swallowing difficulties, postural difficulties that create the need for external support of posture at mealtime, or fine motor difficulties that limit self-feeding skills. The nurse may take the lead in the evaluation process if the child exhibits behavioral difficulties, if the parent's caregiving skills appear limited, or if parent-child interactions are at-risk. The nutritionist may take the lead if the child's diet needs careful analysis and if the family would benefit from specific information on types and amounts of food that the child should eat.

The benefit of an arena assessment of feeding is that the child and caregiver are subjected to the mealtime evaluation only once rather than multiple times. The arena assessment provides an opportunity for collaboration among parents and professionals to observe, discuss, and solve problems in critical areas together.

Selecting Appropriate Evaluation Measures and Methods

Before appropriate evaluation methods and measures can be selected for a child, the therapist must consider several factors. Box 7-5 provides a checklist of the important steps that therapists take in the process of selecting appropriate methods and measures when evaluating children.

STUDY QUESTIONS

CASE STUDY 1

Chelsea is an 8-month-old (corrected age) infant who was born at 32 weeks' gestation. Primary problems in the neonatal intensive care unit (NICU) included infant respiratory distress syndrome and neonatal abstinence syndrome secondary to maternal drug use. Cranial ultrasounds in the NICU indicated intraventricular hemorrhage. Chelsea is living with her mother, who is single, and her 2-year-old brother in a one-room studio apartment. Her mother is concerned because Chelsea is irritable throughout the day. She does not like her bath, nor does she enjoy being cuddled. Chelsea's pediatrician referred her for a therapy evaluation because she has some increased tone in her legs and has not yet achieved independent sitting.

1. Discuss the purpose of the therapy evaluation for Chelsea.

2. Describe what evaluation methods would be appropriate for an initial evaluation of Chelsea and her family, and list two to three specific instruments.

3. What other professionals might be involved with Chelsea?

CASE STUDY 2

Tin is a 2-year-old toddler with developmental delay of unknown cause. He is the firstborn of a newly immigrated South Vietnamese family. The public health nurse administered the Denver Developmental Screening Test–II, which showed that Tin was functioning around the 18-month-old level in gross motor skills, near the 12-month-old level in fine motor and adaptive skills, and at the 10-month-old level in language skills. Tin and his family were referred to a community-based early intervention program. The occupational therapist working in the early intervention program serves on a team that includes a physical therapist, a speech pathologist, and an early childhood special educator. The team is preparing to meet with the family to develop the Individual Family Service Plan.

1. What are some of the major points that the early intervention team should consider when assessing Tin and reporting evaluation information to the family?

2. Discuss the advantages and disadvantages of an arena assessment for Tin.

CASE STUDY 3

Eva is a 6-year-old girl with mild cerebral palsy who has participated in early intervention and preschool programs since she was 2 years of age. Her cognitive abilities appear to be within the normal range. The early intervention staff reports that Eva has some difficulty following adult-directed activities and playing with her peers. Her parents are interested in enrolling her in a regular kindergarten class this year. She is currently being evaluated by the public school occupational therapist to determine if she is eligible for therapy in the school setting. Eva's previous therapist at the early intervention program administered the Peabody Developmental Motor Scales last year.

1. Given the primary purpose of the school occupational therapy evaluation, what methods and measures would be most appropriate for Eva's evaluation?

2. Discuss whether a norm-referenced or a criterion-referenced assessment should be used in this situation.

3. Discuss some important behavioral strategies effective in evaluating Eva when using a standardized assessment.

4. In which natural environments should the therapist observe Eva to gain a better understanding of her occupational performance skills?

CASE STUDY 4

Michael is a 9-year-old boy with sensory processing deficits and a learning disability. His mother reports that Michael has difficulty making friends in the neighborhood and following through with simple chores at home. Michael's teacher indicates that Michael continues to have difficulty in completing his written assignments and frequently disrupts his classmates while they are working. He has recently been referred to the school's occupational therapist to determine if he would benefit from therapy.

1. What are the activities and occupations should the therapist assess in this case?

2. Which measurements would be most appropriate for Michael's initial evaluation?

3. Write two functional, measurable therapy goals for Michael for this school year.

box 7-5 *Checklist for selection of methods and measures*

- Start with reasons for referral.
- Gather relevant medical, educational, and family histories (e.g., precautions for testing, need for interpreter, and previous tests results).
- Consider the caregiver's priorities regarding the child's functional skills.
- Consider the developmental and chronologic age of the child.
- Determine the theoretic frames of reference most appropriate for the evaluation of the child.
- Consider the purpose of the evaluation, and select the most appropriate methods for the evaluation (see Table 7-4).
- Consider the requirements of the testing agency.
- Identify available resources (e.g., child's caregiver, other professionals, instruments and test materials, time, and space).

■ SUMMARY

The provision of accurate, reliable evaluations of children is one of the most challenging and rewarding services that a pediatric occupational therapist can offer. This chapter describes the purposes, process, and methods of evaluation in pediatric occupational therapy. Understanding the many purposes of evaluation and carefully matching appropriate methods and measures with those purposes are critical skills of the pediatric occupational therapist. Observing the details of children's performance on tasks and recognizing the importance of the context in which the child performs those tasks are also essential evaluation skills. Equally important in the evaluation process are the therapist's collaborative skills when working with the child's caregiver and other team members to gain an in-depth understanding of the child and his or her environments. This understanding, shared among team members, leads to the development of relevant, appropriate intervention plans and effective intervention strategies.

References

Achenbach, T.M., & Edelbrock, C.S. (1983). *Manual for the Child Behavior Checklist and Revised Child Behavior Profile.* Burlington: University of Vermont, Department of Psychiatry.

Alpern, G., Boll, T., & Shearer, M. (1986). *Developmental Profile II.* Los Angeles: Western Psychological Services.

Als, H., Lester, B.M., Tronick, E.Z., & Brazelton, T.B. (1982). Toward a research instrument for the Assessment of Preterm Infants' Behavior (APIB). In H. Fitzgerald, B.M. Lester, & M.S. Yogman (Eds.), *Theory and research in behavioral pediatrics* (Vol. 1). (pp. 35-132). New York: Plenum.

American Occupational Therapy Association. (1986). Guidelines for occupational therapy documentation. *American Journal of Occupational Therapy, 40,* 830-832.

American Occupational Therapy Association. (1994). Uniform terminology for occupational therapy, third edition. *American Journal of Occupational Therapy, 48,* 1047-1054.

Amundson, S.J. (1995). *Evaluation Tool of Children's Handwriting (ETCH).* Homer, AK: O.T. KIDS, Inc.

Ayres, A.J. (1989). *Sensory Integration and Praxis Tests.* Los Angeles: Western Psychological Services.

Bailey, D.B., & Simeonsson, R.J. (1988). Family Needs Survey. *Journal of Special Education, 22,* 117-127.

Bailey, D.B., & Wolery, M. (1989). *Assessing infants and preschoolers with handicaps.* Columbus, OH: Merrill.

Bayley, N. (1993). *Bayley Scales of Infant Development* (2nd ed.). San Antonio, TX: The Psychological Corporation.

Berk, R.A., & DeGangi, G.A. (1983). *Degangi-Berk Test of Sensory Integration.* Los Angeles: Western Psychological Services.

Brammer, L.M. (1988). *The helping relationship: Process and skills.* Englewood Cliffs, NJ: Prentice Hall.

Brazelton, T.B. (1984). *Neonatal Behavioral Assessment Scale: Clinics in developmental medicine.* (2nd ed.). Philadelphia: J.B. Lippincott.

Bricker, D., Bailey, E.J., Gumerlock, S., Buhl, M., & Slentz, K. (1986). *Assessment and Programming Systems for Infants and Young Children.* Eugene, OR: Center on Human Development.

Bricker, D., & Squires, J. (1989). *Infant monitoring system.* Eugene, OR: University of Oregon.

Bronfenbrenner, V., Moen, P., & Garbarino, J. (1984). Child, family, and community. In R.D. Parke (Ed.), *Review of child development research* (Vol. 7). (pp. 283-328). Chicago: University of Chicago Press.

Bruininks, R. (1978). *Bruininks-Oseretsky Test of Motor Proficiency.* Circle Pines, MN: American Guidance Service.

Bundy, A. (1997). Play and playfulness: What to look for. In L.D. Parham & L.S. Fazio (Eds.), *Play in occupational therapy for children.* (pp. 52-66). St. Louis: Mosby.

Bundy, A. (1991). Writing functional goals for evaluation. In C.B. Royeen (Ed.), *AOTA self-study series: School-based practice for related services.* (pp. 7-30). Bethesda, MD: American Occupational Therapy Association.

Caldwell, B.M., & Bradley, R.H. (1984). *Home Observation and Measurement of the Environment—Revised.* Little Rock, AR: HOME Inventory, University of Arkansas.

Campbell, S.K., Osten, E.T., Kolobe, T.H.A., & Fisher, A.G. (1993). Development of the Test of Infant Motor Performance. In C.V. Granger & G.E. Gresham (Eds.), *New developments in functional assessments in rehabilitation medicine.* Philadelphia: W.B. Saunders.

Carkhuff, R.R., & Anthony, W.A. (1979). *The skills of helping.* Amherst, MA: Human Resource Development Press.

Clark, G.F., & Miller, L.E. (1996). Providing effective occupational therapy services: Data-based decision making in school-based practice. *American Journal of Occupational Therapy, 50* (9), 701-708.

Colarusso, R.P., & Hammill, D.D. (1972). *Motor Free Visual Perception Test.* Novato, CA: Academic Therapy Publications.

Collier, T. (1991). The screening process. In W. Dunn (Ed.), *Pediatric occupational therapy: Facilitating effective service provision* (pp. 11-33). Thorofare, NJ: Slack.

Cook, D.G. (1991). The assessment process. In W. Dunn (Ed.), *Pediatric occupational therapy: Facilitating effective service provision* (pp. 35-72). Thorofare, NJ: Slack.

Coster, W. (1998). Occupational-centered assessment of children. *American Journal of Occupational Therapy, 52* (5), 337-344.

Coster, W., Deeney, T., Haltiwanger, J., & Haley, S. (1998). *School Function Assessment.* San Antonio: The Psychological Corporation.

DeGangi, G.A., & Greenspan, S.I. (1989). *Test of Sensory Functions in Infants.* Los Angeles: Western Psychological Services.

Dunn, W. (1997). *Sensory Profile.* Kansas City, KS: Sensory Profile Project. OT Education, University of Kansas Medical Center.

Dunn, W., Brown, C., & McGuigan, A. (1994). The ecology of human performance: A framework for considering the effect of context. *American Journal of Occupational Therapy, 48* (7), 595-607.

Dunn, W., & Campbell, P.H. (1991). Designing pediatric service provision. In W. Dunn (Ed.), *Pediatric occupational therapy: Facilitating effective service provision* (pp. 139-159). Thorofare, NJ: Slack.

Dunn-Klein, M. (1983). *The Developmental Checklist for Pre-Dressing Skills.* Tucson, AZ: Therapy Skill Builders.

Dunst, C.J., Trivette, C., & Deal, A.G. (1994). *Supporting and strengthening families, Vol.1: Methods, strategies and practices.* Cambridge, MA: Brookline Books.

Erhardt, R.P. (1994). *Erhardt Developmental Prehension Assessment (Revised).* San Antonio, TX: Therapy Skill Builders.

Erhardt, R.P. (1988). *Erhardt Developmental Vision Assessment.* San Antonio, TX: Therapy Skill Builders.

Exner, C.E. (1993). Content validity of the In-Hand Manipulation Test. *American Journal of Occupational Therapy, 47,* 505-513.

Farran, D.C. (1990). Effects of intervention with disadvantaged and disabled children: A decade review. In S.J. Meisels & J.P. Shonkoff (Eds.), *Handbook of early childhood intervention* (pp. 501-539). Cambridge, MA: Cambridge University Press.

Farran, D., Kasari, C., & Jay, S. (1986). *Parent and Caregiver Involvement Scale.* Greensboro, NC: University of North Carolina.

Folio, M.R., & Fewell, R.R. (2000). *Peabody Developmental Motor Scales* (2nd Ed.), Austin, TX: Pro-Ed.

Frankenburg, W., Dodds, J., Archer, P., Bresnick, B., Maschka, P., Edelman, N., & Shapiro, H. (1990). *Denver Developmental Screening Test-II.* Denver: Denver Developmental Materials, Inc.

Furuno, S., O'Reilly, K., Hosaka, C.M., Zeisloft, B., & Allman, T. (1984). *The Hawaii Early Learning Profile.* Palo Alto, CA: VORT.

Gardner, M.F. (1995). *Test of Visual-Motor Skills (Revised).* Burlingame, CA: Psychological & Educational Publications.

Gardner, M.F. (1996). *Test of Visual-Perceptual Skills (non-motor) (Revised).* Burlingame, CA: Psychological & Educational Publications.

Gibbs, E.D., & Teti, D.M. (1990). *Interdisciplinary assessment of infants: A guide for early intervention professionals.* Baltimore: Brookes.

Glascoe, F.P., Martin, E.D., & Humphrey, S. (1990). A comparative review of developmental screening tests. *Pediatrics, 86* (4), 547-554.

Granger, C.V., Brown, S., Griswold, K., Heyer, N., McCabe, M., Msall, M., & Hamilton, B. (1991). *Functional Independence Measure for Children (WeeFIM).* Buffalo, NY: Center for Functional Assessment Research.

Haley, S.M., Coster, W.J., Ludlow, L.H., Haltiwanger, M.A., & Andrellos, P.J. (1992). *Pediatric Evaluation of Disability Inventory.* San Antonio, TX: Psychological Corporation.

Hammill, D.D., Pearson, N.A., & Voress, J.K. (1993). *Developmental Test of Visual Perception* (2nd ed.). Austin, TX: Pro-Ed.

Hanft, B. (1989). How words create images. In B. Hanft (Ed.), *Family-centered care: An early intervention resource manual* (Unit 2). (pp. 77-78). Bethesda, MD: American Occupational Therapy Association.

Hanft, B. (1994). The good parent: A label by any other name would not smell as sweet. *Developmental Disabilities Special Interest Section Newsletter, 17* (2), 5.

Huber, C.J., & King-Thomas, L. (1987). The assessment process. In L. King-Thomas & B. Hacker (Eds.), *A therapist's guide to pediatric assessment.* Boston: Little, Brown.

Individuals with Disabilities Education Act Amendments of 1991. (1991). (Public Law 102-119). Washington, DC: U.S. Government Printing Office.

Individuals with Disabilities Education Act Amendments of 1997. (1997). (Public Law 105-17). #20 USC 1400.

Ivey, A. (1971). *Microcounseling: Innovations in interview training.* Springfield, IL: Charles C. Thomas.

Johnson-Martin, N.M., Jens, K.G., Attermeier, S.M., & Hacker, B.J. (1991). *The Carolina Curriculum for Infants and Toddlers with Special Needs* (2nd ed.). Baltimore: Brookes.

Knox, S. (1997). Development and current use of the Knox Preschool Play Scale. In L.D. Parham & L.S. Fazio (Eds.), *Play in Occupational Therapy for Children.* (pp. 35-51). St Louis: Mosby.

Law, M.C. (1999). *All about outcomes: A program to help you organize your thinking about pediatric outcome measures.* Thorofare, NJ: Slack.

Law, M.C., Baptiste, S., McColl, M., Carswell, A., Polatajko, H., & Pollock, N. (1994). *Canadian Occupational Performance Measure* (2nd ed.). Ottawa, ON: Canadian Association of Occupational Therapy Publications.

Linder, T.W. (1990). *Transdisciplinary Play-Based Assessment: A functional approach to working with young children.* Baltimore, MD: Paul H. Brookes.

McClain, L.H. (1991). Documentation. In W. Dunn (Ed.), *Pediatric occupational therapy: Facilitating effective service provision* (pp. 35-72). Thorofare, NJ: Slack.

Miller, L.J. (1988). *Miller Assessment for Preschoolers.* San Antonio, TX: Psychological Corporation.

Miller, L.J. (1993). *First STEP Screening Tool.* San Antonio, TX: Psychological Corporation.

Miller, L.J., & Roid, G.H. (1994). *Toddler and Infant Motor Evaluation.* San Antonio: Psychological Corporation.

Mutti, M., Sterling, H.M., & Spalding, N.V. (1978). *Quick Neurological Screening Test.* Novato, CA: Academic Therapy Publications.

Neisworth, J.T., & Bagnato, S.J. (1988). Assessment in early childhood special education: A typology of dependent measures. In S.L. Odom & M.B. Karnes (Eds.), *Early intervention for infants and children with handicaps: An empirical base* (pp. 23-49). Baltimore: Paul H. Brookes.

Notari, A., & Bricker, D. (1990). The utility of a curriculum-based assessment instrument in the development of individualized education plans for infants and young children. *Journal of Early Intervention, 14,* 117-132.

Palisano, R.J, Haley, S.M., & Brown, D.A. (1992). Goal attainment scaling as a measure of change in infants with motor delays. *Physical Therapy, 72* (6), 432-437.

Piers, E.V., & Harris, D.B. (1984). *The Piers-Harris Children's Self-Concept Scale (Revised).* Los Angeles: Western Psychological Services.

Piper, M.C., & Darrah, J. (1994). *Alberta Infant Motor Scale (AIMS).* Philadelphia: W.B. Saunders.

Rogers, S.J., D'Eugenio, D.B., Brown, S.L., Donovan, C.M., & Lynch, E.W. (1981). *Early Intervention Developmental Profile.* Ann Arbor: University of Michigan Press.

Russell, D.J., Rosenbaum, P.L., Gowland, C., Hardy, S., Lane, M., Plews, N., McGavin, H., Cadman, D.T., & Jarvis, S. (1993). *The Gross Motor Function Measure* (2nd ed.). Owen Sound, Ontario: Pediatric Physiotherapy Services.

Sameroff, A.J. (1986). Environmental context of child development. *Journal of Pediatrics, 109,* 192-200.

Sameroff, A.J., & Chandler, M.J. (1975). Reproductive risk and the continuum of caretaking casualty. In F.D. Horowitz, M. Hetherington, S. Scarr-Salapatek, & G. Siegel (Eds.), *Review of child development research* (Vol. 4). (pp. 187-244). Chicago: University of Chicago Press.

Sameroff, A.J., & Fiese, B.H. (1990). Transactional regulation and early intervention. In S.J. Meisels & J.P. Shonkoff (Eds.), *Handbook of early childhood intervention* (pp. 119-145). Cambridge, MA: University of Cambridge Press.

Sanford, A.R., & Zelman, J.G. (1981). *Learning Accomplishment Profile.* Winston-Salem, NC: Kaplan.

Schafer, D.S., & Moersch, M.S. (1981). *Developmental Programming for Infants and Young Children.* Ann Arbor, MI: University of Michigan Press.

Sparrow, S.S., Balla, D.A., & Cicchetti, D.V. (1984). *Vineland Adaptive Behavior Scales*. Circle Pines, MN: American Guidance Service.

Sumner, G., & Spietz, A. (1994). *NCAST Caregiver/Parent-Child Interaction Scales*. Seattle: NCAST Publications, University of Washington, School of Nursing.

Vulpe, S.G. (1994). *Vulpe Assessment Battery—revised*. East Aurora, NY: Slosson Educational Publications.

Washington Administrative Code. (1990). *Rules and regulations for programs providing services to children with handicapping conditions* (W.A.C. 392-171, Section 381). Olympia, WA: Office of Superintendent of Public Instruction.

Werner E.E., & Smith, R.S. (1982). *Vulnerable but invincible: A longitudinal study of resilient children and youth*. New York: McGraw-Hill.

Williamson, G.G., & Szczepanski, M. (1999). Coping frame of reference. In P. Kramer & J. Hinojosa (Eds.), *Frames of reference for pediatric occupational therapy* (pp. 432-468). Baltimore: Williams & Wilkins.

Winton, P.J. (1988). The family-focused interview: An assessment measure and goal setting mechanism. In D.B. Bailey & R.J. Simeonsson (Eds.), *Family assessment in early intervention* (pp. 185-205). Columbus, OH: Merrill.

World Health Organization (WHO). (1997). *ICIDH-2: International classification of impairments, activities, and participation* (Beta-1 draft for field trials). Geneva, Switzerland: Author.

Young, N.L. (1997). *Activities Scale for Kids*. Toronto, ON: Pediatric Outcomes Research Team, Hospital for Sick Children.

Zeitlin, S. (1985). *Coping Inventory*. Bensenville, IL: Scholastic Testing Service.

Zeitlin, S., Williamson, G.G., & Szczepanski, M. (1988). *Early Coping Inventory*. Bensenville, IL: Scholastic Testing Service.

Suggested Readings

American Occupational Therapy Association. (1994). *Pediatric resource guide*. Bethesda, MD: The Association.

Asher, I. (1996). *Occupational therapy evaluation tools: An annotated index*. (2nd ed.). Bethesda, MD: American Occupational Therapy Association.

Clancy, H., & Clark, M.J. (1990). *Occupational therapy with children*. Melbourne, Australia: Churchill Livingstone.

Common Pediatric Evaluation Tools*

Alberta Infant Motor Scales (AIMS)
Piper, M.C., & Darrah, J. (1994). *Motor assessment of the developing infant.*
W.B. Saunders Company
Philadelphia, PA 19106

Battelle Developmental Inventory
Newborg, J., Stock, J.R., Wnek, L., Guidubaldi, J., & Svinicki, A. (1988)
Riverside Publishing
8420 West Bryn Mawr Avenue
Chicago, IL 60631
(800) 767-8378

Bayley Scales of Infant Development, second edition
Bayley, N. (1994)
The Psychological Corporation
555 Academic Court
San Antonio, TX 78204
(210) 299-1061

Beery Developmental Test of Visual Motor Integration, third revision
Beery, K.E. (1989)
Modern Curriculum Press
13900 Prospect Road
Cleveland, OH 44136
(216) 572-0690

Brigance Diagnostic Inventories
Brigance, A.H. (1978)
Curriculum Associates
5 Esquire Road, N
Billerica, MA 01862

Bruininks-Oseretsky Test of Motor Proficiency
Bruininks, R. (1978)
American Guidance Service
4201 Woodland Road
Circle Pines, MN 55014
(612) 786-4343

Coping Inventory
Zeitlin, S. (1991)
Scholastic Testing Service
Bensenville, IL 60106-8056

DeGangi-Berk Test of Sensory Integration
Berk, R.A., & DeGangi, G.A. (1983)
Western Psychological Services
1203 Wilshire Boulevard
Los Angeles, CA 90025
(310) 478-2061

Denver Developmental Screening Test (Revised)
Frankenburg, W., Dodds, J., Archer, P., Bresnick, B., Maschka, P., Edelman, N., & Shapiro, H. (1990)
Denver Developmental Materials, Inc.
P.O. Box 6919
Denver, CO 80206

Developmental Programming for Infants and Young Children
Schafer, D.S., & Moersch, M.S. (1981)
The University of Michigan Press
Ann Arbor, MI 48106
(313) 764-4392

Developmental Test of Visual Perception, 2nd ed.
Hammill, D.D., Pearson, N.A., & Voress, J.K. (1993)
Pro Ed
8700 Shoal Creek Boulevard
Austin, TX 78757-6897
(512) 451-3246

Early Coping Inventory
Zeitlin, S., Williamson, G.G., & Szczepanski, M. (1988)
Scholastic Testing Service
Bensenville, IL 60106-8056

Early Intervention Developmental Profile
Rogers, S.J., Donovan, C.M., D'Eugenio, D.B.,
    Brown, S.L., Lynch, E.W., Moersch, M.S., &
    Schafer, D.S. (1981)
University of Michigan Press
Ann Arbor, MI 48106
(313) 764-4392

Erhardt Developmental Prehension Assessment (Revised)
Erhardt, R.P. (1994)
Psychological Corporation
555 Academic Court
San Antonio, TX 78204-2498

Erhardt Developmental Vision Assessment
Erhardt, R.P. (1988)
555 Academic Court
San Antonio, TX 78204-2498

Evaluation Tool of Children's Handwriting (ETCH)
Amundson, S.J. (1995)
O.T. KIDS, Inc.
P.O. Box 1118
Homer, AK 99603

The First STEP
Miller, L.J. (1993)
The Psychological Corporation
555 Academic Court
San Antonio, TX 78204
(210) 299-1061

Gesell Preschool Test
Ames, L.B., Gillespie, C., Haines, J., & Ilg, F.L.
    (1980)
Programs for Education, Inc.
P.O. Box 167
Rosemont, NJ 08556
(609) 397-2214

The Gross Motor Function Measure (GMFM) (Revised)
Russell, D., Rosenbaum, P., Gowland, C., Hardy, S.
    Lane, M., Plews, N., McGavin, H., Cadman, D., &
    Jarvis, S. (1993)
Pediatric Physiotherapy Services
RR #4
Owen Sound, ON Canada N4K 5N6
(519) 371-2792

Hawaii Early Learning Profile (HELP)
Furuno, S., O'Reilly, K.A., Hosaka, C.M., Inatsuka,
    T.T., Allman, T.A., & Zeisloft, B. (1984)
Vort Corporation
P.O. Box 60123
Palo Alto, CA 94306
(415) 322-8282

Home Observation and Measurement of the Environment (HOME)
Caldwell, B. (1984)
Center for Early Development and Education
University of Arkansas
Little Rock, AR 77204

In-Hand Manipulation Test
Exner, C.E. (research edition only)
Occupational Therapy Department
Towson State University
Towson, MD 21204

Miller Assessment for Preschoolers (MAP)
Miller, L.J. (1988)
The Psychological Corporation
555 Academic Court
San Antonio, TX 78204
(210) 299-1061

Motor-Free Visual Perception Test (MVPT)
Colarusso, R.P., & Hammill, D.D. (1983)
Academic Therapy Publications
20 Commercial Boulevard
Novato, CA 94947-6191
(800) 422-7249

NCAST Parent-Child Interaction Scales
Sumner, G., & Spietz, A. (1994)
NCAST Programs
University of Washington
Box 357920
Seattle, WA 98195-7920
(206) 543-9528

Peabody Developmental Motor Scales
Folio, R., & Fewell, R.
Pro-Ed
8700 Shoal Creek Boulevard
Austin, TX 78757

Pediatric Evaluation of Disability Inventory (PEDI)
Haley S.M., Coster W.J., Ludlow, L.H.,
    Haltiwanger, J.T., & Andrellos, P.J. (1992)
Psychological Corporation
555 Academic Court
San Antonio, TX 78204-2498.

Pediatric Examination of Educational Readiness
Levine, M.D., & Schneider, E.A.
Educators Publishing Service, Inc.
75 Moulton Street
Cambridge, MA 02238-9101

Pediatric Extended Examination at Three
Blackman, J.A., Levine, M.D., & Markowitz, M.
Educators Publishing Service, Inc.
75 Moulton Street
Cambridge, MA 02238-9101

Quick Neurological Screening Test (QNST)
Mutti, M., Sterling, H.M., & Spalding, N.V. (1978)
Academic Therapy Publications
20 Commercial Boulevard
Novato, CA 94949
(415) 883-3314

School Function Assessment (SFA)
Coster, W., Deeney, T., Haltiwanger, J., & Haley, S.
  (1998)
Psychological Corporation
555 Academic Court
San Antonio, TX 78204-2498
(800) 228-0752

Sensory Integration and Praxis Tests (SIPT)
Ayres, A.J., et. al. (1989)
Western Psychological Services
1203 Wilshire Boulevard
Los Angeles, CA 90025-1251
(310) 478-2061

Test of Infant Motor Performance (TIMP)
Cambell, S.K., Osten, E.T., Kolobe, T.H.A., & Fisher,
  A.G. (1993). Development of the Test of Infant
  Motor Performance. In C.V. Granger & G.E.
  Gresham (Eds.), *New developments in functional
  assessment*
W.B. Saunders Company
Philadelphia, PA 19106

Test of Sensory Functions in Infants (TSFI)
DeGangi, G.A., & Greenspan, S.I. (1989)
Western Psychological Services
1203 Wilshire Boulevard
Los Angeles, CA 90025-1251
(310) 478-2061

Test of Visual-Motor Skills (TVMS) (Revised)
Gardner, M.F. (1995)
Psychological and Educational Publications, Inc.
1477 Rollins Road
Burlingame, CA 94010
(800) 523-5775

**Test of Visual-Perceptual Skills (non-motor)
  (TVPS)(Revised)**
Gardner, M.F. (1996)
Psychological and Educational Publications, Inc.
1477 Rollins Road
Burlingame, CA 94010

Toddler and Infant Motor Evaluation (TIME)
Miller, L.J., & Roid, G.H. (1994)
Psychological Corporation
555 Academic Court
San Antonio, TX 78204-2498

Transdisciplinary Play-Based Assessment
Linder, T.W. (1993)
Paul H. Brookes Publishing Co.
P.O. Box 10624
Baltimore, MD 21285-0624
(800) 638-3775

chapter 8

Use of Standardized Tests in Pediatric Practice

Pamela K. Richardson

key terms

Standardized test
Reliability
Norm-referenced test
Criterion-referenced test
Normative sample
Measures of central tendency

Measures of variability
Standard score
Correlation coefficient
Validity
Ethics in testing

■ CHAPTER OBJECTIVES

1. Recognize the characteristics of commonly used standardized pediatric tests.
2. Describe the differences between norm-referenced and criterion-referenced tests and the purpose for each type of test.
3. Understand the descriptive statistics used in standardized pediatric tests.
4. Know the types of standard scores used in standardized pediatric tests.
5. Discuss the concept of reliability.
6. Explain the importance of test validity.
7. Describe the procedures necessary to become a competent user of standardized tests.
8. Understand the ethical considerations when using standardized tests.
9. Apply knowledge of standardized-test applications to information found in a case study.

What are standardized tests, and why are they important to occupational therapists? A test that has been standardized has uniform procedures for administration and scoring (Anastasi, 1988). This means that examiners must use the same instructions, materials, and proce-

dures each time they administer the test, and they must score it using criteria specified in the test manual. A number of standardized tests are in common use. Most schoolchildren have taken standardized achievement tests that assess how well they have learned the required grade-level material. College students are familiar with the Scholastic Aptitude Test (SAT), the results of which are used by many colleges and universities to make decisions about admission. Intelligence tests, interest tests, and aptitude tests are other examples of standardized tests that are used frequently with the general public.

Pediatric occupational therapists use standardized tests to determine eligibility of children for therapy services, to monitor their progress in therapy, and to make decisions about what type of treatment intervention is most appropriate and effective for them. Standardized tests provide precise measurements of a child's performance in specific areas and describe the performance as a standard score. This score can be used and understood by other occupational therapists and child development professionals who are familiar with standardized testing procedures.

Using anthropometric measurements and psychophysical testing to measure intelligence, Galton and Cat-tell developed the initial concept of standardized assessments of human performance late in the nineteenth century. The first widespread use of human performance testing was initiated in 1904, when the minister of public education in Paris formed a commission to create tests that would help to identify "mentally defective children," with the goal of providing them with an appropriate education. Binet and Simon developed the first intelligence test for this purpose. Terman and Merrill (1937) incorporated many of Binet and Simon's ideas in constructing the Stanford-Binet Intelligence Scale that remains widely used today (Sternberg, 1990). Although intelligence was the first human attribute to be tested in a standardized manner, tests have been developed in the past 30 years that assess children's developmental status, cognition, gross- and fine-motor skills, language and communication skills, school readiness, school achievement, visual-motor skills, visual-perceptual skills, social skills, and other behavioral domains. Although the number and types of tests have changed radically since the time of Simon and Binet, the basic reason for using standardized tests remains the same: to identify children who may need special intervention or programming because their performance in a given area is outside the "norm," or average, for their particular age.

The use of standardized tests requires a high level of responsibility on the part of the tester. The occupational therapist who uses a standardized test must be knowledgeable about scoring and interpreting the test, must be aware for whom the test is and is not appropriate, and must understand how to report and discuss a child's scores on the test. The tester must also be aware of the limitations of standardized tests in providing information about a child's performance deficits. This, in turn, requires a working knowledge of standardized testing concepts and procedures, familiarity with the factors that can affect performance on standardized tests, and awareness of the ethics and responsibilities of testers when using standardized tests.

The purpose of this chapter is to introduce pediatric standardized testing that is used by occupational therapists. Purposes and characteristics of standardized tests are discussed, technical information about standardized tests is presented, practical tips for becoming competent users of standardized assessments are given, and ethical considerations are explained. The chapter concludes with a summary of the advantages and disadvantages of standardized tests and a case study that incorporates the concepts presented in the chapter into a "real-life" testing scenario. Throughout the chapter, several standardized assessments that are commonly used by pediatric occupational therapists are highlighted to illustrate the concepts of test administration, scoring, and interpretation.

■ PURPOSES

Standardized tests are used for several reasons. First, a standardized test may be used as a screening tool to assess large numbers of children quickly and briefly and identify those who may have delays and are in need of more in-depth testing. Some examples of screening tests frequently used by occupational therapists include the Miller Assessment for Preschoolers (MAP) (Miller, 1982), the Denver Developmental Screening Test, revised (Denver-II) (Frankenburg, et. al., 1990), and the First STEP (Screening Test for Evaluating Preschoolers) (Miller, 1990).

Screening tests typically assess several developmental domains, with each domain represented by a small number of items (Table 8-1). Screening tests generally take 20 to 30 minutes and can be administered by professionals or by paraprofessionals such as classroom aides, volunteers, or parents. Therapists who work in settings that primarily serve typically developing children (e.g., a public school system or Head Start program) may become involved in developmental screening activities. In addition, occupational therapists frequently use assessment tools to evaluate children with specific developmental

table 8-1 **Developmental Domains Assessed in Four Screening Tools**		
Screening Tool	**Age Range**	**Domains Assessed**
Denver Developmental Screening Test, revised	1 month to 6 years	Personal-social, fine-motor adaptive, language, gross motor
Developmental Indicators for Assessment of Learning, revised	2½ to 6 years	Motor, language, concepts
First STEP: Screening Test for Evaluating Preschoolers	2 years, 9 months to 6 years, 2 months	Cognition, communication, physical, social and emotional, adaptive functioning
Miller Assessment for Preschoolers	2 years, 7 months to 5 years, 8 months	Foundations, coordination, verbal, nonverbal, complex tasks

problems. Therefore it is important for all therapists to be aware of the strengths and weaknesses of specific tests used in their settings. Although the screening tools mentioned are not discussed in greater depth, the concepts of developing, administering, scoring, and interpreting standardized tests (discussed later in this chapter) should also be considered when using screening tools.

Occupational therapists most frequently use standardized tests as in-depth assessments of various developmental or functional domains. Standardized tests are used for three main purposes: (1) to determine a medical or educational diagnosis, (2) to document the child's developmental or functional status, and (3) to plan intervention programs.

Determine a Medical or Educational Diagnosis

The first purpose for standardized tests is to diagnose through use of normative scores that compare the child's performance with that of an age-matched sample of children. Standardized tests are frequently used to determine if a child has developmental delays or functional deficits that are significant enough to qualify for remedial services such as occupational therapy. Many funding agencies, early intervention programs, and public school programs use the results of standardized testing as a primary criterion for making the decision about whether a child will receive special education services or therapy intervention. Funding approval for special services is generally dependent on documentation of a predetermined amount of delay in one or more developmental domains, and standardized test results are an important component of this documentation. The results of standardized testing performed by occupational therapists, when used in conjunction with testing done by other professionals, assist physicians or psychologists in arriving at a medical or educational diagnosis.

Document Child's Developmental and Functional Status

A second purpose for standardized testing is to document a child's status. Many funding agencies and service agencies require periodic reassessment to provide a record of a child's progress and to determine if the child continues to qualify for services. Standardized tests are often a preferred way of documenting progress because the results from the most current assessment can be compared with the results of earlier assessments. Periodic formal reassessment can also provide valuable information to the treating therapist. Careful scrutiny of a child's test results can help identify areas of greatest and least progress. This can assist the therapist in prioritizing treatment goals. Many parents are also interested in seeing the results of their child's periodic assessments. However, care must be taken to put standardized test scores in perspective because gains in functional skills, such as feeding, dressing, and toilet training, may not be reflected in the child's scores on a comprehensive developmental or motor assessment.

A discussion about the child's progress in areas that may not be measured by standardized testing should accompany the discussion of test performance. Structured or unstructured observations of the child's play and self-care behavior and interviews with the caretaker about the child's home routine, developmental, and medical history, as well as review of pertinent medical or educational records, are equally important components of the assessment process. (See Chapter 7 for more information about the assessment process.)

Plan Intervention Programs

A third purpose for standardized testing is program planning. Standardized tests provide information about a child's level of function, and they help therapists to determine the appropriate starting point for therapy intervention. Most commonly, criterion-referenced standardized tests are used as the basis for developing goals and objectives for individual children and for measuring progress and change over time. Criterion-referenced tests are used extensively in educational settings and include such tools as the Hawaii Early Learning Profile (HELP) (Furuno, et. al., 1997); the Assessment, Evaluation, and Programming System for Infants and Children (Bricker, 1993); and the School Function Assessment (SFA) (Coster, Deeney, Haltiwanger, & Haley, 1998). Criterion-referenced tests are described in more detail in the following section.

■ CHARACTERISTICS

As stated earlier, standardized tests have uniform procedures for administration and scoring. These standard procedures are what permit the results of a child's testing to be compared with either the child's performance on a previous administration of the test or with the test norms developed by administering the test to a large number of children.

A first characteristic of standardized tests is that they include a test manual that describes the purpose of the test (i.e., What the test is intended to measure.) The manual should also describe the intended population for the test. For pediatric assessments, this generally refers to the age range of children for whom the test was intended, but it may also refer to specific diagnoses or types of functional impairments. Test manuals also contain technical information about the test, such as a description of the test development and standardization process, characteristics of the normative sample, and

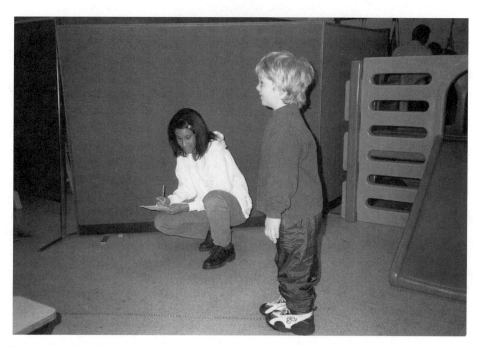

figure **8-1**   A therapist prepares to test a child on the broad jump item from the Bruininks-Oseretsky Test of Motor Proficiency.

studies done during the test development process to establish reliability and validity data. Finally, test manuals contain detailed information about administration, scoring, and interpretation of the test scores.

A second characteristic of standardized tests is that they are composed of a fixed number of items. Items may not be added or subtracted without affecting the standard procedure for test administration. Most tests have specific rules regarding how many items should be administered to ensure a standardized test administration. These may differ significantly from test to test. For instance, the *Bruininks-Oseretsky Test of Motor Proficiency* (BOTMP) (Bruininks, 1978) specifies that the entire item set be administered regardless of the age of the child. In contrast, *the Bayley Scales of Infant Development, revised* (BSID-II) (Bayley, 1993) has a number of item sets corresponding to age bands (e.g., 22 to 24 months). Testers are instructed to begin testing at the age band corresponding to the child's chronologic age (or corrected age, if the child was born prematurely) and to move either to higher or lower age band if necessary, depending on the child's performance. The decision to move on to a different age band is made according to the number of items passed and failed at the initial age band, and the decision rules are stated in the test manual. Below is a description of how to compute ages corrected for prematurity (Box 8-1).

The third characteristic of standardized tests is a fixed protocol for administration. A fixed protocol for administration refers to how each item is administered as well as

how many items are administered. Generally, the protocol for administration specifies what verbal instruction or demonstration is provided, how many times the instructions can be repeated, and how many attempts the child is allowed at the item. For some tests, instructions for each item are printed in the manual and the tester is expected to read the instructions verbatim to the child without deviating from the text. However, other tests allow for more freedom of instruction, especially when the test involves a physical activity (Figure 8-1).

The fourth characteristic of standardized tests is a fixed guideline for scoring. Scoring guidelines usually accompany the administration guidelines and specify what the child's performance must look like to receive a passing score on the item. Depending on the nature of the item, passing performance may be described using text, a picture, or a diagram. The administration and scoring guidelines for two test items are illustrated (Figures 8-2 and 8-3). Figure 8-2 is an item from the BOTMP. In this example, the instructions to be given to the child are printed in bold type. Also included are the criteria for a passing score on the item, examples of incorrect responses, and the number of trials and time allowed to complete the item. This example describes how to present the item and what constitutes a passing score, as well as a diagram of what a passing performance looks like. The BSID-II also includes scoring notes that provide cues to examiners when scoring a series of related items.

box 8-1 *Calculating chronologic and corrected age*

Many standardized tests require that the examiner calculate the child's exact age on the date of testing. The method for calculating chronologic and corrected age is described below:

Calculating chronologic age

First, the date of testing and the child's birth date must be completed in the following order:

	Year	Month	Day
Date of testing:	99	6	15
Birth date:	95	3	10
Chronologic age:	4	3	5

Begin on the right (Day category). The day, month, and year of the child's birth date is subtracted from the date of testing. In the above example, the child's chronologic age is 4 years, 3 months, 5 days at the time of testing.

The convention when calculating age is if the number of days in the chronologic age is 15 or less, the month is *rounded down*. Therefore in the above example, the child's age would be stated as 4 years, 3 months, or 4-3. If the number of days in the chronologic age is between 16 and 30, the month is *rounded up*. If the above child's chronologic age had been 4 years, 3 months, 16 days, the chronologic age would be expressed as 4 years, 4 months, or 4-4.

Sometimes, "borrowing" is necessary to subtract correctly the birth date from the date of testing:

	Year	Month	Day
Date of testing:	99	6	15
Birth date:	95	10	22
Chronologic age:	3	7	23

Begin with the Day category. Twenty-two cannot be subtracted from 15 without borrowing from the Month category. One month must be borrowed and placed in the Day category. One month equals 30 days; 30 is added to the 15 days in the Date of testing, giving a total of 45. Twenty-two is subtracted from 45, leaving 23 days. Moving to the Month category, one month has been borrowed by the Day category, leaving 5 months. Ten cannot be subtracted from 5, so one year must be borrowed from the Year category. One year equals 12 months, so 12 will be added to the 5 in the Month cat-

egory for Date of testing, totaling 17. Ten is subtracted from 17, leaving 7 months. Moving to the Year category, 1 year has been borrowed by the Month category, leaving 98. Ninety-five can be subtracted from 98, leaving 3 years. Therefore this child's chronologic age is 3 years, 7 months, 23 days. Using the rounding convention discussed above, the month will be rounded up, giving a chronologic age of 3 years, 8 months.

Calculating corrected age

Corrected age is used for children who were born prematurely to "correct" for the number of weeks they were born prior to before the due date. Generally, the age is corrected until the child turns 2 years old, although this convention can vary. Given 40 weeks gestation as full-term, the amount of correction is the difference between the actual gestational age at birth and the 40 weeks full-term gestational age. Therefore a child born at 30 weeks gestation is 10 weeks premature. Many practitioners consider 36 or 37 weeks and above to be full-term gestation, so children with a gestational age of 36 weeks and above do not receive a corrected age. Because there is some variation in how and when corrected age is used, it is wise for the therapist to learn the procedures of his or her facility and adhere to them when calculating corrected age.

If the expected due date and birth date are both known, subtracting the birth date from the due date will yield an exact measurement of prematurity:

	Year	Month	Day
Due date:	98	9	20
Birth date:	98	6	12
		3	8

This child is 3 months, 8 days premature. To calculate corrected age, subtract the amount of prematurity from the chronologic age:

	Year	Month	Day
Chronologic age:	1	1	25
Prematurity:		3	8
		10	17

The child's corrected age is 10 months, 17 days, or, when rounded, 11 months.

Touching Thumb to Fingertips — Eyes Closed

With eyes closed, the subject touches the thumb of the preferred hand to each of the fingertips on the preferred hand, moving from the little finger to the index finger and then from the index finger to the little finger, as shown below. The subject is given 90 seconds to complete the task once. The score is recorded as a pass or a fail.

Trials: 1

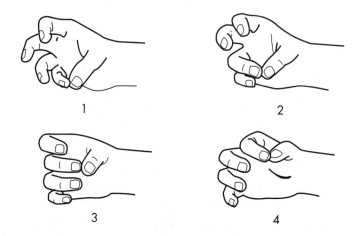

Administering and Recording

Have the subject sit beside you at a table. Have the subject extend the preferred arm. Then say, **You are to touch your thumb to each of the fingertips on this hand. Start with your little finger and touch each fingertip in order. Then start with your first finger and touch each fingertip again as you move your thumb back to your little finger** (demonstrate). **Do this with your eyes closed until I tell you to stop. Ready, begin.**

Begin timing. If necessary provide additional instruction. During the trial correct the subject and have the subject start over if he or she:
    a. Fails to maintain continuous movements
    b. Touches any finger except the index finger more than once in succession
    c. Touches two fingers at the same time
    d. Fails to touch fingers above the first finger joint
    e. Opens eyes

Allow no more than 90 seconds, including time needed for additional instruction, for the subject to complete the task once. After 90 seconds, tell the subject to stop.

On the Individual Record Form, record pass or fail.

figure8-2   Administration and scoring protocol for Bruininks-Oseretsky Test of Motor Proficiency subtest 5, item 8. *(From Bruininks, R.H. [1978]. Bruininks-Oseretsky Test of Motor Proficiency. Circle Pines, MN: American Guidance Service.)*

■ TYPES OF STANDARDIZED TESTS

There are two main types of standardized tests: *norm-referenced* and *criterion-referenced*. Many pediatric occupational therapists use both norm-referenced and criterion-referenced tests in their practices. Each type of test has a specific purpose, and it is important for testers to be aware of the purpose for the test they are using.

A norm-referenced test is developed by giving the test in question to a large number of children, usually several hundred or more. This group is called the *normative sample,* and "norms," or average scores, are derived from this sample. When a norm-referenced test is administered, the performance of the child being tested is compared with this normative sample. The purpose of

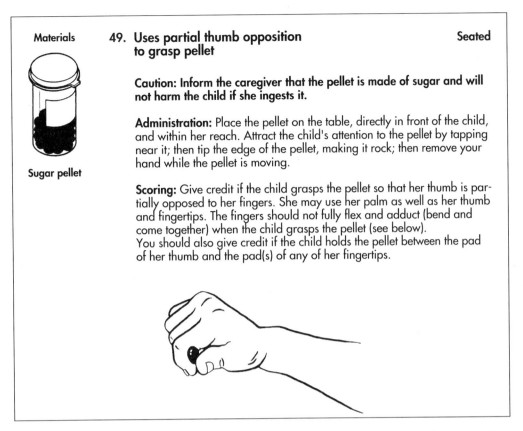

Materials

49. Uses partial thumb opposition to grasp pellet

Seated

Caution: Inform the caregiver that the pellet is made of sugar and will not harm the child if she ingests it.

Administration: Place the pellet on the table, directly in front of the child, and within her reach. Attract the child's attention to the pellet by tapping near it; then tip the edge of the pellet, making it rock; then remove your hand while the pellet is moving.

Scoring: Give credit if the child grasps the pellet so that her thumb is partially opposed to her fingers. She may use her palm as well as her thumb and fingertips. The fingers should not fully flex and adduct (bend and come together) when the child grasps the pellet (see below). You should also give credit if the child holds the pellet between the pad of her thumb and the pad(s) of any of her fingertips.

Sugar pellet

figure 8-3   Administration and scoring protocol for Bayley Scales of Infant Development—II motor scale item 49. *(From Bayley, N. [1993]. Bayley Scales of Infant Development [2nd ed.]. San Antonio: The Psychological Corporation.)*

norm-referenced testing, then, is to determine how a child performs in relation to the average performance of the normative sample.

Test developers generally attempt to include children from a variety of geographic locations, ethnic and racial backgrounds, and socioeconomic levels so that the normative sample is representative of the population of the United States, based on the most recent U.S. Census data. Generally, the normative sample is composed of children who have no developmental delays or conditions, although some tests include smaller subsamples of clinical populations as a way to determine whether the test discriminates between children whose development is proceeding normally and children who have known developmental delays.

Norm-referenced tests tend to be rather general in content and cover a wide variety of skills. Some of the items may not have functional significance but give an indication of the child's ability level in a particular domain. For example, the BOTMP contains a subtest entitled *Bilateral Coordination.* Items in this subtest involve tapping fingers and feet simultaneously, jumping and touching the feet, and performing running patterns with armsand legs. Although none of these activities are particularly functional in and of them-

selves, the standard score obtained from this subtest can tell the therapist whether a child is having difficulties with bilateral coordination. The therapist can then select related functional activities to address the child's performance deficits.

Norm-referenced tests have standardized protocols for administration and scoring. The tester must adhere to these protocols so that each test administration is as similar as possible to that of the normative sample. This is necessary to compare any child's performance fairly with that of the normative sample.

Sometimes the examiner must deviate from the standard protocol because of special needs of the child being tested. For instance, a child with visual impairments may need manual guidance to cut with scissors, or a child with cerebral palsy may need assistance in stabilizing the shoulder and upper arm to reach and grasp a crayon. If changes are made in the standardized procedures, the examiner must indicate this in the summary of assessment, and standard scores cannot be used to describe that child's performance in comparison with that of the normative sample.

Descriptive scores, such as *age-equivalent scores,* can be used on tests such as the Peabody Developmental Motor Scales (PDMS) (Folio & Fewell, 2000) and the BSID-II when the standardized protocol has been altered. In this way the examiner can obtain an approximate measurement of the child's developmental level. Age-equivalent scores are discussed in more detail in the section on standard scores.

Norm-referenced tests have specific psychometric properties. They have been analyzed by statisticians to obtain score distributions, mean or average scores, and standard scores. This is done to achieve the primary objective of norm-referenced tests: comparability of scores with the normative sample. A test under development initially has a much larger number of items than what ends up on the final version of the test. Through pilot testing, items are chosen or rejected based partially on how well they statistically discriminate between children of different ages and abilities. Items are not primarily chosen for their relevance to functional skills or developmental milestones. Consequently, norm-referenced tests are generally not intended to link test performance with specific objectives or goals for intervention.

Criterion-referenced tests, by contrast, are designed to provide information on how children perform on specific tasks. The term criterion-referenced refers to the fact that a child's performance is compared with a particular criterion, or level of performance of a particular skill. The goal of a criterion-referenced test is to determine which skills a child can and cannot accomplish, providing a focus for intervention. In general, the content of a criterion-referenced test is detailed and, in some cases, may relate to specific behavioral or functional objectives. The intent of a criterion-referenced test is to measure a child's performance on specific tasks, rather than to compare the child's performance with that of his or her peers.

Many developmental checklists have been field tested and then published as criterion-referenced tests. The HELP is a good example of a developmental checklist designed to be used with children from the ages of birth to 3 years. It contains a large number of items in each of the domains of gross-motor, fine-motor, language, cognitive, social-emotional, and self-help skills. Each item is correlated to specific intervention objectives. For instance, if a child is not able to pass Fine-Motor item 4.81, *Snips with Scissors,* a list of intervention ideas are

A

4.81 Snips with scissors (23 to 25 months)
Definition: The child cuts a paper edge randomly one snip at a time, rather than using a continuous cutting motion. **Example observation opportunities:** <u>Incidental</u>—may observe while child is preparing for a tea party with stuffed animals or dolls. Demonstrate making fringe on paper placemats and invite the child to help. <u>Structured</u>—using a half piece of sturdy paper and blunt scissors, make three snips in separate places along the edge of the paper while the child is watching. Exaggerate the opening and closing motions of your hand. Offer the child the scissors and invite him or her to make a cut. Let the child explore the scissors (if interested), helping him or her position the scissors in his or her hand, as needed. **Credit:** (see also Credit Notes in this strand's preface) plus snips paper in one place, holding the paper in one hand and scissors in the other.

B

4.81 Activity guide suggestions
The child cuts with the scissors, taking one snip at a time rather than doing continuous cutting. 1. Let the child use small kitchen tongs to pick up objects and to practice opening and closing motions. 2. Let the child use child-sized scissors with rounded tips. 3. Demonstrate by placing your finger and thumb through the handles. 4. Position the scissors with the finger holes one above the other. Position the child's forearm in midsupination (i.e., thumb up). Let the child place his or her thumb through the top hole and the middle finger through the bottom hole. If the child's fingers are small, place the index and middle fingers in the bottom hole. The child will adjust his or her fingers as experience is gained. 5. Let the child open and close the scissors. Assist as necessary by placing your hand over the child's hand. 6. Let the child snip narrow strips of paper and use it for fringe in art work. 7. The different types of scissors that are available for children are a scissors with reinforced rubber coating on the handle grips, a scissors with double handle grips for your hand and the child's hand, a left-handed scissors, and a scissors for a prosthetic hook. Use these different types of child's scissors appropriately as required.

figure 8-4   **A,** Administration and scoring protocol for Hawaii Early Learning Profile item 4.81 and, **B,** item 4.81 activity guide suggestions. *(Part A From Parks, S. [1992]. Inside HELP: Administration and reference manual for the Hawaii Early Learning Profile. Palo Alto, CA: Vort)(Part B From Furuno, S., O'Reilly, K.A., Hosaka, C.M., Zeisloft, B., & Allman, T. [1985]. HELP activity guide. Palo Alto, CA: Vort.)*

presented in the HELP activity guide (Furuno et. al., 1997). The activity guide is meant to accompany the test and is designed to help the therapist or educator by providing ideas for developmentally appropriate activities to address areas of weakness identified in the criterion-based assessment. The administration protocol for this item and the associated intervention activities are illustrated in Figure 8-4.

Administration and scoring procedures may or may not be standardized on a criterion-referenced test. The HELP has standard procedures for administering and scoring each item. In addition, many other criterion-referenced tests take the form of checklists in which the specific performance needed to receive credit on an item is not specified. Many therapist-designed tests for use in a particular facility or setting are nonstandardized, criterion-referenced tests.

Criterion-referenced tests are not subjected to the statistical analyses that are performed on norm-referenced tests. No mean score or normal distribution is calculated; a child may pass all items or fail all items on a particular test without adversely affecting the validity of the test results. The purpose of the test is to learn exactly what a child can accomplish, not to compare the performance of the child with that of the peer group. This goal is also reflected in the test development process for criterion-referenced tests. Items are generally chosen based on a process of task analysis or identification of important developmental milestones, rather than for their statistical validity. Therefore the specific items on a criterion-referenced test have a direct relationship with functional skills and can be used as a starting point for generating appropriate goals and objectives for therapy intervention. The summary scores from criterion-referenced tests should relate closely to the child's current pattern of performance in order to be useful for intervention planning (Fisher, 1993).

The characteristics of norm-referenced and criterion-referenced tests are compared below (Table 8-2). As Table 8-2 indicates, some tests are both norm-referenced and criterion-referenced. This means that although the items have been analyzed for their ability to perform statistically, they also reflect functional or developmental skills that are appropriate for intervention. These tests permit the therapist to compare a child's performance with that of peers in the normative sample while, providing information about specific skills that may be appropriate for remediation.

The PDMS is one example of both a norm-referenced and a criterion-referenced test. Although the PDMS has been subjected to the statistical analyses used in norm-referenced tests, many individual items on the PDMS also represent developmental milestones that are frequent areas of focus for intervention. The SFA, while primarily a criterion-referenced test, provides a criterion score and standard error for each raw score based on a national standardization sample.

■ TECHNICAL ASPECTS OF STANDARDIZED TESTS

The following discussion of the technical aspects of standardized tests focuses on the statistics and test development procedures used for norm-referenced tests. Information on how standard scores are obtained and reported is included, as well as how the reliability and validity of a test are determined.

table 8-2   Comparison of Norm-Referenced and Criterion-Referenced Tests

Characteristic	Norm-Referenced Test	Criterion-Referenced Test
Purpose	Comparison of child's performance with normative sample	Comparison of child's performance with a defined list of skills
Content	General; usually covers a wide variety of skills	Detailed; may cover specific objectives or developmental milestones
Administration and scoring	Always standardized	May be standardized or nonstandardized
Psychometric properties	Normal distribution of scores; means, standard deviations, and standard scores computed	No score distribution needed; a child may pass or fail all items
Item selection	Items chosen for statistical performance; may not relate to functional skills or therapy objectives	Items chosen for functional and developmental importance; provides necessary information for developing therapy objectives
Examples	BSID-II; PDMS; BOTMP; PEDI	PDMS, PEDI, HELP, Gross-Motor Function Measure, SFA

BOTMP, Bruininks-Oseretsky Test of Motor Proficiency; *BSID-II,* Bayley Scales of Infant Development (revised); *HELP,* Hawaii Early Learning Profile; *PDMS,* Peabody Developmental Motor Scales; *PEDI,* Pediatric Evaluation of Disability Inventory; *SFA,* School Function Assessment.

1. Therapists need to be able to analyze and select standardized tests appropriately, according to the child's age, functional level, and purpose of testing.
2. Therapists need to be able to interpret and report scores accurately from standardized tests.
3. Therapists need to be able to explain test results to caregivers and other professionals working with the child in a clear and understandable manner.

The following discussion of technical aspects of standardized tests focuses on the statistics and test-development procedures used for norm-referenced tests. It includes information on (1) descriptive statistics, (2) standard scores, (3) correlation coefficients, (4) reliability, and (5) validity.

Descriptive Statistics

Descriptive statistics inform us about the characteristics of a particular group. Many human characteristics, such as height, weight, head size, and intelligence, are represented by a distribution called the *normal curve* (or bell-shaped curve) (Figure 8-5). The pattern of performance on most norm-referenced tests also follows this curve.

The largest number of people receives a score in the middle part of the distribution, with progressively smaller numbers of people receiving scores at either the high or the low end of the distribution. Descriptive statistics provide information about where members of a group are located on the normal curve. The two types of descriptive statistics are the *measure of central tendency* and the *measure of variability*.

The measure of central tendency indicates where the middle point of the distribution is for a particular group, or sample, of children. The most frequently used measure of central tendency is the *mean*. The mean is the sum of all the scores for a particular sample divided by the number of scores. It is computed mathematically through a simple formula:

$$\overline{X} = \frac{\Sigma X}{n}$$

In this formula, Σ means to sum, X = each individual score, and n = the number of scores in the sample (the mean is also often called the average score).

A second measure of central tendency is the *median*.

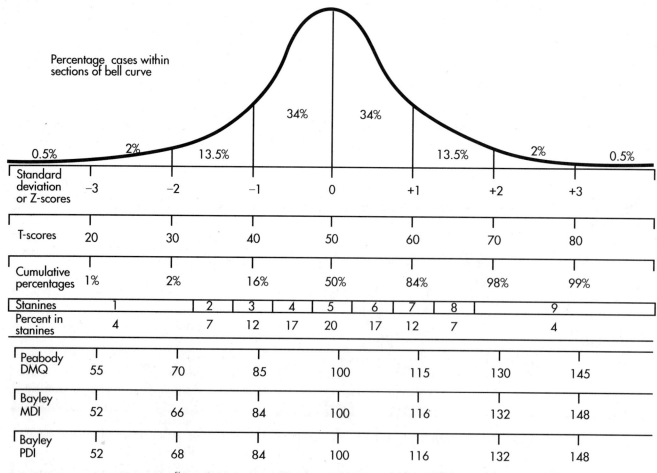

figure 8-5 The normal curve and associated standard scores.

The median is simply the middle score of a distribution. Half the scores lie below the median and half the scores lie above the median. The median is the preferred measure of central tendency when there are outlying or extreme scores in the distribution. For instance, look at the following distribution of scores:

2   3   13   14   17   17   18

The mean score is $(2 + 3 + 13 + 14 + 17 + 17 + 18) \div 7 = 12$. The median, or middle score, is 14. In this case the score of 14 is a more accurate representation of the middle point of these scores than is the score of 12. This is because the two low scores, or outliers, in the distribution pulled down the value of the mean.

A second type of descriptive statistic is a *measure of variability* in a sample. These statistics determine how much the performance of the group as a whole deviates from the mean. These measures of variability are used to compute the standard scores used in standardized tests. As with the measures of central tendency, the measures of variability are derived from the normal curve. The two measures of variability discussed are the *variance*, and the *standard deviation* (SD).

The variance is defined as the average of the squared deviations of the scores from the mean. In other words, it is a measure of how far the score of an average individual in a sample deviates from the group mean. The variance is computed using the following formula:

$$S^2 = \frac{\Sigma(X - \overline{X})^2}{n}$$

Where S^2 is the variance, $\Sigma(X - \overline{X})^2$ is the sum of each individual score minus the mean score, and n is the total number of scores in the group. The standard deviation is simply the square root of the variance. To illustrate, calculations are provided for the mean, the variance, and the standard deviation for the following set of scores from a hypothetical test:

17   19   21   25   28

To calculate the mean, the following equation is used:

$$\frac{(17 + 19 + 21 + 25 + 28)}{5} = 22$$

To calculate the variance, the mean must be subtracted from each score and then that value must be squared:

$$17 - 22 = (-5)^2 = 25$$
$$19 - 22 = (-3)^2 = 9$$
$$21 - 22 = (-1)^2 = 1$$
$$25 - 22 = (3)^2 = 9$$
$$28 - 22 = (6)^2 = 36$$

The squared values are then summed and then divided by the total number of scores:

$$25 + 9 + 1 + 9 + 36 = 80$$
$$\frac{80}{5} = 16$$

The variance of this score distribution is 16. The standard deviation is simply the square root of the variance, or 4.

The standard deviation is an important number because it is the basis for computing many standard scores. In a normal distribution (Figure 8-5), 68% of the people in the distribution score within 1 *SD* of the mean (± 1 *SD*), 95% score within 2 *SD* of the mean (± 2 *SD*), and 99.7% score within 3 *SD* of the mean (± 3 *SD*). In the score distribution with a mean of 22 and a standard deviation of 4, three of the five scores were within 1 *SD* of the mean (22 ± 4; a score range of 18 to 26), and all five scores were within 2 *SD* of the mean (22 ± 8; a score range of 14 to 30). The standard deviation, then, determines the placement of scores on the normal curve. By telling us the amount of variability in the sample, the standard deviation reveals how far the scores can be expected to range from the mean value.

Standard Scores

Standardized tests are scored several different ways. Scoring methods include: *Z-scores T-scores, deviation IQ scores* and *developmental index scores, percentile scores* and *age-equivalent scores.*

The Z-score is computed by subtracting the mean for the test from the individual's score and dividing it by the standard deviation, using the following equation:

$$Z = \frac{X - \overline{X}}{SD}$$

Using the score distribution above, the person receiving the score of 17 would have a Z-score of $(17 - 22) \div 4 = -1.25$. The person receiving the score of 28 would have a Z-score of $(28 - 22) \div 4 = 1.5$. Note that the first score has a negative value. This indicates that the Z-score value is below the mean for the test. The second score has a positive value, indicating that the Z-score value is above the mean. Generally, a Z-score value of -1.5 or less is considered indicative of delay or deficit in the area being measured, although this can vary depending on the particular test.

The T-score is derived from the Z-score. In a T-score distribution, the mean is 50 and the standard deviation is 10. The T-score is computed using the following equation:

$$T = 10(Z) + 50$$

For the two Z-scores computed above, the T-score

values are as follows: For the first Z-score of −1.25, the T-score is 10(−1.25) + 50 = 37.50. For the second Z-score of 1.5, the T-score is 10(1.5) + 50 = 65. Note that all T-scores have positive values, but because the mean of a T-score distribution is 50, any number below 50 indicates a score below the mean. Because the standard deviation of the T distribution is 10, the first score of 37.50 is slightly more than 1 *SD* below the mean. The second score of 65 is 15 points, or 1.5 *SD* above the mean.

Two other standard scores that are frequently seen in standardized tests include the Deviation IQ score and developmental index score. Deviation IQ scores have a mean of 100 and a standard deviation of either 15 or 16. These are the intelligence quotient (IQ) scores obtained from such tests as the Stanford-Binet (Thorndike, Hagen, & Sattler, 1986) or the Wechsler Intelligence Scale for Children (WISC) (Wechsler, 1974). On these tests, individuals who have IQ scores that are 2 *SD* below the mean (IQs of 70 and 68, respectively) are considered to be mentally retarded. Individuals who have IQ scores that are 2 *SD* above the mean (IQs of 130 and 132, respectively) are considered gifted.

Two other types of scores are frequently used in standardized tests. These are not standard scores in the strictest sense, because they are computed directly from raw scores rather than through the statistically derived measures of central tendency and variability. However, they give an indication of a child's performance relative to that of the normative sample. The first of these scores is the percentile score. A percentile score is the percentage of people in a standardization sample whose score is at or below a particular raw score. A percentile score of 60, for instance, indicates that 60% of the people in the standardization sample received a score that was at or below the raw score corresponding to the 60th percentile. Tests that use percentile scores generally include a table in the manual by which raw scores can be converted to percentile scores. These tables usually indicate at what percentile rank performance is considered deficient. Raw scores can be converted to percentile rank (PR) scores by a simple formula:

$$PR = \frac{(\text{Number of people below score} + \frac{1}{2} \text{ of people at score})}{\text{Total number of scores}} \times 100$$

Using the sample data from the previous page, percentile ranks for the highest and lowest scores can be computed. The raw score of 17 is the lowest score in the distribution and is the only score of 17. Consequently, the equation is as follows:

$$\frac{(0 + \frac{1}{2})}{5} \times 100 = \frac{0.5}{5} \times 100 = 10$$

The highest score in the distribution is 28. Consequently, four people have lower scores and one person received a score of 28. The equation is as follows:

$$\frac{(4 + \frac{1}{2})}{5} \times 100 = \frac{4.5}{5} \times 100 = 90$$

In this distribution, then, the lowest score is at the 10th percentile and the highest score is at the 90th percentile.

Although percentile-rank scores can be easily calculated and understood, they have one significant disadvantage. The percentile ranks are not equal in size across the score distribution. Distances between percentile ranks are much smaller in the middle of the distribution than at the ends of the distribution, so improving a score from the 50th to the 55th percentile entails much less effort than improving a score from the 5th to the 10th percentile (see Figure 8-4). Therefore an improvement in performance by a child who is functioning at the lower end of the score range may not be reflected in the percentile-rank score the child achieves. Other standard scores are more sensitive in measuring changes in the performance of children who fall at the extreme ends of the score distribution.

Another score that is derived directly from the raw score is the *age-equivalent score*. The age-equivalent score is the age at which the raw score is at the 50th percentile. The age-equivalent score is generally expressed in years and months, for example, 4-3 (i.e., 4 years, 3 months). It is a score that is easily understood by parents and caregivers who may not be familiar with testing concepts or terminology. For this reason it is used frequently.

However, age-equivalent scores have some disadvantages. Although they may provide a general idea of a child's overall developmental level, saying, for instance, that a 4-year-old child is functioning at the 2½-year level may be misleading. The age-equivalent score may be more or less an average of several developmental domains, some of which may be at the 4½-year level and some of which may be at the 1½-year level. Therefore the child's performance may be highly variable and may not reflect that of a typical 2½-year-old child. Additionally, because the age-equivalent score only represents what a child of a particular age who is performing at the 50th percentile would receive, a child who is performing within normal limits for his or her age, but whose score is below the 50th percentile, would receive an age-equivalent score below his or her chronologic age. This can cause parents or caregivers to conclude incorrectly that their child has delays. Age equivalents, then, can be a useful way to describe a child's performance, but they should be used with caution.

Correlation Coefficients

Test manuals often report *correlation coefficients* when describing the test's reliability and validity. A correlation coefficient tells the degree or strength of the relationship between two scores or variables. Although the standard scores are used to compute individual scores, correlation coefficients are used to determine the relationship between scores on one measurement and scores on another. Correlation coefficients range from -1.00 to $+1.00$. A correlation coefficient of 0.00 indicates that there is no relationship between the two variables measured. Any relationship that occurs is strictly by chance. The closer the correlation coefficient is to either -1.00 or $+1.00$, the stronger the relationship is between the two variables. A negative correlation means that a high score on one variable is accompanied by a low score on the other variable. A positive correlation means that a high score on one variable is accompanied by a high score on the other variable and that a low score on one variable is accompanied by a low score on the other variable.

Examples of two variables that generally have a fairly high positive correlation are height and weight. Taller individuals are also generally heavier than shorter individuals. However, this is not always true. There are tall individuals who are light and short individuals who are heavy. Consequently, the correlation between height and weight for a given population is a positive value, but it is not a perfect 1.00. Examples of two variables that are unrelated are eye color and height. The correlation coefficient for these two variables for any population is close to zero, because you cannot predict what a person's eye color is by knowing their height.

An example of two variables that have a negative correlation might be hours spent studying and hours spent watching television. A student who spends many hours studying probably watches fewer hours of television, and a student who watches many hours of television probably spends fewer hours studying. Hence, there is a negative relationship between these two variables. As one variable increases, the other decreases. Several different correlation coefficients may be calculated, depending on the type of data used. Some correlation coefficients commonly used in test manuals include the Pearson Product-Moment Correlation Coefficient or Pearson **r;** the Spearman Rank-Order Correlation Coefficient, and the Intraclass Correlation Coefficient (ICC). Why are correlation coefficients important? As the following sections on reliability and validity illustrate, correlation coefficients are important tools for evaluating the properties of a test. Knowledge of test characteristics helps testers know how best to use a test and be aware of the strengths and limitations of individual tests.

Reliability

The *reliability* of a test describes the consistency or stability of scores obtained by one individual when tested on two different occasions with different sets of items or under other variable examining conditions (Anastasi, 1988). For instance, if a child is given a test and receives a score of 50 and 2 days later is given the same test and receives a score of 75, the reliability of the test is questionable. The difference between the two scores is called the *error variance* of the test, which is a result of random fluctuations in performance between the two testing sessions. It is expected that there is always some amount of random error variance in any test situation because of variations in such things as the child's mood, fatigue, or motivation. Error variance can also be caused by environmental characteristics such as light, temperature, or noise. However, it is important that error variance caused by the variations in the examiner, or by the characteristics of the test itself, be minimal. To have confidence in the scores obtained on a test, the test must have adequate reliability over a number of administrations and low error variance.

Most standardized tests evaluate two or three forms of reliability. The three forms of reliability most commonly used in pediatric standardized tests are (1) *test-retest reliability*, (2) *interrater reliability*, and (3) *standard error of measurement* (SEM).

Test-retest reliability

Test-retest reliability is a measurement of the stability of the test over time. It is obtained by giving the test to the same individual on two different occasions. When evaluating test-retest reliability for a pediatric test, the time span between test administrations must be short to minimize the possibility of developmental changes occurring between the two test sessions. However, the time span between tests should not be so short that the child may recall items administered during the first test session, thereby improving his or her performance on the second test session (this is called the learning, or practice, effect).

Generally, the time span between testings is no more than 1 week for infants and very young children and no more than 2 weeks for older children. During the process of test development, test-retest reliability is evaluated on a subgroup of the normative sample. The size and composition of the subgroup should be specified in the manual. The correlation coefficient between the scores of the two test sessions is calculated. This coefficient is the measure of the test-retest reliability of the test. A test that has a high test-retest reliability coefficient is more likely to yield relatively stable scores over time. That is, it is affected less by random error variance than a test that has a low test-retest reliability coefficient. The problem with a test that has a low test-retest reliability coefficient is that one has less confidence that the score obtained from testing a child is a true reflection of that child's abilities. If the child were tested at a different time of day or in a different setting entirely, different results might be obtained.

A sample of 175 infants was evaluated twice within 2 weeks (about 4 days apart) to assess the test-retest reliability on the BSID-II. Correlation coefficients were high but not perfect (0.83 for the Mental Scale and 0.77 for the Motor Scale). The performance of a young child often varies within short periods, because it is highly influenced by variables such as mood, hunger, sleepiness, and irritability. The test-retest reliability for the PDMS was high (0.95 for Gross Motor and 0.80 for Fine Motor) when 38 children were tested within 1 week's time.

To evaluate test-retest reliability of the Developmental Test of Visual Perception, Second Edition (DTVP-II) (Hammill, Pearson, & Voress, 1993), 88 students were tested twice within 2 weeks. The correlation coefficients for the test's subsections ranged from 0.80 to 0.93. The reliability for the total test scores was 0.95. These three examples of good to excellent test-retest reliability are typical examples of pediatric sensorimotor tests. The rapid and variable development of young children and the practice effect are two factors that negatively influence the tests' stability over time. This test characteristic is critical to using the results as a measure of progress or intervention efficacy.

Interrater reliability

A second form of reliability is interrater reliability. This refers to the ability of two independent raters to obtain the same scores when scoring the same child simultaneously. Interrater reliability is generally measured on a subset of the normative sample during the test-development process. This is often accomplished by having one rater administer and score the test while another rater observes and scores at the same time. The correlation coefficient calculated from the two raters' scores is the interrater reliability coefficient of the test. It is particularly important to measure interrater reliability on tests where the scoring may require some judgment on the part of the examiner.

Although the scoring criteria for many test items are specific on most tests, to a certain extent, scoring depends on individual judgment, and scoring differences can arise between different examiners. A test that has a low interrater reliability coefficient is especially sensitive to differences in scoring by different raters. This may mean that the administration and scoring criteria are not stated explicitly enough, requiring examiners to make judgment calls on a number of items. Alternatively, it can mean that the items on the test call for responses that are too broad or vague to permit precise scoring.

What is an acceptable coefficient for test-retest and interrater reliability? There is no universal agreement regarding the minimum acceptable coefficient. The context of the reliability measurement, the type of test, and the distribution of scores are some of the variables that

can be taken into account when determining an acceptable reliability coefficient. One standard suggested by Anastasi (1988) and used by a number of examiners is 0.80. The examples reported meet this criterion.

Not all tests have test-retest or interrater reliability coefficients that reach the 0.80 level. For example, the BSID-II Motor Scale has an interrater reliability of 0.75. This coefficient may indicate variability in scores by different raters. When examiners use a test that has a reliability coefficient below 0.80, scores must be interpreted with great caution. For example, if one subtest of a test of motor development has test-retest reliability of 0.60, care must be exercised when using it to measure change over time, recognizing that a portion of the apparent change between the first and second test administration is a result of error variance of the test.

Interrater reliability was assessed for the BSID-II using 51 children of ages 2 to 30 months. Items were administered and scored by one examiner and were simultaneously scored by an observer. Interrater reliability coefficients were 0.96 for the Mental Scale and 0.75 for the Motor Scale. The correlation coefficient for the Motor Scale seemed to be lower because these items involved manipulation of the infant to score, placing the observer at a disadvantage (Bayley, 1993). Interrater reliability for the PDMS was evaluated using the same method: one tester administering and one observing the items. The resulting correlation coefficients were 0.97 for Gross Motor and 0.94 for Fine Motor, giving the tester strong confidence in the reliability of the scores across raters (Folio & Fewell, 1983). In a test such as the DTVP-II, where scores are based on a written record of the child's response, interrater reliability is excellent. When two individuals scored 88 completed DTVP-II protocols, the inter-scorer reliability was 0.98 (Hammill, et. al., 1993).

When individual subtests of a comprehensive test have a low reliability coefficient, it is generally not recommended that the standard scores from the subtests be reported. Often the reliability coefficient of the entire test is much higher than that of the individual subtests. One reason for this is that reliability increases with the number of items on a test. Because subtests have fewer items than the entire test, they are more sensitive to fluctuations in the performance or scoring of individual items. When this occurs, it is best to describe subtest performance qualitatively but not to report standard scores.

Standard scores can be reported for the total, or comprehensive, test score. Examiners should consult the reliability information in the test manual before deciding how to report test scores for individual subtests and for the test as a whole. The interrater reliability coefficients reported in the manual are estimates based on the context and conditions under which they were studied by the test developers. This reliability coefficient is an estimate; interrater reliability may vary when children are tested in different contexts or when examiners have differing levels of training and experience.

Examiners can exert some control over the interrater reliability of tests that they use frequently. It is good practice to check interrater reliability with more experienced colleagues when learning a new standardized test before beginning to administer the test to children in the clinical setting. Additionally, periodically checking interrater reliability with colleagues who are administering the same standardized tests is a good practice. There are some simple methods for assessing interrater reliability. These are discussed in more depth later in the chapter.

Standard error of measurement

A third form of reliability is the SEM. This statistic is used to calculate the expected range of error for the test score of an individual. It is based on the range of scores that an individual might obtain if the same test were administered a number of times simultaneously, with no practice or fatigue effects. Obviously, this is impossible; therefore the SEM is a theoretic construct. It is, however, an indication of the possible error variance in individual scores.

The SEM creates a normal curve for the individual's test scores, with the obtained score in the middle of the distribution. The child has a higher probability of receiving scores in the middle of the distribution than scores at the extreme ends of the distribution. The SEM is based on the standard deviation of the test, as well as the test's reliability (usually test-retest reliability). The SEM can be calculated using the following formula:

$$SEM = SD\sqrt{1 - r}$$

Once the SEM is calculated for a test, the value is added to and subtracted from the child's obtained score. This gives the range of expected scores for that child. This range is known as the *confidence interval*. The SEM corresponds to the standard deviation for the normal curve: 68% of the scores in a normal distribution fell within 1 SD on either side of the mean, 95% of the scores fell within 2 SD on either side of the mean, and 99.7% of the scores fell within 3 SD on either side of the mean. Similarly, a child receives a score within 1 SEM on either side of his or her obtained score 68% of the time, a score within 2 SEM of the obtained score 95% of the time, and a score within 3 SEM of the obtained score 99.7% of the time.

Generally, test manuals report the 95% confidence interval. As you can see by the equation, when the standard deviation of the test is high or the reliability is low, the SEM increases. A larger SEM value means that there is potentially a much larger range of possible scores for an individual child (i.e., a larger confidence interval) and,

consequently, a greater amount of possible error variance for the child's score. This means that an examiner can have less confidence that any score obtained for a child on that test represents the child's true score.

An example may help to illustrate this point. Consider two tests, both consisting of 50 items and both testing the same skill area. One test has a standard deviation of 1.0 and test-retest reliability coefficient of 0.90. The SEM for that test is calculated as follows:

$$SEM = 1\sqrt{1 - 0.90}$$
$$SEM = 0.32$$

The second test has a standard deviation of 5.0 and a test-retest reliability coefficient of .75. The SEM for that test would be calculated as follows:

$$SEM = 5\sqrt{1 - 0.75}$$
$$SEM = 2.5$$

Using the SEM, a 95% confidence interval can be calculated for each test. A 95% confidence interval is 2 *SEM,* so Test 1 has a confidence interval of ±0.64 points from the obtained score, or a total of 1.28 points. Test 2 has a confidence interval of ±5 points, or a total of 10 points. If both Tests 1 and 2 were available for a particular client, an examiner could use Test 1 with much more confidence that the obtained score is truly representative of that individual's abilities and is not caused by random error variance of the test.

Occupational therapists who use standardized tests should be aware of how much measurement error a test contains so that the potential range of performance can be estimated for each individual. Currently, the trend is to report standardized test results as confidence intervals rather than as individual scores (Deitz, 1989). The score tables for the BSID-II include confidence intervals for each index score. "The reporting of confidence intervals also serves as a reminder that the observed score contains some amount of measurement error" (Bayley, 1993, p. 192).

The SEM is especially important to consider when evaluating the differences between two scores (e.g., when evaluating the progress a child has made over time with therapy) (Anastasi, 1988). If the confidence intervals of the two test scores overlap, it may be incorrect to conclude that any change has been made. For instance, a child is tested in September and receives a raw score of 60. The child is tested again in June with the same test and receives a raw score of 75. After comparing the two raw scores, it appears that the child has made substantial progress. However, the scores should be considered in light of an *SEM* of 5.0. Using a 95% confidence interval (the 95% confidence interval is 2 *SEM* on either side of the obtained score), the confidence interval for the first score is from 50 to 70, and the confidence interval of the second score is from 65 to 85.

Based on the two test scores, it cannot be conclusively stated that the child has made progress because the confidence intervals overlap. It is conceivable that a substantial amount of the difference between the first and second scores is a result of an error variance of the test rather than of actual change in the child's abilities. (See Cunningham-Amundson, & Crowe [1993] for a more in-depth discussion of the use of SEM in pediatric assessment, particularly the effect of SEM on interpretation of test scores and qualifying children for remedial services).

Validity

Validity is the extent to which a test measures what it says it measures (Anastasi, 1988). It is important for testers to know that a test of fine-motor development, for instance, actually measures fine-motor skills and not gross-motor or perceptual skills. The validity of a test must be established with reference to the particular use for which the test is being considered (Anastasi, 1988). For instance, the test of fine-motor development is probably highly valid as a measure of fine-motor skills. It is less valid as a measure of visual-motor skills, and has low validity as a measure of gross-motor skills.

Test manuals report information about test validity that has been obtained during the test development process. Additionally, once a test is available commercially, clinicians and researchers continue to evaluate validity and publish the results of their validation studies. This information about test validity can help examiners make decisions about appropriate uses of standardized tests. Four categories of validity: (1) *construct-related validity*, (2) *content-related validity*, (3) *criterion-related validity*, and (4) *rasch analysis are described in the following section.*

Construct-related validity

Construct-related validity refers to the extent to which a test measures a particular theoretic construct. Some constructs frequently measured by pediatric occupational therapists include fine-motor skills, visual-perceptual skills, self-care skills, gross-motor skills, and sensory integration. There are many ways to determine construct validity and only a few are discussed in this chapter.

One method of establishing construct validity is by investigating how well a test discriminates between different groups of individuals. For instance, in a developmental test, such as the BSID-II, the PDMS, and the BOTMP, it is expected that the test differentiates between the performance of older and younger children. Older children should receive higher scores than younger children, providing clear evidence of developmental progression with increasing age. Because these tests are also intended to discriminate normally developing children from children with developmental delays, children in specific diagnostic categories should receive lower scores than children who have no documented deficits.

For example, during the development process of the BSID-II, the performance of children in the following clinical groups was evaluated: premature birth, HIV-positive, prenatal drug exposure, perinatal asphyxia, Down syndrome, autism, developmental delay secondary to medical complications, and chronic otitis media. Performance of children of comparable ages in each of these groups was significantly lower than that of the standardization sample. Therefore the BSID-II was found to discriminate between children in the clinical groups and in the standardization sample, indicating that the BSID-II is able to differentiate the performance of children who have differing ability levels.

A second method of establishing construct validity is by the use of factor analysis. Factor analysis is a statistical procedure for determining relationships between test items. In a test of motor skills that includes gross-motor items and fine-motor items, factor analysis is expected to identify two factors where items showed the strongest correlation: one composed mostly of gross-motor items, and one composed mostly of fine-motor items. The factor analysis of the Sensory Integration and Praxis Tests (SIPT) resulted in identification of four primary factors. The constructs that emerged from the analysis demonstrated that the test primarily measures praxis (motor planning). One construct measures visual-perceptual skills (related to praxis); one somatosensory-praxis skills; one, bilateral integration and sequencing of movements; and one, praxis on verbal command (Ayres & Marr, 1991). The factor analysis helped establish what functions are measured by the SIPT and can be used to interpret the results of testing individual children.

The third method of establishing construct-related validity is by repeated administration of a test before and after a period of intervention. For example, a group of children is given a test of visual-perceptual skills and then receives intervention focused on improving their visual-perceptual skills. They are then retested using the same test to determine if test scores improve. An increase in test scores supports the assertion that the test measured visual perceptual skills and provides evidence for construct-related validity.

Content-related validity

Content-related validity is the extent to which the items on a test accurately sample a particular behavior domain. For instance, to test self-care skills, it is impractical to ask a child to perform every conceivable self-care activity. A sample of self-care activities must be chosen to be included on the test, and conclusions then can be drawn about the child's abilities on the basis of the selected items. Examiners must have confidence that self-care skills are adequately represented so that accurate conclusions regarding the child's self-care skills can be made. Test manuals should show evidence that the authors have systematically analyzed the domain that is being tested. Content validity is established by review of the test content by experts in the field who reach some agreement that the content is, in fact, representative of the behavioral domain to be measured.

Criterion-related validity

Criterion-related validity refers to the ability of a test to predict how an individual performs on other measurements or activities. To establish criterion-related validity, the test score is checked against a criterion, an independent measure of what the test is designed to predict. The two forms of criterion-related validity are (1) *concurrent validity* and (2) *predictive validity*.

Concurrent validity describes how well test scores reflect present performance. The degree of the relationship between concurrent validity and predictive validity, which describes how well test scores predict future performance, is described with a correlation coefficient. Most validity correlation coefficients range from 0.40 to 0.80; a coefficient of 0.70 or above indicates that performance on one test can predict performance on a second test.

How is concurrent validity assessed? Concurrent validity is examined in the test-development process to determine the relationship between a new test and existing tests that test a similar construct. For instance, during the development of the original PDMS, children were tested with both the PDMS and the BSID (Bayley, 1969). The scores on the two tests were compared. Portions of the concurrent validity data are reproduced (Table 8-3).

As Table 8-3 shows, there are some areas of moderate-to-high correlation and one area of low correlation between the two tests. The BSID Mental Scale, which as-

sesses a broad range of mental functions that include receptive and expressive language, problem solving, and attention, also includes a number of items involving fine-motor skills, visual-perceptual skills, and visual-motor skills. Not surprisingly, it has almost no relationship with the PDMS Gross Motor Scale, which assesses an entirely different developmental area. However, the BSID Mental Scale correlates highly with the PDMS Fine Motor Scale, which is composed of fine-motor items. The BSID Psychomotor Scale, which is composed of both gross-motor and fine-motor items, has moderate correlation with the PDMS Gross Motor and Fine Motor Scales. This pattern of correlation coefficients is an expected finding when comparing the two tests, and it supports the concurrent validity of the PDMS as a measure of gross-motor and fine-motor skills.

In contrast to concurrent validity, predictive validity identifies the relationship between a test given in the present and some measure of performance in the future. Establishing predictive validity is a much lengthier process than other forms of validity because several years must often elapse between the first and second testing sessions. Often, the predictive validity of a test is not well documented until it has been in use for several years.

An area of interest to many pediatric occupational therapists working in early intervention has been the ability of developmental tests to predict which infants and young children, who are identified as "high-risk" because of premature birth or perinatal medical complications, will have cerebral palsy or other developmental disabilities as they become older. Predicting outcomes necessitates testing the children as infants and then testing their developmental, physical, or cognitive status several months or years later. The second testing can use the same test if the child is still within the intended age range of that test, or another test that presumably tests the same construct as the first test (but is appropriate for the child's current age) may be used. When infants are born prematurely, corrected, or adjusted, ages should be used until 2 years of age (see Box 8-1 on adjusting age for prematurity).

Palisano (1986) investigated the predictive validity of the PDMS and the BSID for full-term and premature infants who were given both tests at 12, 15, and 18 months. He found that scores obtained for either test at 12 months did not predict 18-month scores (i.e., the correlation between scores was low). Palisano concluded that the BSID and PDMS can only be used to describe current developmental status and should not be used for predictive purposes. Therefore an infant who achieves a low score on either of these tests will not necessarily go on to have developmental delays. In contrast, BSID scores obtained at 12 months of age for infants with biologic risk factors correlated with verbal and motor performance at 4½ years of age (Crowe, Deitz, & Bennett, 1987). Also, 6-month

table 8-3	**Correlation Coefficients Between the Peabody Developmental Motor Scales and the Bayley Scales of Infant Development**	
	Bayley Mental Scale	**Bayley Motor Scale**
Peabody Gross Motor Scale	−0.03	0.37
Peabody Fine Motor Scale	0.78	0.36

Modified from Folio, M.R., & Fewell, R.R. (1983). *Peabody Developmental Motor Scales and Activity Cards* (p. 118). Austin, TX: Pro Ed.

BSID Mental Scale scores for infants at risk because of environmental deprivation predicted Stanford-Binet IQ at 24 and 48 months for children who did not receive intervention (Farran & Harber, 1989). Thus the question of predictive validity of early developmental assessments for children at biologic or environmental risk remains unresolved. Therapists should conduct repeated testings when the child is at risk for developmental delays.

One final point about criterion-related validity: The meaningfulness of the comparison between a test and its criterion measure depends on both the quality of the test and the quality of the criterion. In the example of concurrent validity previously cited, the comparison of the PDMS and the BSID rests on the assumption that the BSID is an adequate measure of the criteria of gross- and fine-motor development. If the BSID was found to measure these criteria inaccurately, the validity of the PDMS would also be in question. Because no measure of criterion-related validity provides conclusive evidence of the test's validity, multiple investigations should be undertaken. Important developmental assessments, such as the BSID, undergo extensive evaluation of validity after publication. The resulting information helps the test user decide when and with whom the test results are most valid.

In summary, validity is an important but sometimes elusive concept that rests on a number of judgments by authors of the tests, users of the tests, and experts in the field occupational therapy. It is important to remember that validity is not an absolute, and that a test that is valid in one setting or with one group of children may not be valid for other uses. Test users must not assume that because a test has been developed and published for commercial distribution, it is universally useful and appropriate. An examiner must apply his or her clinical knowledge and experience, knowledge of normal and abnormal development, and understanding of an individual child's situation when deciding whether a test is a valid measure of the child's abilities.

Rasch analysis: an emerging model of test development

The Rasch models of measurement (Andrich, 1988) have been used to develop item scaling for several tests developed recently in the field of occupational therapy. The SFA, the PEDI, and the Assessment of Motor and Process Skills (Fisher, 1997) have used Rasch methodology in the test-development process. A test instrument developed using Rasch methodology must meet several assumptions (Coster et. al., 1998). The construct being measured (e.g., self-help skills) can be represented as a continuous function with measurement covering the full range of possible performance from dependent to independent. The instrument (or individual scale of the instrument) measures one characteristic (or construct) of performance, and each item represents a sample of the characteristics being measured. The scale provides estimates of item difficulty that are independent of the sample of persons tested, and an individual's ability estimate is independent of the specific items tested.

The Rasch model generates a hierarchical ranking of items on the test from easiest to most difficult, creating a linear scale of items from ordinal observations. With the items ranked along the continuum within each skill area, an individual's performance can be compared to an item's difficulty, rather than against a normative sample. The ranking of items creates an expected pattern of mastery of items; the model predicts that mastery of more difficult items on the continuum will occur only after easier items are mastered. Therefore therapists using an assessment tool developed using Rasch methodology can generally assume that the most appropriate goals for intervention will be the items and/or skills immediately above the items successfully passed by the client.

Tests developed using the Rasch model are not considered norm-referenced because individual performance is not compared against that of a normative sample. However, the Rasch model provides an objective measure of performance that can be linked directly to desired functional outcomes. The Rasch model has been applied to a variety of rating scales and traditional measurement instruments to assess disablement and functional status (Grimby et. al., 1996; Roth, et. al., 1998). It shows promise as a model that can be used alone or in conjunction with traditional test development and measurement theory to produce measurement tools that provide a clearer connection between the assessment process and intervention planning.

■ BECOMING A COMPETENT USER

The amount of technical information presented here might make the prospect of learning to administer a standardized test seem daunting. However, potential examiners can take a number of specific steps to ensure that they will be able to administer and reliably score a test. These steps will also help examiners to interpret test results accurately so that they provide a valid representation of each child's abilities. This section discusses what is necessary to learn to administer and interpret any standardized test, whether it is a screening tool or a comprehensive assessment.

Decide which Test to Learn

The first step is to decide which test, or tests, to learn. A number of standardized tests used by pediatric occupational therapists address a wide age span and a number of different performance components and performance areas. A potential examiner must decide which tests will most likely meet the assessment needs for his or her particular work setting. For instance, an occupational therapist working in an early intervention setting might use the BSID-II or the Alberta Infant Motor Scale (AIMS) (Piper, 1998). A therapist working in preschools might use the MAP (Miller, 1982) or the PDMS. A therapist working in a school-based setting might use the BOTMP. Selected pediatric standardized assessments are summarized below (Table 8-4).

A number of other standardized tests are available that assess more specialized areas of function, such as the SIPT (Ayres, 1989), the Developmental Test of Visual-

Motor Integration (Beery, 1997), or the DTVP-II (Hammill, et. al., 1993). Potential examiners should consult with other therapists working in their practice settings to determine which tests are most commonly used. In addition, they should examine the characteristics of the children referred to them for assessment to determine which tests are most appropriate.

Study Test Manual

Once a decision is made about which test to learn, the therapist should thoroughly read the test manual. In addition to becoming familiar with administration and scor-

table 8-4 Summary of Selected General Pediatric Standardized Tests

Test Name	Age Range	Domains Tested	Standard Scores Used	Time to Administer
Bayley Scales of Infant Development—II	1 to 42 months	Mental scale: cognitive, language and personal-social. Psychomotor scale: gross-motor skills, fine-motor skills, quality of movement, sensory integration, perceptual-motor integration. Behavior rating scale: social interactions, orientation toward environment and objects, interests, activity level, and need for stimulation	Developmental index scores. Percentile-rank scores. Developmental age-equivalent scores	25 to 60 minutes, depending on child's age
Peabody Developmental Motor Scales-II	1 to 84 months	Gross-motor scale: reflexes, balance, locomotor, nonlocomotor, receipt, and propulsion. Fine-motor scale: grasping, hand use, eye-hand coordination, manual dexterity	Percentile-rank scores. Z-scores. T-scores. Age-equivalent scores. Developmental motor quotient scores. Scaled scores	45 to 60 minutes for total test; 20 to 30 minutes for each scale
Bruininks-Oseretsky Test of Motor Proficiency	4½ to 14½ years	Gross-motor subtest: running speed and agility, balance, bilateral coordination, strength, and upper-limb coordination. Fine-motor subtest: response speed, visual-motor control, upper limb speed, and dexterity	Subtest and total test. Standard score. Percentile-rank score. Stanine score. Age-equivalent scores	45 to 60 minutes for long form; 15 to 20 minutes for short form
Pediatric Evaluation of Disability Inventory	6 months to 7 years	Social function, self-care, mobility. Each domain is scored in each of the following areas: functional skills, caregiver assistance, and modifications	Normative standard score. Scaled score	45 to 60 minutes when scoring by parent report
School Function Assessment	Grades K to 6	Participation, Task Supports (divided into 5 assistance and 5 adaptations scales), and Activity Performance, which is divided into physical tasks (12 scales) and cognitive and/or behavioral tasks (9 scales)	Criterion scores for each scale; cut-off scores identified for K to 3 and 4 to 6 grade levels for each scale	Varies; can be completed by one or more respondents. Total time 1½ to 2 hours; 5 to 10 minutes per scale

ing techniques, the technical attributes of the test should be studied. Particular attention should be paid to the size and composition of the normative sample, the reliability coefficients, the validation data, and the intended population for the test. What are the standardized administration procedures, and can they be altered for children with special needs? How should the scores be reported and interpreted if the standardized procedure is changed?

It may also be appropriate to consult other sources for information about a test. *The Twelfth Mental Measurements Yearbook* (Conoley & Impara 1995), or *Tests in Print IV* (Murphy, Impara, & Conoley, 1994) publish descriptions and critical reviews of commercially available standardized tests written by testing experts. In addition, published studies of validity or reliability of tests relevant to pediatric occupational therapists appear throughout the occupational therapy literature.

Observe the Test Being Administered

The next step in learning a test is to observe it being administered by an experienced examiner. If possible, the therapist should also discuss administration, scoring, and interpretation of the test results. One observation may suffice; however, it may be helpful to see several administrations of the test given to children of different ages and abilities. Observation provides an excellent way to see how other examiners manage the practical aspects of testing, such as arrangement of test materials, sequencing of test items, handling unexpected occur-

rences, and managing behavior. A discussion with the examiner regarding how a child's performance is interpreted can also be extremely helpful in understanding how observed behaviors are translated into conclusions and recommendations.

Practice Administering the Test

Once these preparatory activities are completed, the learner should practice administering the test. Neighborhood children, friends, or relatives can be recruited to be "pilot subjects." It is a good idea to test several children who are of similar ages to those with whom the test will be used. Testing children, rather than adults, provides the realism of the mechanical, behavioral, and management issues that will be faced with a clinical population (Figure 8-6).

Have an Observer Check Interrater Reliability

When possible, an experienced examiner should observe the testing and simultaneously score the items as a check of interrater reliability. A simple way to assess interrater agreement is by the use of *point-by-point agreement* (Kazdin, 1982). Using this technique, one examiner administers and scores the test while the other observes and scores. The two examiners then compare their scores on each item (Figure 8-7). The number of items on which the examiners agreed on the score is calculated.

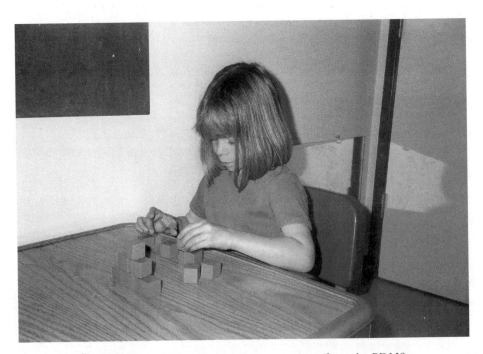

figure**8-6** A child performs a fine-motor item from the PDMS.

The interrater agreement is then computed using the following formula:

$$\text{Point-by-point agreement} = \frac{A}{A + D} \times 100$$

In the formula above, A equals the number of items where there was agreement and D equals the number of items where there was disagreement.

The following is an example of point-by-point agreement: Two examiners score a test of 10 items. The child receives either a pass ($+$) or fail ($-$) for each item. Scores for each examiner are shown (Table 8-5). According to Table 8-5, the raters agreed on 7 of the 10 items. They disagreed on items 2, 7, and 9.

Their point-by-point agreement would be calculated as follows:

$$\frac{7}{(7 + 3)} = 0.70 \times 100 = 70\% \text{ point-by-point agreement}$$

This means that they agreed on the scores for 70% of the items. To benefit from this exercise, the two examiners should discuss the items on which they disagreed and their reasons for giving the scores that they did. A new examiner may not understand the scoring criteria and may be making scoring errors as a result. The experienced examiner can help clarify scoring criteria. This procedure helps bring the new examiner's administration and scoring techniques in line with the standardized procedures.

The point-by-point agreement technique can also be used for periodic reliability checks by experienced examiners, and it is particularly important if the examiners may be testing the same children at different times. What is a minimum acceptable level for point-by-point agreement? No universally agreed-on standard exists. However, 80% is probably a good guideline for the minimum acceptable agreement. Examiners would be well advised to aim for agreement in the range of 90%, if possible. Organization of the testing environment and the materials can improve reliability by creating a standard structured environment.

table 8-5	Rater's Scores for Point-by-Point Agreement	
Item	Rater 1	Rater 2
1	+	+
2	+	−
3	+	+
4	−	−
5	−	−
6	+	+
7	−	+
8	−	−
9	−	+
10	+	+

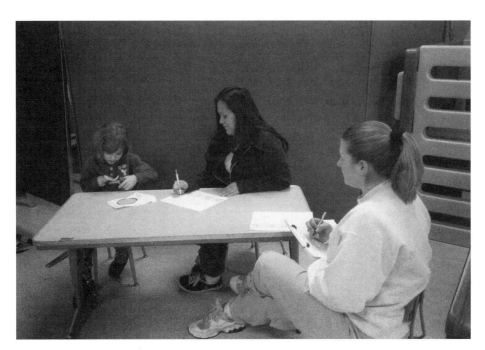

figure 8-7   Two therapists check their interrater reliability by scoring the same testing session.

Selecting and Preparing an Optimal Testing Environment

The testing environment should meet the specifications stated in the test manual. Generally, the manual specifies a well-lighted room free of visual or auditory distractions. If a separate room is not available, a screen or room divider can be used to partition off a corner of the room. Below you'll find an example of appropriate test set-up (Figure 8-8).

Testing should be scheduled at a time when the child is able to perform optimally. For young children, caregivers should be consulted about the best time of day for testing so that the test session does not interfere with naps or feedings. Older children's school or other activities should be considered when scheduling assessments. For instance, a child who has just come from recess or a vigorous physical education session may have decreased endurance for gross-motor activities.

The test environment should be ready before the child arrives. Furniture should be appropriately sized so that children sitting at a table can rest their feet flat on the floor and can comfortably access items on the table. If a child uses a wheelchair or other adaptive seating, he or she should be allowed to sit in the equipment during testing. Infants or young children are generally best seated on the caregiver's lap, unless particular items on the test specify otherwise. The examiner should place the test kit where he or she can easily access the items but not

where the child can see it or get into it. Often a low chair placed next to the examiner's chair is a good place to locate a test kit.

Each examiner should consider what adaptations are necessary to administer the test efficiently. In many cases a test manual is too large and unwieldy to have at hand during testing, and the score sheet does not provide enough information about administration and scoring criteria. Examiners have developed many ways to accommodate this need. One common method is a cue card, on which the examiner records specific criteria for administration and scoring, including the instructions to be read to the child. This can be accomplished by making a series of note cards, putting color codes on a score sheet, or developing a score sheet with administration information (see Hinderer, Richardson, and Atwater [1989]).

Item Administration

Most importantly, the examiner has to be familiar enough with the test that attention can be focused on the child's behavior, not on the mechanics of administering the test. This is a critical part of preparation because much valuable information can be lost if the examiner is not able to observe carefully the quality of the child's responses, he or she must instead devote energy to finding test materials or looking through the test manual. Additionally, young children's attention spans can be short,

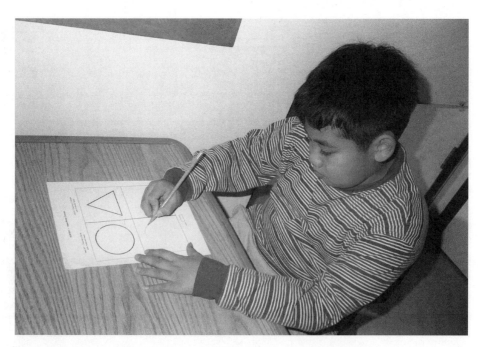

figure 8-8   A child completes a portion of the visual-motor subtest of the Bruininsky-Oseretsky Test of Motor Proficiency.

and the examiner must be able to take full advantage of the limited time that the child is able to attend to the activities.

Familiarity with the test also allows the examiner to change the pace of activities, if necessary. It also allows the examiner to give the child a brief break to play, have a snack, or use the bathroom, while the examiner interviews the caregiver or jots down notes. Most standardized tests have some flexibility about the order or arrangement of item sets, and an examiner who knows the test can use this to his or her advantage. Sometimes, because of the child's fatigue, behavior, or time constraints, it is impossible to administer a test completely in one session. Most tests provide guidelines about how the test can be administered in two sessions, and examiners should be familiar with these guidelines before starting to test.

Evaluate Clinical Usefulness

The final area of preparation is to evaluate the clinical usefulness of the test. Discuss the test with colleagues: What are its strengths and weaknesses? What important information does it give? What information needs to be collected through other techniques? For which children does it seem to work especially well or especially poorly? Can it be adapted for children with special needs? Does it measure what it says it measures? Are there other tests that do a better job of measuring the same behavioral domain? Is it helpful for program planning or program evaluation? An ongoing dialogue is an important way to ensure that the process of standardized testing meets the needs of the children, families, therapists, and service agencies that make use of the tests. The steps to becoming a competent user of standardized tests are summarized (Box 8-2).

---

box 8-2 *Steps to becoming a competent test user*

1. Study the test manual.
2. Observe experienced examiners; discuss observations.
3. Practice using the test.
4. Check interrater agreement with experienced examiner.
5. Prepare administration and scoring cue sheets.
6. Prepare the testing environment.
7. Consult with experienced examiners about test interpretation.
8. Periodically recheck interrater agreement.

■ ETHICAL CONSIDERATIONS IN TESTING

All pediatric occupational therapists who use standardized tests in their practice must be aware of the responsibilities they have to the children they evaluate and their families. Anastasi (1988) found several ethical issues are relevant to standardized testing. These include (1) *examiner competency,* (2) *subject privacy,* (3) *communicating test results,* and (4) *cultural bias.*

Examiner Competency

The first ethical issue is that of examiner competency. This has been discussed in detail in the previous section, but it is important to reemphasize here that examiners need to achieve a minimal level of competency with a test before using it in practice. Along with knowing how to administer and score a test, a competent examiner should know who the test should be used with and for what purpose. This also means knowing when it is *not* appropriate to use a particular standardized instrument. The examiner should be able to evaluate the technical merits of the test and know how these characteristics may affect the administration and interpretation of the test. The examiner should also be aware of the many things that can affect a child's performance on a test, including factors such as hunger, fatigue, illness, or distractions, as well as sources of test or examiner error.

Finally, the competent examiner draws conclusions about a child's performance on a standardized test only after considering all available information about the child. This can include nonstandardized testing, informal observations, caregiver interviews, and reviews of documentation from other professionals. It is extremely important to put a child's observed performance on standardized testing within the context of all sources of information about the child. This provides a more accurate and meaningful interpretation of standard scores.

Subject Privacy

The second ethical issue is the protection of subject privacy. Informed consent must be obtained from the child's legal guardian before testing is initiated. Agencies have different guidelines regarding how consent is obtained, and examiners should be aware of the guidelines for their particular institution. Informed consent is generally obtained in writing and consists of an explanation of the reasons for testing, the types of tests that will be used, the intended use of the tests and their consequences (refers to program placement or qualification for remedial services), and what testing information will be released and to whom it will be released. Caregivers should be given a copy of the summary report and should be informed about whom will receive the additional copies.

Verbal exchanges about the child should be limited. Although it is often necessary to discuss a case with a colleague for the purposes of information sharing and consultation, it is not acceptable to have a casual conversation about a particular child in the elevator, lunchroom, or hallway. If others overhear the conversation, this could result in a violation of confidentiality.

Communicating Test Results

The third ethical issue is that of communicating test results. Reports should be written in a manner that is understandable to a nonprofessional, with a minimum of jargon. Each report should be objective in tone, and the conclusions and recommendations should be clearly stated. When discussing the results of testing, the characteristics of the recipient should be taken into account.

Different communication techniques are needed for speaking to other professionals and for speaking to family members. When sharing assessment results with family members, the examiner should be aware of the general level of education and, in the case of bilingual families, the level of proficiency with English. Even when family members have some fluency with the English language, it may be a good idea to have an interpreter available. Often the family members who are most skilled in English will act as an interpreter. This may not be an optimal arrangement for sessions where test results are being discussed because of the technical nature of some of the information. An ideal interpreter is one who is familiar with the agency, the kinds of testing and services it offers, and techniques for helping the examiner offer information in an understandable and culturally meaningful way.

When presenting information to family members, examiners must also consider the anticipated emotional response. A parent who hears that his young child has developmental delays may be emotionally devastated. Therefore the information should be sensitively communicated. Every child has strengths and attributes that can be highlighted when discussing overall performance. The examiner should also avoid any appearance of placing blame on the parent for the child's difficulties, because many parents are quick to blame themselves for their child's problems. The tone of any discussion should be objective, yet positive, with the emphasis placed on sharing information and making joint decisions about a plan of action.

Cultural Bias

The final ethical issue relates to cultural bias. In recent years there has been a great deal of criticism about cultural bias in standardized tests. These criticisms raise many important points about the validity of tests developed primarily on a white, middle-class population, when they are used with children from different cultural backgrounds. It is important for examiners to be aware of the factors that may influence how children from diverse cultures perform on standardized tests.

First, children who do not have experience with testing may not understand the unspoken rules about test taking. They may not understand the importance of doing a task within a time limit or following the examiner's instructions. They may not be motivated to perform well on tasks because the task itself has no intrinsic meaning to them. The materials or activities may be seen as irrelevant or, having had no experience with the kinds of materials used in the tests, they may not know how to interact with the materials. Establishing rapport may be difficult either because of language barriers or because there is a cultural mismatch between the social interaction patterns of the child and the examiner. If the examiner is aware of these potential problems, some steps can be taken to minimize possible difficulties.

The caregiver or an interpreter can be present to help the child feel more at ease. The caregiver can be questioned regarding the child's familiarity with the various test materials. This can give the examiner some information about whether the child's failure to perform individual items is caused by unfamiliarity with the materials or by inability to complete the task. The caregiver can also be shown how to administer some items, particularly those involving physical contact or close proximity to the child. This may make the situation less threatening for the child. However, if these adjustments are made, standard procedure has been violated and it may be inappropriate to compute a standard score. Even so, the test can provide a wealth of descriptive information about the child's abilities.

Clearly, occupational therapists must possess a number of skills beyond the ability to simply administer test items when using standardized tests. Professional communication skills are essential when administering tests and reporting information. Awareness of family and cultural values helps to put the child's performance within a contextual framework. An understanding of the professional and ethical responsibilities involved in dealing with sensitive and confidential information is also extremely important. A competent examiner brings all of these skills into play when administering, scoring, interpreting, and reporting the results of standardized tests.

■ ADVANTAGES AND DISADVANTAGES OF STANDARDIZED TESTING

Standardized tests have permitted occupational therapists and other professionals to develop a more scientific approach to assessment. The use of tests that give statistically valid numeric scores has helped give more credibility to the assessment process. However, standardized tests are not without their drawbacks. The following section discusses the advantages and disadvantages of using standardized tests, along with suggestions concerning how to make test results more accurate and meaningful.

Advantages

Standardized tests possess several characteristics that make them a unique part of the assessment inventory of pediatric occupational therapists. First, they are tests that are, in general, well known and commercially available. This means that a child's scores on a particular test can be interpreted and understood by therapists in other practice settings or geographic locations.

Standard scores generated by standardized tests allow testers from a variety of professional disciplines to "speak the same language" when it comes to discussing test scores. For instance, a child is tested by an occupational therapist for fine-motor skills, a physical therapist for gross-motor skills, and a speech pathologist for language skills. All three tests express scores as T-scores. An average T-score is 50. The child receives a fine-motor T-score of 30, a gross-motor T-score of 25, and a language T-score of 60. It is apparent that although this child is below average in both gross- and fine-motor skills, language skills are an area of strength; in fact, they are above average. These scores can be compared and discussed by the assessment team, and they can be used to identify areas requiring intervention and areas in which the child has particular strengths.

Standardized tests can be used to monitor developmental progress. Because they are norm-referenced according to age, the progress of a child with developmental delays can be measured against expected developmental progress as compared with the normative sample. In this way, occupational therapists can determine if children receiving therapy are accelerating their rate of development because of intervention. Similarly, children who are being monitored after being discharged from therapy can be assessed periodically to determine if they are maintaining the expected rate of developmental progress or if they are beginning to fall behind their peers without the assistance of intervention.

Disadvantages

Standardized tests have been criticized for giving therapists a false sense of accountability and security (Royeen, 1992). Much of the criticism centers on using standardized tests as a substitute for functional performance assessments. Additionally, the 1997 amendments to the Individuals with Disabilities Education Act (IDEA) place a greater emphasis on functional assessments than did the original legislation, and the standard scores obtained from norm-referenced tests do not assist in developing functional goals (Clark & Coster, 1998).

Because most standardized tests assess performance components (e.g., balance, bilateral coordination, and visual-motor skills) rather than occupational performance areas (e.g., play, activities of daily living, and educational or prevocational activities), the intervention goals that are generated because of standardized assessment frequently address these performance components instead of the child's functional performance within the environmental context. As a result, occupational therapy intervention may not adequately address a child's occupational performance in a meaningful way.

Stewart (Chapter 7) discusses the importance of placing standardized testing within the child's performance context. A standardized test cannot stand alone as a measure of a child's abilities. Clinical judgment, informal or unstructured observation, caregiver interview, and data gathering from other informants are all essential parts of the assessment process. These less-structured evaluation procedures are needed to provide meaning and interpretation to the numeric scores obtained by standardized testing.

There are several other considerations that testers must take into account when using standardized tests. First, a test session provides only a brief "snapshot" of a child's behavior and abilities. The performance that a therapist sees in a 1-hour assessment in a clinic setting may be different from that seen on a daily basis at home or at school. Illness, fatigue, anxiety, or lack of familiarity with the test materials, the room, or the tester, can adversely affect a child's performance. The tester must be sensitive to the possible impact of these factors on the child's performance.

A competent tester can do a great deal to alleviate a child's anxiety about testing and to ensure that the experience is not an unpleasant one. However, any test situation is artificial and usually does not provide an accurate indication of how the child performs on a daily basis. Therefore it is important for the therapist to speak to the child's parent, caregiver, or teacher at the time of testing to determine if the observed behavior is truly representative of the child's typical performance. The representativeness of the behavior must then be taken into account in interpreting and reporting the child's test scores.

Another concern about standardized tests is the rigidity of the testing procedures themselves. Standardized tests specify both particular ways of administering test items and, in many cases, exactly what instructions the tester must give. Children with problems as diverse as hearing impairment, attention deficit, muscle weakness, or lack of coordination may not have an opportunity to perform optimally given these administration requirements. Many therapists believe that the standard score obtained by a standardized test administration is strongly affected by the child's particular deficits and does not accurately reflect the child's true abilities.

Although this issue is not addressed by all standardized tests, some tests provide guidelines to use when attempting to administer the test under nonstandard conditions. For example, the PDMS provides case illustrations of how the test can be adapted for testing children with vision impairment and cerebral palsy. This provides testers with some guidance in the use of the test when special accommodations may need to be made. The BSID-II provides normative data for several clinical groups. Piper and Darrah, in developing the AIMS, used infants who were preterm or born with congenital anomalies as well as those who were full-term and without any diagnosis.

It is important to reiterate that although it is permissible to alter the administration procedures of most tests to accommodate children's individual needs, the child's performance cannot be expressed as a standard score. Rather, the purpose of the testing is to provide a structured format for describing the child's performance. The test manual should always be consulted for guidelines related to alterations in test procedures.

Three standardized tests are available that have been developed specifically for use with children who have physical disabilities: the PEDI (Haley et. al., 1992), the Gross Motor Function Measure (GMFM) (Russell et. al., 1990), and the SFA (Coster et. al., 1998). A unique characteristic of the PEDI is that it measures the amount of caregiver assistance and environmental modifications required for children to perform specific functional tasks. This provides a way to assess the level of independence and the quality of performance for children whose disabilities may prevent them from ever executing a particular task normally. The GMFM is a criterion-referenced test that measures the components of a gross-motor activity that a child with cerebral palsy can accomplish. It is meant to provide information necessary for designing therapy programs and measuring small increments of change. The SFA is a criterion-referenced test that is to be used with children who have a variety of disabling conditions. Unlike most pediatric tests that assess performance components, the SFA approaches assessment from a top-down approach. It evaluates the child's performance of occupational roles within the daily context; in this case the performance of functional tasks that support participation in the academic and social aspects of an elementary school program. These tests are among a new wave of tests designed by and for occupational and physical therapists, and they show promise in addressing the specific assessment and program-planning needs of pediatric therapists.

Case Study
Background information

Caitlin is a 5½-year-old kindergarten student referred for occupational therapy assessment by her teacher, Mrs. Clark. Mrs. Clark notes that Caitlin appears to be having a great deal of difficulty in learning to write; she holds her pencil awkwardly and either exerts too much or not enough pressure on the paper. She complains of fatigue during writing and coloring activities. On the playground and in physical education (PE) classes she has difficulty keeping up with the rest of the class. She falls frequently, appears uncoordinated, and has difficulty learning new motor skills. On several occasions she has complained of minor ailments; Mrs. Clark believes that she does this to avoid participating in PE. Mrs. Clark would like to know whether there are any underlying problems that may be causing Caitlin's school difficulties and if any special help is needed.

Debra received the occupational therapy referral. She spoke to Caitlin's parents before initiating her assessment and obtained additional information. She discovered that Caitlin received physical therapy briefly as an infant because of low muscle tone and slow achievement of developmental milestones. Although she appeared to make good progress in therapy, she continued to lag behind her peers. Her parents were particularly worried about Caitlin's ability to cope with the increased written requirements of first grade and how other children would accept her if she continued to struggle in school. They did not have much free time but were willing to consider some home activities to help Caitlin develop additional skills. They declined Debra's offer for them to be present at the testing session, citing concerns about Caitlin's behavior when they were present. However, they asked to meet with Debra after Caitlin's evaluation.

Debra considered Caitlin's age (5½ years) and the areas of concern expressed by Mrs. Clark and Caitlin's parents (gross- and fine-motor skills and social adjustment) in choosing which standardized test to use. She decided to administer the PDMS, along with clinical observations of Caitlin's posture, muscle tone, strength, balance, motor planning, hand use and hand preference, attention, problem-solving skills, and visual skills. She also asked Caitlin's teacher to complete the School Function Assessment (SFA) to provide information on performance of functional school-related behaviors.

Test results

Caitlin came enthusiastically to the testing session, which was scheduled at a midmorning to avoid possible effects of fatigue or hunger. She attended well, although she needed encouragement for the more challenging items. By the end of the session she complained of fatigue, but Debra believed she was able to get a representative sample of Caitlin's motor skills and that the scores obtained were reliable.

On the PDMS Caitlin received a total gross-motor raw score of 313, placing her in the 13th percentile for her age. Her total fine-motor raw score was 205, placing her at the 5th percentile. These scores translate into Z-scores of -1.13 for gross motor and -1.64 for fine motor. In the gross motor area, ball skills were an area of relative strength for Caitlin, but she had difficulty with balance activities and activities involving hopping, skipping, and jumping. In the fine-motor area, Caitlin used a static tripod grasp on the pencil, frequently shifting into a fisted grasp if the writing task was challenging. Based on the small number of visual-motor items on this test, visual-perceptual skills appeared to be an area of strength, whereas tasks involving speed and dexterity were particularly difficult.

Debra found that Caitlin had low muscle tone overall, particularly in the shoulder girdle and hands, and strength was somewhat decreased overall. Caitlin's endurance was poor; for many tasks she performed well initially, but her performance deteriorated as she continued. Motor planning difficulties were evident in the way she handled test materials and moved about the environment. She had difficulty devising alternate ways to accomplish tasks that were challenging for her and required Debra's manual guidance to complete some tasks. She became frustrated to the point of tears on two occasions, and she needed encouragement to continue when this occurred.

Debra obtained a functional profile on the SFA based on Mrs. Clark's responses to the items on the test. On the scales of recreational movement, using materials, clothing management, written work and task behavior and/or completion Caitlin received scores below the cutoff for her grade level. Other scales were within grade-level expectations, with strengths in the scales of memory and understanding, following social conventions, and personal-care awareness.

Observations and recommendations

According to her scores on the PDMS, Caitlin had mild delays in her gross-motor skills and mild to moderate delays in her fine-motor skills. Although Debra believed that the PDMS gave a good indication of what Caitlin could do under optimal circumstances (i.e., a nondistracting environment, individual attention and encouragement, and structuring of tasks to maximize success and minimize frustration), she also thought it did not represent the level of performance that would be seen over the course of a typical day.

She observed Caitlin in her classroom and discovered that Caitlin avoided fine-motor and gross-motor activities whenever possible and completed writing and drawing activities rapidly, resulting in poor quality of the end-product. She was near tears after experiencing frustration with her attempts at an art activity. SFA results indicated that her performance of tasks involving fine- and gross-motor coordination and task organization was below grade-level expectations.

In Caitlin's school district, a child did not qualify for special education or related services unless scores in two or more developmental domains were below a Z-score of -1.5. In Caitlin's case only one Z-score (fine-motor) was below this level. Because both Debra and Mrs. Clark felt strongly that Caitlin would not be successful without intervention, they met with the school psychologist, the school principal, and Caitlin's parents to determine a plan of action. The SFA was used to facilitate collaborative problem solving by helping to identify which specific areas of school function could be targeted in the classroom, and which skills should be identified as functional outcomes.

The team determined that Debra would provide recommendations to Mrs. Clark about classroom modifications and activities that would increase Caitlin's success and build her motor skills. The team members also collaborated to design strategies and routines that could be used at school and at home to improve Caitlin's on-task behavior and ability to manage daily tasks at school.

Debra provided a pencil gripper and a chair that fit Caitlin better and provided better positioning for writing. She provided Mrs. Clark with ideas for appropriate activities and ways of teaching Caitlin new motor skills. Debra provided Caitlin's parents with suggestions for family-oriented activities that would improve general strength and endurance (e.g., bicycle riding and swimming) and provided specific ideas for ways they could build Caitlin's fine-motor skills at home. She also agreed to be available to Mrs. Clark for periodic informal consultation. It was agreed that a reassessment would be scheduled at the end of the school year so that the team could make a decision about further intervention and program planning for next school year.

Summary

Standardized testing, specifically the PDMS and SFA, provided a helpful framework for Debra's assessment of Caitlin and gave specific information about areas of strength and difficulty. In this case Caitlin did not qualify for occupational therapy intervention because her standard scores did not satisfy the school's eligibility criteria.

Debra made use of her clinical observations and information gathering from a variety of sources to make a decision about what type of intervention was both necessary and feasible, given the constraints of the school district regulations. Clearly, if she had simply relied on standardized test scores, she would not have developed the breadth of knowledge that led to her decision-making process about intervention options. This example illustrates the important roles of both standardized testing and other methods of data collection in arriving at meaningful and realistic conclusions about children's intervention needs and modes of service delivery.

STUDY QUESTIONS

1. For what testing purposes is a criterion-referenced test preferred? A norm-referenced test?

2. Brandon, who is 2 years old, is being evaluated using a standardized test. He refuses to attempt several items, throws test materials, and repeatedly tries to leave the test area. Brandon's mother states that this behavior is not typical, and that she knows that he is able to do many of the tasks that were presented to him. What statement can be made about the reliability of the test results? What strategies might be used to maximize the quantity and quality of information obtained during the test session?

3. Carmen, who is 9 years old, is scheduled for her periodic, formal school reassessment. Previous testing was done when Carmen was 6, using the PDMS. Now that Carmen is beyond the age range of the PDMS, what tests can be used and how can the scores from these tests be compared with her previous test scores?

4. Jared, who is 7 years old, is given a standardized test and receives a raw score of 83. Therapy services are then provided to Jared for 6 months. On reevaluation he receives a score of 98 on the same standardized test. The SEM of the test is 4.0. Using the 95% confidence interval, what is the potential range of scores for Jared for each testing? What can be concluded about the effect of the therapy he has been given?

5. A therapist has just purchased a newly published test of visual-motor skills and is interested in how a child's performance on this test will relate to his or her handwriting skills. What information would the therapist look for in the test manual to answer this question?

6. A therapist is learning to administer a standardized test. He or she checks the interrater agreement on the test with another therapist who frequently uses the test. Their point-by-point agreement on the test is 65%. What strategies can they use to improve interrater agreement, and what level of agreement should they aim to achieve?

7. A child is referred to a therapist for assessment. When the child and her mother arrive, the therapist discovers that their English skills are extremely limited. Knowing that the test the therapist plans to use requires the child to be given verbal instructions, how should he

or she proceed? How should the therapist discuss the results?

8. A therapist is reviewing a new test. The test manual reports concurrent validity of 0.85 with another well-known and well-regarded test that is used frequently by the therapist's department and other agencies in the area. What additional information should the therapist look for when deciding which of these two tests to administer?

9. A 3-year-old boy with possible developmental delays is referred to a therapist. No other information is available on the referral note, but the therapist knows that he was recently screened in his preschool program. What information can the therapist obtain that would help him or her to decide what areas to test and at what approximate developmental level to begin testing?

10. Given the following referral information, state what standardized tests and nonstandardized evaluation techniques should be used to assess this child.

Natalie was 3 years, 3 months old at the time of her referral. She was born at 35 weeks' gestation to a mother who used cocaine and marijuana throughout her pregnancy. She had mild respiratory distress in the first few days of life. Natalie has had chronic middle ear infections and currently has ear tubes. She had early difficulties with sucking and is a picky eater.

Her mother entered a drug treatment program during a subsequent pregnancy and has been clean and sober for 1½ years. Natalie lives with her mother and two siblings in a small apartment. Her mother states that Natalie is "different" than her other children, and that she has difficulty controlling Natalie's behavior. Natalie seems to be bright, but she is active and easily frustrated with fine-motor activities. She has frequent temper tantrums, refuses to nap, and wakes several times during the night.

A public health nurse has been involved with the family since Natalie's birth, and she and Natalie's mother agree that some additional intervention may be necessary. Natalie is scheduled to enter a Head Start preschool program, and they would like recommendations for both home and school.

References

American Occupational Therapy Association. (1994). *Occupational Therapy Code of Ethics 48* (11), 1037-1038.

Anastasi, A. (1988). *Psychological testing* (6th ed.). New York: Macmillan.

Andrich, D. (1988). *Rasch models for measurement.* Beverly Hills, CA: Sage.

Ayers, A.J. (1989). *Sensory Integration and Praxis Test manual.* Los Angeles: Western Psychological Corporation.

Ayres, A.J., & Marr, D. (1991). Sensory integration and praxis tests. In A. Fisher, E. Murray, & A. Bundy (Eds.), *Sensory integration: Theory and practice* (pp. 201-233). Philadelphia: F.A. Davis.

Bayley, N. (1969). *Bayley Scales of Infant Development.* New York: The Psychological Corporation.

Bayley, N. (1993). *Bayley Scales of Infant Development* (2nd ed.). San Antonio, TX: The Psychological Corporation.

Beery, K.E. (1997). *Developmental Test of Visual-Motor Integration: Administration, scoring, and teaching manual—4th revision.* Los Angeles: Western Psychological Services.

Bricker, D. (Ed.). (1993). *AEPS measurement for birth to three years.* Baltimore: Brookes.

Bruininks, R.H. (1978). *Bruininks-Oseretsky Test of Motor Proficiency.* Circle Pines, MN: American Guidance Service.

Clark, G.F., & Coster, W.J. (1998). Evaluation, problem solving and program evaluation. In J. Case-Smith (Ed.), *Occupational therapy: Making a difference in school system practice.* Bethesda, MD: American Occupational Therapy Association, Inc.

Conoley, J.C., & Impara, J.C. (Ed.). (1995). *The twelfth mental measurements yearbook.* Lincoln, NE: Buros Institute of Mental Measurements.

Coster, W., Deeney, T., Haltiwanger, J., & Haley, S. (1998). *School function assessment.* San Antonio, TX: Psychological Corporation.

Crowe, T.K., Deitz, J.C., & Bennett, F.C. (1987). The relationship between the Bayley Scales of Infant Development and preschool gross motor and cognitive performance. *The American Journal of Occupational Therapy, 41,* 374-378.

Cunningham-Amundson, S.J., & Crowe, T.K. (1993). Clinical applications of the standard error of measurement for occupational and physical therapists. *Physical and Occupational Therapy in Pediatrics, 12* (4), 57-71.

Deitz, J.C. (1989). Reliability. *Physical and Occupational Therapy in Pediatrics, 9* (1), 125-147.

Farran, D.C., & Harber, L.A. (1989). Responses to a learning task at 6 months and IQ test performance during the preschool years. *International Journal of Behavioral Development, 12,* 101-114.

Fisher, A.G. (1997). *Assessment of motor and process skills.* Fort Collins, CO: Three Star Publishing.

Fisher, W.P. (1993). Measurement-related problems in functional assessment. *American Journal of Occupational Therapy, 47,* 331-338.

Folio, M.R., & Fewell, R.R. (1983). *Peabody Developmental Motor Scales.* Austin, TX: Pro-Ed.

Folio, M.R., & Fewell, R.R. (2000). *Peabody Developmental Motor Scales,* (2nd ed.). San Antonio, TX: Psychological Corporation.

Frankenburg, W.K., Dodds, J.B., Archer, P., Bresnick, B., Maschka, P., Edelman, N., & Sapiro, H. (1990). *Denver II Developmental Screening Test.* Denver: Denver Developmental Materials.

Furuno, S., O'Reilly, K.A., Hosaka, C.M., Inatsuka, T.T., Allman, T.L., & Zeisloft, B. (1997). *The Hawaii Early Learning Profile.* Palo Alto, CA: Vort.

Furuno, S., O'Reilly, K.A., Hosaka, C.M., Inatsuka, T.T., Allman, T.L., & Zeisloft, B. (1997). *Hawaii Early Learning Profile activity guide.* Palo Alto, CA: Vort.

Gardner, M.F. (1982). *Test of Visual-Perceptual Skills (non-motor).* Burlingame, CA: Psychological and Educational Publications.

Grimby, G., Andren, E., Holmgren, E., Wright, B., Linacre, J.M., & Sundh, V. (1996). Structure of a combination of functional independence measure and instrumental activity measure items in community-living persons: A study of individuals with cerebral palsy and spina bifida. *Archives of Physical Medicine and Rehabilitation, 77,* 1109-1114.

Haley, S.M., Coster, W.J., Ludlow, L.H., Haltiwanger, J.T., & Andrellos, P.J. (1992). *Pediatric Evaluation of Disability Inventory: Development, standardization and administration manual.* San Antonio, TX: Psychological Corporation.

Hammill, D.D., Pearson, N.A., & Voress, J.K. (1993). *Developmental Test of Visual Perception* (2nd ed.). Austin, TX: Pro Ed.

Hinderer, K.A., Richardson, P.K., & Atwater, S.W. (1989). Clinical implications of the Peabody Developmental Motor Scale: A constructive review. *Physical and Occupational Therapy in Pediatrics, 9* (2), 81-106.

Kazdin, A.E. (1982). *Single-case research designs.* New York: Oxford University Press.

Miller, L.J. (1990). *First STEP screening tool.* San Antonio, TX: Psychological Corporation.

Miller, L.J. (1982). *Miller Assessment for Preschoolers.* San Antonio, TX: Psychological Corporation.

Murphy, L.L., Impara, J.C., & Conoley, J.C. (Eds.). (1994). *Tests in print IV.* Lincoln, NE: Buros Institute of Mental Measurements.

Palisano, R. (1986). Concurrent and predictive validities of the Bayley Motor Scale and the Peabody Developmental Motor Scales. *Physical Therapy, 66* ,1714-1719.

Parks, S. (1992). *Inside HELP: Administration and reference manual for the Hawaii Early Learning Profile.* Palo Alto, CA: Vort.

Piper, E.J., Heinemann, A.W., Lowell, L.L., Harvey, R.L., McGuire, J.R., & Dias, S. (1998). Impairment and disability. Their relation during stroke rehabilitation. *Archives of Physical Medicine and Rehabilitation, 79,* 329-335.

Roth, E.J., Heinemann, A.W., Lovell, L.L., Harvey, R.L., McGuire, J.R., & Diaz, S. (1998). Impairment and disability: Their relation during stroke rehabilitation. *Archives of Physical Medicine and Rehabilitation, 79,* 329-335.

Royeen, C.B. (1992). Measuring and documenting all services. In C.B. Royeen (Ed.), *AOTA self study series: School-based practice for related services.* Rockville, MD: American Occupational Therapy Association.

Russell, D., Rosenbaum, P., Gowland, C., Hardy, S., Lane, M., Plews, N., McGavin, H., Cadman, D., & Jarvis, S. (1993). *Gross Motor Function Measure (revised).* OH, Canada: Pediatric Physiotherapy Services.

Sternberg, R.J. (1990). *Metaphors of mind: Conceptions of the nature of intelligence.* Cambridge, England: Cambridge University Press.

Terman, L.M., & Merrill, M.A. (1937). *Measuring intelligence.* Boston, MA: Houghton Mifflin.

Thorndike, R.L., Hagen, E.P., & Sattler, J.M. (1986). *Technical manual, Stanford-Binet Intelligence Scale,* (4th edition). Chicago: Riverside Publishing Company.

Wechsler, D. (1974). *Wechsler Intelligence Scale for Children—revised.* San Antonio, TX: Psychological Corporation.

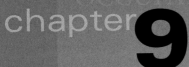

chapter 9

Planning and Implementing Services

Pamela K. Richardson
Winifred Schultz-Krohn

key terms

Intervention planning
Clinical reasoning
Frames of reference
Performance contexts
Long-term goals
Short-term goals
Service delivery models
Implementation plan

■ CHAPTER OBJECTIVES

1. Explain the process of clinical reasoning when planning and implementing therapy programs with children and families.
2. Understand the role of frames of reference in developing intervention plans.
3. Describe the component parts of measurable short- and long-term goals.
4. Apply intervention planning procedures to selected case studies.
5. Understand the structure of the service delivery models used most frequently in pediatric therapy.
6. Describe the knowledge and skills necessary for successful management of implementation programs.
7. Apply intervention management strategies to selected case studies.

The *intervention planning* process links evaluation and treatment. Through this process, the occupational therapist interprets evaluation findings and uses this information to make decisions about the type, amount, and duration of occupational therapy services to be provided for the client. Priorities of the family and child are an essential component in the intervention planning process. Other services received; medical and educational concerns; and financial, transportation, and scheduling constraints influence where, when, and how therapy services will be provided. The success of any treatment program hinges on the ability of the occupational therapist to integrate information from a variety of sources to develop a treatment program that considers the child's strengths and needs in the context of environmental demands, child and family priorities, and time and funding considerations.

This chapter discusses the process of treatment planning and implementation. The chapter is divided into two main sections: the intervention plan, in which the process of generating short- and long-term goals is discussed, and the implementation plan, in which *service delivery models* are presented. Throughout the chapter the clinical reasoning process is emphasized. Parameters to consider when making various treatment decisions are discussed at each step. Additionally, specific questions to ask to facilitate decision making are presented. The clinical reasoning process is illustrated through descriptions of children and the decision-making process used in evaluation and intervention.

■ EVALUATION TO INTERVENTION PLANNING

As described in Chapter 7, evaluation of a child involves examination of impairments, performance of daily activities, and participation in a variety of social, temporal, and physical contexts.

Performance components or impairments—sensorimotor, cognitive, and psychosocial—are often the basis for the short-term goals established for the child's intervention plan. Subsequently, specific activities are designed to help remediate the impairments identified.

Performance activities (work, play, and daily living) describe the desired functional outcomes and are often the basis of the child's long-term goals.

Performance contexts, physical, temporal, and environmental, address the how, when, and why of functional performance. Knowledge of the performance context of a particular activity is an essential part of the treatment-planning process (Schkade & Schultz, 1992; Schultz & Schkade, 1992). For instance, developmental aspects of the temporal context are always an important consideration when working with children. The expected functional outcomes for an 18-month-old child identified with decreased fine motor dexterity are different than those for a 10-year-old child with the same problem.

Disability status is another important aspect of the temporal performance context. Expectations for functional outcomes differ according to whether the identified disability is acute or chronic. In an acute injury the frequency and intensity of treatment intervention is often greater than in a chronic disability. Depending on the nature and severity of the injury, long-term goals may reflect an expectation of full or partial recovery of function. In the case of a chronic disability, *habilitation* rather than *rehabilitation* may be the therapeutic emphasis. Rather than assisting children to regain lost function, therapists working with children who have chronic disabilities often help children acquire functional skills that they cannot achieve on their own. Adaptations to the task process, the equipment used for the task, and/or the environment may be necessary for the child to achieve a level of independence with the task. This approach is reflected in the occupational adaptation frame of reference (Schkade & Schultz, 1992; Schultz & Schkade, 1992).

The therapist considers the physical, social, and cultural aspects of the child's environment. Input from the child, the family, and others in the child's school or home environment is essential to developing an intervention plan that is meaningful to the child and those around him or her. For instance, when evaluating a 7-year-old child

with delayed fine-motor skills, the therapist discusses with the mother the child's difficulty with skills such as buttoning, snapping, and tying. The mother replies that these are not currently a priority because she has chosen a wardrobe of pullover clothing and shoes with Velcro fasteners. The mother believes that school-related skills such as cutting, coloring, and writing are more problematic and create functional limitations that are more significant for her child. The therapist works with the mother and teacher to develop long- and short-term goals to address these concerns.

An example of intervention planning in which both the physical and social performance contexts are integral is a 9-year-old child with cerebral palsy who ambulates for short distances but has significant energy expenditure. When investigating alternative modes of mobility for this child, the therapist, parent, and child identify the following priorities: ability to move independently around the school campus, especially the playground, and ability to keep up with the child's Cub Scout group, which participates in numerous outdoor activities and excursions. These priorities lead the therapist to consider powered mobility as the option that best supports the child's social interactions while conserving energy for other important daily activities. Together the therapist, parent, and child investigate power mobility systems that are suitable for outside terrain to find the best match for the child. This example illustrates the importance of person-environment fit (Christiansen & Baum, 1997). The therapist must always consider the influence of the family, school, and home contexts on the child's performance when designing an intervention plan.

■ CLINICAL REASONING

How does the occupational therapist make decisions about what goals are most important to address? What frames of reference or practice models are most appropriate in the implementation plan? What activities provide the greatest therapeutic value? The answers to these questions are determined individually for each child through a *clinical reasoning* process. The therapist employs clinical reasoning to analyze important aspects of the child's behavior and the environment and to use this analysis to make decisions about intervention. The four types of clinical reasoning are procedural, interactive, intuitive, and conditional (Table 9-1).

Procedural Reasoning

In a qualitative study of clinical reasoning, Mattingly and Fleming (1994) described several strategies used by occupational therapists to make intervention decisions. The strategies are used concurrently as the therapist contemplates the needs of the whole child. *Procedural* and *interactive reasoning* are employed to make the decisions

table 9-1	Summary of Clinical Reasoning Strategies
Clinical Reasoning Strategies	**Purposes**
Procedural	• Problem identification and development of an intervention plan • Identification of specific methods to improve function
Interactive	• Development of an understanding of the child and family as individuals • Selection and adaptation of interventions to maintain the child's interest and attention • Communication of acceptance, trust, and hope
Intuitive	• Interpretation of interactive cues to gain the child's engagement and participation • Matching activity selection to program goals and the child's interests
Conditional	• Selection of activities based on the child's problem and therapist's vision for the child in the future • Creating intentionality in the child by offering choices and promoting the child's sense of purpose and desire to accomplish the goal

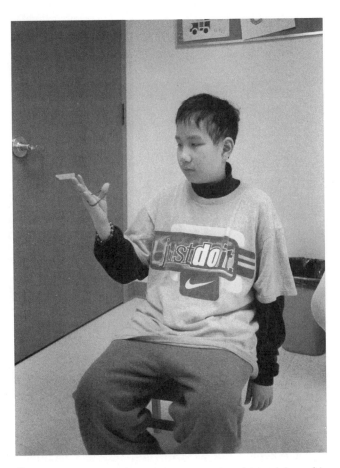

figure 9-1   A boy learns a new magic trick to show his friends.

that result in recommendations for an intervention plan. Given an understanding of the child's limitations and needs, *procedural reasoning* is used to identify specific methods designed to improve function. The therapist matches his or her understanding of the child's problems to the range of intervention approaches that appropriately address that problem. Procedural reasoning defines the process that the therapist employs to identify the problems and logically develop a goal and plan. This analysis is similar to the medical problem-solving model in which a problem is identified, different solutions are tested, and intervention is defined.

Interactive Reasoning

Therapists also employ *interactive reasoning* to gain understanding of the child and family as individuals (Mattingly & Fleming, 1994). This reasoning is used to help the therapist understand the perspectives and experiences of the child and family from their individual and collective points of view. Mattingly and Fleming list several purposes for using interactive reasoning, some of which are listed below:
■ To engage the child in the treatment session

■ To know the child and family as individuals
■ To understand the disability from the family's perspective
■ To finely match the treatment goals and strategies to the particular child with his or her disability and experience
■ To communicate a sense of acceptance, trust, and hope

Positive and meaningful interactions are essential to intervention (Kalmanson & Seligman, 1992). Therapists use interactive reasoning to assimilate the whole individual, including values and beliefs (Mattingly & Fleming, 1994). The therapist then employs this understanding to guide decision making about intervention. In this form of reasoning the therapist responds to subtle cues of the child to select specific intervention activities and then adapts those activities to maintain the child's interest and attention. The result of interactive reasoning is that intervention activities are individualized to each child. Figures 9-1 and 9-2 are examples of therapy activities that evidence procedural and interactive reasoning. The movements required for the magic trick are similar to those required in tying shoelaces. The therapist se-

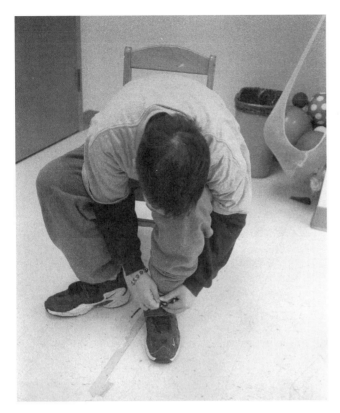

figure 9-2   The boy in Figure 9-1 practices isolated finger movements to improve his efficiency in tying shoelaces.

lected a magic trick because it elicits the needed isolated finger movements and because this boy revealed to the therapist his interest in magic tricks and his reputation for performing magic tricks for his peers.

Intuitive Reasoning

The therapist's thorough understanding of the child and the child's preferences and interests guides the selection of toys and activities that will engage the child in play and that will meet identified intervention goals. This process is intuitive rather than analytic (Mattingly & Fleming, 1994). Although the therapist's *intuitive reasoning* often defies definition, the therapist's interpretation of the complex, subtle interactive cues is core to the effectiveness of intervention. When the occupational therapist accurately "reads" the child's mood, interests, and intentions, he or she can match these by offering appropriate activity choices that gain the interest and participation of the child. This intuitive activity selection is as important to the success of intervention as the analytic, procedural reasoning in which an activity was selected to address directly the established goals. Once engaged in an activity with the child, the therapist continues to use his or her knowledge of intervention procedures and techniques to remediate the problem and

his or her interactive abilities to individualize the activities to motivate and capture the child's attention.

Conditional Reasoning

Many therapists use conditional reasoning to develop holistic long-term intervention plans (Mattingly & Fleming, 1994). In *conditional reasoning*, the therapist thinks about the child's condition in three ways:

■ The therapist views the whole (i.e., the child and his or her disability, the family, and the environment).

■ The therapist contemplates how the condition can change. He or she envisions a different child who can perform a skill at a higher level.

■ The therapist considers ways to ensure the child's participation and decision making, to help the child engage in a change process, and to create his or her own picture of the future. The therapist develops activities that create ongoing interest and motivate the child to initiate those activities in other contexts. The therapist realizes that the success of intervention is based on the child's participation and motivation to make changes.

In conditional reasoning the therapist selects appropriate intervention activities based on the child's problem and his or her vision for the child in the future (Mattingly & Fleming, 1994). This vision guides the therapist's decision to continue an emphasis on promoting developmental skills or to explore possible adapted methods for the child to compensate for functional limitations. The family's and the child's visions of the future also determine whether therapy should emphasize compensatory, functional strategies in lieu of developmental goals. Intervention is at high risk for failure when the therapist and family hold different visions for the future and therefore believe that different strategies should be employed.

For example, the parents of a 2 year old with severe neuromotor delays envision that their child, Mike, will walk within a year. The occupational therapist believes that Mike will not achieve this goal but is a good candidate for a power wheelchair. The family prefers that therapy sessions focus on standing and walking activities, but the occupational therapist prefers to focus on the hand-eye coordination needed to use a joystick to control a wheelchair. If both the family and the therapist insists on pursuing their vision, it is likely that neither goal will be achieved.

Through the interactive reasoning process, the therapist must develop an understanding of the family's vision and consider their perspectives of the child's problems. The therapist also needs to convey his or her vision and the rationale for such a vision. By sharing their individual goals for Mike, Mike's parents and the therapist can negotiate an intervention plan that clearly addresses the family's priorities and values and engages their participation in intervention. The occupational therapist and the parents reach a consensus on the goal of improved trunk stability as a prerequisite skill for independent standing and for upright sitting in a wheelchair. By setting a common goal that both parties believe to be a priority, a basis for communication about the child's progress is established that helps the parents and the occupational therapist develop additional appropriate goals.

■ INTERVENTION PLAN

An evaluation provides specific data regarding the child's performance abilities, but the occupational therapist must synthesize these data to develop an effective intervention plan. Box 9-1 lists the four components of an intervention plan as defined by the Standards of Practice for Occupational Therapy (AOTA, 1994). Although most pediatric assessment instruments measure performance components, the occupational therapist must identify how specific impairments compromise performance of daily activities. An effective intervention plan must always address functional performance. It is not sufficient to merely remediate impairments, such as sitting balance or limited bilateral coordination if these performance improvements do not result in increased functional skills and occupations.

The development of an intervention plan requires the therapist to answer several questions. Clinical reasoning is required whenever an intervention plan is developed (Crepeau, 1991; Fleming, 1991a, 1991b; Mattingly, 1991a, 1991b). Following is a set of questions that can be used to facilitate the clinical reasoning process and provide guidance for development of the intervention plan. A more concise list of the questions is presented in Box 9-2.

1. *What are the priorities of the family and child?* An intervention plan must consider the social and cultural background of the family. Development of specific grooming skills or self-feeding skills may not be emphasized within a family. The family may be much more concerned with a child's ability to engage socially with other family members rather than perform self-care tasks.

2. *What is the next set of skills and occupational roles that this child will need to develop to meet environmental demands?* Although many developmental assessment tools measure a child's ability to stack blocks, this skill may not significantly influence the child's ability to interact effectively within his or her environment. A therapist needs to consider carefully what skills the child currently possesses and what set of skills will allow the child to meet environmental demands successfully.

3. *What developmental trajectory has this child demonstrated?* Acquisition of previous developmental skill is often an indicator of future growth. A 5-year-old child

---

box 9-1 *American Occupational Therapy Association standards of practice*

Standard V: intervention plan

1. An occupational therapist shall develop and document an intervention plan based on analysis of the occupational therapy assessment data and the individual's expected outcome after the intervention. A certified occupational therapist assistant may contribute to the intervention plan under the supervision of the therapist.

2. The intervention plan is stated in goals that are clear, measurable, behavioral, functional, and appropriate to the individual's needs, personal goal, and expected outcome after intervention.

3. The plan shall reflect the philosophic base of occupational therapy and be consistent with its established principles and concepts of therapy and practice. The intervention plan shall include the following:
   a. Formulating a list of strengths and weaknesses
   b. Estimating rehabilitation potential
   c. Identifying measurable short-term and long-term goals
   d. Collaborating with the individual, family members, other caregivers, professionals, and community resources
   e. Selecting the media, methods, environment, and personnel needed to accomplish the intervention goals
   f. Determining the frequency and duration of occupational therapy services
   g. Identifying a plan for reevaluation
   h. Planning discharge

4. An occupational therapist shall prepare and document the intervention plan within the timeframes and according to the standards established by the employing practice settings, government agencies, accreditation programs, and third-party payers.

AOTA. (1994). Standards of Practice, *AJOT, 48*, 1047-1054.

---

who displays gross motor skills commensurate to a 7-month-old child may never reach age-appropriate skills of walking, running, or hopping. The occupational therapist must consider what modifications will allow this child to compensate for limited gross motor skills instead of only focusing the intervention plan on the development of a specific skill.

4. *What are the specific environmental demands that are placed on this child?* The therapist must consider the physical environment (e.g., an apartment located on

box **9-2** *Guiding questions for intervention planning*

1. What are the priorities of the family and child?
2. What is the next set of skills and occupational roles that this child will need to develop to meet environmental demands?
3. What developmental trajectory has this child demonstrated?
4. What are the specific environmental demands that are placed on this child?
5. What is the service delivery setting and model and how does it influence the intervention plan?
6. Which theoretic model of practice or frame of reference provides a template for the occupational therapist to develop an intervention plan?
7. What is the nature of the disabling condition?

the third floor of a building without an elevator) and the social environment (e.g., whether a child is able to engage a peer in a play activity). Although adaptive equipment may be useful in promoting a specific skill, the environment may not support the use of such equipment. A teenage girl with cerebral palsy may find dressing easier if she uses loose fitting elastic-waist pants, but this type of clothing may compromise her ability to join a peer group successfully.

5. *What is the service delivery setting and model and how does it influence the intervention plan?* Early intervention services provided under the Individuals with Disabilities Education Act (IDEA, 1997) are to be family centered. This requires an occupational therapist to develop a plan for the child with special needs that incorporates family concerns. This is contrasted with services provided in a school system under the IDEA. Occupational therapy services are provided in this setting to assist a child in specific educational pursuits. Hospital-based occupational therapy services are influenced by the limited time that a child will stay in the hospital.

6. *Which theoretic model of practice or frame of reference provides a template for the occupational therapist to develop an intervention plan?* Selection and application of the frame of reference becomes an integral part of the clinical reasoning process and provides a flexibility of approaches to meet the needs of each child's unique situation. Often a therapist will combine several *frames of reference* when working with a child (Kramer & Hinojosa, 1999). A child with autism may benefit from an intervention plan that combines aspects of the sensory integration, human occupation, and behavioral

practice models. A therapist may use behavioral constructs to help a child with an autistic disorder comply with parental requests (Gerlach, 1996). Sensory integration provides the therapist with an orientation with which to view the child's tactile hypersensitivity and helps the therapist determine which interventions to select (Ayres, 1979). The model of human occupation provides a framework for understanding the child's personal motivation and the interaction between the child and the environment (Kielhofner & Burke, 1985).

7. *What is the nature of the disabling condition?* A child with an acute illness or injury, such as a burn or encephalitis, requires the therapist to address the resultant problems aggressively while the child is hospitalized. As the child becomes medically stable, the focus of intervention expands to include functional skill development such as self-feeding or dressing skills as appropriate. The intervention plan is to regain previous functional skills and promote future skill development. This type of intervention plan is contrasted to a plan developed for a child with a chronic, progressive disorder, such as Rett syndrome or Duchenne's muscular dystrophy, in which children present with a deterioration of skills. Children with degenerative conditions often require the therapist to focus the intervention on environmental modifications and coping strategies because previous skills are lost.

Case Study 1

This case study illustrates the intervention planning process applied to a case in which rapid change in the functional status of the child occurs. This requires frequent adjustments to the intervention plan throughout the course of occupational therapy services.

Justin is a 15-year-old male adolescent who sustained a traumatic brain injury and a brachial plexus injury on his right side during a gang-related fight. Police stopped the fight and Justin was rushed to a hospital where he was comatose and unresponsive to painful stimuli. He was intubated, and a nasogastric tube was inserted.

The day after the injury, Justin displayed responses to painful stimuli and randomly moved his left arm. He continued to be fed through a nasogastric tube. He was medically stable and was transferred to the intensive rehabilitation floor for a comprehensive team evaluation. Members of the team included nurses, an occupational therapist, a physical therapist, a speech and language pathologist, and a psychiatrist.

The occupational therapy evaluation included assessment of activities of daily living skills (ADLs), cognitive status, range of motion, oral motor skills, postural control, and sensation. The therapist found Justin to have limited active range of motion in his right arm, random movement of his left arm in all planes of motion, poor oral motor control, and inability to swallow his own saliva. He did not display purposeful movement and was nonambulatory. Justin was at a Glasgow level of 10. The Glasgow Coma Scale evaluates a client's level of coma using eye opening, motor responses, and verbal responses on a scale of 1 to 15, with 15 being the highest functional level (Teasdale & Jennett, 1974). At this time, Justin opens his eyes spontaneously, displayed a flexion-withdrawal response to painful stimuli, and made incomprehensible sounds. He did not actively engage in any self-care tasks.

The therapist used several practice models in developing a treatment plan. Clinical reasoning skills were used to select which practice models offer the best foundation for intervention (Mattingly, 1991b). Sensory integration theory provides a foundation for the therapist to use familiar olfactory stimuli with Justin before attempting to facilitate the oral motor skills needed for feeding (Kimball, 1999). Using biomechanical principles, the therapist provides a positioning device to support Justin's right shoulder and decrease the risk of subluxation (Colangelo, 1999). The therapist was also concerned about Justin's lack of appropriate responses within the environment. Concepts from the occupational adaptation frame of reference provided the therapist with a guide for intervention strategies directed at the interaction between Justin and his environment (Schkade & Schultz, 1992; Schultz & Schkade, 1992). The therapist suggested to Justin's mother that pictures of family members and friends be posted around the room. The therapist also asked Justin's mother to bring a few of his own clothes to the hospital. Even though Justin was unable to dress himself, the therapist suggested that wearing familiar clothing can assist Justin in regaining his memory and sense of self-identity.

Justin received direct occupational therapy services twice a day with a focus on promoting responsiveness to the environment, fostering oral motor skills for a transition to oral feeding, and regaining functional movement of his right arm. The therapist synthesized the practice models of sensory integration, biomechanics, and occupational adaptation in developing Justin's intervention plan.

Within 10 days of the injury, Justin progressed from a deep coma and became more responsive to his environment but also more combative and verbally abusive to hospital staff. This change required an alteration to the intervention plan. Again clinical reasoning skills were employed to select a theoretic practice model to address the newly emerging problems (Fleming, 1991b; Mattingly, 1991a). The occupational therapist selected a behavioral frame of reference to decrease the behavioral outbursts during therapy sessions. Praise and verbal encouragement were used as positive reinforcement, and loss of time with friends was used as negative reinforce-

ment. If Justin engaged in abusive language or combative actions against staff, specific consequences occured, such as restricting visitation by friends.

Justin continued to receive direct occupational therapy service, and the frequency was increased to three times a day. One session was a group session jointly conducted by the occupational therapist and speech and language pathologist with a focus on orientation skills and recovery of cognitive abilities. The other two sessions continued to focus on rehabilitation of functional ADLs such as self-feeding and dressing.

Justin's physical and cognitive skills continued to progress. He regained the ability to ambulate independently and to move his right elbow through approximately half of the available range, but he continued to lack functional shoulder and hand motion. He displayed severe memory loss and poor problem-solving ability. He was unable to dress himself independently because of sequencing problems. Justin's ability to initiate an activity was significantly impaired, and he depended on others to prompt him verbally to complete the next task in a sequence. Justin's behavior had substantially improved, and he was cooperative with members of the rehabilitation team. Although verbal, Justin continued to have great difficulties following verbal instructions and was unable to continue a topic of conversation that lasted more than two or three sentences.

Before his traumatic brain injury, Justin lived at home with his mother, grandmother, and two younger siblings. Although he had been enrolled in school, he seldom attended. His fellow gang members provided most of his social support. The occupational therapist considered the influence of his social environment as she revised her treatment plan. The rehabilitation team and Justin's mother wanted him to return to school. Justin's previous peer group had not supported his participation in school. Both Justin's mother and the occupational therapist were concerned about his ability to develop new peer relationships in the school environment. It was hoped that services provided in a school setting would help Justin as he continued to recover functional skills.

As discharge plans were finalized, Justin continued to display significant cognitive deficits that compromised his completion of school-related tasks. A plan that included supportive services in his school setting was developed. He continued to receive occupational therapy services within his classroom setting to address his deficits in memory, initiation of activities, perceptual-motor skills, and problem-solving abilities that compromise completion of schoolwork. Direct speech and language services were provided within his school setting. The occupational therapist and speech and language pathologist in the school agreed that a peer social skills group would be helpful. This group would focus on developing supportive peer relationships within the school environment.

The team felt that an educational aide was necessary to provide support to Justin during the first few months after he returns to school. The need for an aide would be re-evaluated by the educational team after 4 months.

Writing Goals and Objectives

Goals or objectives guide intervention and provide a measure of intervention efficacy. The intervention goal reflects a specific, clear change in the child's behavior. The development of a goal must reflect the needs of the child within the demands of the environment. A well-written goal consists of three parts (Zimmerman, 1988):
1. A behavioral statement of what the child is expected to complete or perform
2. A criterion that stipulates the measure of the stated behavior
3. The conditions for the performance of the stated behavior

Goals are divided into two classifications: long-term and short-term goals. In some settings the term *goal* represents a long-term goal and the term *objective* represents a short-term goal. Long-term goals generally reflect a terminal behavior for the child. These goals must address a performance of activities and participation in occupations. Occupational therapists are committed to fostering a child's ability to perform tasks in the areas of ADLs, school-related tasks, or play and leisure activities. The behavioral statement for a long-term goal must identify a child's skill in a performance area that will be gained or improved through the course of treatment.

Short-term goals or objectives can be documented in written behavioral statements as steps that lead to the targeted performance or focus on developing the underlying performance components necessary to complete a task related to self-care, school, or play. A long-term goal stating that *the child will independently feed himself breakfast while seated in an adapted highchair* suggests that several short-term goals need to be accomplished first. A short-term goal can state that *the child will independently hold a built-up handled spoon while eating applesauce.* Another short-term goal can state that *the child will use a radial digital grasp to self-feed dry cereal.* In the first example, a step within the process of self-feeding, holding the spoon, was identified as the behavior addressed in the short-term goal. The second identifies the performance component of grasp as a necessary skill to achieve the long-term goal of self-feeding.

Behavioral statements can be graded in complexity. A long-term goal that identifies self-feeding as the desired outcome involves many underlying skills. The long-term goal can be stated that by *January, the child will independently feed self all meals.* Here the criterion is *independently* and the condition is *all meals.* A timeframe specifies a target date when the child is expected to meet the goal. The following are examples of underlying skills that need to be addressed to meet a goal successfully:
1. The child will exhibit the fine motor skills to handle utensils efficiently.
2. The child will exhibit the oral motor skills necessary to eat various textures of foods.
3. The child will exhibit the ability to initiate and terminate the behavior appropriately.
4. The child will exhibit the postural control to maintain an upright sitting position.

This same area of self-feeding can be further focused as appropriate for a younger child. The condition and criteria can be narrowed to state that *the child will independently drink a 6-ounce bottle while holding the bottle and remaining seated in a feeder seat.* Here the behavioral statement is focused on the performance area of feeding but limited in how the behavior is to be performed. The criteria of this task are *independently* (how) and *a 6-ounce bottle* (what). The two conditions are *while holding the bottle* and *remaining seated in a feeder seat.*

Box 9-3 provides examples of behavioral statements that can be used to formulate long-term goals. These statements specifically address performance areas.

Box 9-4 provides examples of behavioral statements that can be used to formulate short-term goals. These statements specifically address performance components.

box 9-3 *Possible behavioral statements for long-term goals*

Activities of daily living
Feeding skills
- Drink from bottle
- Drink from cup
- Eat with spoon
- Finger-feed self
Grooming skills
- Brush teeth
- Wash face
- Wash hands
- Wipe self after toileting
Dressing skills
- Don and doff shirt
- Don and doff pants
- Tie shoes
- Button jacket

Educational activities
- Complete written assignments for English (or another specified class)
- Copy assignments from board
- Participate in class discussion

box **9-4** *Possible behavioral statements for short-term goals*

Sensorimotor performance
- Use fine pincer grasp
- Sit on chair
- Use both hands

Cognitive performance
- Attend to task
- Sequence three steps
- Follow two-step directions
- Initiate activity

Psychosocial performance
- Display eye contact
- Identify preferences
- Transition between activities

box **9-5** *Possible criteria used to determine how well a child performs a task*

Frequency of specified behavior
- 1 of 4 trials
- 2 of 4 trials
- 3 of 4 trials
- Percentage of given opportunities during the treatment session

Duration of a specified behavior during the treatment session
- 5 seconds
- 10 seconds
- 2 minutes
- 5 repetitions

Amount of assistance provided to complete the task
- Independently
- With supervision
- With standby assistance
- Minimal assistance (verbal or physical assistance provided for 25% of task)
- Moderate assistance (verbal or physical assistance provided for 50% of task)
- Maximum assistance (verbal or physical assistance provided for 75% of task)

Adapted from Zimmerman, J. (1988). *Goals and objectives for developing normal movement patterns.* Rockville, MD: Aspen Publishing.

An example of a long-term goal for Justin while he is hospitalized is as follows: *In 4 weeks, Justin will feed himself lunch with intermittent verbal cues from the therapist while seated in the hospital dining room.*

In this goal the behavioral statement is *Justin will feed himself lunch.* The criterion is *with intermittent verbal cues from the therapist.* The condition is *seated in the hospital dining room.* This goal reflects the level of task performance that Justin will need to function within his school setting. Since an educational aide will initially be assigned to Justin as he returns to school, that individual can provide verbal cues as needed to prompt Justin to complete his meal. When this goal is evaluated, if Justin requires physical assistance to complete the activity, then he has not met the criteria for that goal, but if Justin completes his lunch independently (with no verbal prompts) then he exceeds the criteria. The setting of a hospital dining room provides a level of distraction comparable with a school cafeteria. Justin must accommodate to the extra noise and distractions and complete the task of feeding himself. He must also display the fine motor and bilateral motor skills to carry a tray in the dining room and be able to open cartons.

The occupational therapist must assess whether recovery of function in the right arm will be sufficient to perform such an activity or whether Justin must be instructed in an alternate method of opening cartons and provisions must be made for the aide to carry Justin's tray. Considering where he would complete this activity in the near future (i.e., to participate in the social setting of a high school cafeteria), the preferred outcome was Justin's ability to complete this entire task independently. Although this goal had merit, the therapist expressed that this outcome was unrealistic given the prescribed length of his inpatient rehabilitation.

Each goal must have a clear measure of the stated behavior. These measures are the criteria by which the therapist can determine if the goals have been met. The criteria establish how well the behavior is to be performed. Box 9-5 provides typical measures used to determine how well a child performs a task.

The *condition* refers to the environmental situation in which the behavior will be performed. This includes the physical environment, the equipment necessary for completion of the task, and the social context for the performance of the specified behavior. Conditions must be stated to clarify the range of the child's behavior. An example of conditions for a task such as self-feeding includes the specific meal, the type of foods, the equipment used, or the social setting. These conditions dramatically alter the child's performance and must be included in every goal to clarify the extent of the child's performance. A child who is expected to self-feed only at home while positioned in a feeder seat and with only his

box 9-6 *Categories of conditions for long- and short-term goals*

Equipment used to complete the task
- Specific positioning device
- Specific adapted utensil
- Modified classroom equipment such as slant boards or pencil grips

Physical environment
- Specific location (demands to eat at home in quiet environment are different than in school cafeteria)

Social environment
- Specific persons are present (persons included in environment and social context; behavior demonstrated within structured classroom may not be exhibited in free play setting because of child's lack of organization)

or her mother present is eliciting a different behavioral expectation than a child expected to self-feed while seated at a table in a school cafeteria with peers.

Box 9-6 provides examples of categories of conditions to be incorporated into a long- or short-term goal.

Goals can be constructed easily by stating the specific behavior that the child will perform and selecting a measure of that behavior followed by the condition for performance. An example from the case of Justin is: *In 4 weeks, Justin will sign his name within 5 seconds using narrow-lined paper.* In this example the behavior identified is: *sign his name in cursive,* the criteria is a time limit of *5 seconds,* and the condition is *using narrow-lined paper.* If Justin were using unlined or wide-lined paper, it may alter his performance. The advantage of constructing clear, measurable goals can be seen when progress notes are required and the therapist can quickly identify whether the targeted behavior was observed. When a goal is not achieved, the therapist makes a decision to continue with, alter, or terminate the intervention plan. The therapist may select an alternate frame of reference or practice model or may change the performance condition or task criteria.

Case Study 2

This case study provides an example of a child with a chronic condition requiring management and treatment of a variety of problems over a long period. Several practice models and service delivery roles are illustrated.

Michelle is a 7-year-old girl with a diagnosis of spina bifida. She has received occupational therapy services pe-

riodically for most of her life. She was referred for her current round of occupational therapy after undergoing surgery to release her tethered spinal cord, a condition that caused progressive weakness and incoordination of her upper extremities and loss of previously attained skills. After surgery, she had difficulty managing buttons and tying her shoes and became quickly fatigued when writing. She also became fatigued when pushing her manual wheelchair and complained of shoulder pain after a typical day at school. The occupational therapist collaborated with Michelle, her parents, her teacher, and the physical therapist on the intervention team in designing an intervention plan for Michelle. The following short- and long-term goals were written:

1. By the end of the school year, Michelle will independently complete all academic tasks at school without accommodations.
   a. She will complete a 10-minute printing activity using wide-lined paper without stopping, 90% of the time, by her first report card.
   b. When coloring with crayons, she will stay within the lines of a 2-inch figure, three of four times, by her second report card.
   c. She will complete a math worksheet in the allotted time using a primary pencil, 90% of the time, by her third report card.
2. By the end of the school year, Michelle will independently manage all clothing fastenings.
   a. She will button a front-buttoning sweater within 2 minutes, 90% of the time, while sitting on the floor, by her first report card.
   b. She will tie both shoes independently within 3 minutes, 90% of the time, while sitting on the floor, by her second report card.
   c. She will zip and button jeans independently within 1 minute, 90% of the time, while lying on the bed, by her third report card.
3. By the end of the school year, Michelle will attain independent wheelchair mobility for a typical day of activities without complaints of pain or fatigue.
   a. She will independently wheel from classroom to playground, 90% of the time, with her peers (classmates), by her first report card.
   b. She will go up the wheelchair ramp into her house within 30 seconds, 4 to 5 days, with her mother present for standby assistance, by her second report card.

After these goals are written, the occupational therapist designed an implementation plan with three components:

1. The first component consisted of direct therapy services twice a week at the therapy clinic, where the occupational therapist worked with Michelle on progressive graded activities to increase upper-extremity strength and endurance and fine motor strength and dexterity. The occupational therapist also worked with

Michelle on functional skills such as writing, dressing, and wheelchair mobility.

2. The second component of the intervention plan was a home program involving consultation with Michelle's parents and provision of activities that provided opportunities for practice and carryover of the goals during interactions with her parents and siblings.

3. The third component of the intervention plan was a school consultation program. The occupational therapist visited the school to observe Michelle and to educate the school staff regarding her medical condition and her functional status at school. The occupational therapist provided suggestions for ways to grade activities to match Michelle's capabilities as her skills improve and offered ideas for ways to maximize her participation in school activities.

As part of the intervention plan, an orthopedic consult was recommended because of Michelle's complaints of shoulder pain. The occupational therapist and physical therapist also collaborated on evaluating the appropriateness and fit of Michelle's wheelchair, since an improperly fitting wheelchair can contribute to shoulder pain. Based on this evaluation, the therapists recommended adjustments to the wheelchair to make it more ergonomically efficient for Michelle. In addition, they provided information to Michelle's parents on ultralight wheelchairs and suggested that they consider an ultralight chair for Michelle when she outgrows her current wheelchair.

After 3 months of occupational therapy intervention, Michelle attained most of her goals, and her parents and teacher reported that her strength, coordination, and dexterity were adequate for daily tasks at home and school. Direct occupational therapy intervention was discontinued, but the team agreed that Michelle needed to remain on monitor status, with a semiannual reevaluation of upper-extremity strength and coordination. This was done to observe her functional status and provide documentation of a decrease in function if spinal cord tethering reoccurs.

At that time, the team agreed that it was appropriate to address the self-care goal of independent self-catheterization. The role of the occupational therapist in this process was evaluative and consultative.

Before initiating training in self-catheterization, the occupational therapist was asked to evaluate whether fine-motor, perceptual-motor, and sequencing skills were adequate to perform the component steps of the catheterization procedure. The occupational therapist's knowledge of Michelle's fine-motor skills was important here. In addition, the occupational therapist assessed Michelle's ability to perform fine-motor tasks while looking in a mirror rather than directly at the objects. This perceptual skill was important in the initial stages of learning self-catheterization because the child must use a mirror to guide the insertion of the catheter into the urethra.

Upon satisfactory completion of these activities, Michelle was ready to begin training in self-catheterization. The school nurse, who trained the school health aide and Michelle's mother on how to teach Michelle to catheterize herself, carried out the instruction. The occupational therapist visited the nurse's office at school and Michelle's home to provide consultation regarding setup for transfers and placement of the mirror and catheterization supplies. The occupational therapist recommended the use of a transfer board at school and wall-mounted extendable mirrors at school and at home so that Michelle could perform the process independently. Additionally the occupational therapist consulted with the nurse, Michelle, and her mother to devise a method for Michelle to change her diaper independently after catheterization. The following occupational therapy goals were written for this intervention:

1. By the end of the school year, Michelle will independently perform self-catheterization at home and at school.
   a. She will independently transfer from wheelchair to toilet and back to wheelchair using safe technique, 100% of attempts, by her first report card.
   b. She will use a wall-mounted mirror to perform the catheterization procedure independently, 100% of attempts, by her second report card.
   c. She will independently manage lower-extremity clothing (off and on), including changing her diaper, 100% of attempts, in the nurses station bathroom, by her third report card.

The criterion for successful completion of each goal is 100% of attempts, because for Michelle to be considered independent and safe for this task, it was necessary that she perform each step correctly each time she attempted it. In the previous set of goals for upper-extremity and fine-motor function, a criterion of 90% of attempts was considered adequate. The criteria for these goals indicated mastery of the task while taking into account potential day-to-day performance fluctuations that were due to a variety of factors.

▪ IMPLEMENTATION PLAN

Once short- and long-term goals have been agreed upon, an *implementation plan* must be made regarding how to provide services to meet these goals most effectively. Many factors influence the method of service delivery. The setting or practice arena is a major determinant, both in what types of goals are written and in how services are provided. For instance, a therapist working in an inpatient hospital setting addresses goals that are primarily health- or medical-related, whereas a therapist working in a school setting addresses primarily educationally oriented goals. The frame of reference used also influences the service delivery model. A therapist using a neurodevelopmental approach when working with a young child primarily provides direct one-on-one intervention. Consultation may involve recommendations for handling techniques or purchase of positioning or mobility equipment. A therapist using the coping frame of reference may provide some direct intervention, and consultation to the parents and/or teacher focuses on providing appropriate environmental adaptations and challenges for the child.

The child's age and characteristics of the disabling condition are often considered together in selecting a service delivery model. Frequently, young children are considered candidates for intensive direct services because of their neural plasticity and capacity for change. Older children are often seen to benefit more from consultation or monitoring that emphasizes environmental adaptation, training of parents and teachers, and provision of adaptive equipment. However, this general rule varies significantly according to specific characteristics of the child. A 1-year-old child with an upper-extremity limb deficiency may be best served by a combination of consultation and monitoring as the therapist, physician, and family watch to see how the child progresses through the developmental sequence. Conversely, an adolescent may require an intensive course of direct therapy after a muscle transfer surgery. In general, an injury or disease process in the acute stage must be handled according to appropriate medical and therapeutic guidelines regardless of the child's age.

Other considerations in the selection of the service delivery model are related to the child's environment, including the constellation of services the child receives, the performance context, and the pragmatic considerations of funding, transportation, and scheduling. Often children who receive occupational therapy services also receive other services such as speech therapy, physical therapy, counseling, nursing care, special education or tutoring. Occupational therapy services must be placed within this service structure, and the importance of these services must be prioritized. At times occupational therapy services may merit a large investment of time, energy, and funding. Examples of this include implementation of an oral feeding program for a young infant or training in the use of a prosthetic limb. At other times, it may be most appropriate for occupational therapy to take a less prominent role. A child whose motor delays and sensory integrative dysfunction have improved as a result of direct occupational therapy services may reach a point where participating in community activities, such as horseback riding, swimming, or T-ball, will provide greater opportunities for growth than will continued therapy intervention. The therapist may monitor the child's progress or act as a consultant to others in the community who work with the child. Alternatively, the therapist may discharge the child from therapy services with suggestions for appropriate activities.

The performance context also guides the selection of the service delivery model. For example, when working with a child in a school-based setting, a therapist must decide if services would be most effective when carried out on an individual or small group basis or in consultation with the classroom teacher. Initially a child with handwriting difficulties may require direct one-on-one intervention, but as the child acquires the necessary skills, the program can be transferred to the classroom as part of the daily school routine. A student with ataxia who is taking a high school art class may require consultation from the occupational therapist to provide adaptive devices and to instruct the teacher on how to facilitate the student's full participation. The same student may subsequently require direct intervention from the occupational therapist when working on cooking and housekeeping skills in preparation for moving into an apartment.

Family considerations are always an important part of the child's environment. A working parent with other small children may not have the time to bring a child three times weekly to a therapy session. The family's medical insurance may cover only a limited course of therapy, or there may be no insurance coverage at all. The family may not have reliable transportation. Factors such as these may necessitate an alteration in the service delivery plan. The occupational therapist may need to coordinate with social workers or caseworkers to assist the family in accessing resources. Additionally the therapist may need to change the location, frequency, or duration of therapy, emphasizing home-based consultation, for instance, rather than center-based direct intervention. The method of service delivery can be changed if at any time the family circumstances or the child's needs change. Certain factors to consider when choosing a service delivery model are summarized in Box 9-7.

Three primary models of service delivery for children have been identified by the AOTA (1997). As the ex-

---

box **9-7** *Factors to consider when selecting a service delivery model*

1. Practice arena
2. Appropriate frames of reference or practice models
3. Age of child
4. Type of disabling condition
5. Acuity and chronicity of condition
6. Coordination with other service providers
7. Performance context
8. Pragmatic considerations, including funding, transportation, and time

amples in Box 9-7 show, the models can be used sequentially or together with a variety of options as to how they can be combined.

■ DIRECT SERVICES

In direct services the therapist works in one-on-one interaction with the child or leads a small group of children in intervention activities. Therapists select direct service models when specialized occupational therapy approaches and techniques are needed that are individualized to the child and require specific skills to administer. Direct services are appropriate when the intervention techniques cannot be safely administered by others or when the success of the techniques relies on continually adjusting and adapting the input according to the child's unique responses. For example, the therapy approaches that require constant and ongoing monitoring of the child's autonomic nervous system and postural responses need to be implemented directly by the occupational therapist (Dunn & Campbell, 1991). Most often direct hands-on therapy involves use of motor learning, sensory integration, or play therapy, which are individually based techniques that require close monitoring of the child's responses and frequent adaptation of the method. Each action of the occupational therapist is closely tied to the child's responses and reactions. In addition to critical observation skills, the occupational therapist uses clinical reasoning to adapt or modify each activity or piece of equipment to ensure its therapeutic benefit. Activities are adapted so that a "just right" challenge is presented, the child effectively copes with that challenge, and the activity is intrinsically rewarding. Direct therapy is the best model when specific physical or behavioral handling is required and when a combination of verbal, visual, and physical cues is needed to assist in the child's performance (Case-Smith, 1996).

Direct services are frequently provided in the child's natural environments (e.g., at home or in the classroom). Figure 9-3 provides an example of therapy activities in the classroom. Although services in the child's everyday environment promote generalization of the skills learned, an isolated environment (e.g., the therapy clinic) is sometimes useful when the full attention of the child is needed, when a more intimate interaction is desirable, or when certain types of equipment are to be used. Direct services may be provided with intense frequency for a short period, then later with less frequency and with greater reliance on family members, teachers, and assistants to carry out the program.

■ MONITORING

When the occupational therapist monitors the intervention program, he or she evaluates the child, develops a program, and teaches others in the child's environment to implement the program. The therapist remains responsible for the outcome of the plan and oversees the

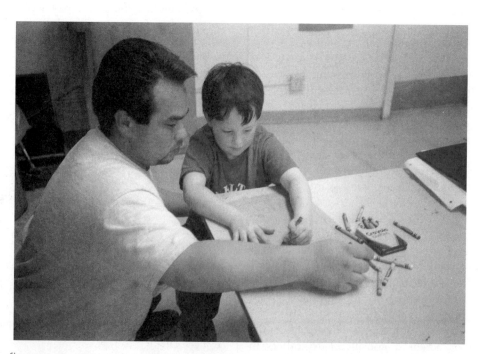

figure 9-3 This child is tracing a football play that will be used during the game at recess. The therapist provides visual and verbal assistance to promote his accuracy in tracing.

program to ensure that the procedures are implemented on a consistent basis. Although the therapist may not directly interact with the child on an ongoing basis, he or she remains in regular contact with the persons who carry out the program, evaluates their verbal feedback about the child's progress, and suggests modifications of the program if needed.

Dunn and Campbell (1991) recommend that monitoring is an appropriate model of service delivery when three criteria are met: (1) the health and safety of the child are protected when the plan and procedures are carried out by the implementor, (2) the implementor correctly demonstrates the procedure, and (3) the implementor demonstrates knowledge of child cues that indicate that the procedure needs to be discontinued or modified.

To effectively use monitoring, the occupational therapist must demonstrate the ability to teach other adults and to share his or her knowledge in ways that enable the performance of others. Because the therapist remains responsible for the child's program, although he or she is not the daily implementor, monitoring involves trust in other team members, the ability to articulate intent and specific activities clearly, and skill in motivating, encouraging, and coaching other adults (Rainforth & York-Barr, 1997).

■ CONSULTATION

Consultative services are designed to enable others to meet their expressed goals (Dunn, 1991; Dunn & Campbell, 1991). In consultation the therapist uses his or her knowledge to enable another person to interact with the child or group of children successfully in a way that promotes functional skills. Often the therapist provides consultation when a student or child's problem arises, suggesting that the expertise of the occupational therapist would be helpful. On request for consultation the therapist typically confers with the teacher to gain his or her perspective, observes the student or evaluates the student, and makes recommendations. Consultation is an effective choice when skills need to be generalized to the natural environment or when the environment can be adapted to support improved functional skills. The therapist uses consultation with the teacher or other members of the team to establish therapeutic routines or to adapt specific tasks and activities expected of the child.

Dunn (1991) listed two goals in consultation: (1) to create solutions that remediate the immediate problems that the child is experiencing, and (2) to increase the consultee's skills so that he or she can respond more effectively to similar problems that arise in the future. Commitment to the second goal implies that the occupational therapist helps the consultee learn and generalize new skills. By promoting the consultee's skills, this model of service delivery holds benefits beyond the specific child's problem, which was the original basis of the occupational therapy consultation.

Most of the work in developing consultative models has been done in the fields of education, psychology, and social work. Idol, Paolucci-Whitcomb, and Nevin (1987) described a model of collaborative consultation that meets the goals listed previously. This model helps remediate the student's problems and enables the consultee to manage future situations that involve similar problems.

In collaborative consultation, teams of professionals meet to solve problems and develop solutions (Figure 9-4). The team members work together to identify the problem and solution, to formulate a plan, and to evaluate the recommendation. It is characterized by a trusting relationship in which each partner appreciates and respects the skills and ideas of the other. Each partner is committed to the plan, taking responsibility for portions of the plan. Because of the collaboration, new strategies are tried, responses are evaluated, and adaptations to the strategies are made (Case-Smith, 1996).

To provide effective consultation, the occupational therapist directly interacts with the child. Opportunities to observe (and handle, when appropriate) the child help the therapist develop an understanding of strengths and limitations that guide his or her decision making (clinical reasoning). Once the occupational therapist and consultee have formulated a plan and the recommendations are implemented, the occupational therapy consultant regularly observes and interacts with the child to evaluate the effectiveness of the recommendations and to monitor changes in the child. Extensive follow-up and evaluation are important for effective results. An ongoing collaborative relationship between the occupational therapist and the consultee helps ensure that the plan is implemented and, when needed, revised. The relationship also ensures that the consultee gains new skills in working with the child and solving similar problems that may arise.

■ KNOWLEDGE AND SKILLS FOR EFFECTIVE TREATMENT IMPLEMENTATION

Once the service delivery model has been determined, the therapist must decide what activities, procedures, and techniques will best facilitate success in meeting the goals. This is where the art and science of occupational therapy converge. The effective therapist uses knowledge gained through scientific inquiry and study along with creativity and problem-solving skills to implement a treatment program that will meet each child's unique needs. Several types of knowledge and skills are needed.

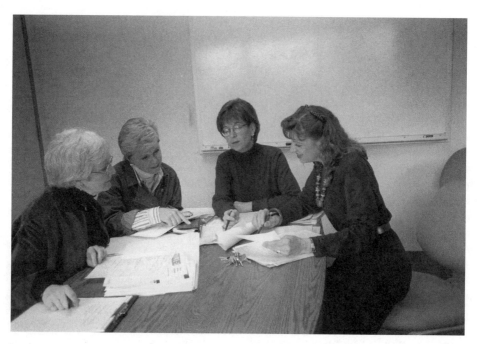

figure**9-4**   The assessment team meets to review their test results, share their perceptions, and develop program recommendations.

Some are specific to the profession of occupational therapy. Many of these are thoroughly discussed in subsequent chapters of this book. Other knowledge is relevant to all professionals who work with children. Some of the most important areas of knowledge and skills are highlighted in this section, with case studies used to illustrate the practical application of these skills.

Child management skills, such as the ability to deal with behavior effectively and motivate children for optimal performance, are important in all professions and in all types of service delivery but are especially critical when providing direct intervention. The most effective way of managing and motivating children is to focus the intervention on an occupation that is developmentally appropriate and functionally relevant, using activities that are interesting and meaningful to the child. Activities are most often presented in a playful context.

At the same time, behavioral and performance expectations must be made clear in a way that is appropriate to the child's level of understanding. When possible, the therapist takes the child's lead and follows activity ideas that the child has initiated. An understanding of the psychosocial and cognitive development of children is essential to do this effectively. Additionally, techniques such as limit setting and creative presentation of activities assist the therapist in maintaining control over the flow of the session. At the same time, the child is presented with choices and allowed to have a voice in the process. In older children, decision making during intervention ac-

tivities becomes vital to their participation and interest in the therapy process.

Another important skill for treatment success is the ability to work effectively with adults, including caregivers, family members, teachers, and others involved in the child's life. In Figure 9-5, the therapist has designed a therapeutic play activity that both the mother and daughter enjoy. The therapist must be willing to solicit and listen to the concerns and priorities of others. He or she must then take this information and understand how it relates to assessment findings, environmental characteristics, and child needs and priorities. In most treatment settings the therapist functions as a member of a professional team. Many decisions regarding assessment and programming are made as a team. These skills are essential to participate in the group problem-solving process. The therapist must also develop skills in teaching adults so that ideas and suggestions for home programs and environmental adaptations are effectively communicated (Rainforth & York-Barr, 1997).

The following case studies illustrate the relationship between the knowledge of psychosocial development and successful implementation of a therapy program at different developmental stages.

Case Study 3

Charles was a corrected age of 4 months at the time of referral to occupational therapy for a feeding assessment. His history included prematurity and respiratory distress.

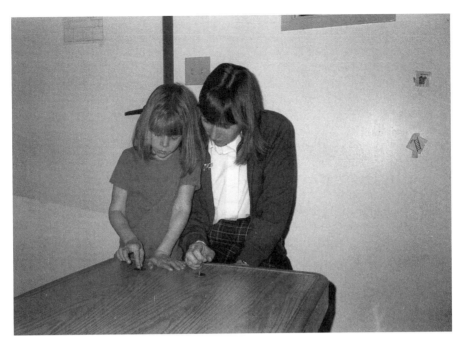

figure 9-5 The occupational therapist suggests a play activity that both the mother and her daughter can enjoy and play at home.

He made a poor transition from tube feeding to oral feeding and demonstrated poor weight gain since oral feedings were initiated. Feedings were time and energy consuming for Charles and his mother, and she expressed frustration to the occupational therapist that she did not adequately provide for her infant's most basic need. Acknowledging that the infant's primary relationship is with the parents or primary caregivers, the therapist centered her intervention on techniques that would facilitate the development of this relationship (Schultz-Krohn, 1997). She taught Charles' mother how to read his physiologic and behavioral cues so that she would time her interactions with him to correspond with his level of readiness. She also demonstrated techniques such as jaw and cheek support and positioning techniques to facilitate feeding efficiency. Additionally, she helped Charles' mother discover ways to use feeding time as an opportunity for social interaction. After the occupational therapy intervention, efficiency of feeding improved, rate of weight gain increased, and Charles' mother reported increased satisfaction with the quality of her interactions with her infant.

Case Study 4

Maria was 4 years old at the time of her referral for occupational therapy services to improve self-care function. Her diagnosis was arthrogryposis that resulted in severe limitation in strength and mobility of all joints. At the time of referral, Maria's mother expressed that Maria was

ready to do more for herself but was fearful of movement and preferred to have things done for her.

Maria arrived at the evaluation dressed in a lacy pink tutu and a tiara. In commenting on this striking outfit, the therapist discovered that Maria was involved in a fantasy of being a fairy princess. The therapist knew that preschool children are often fascinated by the activities of favorite cartoon, television, or movie characters and that they enjoyed fantasy games involving these characters. Impersonation of a powerful or glamorous "superhero" can help children of this age feel that they have more control over their world and practice roles that they will assume as adults (Haight & Miller, 1993). The therapist can use this developmental stage effectively to encourage participation in activities that the child may perceive as difficult, challenging, and potentially threatening by encouraging this fantasy play. This encouragement motivates and engages the child in therapeutic activities and facilitates repetition and practice to promote skill development. When activities match the child's developmental stage and interest, the child often readily attempts the activity without adult prompting, further extending opportunities for practice and mastery.

The therapist used this knowledge to set up fantasy dress-up activities during Maria's therapy sessions. With the help of Maria's mother, the therapist collected hair ornaments, dress-up clothing, and play makeup and set up a "vanity table" in front of a wall mirror. The therapist also adapted the environment to provide necessary supports and provided physical assistance when needed for success. While Maria engaged in repeatedly donning and doffing articles of clothing and arranging and rearranging her hair and makeup, she was practicing the skills needed for independence in self-care.

This activity was so successful that Maria asked if she could invite two neighborhood friends along for a dress-up party. When her two friends accompanied her to therapy, the three children interacted on a reciprocal basis and Maria was as actively involved in the play activity as her peers. Maria's mother stated that Maria's dependence on her mother and her fearfulness to attempt new activities had limited her ability to interact with other children. She was thrilled to see Maria interacting with other children on an equal basis and planned to continue similar activities at home.

Case Study 5

Brian has autism and attended third grade in a full inclusion program. He received school-based occupational therapy services for sensory processing and motor coordination deficits. Brian's teacher asked for the occupational therapist's advice because the children in the class refused to allow Brian to participate in playground games, complaining that "he messes up their games." From her observation of Brian on the playground, the therapist knew that Brian had poor body awareness and frequently intruded into others' personal space, a practice that irritates other children. He did not appear to attend to the rules of the games, running onto the playing field at inappropriate times, and does not focus on the game when it is his turn. His poor coordination also affected his performance, but the teacher and therapist agree that if Brian's behavior was more appropriate, the other children would be more forgiving of his poor motor skills and allow him to participate.

The therapist knew that school-age children are interested in organized games and sports involving rules and are concerned with fairness and equity. They also are occupied with peer interactions and the rules of behavior (Parker & Gottman, 1989). This is why Brian's behavior is so upsetting to his classmates. The therapist can use these characteristics effectively to address therapeutic goals. Therapy in groups is often appropriate for children of this age. Both cooperative and competitive activities can be used to motivate children to engage in activities that address intervention goals. At this age, children's desire to have power over their world is often manifested as a desire to help others. This can be used effectively in therapy by working with mixed age groups, having children assist younger or less able children, and integrating children into age-appropriate activities involving typically developing children.

Children with autism often require specific training in the behaviors appropriate to a specific social setting for them to participate appropriately in that setting. Haring and Lovinger (1989) observed a group of preschoolers at play, identified the social roles assumed by the children in the play activities, and coached a group of preschoolers with autism so that they could assume a social niche in the play activities. The children with autism began to use the social initiation skills taught to them by the examiners to take a role in the play without further adult intervention.

Using this knowledge, the therapist enlisted the cooperation of Brian, his teacher, and his classmates in helping Brian learn the rules of kickball, a popular game in his class. The therapist coaches Brian on the rules of play by working with him individually and with one or two other children in the therapy clinic. After Brian began to demonstrate a basic understanding of the game, the therapist moved the therapy session to the playground and worked with Brian and his classmates to coach him in an actual game situation. The other children, feeling an investment in this process, actively assisted in cueing Brian and in cheering him on when he played by the rules. The therapist demonstrated positive cueing and feedback strategies to help Brian succeed, and on subsequent days the children used these strategies to continue to help Brian learn the game and interact more appropriately. The combination of cooperation and competition applied in Brian's real-life setting (the playground) by the participation of Brian's peers, provided a far more powerful intervention than the therapist could provide individually, and facilitated the acceptance of Brian's into his peer group.

Case Study 6

At 16 years of age, Jennifer, diagnosed with spastic quadriplegic cerebral palsy, had received direct occupational and physical therapy throughout most of her childhood. She had not received direct services since she was 12 years of age, when her resistance to therapy and lack of progress caused Jennifer, her therapists, and her parents to decide to discontinue direct therapy. She had been monitored since that time with periodic reassessments. During one of these assessments, Jennifer stated that her friends were beginning to get their driver's licenses and that she would like to do so also. She also voiced her concern that decreased coordination made it difficult for her to manage fastenings on the type of clothing that she likes to wear, to style her hair to her satisfaction, and to apply makeup. However, she was reluctant to begin therapy sessions again, because she felt that this would isolate her from her friends. The therapist was aware that these concerns represent an age-appropriate interest in achieving independence and fitting in with the peer group. The therapist was also aware that a short-term therapy program specifically directed toward these goals would most likely have a high rate of follow through and motivation on Jennifer's part and would possibly override her concerns about appearing different to her friends.

With this awareness the therapist, in cooperation with Jennifer and her parents, set up a two-part program. First, she communicated with the adapted driving program in the rehabilitation department of a nearby university, providing information on Jennifer's motor, cognitive, and functional status. Once Jennifer was deemed an appropriate candidate for adapted driving instruction, the therapist contacted Jennifer and her family so that they could make an appointment with the occupational therapist in the adapted driving program.

After the adapted driving program was initiated, the therapist discussed desired self-care outcomes with Jennifer. The therapist described to Jennifer the types of intervention and adapted equipment that could be provided to facilitate her independence in self-care, allowing her to make informed choices about the direction of her occupational therapy program. The therapist also discussed possible service delivery options so that Jennifer would not miss important academic and social activities to receive intervention. Jennifer identified three priorities for her self-care independence and selected a preferred schedule and location for her therapy program. She and the therapist then proceeded to work directly on the functional outcomes that Jennifer identified.

By allowing Jennifer to take the lead in identifying treatment priorities, the therapist validated her growing maturity and desire for independence while acknowledging her need to feel like a part of the group. The therapist also provided a reality check, informing Jennifer about realistic expectations for therapy outcomes. This increased the likelihood that the therapy program would result in outcomes that are achievable, meaningful, and functional for Jennifer at this stage in her life.

■ SUMMARY

Intervention planning requires careful interpretation of assessment information, clear communication of concerns about the child, and willingness to consider creative options for helping the child. The key to the process is the therapist's and team's ability to develop consensus around a plan that meets the child's needs, builds on cur-

rent child and family strengths, addresses family priorities, and reaches toward a future vision for the child. An intervention plan that specifies the desired functional outcomes in the child's performance context is an essential tool for communicating occupational therapy goals, ensures accountability for services provided, and becomes a basis for measuring the effectiveness of intervention services. The therapist uses clinical reasoning to develop the intervention and implementation plan and to adapt the intervention program to meet the child's changing needs. Use of creative problem-solving skills and knowledge of children's cognitive and psychosocial development allows therapists to base decisions regarding intervention planning and management of the intervention program on sound developmental principles and a holistic understanding of the child. This basis for intervention and development of an open relationship with the adults who surround the child facilitates optimal functional outcomes.

STUDY QUESTIONS

1. Use each of the case studies to identify clinical reasoning strategies used in the intervention and implementation planning processes.

2. Apply the short- and long-term goal writing process to the case study of Justin to generate additional goals that are measurable, behaviorally specific, and contextually specific.

3. Identify which practice models and frames of reference the occupational therapist used in the case study of Michelle.

4. Describe the service delivery models used in the case studies of Charles, Maria, Brian, and Jennifer. Write at least one long-term and two short-term goals based on the service delivery model, frame of reference, and background information provided.

5. List at least three therapy activities that are appropriate for the children in each of the case studies. Use the background information and guiding questions in Boxes 9-2 and 9-7 to help you.

References

American Occupational Therapy Association. (1994). Standards of practice. *American Journal of Occupational Therapy, 48,* 1047-1054.

American Occupational Therapy Association. (1997). *Occupational therapy services for children and youth under the Individuals with Disabilities Education Act.* Bethesda, MD: American Occupational Therapy Association.

Ayres, A.J. (1979). *Sensory integration and the child.* Los Angeles: Western Psychological Services.

Case-Smith, J. (1996). Planning and implementing services. In J. Case-Smith, A. Allen, & P. Pratt (Eds.), *Occupational therapy for children* (3rd ed.). (pp 225-246). St. Louis: Mosby.

Christiansen, C., & Baum, C. (1997). Person-environment occupational performance. In C. Christiansen & C. Baum (Eds.), *Occupational therapy: Enabling function and well-being* (2nd ed.). (pp.46-70). Thorofare, NJ: Slack.

Colangelo, C. (1999). Biomechanical frame of reference. In P. Kramer & J. Hinojosa (Eds.), *Frames of reference for pediatric occupational therapy* (2nd ed.). (pp. 233-305). Baltimore, MD: Lippincott Williams & Wilkins.

Crepeau, E. (1991). Achieving intersubjective understanding: Examples from an occupational therapy treatment session. *American Journal of Occupational Therapy, 45,* 1016-1025.

Dunn, W. (1991). Consultation as a process: How, when, and why? In C. Royeen (Ed.), *AOTA self study series: School-based practice for related services.* Rockville, MD: American Occupational Therapy Association.

Dunn, W., & Campbell, P. (1991). Designing pediatric service provision. In W. Dunn (Ed.), *Pediatric occupational therapy.* Thorofare, NJ: Slack.

Fleming, M. (1991a). Clinical reasoning in medicine compared with clinical reasoning in occupational therapy. *American Journal of Occupational Therapy, 45,* 988-996.

Fleming, M. (1991b). The therapist with the three track mind. *American Journal of Occupational Therapy, 45,* 1007-1014.

Gerlach, E.K. (1996). *Autism treatment guide.* Eugene, OR: Four Leaf Press.

Haight, W., & Miller, P. (1993). *The ecology and development of pretend play.* Albany: State University of New York Press.

Haring, T.G., & Lovinger, L. (1989). Promoting social interaction through teaching generalized play initiation responses to preschool children with autism. *Journal of the Association for Persons with Severe Handicaps, 14* (1), 255-262.

Idol, L., Paolucci-Whitcomb, P., & Nevin, A. (1987). *Collaborative consultation.* Austin, TX: Pro Ed.

Kalmanson, B., & Seligman, S. (1992). Family-provider relationships: The basis of all interventions. *Infants and Young Children, 4,* 46-52.

Kielhofner, G., & Burke, J. (1985). Components and determinants of human occupation. In G. Kielhofner (Ed.), *A model of human occupation* (pp. 12-36). Baltimore, MD: Williams & Wilkins.

Kimball, J. (1999). Sensory integrative frame of reference. In P. Kramer & J. Hinojosa (Eds.), *Frames of reference for pediatric occupational therapy* (2nd ed.) (pp. 87-175). Baltimore, MD: Lippincott Williams & Wilkins.

Kramer, P., & Hinojosa, J. (1999). Structure of the frame of reference. In P. Kramer & J. Hinojosa (Eds.), *Frames of reference for pediatric occupational therapy* (2nd ed.). (pp. 37-48). Baltimore, MD: Lippincott Williams & Wilkins.

Mattingly, C. (1991a). The narrative nature of clinical reasoning. *American Journal of Occupational Therapy, 45,* 1016-1025.

Mattingly, C. (1991b). What is clinical reasoning? *American Journal of Occupational Therapy, 45,* 979-986.

Mattingly, C., & Fleming, M.H. (1994). *Clinical reasoning: Forms inquiry in a therapeutic practice.* Philadelphia: F.A. Davis.

Parker, J.G., & Gottman, J.M. (1989). Social and emotional development in a relational context: Friendship interaction from early childhood to adolescence. In T.J. Berndt & G.W. Ladd (Eds.), *Peer relationships in child development.* New York: Wiley.

Rainforth, B., & York-Barr, J. (1997). *Collaborative teams for students with severe disabilities: Integrating therapy and educational services.* Baltimore: Brookes.

Schkade, J., & Schultz, S. (1992). Occupational adaptation: Toward a holistic approach for contemporary practice, part 1. *American Journal of Occupational Therapy, 46,* 829-837.

Schultz, S., & Schkade, J. (1992). Occupational adaptation: Toward a holistic approach for contemporary practice, part 2. *American Journal of Occupational Therapy, 46,* 998-1005.

Schultz-Krohn, W. (1997). Early intervention: Meeting the unique needs of parent-child interaction. *Infants and Young Children, 10,* 47-60.

Teasdale, G., & Jennett, B. (1974). Assessment of coma and impaired consciousness: A practical scale. *Lancet, 2,* 81-84.

Zimmerman, J. (1988). *Goals and objectives for developing normal movement patterns.* Rockville, MD: Aspen Publishing.

section **III**

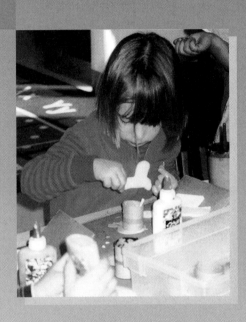

OCCUPATIONAL THERAPY INTERVENTION: PERFORMANCE AREAS

chapter 10

Development of Postural Control

Deborah S. Nichols

■ CHAPTER OBJECTIVES

1. Describe the development of postural control systems and the influence of that development on gross and fine-motor development.
2. Discuss atypical development of postural control and its influence on the development of gross and fine-motor skills.
3. Identify appropriate assessment tools available for the evaluation of postural control.
4. Identify appropriate treatment techniques for facilitating reactive and anticipatory postural control.
5. Apply the knowledge gained in this chapter to specific case studies of children with postural control deficits.

Early child development is characterized by the emergence of a series of motor milestones (rolling, crawling, creeping, and walking), which parents track and brag about to their friends and which therapists use to identify developmental delays. However, underlying these observable milestones is the emergence of postural control, which is the ability to maintain body alignment while upright in space. Thus postural development and motor development are inextricably linked.

Postural control requires the development of both muscle strength that allows for *antigravity movements* and proximal-axial muscle control, which results in dynamic patterns of cocontraction and mature equilibrium responses. In the past, therapists conceptualized postural and motor development as a hierarchy in which high-level brain structures (i.e., the cortex) control and mediate the functions of lower-level brain structures (i.e., the brainstem). Under the hierarchic model of *neuromotor control*, postural and motor development was thought to be determined by maturation of the nervous system, resulting in the emergence of increasingly advanced reflex patterns and eventually voluntary movement as higher levels of the nervous system developed (Woollacott, Shumway-Cook, & Williams, 1989). In addition, postural control was considered to mirror motor development and proceed in a cephalocaudal and proximodistal manner (Bly, 1983; Connor, Williamson, & Siepp, 1978).

Recent research suggests (1) an interplay between higher and lower system control; (2) control of complex movements, not just reflexes, at low levels of the nervous system; and (3) an overlap in the emergence of proximal versus distal control as well as head and trunk control. All of these contradict the hierarchic model. Furthermore, the hierarchic model of motor development does not adequately explain the high level of variability in child development (e.g., why some babies roll at 4 months and others at 6 months or why some babies roll leading with their head and others leading with their legs).

Recently, system theories of motor control have been used to explain motor development, influencing the way that therapists view development. System theories recognize that postural and motor development result from more than maturation of a hierarchically organized nervous system. These theories acknowledge the importance of muscle strength, body mass, sensory system function, behavioral systems, and environmental constraints on motor and postural development. They also begin to answer the question of why babies develop at such variable rates (e.g., why a baby born weighing 10 pounds acquires motor milestones at a later age than a baby born weighing 7 pounds or why active babies acquire motor milestones faster than less active babies). Systems theories begin to provide explanations of these phenomena.

This chapter uses these recently developed theories to explain assessment and intervention for postural and motor function in children. It includes descriptions of the development of antigravity movement, postural reactions and control, sensory processing associated with postural control and anticipatory postural control, and the interaction of postural control development and motor milestone acquisition. Evaluations of all of these components of posture are described, and intervention strategies for improving postural control, and indirectly motor development, are provided.

■ DEVELOPMENT OF ANTIGRAVITY MOVEMENT

An important aspect of postural control is the development of antigravity movement. Margaret Rood proposed a four-stage sequence in the development of movement: (1) mobility, (2) stability, (3) mobility superimposed on stability, and (4) skill (Stockmeyer, 1967) (Figure 10-1). The stage of mobility is characterized by the development of antigravity movement. This stage is followed by the development of muscle cocontraction at the proximal joints, producing stability sufficient for the maintenance of weight-bearing postures. Once stability is achieved, the child superimposes movement on this stability, characterized by Rood as proximal movement on a fixed distal limb component. An example of this behavior is the infant who assumes a quadruped position and then begins to rock back and forth (proximal movement on a fixed distal limb component, the hands and knees). The last stage is characterized by skill or the ability to combine stability and mobility in non–weight-bearing postures (e.g., reach, grasp, and

manipulation) (Stockmeyer, 1967). Rood's model suggests that the development of postural control and movement are integrated.

An important component of the development of mobility and stability is the development of antigravity movement. Pountney, Mulcahy, and Green (1990) identified six levels in the development of antigravity movement, which were associated with more mature movement patterns, in both the prone and supine positions (Figures 10-2 and 10-3). Using this sequence, the child develops an increased ability to move against gravity with all body parts, demonstrated by a shift from lateral movements to midline movements as antigravity muscle strength is achieved. The newborn infant is asymmetric, with the head turned to the side and arm and leg movements occurring in the lateral plane. Furthermore, the progression involves movement of the center of gravity from the upper body toward the pelvis, which is associated with increased freedom of movement of the head and extremities, allowing head control and extremity weight bearing to develop. Also, this progression includes a dissociation of the body segments so that the infant can roll segmentally, lift one leg, and reach across midline with one hand. Accordingly, the progression from one level to the next involves changes in head control, trunk control, and extremity movement and therefore does not follow a strict cephalocaudal progression. In addition, the change from one level to the next coincides with the integration of the preceding level in both prone and supine positions.

Similar changes in neck and trunk extension, including increased scapular stabilization, occur in the acquisition of independent sitting. The posture of an infant when placed in a sitting position is one of total trunk flexion. This stage is followed by one in which the child exhibits increasing trunk extensor strength but has difficulty grading the activation of the back extensor muscles. When placed in a sitting position, the child frequently activates the back extensors without sufficient coactivation of the trunk flexors and, as a result, falls backward. At this time the child uses upper-extremity weight bearing (propping) to maintain a sitting position. Finally, the child develops sufficient strength of the trunk muscles to allow upright sitting. These changes in the development of antigravity trunk extension with reciprocal trunk flexion and the emergence of sitting stability are depicted in Figure 10-4 on page 271.

As stated previously, the *development of postural control* is tightly linked to the acquisition of motor milestones. The center of gravity is initially located toward the head and then moves toward the pelvis. This shift frees the upper body from providing static stability to demonstrating dynamic mobility as the child moves in and out of upper-extremity weight-bearing positions. As the center of gravity moves to the pelvis, the child dem-

PROGRESSION OF MOTOR DEVELOPMENT

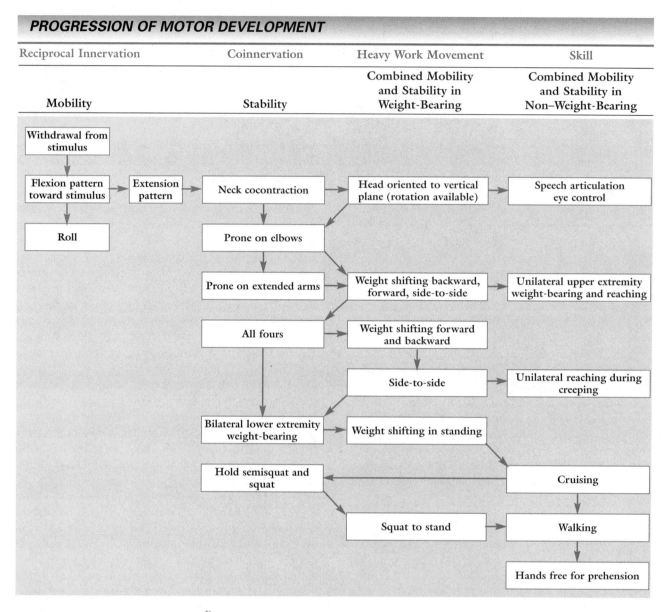

Reciprocal Innervation	Coinnervation	Heavy Work Movement	Skill
Mobility	Stability	Combined Mobility and Stability in Weight-Bearing	Combined Mobility and Stability in Non–Weight-Bearing

figure **10-1** Rood's developmental progression.

onstrates increased independence in extremity movement and dissociation of body parts, including rotation through the trunk and pelvis. When the child first attempts new postures against gravity, he or she tends to stiffen the trunk to achieve the stability needed. For example, when the child begins to sit and stand, he or she shows minimal rotation. With practice and experience the child uses rotation in each new posture. This rotation increases movement opportunities for the child and enables him or her to make transitions from one posture to another (e.g., sitting to quadruped) (Connor et. al., 1978). The approximate ages of motor milestone acquisition are depicted in Table 10-1. Although an age range is provided for each skill, individual development is highly variable, and thus many factors should be taken into account when using age ranges to evaluate motor development.

The development of antigravity muscle strength has also been found to coincide with the development of higher-level balance and motor skills. In addition, there is an interaction between the posture of the child, the weight of the limb and body, and the emergence of antigravity movement. Newborns demonstrate infantile stepping, involving antigravity hip flexion, which "disappears" typically during the second month and reemerges during the fifth or sixth month before the emergence of cruising and walking. Hierarchic theorists explained this change in behavior as secondary to maturation of higher

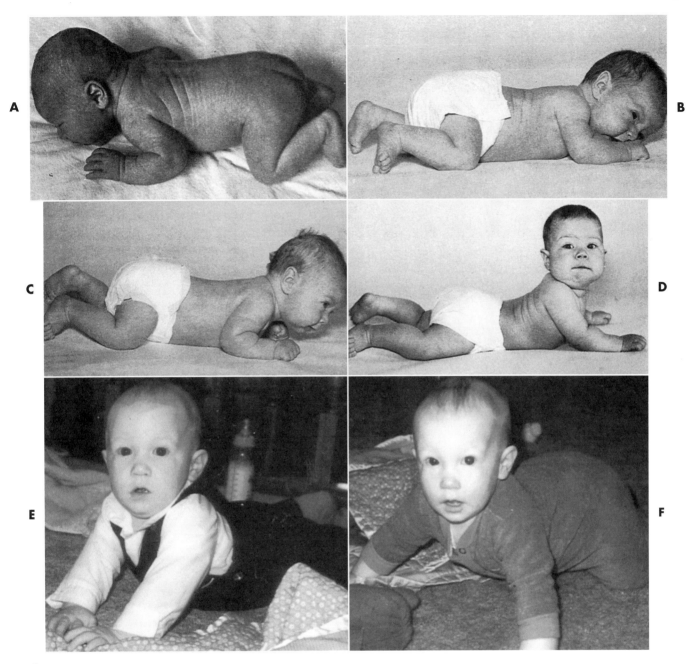

figure 10-2   Prone development of antigravity movement. **A,** Level 1: "Top heavy." Weight-bearing is through chest, shoulders, and face. Pelvis is posteriorly tilted, hips and knees are flexed, and shoulder girdle is retracted. Posture is asymmetric, and head is to one side. **B,** Level 2: Child settles when placed. Weight-bearing is through chest and upper abdomen. Shoulder girdle is retracted, shoulders are flexed and adducted, head is to one side, and child is beginning to lift head from floor but not sustaining. Posture is asymmetric, and bottom is moving laterally as head turns side-to-side. **C,** Level 3: Child maintains prone position with neutral pelvis, and shoulder girdle is beginning to protract. Symmetric weight-bearing is through abdomen, lower chest, knees, and thighs. Child maintains head lift from floor. Child has no lateral weight shift and therefore often topples into supine position when lifting head and chest. **D,** Level 4: Pelvis is anteriorly tilted but not "anchoring." Shoulder girdle is protracted, and child bears weight through abdomen and thighs, varying between forearm and hand propping with shoulders elevated. Head and upper trunk movement is dissociated from lower trunk, allowing lateral trunk flexion with lateral weight shift (a beginning of pivoting). Unilateral leg is kicking, and hand and foot play is midline. **E,** Level 5: Pelvis is anteriorly tilted, shoulder girdle is protracted with hand propping, extended elbows, and lumbar spine extension. Weight-bearing is through iliac crest, thighs, and lower abdomen. Deft pivoting with lateral trunk flexion and moving backward on floor. Child rolls purposefully from prone to supine position. **F,** Level 6: Free movement of pelvis and shoulder girdle. Child begins to bear weight on all fours, rocking on all fours.

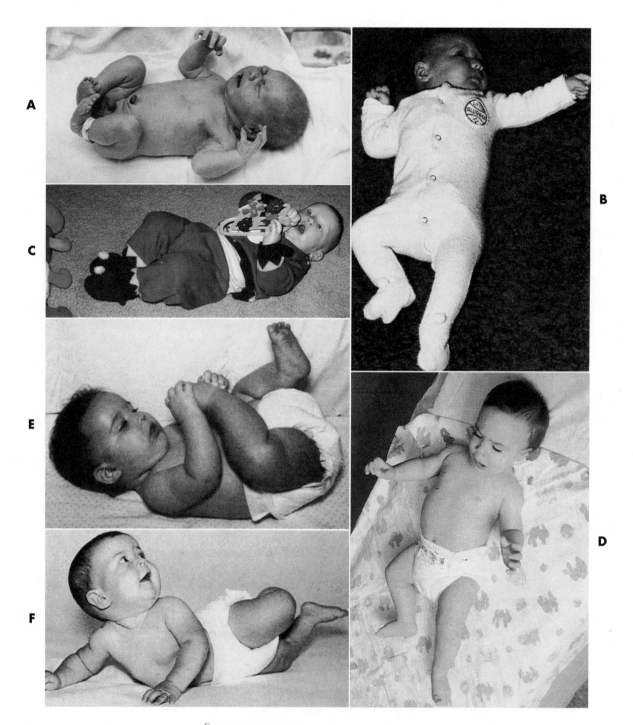

figure**10-3**   For legend see opposite page.

figure**10-3**   Supine development of antigravity movement. **A,** Level 1: Child is unable to maintain supine position when placed, except momentarily, and then position is asymmetric. Child rolls into and maintains side-lying position (body follows head, turning in a total body movement). Weight-bearing is through lateral aspect of head, trunk, and thigh. **B,** Level 2: Child settles when placed on back ("top heavy"). Weight-bearing is through upper trunk and head. Posture is asymmetric (head is to one side), and child has difficulty turning it side-to-side. Bottom moves laterally as the head is turned, resulting in a "corkscrew" appearance. **C,** Level 3: Child maintains supine position with neutral pelvic tilt, hip abduction, and shoulder girdle in neutral position. Posture is symmetric but "top heavy." Chin is tucked (not retracted) and head is in midline and able to move freely from side-to-side without lateral movement of bottom. Child is able to track objects visually and make eye contact. Child begins unilateral grasp to side of body and takes fist and objects to mouth. Child may roll into prone position. **D,** Level 4: Symmetry of posture and movement is first seen at level 4. Shoulders are flexing and adducting, allowing midline play above chest with hands and feet together. Posture is symmetric, and weight-bearing is through upper trunk and pelvis. "Free" pelvic movement is beginning, allowing child to touch knees with flexed hips (but not toes). Child begins to be able to shift weight laterally and raise leg unilaterally, indicating independence of limbs from trunk. Adept finger movements toward end of this stage. **E,** Level 5: Free movement of shoulder girdle and pelvis on trunk. Pelvis has full range of movement, allowing child to play with toes with legs extended and to roll into side-lying position. Child is functional in side-lying position and can return to supine position. Child plays between these postures. Efficient limb movement (hand play and prehensile feet) crossing midline. **F,** Level 6: Pelvic and shoulder girdle move freely. Child is able to roll into prone position by achieving side-lying position (level 5) and then anteriorly tilting pelvis on trunk and extending hips.

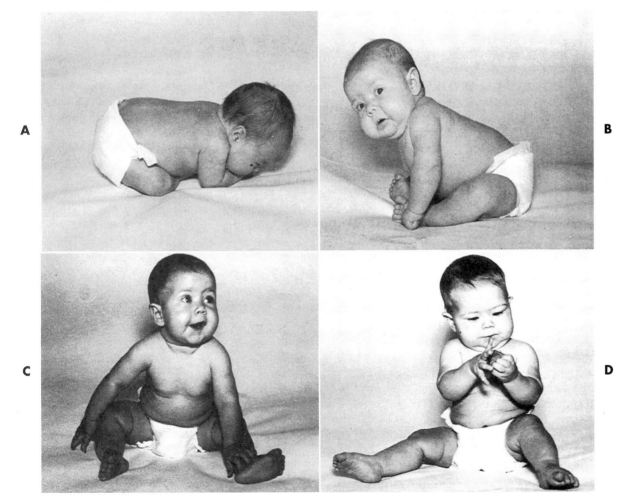

figure**10-4**   Development of antigravity movement in sitting. **A,** Total flexion posture of infant. **B,** Bursts of back extensor activity results in falling backward. **C,** Increased upper extremity strength allows stability in sitting with upper-extremity weight bearing. **D,** Mature sitting posture associated with antigravity trunk and neck extensor strength.

table 10-1	Ages of Motor Milestone Acquisition	
Motor Milestone	**Age in Months**
HEAD CONTROL	
Prone	
Lifts head to 45 degrees	2
Lifts head to 90 degrees	4
Supine	
Maintains in midline	2
Lifts	6
ROLLING	
Prone to supine	
Without rotation	4-6
With rotation	6-9
Supine to prone	
Without rotation	5-7
With rotation	6-9
SITTING	
Unsustained with arm support	4-5
Sustained with arm support	5-6
Unsustained without arm support	6-7
Sustained without arm support	7-9
MOBILITY	
Crawling	7-9
Creeping	9-11
Cruising	9-13
Walking	12-14

brain centers with the subsequent inhibition of lower brain centers. Thelen and Fisher (1982) related the loss of stepping behavior to an increase in the weight of the legs (primarily because of an increase in subcutaneous fat, not muscle), which prevents the demonstration of stepping during these early months. As further evidence of this relationship, they found that infants supported in a standing position in water continued to display stepping. In addition, they explored the relationship between supine kicking and infantile stepping and identified that the pattern of movement was the same (Thelen & Fisher, 1983). Thus the inability of 2- to 5-month-old infants to step seems to be because of the increased weight of the legs and not to a reorganization or maturation of the nervous system.

Additional support for the interaction of antigravity muscle strength and motor development was found in a study of children between 4 and 5½ years of age (Sellers, 1988). The children's abilities to maintain the antigravity postures of prone extension and supine flexion, which require substantial antigravity muscle strength, were highly correlated with static balance (e.g., single limb stance) and dynamic balance capabilities (e.g., balance beam activities). Therefore the development of antigravity movement is strongly associated with the development of higher levels of postural control, balance and movement. Furthermore, the weight of the children was related to the acquisition of antigravity movement. These associations have relevance when asking why the motor development of a baby born weighing 10 pounds might be slower than that of a baby born weighing 7 pounds.

■ EMERGENCE OF POSTURAL REACTIONS

The development of postural reactions (i.e., righting, protective, and equilibrium) has been reported to occur in a predictable sequence with reactions first appearing in the prone position, followed by supine, sitting, quadruped, and standing. Success in the development of these reactions in earlier positions may be a prerequisite for their development in later positions (Connor et. al., 1978).

A series of righting reactions develops in the first year of life and serves to maintain head alignment with the body and upper-body alignment with the lower body. When rotation is imposed on the body, these reactions realign the segments of the body. These reactions also maintain body alignment during forward flexion of the trunk and prone suspension (Barnes & Crutchfield, 1990).

The neck on body righting reaction is observed in two forms. In the immature infant, turning of the head to the side results in a log roll to the side-lying position; in the mature form, turning of the head produces a segmental roll. The body on body righting reaction is similar; rotation of the infant's hips stimulates a log roll of the upper body in the immature form and a segmental roll of the upper body in the mature form to realign the body segments. The body on head righting reaction, serves to influence head position in response to a part of the body touching a support surface (e.g., in the prone position, the tactile input from the stomach touching the support surface stimulates head lifting).

Two other righting reactions give the infant experiences of full body extension and full body flexion. The Landau reaction results in maintenance of body alignment during prone suspension, produced by neck, trunk, and leg extension. When the child is pulled to a sitting position, the development of antigravity neck flexion is associated with the child's ability to maintain head and trunk alignment against the pull of gravity, which is sometimes referred to as the *flexion righting reaction* and

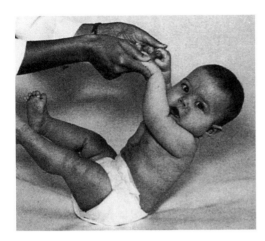

figure**10-5** Flexion response. The development of antigravity neck strength is first associated with the ability to maintain the head aligned with the body when pulled to a sitting position.

table **10-2** *Age of Postural Reactions Acquisition*	
Balance Reactions	**Age (months)**
RIGHTING REACTIONS	
Neck on body	
Immature	Birth
Mature	4-5
Body on body	
Immature	Birth
Mature	4-5
Body on head	
Prone (partial)	1-2
Mature	4-5
Supine	5-6
Landau	
Immature	3
Mature	6-10
Flexion	
Partial (head in line)	3-4
Mature (head forward)	6-7
Vertical	
Partial (head in line)	2
Mature (head to vertical)	6
PROTECTIVE REACTIONS	
Forward	6-7
Lateral	6-11
Backward	9-12
EQUILIBRIUM REACTIONS	
Prone	5-6
Supine	7-8
Sitting	7-10
Quadruped	9-12
Standing	12-21

is demonstrated in Figure 10-5. Table 10-2 provides approximate ages when righting reactions emerge.

Orientation of the body in space involves the maintenance of an upright posture under both static and dynamic conditions. This ability is often called *balance*. The earliest form of body orientation is observed in two vertical righting reflexes: the optical righting reflex and the labyrinthine righting reflex. These two reflexes serve to realign the head vertically when the body is displaced and are mediated, respectively, by the visual and vestibular systems. The maintenance of balance also involves the child's ability to respond adequately to external disturbances (e.g., a push or trip) or self-generated movements (e.g., reaching).

Responses to external disturbances are reactive or compensatory and are classified as equilibrium or protective reactions. These reactions emerge in lower-level positions (supine and prone) when the infant is 4 to 6 months of age. They continue to develop in more upright positions throughout the first 5 years. Equilibrium reactions, often called *tilting reactions* because of the way they are tested, serve to return the child's body to a vertical position after displacement. When the child is supine on a tiltboard, a lateral tilt to the right elicits trunk incurvation to the left, righting of the head, and abduction of the left arm and leg. These same movements are associated with equilibrium reactions in prone, sitting, quadruped, and standing to lateral tilt positions. Figure 10-6 demonstrates equilibrium reactions to lateral displacements in sitting, quadruped, and standing positions. In addition, when the child is in upright postures (e.g., sitting or kneeling), tilting anteriorly or posteriorly results in a corrective movement in the opposite direction to the tilt (i.e., posterior

to an anterior displacement), returning the body to an upright position. Protective reactions differ from equilibrium reactions in that they protect the infant from a fall rather than correct a displacement. Therefore these reactions are characterized by extension of the extremities to "catch" the child as he or she falls, and they occur in the direction of the fall.

Haley (1986) assessed the emergence of a series of righting, protective, and equilibrium reactions in infants between 2 and 10 months of age. Righting reactions emerged first in all positions, at least in their immature forms, before the development of any protective or equilibrium reactions in these postures. However, the development of protective and equilibrium reactions was overlapping within a given posture and between postures. For example, protective reactions in the sitting position developed at the same time as the equilibrium reactions. In addition, equilibrium reactions began to develop in higher-level positions (e.g., quadruped) and continued to be refined in lower-level positions (e.g., supine) simultaneously (Haley, 1986). These findings are inconsistent with a hierarchic explanation of motor development but are easily explained through systems theories, which posit simultaneous and overlapping development of higher and lower level brain areas and corresponding motor functions.

■ NATURE VERSUS NURTURE IN THE EMERGENCE OF POSTURAL CONTROL AND MOTOR MILESTONES

Historically, the emergence of postural reactions was attributed to the maturation of the nervous system as predicated on the hierarchic model of motor control. Although the debate on the effects of nature and nurture raged in the areas of psychologic and language development, little attention was paid to the role of experience on motor development. However, recent research provides substantial evidence for the role of experience in development of postural control and acquisition of motor milestones.

First, the amount of experience that a child has in a given posture has been found to influence the development of mature postural reactions as evidenced by patterns of muscle activation. Woollacott, Debu, and Mowatt (1988) found that infants younger than 5 months of age demonstrated inadequate or absent neck and trunk muscle activation patterns to linear translations in supported sitting. However, infants 6 to 8 months of age who had experience in independent sitting demonstrated appropriate activation patterns of the neck and trunk muscles to the same translations. Similar differences in the standing position were identified between infants who had not yet developed independent stance and those who had. In addition, young children tend to demonstrate larger amplitude of muscle activation and greater variability in the activation patterns (Shumway-Cook & Woollacott, 1985a; Williams, Fisher, & Tritschler, 1983). Thus the maturation of the nervous system can set the foundation for the emergence of these reactions, and postural reactions relate to experience in a given position and to neuronal maturation.

Similarly, the development of motor skills appears dependent on experience in given postures. Recent research has found that infants who sleep in the prone position roll from prone to supine earlier than infants who sleep in either the side-lying or supine position. Additionally,

some infants whose primary sleeping position was supine rolled from supine to prone before rolling from prone to supine (Jantz, Blosser, & Fruechting, 1997). Thus the sleeping position of an infant, or more likely the time that the child spends in either the prone or supine position, influences the emergence of rolling.

Evidence of the influence of experience on motor development suggests that training, practice, and experience can affect motor skill acquisition. Practicing reaching, with emphasis on reaching to the side and semibackward, facilitates the development of postural muscle activity in sitting in infants between 5 and 9 months of age (Hadders-Algra, Brogren, & Forssberg, 1997). Similarly, infants who practiced stepping on a treadmill between 3 and 7 months of age were found to demonstrate an increase in stepping behavior (Vereijken & Thelen, 1997). Findings such as these support the interactive nature of neuromotor maturation and environmental experience.

■ SENSORY SYSTEMS ASSOCIATED WITH POSTURAL CONTROL

Three sensory systems contribute to the child's awareness of orientation in space: the visual system, the vestibular system, and the somatosensory system. The visual system provides a representation of the vertical plane that is dependent on the objects in the visual field. The child's somatosensory system provides input from proprioceptors, mechanoreceptors, and cutaneous receptors, which supply information about limb position and support surface characteristics. The vestibular system provides a constant gravitational reference for postural orientation with which the child compares visual and somatosensory input. When the three sensory systems provide disparate information, a feeling of disequilibrium results. Discrepancies between the visual and somatosensory cues are decided in favor of the vestibular system (Horak & Nashner, 1986; Nashner, 1990).

As the infant matures, the relative influence of the sensory systems on postural control changes. Newborns demonstrate the ability to orient to a visual stimulus and are capable of tracking a moving object by turning the head if it is supported (Bullinger, 1981). Initially, infants appear to rely more on visual than somatosensory information in developing postural control. Eventually, and with experience in each new posture, this reliance on vision is transferred to reliance on somatosensory cues (Woollacott, 1988; Woollacott et. al., 1989). Studies document that the vestibular system is able to detect accurately postural disturbances at an early age (Jouen, 1984). Infants as young as 4 months of age make appropriate postural responses when they are tilted with their vision occluded. This early maturation of the vestibular system seems to be critical to the development of postural control. However, despite the integrity of the vestibular system early in life, when visual inputs are available, infants and young children tend to rely on them. This dominance of visual input is seen in each transitional state as the child acquires motor milestones. Thus the child first uses visual information to make postural adjustments in sitting. He or she later relies on vestibular and somatosensory input. Similar changes occur in the quadruped and standing positions (Woollacott, 1988). The time course of this transition in standing is long; it is not until 6 or 7 years of age that children appear to switch from a reliance on visual inputs to a reliance on somatosensory inputs similar to that of adults (Shumway-Cook & Woollacott, 1985b).

■ EMERGENCE OF ANTICIPATORY POSTURAL CONTROL

In addition to the automatic reactions described in the preceding paragraphs, postural control also involves the programming of postural muscle activation in association with volitional movement. This activation occurs in a feed-forward manner. *Feedforward* refers to the anticipatory strategies that are observed in the postural adjustments that the individual makes before voluntary movements. These postural adjustments can be observed before the onset of arm, hand, or whole-body movements. This type of anticipatory control is dependent on the child's experience with the task and the environment in which the task takes place. It is also dependent on adequate postural muscle strength. The effect of anticipatory muscle activation is the creation of a stable base on which movement can take place (Bouisset & Zattara, 1981; Forssberg & Nashner, 1982).

Infants as young as 10 months of age demonstrate anticipatory responses to an arm reach in the sitting position, yet these responses are inconsistent until the infant is independent while sitting and has had considerable experience with reaching in this position (von Hofsten, 1986). Investigations of reaching have identified the emergence of anticipatory postural activation in the standing position by 12 to 15 months of age (Forssberg & Nashner, 1982). By 4 years of age, children demonstrate a pattern similar to that found in adults when reaching while standing (Hayes & Riach, 1989). Again, there is an interaction between development and experience. Children must play within a given posture, disturbing their own balance as they reach for toys, lean in all planes, and right themselves for feed-forward control to develop. In therapy sessions, anticipatory control may be facilitated through practice activities.

■ DEVELOPMENTAL CHANGES IN POSTURAL SWAY AND MUSCLE ACTIVATION

Postural sway is the natural movement of the center of gravity within the base of support in any upright position. When standing, a child or an adult is not perfectly still but demonstrates a normal oscillatory movement from side-to-side and forward and back. With recent advances in technology, this postural sway has been evaluated and quantified by using several different techniques. Several studies have examined postural sway in children and have identified a developmental progression. Young children demonstrate significantly more postural sway than older children, with more variability between children and with less influence from closing the eyes (Forssberg & Nashner, 1982; Foudriat, DiFabio, & Anderson, 1993; Riach & Hayes, 1987). In studies that used the Pediatric Clinical Test of Sensory Integration for Balance (P-CTSIB) (Crowe, Deitz, Richardson, & Atwater, 1990; Deitz, Richardson, Atwater, Crowe, & Odiorne, 1991; Richardson, Atwater, Crowe, & Deitz, 1992), mature levels of postural sway in static standing emerge somewhere around 13 years of age. Children between 5 and 7 years of age demonstrate greater sway than younger children, which may be attributable to the transition that occurs at this age between dominance of the visual system and dominance of the somatosensory system for the control of balance in standing (Deitz et. al., 1991; Riach & Hayes, 1987; Shumway-Cook & Woollacott, 1985b).

The muscle activity elicited also varies with age in children. In young children, significantly greater amplitudes of muscle activity are used to maintain a posture than in older children (Berger, Quintern, & Dietz, 1985; Haas, Diener, Bacher, & Dichgans, 1986). Thus young children tend to use more muscles than do older children to maintain balance, and they require a greater degree of muscle contraction than do older children. With experience in a given posture, there is a natural refinement in the muscle activity needed to maintain the posture (Shumway-Cook & Woollacott, 1985b; Williams et. al., 1983; Woollacott & Sveistrup, 1992).

■ OTHER INFLUENCES ON MOTOR AND POSTURAL CONTROL DEVELOPMENT

Systems theorists and motor learning theorists have sparked interest in the influence of other systems, outside of the neuromotor system, on the development of postural control and motor milestones. As mentioned previously, maturation of the musculoskeletal system influences the development of posture and movement because antigravity muscle strength and muscle cocontraction are necessary for the emergence of upright postures and higher-level motor skills. There also is an interaction between the weight of a body segment and the ability to move against gravity (Thelen & Fisher, 1982, 1983).

■ ASSESSMENT OF POSTURAL CONTROL

The assessment of postural control takes different forms, depending on the age of the child and the nature of the postural control dysfunction. In young children, postural assessment is linked to motor milestones and the development of antigravity movement and appropriate postural reactions. In children who have acquired ambulation, postural assessment has typically focused on higher-level balance capabilities, such as single-limb stance and balance beam activities, and the acquisition of play skills (ball throwing, kicking, and jumping). Although an indirect measure of postural control, these milestones are dependent on the development of adequate feed-forward postural control. More recently, evaluations of standing balance have begun to examine the functioning of sensory systems associated with balance function, the development of appropriate muscle synergies in response to perturbations, and the development of stability under various testing conditions.

Assessment of Righting, Equilibrium, and Protective Reactions

Righting reactions

The *righting reactions* (neck on body, body on body, body on head, Landau, flexion, and vertical) are assessed through handling of the infant. The relative ages of emergence of these reflexes in their mature form are depicted in Table 10-2.

1. To elicit the *neck on body reaction*, the child's head is manually turned to the side and the rolling response is observed. As stated previously, the immature response is a log roll to realign the body, and the mature response is a segmental roll.
2. The *body on body reaction* is evaluated in a similar fashion; the child's hips are rotated to the side and the upper body is observed. The immature response is a log roll, and the mature response is a segmental roll.
3. The *body on head reaction* is observed, as the child is placed prone on a support surface. In the partial response the child lifts his or her head vertically 45 degrees, and in the full response the child raises the head vertically in midline to face (90 degrees) and is able to maintain this upright position.

4. The *Landau reaction* is observed in prone suspension; the examiner supports the child under the abdomen and looks for extension of both the neck and lower extremities. An immature response may be noted for the Landau; young infants may keep the head in line with the body before being able to demonstrate the mature response of head, trunk, and lower-extremity extension.
5. The *flexion response* is assessed by pulling the child to sitting from the supine position and is considered present if the child can maintain the head in alignment with the body without any initial head lag.
6. The *vertical reactions (labyrinthine and optical)* are typically evaluated by supporting the infant under the arms and suspending him or her vertically. Then the infant is laterally tilted about 45 degrees; the reaction is considered present if the infant rights his or her head vertically. The *labyrinthine reaction* is tested either with a blindfold covering the eyes or in a dark room. Testing with the eyes open is considered to evaluate *optical righting* because vision dominates vestibular input in young infants (see previous section on sensory development). A partial response to vertical righting is often observed, characterized by the maintenance of the head in line with the body, which is considered an immature response (Barnes & Crutchfield, 1990).

Recently therapists and researchers have begun to question the relative importance of evaluating righting reactions and what the presence or absence of righting reactions indicates. Although the emergence of mature responses is associated with a normally developing nervous system, delay in developing these reactions provides little insight into the cause. Delayed or deficient reactions can be secondary to neuromotor dysfunction, musculoskeletal abnormalities, or sensory system dysfunction.

Equilibrium reactions

Testing *equilibrium* and protective reactions has typically taken the form of placing the child on a tiltboard or other unstable surface (e.g., ball or bolster). The child's responses to displacement are observed in lateral, anterior, posterior, and diagonal directions. All appropriate developmental positions are used (prone, supine, sitting, quadruped, kneeling, and standing).

An alternate form of testing involves observation of the child's response to manual displacement from a stationary support surface (i.e., the child is pushed in a given direction). A typical equilibrium reaction is characterized by movements of the trunk and extremities that oppose the imposed displacement and bring the center of gravity back within the base of support. For example, when the child is sitting, a posterior displacement results in contraction of the abdominal, neck flexor, hip flexor, and hamstring muscles to produce a forward movement

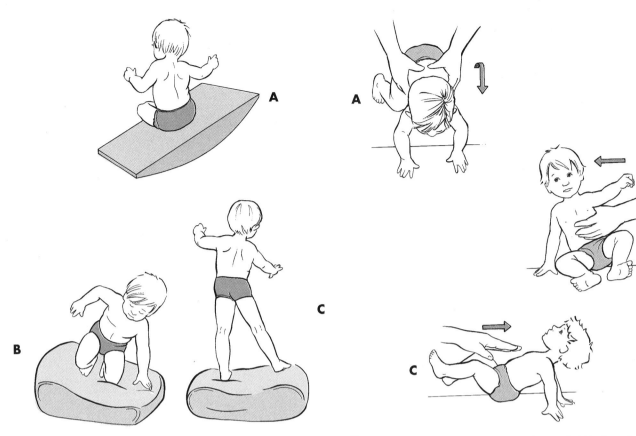

figure 10-6   Equilibrium reactions in sitting (A), quadruped (B), and standing (C).

figure 10-7   Protective reactions forward (A), lateral (B), and backward (C).

of the body. Conversely, an anterior push or tilt is associated with neck, trunk, and hip extension; and hamstrings may activate to maintain the seated position. Similarly, lateral displacements are associated with trunk incurvation toward the elevated side if tilted or toward the pushed side if pushed. The child should rotate the upper body toward the elevated (pushed) side and often will extend the extremities on the elevated or pushed side (Figure 10-6). These responses to lateral tilting are consistent with those seen in all positions. Tilting in a diagonal direction is associated with increased trunk and neck rotation to oppose the movement. These rotary movements combine with trunk flexion when the child is tilted backward and trunk extension when he or she is tilted forward.

Adequate flexibility, muscle strength, and experience with postural disturbance in a given position are necessary for mature equilibrium responses. Thus neuromotor maturation alone does not account for the emergence of these responses.

Protective reactions

Protective reactions, sometimes called *parachute reactions,* are also elicited by displacement on a tilting surface or manual displacement on a stable surface. These reactions differ from equilibrium reactions in that they are designed to protect the infant from a fall rather than to correct the displacement. Therefore these reactions are characterized by extension of the extremities to "catch" the child as he or she falls and occur in the direction of the fall. Forward protective reactions can be tested by suspending the child and then moving him or her forward toward a support surface. A positive response includes arm extension and abduction sufficient to stop the forward movement. Testing while the child is sitting also involves displacement in any direction sufficient to elicit arm extension to stop the movement. The amount of displacement needed to elicit a protective reaction must be greater in degree than that used to elicit an equilibrium reaction (Figure 10-7).

Neuromotor assessment

Neuromotor assessments have been designed to evaluate the emergence and progression of postural reactions. The Milani-Comparetti Motor Development Screening Test tracks the emergence of these reactions, the emergence of antigravity movement, and the integration of primitive reflexes (Milani-Comparetti & Gidoni,

1967). The Movement Assessment of Infants (MAI) (Chandler, Andrews, & Swanson, 1980) also examines postural reactions, or *automatic reactions* as they are referred to in the assessment, with an emphasis on examining asymmetries and the emergence of the reactions. Other neuromotor assessments include some, but not all, of the postural reactions in their assessment of motor milestones. Examples include the Infant Neurological International Battery (INFANIB) (Ellison, 1994), Alberta Infant Motor Scale (AIMS) (Piper & Darrah, 1994), and the Postural and Fine Motor Assessment (Case-Smith & Bigsby, 2000).

Assessment of Antigravity Movement

The emergence of antigravity movement is assessed in most developmental tests through the appearance of motor milestones such as prone and supine head control and reaching. The six levels of prone and supine postural development described by Pountney and others (1990) can be used to plot an infant's progression. In addition, the Milani-Comparetti Motor Development Screening Test (Milani-Comparetti & Gidoni, 1967), AIMS (Piper & Darrah, 1994), and MAI (Chandler et. al., 1980) each have sections that address antigravity movement and the emergence of antigravity postures.

Assessment of Sensory Organization

The initial evaluation of the child should include testing of sensory systems to determine function. The testing of optical and labyrinthine righting in infants begins to explore the integrity of these systems for use in the control of balance. As described previously, these reactions are typically tested with the infant vertically suspended because this position is believed to assess vestibular system function while eliminating somatosensory input. However, in optical righting, with the eyes open, the vestibular system operates in conjunction with the eyes and may provide the essential input for balance control. Therefore the testing procedure for optical righting does not effectively evaluate the infant's ability to use visual information to orient his or her body in space.

Several tests have been designed for evaluation of sensory integrative function, including sensory organization, balance, and coordination. These tests are the DeGangi Berk Test of Sensory Integration (Berk & DeGangi, 1983) and the Sensory Integration and Praxis Tests (Ayres, 1989), which are described in Chapter 12.

Primarily developed for research purposes, posturography provides a method for analyzing the separate and combined influences of the sensory systems on standing balance (Nashner, 1990). Although this sophisticated test is not often available to clinicians, the method of analysis is helpful in understanding how the interactions of the sensory systems contribute to postural stability and upright stance.

Posturography typically involves testing under six conditions, also involving sensory deprivation and conflict, using a computerized force platform system on which the child stands. The platform can be stable or sway-referenced (moves as child sways such that the ankle joint remains in the same position). A curtainlike structure surrounds the child's entire visual field and can also be sway-referenced. The six testing conditions are (1) eyes open, stable platform; (2) eyes closed, stable platform; (3) sway-referenced visual surround, stable platform; (4) eyes open, sway-referenced platform; (5) eyes closed, sway-referenced platform; and (6) sway-referenced visual surround and platform (Nashner, 1990). This type of evaluation requires expensive equipment, but it is often used to assess vestibular dysfunction in adults and has been used with children (Forssberg & Nashner, 1982; Horak, Shumway-Cook, Crow, & Black, 1988; Nashner, Shumway-Cook, & Marnin, 1983; Shumway-Cook, Horak, & Black, 1987).

Interpretation of posturography involves the examination of sway and the duration of time that the child can maintain each position. Children who have difficulty with a given condition demonstrate increased sway or lose their balance. Difficulty with condition 2 reflects an overreliance on the visual system. Although children and adults demonstrate a slight increase in sway in this condition, children as young as 4 years of age have had no difficulty in maintaining stance for 30 seconds. Condition 3 examines the child's ability to remain standing in the presence of inaccurate visual cues but with accurate somatosensory and vestibular cues. Conditions 4 through 6 require stance in the presence of inaccurate somatosensory cues and varying visual input (present, absent, or conflicting). Individuals with sensory organization problems have difficulty with all conditions in which conflicting sensory cues are present (conditions 3 through 6). However, the last two conditions require the individual to rely on vestibular information only; therefore difficulties with only conditions 5 and 6 are typical of individuals with vestibular disorders. In testing with young children, a developmental progression occurs with an increase in stability between 3 and 6 years of age; 6-year-old children responded similarly to adults across conditions (Foudriat et. al., 1993). However, even 3- and 4-year-old children were able to disregard misleading sensory inputs to maintain stance but with increased sway (Foudriat et. al., 1993; Richardson et. al., 1992).

Assessment of Higher-Level Balance Skills

More advanced balance skills are typically evaluated through parts of gross motor tests. Typical test items include single-limb stance (standing on one foot), balance beam activities involving stance and ambulation, and other walking balance activities (walking heel-to-toe or walking in a straight line). For the most part, assessment of these skills involves timed tests of static stance capabilities (how long the child can stand on one foot) or frequency counts (how many consecutive heel-to-toe steps the child can take). The Bruininks-Oseretsky Test of Motor Proficiency can be used to examine these areas in children 4½ to 14½ years of age (Bruininks, 1978). The Gross Motor Scale of the Peabody Development Motor Scales (PDMS) (Folio & Fewell, 2000) includes several items for children between 4 and 6 years of age that rate balance reactions in higher-level positions (e.g., on the balance beam, in single-limb stance, or hopping).

Assessment of Anticipatory Postural Control

Assessment of anticipatory postural control is accomplished through the observational skills of the therapist. Children who have delays in anticipatory postural control likely exhibit general delays in motor control. Children with limited anticipatory control have difficulty reaching, catching, or throwing in any posture. These activities involve sequential displacements of the child's center of gravity and require that postural tone remain activated (preset) for the child to be successful. An overreliance on protective reactions is another indication that anticipatory control is ineffective or limited. For example, a child who loses his or her balance when he or she attempts a reach may be demonstrating poor feed-forward control.

■ ATYPICAL POSTURAL DEVELOPMENT

Postural development is associated with maturational and experiential changes in the sensorimotor, musculoskeletal, and cognitive systems. Therefore abnormal functioning of any of these systems can result in atypical postural development.

Persistence of Primitive Reflexes

Primitive reflexes are present at or soon after birth and disappear during the first year of life. The traditional hierarchic model proposed that these reflexes were controlled at lower levels of the central nervous system (CNS) and that reflex integration was associated with maturation of patterns mediated by higher centers (i.e., the higher centers inhibited the expression of these reflexes by the lower centers) (Bobath & Bobath, 1954; Taylor, 1931; VanSant, 1993). The reemergence of these reflex patterns after brain injury in children and adults lend support to this concept.

The movement patterns of many children with cerebral palsy and children who have incurred traumatic brain injury are influenced by primitive reflex activity, including the asymmetric tonic neck, symmetric tonic neck, and tonic labyrinthine reflexes. The persistence of these reflexes or their reemergence after brain injury has been associated with delayed postural reflex development (i.e., righting, protective, and equilibrium reactions) (Bobath & Bobath, 1954; Shumway-Cook, 1989). However, in a study of 156 typically developing children, Bartlett (1997) found that the emergence of motor milestones did not relate to the presence or absence of primitive reflexes. Thus in the typically developing infant the emergence of motor milestones can be independent of the integration of primitive reflexes. However, damage to the developing nervous system may result in persistence of primitive reflexes and disrupted neuromotor control, both of which may influence the acquisition of postural reactions and motor milestones.

Abnormal Muscle Tone, Motor Control, and Force Generation

Damage to the CNS is associated with many changes in motor control, including changes in muscle tone, motor planning, and patterns of movement. The adequate development of postural reactions has also been linked to the presence of normal muscle tone (Bobath, 1966). Conversely, the presence of abnormal muscle tone in the form of hypertonia, hypotonia, athetosis, or rigidity (i.e., in cerebral palsy) has been associated with deficits in postural control mechanisms. Children with cerebral palsy demonstrate limitations in postural reactions, antigravity movement, proximal muscle cocontraction, and stability in upright postures (Bly, 1983; Bobath, 1966; Perin, 1989).

According to Bly (1983), the inability to develop antigravity movement and stability combined with the need to move result in fixing, or locking, of various body segments, which provides some stability but also blocks more mature movement patterns, such as head control, extremity mobility, and dynamic weight bearing. Repeatedly using limited patterns of movement suggests that children with poor stability limit the degrees of freedom within the system by stabilizing, or locking, certain body segments. Furthermore, the continued use of this type of movement pattern can increase the stability of the pattern and limit the acquisition of other patterns of movement (Kamm, Thelen, & Jensen, 1990).

Children, who lack antigravity muscle strength and therefore stability, learn to provide stability through the fixing (blocking) of certain joints (e.g., the neck in hyperextension to maintain the head upright in sitting). This fixing, in turn, limits the variety of movements that the child can produce. The child who achieves upright head control by hyperextending the neck and elevating the shoulders while sitting limits his or her ability to develop protection and equilibrium reactions, reaching skill in sitting, and independent neck and trunk movements. Over time the abnormal movement pattern becomes more stable, limiting the development of more mature patterns of movement and making the pattern difficult to change.

In addition to the delay or inability to develop antigravity movement and stability, many children with abnormal tone associated with cerebral palsy demonstrate hyperreflexia, which is characterized by exaggerated monosynaptic reflexes (e.g., deep tendon reflexes such as the patellar tendon reflex). These reflexes are hyperexcitable and are associated with activation of both the agonist and antagonist muscles. In response to tapping of the patellar tendon, both the quadriceps muscle and hamstrings would be activated. As a result the child is unable to make a selective, graded movement.

In many children with cerebral palsy, muscle groups adjacent to those stimulated are activated as well; this response is termed *overflow*. Overflow is often seen in young, typically developing children and decreases after the first year of life. Normal overflow is not as widespread and does not involve as many muscles as the atypical overflow observed in children with cerebral palsy (Leonard, Hirschfeld, & Forssberg, 1988). Because stretching of a spastic muscle activates this same monosynaptic reflex, this overflow pattern can be expected to occur in such activities as extending the arm quickly to protect from a fall. In the child with cerebral palsy the reflex activates the biceps, shoulder, and wrist muscles and results in failure to stop the fall effectively. In children with spasticity, the development of effective protective reactions is typically delayed and often absent (Bobath & Bobath, 1954).

Although abnormal tone and changes in reflex activity are often the most observable alterations in motor function associated with brain injury, adults and children with CNS injuries also demonstrate alterations in motor planning and force generation. Motor planning requires the ability to use sensory feedback from a movement to determine its effectiveness and the efficiency of the muscles activated and the movement produced. In addition, motor planning requires that the child be able to interpret the demands of the task accurately, using sensory and cognitive systems. Deficits in sensory systems and the interpretation of sensory feedback also accompany CNS damage (see section on alterations in sensory function). Furthermore, successful movements require sufficient antigravity control, appropriate motor unit recruitment, and grading of muscle contraction in both agonistic and antagonistic muscles. Children with CNS damage display difficulties in motor unit recruitment and grading of muscle contractions (see the later section on the organi-

zation of the motor response). Thus the presence of abnormal muscle tone coupled with motor planning and force generation difficulties may delay or prevent the development of antigravity control necessary for mature movement patterns.

Delays in the development of postural control have been described in conjunction with ligamentous laxity and decreased muscle strength in children with Down syndrome (Fetters, 1991). Musculoskeletal abnormalities are also associated with cerebral palsy and other developmental disabilities (e.g., arthrogryposis and muscular dystrophy). Contractures secondary to spasticity or soft tissue abnormalities can restrict movement and thereby disrupt the efficacy of postural reactions; thus changes in musculoskeletal alignment and joint biomechanics can reduce the child's ability to exhibit adequate protective reactions. Adequate muscle strength is also necessary to produce joint stability and adequate equilibrium reactions; therefore conditions that result in diminished muscle strength (e.g., muscular dystrophy and cerebral palsy) may be associated with deficits in postural control.

The development of equilibrium reactions is affected by the presence of musculoskeletal abnormalities, and the need for these reactions is altered. In any position there are limits to how far the child can lean before a fall occurs. These limits are referred to as *the limits of stability* (Nashner, 1990). Because these limits of stability are decreased in children or adults with musculoskeletal limitations, it takes a smaller movement to elicit a loss of balance. A movement such as lifting the arm to reach for a toy may be sufficient to displace the child's center of gravity outside of the limits of stability and thereby elicit a fall. If the musculoskeletal change is asymmetric (e.g., in the child with hemiplegia), the decrease in the limits of stability occurs only on the side of the musculoskeletal abnormality (Nashner, 1990). Thus in a child with unilateral weakness, the limits of stability on the involved side are decreased. To compensate for this, the child moves his or her center of gravity toward the sound side to minimize the chance of falling, resulting in asymmetric postures.

Altered Sensory Function or Integration

Postural control, according to Horak and Shumway-Cook (1990), "relies on (1) intact peripheral sensory pathways, and (2) the ability of the CNS to extract appropriate sensory information relevant to gravity, the surface, and visual environments" (p. 110). Postural control requires intact perception of visual, vestibular, and somatosensory stimulation and the ability to determine the best source of information under the existing environmental conditions, particularly when conflicting sensory inputs are presented (e.g., unstable support surface resulting in inaccurate somatosensory inputs). When children with impairments in visual, somatosensory, or vestibular processing are required to resolve conflicting sensory input, they demonstrate deficits in postural control. Children with visual impairments typically demonstrate deficits in both static and dynamic balance skills when compared with sighted children (Johnson-Kramer, Sherwood, Frech, & Canabal, 1992; Ribaldi, Rider, & Toole, 1987). Similarly, about 60% of children with hearing impairments also demonstrate abnormal vestibular function and deficits in balance activities that rely on vestibular integrity. However, children with loss of one sensory system are able to compensate in most conditions by use of the two remaining systems (Horak et. al., 1988).

Shumway-Cook (1989) reported that children with impaired hearing and hypothesized vestibular dysfunction demonstrated normal postural reactions under conditions in which the sensory inputs were consistent but had difficulty in situations in which the sensory inputs were conflicting (e.g., on a moving platform with visual input that remained unchanged despite postural sway). This inability to interpret conflicting inputs and organize an appropriate response appears to be secondary to abnormalities within the central processes at the level of the cerebellum, brainstem, or cortex (Shumway-Cook, 1989). Children with a variety of other diagnoses, including cerebral palsy and learning disabilities, have been reported to have deficits in the selection of appropriate sensory inputs for postural control (Horak et. al., 1988; Nashner et. al., 1983; Shumway-Cook, et. al., 1987). Children with ataxic or diplegic cerebral palsy have demonstrated similar deficits in sensory organization under conditions of conflicting sensory cues (Nashner et. al., 1983). Since the accurate interpretation of sensory cues from the environment is necessary for effective motor planning to occur, deficits in sensory processing and integration are expected to affect the acquisition of mature postural control and mature patterns of movement necessary for motor milestone acquisition.

Organization of the Motor Response

The child's motor response to tilt on an unstable surface or displacement of his or her center of gravity results in activation of the appropriate muscle groups to compensate for the loss of balance. An effective response to this displacement requires muscle activation that is accurately timed and of sufficient amplitude to reestablish the child's center of gravity. Abnormalities in the motor response result in inaccurate patterns of muscle activation and errors in the timing or amplitude, limiting the child's ability to maintain an upright posture.

A delay in the onset of muscle activity has been reported in children with Down syndrome (Shumway-Cook & Woollacott, 1985a) and children with cerebral palsy (both hemiplegic and ataxic) (Nashner et. al., 1983; Shumway-Cook, 1989). This delay can result in use of an ineffective movement strategy when the child's center of gravity is displaced. In addition to a delay in the onset of muscle activity, children with cerebral palsy demonstrate patterns of muscle activation that are ineffective for maintaining postural control. The child may activate distal rather than proximal muscles, resulting in a stiffening of extremities instead of dynamic axial cocontraction. Additionally, overflow contractions that do not effectively contribute to the equilibrium response are observed (Leonard et. al., 1988; Nashner et. al., 1983).

High-level motor skills require appropriate anticipatory control in addition to the selection of appropriate movement strategies. Thus when a child wants to throw a ball, he or she needs to activate appropriate muscles on the back of the body to counteract the forward momentum created by the throw, or he or she will fall forward as the ball is released. Again, children with CNS damage may demonstrate ineffective anticipatory control, thus limiting the effectiveness of their movements. Similar to the preceding discussion of postural reactions, children with CNS damage may activate too many muscles, select the wrong muscles for activation, or have difficulty with matching the strength of the postural muscle activation needed for the ongoing movement. They may also demonstrate poor motor unit recruitment when trying to move postural muscles resulting in timing of the anticipatory response that is not tied to the ongoing movement. These deficits in the planning or implementation of anticipatory control may limit the child's ability to acquire advanced motor skills. In the case of a child throwing a ball, too little postural activity or inaccurately timed trunk extension results in him or her falling forward as the ball is released; too much postural activity may result in limited shoulder excursion during the throw and thus an unsuccessful throw. Evaluation of advanced motor skills should also take into account the presence and effectiveness of anticipatory postural control.

■ INTERVENTION

This chapter describes intervention as it relates to basic posture and movement. Subsequent chapters address the integration of postural control as a foundation for skilled activity performance. Specific occupational therapy approaches to intervention with children who have neuromotor or musculoskeletal problems are presented elsewhere in this text.

Intervention, based on a systems view of motor development, should take into account the many influences contributing to the movement, including the task requirements, the neuromotor system, the environment in which the intervention takes place, and the motivation of the child. Motor learning theories acknowledge that motor skills do not simply develop as a course of maturation and that motor function involves more than subcortical sensory experiences. A motor pattern is the result of learning and practice with a permanent change in skill. Therapists who use motor learning theories stress the important role of motivation and volition in learning new skills (VanSant, 1994).

An individual learns a new motor skill from the intrinsic and extrinsic feedback received in association with the movement (Adams, 1971). *Intrinsic feedback* refers to the sensory information generated from the action or the perceptual experience. *External feedback* refers to the response of the environment produced because of the action (knowledge of results). The therapist's response to the child's accomplishment or achievement reinforces the learner's "knowledge of results." The child's knowledge of the effects and results of his or her own movements is critical to learning and generalizing motor skills.

Although feedback appears important to learning new movements, not all movement is based on somatosensory feedback. Some is generated and carried out without feedback (e.g., rapid movements such as throwing a ball). Schmidt (1988) hypothesized that recall and recognition schema are the basis for learning new motor skills. The schema are a set of rules learned about movement that are applied and generalized to new situations. The learner recognizes the relationships between the environment conditions, task requirements, and previously learned movements. In this theoretic context, movement is the solution to a motor problem; skill allows the generalization of this solution to multiple problems similar to the original. The outcome of performance and the sensory feedback help the learner establish new motor skills based on an understanding of the relationships between environmental conditions, task requirements, and previously learned movements. Thus although sensory feedback may not be required as the movement is carried out, it is used in the production of the "next" movement.

Motor learning theories emphasize the importance of practice and sensory feedback combined with knowledge of results. Implications of these theories on practice have been postulated and are currently topics of research. One implication is that random practice reinforces learning more than blocked practice. Blocked practice involves extended periods of repetitious movements with consistent reinforcement provided throughout the practice session. In random practice, an activity is practiced under constantly changing conditions (e.g., therapist changes direction and distance in practice of reach), and practice of one task (e.g., reaching) is interspersed with practice of other tasks (e.g., in-hand manipulation, placing of the object). Performance is reinforced on an intermittent or random schedule.

Feedback during practice is also important to learning. High levels of feedback appear to be detrimental rather than helpful when learning a new motor task. Giving intermittent feedback and reducing feedback as the skill is achieved are ideal ways to reinforce learning (feedback frequency should be higher early in skill acquisition and taper as the child learns the task). Another tenet of motor learning theory is that errors during practice are important for learning, allowing the learner to compare the internal and external feedback from the unsuccessful movement with those of the successful movement.

When applying a motor learning practice model, handling of the child is viewed from several aspects:
1. Handling becomes a type of feedback by providing sensory cues for the movement. Early in the acquisition of a motor skill, higher levels of feedback are thought to facilitate movement, and therapist input, such as tapping a muscle to focus attention on its recruitment, may facilitate the development of the movement. However, feedback during every attempt, including handling, is thought to be detrimental because it may encourage the child to rely on that input rather than his or her own sensory feedback for planning and performing the movement.
2. Handling the child changes the demands of the task (i.e., decreasing the need for anticipatory control or changing the amount of force needed to produce the movement) and may result in ineffective motor learning. If the child learns to move only with assistance of the therapist's hands, he or she may not be able to produce the same movement in the absence of handling.
3. Handling typically decreases the number of errors produced by the child in attempting to move. If errors are important to learning, then preventing errors through too much handling may impair motor learning.

Handling should be used judiciously. A small number of assisted repetitions may allow the child to "feel" the movement and facilitate motor learning. Thus although handling should be done with caution, it may still play a roll in facilitating movement acquisition.

Another aspect of motor learning is the role of part versus whole practice. In tasks that have identifiable components (e.g., picking up a block and placing it in a container), the individual parts can be practiced; however, the practice of parts of a skill should be followed by practice of the entire skill for motor learning to occur. In many skills the parts are interrelated and therefore inseparable. Thus practicing components of the task appears to be ineffective. For example, when reaching for a glass, the amount of finger opening, the force of the grip, and the force of the arm movement are predicated on the expected weight of the glass and how full it is. Thus practicing opening the hand in the absence of gripping the glass may not facilitate the task of grasping the glass and bringing it to the mouth. Therefore the learning of the skill parts may best occur within the context of whole skill practice. These principles regarding learning and the system theories that relate postural development to the function of neurophysiologic and biomechanical variables in the child are the basis for the intervention activities described in the following section.

Treatment of Musculoskeletal Abnormalities

To prepare the child to work on postural control, limitations in joint range of motion and problems in postural alignment need to be addressed (Effgen, 1993). Contractures or joint limitations secondary to spasticity or soft tissue changes often result in poor postural alignment (e.g., anterior or posterior pelvic tilt that blocks trunk rotation). Decreased range of motion limits mobility and decreases the base of support. As a result, adequate equilibrium and protective reactions do not develop, and the child is limited in everyday play, self-care, and school activities.

A variety of inhibition techniques can be used to reduce muscle tone and improve range of motion. Most techniques focus on improving the child's range of motion and flexibility of the spine with the expected result of improved postural alignment and increased postural flexibility. Therapeutic techniques to increase muscle elongation are also used to help the child achieve extension of the extremities. Adequate arm and leg extension are needed for the development of protective extension responses. In particular, full knee and hip extension are required as a base for effective equilibrium responses in stance.

Facilitation of Antigravity Movement

As previously described, normal postural control requires antigravity control in prone, supine, and upright postures. With the development of antigravity trunk flexion and extension, the child achieves upright positions that allow for the development of skilled movements. When a child has not developed sufficient strength in the neck and trunk musculature to move against gravity, he or she is limited in activities such as prone extension and coming to sitting. These movements can be modified to diminish the pull of gravity so that the child can successfully practice the positions and movements to increase neck and trunk strength. Use of a therapeutic ball or a wedge provides some assistance against gravity and reduces the range in which the child must move against gravity. A pull-to-sit activity can then be done from an incline or a ball (Figure 10-8). With the child's head and trunk positioned on an inclined surface, less neck and trunk flexion is required to accomplish pull-to-sit activity. The degree of incline is gradually decreased as the child gains neck flexor strength.

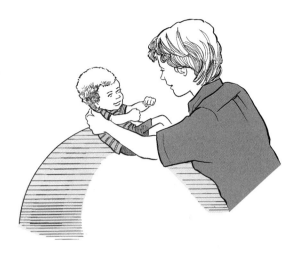

figure 10-8 Facilitation of head righting from therapeutic ball. Other inclined surface could be used. Therapist supports child's shoulders, scapula, and trunk to encourage isolated activation of neck muscles.

An alternative method for eliciting neck flexion is to help the child move from sitting toward the supine position. The therapist gradually lowers the child backward from the sitting position until the child starts to lose head control. The therapist then assists the child in returning to a sitting position. This activity requires neck flexor control in both directions (lowering from and returning to the sitting position). If the child does not have sufficient strength to perform either of these activities, neck and trunk flexion can be initiated in the side-lying position where gravity is eliminated and then progressed to the coming-to-sitting activities. Moving the child in lateral weight shifts while sitting also increases neck strength in a gravity-reduced plane. The therapist's support at the shoulders, trunk, and pelvis is necessary to allow isolation of the neck and trunk flexors. As the child's strength increases, the therapist introduces diagonal weight shifts that produce rotation. Diagonal or angular movements activate the transverse neck and trunk muscles (e.g., the oblique abdominal muscles) that are required in mature equilibrium responses.

Similarly, neck and trunk extension can be elicited by working with the child in a variety of activities in the prone position over a ball, bolster, or wedge. When the child is positioned in a prone position on an inclined surface, the pull of gravity is reduced, allowing for more effective use of neck and trunk extension. Toys or the parent's voice is used to motivate the child to raise his or her head while the therapist moves him or her in small ranges of anterior and posterior weight shift to stimulate a righting response. As the child's control of head and trunk extension improves, the degree of incline is gradually decreased. Engaging the child in reaching activities with one or both hands can facilitate antigravity trunk exten-

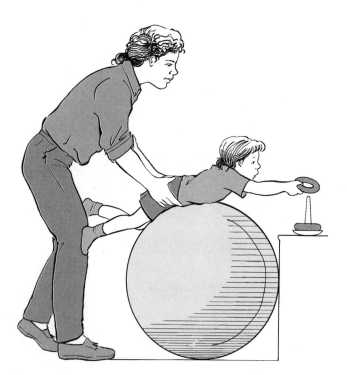

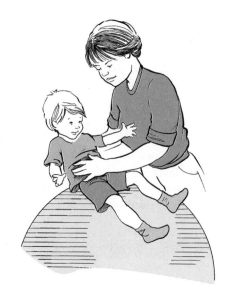

figure**10-9** Facilitation of prone extension over therapeutic ball. Key point of control is at pelvis.

figure**10-10** Facilitation of protective and equilibrium reaction to displacement on therapeutic ball.

sion in the prone position (Figure 10-9). The therapist's handling should again provide stability so that specific extensor muscle activity is elicited and overflow contractions are inhibited (Bobath & Bobath, 1964; Perin, 1989; Sternat, 1993).

In addition to the traditional activities described previously, biofeedback devices are increasingly used with children who have muscular and neuromuscular disorders. Biofeedback can provide the needed feedback to the child about successful and unsuccessful muscle activation or positioning. In addition, it can provide the motivation for the child to attempt the activity. One example of biofeedback is a mercury switch strapped to the child's head and activated with upright head movement. Using this switch, the child can turn on the radio, tape recorder, or other battery-powered toy using simple head movements. Kramer, Ashton, and Brander (1992) found the mercury head switch to be effective in improving head control in prone and sitting positions over an 8-week period. Thus for some children, biofeedback can be used during therapy sessions or in a home-based program as a tool to increase the child's motivation and improve antigravity movement.

Facilitation of Postural Reactions

The therapist can facilitate postural reactions using activities that displace the center of gravity and require corrective or protective responses. The speed, range, and direction of displacement determine whether righting or equilibrium responses are elicited. As mentioned previ-

ously, rapid movements in greater ranges elicit protective extension responses. These activities can also be performed on therapeutic balls, bolsters, equilibrium boards, or any other unstable surfaces (Figure 10-10). Reaching activities with the child positioned on an unstable surface can facilitate the development of these reactions because the child will displace his or her center of gravity during the reach, requiring a compensatory response. Initially, the therapist provides pelvic stability (e.g., with his or her hands) as a base from which the child can begin to produce the desired response. As postural reactions improve, this support is reduced and finally eliminated. Then the child practices skills unsupported on a stable surface, using first a wide base of support (most of his or her legs and buttocks are in contact with the supporting surface) and later a smaller base of support (only the buttocks are in contact with the surface). Placing the child in a sitting position on an unstable surface will refine postural reactions. During advanced practice of these activities, the therapist moves the surface using a variety of speeds, ranges (degrees of tilt), and rhythms. Safety and protection of the child's fall become increasingly important as greater challenges to balance are imposed on the child. In addition to activities on an unstable surface, reaching activities that require the child to shift weight facilitate the development of equilibrium and righting reactions (Bobath & Bobath, 1964; Effgen, 1993; Perin, 1989). During all of these activities, a high level of task variability can facilitate the learning process.

Mature postural control and the motor patterns associated with these abilities develop through experience with the conditions in which they are required. Therefore the therapist provides the child with a variety of experiences that demand the use of postural reactions (VanSant, 1991). The therapist's role is to present a task that is sufficient for these motor patterns to be expressed, motivate the child such that the activity is fun and meaningful, and provide feedback to the child about the appropriateness of the motor response. As skills develop, the child is encouraged to evaluate his or her own responses (Effgen, 1993). As described in the section on facilitating antigravity movement, biofeedback can be used as a method for reinforcing postural responses by providing additional feedback to the child. Research has demonstrated its successful use to increase head righting and control in the prone and supine positions (Kramer et. al., 1992) and to improve weight shift and ankle motion during walking (Conrad & Bleck, 1980; Seeger & Caudrey, 1983).

Facilitation of Sensory Organization

As discussed previously, many children with developmental disorders demonstrate deficits in the organization of sensory inputs for use in balance. When sensory organization seems to be the basis for difficulty in postural control, it also becomes the focus of intervention. The therapist creates experiences with altered surfaces or visual contexts that match the identified needs of the child (Shumway-Cook et. al., 1987). For example, children who demonstrate immature equilibrium responses when relying only on the somatosensory system benefit from activities that challenge this system, such as ball, bolster, or tilt board activities in a darkened room or with vision occluded (e.g., with the use of a blindfold). These activities should be designed so that the child does not feel threatened by the disruption of his or her vision and by the progress from easier positions to more complex positions (e.g., sitting to standing). Conversely, children with difficulty balancing when relying on visual information in the presence of conflicting somatosensory cues should benefit from practice of activities on unstable surfaces that challenge the somatosensory system. Movement on a surface padded with foam or covered with sand challenges balance with ambiguous information to the proprioceptive system. Combining the conflicting visual and somatosensory cues should require reliance on the vestibular system and would be appropriate to facilitate vestibular function in children with deficits in this area.

Facilitation of Anticipatory Postural Control

Facilitation of anticipatory postural control requires that the child experience the need for this control. Reaching, catching, and throwing activities can be used to identify deficits in anticipatory control and to facilitate its use. Again, the therapist needs to set up a task that requires anticipatory control. Practice with weight shifting may be necessary before practice of the displacing activity. Initially, this may be enhanced by handling, but as soon as possible the handling must be diminished and then curtailed. When the child experiences success or failure in independent performance of the task, the knowledge of results reinforces learning of the task (Schmidt, 1988). Experiences in reaching with and without handling allow the child to evaluate and learn from the sensory input during anticipatory weight shift (e.g., to recognize errors in anticipatory postural control). Varying the direction, speed, and magnitude of the displacing activity is also important so that the child is required to reassess the intended movement and impose the appropriate anticipatory response (Van Sant, 1994). Reaching for a variety of objects of different size and weight at a variety of positions with a different goal (throwing, placing, bringing to the mouth) should provide sufficient variability to facilitate motor learning.

■ SUMMARY

This chapter described the development of postural control as influenced by the neuromotor, somatosensory, vestibular, and musculoskeletal systems. The importance of experience, sensory feedback, and practice to the development of effective postural control was explained using motor learning theories. Through in-depth understanding of the influence of multiple systems and experience to a child's development of dynamic upright postures, the therapist can successfully design interventions for children with postural instability.

Case Study 1

Marcy was diagnosed with spastic diplegic cerebral palsy. She was born at 32 weeks' gestation, weighing 2 pounds 11 ounces. Her hospital stay was complicated by respiratory distress syndrome and a grade II intraventricular hemorrhage.

Assessment

At 2½ years of age, Marcy presented with spasticity in all four extremities, greater in the legs than in the arms. She demonstrated hypotonicity in the trunk. Her head control was good in all positions, but she continued to demonstrate an immature neck flexion response when pulled to sit. While sitting, she demonstrated a posterior pelvic tilt with weight bearing primarily on her sacrum and her trunk flexed forward. She could free one hand for play but required one hand for support to maintain sitting. She lacked antigravity back extension sufficient for sitting without arm support. Forward protective reactions were present, and lateral protective reactions were developing (i.e., they remained inconsistent). Protective and equilibrium reactions backward were absent. Marcy was motivated to move about her environment using a type of commando crawl movement of the arms with her legs tightly scissored. She was unable to assume or maintain the quadruped position.

Interpretation

Marcy demonstrated gross motor skills at the 6- to 7-month age level. She also demonstrated delayed development of antigravity head and trunk control and delayed development of protective and equilibrium reactions. Her movement patterns were influenced by spasticity with overflow into synergistic and antagonistic muscles.

Intervention

Intervention focused on developing antigravity neck and trunk strength, facilitating protective and equilibrium reactions, and developing independent sitting without arm support. Antigravity neck flexion was facilitated by lowering from a sitting to a supine position and practicing small lateral weight shifts in sitting. Antigravity neck and trunk extension were promoted through activities that involve moving from a side-lying to a prone position on a large therapy ball. The movement of the ball was used to facilitate postural extension. Reaching activities while sitting on a ball or bolster were used to facilitate trunk strength and the development of trunk righting and equilibrium and protective reactions.

Case Study 2

John, who has Down syndrome, was enrolled in a preschool program at 5 years of age. His teacher reported that he frequently fell and had difficulty keeping up with the other ambulatory children in the class. He avoided situations that required walking on unstable surfaces such as gravel or stepping over obstacles. Prior testing found vision and vestibular function to be within normal limits.

Assessment

John presented with a mild degree of hypotonia, ligamentous laxity, and joint hypermobility at all peripheral joints. He walked with a stiff-legged, flat-foot gait characterized by minimal hip and knee flexion, knee recurvatum during stance, and an absent heel-strike. He did not achieve either a prone extension or supine flexion posture. On the Gross Motor Scale of the PDMS, John scored at the 30-month age level. Testing using posturography revealed that John had difficulty with balance when conflicting sensory input was given and seemed to over-rely on vision to maintain his balance.

Interpretation

John exhibited generalized hypotonia and immature movement patterns while standing associated with decreased antigravity muscle strength. John demonstrated a gross motor delay with function limited in activities of jumping and single-limb stance such as hopping, skipping, and alternating feet on walking up or down steps (the activities that John failed on the PDMS). The results of the posturography suggested that John had difficulty with the organization of sensory cues for use in balance, resulting in difficulty under conditions of conflicting sensory cues from either the visual or somatosensory system.

Intervention

Intervention focused on developing antigravity muscle strength and facilitating the organization of sensory cues. Activities to increase antigravity extension included (1) reaching while prone on a ball or bolster, (2) pushing from a wall and holding onto rubber tubing while being pulled around the room prone on a scooter board, and (3) reaching and throwing while lying prone in a hammock swing. Activities to increase supine flexion included (1) moving from the supine position to sitting on an inclined surface and (2) reaching while sitting on the therapy ball.

Activities that challenged the sensory organization system were helpful in facilitating the ability to deal with conflicting sensory cues, including walking on foam, sand, grass, or thick carpet in various visual conditions such as eyes closed, dim lighting, and conflicting conditions (e.g., the conflict dome). In addition, standing activities that challenged the postural system facilitated more mature balance reactions. These activities included walking up and down stairs with an alternating step pattern, stepping over obstacles of various heights and widths, and kicking a ball.

STUDY QUESTIONS

1. What are the roles of the visual, vestibular, and somatosensory systems in balance control? How do these roles change in the developing child?

2. What is the difference between compensatory postural reactions and anticipatory postural control? How can each of these be evaluated?

3. How is postural control affected by abnormalities of the musculoskeletal system, alterations in muscle tone, and abnormal motor pattern selection? How can intervention address these limitations?

Development of Postural Control ■ chapter 10 287

References

Adams, J.A. (1971). A closed loop theory of motor learning. *Journal of Motor Behavior, 3,* 110-150.

Ayres, A. (1989). *Sensory Integration and Praxis Tests.* Los Angeles: Western Psychological Services.

Barnes, M., & Crutchfield, C. (1990). *Reflex and vestibular aspects of motor control, motor development and motor learning.* Atlanta: Stokesville.

Bartlett, D. (1997). Primitive reflexes and early motor development. *Developmental and Behavioral Pediatrics, 18* (1), 151-156.

Berger, W., Quintern, J., & Dietz, V. (1985). Stance and gait perturbation in children: developmental aspects of compensatory mechanisms. *Electroencephalographic Clinical Neurophysiology, 61,* 385-395.

Berk, R., & DeGangi, G. (1983). *DeGangi-Berk Test of Sensory Integration.* Circle Pines, MN: American Guidance Service.

Bly, L. (1983). *The components of normal movement during the first year of life and abnormal development.* Oak Park, IL: Neurodevelopmental Treatment Association.

Bobath, B., & Bobath, K. (1954). A study of abnormal postural reflex activity in patients with lesions of the central nervous system. *Physiotherapy, 40,* 1-30.

Bobath, K. (1966). The motor deficit in patients with cerebral palsy. *Clinics in Developmental Medicine, 23,* 1-54.

Bobath, K., & Bobath, B. (1964). The facilitation of normal postural reactions and movements in the treatment of cerebral palsy. *Physiotherapy, 21,* 3-19.

Bouisset S., & Zattara, M. (1981). A sequence of postural movements precedes voluntary movement. *Neuroscience Letters, 22,* 263-270.

Bruininks, R. (1978). *Bruininks-Oseretsky Test of Motor Proficiency.* Examiners Manual, Circle Pines, MN: American Guidance System.

Bullinger, A. (1981). Cognitive elaboration of sensorimotor behavior. In G. Buttorworth (Ed.), *Infancy and epistemology: An evaluation of Piaget's theory.* London: Harvester Press.

Case-Smith, J., & Bigsby, R. (2000). *Posture and Fine Motor Assessment of Infants: Parts I and II.* San Antonio, TX: Psychological Corporation.

Chandler, L., Andrews, M., & Swanson, M. (1980). *Movement assessment of infants manual.* Rolling Bay, WA.

Connor, F., Williamson, G., & Siepp, J. (1978). *Program guide for infants and toddlers with neuromotor and other developmental disabilities.* New York: Teachers College Press.

Conrad, L., & Bleck, E. (1980). Augmented auditory feedback in the treatment of equinus in children. *Developmental Medicine and Child Neurology, 22,* 713-718.

Crowe, T., Deitz, J., Richardson, P., & Atwater, S. (1990). Interrater reliability of the pediatric clinical test of sensory interaction for balance. *Physical and Occupational Therapy in Pediatrics, 10* (4), 1-27.

Deitz, J., Richardson, P., Atwater, S., Crowe, T., & Odiorne, M. (1991). Performance of normal children on the Pediatric Clinical Test of Sensory Interaction for Balance. *Occupational Therapy Journal of Research, 11* (6), 336-356.

Effgen, S. (1993). Developing postural control. In B. Connolly, & P. Montgomery (Eds.), *Therapeutic exercise in developmental disabilities.* Hixson, TN: Chattanooga Group.

Ellison, P. (1994). *The INFANIB: A reliable method for the neuromotor assessment of infants.* Tucson: Therapy Skill Builders.

Fetters, L. (1991). Cerebral palsy: Contemporary treatment concepts. In M. Lister (Ed.), *Contemporary management of motor control problems proceedings of the II step conference.* Alexandria, VA: Foundation for Physical Therapy.

Folio, M., & Fewell, R. (1999). *Peabody developmental motor scales* (2nd ed.). Austin, TX: Pro Ed.

Forssberg, H., & Nashner, L. (1982). Ontogenetic development of postural control in man: Adaptation to altered support and visual conditions during stance. *Journal of Neuroscience 2* (5), 545-552.

Foudriat, B., DiFabio, R., & Anderson, J. (1993). Sensory organization of balance responses in children 3-6 years of age: A normative study with diagnostic implications. *International Journal of Pediatric Otorhinolaryngology, 27,* 255-271.

Haas, G., Diener, H., Bacher, M., & Dichgans, J. (1986). Development of postural control in children: Short-, medium-, and long-latency EMG responses of leg muscles after perturbation of stance. *Experimental Brain Research, 64,* 127-132.

Hadders-Algra, M., Brogren, E., & Forssberg, H. (1997). Nature and nurture in the development of postural control in human infants. *Acta Pediatric Supplement 422,* 48-53.

Haley, S. (1986). Sequential analyses of postural reactions in nonhandicapped infants. *Physical Therapy, 66* (4), 531-536.

Hayes, K., & Riach, C. (1989). Preparatory postural adjustment and postural sway in young children. In M. Woollacott & A. Shumway-Cook (Eds.), *Development of posture and gait across the life span.* Columbia: University of South Carolina Press.

Horak, F., & Nashner, L. (1986). Central programming of posture control: Adaptation to altered support-surface configurations. *Journal of Neurophysiology, 55,* 1368-1381.

Horak, F., & Shumway-Cook, A. (1990). Clinical implications of posture control research. In P. Duncan (Ed.), *Balance proceedings of the APTA forum.* Alexandria, VA: American Physical Therapy Association.

Horak, F., Shumway-Cook, A., Crow, T., & Black, F. (1988). Vestibular function and motor proficiency in children with hearing impairments and in learning disabled children with motor impairments. *Developmental Medicine and Child Neurology, 30,* 64-79.

Jantz, J., Blosser, C., & Fruechting, L. (1997). A motor milestone change noted with a change in sleep position. *Archives of Pediatric and adolescent Medicine, 151,* 565-568.

Johnson-Kramer, C., Sherwood, D., Frech, R., & Canabal, M. (1992). Performance and learning of a dynamic balance task by visually impaired children. *Clinical Kinesiology, 1,* 3-6.

Jouen, F. (1984). Visual-vestibular interactions in infancy. *Infant Behavior and Development, 7,* 135-145.

Kamm, K., Thelen, E., & Jensen, J. (1990). A dynamical systems approach to motor development. *Physical Therapy, 70* (12), 763-775.

Kramer, J., Ashton, B., & Brander, R. (1992). Training of head control in the sitting and semi-prone position. *Child Care, Health, and Development, 18,* 365-376.

Leonard, C., Hirschfeld, A., & Forssberg, H. (1988). Gait acquisition and reflex abnormalities in normal children and children with cerebral palsy. In B. Amblard, A. Berthoz, & F. Clarae (Eds.), *Posture and gait development, adaptation, and modulation.* New York: Elsevier Science.

Milani-Comparetti, A., & Gidoni, E. (1967). Routine developmental examination in normal and retarded children. *Developmental Medicine and Child Neurology, 9,* 631-638.

Nashner, L. (1990). Sensory, neuromuscular, and biomechanical contributions to human balance. In P. Duncan (Ed.), *Balance proceedings of the APTA forum.* Alexandria, VA: American Physical Therapy Association.

Nashner, L., Shumway-Cook, A., & Marin, O. (1983). Stance posture control in selected groups of children with cerebral palsy: Deficits in sensory organization and muscular coordination. *Experimental Brain Research, 49,* 393-409.

Perin, B. (1989). Physical therapy for the child with cerebral palsy. In J. Techlin (Ed.), *Pediatric physical therapy.* Philadelphia: J.B. Lippincott.

Piper, M., & Darrah, J. (1994). *Motor assessment of the developing infant.* Philadelphia: W.B. Saunders.

Pountney, T., Mulcahy, C., & Green, E. (1990). Early development of postural control. *Physiotherapy, 76* (12), 799-802.

Riach, C., & Hayes, K. (1987). Maturation of postural sway in young children. *Developmental Medicine and Child Neurology, 29,* 650-658.

Ribaldi, H., Rider, R., & Toole, T. (1987). A comparison of static and dynamic balance in congenitally blind, sighted, and sighted blindfolded adolescents. *Adapted Physical Activity Quarterly, 4,* 220-225.

Richardson, P., Atwater, S., Crowe, T., & Deitz, J. (1992). Performance of preschoolers on the pediatric clinical test of sensory interaction for balance. *American Journal of Occupational Therapy, 46* (9), 793-800.

Schmidt, R. (1988). *Motor control and learning* (2nd ed.). Champaign, IL: Human Kinetics.

Seeger, B., & Caudrey, D. (1983). Biofeedback therapy to achieve symmetrical gait in children with hemiplegic cerebral palsy: Long term efficacy. *Archives of Physical Medicine and Rehabilitation, 64,* 160-162.

Sellers, J. (1988). Relationship between antigravity control and postural control in young children. *Physical Therapy, 68* (4), 486-430.

Shumway-Cook, A. (1989). Equilibrium deficits in children. In M. Woollacott & A. Shumway-Cook, A. (Eds.), *Development of posture and gait across the life span.* Columbia: University of South Carolina Press.

Shumway-Cook, A., & Horak, F. (1986). Assessing the influence of sensory interaction on balance. *Physical Therapy, 66,* 1548-1550.

Shumway-Cook, A., Horak, F., & Black, F. (1987). A critical examination of vestibular function in motor impaired learning disabled children. *International Journal of Otorhinolaryngology, 14,* 21-30.

Shumway-Cook, A., & Woollacott, M. (1985a). Dynamics of postural control in the child with Down syndrome. *Physical Therapy, 9,* 1315-1322.

Shumway-Cook, A. & Woollacott, M. (1985b). The growth of stability: Postural control from a developmental perspective. *Journal of Motor Behavior, 17* (2), 131-147.

Sternat, J. (1993). Developing head and trunk control. In B. Connolly, & P. Montgomery (Eds.), *Therapeutic exercise in developmental disabilities.* Hixson, TN: Chattanooga Group.

Stockmeyer, S. (1967). An interpretation of the approach of Rood to the treatment of neuromuscular dysfunction. *American Journal of Physical Medicine, 46,* 900-956.

Taylor, J. (1931). *Selected writings of John Hughlings Jackson* (Vol. II). London: Holder & Stoughton.

Thelen, E., & Fisher, D. (1982). Newborn stepping: An explanation for a "disappearing reflex." *Developmental Psychology, 18,* 760-775.

Thelen, E., & Fisher, D. (1983). The organization of spontaneous leg movements in newborn infants, *Journal of Motor Behavior, 15,* 353-377.

VanSant, A. (1991). Neurodevelopmental treatment and pediatric physical therapy: A commentary. *Physical Therapy, 3* (3), 137-140.

VanSant, A. (1993). Concepts of neural organization and movement. In B. Connolly & P. Montgomery (Eds.), *Therapeutic exercise in developmental disabilities.* Hixson, TN: Chattanooga Group.

VanSant, A. (1994). Motor control and motor learning. In D. Cech, & S. Martin (Eds.), *Functional movement development across the life span.* Philadelphia: W.B. Saunders.

Vereijken, B., & Thelen, E. (1997). Training infant treadmill stepping: The role of individual pattern stability. *Developmental Psychobiology, 30,* 89-102.

Von Hofsten, C. (1986). The emergence of manual skills. In M. Wade & A. Whiting (Eds.), *Motor development in children: Aspects of coordination and control.* Boston: Martinus Nijhoff.

Williams, H., Fisher, J., & Tritschler, K. (1983). Descriptive analysis of static postural control in 4, 6, and 8 year old normal and motorically awkward children. *American Journal of Physical Medicine, 62* (1), 12-26.

Woollacott, M. (1988). Posture and gait from newborn to elderly. In B. Amblard, A. Berthoz, & F. Clarae (Ed.), *Posture and gait development, adaptation, and modulation.* New York: Elsevier Science.

Woollacott, M., Debu, B., & Mowatt, M. (1988). Neuromuscular control of posture in the infant and child: Is vision dominant? *Journal of Motor Behavior, 19* (2), 167-186.

Woollacott, M., Shumway-Cook, A., & Williams, H. (1989). The development of posture and balance control in children. In M. Woollacott & A. Shumway-Cook (Eds.), *Development of posture and gait across the lifespan.* Columbia: University of South Carolina Press.

Woollacott, M., & Sveistrup, H. (1992). Changes in the sequencing and timing of muscle response coordination associated with developmental transitions in balance abilities. *Human Movement Science, 11,* 23-36.

chapter **11**

Development of Hand Skills

Charlotte E. Exner

key terms

Visual-motor
   integration
Fine motor
   coordination
Dexterity
Hand skills
Reach
Grasp

Carry
Voluntary release
In-hand manipulation
Bilateral hand use

■ CHAPTER OBJECTIVES

1. Describe typical development of hand skills in children.
2. Identify factors that contribute to typical or atypical development of hand skills.
3. Explain the implications of hand skill problems for play, self-care, and school performance.
4. Describe typical problems with children's development of hand skills.
5. Describe frames of reference and theories that the therapist can use in structuring intervention plans for children who have problems with hand skills.
6. Identify evaluation tools and methods useful in assessing hand skills in children.
7. Describe intervention strategies for assisting children in improving or compensating for problems with hand skills.

Hand skills are critical to interaction with the environment. The hands allow action through human contact and through contact with objects. Hands are the "tools" most often used to accomplish work, play, and perform self-maintenance tasks. The child who has a disability affecting hand skills has less opportunity to take in sensory information from the environment and experience the effect of his or her actions on the world.

■ COMPONENTS OF HAND SKILLS

Effective use of the hands to engage in activities of daily occupations depends on a complex interaction of hand skills, postural mechanisms, cognition, and visual perception. The term *visual-motor integration* refers to the interaction of visual skills, visual perceptual skills, and motor skills. The term *hand skills* is used interchangeably with the terms *fine motor coordination, fine motor skills,* and *dexterity*. Because this chapter refers to only those skills accomplished with hands to attain and manipulate objects, the more specific term *hand skills* is used.

Although most therapists assume that the development of hand skills depends on adequate somatosensory and postural functions and sufficient visual perceptual and cognitive development, these areas are not discussed in detail in this chapter. Hand skills are patterns that normally rely on both tactile-proprioceptive and visual information for accuracy. However, the child can accomplish these skills without visual feedback if somatosensory functions provide adequate information. The patterns include basic reach, grasp, carry, release, and the more complex skills of in-hand manipulation and bilateral hand use. Brief definitions of these patterns follow:

- *Reach.* Movement of the arm and hand for the purpose of contacting an object with the hand
- *Grasp.* Attainment of an object with the hand
- *Carry.* Transportation of a hand-held object from one place to another
- *Voluntary release.* Intentional letting go of a hand-held object at a specific time and place
- *In-hand manipulation.* Adjustment of an object within the hand after grasp
- *Bilateral hand use.* Use of two hands together to accomplish an activity

In this discussion, *hand-arm* refers to the interactive movement and stabilization of different parts of the hand and arm to accomplish a fine motor task.

Visual skills are the use of extraocular muscles to direct eye movements. These include the ability to visually fix on a stationary object and the smooth, accurate tracking of a moving target. *Visual perceptual skills* are the recognition, discrimination, and processing of sensory information through the eyes and related central nervous system (CNS) structures. Visual perceptual skills include the identification of shapes, colors, and other qualities; the orientation of objects or shapes in space; and the relationship of objects or shapes to one another and to the environment (see Chapter 13).

■ CONTRIBUTIONS OF OTHER PERFORMANCE COMPONENTS TO HAND SKILLS

As children mature, they begin to effectively coordinate visual skills with hand skills, and later they combine hand-eye coordination with visual perceptual skills (Ayres, 1958). These skills, in conjunction with cognitive and social development, allow the child to engage in increasingly complex activities. Although therapists usually give motor issues the most attention, many dimensions of development significantly influence effective hand use, including the child's visual skills, somatosensory functions, sensory integration (SI), visual perception, cognition, social factors, and culture.

Visual Skills

Visual skills have a major role in the development of hand function (Bertenthal & von Hofsten, 1998; Jeannerod, 1994; von Hofsten, 1991). Vision is particularly important in learning new motor skills. At about 4 months of age, infants begin to move their hands under visual control as they reach for an object and make differentiated finger movements. The visuomotor development required for accurate reach matures by approximately 6 months of age. The infant's visual motor coordination continues to refine, and by 9 months of age the infant guides his or her hand movements using visual-somatosensory integration (i.e., these sensory inputs are combined and compared as he or she anticipates and plans movement). Vision remains important when the infant learns new fine motor skills or when an activity requires highly precise and accurate movements (e.g., stringing small beads or putting together a puzzle).

Somatosensory Functions

The relationship between somatosensory functions of the hands and hand skills is strong. Good hand skills are associated with good somatosensory functioning. However, good somatosensory functioning does not necessarily yield good hand skills.

The role of somatosensory information and feedback is critical to the development of children's hand skills, particularly those that involve isolated movements of the fingers and thumb. Typical infants develop the ability to match haptic (knowledge of objects gathered via active) touch perception of some three-dimensional objects with visual perception within the first 6 months of life (Stillwell & Cermak, 1995). Bushnell and Boudreau (1998) reported that children as young as 2½ years of age can identify common objects by touch alone and children 5 years of age demonstrate good haptic recognition of unfamiliar objects. Many aspects of haptic perception, such as identification of three-dimensional common objects and perception of spatial orientation, are well developed by 6 years of age. By adolescence the child fully develops the refinement of haptic perception and the ability to discriminate all aspects of object characteristics through touch (Stillwell & Cermak, 1995).

The fingertips gather precise information about many types of object qualities. Children who lack the ability to use finger control have limited access to somatosensory information. Initiating and sustaining grasp force requires tactile and proprioceptive input and integration (Johansson & Westling, 1988). The ability to sustain objects in the hand (i.e., to prevent objects from dropping) is primarily related to intact somatosensory functioning (Gordon & Forssberg, 1997).

Somatosensory problems can produce significant problems with hand function, even when motor control is good (Pehoski, 1995), and poor hand skills can contribute to the child obtaining a limited amount of somatosensory information. Children who have poor tactile discrimination receive less feedback about how their fingers move together and independently of one another.

Children with cerebral palsy are likely to have tactile discrimination problems and motor control problems. Between the 1950s and 1960s, several studies of tactile dysfunction in children with cerebral palsy were conducted. These studies verified the presence of a variety of tactile discrimination problems in the hands of a high percentage of children with cerebral palsy (Kenney,

1963; Monfraix, Tardieu, & Tardieu, 1961; Tachdjian & Minear, 1958; Twitchell, 1965). Although the degree of tactile problems was not always associated with the degree of motor impairment, children with cerebral palsy tend to need more trials than nondisabled children to match tactile and proprioceptive information with force for grasp and lift of objects (Eliaason, 1995). Children with cerebral palsy also have difficulty anticipating how much force will be needed.

Children with milder problems also are at risk for somatosensory problems that affect hand skills. Case-Smith (1991) studied the relationship between both tactile defensiveness and tactile discrimination and in-hand manipulation skills in 50 children between 4 and 6 years of age. In this sample, which included 80% nondysfunctional children, those having problems with either tactile defensiveness or decreased tactile discrimination showed no significant problems with performing the in-hand manipulation tasks presented. However, those who had both tactile discrimination problems and tactile defensiveness had difficulty with performance of the in-hand manipulation tasks that were timed. Their performances were significantly less efficient than those of the children in the other groups.

Somatosensory functioning is difficult to study in children, particularly in young children and those with disabilities. In testing, the performance of these children varies from one session to another, which further complicates the assessment process. Knowledge of a child's perception of an object's shape does not provide information about the child's perception of other object qualities (Stillwell & Cermak, 1995). Given that the link between somatosensory functioning and hand skills is a strong one, further investigation of the relationship between tactile functioning and various hand skills will support intervention approaches with these children.

Sensory Integration

The types of SI problems that are most likely to influence hand use are sensory registration problems, tactile hypersensitivity, poor tactile discrimination, and dyspraxia. Children who have poor sensory registration engage in few activities involving hand skills. The child with tactile defensiveness is likely to avoid contact with certain materials, thus limiting exposure to various objects. Motor-planning deficits and clumsiness are associated with poor tactile and proprioceptive functioning. Praxis problems based on poor tactile and proprioceptive processing are referred to as *somatodyspraxia* (Ayres, 1989).

Visual Perception and Cognition

Perceptual development and cognitive development are difficult to isolate from each other, particularly as they relate to object-handling skills in children; therefore these areas are addressed together in this section. Development of hand skills allows for more complex interaction with objects, and perceptual and cognitive development allows the child to know the possibilities available for object use and interactions.

The child's perception of object characteristics, movement speed required, and power needed affects his or her ability to effectively control objects (Elliott & Connolly, 1984). The child acquires knowledge about objects through object manipulation.

During the first 6 months, the infant uses visual and tactile stimuli to guide fine motor development and begins to develop an awareness of object placement in space. In the second half of the first year, the infant adjusts actions of the hand in response to object characteristics such as size, shape, and surface qualities (Corbetta & Mounoud, 1990). Ruff, McCarton, Kurtzber, and Vaughan (1984) emphasized the importance of object manipulation in infants between 6 and 12 months of age for learning of object characteristics because this learning was believed to be important for concept and language development. Infants reflect their perceptual and cognitive skills in preparation for object contact. By 9 to 10 months of age, infants adapt their arm positions to horizontal versus vertical object presentations and shape their hands appropriately for convex and concave objects.

During the second year, infants learn to relate objects to one another with more accuracy and purpose. Before 18 months of age, infants modify their movement approach to the anticipated weight of the object (Bushnell & Boudreau, 1998; Corbetta & Mounoud, 1990).

Exner and Henderson (1995) discussed the interaction of cognition and hand skill development. Like perceptual development, cognitive development influences and is supported by development of hand skills. For example, changes in attentional control and development of problem-solving strategies are seen in the gradual improvement in infants' ability to handle two objects simultaneously. Without this development in cognition, bilateral skills would not be possible. The infant must be able to attend to two objects simultaneously to be able to bang objects together, stabilize an object with one hand while manipulating with the other, and manipulate two or more objects simultaneously (e.g., in buttoning or tying). Attention and planning demands are greater for two-handed activities than for one-handed activities; thus bilateral skill development lags behind unilateral skill development (Bushnell & Boudreau, 1998; Corbetta & Mounoud, 1990).

Social Factors

Social factors that can affect the development of hand skills include socioeconomic status, gender, and role expectations. Like culture, social factors are less likely to affect development of more basic hand skills but may have a greater influence on skills needed for the complex manipulation of objects and tool use. For example, children in conditions of poverty may not have exposure to writing utensils, scissors, and other materials common to children from middle class environments.

Verdonck and Henneberg (1997) studied differences in performance on the Box and Block Test of Manual Dexterity in two groups of South African children between 6 and 17 years of age. The groups reportedly differed only in socioeconomic status and rural versus urban living environments. Children from the middle class urban area performed significantly better than those from the poor rural area.

Cultural Factors

The objects that are important to the child's cultural group influence development of object manipulation. The tools important in one culture may not be available in another culture; therefore children may not have the opportunity to develop some tool-specific skills. For example, eating utensils vary from chopsticks to forks and spoons. Scissors use may be important for school performance in some cultures but not in others.

In addition, the age at which children are expected to achieve skill in object manipulation can vary. Safety concerns influence parents in some cultural groups to delay the introduction of a knife to their child, whereas other parents encourage independence in knife use. Some cultures introduce the use of writing materials to children before 1 year of age. Other families do not provide children with these materials until they are expected to adhere to requirements such as only using them on paper (versus on the wall or on clothing).

Culture also influences the perception of children's need for manipulative materials. Linked to this is the cultural group's view of the importance of play. Play materials that provide opportunities for development of manipulative skills (such as building sets, beads, puzzles, and table games) are highly valued in some cultural groups, whereas in other groups, play with gross motor objects such as balls and riding toys or play with animals is more valued. Some cultural groups view children's play as highly important; thus few play materials of any type are available.

Although types of activities encouraged can promote the development of specific skills, acquisition of basic hand skills of reach, grasp, release, and manipulation does not rely on the availability of any particular materials. It relies on reasonable exposure to a variety of materials with the opportunity to handle them.

■ MOTOR AND PHYSICAL FACTORS

Integrity of the Hand

The integrity of the hand is an important consideration in hand function. Children with congenital hand anomalies may be missing one or more digits, thus sig-

nificantly affecting the variety of possible prehension patterns. Refined finger movements and in-hand manipulation skills may also be limited or absent. Severe congenital anomalies can affect bilateral hand use. Involvement of the thumb has a more significant effect on hand function development than impairment of any other digit.

Range of Joint Motion

Range of joint motion has a significant effect on positioning the arm for hand use and reaching and carrying skills. Effective hand function also depends on adequate mobilization of distal muscle groups that control palmar arches. Limitations in range can occur as a result of abnormal joint structure, muscle weakness, or joint inflammation. Any of the problems that decrease range of motion are likely to affect the child's ability to grasp larger objects or to flatten the hand for use in stabilizing materials.

Strength

Sufficient strength is necessary to initiate all types of grasp patterns and to maintain these patterns during carrying. Children's strength in grasp gradually increases through the preschool years (Link, Lukens, & Bush, 1995) and through adolescence (Mathiowetz, Weimer, & Federman, 1986), which allows them to engage in activities with objects of increasing weight. Children with poor strength may be unable to initiate the finger extension or the thumb opposition pattern necessary before grasp. They also may not have the flexor control to hold a grasp pattern. Many children with decreased strength are unable to use patterns that rely on the intrinsic muscles for control and are therefore unable to use thumb opposition or metacarpophalangeal (MCP) joint flexion with interphalangeal (IP) joint extension. Children with fair strength may be able to initiate a grasp pattern but may be unable to lift an object against gravity while maintaining the grasp. Endurance during an activity can be a problem for children with mildly decreased strength, particularly in situations in which they must use a sustained grasp pattern or hold an object against resistance (e.g., during eating with utensils, coloring, handwriting, and scissors activities).

Tone

Tone within muscle groups affects the stability of parts of the arms and hands during activities and the types of movements possible. Damage to the CNS causes tone abnormalities, which can affect range of joint motion and, in general, decrease speed of movement. Increased tone results in loss of range, whereas decreased tone results in exaggerated joint range and decreased stability. Children with fluctuating tone typically have full range, but they can maintain joint stability only at the extreme end of a joint position (full flexion or full extension). In addition, movements are less controlled and often are random or unrelated to the task.

■ GENERAL DEVELOPMENTAL CONSIDERATIONS

Developmental principles are further described in Chapter 4. Two principles with particular application to hand skill development are mass-to-specific and proximal-to-distal.

The mass-to-specific principle indicates that less-differentiated movement patterns precede discrete, highly specialized skills. For example, the infant uses all fingers in early grasping and later uses only the specific number of fingers needed for object contact.

The proximal-to-distal principle of development suggests that development initially occurs proximally (in the head and trunk) and then gradually progresses toward the distal parts of the body (hands and feet). In using this principle to guide treatment, some therapists suggest that intervention for hand skills should be deferred until postural control matures. Clinicians have interpreted this relationship to mean that improvement in postural control results in hand skills improvement and/or that intervention should be sequential from proximal to distal control.

However, several clinical research studies (Case-Smith, Fisher, & Bauer, 1989; Wilson & Trombly, 1984) and Pehoski (1992, 1995), in her chapters addressing CNS control of precision movements of the hand, have questioned this principle. The clinical studies have yielded weak correlations between postural or proximal control and hand function (approximately r = 0.20 to 0.35). Case-Smith and others (1989) stated that "the correlations between the proximal and distal motor functions would be markedly higher if proximal motor control was necessary for the development of distal motor skill" (p. 661). The relationship between proximal and distal control is a functional or biomechanical one in which postural control is necessary for placement of the hand in space and support of the hand during its execution of skills. Case-Smith and others (1989) emphasized that "therapists should not assume that proximal control is a necessary precursor to fine motor skill; they should, however, assume that treating proximal weakness may affect distal function" (p. 661). However, the degree of proximal control does not necessarily determine the child's degree of distal control.

Pehoski (1992, 1995) used work by Lawrence and Kuypers (1968) to explain why distal control is not directly linked to proximal control. Two motor systems are used in upper extremity control. One system is responsible for postural control and proximal control, including integrated body-limb and body-head movements. This system comprises primarily the ventral-medial brainstem

pathways; that synapse primarily with interneurons to trunk and proximal muscles (Pehoski, 1992, 1995). In contrast, the corticospinal track system originates in the primary motor cortex, and its fibers directly synapse with the motoneurons for hand muscles. The latter system allows for isolated finger movements, which are needed for a precise pincer grasp and fine manipulation (Pehoski, 1992, 1995). Thus development of upper extremity skills and hand skills occurs because of proximal *and* distal control mechanisms, rather than one proximal *to* distal mechanism.

Refined movements also depend on the ability to effectively combine *patterns of stability and mobility* (Bobath, 1978). The child must develop the ability to stabilize the trunk effectively and maintain it in an upright position without relying on frequent use of one or both arms to maintain balance. Additionally, the child sequentially develops patterns of stability and mobility in the scapulohumeral, elbow, and wrist joints. This permits arm use that is independent from, but effectively used with, trunk movement. Eventually the ability to use stability and mobility in the hand emerges.

For normal functioning, joints must be able to stabilize at any point within the normal range of movement and to move within small, medium, or large segments of range. At times during arm-hand activities, the proximal joints are more stable. Grasp is an example of this because the arm is stable while the fingers are moving. However, in carrying, the distal joints are stable while the arm is moving. In mature handwriting, the elbow, forearm, and wrist joints are relatively stable and the shoulder and finger joints are mobile.

An important sequence in the development of motor control is the use of straight movement patterns before the emergence of controlled rotation patterns. For example, the infant first develops controlled stability and mobility in basic flexion and extension of the shoulder, elbow, and wrist. This is followed by control of internal and external rotation of the shoulder and pronation and supination of the forearm.

In normal development the infant gradually learns to use both sides of the body well together and to use each side of the body independently from the other. Initially the infant uses his or her arms in asymmetric patterns that are not coordinated. Movements of one arm often elicit reflexive, nonpurposeful reactions in the other arm. Gradually, the infant develops the ability to move the two arms together in the same pattern. As skilled use of symmetric hand and arm patterns is refined, the infant begins to use the two arms independently of one another for different parts of an activity. For example, an one hand stabilizes an object while the other hand manipulates it. Overflow and associated movements gradually decrease to allow separate but coordinated action of the two hands.

■ DEVELOPMENT OF HAND SKILLS

As in all areas of occupational therapy, the therapist must supplement academic study of hand skill development and treatment with observations of typical infants and children and of children with differences in development. In addition, imitating each of the normal and abnormal movements and patterns described in the following text is helpful in clarifying the descriptions provided.

Reach

Rosblad (1995) states that "in a reaching movement the goal is to transport the hand to the target, with precision in both time and space" (p. 81). Thus the development of reaching is described in terms of the changes that take place in the control and speed of the hand's movement toward the object and the preparation of the hand for grasp.

The arm movements of the newborn are asymmetric. However, even within the first several days of life, the infant shows increasing visual regard of objects close to him or her and activation of the arms in response to objects (von Hofsten, 1982). Within the next few months, the general arm activation becomes active swiping or batting at objects, with the arm abducted at the shoulder. Objects are rarely grasped, and then only by accident. If grasped, they are released at random, generally in association with arm movements.

Gradually a midline orientation of the hands develops. Initially the hands are held close to the body. Soon, with an increased desire for visual regard of the hands and greater proximal arm stability, the child holds the hands further away to view them. This pattern precedes the onset of symmetric bilateral reaching, which usually occurs first in the supine and then in the sitting position. At this stage, the child initiates reach with humeral abduction, partial shoulder internal rotation, forearm pronation, and full finger extension.

As the infant shows increasing disassociation of the two body sides during movement, unilateral reaching begins. Abduction and internal rotation of the shoulder are less prominent in reach. The hand opens in preparation for grasping the object and is usually more open than necessary for the size of the object.

As scapular control and trunk stability mature, the infant begins to use shoulder flexion, slight external rotation, full elbow extension, forearm supination, and slight wrist extension during reaching. Active supination of the forearm is not seen until some external rotation is used to stabilize the humerus. In addition, well-controlled elbow extension evolves as the rotation elements are developing. Mature reach is usually seen with sustained trunk extension and a slight rotation of the trunk toward the object of interest. Over the next few years the child refines this unilateral reaching pattern, increasing accuracy of arm placement and grading of finger extension as appro-

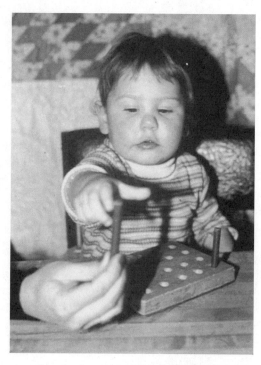

figure**11-1** This typical child demonstrates reach with trunk rotation, full elbow extension, slight forearm rotation, and wrist stability, yet some degree of excess finger extension before grasp. *(Photograph by Ed Exner.)*

priate to the size of the object (Figure 11-1), as well as timing of the various movement elements.

Grasp
Classifications of grasp patterns

Napier (1956) proposed two basic terms to describe hand movements: prehensile and nonprehensile. *Nonprehensile movements* involve pushing or lifting the object with the fingers or the entire hand. In contrast, *prehensile movements* involve grasp of an object and may be further divided according to purpose of the grasp: precision or power. *Precision grasps* involve opposition of the thumb to fingertips. *Power grasps* involve use of the entire hand. In a power grasp, the thumb is held flexed or abducted to other fingers, depending on control requirements.

In most cases, the activity and the object's characteristics determine the grasp pattern used. Small objects are generally held in a precision grasp primarily because of the large amount of sensory feedback that is available through the fingertips and the control that is used to move them. Medium objects can be held with either pattern, and large objects are held with a power grasp. Napier (1956) noted a frequent interplay between precision and power handling of different objects based on needs within an activity.

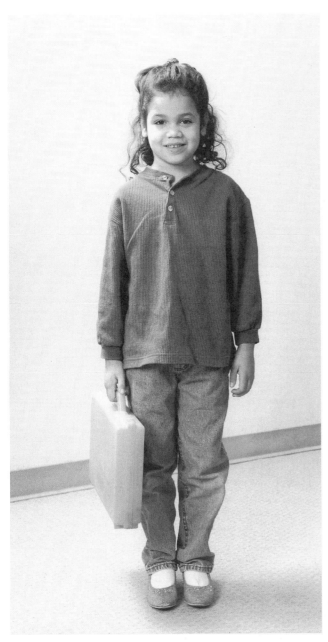

figure**11-2**   Hook grasp used to carry a child's art case. *(Photo by Kanji Takeno.)*

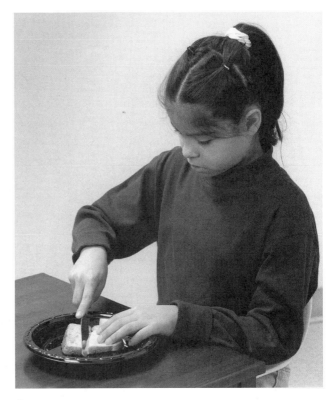

figure**11-3**   Power grasp with the right hand used in cutting bread. *(Photo by Kanji Takeno.)*

Weiss and Flatt (1971) described a slightly different method of classification. Grasps with no thumb opposition include hook grasp, power grasp, and lateral pinch. The patterns that use thumb opposition include tip and palmar pinches. The palmar pinch category is divided into standard, spherical, cylindrical, and disc grasps.

The *hook grasp* is used when strength of grasp must be maintained to carry objects. The transverse metacarpal arch is essentially flat, fingers are adducted with flexion at the IP joints, and flexion or extension occurs at the MCP joints (Weiss & Flatt, 1971) (Figure 11-2). The thumb

can be flexed over the fingers if additional power is needed. Observation of this pattern provides an indication of the child's ability to sustain wrist extension during finger flexion.

In contrast, the *power grasp* is often used to control tools or other objects. Oblique object placement in the hand, flexion of the ulnar fingers, less flexion with the radial fingers, and thumb extension and adduction facilitate precision handling with this grasp (e.g., for brushing hair). Thus the child stabilizes the object with the ulnar side of the hand and controls the object for position and use with the radial side of the hand (Weiss & Flatt, 1971) (Figure 11-3). Observation of this pattern allows for notation of the degree of radial/ulnar disassociation in the hand that the child can use and his or her control of thumb adduction with extension.

Lateral pinch is used to exert power on or with a small object. Partial thumb adduction, MCP flexion, and slight IP flexion are characteristics of this pattern. Although the index finger is slightly flexed, it is more extended than the other fingers. The pad of the thumb is placed against the radial side of the index finger at or near the distal interphalangeal (DIP) joint (Figure 11-4). This pattern involves control of the index finger while adducting and flexing the thumb.

There are two types of *standard* pinches. Opposition of the thumb to the index finger pad only, describes *pad*

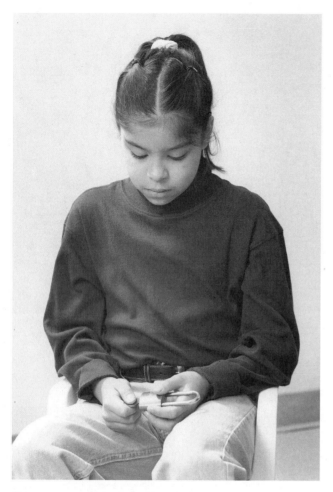

figure**11-4**   Lateral pinch with the right hand to open a padlock. *(Photo by Kanji Takeno.)*

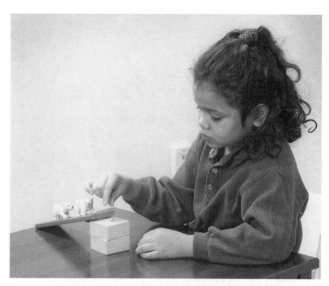

figure**11-5**   Pincer grasp used to place "food" for the climbing polar bears. *(Photo by Kanji Takeno.)*

to pad, two-point pinch (Smith & Benge, 1985), or *pincer grasp* (Gesell & Amatruda, 1947) (Figure 11-5). Opposition of the thumb simultaneously to the index and middle finger pads, which provides increased stability of prehension, describes *three-point pinch* (Smith & Benge, 1985), or *three-jaw chuck* (Erhardt, 1982) (Figure 11-6). In both cases the thumb forms an oval shape or a modified oval shape with the fingers. In addition, the forearm is slightly supinated, which frees the thumb and radial fingers from contact with the surface and allows for an optimal view of the object. Observation of this pattern allows for notation of the child's ability to control objects with the radial finger pads while controlling thumb opposition.

Opposition of the thumb tip and index fingertip so that a circle is formed describes *tip pinch* (Figure 11-7). All joints of the index finger and thumb are partially flexed. This pinch pattern is used to obtain small objects. Observation of this grasp provides information about the child's ability to disassociate the two sides of the hand and use the tips of the index finger and thumb.

Differences in hand posture characterize the other palmar grasps. Significant wrist extension, finger abduction, and some degree of flexion at the MCP and IP joints describe *spherical grasp* (Figure 11-8). Stability of the longitudinal arch is necessary to use this pattern to grasp large objects. The hypothenar eminence lifts to assist the cupping of the hand for control of the object (Weiss & Flatt, 1971). Observation of this grasp pattern suggests the child's ability to balance muscle control of the intrinsic and extrinsic hand muscles.

In the *cylindrical grasp* the transverse arch is flattened to allow the fingers to hold against the object. The fingers are only slightly abducted, and IP and MCP joint flexion is graded according to the size of the object. When additional force is required, more of the palmar surface of the hand contacts the object (Weiss & Flatt, 1971) (Figure 11-9). Observation of this pattern allows for observation of palmar arch control during handling of a relatively large object.

Finger abduction that is graded according to the size of the object held, hyperextension of the MCP joints, and flexion of the IP joints (see Figure 11-9) describe *disc grasp* (Weiss & Flatt, 1971). The wrist is more flexed when objects are larger, and only the pads of the fingers contact the object. The amount of thumb extension also increases with object size. The transverse metacarpal arch is flattened in this prehension pattern. This pattern involves disassociation of flexion and extension movements and use of a combination of wrist flexion with MP extension and IP flexion.

Sequential development of grasp patterns

Several developmental trends affect the particular type of grasp pattern that an infant is able to use at any time.

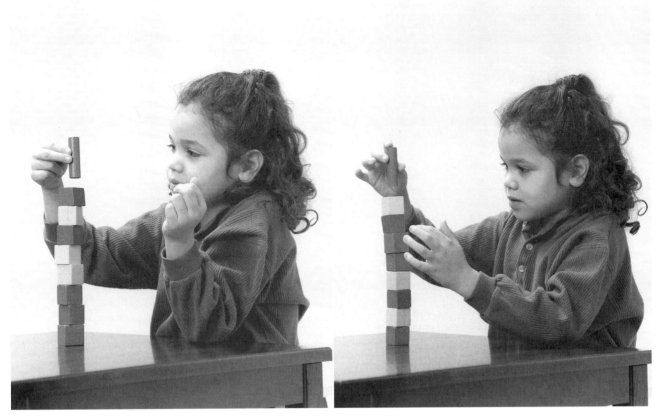

figure**11-6** This child uses variations of a three-jaw chuck grasp with her right hand, depending on task demands. *(Photo by Kanji Takeno.)*

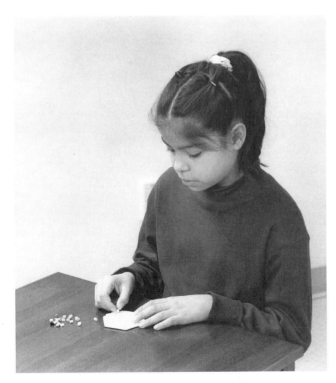

figure**11-7** Tip pinch with the right hand used to complete a bead craft project. Normal radial grasps, such as tip pinch, are accompanied by slight forearm supination. The left hand uses stabilization without grasp on the board. *(Photo by Kanji Takeno.)*

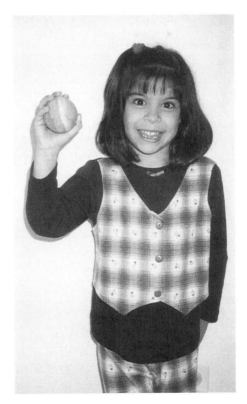

figure**11-8** Spherical grasp used in preparation for ball throwing.

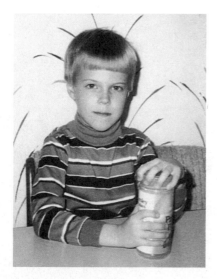

figure**11-9** The child uses a cylindrical grasp with his right hand and a disc grasp with his left to open a jar.

The sequences shown in Box 11-1 interact and overlap. The infant's growing interest in objects, desire to attain them, and desire to explore them and relate them to other objects influence these motor sequences. Haptic and visual perceptual development contributes to the infant's ability to shape the hand appropriately for the object and to approach the object with optimal orientation of the arm and hand.

Another aspect of motor development that contributes to the infant's use of increasingly mature and more varied patterns is the ability to use internal stability throughout the upper extremity, forearm supination, and thumb opposition. Thumb activity and control are necessary to allow for patterns other than palmar grasp. Hirschel, Pehoski, and Coryell (1990) discussed the influence of increasing arm stability on the infant's use of a mature pincer grasp. The ability to stabilize the wrist in a slightly extended position is important for grasp patterns that use distal (fingertip) control. Slight forearm supination is important because it positions the hand so that the thumb and radial fingers are free for active object exploration, and it allows the infant to view his or her fingers and thumb during grasp.

The following sequence is typical during the infant's first 6 months. Initially the infant has no voluntary hand use. The hands alternately open and close in response to various sensory stimuli. Gradually, the traction response and grasp reflex decrease and a voluntary ulnar grasp begin to emerge. By approximately 6 months the infant progresses to being able to use a palmar grasp. Case-Smith, Bigsby, and Clutter (1998) found a marked increase in grasp skill between 4 and 5 months of age. They noted less change between 5 and 6 months of age.

The second 6 months is a key period for development of hand skills. The ability to grasp a variety of objects increases significantly between 6 and 9 months of age. During this time, grasp patterns with active thumb use emerge. Crude raking of a tiny object is present by about 7 months of age, and by 9 months of age the infant is able to attain a tiny object on the finger surface and with the thumb. However, with larger objects the infant's grasp is much more mature. By 8 to 9 months of age the infant holds an object between the thumb and the two radial fingers (i.e., uses a radial digital grasp) and readily varies the grasping pattern according to the shape of the object. Case-Smith and others (1998) noted a particularly dramatic increase in skill between 8 and 9 months of age. However, at this time intrinsic muscle control is not effective because the infant does not use grasp with MCP flexion and IP extension. Between 9 and 12 months of age, refinement occurs in the ability to use thumb and finger pad control for tiny and small objects. More precise preparation of the fingers before initiating grasp, more inhibition of the ulnar fingers, and slight wrist extension and forearm supination are characteristics of this refinement.

After 1 year of age, further refinement occurs in grasp patterns that were seen earlier and more sophisticated patterns emerge. Between 12 and 15 months of age the infant's ability to hold crackers, cookies, and other flat objects identifies an increasing control of the intrinsic muscles. Although studies are limited in terms of grasp development for patterns other than the pincer grasp, between 18 months and 3 years of age most children with typical development acquire the ability to use a disc grasp, a cylindrical grasp, and a spherical grasp with control. Control of a power grasp continues to develop through the preschool years. The pattern for a lateral pinch may be present by 3 years of age, but children generally do not use this pattern with power until later in the preschool years. Overall grasp patterns for a variety of objects is well developed by 5 years of age, but those involving tools may continue to mature into the early school years.

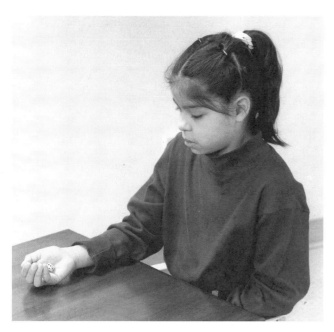

figure**11-10**   The child shows the ability to hold the palm in a cupped position while shaking dice. *(Photo by Kanji Takeno.)*

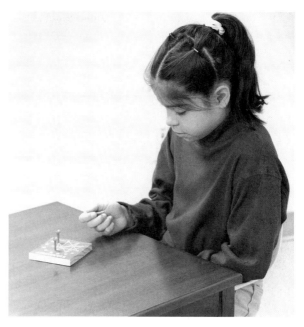

figure**11-11**   Palm-to-finger translation used in handling pieces for a game. *(Photo by Kanji Takeno.)*

In-Hand Manipulation Skills
Classifications

In-hand manipulation includes five basic types of patterns: finger-to-palm translation, palm-to-finger translation, shift, simple rotation, and complex rotation (Exner, 1992). All skills require the ability to control the arches of the palm (Figure 11-10). Long, Conrad, Hall, and Furler (1970) described translation as a linear movement of the object from the palm to the fingers or from the fingers to the palm; the object stays in constant contact with the thumb and fingers during this pattern. The fingers and thumb maintain grasp but then move into and out of MCP and IP flexion and extension. In contrast, Exner's description of the pattern of finger-to-palm translation notes that the object is grasped with the pads of the fingers and thumb and then is moved into the palm (Exner, 1992). The finger pad grasp is released so that the object rests in the palm of the open hand or is held in a palmar grasp at the conclusion of the pattern (Figure 11-11). The object moves in a linear direction within the hand, and the fingers move from an extended position to a more flexed position during the translation. An example of this skill is picking up a coin with the fingers and thumb and moving it into the palm of the hand.

Palm-to-finger translation is the reverse of finger-to-palm translation (Exner, 1992). However, palm-to-finger translation requires isolated control of the thumb and use of a pattern beginning with finger flexion and moving toward finger extension. This pattern is more difficult for the child to execute than finger-to-palm translation. An example of this skill is moving a coin from the palm of the hand to the finger pads before placing the coin in a vending machine.

Shift involves a linear movement of the object on the finger surface (Exner, 1992) to allow for repositioning of the object on the pads of the fingers. In this pattern the fingers move just slightly at the MCP and IP joints, and the thumb typically remains opposed or adducted with MCP and IP extension throughout the shift. The object usually is held solely on the radial side of the hand. Examples of this skill include separating two pieces of paper when they are slightly stuck together, moving a coin from a position against the volar aspect of the DIP joints to a position closer to the fingertips (e.g., so that the coin can be placed easily into the slot on the vending machine), and adjusting a pen or pencil after grasp so that the fingers are positioned close to the writing end of the tool. This skill is used frequently in dressing tasks such as buttoning, fastening snaps, putting laces through the holes on shoes, and putting a belt through beltloops.

The two patterns of rotation are simple and complex. Simple rotation involves the turning or rolling of an object held at the finger pads approximately 90 degrees or less (Exner, 1992). The fingers act as a unit (little or no differentiation of action is shown among them), and the thumb is in an opposed position. Unscrewing a small bottle cap, reorienting a puzzle piece within the hand by turning it slightly before placing it into the puzzle, and picking up a small peg from a surface and rotating it from a horizontal to a vertical position for placement into a pegboard are examples of simple rotation.

Complex rotation involves the rotation of an object 180 to 360 degrees once or repetitively (Exner, 1992). During complex rotation the fingers and thumb alternate in producing the movement, and the fingers typically move independently of one another. An object may be moved end over end, such as in turning a coin or a peg over or in turning a pencil over to use the eraser.

In-hand manipulation skills with and without stabilization

In-hand manipulation skills can occur with only one object in the hand or with two or more objects in the hand. (The skills with only one object in the hand are described in a previous section.) For example, a child typically unscrews a bottle lid with no other objects in his or her hand. However, these skills may be used when the child is holding other objects in the hand. For example, a child may have two or more pieces of cereal in his or her hand but only brings one piece out to the finger pads before placing in the mouth. The term *with stabilization* refers to the use of an in-hand manipulation skill while other objects are being stabilized in the hand. Therefore this activity is described as involving palm-to-finger translation with stabilization, whereas unscrewing the bottle lid is simple rotation. In-hand manipulation skills done with stabilization are more difficult than the same skill done without the simultaneous stabilization of other objects in the hand.

Developmental considerations

Motor skill prerequisites for in-hand manipulation include the following:
■ Movement into and stability in various degrees of supination
■ Wrist stability
■ Opposed grasp with thumb opposition and object contact with the finger surface (not in the palm)
■ Isolated thumb and radial finger movement
■ Control of the transverse metacarpal arch
■ Disassociation of the radial and ulnar sides of the hand

Children who are unable to use in-hand manipulation skills are likely to substitute other patterns. Substitution patterns are part of the typical strategies used in acquiring in-hand manipulation skills; their use does not necessarily represent abnormal fine motor control. Typical patterns that a child uses when he or she shows no evidence of in-hand manipulation are (1) changing of hands (putting the object in the other hand for use), and (2) transferring from hand to hand (moving the object from one hand to the other and back to the hand that held

it first). The child uses these patterns after the initial grasp when he or she realizes that the object in the hand needs to be repositioned for use, but the child cannot readily adjust the object within that hand. Therefore the child moves the object to the other hand (and perhaps back to the first hand) to adjust the position. An example is when a child picks up a crayon or marker with one hand but is not able to shift it to place the fingers near the writing end, so he or she grasps the object with the other hand with the fingers appropriately positioned. Some children preplan for this by picking up the crayon with the nonpreferred hand and changing it to the preferred hand.

Therapists observe several skills in children who are beginning to use in-hand manipulation skills or are preparing for the use of these skills. The substitutions or precursors involve supporting the object while the hand is changing position on it. The type of support that the child uses depends on the type of in-hand manipulation skill being used. Infants typically engage in bilateral manipulation of objects by moving an object between the two hands. As the child moves the object between the hands, he or she turns and repositions it within the hands. Children use this strategy, called a *hand assist,* to substitute for palm-to-finger translation or rotation. In this case the object does not leave the hand that grasped it initially, but the other hand helps with repositioning of the object. The child uses movement of the fingers to assist with repositioning the object as opposed to only grasp and release of the object. Sometimes children use other surfaces or other parts of their body to provide support for the manipulation. Children commonly use assist strategies for shift and complex rotation.

Ongoing research is directed toward determining a sequence for the development of in-hand manipulation (Exner, 1990a; Pehoski, Henderson, & Tickle-Degnen, 1997a, 1997b). The following is a developmental sequence that researchers have identified. By approximately 12 to 15 months of age, infants use finger-to-palm translation to pick up and "hide" small pieces of food in their hands. By 2 to 2½ years of age, children use palm-to-finger translation and simple rotation with some objects. Complex rotation skills are observed in 2½- to 3-year-olds; however, they often have difficulty. By 4 years of age, children consistently use complex rotation without using an external support (Pehoski et. al., 1997a). Relating these skills to functional abilities, children between 3½ and 5½ years of age develop skills in rotating a marker (regardless of its initial orientation) and shifting it into an optimal position for coloring and writing (Exner, 1990a; Humphry, Jewell, & Rosenberger, 1995). Children begin using shift between 3 and 3½ years of age (Exner, 1990a).

After 3 years of age the child uses in-hand manipulation skills with greater proficiency and consistency. Dropping of objects decreases through the preschool years

(Pehoski et. al., 1997b). By 6 years of age, children develop the ability to use a variety of in-hand manipulation skills with stabilization (Exner, 1990a; Pehoski et. al., 1997b). Children more consistently use combinations of in-hand manipulation skills that must be used within an activity, such as palm-to-finger translation with stabilization followed by complex rotation with stabilization, between 6 and 7 months of age. Ongoing research by Exner and others suggests that children continue to refine in-hand manipulation skills up to approximately 9 to 10 years of age and continue to develop speed of skill use through 12 years of age.

The presence of a skill with one type of object is not always associated with the child being able to use the skill with another size or shape of object. For example, the child may be able to use simple rotation to turn a small peg but may not be able to use simple rotation to orient a crayon for coloring. In general, small objects (e.g., smaller-diameter crayons) are easier for children to manipulate than slightly larger objects (e.g., larger-diameter crayons) or tiny objects. Tiny objects require precise fingertip control, whereas medium and larger objects require control with more fingers than small objects.

In addition to object characteristics and the need for using an in-hand manipulation skill with or without stabilization, other factors can contribute to the child's use of these skills with particular materials. These factors include the cognitive-perceptual demands of the activity, the child's interest in the manipulative materials or the activity, and the child's motor planning skills. Problems in any of these areas, or in processing tactile-proprioceptive information or visual acuity, can affect development of in-hand manipulation skills.

Carry

Carrying involves a smooth combination of body movements while stabilizing an object in the hand. Small ranges of movements are used and adjusted in accordance with the demands of the tasks. Cocontraction in the more distal joints of the wrist and hand often is present. The child must be able to hold the forearm stable while in any position, and he or she must be able to modify the forearm and wrist positions during the carry so that the object remains in an optimal position. Similarly, the child must be able to use shoulder rotation movements simultaneously with shoulder flexion and abduction so that appropriate object orientation is maintained.

Voluntary Release

Voluntary release, like grasp, depends on control of arm and finger movements. To place an object for release, the arm needs to move into position accurately and then stabilize as the fingers and thumb extend. Initially the infant does not voluntarily release an object; objects either drop involuntarily from the hand or must be forc-ibly removed from the infant's hand. As the infant's non-discriminative responses to tactile and proprioceptive stimuli decrease and visual control and cognitive development increase, volitional control of release emerges.

With increased mouthing of objects and bringing both hands to midline and playing with them there, the infant begins to transfer objects from one hand to another. Initially the child stabilizes the object in the mouth during transfers or pulls it out of one hand with the other. Soon the infant begins to freely transfer the object from one hand to another. The receiving hand stabilizes the object, and the releasing hand is fully opened.

By 9 months of age the infant begins to release objects without stabilizing with the other hand. The arm is fairly extended during release (Connor, Williamson, & Siepp, 1978). The infant exhibits increasing humeral control as he or she moves the arm to drop objects in different locations. The next step is development of elbow stability in various positions, and the infant begins to release with the elbow in some degree of flexion. The therapist may stabilize the arm or hand on the surface during release. At about 1 year of age the child can release objects with shoulder, elbow, and wrist stability, but the MCP joints remain unstable during this pattern, so the infant continues to show excess finger extension (Figure 11-12). Gradually the child develops the ability to release objects into smaller containers (Figure 11-13) and to stack blocks (Figure 11-14). The release pattern is refined over the next few years until the child can release small objects with graded extension of the fingers, indicating control over the intrinsic hand muscles. These skills also illustrate the integration of perceptual, cognitive, and sensory skills with motor skills.

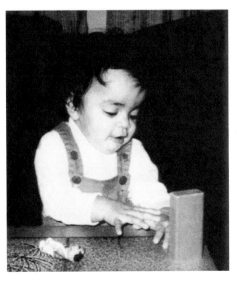

figure**11-12**   Full finger extension and some wrist movement occur with voluntary release.

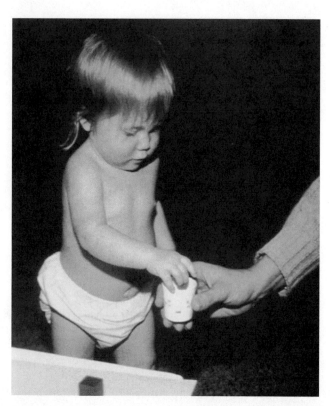

figure**11-13**   Shoulder, elbow, and wrist are stable, and less finger extension occurs with release. The child can release objects into a small container. *(Courtesy Kennedy Kreiger Institute, Baltimore, MD.)*

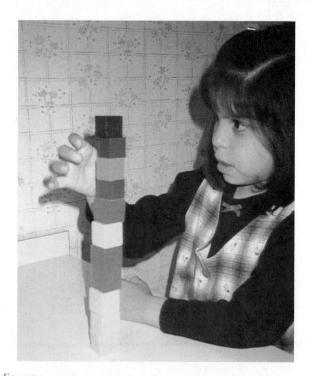

figure**11-14**   Shoulder, elbow, forearm, wrist, and finger stability combines with perceptual development to promote accurate placement of objects.

Bilateral Hand Use

As discussed previously, the normal infant progresses from asymmetry to symmetry to differentiated asymmetric movements, which are used in bilateral hand activities. Asymmetry is a characteristic of movement patterns until almost 3 months of age. Symmetric patterns predominate between 3 and 10 months of age when bilateral reach, grasp, and mouthing of the hands and objects are primary activities. Control for these movements originates proximally at the shoulders, allowing the hands to engage at midline. By 9 to 10 months of age the infant can hold one object in each hand and bang them together. This ability to hold an object in each hand at the same time is critical for further bilateral skill development. By 10 months of age, bimanual action is well differentiated, with one hand grasping the object and the other manipulating parts of it (Fagard, 1998; Fagard & Jacquet, 1989). More complex bilateral skills depend on this ability.

Bimanual activity emerges first as reciprocal or alternating hand movements, then as simultaneous hand movements. By 17 to 18 months of age, infants frequently use role-differentiated strategies (i.e., one hand stabilizes or holds the materials and the other manipulates or activates them) (Ramsey & Weber, 1986). For these skills to emerge, the infant must be able to disassociate the two sides of the body and begin to use the two hands simultaneously for different functions. Effective stabilization of materials also depends on adequate shoulder, elbow, and wrist stability.

Between 18 and 24 months of age the child begins to develop skills that are precursors to simultaneous manipulation. Bilateral skill refinement depends heavily on continuing development of reach, grasp, release, and in-hand manipulation skills. Skills in visual-perceptual, cognitive, and motor areas become more integrated, leading to the child's effective use of motor planning for task performance. The child demonstrates simultaneous manipulation at 2 to 3 years of age (Connor et. al., 1978). The mature stage of bilateral hand use, which is the ability to use opposing hand and arm movements for highly differentiated activities such as cutting with scissors, begins to emerge at about 2½ years of age. The child applies and refines the patterns from each stage of bilateral hand use in a variety of activities throughout childhood.

Ball-Throwing Skills

Ball-throwing skills reflect the child's ability to use voluntary release skills. In throwing a small ball the child must sequence and time movements throughout the entire upper extremity. The child must bring the arm into a starting position, then prepare for projection of the ball into space by moving the trunk with the scapulohumeral joint, stabilizing the shoulder while beginning to extend the elbow, stabilizing the elbow while moving the wrist from extension to a neutral position, and simultaneously forcefully extending the fingers and thumb.

Children progress through a series of skill levels before they can smoothly sequence these movements and project the ball to the desired location. By 2 years of age the child should be able to throw a ball forward and maintain balance so that his or her body also does not move forward (Sheridan, 1975). At this age the child is using extensor movements to fling the ball but is not able to sustain shoulder flexion during the toss (Folio & Fewell, 2000). The child can disassociate trunk and arm movement but cannot disassociate humeral and forearm movements. By 2½ to 3 years of age the child is able to aim the ball toward a target and project the ball approximately 3 feet forward. This ability to control the direction of the ball to some degree implies that the child can control the humerus so that the elbow is in front of the shoulder when the ball is released. Thus the shoulder has sufficient stability to support controlled elbow and finger movement. By 3½ years of age the child is able to throw the ball 5 to 7 feet toward a target with little deviation from a straight line (Folio & Fewell, 2000). To accomplish this accuracy, the child positions his or her elbow in front of the shoulder before the ball is released.

Further refinement of ball-throwing skills continues over the next few years. Distance and accuracy improve as the child gains scapulohumeral control, the ability to sustain the humerus above the shoulder, and the ability to control the timing of elbow, wrist, and finger extension. Thus at approximately 5 years of age the child is able to use an overhand throw to fairly consistently hit a target 5 feet away. Children between 6 and 7 years of age are able to hit a target 12 feet away by using an overhand throw (Folio & Fewell, 2000). Underhand throws to contact a target are also possible in children who are 5 years of age or older. This skill requires the ability to move the humerus into flexion while sustaining full external rotation.

Tool Use

Connolly and Dalgleish (1989) defined a *tool* as "a device for working on something . . . tools serve as extensions of the limbs and enhance the efficiency with which skills are performed" (p. 895). They defined *tool use* as "a purposeful, goal-directed form of complex object manipulation that involves the manipulation of the tool to change the position, condition or action of another object" (p. 895). Tool use skills are more complex than other hand skills since the child must use a tool to act on objects, rather than using the hand to act on objects.

A child's development of skill in using tools is critical for accomplishment of a variety of self-care, play and leisure, and school and work tasks. Skills in tool use for eating and play typically begin to emerge during the second year, after the child has mastered the basic skills of reach, grasp, and release. The skills emerge concurrently with in-hand manipulation skills. In-hand manipulation skills are necessary for the progression of tool use skills beyond grasp and release proficiency. In-hand manipulation skills allow the tool to be adjusted in the hand after it is grasped.

A key factor in acquisition of tool use skills is the high degree of interaction of these skills and cognitive development. Connolly and Dalgleish (1989) emphasized that an individual needs to know both what he or she wants to do (the intentional aspect of the task) and how he or she can accomplish the task (the operational aspect of the task). Both of these elements require development of the child's cognitive skills and operational aspects on the child's motor skills.

Children develop tool use skills in a manner similar to grasp skills and in-hand manipulation skills in that the skills are not present initially. The child accomplishes them with a variety of strategies (a child may show multiple strategies for the same task), and gradually the strategies are limited so that the focus is on efficiency in the skill and accomplishment of the goal.

When the child is developing any new skill, the therapist sees inconsistencies in the child (even within the same session) and with children of the same age. The therapist is likely to record multiple strategies for children who are beginning to use a particular skill. Thus "inconsistency" in the strategy used for performing a skill should be considered an important stage in the skill acquisition process. As skill acquisition progresses, practice allows a skill to move from being performed with a high level of attention to being performed at a more automatic level. With such practice, performance becomes faster, more accurate, and smoother. Practice is typically necessary for a skill to become functional for execution in daily life tasks.

Researchers have studied acquisition of children's skills in using three tools—drawing and writing, scissoring, and eating. The area receiving the most study is in the drawing and writing tool use. See Chapter 18 for a description of this type of tool use.

Schneck and Battaglia (1992) described the development of scissors skills in young children. This skill emerges when the child first learns to place his or her fingers in the holes and to open and close the scissors. Early cutting is actually snipping, a process of closing the scissors on the paper with no movement of the paper and with no ability to repetitively open and close the scissors while flexing the shoulder and extending the elbow to move across the paper. Three-year-old children may use a pronated forearm position or a forearm-in-midposition placement (Schneck & Battaglia, 1992), or they may alternate between the two forearm positions. By 4 years of age children typically hold both forearms in midposition for the cutting activity.

The Peabody Developmental Motor Scales (Folio & Fewell, 2000) has established the following sequence:
- By 2 years of age children can snip with scissors
- By 2½ years of age most children can cut across a 6-inch piece of paper
- By 3 to 3½ years of age they can cut on a line that is 6-inches long
- By 3½ to 4 years of age they can cut a circle
- By 4½ to 5 years of age they can cut a square.

More complex cutting skills develop between 6 and 7 years of age. Other factors that the therapist should consider when assessing the child's skill in cutting include the width of the line to cut on, the size of the paper, the size of the design to be cut, and the complexity of the design.

The child's grasp on the scissors changes over time. The thumb position in one hole remains consistent, but the finger positions change according to the child's level of maturation and the type of scissors used (Schneck & Battaglia, 1992). In a mature grasp, which may not be achieved until after 6 years of age, the child has the middle finger in the lower hole of the handle, the ulnar two fingers flexed, and the index finger positioned to stabilize the lower part of the scissors (Myers, 1992; Schneck & Battaglia, 1992).

The general ages at which a child learns to use various utensils in eating are as follows: spoon by 18 months of age, fork by 2½ years of age, and knife by 6 years of age (Henderson, 1995). However, documentation regarding how these skills are acquired and how various components of movement interact to produce skill is limited. To address this issue, Connolly and Dalgleish (1989) conducted a longitudinal study on development of spoon use skills in infants between 11 and 23 months of age. They analyzed videotapes of the infants' grasp patterns on the spoon; the placement of the spoon within the hand; movements used in filling the spoon, bringing it to the mouth, clearing the spoon, and taking it out of the mouth; and visual monitoring of the pattern, timing, and use of the nonpreferred hand in the eating process. They found that the mean number of grasp patterns decreased between 11 and 17 months of age and that most infants 17 months of age and older showed a clear hand preference for eating.

The infants used 10 different grasp patterns, but none of them used an adult pattern. The most commonly used pattern was a transverse palmar grasp with all four fingers flexed around the handle of the spoon. The next two most commonly used patterns were ones in which the fingers were flexed but the handle was on the finger surface rather than in the palm. In the 17- to 23-month-old infants this pattern was accompanied by some degree of index finger extension, which is a precursor to manipulation of the spoon's orientation within the hand and is similar to a power grasp. The infants became increasingly efficient in spoon use during this period and improved their visual monitoring of the process.

Another component in the development of tool use in children is the role of the assisting hand. In handwriting and coloring, the assisting hand plays an important role in stabilizing the paper. However, in using scissors and eating, the assisting hand is likely to be much more active. In cutting, this hand must hold the paper and orient it through rotation by moving in the same or opposite direction as the hand with the scissors. In eating, the child's assisting hand may be involved in a variety of activities, depending on the child's age and the utensils used. Connolly and Dalgleish (1989) found that infants between 18 and 23 months of age showed significantly more involvement of the assisting hand in stabilizing a dish during spoon feeding than infants between 12 and 17 months of age. Learning to use a knife entails learning to stabilize food with one hand or with another tool while the child uses the preferred hand with the knife for spreading or cutting.

■ RELATIONSHIP OF HAND SKILLS TO FUNCTIONAL PERFORMANCE OF DAILY LIFE SKILLS

Hand skills are vital to the child's interaction with the environment. Functional performance of daily life skills requires object handling, almost all of which is accomplished with the hands. Usually greater impairment of hand use results in the need for increased adaptations if the child is to develop daily life skills.

Play

Although infants engage with people and objects through their visual and auditory senses, these are distant senses and do not readily bring the infant key information, which can only be gained through touch. Ruff (1980) described the importance of object handling with visual exploration as essential for an infant to learn object properties. The interaction of touching and looking helps enhance the infant's ability to integrate sensory information and to learn that objects remain the same regardless of visual orientation. Typically this object handling in infants is called *play* because it is purposeful and done with pleasure.

With increasing age, until at least the early school years, a great deal of play depends on competence in fine motor skills. These skills are reflected in the child's interest in activities such as cutting with scissors, dressing and undressing dolls, putting puzzles together, constructing with various types of building materials and model sets, participating in sand play, completing craft projects, and playing with jacks. Playing video games and using computers also require fine motor control. Some children may pursue play and leisure activities through organized groups such as Girl or Boy Scouts and 4-H clubs, which tend to use projects that require manual skills as a key component of their programs.

Self-Care

Self-care skills also depend on the child's ability to use all types of fine motor skills. Hand skills needed for self-care activity skill development include "(1) abilities in grip, (2) the use of two hands in a complementary fashion, (3) the ability to use the hands in varied positions with and without vision, (4) the execution of increasingly complex action sequences, and (5) the development of automaticity" (Henderson, 1995, p. 181). Case-Smith (1996) found that speed of object rotation using in-hand manipulation skills, grasp strength, motor accuracy, and tool handling were each significantly, positively correlated with self-care skills in preschool-age children who were receiving occupational therapy services.

Dressing skills involve complex grasp patterns and in-hand manipulation skills in the use of fasteners, but the ability to use all types of bilateral skills and a variety of grasp patterns is useful for putting on and removing shirts, shoes, socks, and pants. The ability to handle jewelry relies on the ability to use delicate grasp patterns and in-hand manipulation.

Hygiene skills depend on the child's increasing fine motor skills when handling slippery objects (e.g., soap). In addition, these skills are likely to be done in a standing position, such as when brushing teeth, shaving, and applying makeup. A high level of skill in tool use is needed for complex hygiene activities such as shaving, applying makeup, using tweezers, cutting nails, and styling hair (using barrettes, rubber bands, curling iron, brush, and hair dryer).

Eating skills rely on refinement of the ability to use forearm control with a variety of grasp patterns and tools. The ability to use both hands together effectively is necessary for spreading and cutting with a knife, opening all types of containers, pouring liquids, and preparing food. In-hand manipulation skills are used to adjust eating utensils and finger foods in one's hand, handle a napkin, and manipulate the opening of packaged food and utensils.

School

Functioning within the school environment requires the presence of effective fine motor skills. The preschool classroom presents children with a variety of manipulative activities, including use of crayons, scissors, small building materials, puzzles, and simple cooking and art projects. During kindergarten and the early elementary school years, children should be able to use fine motor skills most of the school day. McHale and Cermak (1992) found that 45% to 55% of the school day for first and second grade children is spent in fine motor activities. Fourth grade children spend approximately 30% of their school day participating in fine motor tasks. The primary fine motor activities in all of these grades are paper-pencil tasks. Any writing activity includes preparing one's paper, using an eraser, and getting writing tools in and out of a box. Other typical fine motor activities in children's classrooms include cutting with scissors, folding paper, using paste and tape, carrying out simple science projects, assuming responsibility for managing one's own snack and lunch items, and organizing and maintaining one's desk. Children also need computer skills in most elementary classrooms.

Older children and adolescents need fine motor skills for science projects, vocational courses (e.g., woodworking, metal shop, and home economics), art classes, music classes (other than vocal music), managing a high volume of written work and notebooks, keyboarding, and maintaining a locker. Adolescents should be able to demonstrate consistent fine motor skills that they can execute quickly in a variety of situations.

■ GENERAL MOTOR PROBLEMS AFFECTING HAND SKILLS

Regardless of the nature of the disability that a child may have, he or she is likely to have impaired hand skills. Impairment of basic hand function (reach, grasp, carry, and release) in early childhood precludes emergence of more advanced hand skill and bilateral hand use. This section presents problems that may be observed as major or minor problems in any child with hand skill difficulties.

One of the more common problems is *inadequate isolation of movements.* Children who demonstrate significant problems in this area tend to use total patterns of flexion or extension throughout the upper extremities, and they are unable to combine wrist extension with finger flexion or elbow flexion with finger extension. Similarly, the child may be unable to perform differentiated motions with each arm and hand. Inadequate isolation of movements is handicapping even in early infancy because it affects the most basic reach and grasp skills. More subtle problems may be seen in children who have difficulty isolating wrist and finger movements.

Another common problem is *poorly graded movements.* Usually the extent of a movement is too great for the task, thus impairing accuracy of performance. This problem occurs when joint stability in the hand or proximal to the hand is not effective. For example, the child may be unable to hold the elbow in approximately 90 degrees of flexion and the wrist in neutral position during a grasp activity. Thus when initiating the grasp, the child may overflex the fingers in an attempt to obtain the object before the arm posture is lost. Children with poorly graded movements lack the ability to effectively use the middle ranges of movement; instead they hold one or more joints in a locked position of full flexion or full extension during attempts at hand use (Figure 11-15). Typical patterns that children use to increase their stability include internal rotation of the shoulder, elbow extension, and hyperextension of the MCP joints. Problems with grading of movement are typically associated with abnormal tone, muscle weakness, or sensory integrative dysfunction. In the latter situation the child has difficulty perceiving and evaluating sensory feedback and so cannot accurately plan the extent of movements needed for a task.

Poor timing of movements can also be a problem. Inadequate timing of muscle contractions leads to the use of movements that are too fast or too slow for the intended purpose. Movements that are too fast also tend to be poorly graded. Disorders of tone or muscle weakness are often the underlying factors in movement that is too slow. Instability at joints causes disordered sequences of hand and arm movements. For example, wrist extension may not be combined with the reach for an object but may occur after the grasp instead.

A fourth problem that affects hand function is a *disorder in bilateral integration of movements*. This affects both the normal symmetric and asymmetric movements needed to develop and use hand functions. Some children are unable to effectively bring both hands to midline or to maintain use of both hands at midline long enough to accomplish a task. Other children can hold objects symmetrically at midline but are unable to dissociate arm movements. Therefore they have difficulty with activities that require reciprocal or simultaneous bilateral hand use.

Many children have difficulty with hand use because of *limitations in trunk movement and control*. CNS dysfunction or generalized muscle weakness can impair development or effective use of equilibrium reactions. Therefore the child may use one or both arms for support in maintaining sitting or standing positions. This significantly limits bilateral hand use and may limit the development of fine motor skills in the hand that the child most often uses for support.

Children with trunk instability or abnormal posture have difficulty with smooth and accurate placement of the hand and arm that is being used for a fine motor task. When the trunk is postured in flexion, functional range of motion in the arm is limited (Figure 11-16). Conversely, arching of the trunk is accompanied by hyperextension of the humerus. The latter pattern typically causes one of three patterns of shoulder and elbow positioning: external rotation with elbow flexion, neutral rotation with elbow flexion, or internal rotation with elbow extension. Posturing in any of these arm patterns affects the development of hand skills. Similarly, lateral trunk flexion causes the child to lean to one side and thus affects the child's ability to use the arm on the flexed side.

The problems discussed in this section can contribute to the child's use of *compensatory patterns of movement*.

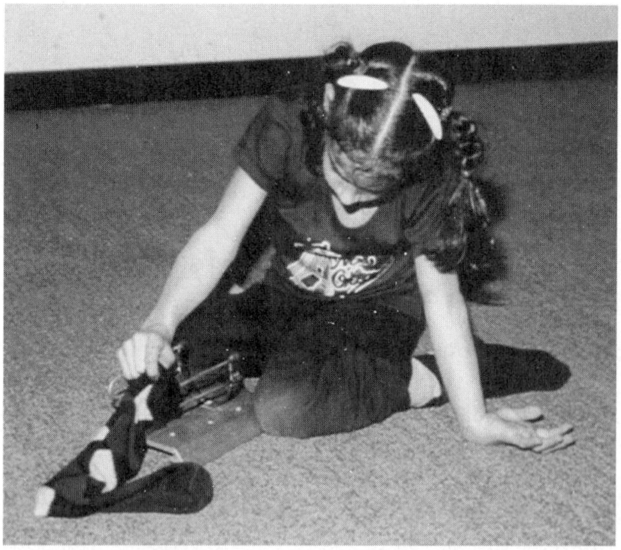

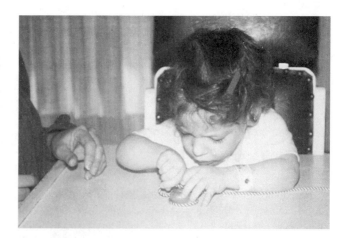

figure 11-15   This child, who has involuntary movement, demonstrates the attempt to find stability by locking her elbows in extension and by elevating her right shoulder during hand use. She also has difficulty isolating upper-extremity movements and using both hands together at midline. *(Courtesy Kennedy Kreiger Institute, Baltimore, MD.)*

figure 11-16   Poor trunk stability affects the upper-extremity range of motion that this child can use. Note her forearm pronation and wrist flexion on the right. She is unable to effectively use a three-jaw chuck or a pincer grasp on the materials. *(Courtesy Kennedy Kreiger Institute, Baltimore, MD.)*

In an effort to increase function, the child seeks another pattern to substitute for movements impaired by the primary problem. For example, the child with weakness or instability may learn to use lateral trunk flexion to increase the height of the arm during reach, or a child with increased tone may compensate for limited finger extension by using a wrist tenodesis action. Although these patterns are functional for certain tasks, continued use of compensatory movements may hinder the development of higher-level skills.

---

box 11-2 *Problem: unable to effectively engage in constructive manipulative play*

Components, subcomponents, and causes

1. No in-hand manipulative skills
   a. Unstable wrist in neutral position or extension, uses wrist flexion; possible causes:
      (1) Decreased tone in wrist extensors
      (2) Increased tone in wrist flexors
   b. Unstable metacarpophalangeal (MCP) joints; possible causes:
      (1) Poor cocontraction in finger joints
      (2) Increased pull of extensor digitorum
   c. Inability to identify finger being touched, resulting from decreased tactile discrimination
   d. Lack of midrange movements of finger joints; possible causes:
      (1) Decreased proprioception
      (2) Poor cocontraction in MCP and interphalangeal (IP) flexors and extensors
      (3) Increased tone in intrinsics and long finger flexors
2. Breaks materials often as a result of dropping and crushing them
   a. Inability to sustain finger pad grasp; possible causes:
      (1) Poor tactile or poor proprioceptive awareness
      (2) Poor cocontraction of muscle groups
   b. Excessive finger flexion in grasp; possible causes:
      (1) Poor proprioceptive awareness of size and weight of object
      (2) Increased finger flexor tone
      (3) Associated reactions
      (4) Inactivity in intrinsics
   c. Ineffective bilateral handling; possible causes:
      (1) Poor spatial relations
      (2) Unstable grasp because of poor wrist extension caused by increased flexor tone
      (3) Overflow in one upper extremity
      (4) Unilateral disregard

▪ ANALYSIS OF A HAND SKILL PROBLEM

A sample analysis of a functional problem that is at least partially caused by hand skill difficulties is presented in Box 11-2. In this example the therapist has identified two main components of this functional or activity level problems: the lack of ability to manipulate materials after grasp and the breakage of materials being handled. The therapist then attempts to determine the motor or other impairments that contribute to these activity limitations. Performance components associated with this problem may include problems with wrist and MCP joint stability, limited midrange movement control, lack of isolated finger movement, and excessive use of flexion. Based on evaluation findings and the therapist's frames of reference, specific impairments are identified. The impairments may include neuromotor, sensory integrative, or cognitive-perceptual disorders.

▪ THEORIES AND FRAMES OF REFERENCE USED IN ASSESSING AND INTERVENING FOR HAND SKILL PROBLEMS IN CHILDREN

Once the therapist has described the child's functioning, he or she needs to determine the probable underlying causes of the child's difficulties. The theory or frame of reference that the therapist is using, delineation of the probable causes of the performance problems, and decisions about how intervention should be structured affect the description of the child's performance. This section refers to the most commonly used theories or frames of reference in assessing children who have problems with hand skills and intervening for those problems.

Biomechanical Frame of Reference

The biomechanical frame of reference is used primarily in assessing and treating children with limitations in range of motion, strength, or endurance that affect their hand skills. It is used to explain difficulties in arm use for reach caused by problems in postural alignment or impaired ability to use the arms against gravity (Colangelo, 1999). Biomechanics helps the therapist understand the principles involved in tenodesis grasping patterns and the relationship of intrinsic and extrinsic muscle control for grasp and in-hand manipulation patterns. Activities are designed based on these principles of hand function. Splinting for hand problems most often relies on the biomechanical frame of reference.

Developmental Frame of Reference

The developmental frame of reference focuses on describing the sequences of skills as they are observed in typically developing children. For example, this frame of reference is used to describe children's grasp progression from an ulnar grasp pattern to a pincer grasp pattern. This frame of reference is also used in developmental curricula that present tasks in a sequential order and are grouped under age levels. In planning intervention for hand skill problems, occupational therapists often rely on an understanding of the developmental sequences of skills that children typically follow; these sequences may be used as a basis for sequencing goals and treatment. At other times the therapist makes a decision not to use the typical sequence of skill acquisition. This frame of reference also helps the therapist understand how hand skills relate to other developmental skills.

Neurodevelopmental Treatment Frame of Reference

The neurodevelopmental treatment frame of reference focuses on understanding the child's difficulties with postural tone, postural control, and stability and mobility and presents interventions to address these areas of difficulty (Schoen & Anderson, 1999). Although the therapist uses this frame of reference most often to address the development of equilibrium and controlled movement against gravity, it also includes methods to improve arm and hand motor control (Boehme, 1988; Danella & Vogtle, 1992). Certain splinting techniques use neurodevelopmental treatment principles.

Sensory Integration Frame of Reference

The SI frame of reference addresses the importance of sensory functioning and the integration of sensory processing to allow for adaptive responses. Occupational therapists can use this frame of reference to describe hand skill problems that are caused by problems with integrating tactile or proprioceptive information. These children function as if they were wearing mittens. Because they have difficulty differentiating among the specific sensory qualities of objects, they lack adaptive hand use. The therapist can use this frame of reference in assessing and treating children who demonstrate somatodyspraxia, a problem that is characterized by difficulties with praxis and processing of tactile and proprioceptive information.

Motor Learning Theory

Therapists are increasingly using motor learning theory in occupational therapy practice. When using this theory, therapists focus on the child's acquisition of specific motor skills and how the learning of these motor skills occurs. The therapist assists children in acquiring these skills through structure and feedback and provide him or her with structured practice to refine the skills. The type of practice that the therapist uses and the feedback that he or she gives the child while practicing are important. The therapist can use motor learning theories in assisting the child with developing a particular grasp pattern or in-hand manipulation skill or with developing speed in a motor skill, such as buttoning.

Behavioral Theory

The behavioral frame of reference focuses on reinforcing children's performances through specific feedback. In contrast to motor learning theory, this acquisitional theory usually focuses on tasks or functional activities that involve more than motor components. Therapists often structure activities by using backward chaining in which the child first performs the last step of the desired skill, then other elements of the skills are added in a backward order so that the first step of the process is learned last. For example, in teaching shoe tying the therapist first directs the child to pull the loops of the bow tight. The therapist eventually adds each step of the process to the sequence until the last step involves beginning to form the bow. In addition, therapists typically provide positive verbal feedback for the child to indicate success with performance of the task or a component of it. Therapists often let the child choose an activity that he or she will complete after doing a nonpreferred activity.

■ EVALUATION OF HAND SKILLS IN CHILDREN

The occupational therapist evaluates a child's hand skills when there is sufficient evidence to suggest that problems with performance of daily life skills are at least partially attributable to the child's problems with hand skills. The therapist should not perform a hand skill evaluation simply to provide information about the child's fine motor skills. The therapist must first have evidence to suggest that the child has at least one problem with daily life skills or limited participation in school. Parents, teachers, and the child are often the best sources of information about difficulties with daily life skills.

Screening for Hand Skill Problems

When the therapist identifies a functional problem with a daily life skill, he or she needs to continue the data-gathering process to determine if it is reasonable to carry out a full evaluation of fine motor and hand skill performance. This information needs to include data about the child's age and general information about motor skills, cognitive and perceptual skills, sensory processing, social situation and skills, and emotional development. The therapist can obtain screening information from parents, teachers, the child, other professionals, or reports of other professionals.

The hand skills part of the screening can include observation of skills noted in Table 11-1. This list of observations of fine motor skills includes reach, grasp, release,

table 11-1 *Hands Skills Screening Activities*

Activities	Age Groups			
	6-12 mos	1-2 yrs	3-5 yrs	6 yrs +
REACH				
Move both arms full ROM	X	X	X	X
Reach to midline, extended elbow	X	X	X	X
Reach across midline		X	X	X
GRASP				
Use full palmar grasp	X	X	X	X
Use radial-digital grasp	9 mo	X	X	X
Use standard pincer grasp	10 mo	X	X	X
Use spherical grasp		X	X	X
Use intrinsic-plus grasp		X	X	X
Use power grasp on tool			X	X
RELEASE				
Release object freely	X	X	X	X
Release 1-inch object into container		X	X	X
Stack 1-inch blocks*		2-6	9-10	10
Release tiny object into small hole		X	X	X
Throw small ball at least 3 feet			X	X
IN-HAND MANIPULATION				
Manipulate object between two hands	X	X	X	X
Use finger-to-palm translation, small object†		X	X	X
Use palm-to-finger translation				
One object†		2 yrs	X	X
Two to three objects†		2 yrs	X	X
With coin			X	X
Unscrew bottle top		2 yrs	X	X
Use shift to separate magazine pages or cards			X	X
Roll piece of clay into a ball‡			X	X
Pick up marker or crayon using rotation			4 yrs	X
Shift on marker or pencil			5 yrs	X
Rotate pencil to use eraser and back				X
BILATERAL SKILLS				
Hold or carry large ball with 2 hands	X	X	X	X
Stabilize paper during coloring or writing			X	X
Hold paper during scissors use			X	X
Manipulate paper during scissors use				X
TOOL USE				
Use scissors to cut				
Line			3 yrs	X
Simple shapes			4 yrs	X
Complex shapes				X
Scribble with marker		X		
Copy appropriate forms			X	X
Handwriting appropriate for grade				X

*Block stacking allows for assessment of arm stability in space, spatial orientation of the objects, and controlled finger extension. Voluntary release of objects other than blocks may be used. Screening should include placement of objects when arm is not supported and placement that requires precision.

†An object that is not flat should be used. Examples include small pieces of cereal (appropriate for children under 3 years or those who still mouth objects), small beads, or small pegs.

‡A piece of clay that is approximately ¼-inch thick and 1-inch in diameter is placed in the palm of the child's hand. The child is asked to form the clay into a ball without using the other hand or the table surface. Palm-to-finger translation, finger-to-palm translation, simple rotation, and sometimes complex rotation may be observed.

ROM, Range of motion.

in-hand manipulation, and bilateral skills. It is not a standardized test or meant to replace administration of standardized tests to a child. However, because few standardized tests include assessment of specific hand skills, the therapist can use this list to record his or her observations about the child's quality of hand skills. The therapist can use sections of this chapter on normal development of the various hand skills as a basis for determining if the child has difficulty with a particular skill.

Information gathered in this screening is useful in determining if further observation of the child's hand skills is necessary or if the therapist should administer a standardized test. In addition, parents or teachers and the child may find that these tasks are useful to them in delineating the areas that are difficult for the child versus those with which the child may be more successful. Discussing observations during or after the screening often serves as a basis for collaborative intervention planning to address the areas of difficulty.

The activities listed in Table 11-1 are appropriate for the therapist' use in screening a child's fine motor abilities. Because some skills are inappropriate for younger children, an "X" designates the age group for which any activity may be used. When a skill emerges within a particular age group, ages are listed rather than an "X." For block stacking, the number represents the number of blocks that a child within that age group should be able to stack. The therapist can vary materials used for some of the items so that he or she can assess many of these skills during a mealtime, dressing, hygiene, or play activity. For all categories except *Bilateral Skills* and *Tool Use,* the therapist should ask the child to perform the activities with right and left hands.

Evaluation Content

The therapist should further evaluate the child with functional problems who shows difficulties on screening for hand skills to carefully delineate the characteristics of the problem and the situations in which the child's performance is optimal. For example, the therapist may need to determine (1) whether the child is able to use any type of functional grasp, (2) if wrist extension is possible in any grasp patterns, (3) the situations under which voluntary release are most feasible for the child, (4) the types of objects that are easiest for the child to handle when using the in-hand manipulation skill of simple rotation, and (5) whether the child is able to stabilize materials better when the materials are closer to or further from his or her body.

When determining the child's performance in the area of hand skills and potential reasons for any problems, the occupational therapist often uses a variety of standardized and nonstandardized assessments. All children should receive an assessment of hand skills in functional activities such as dressing, eating, hygiene skills, school activities, and play activities. The therapist can perform

other standard testing if this testing meets one or more of the following purposes:

1. The test is likely to yield information that will be:
   a. Valuable for documenting the child's current status to later determine whether the child has shown progress in hand skills, maintained the same skills, or lost skills
   b. Helpful in determining whether the child qualifies for occupational therapy services by clarifying the degree of the child's disability
   c. Helpful in determining the causes of the child's hand skill problems
   d. Helpful in determining the child's potential for improvement in hand skills and in selecting specific intervention goals
   e. Helpful in planning intervention strategies
2. For children with strength or range of motion problems, evaluation should include (Ager, Olivett, & Johnson, 1984; Latch, Freeling, & Powell, 1993; Mathiowetz et. al., 1986; Link et. al., 1995):
   a. Measurement of active and passive range of motion
   b. Evaluation of strength
      (1) Muscle testing
      (2) Grip and pinch strength testing
3. For children with moderate to severe impairment caused by abnormal tone, evaluation should include:
   a. Assessment of range of motion with documentation of contractures
   b. Assessment of tactile and proprioceptive functioning using standard method
   c. Administration of the Erhardt Developmental Prehension Assessment (Erhardt, 1982)
4. For children with mild-to-moderate impairment caused by abnormal tone and sensory processing or SI problems, evaluation should include:
   a. Assessment of range of motion with documentation of contractures
   b. Assessment of tactile and proprioceptive functioning using one of the following:
      (1) Standard method
      (2) Sensory Integration and Praxis Tests
   c. Administration of a standardized developmental test that includes a fine motor section (see Appendix 7-A)
      (1) Hawaii Early Learning Profile (HELP)
      (2) Bayley Scales of Infant Development—Revised
      (3) Battelle Developmental Inventory
   d. Administration of a developmental motor test
      (1) Toddler and Infant Motor Evaluation (TIME)
      (2) Peabody Developmental Motor Scales—Fine Motor
      (3) Bruininks-Oseretsky Test of Motor Proficiency
   e. Administration of a visual-motor integration test
      (1) Test of Visual Motor Skills (TVMS)
      (2) Developmental Test of Visual Motor Integration (VMI)

5. For the adolescent with hand skill problems, evaluation should include:
   a. Assessment of range of motion with documentation of any contractures
   b. Assessment of hand skills in prevocational or work tasks
   c. Administration of a standardized motor test
      (1) Purdue Pegboard Test (Mathiowetz, Rogers, Dowe-Keval, Donohoe, & Rennells, 1986)
      (2) Bruininks-Oseretsky Test of Motor Proficiency

■ GUIDELINES FOR INTERVENTION

Setting Goals

The child's functional problems and types of problems in the hand skill area, the therapist's frame of reference, and the setting in which services are to be provided influence the types of goals that are developed in the area of hand skill and in other areas of the child's functioning. For some children, developmental sequences of skills influence the selection of goals, but for the child with a motor disability, other factors affect the goals established and the strategies selected for intervention. These factors include the types of functional skills that the child needs, the complexity of the child's problems, and the human and nonhuman resources available to support the intervention program.

The therapist must be realistic in the number and types of these goals that he or she can establish relative to any other goals for the child. In addition, the therapist needs to consider hand skill goals that are feasible for the child to accomplish and within the child's behavioral repertoire. Such goals may be limited for children with severe disabilities. In all cases the therapist must link hand skill goals to the child's ability to more effectively engage in daily life skills. For some children the most appropriate focus of intervention is development of skills in using adaptive equipment and strategies for accomplishing functional skills. For children who show readiness to develop better quality or more complex hand skills, intervention can focus on acquisition of these skills. Factors to consider in planning intervention for hand skill problems are discussed in the following sections.

Sequencing Intervention Sessions

When the therapist provides direct services to improve hand and arm function, he or she usually carries it out in the following sequence:
1. Preparation
   a. Positioning the child
   b. Addressing postural tone issues
   c. Improving postural control (pelvic, shoulder, head)
2. Development of hand skills
   a. Promoting isolated arm and hand movements, such as external rotation, supination, and wrist extension
   b. Enhancing reach, grasp, carry, and release skills
   c. Enhancing in-hand manipulation skills
   d. Facilitating bilateral hand use skills
3. Generalization of skills (integrating hand skills into functional activities)

Not all children need all of the steps of this sequence. In addition, intervention for all areas is rarely done in one session.

Preparation for Hand Skill Development

Many children require preparation of the total body in each treatment session before the therapist addresses intervention for specific hand skill problems. In addition to intervention to improve motor function, the therapist should give specific attention to the child's sensory functioning. The therapist can provide tactile and proprioceptive input to the arms and hands to enhance sensory awareness and discrimination. Lotion, toys, the child's own clothing, or preferably, active movements of the child's hands, with or without assistance, can provide stimuli. Children have greater tactile sensitivity when performing an activity that involves active touching rather than being touched (Haron & Henderson, 1985). The therapist should also encourage visual awareness of the hands with tactile and proprioceptive input.

Positioning the child

In selecting positioning of the therapist and the child for fine motor intervention, the therapist must consider the optimal position for eliciting the particular skills desired in that child and the position in which the child will use the skills. When these positions are different, the therapist needs to consider whether to use only one position at this time and to introduce the other position later or whether to use both positions at this time. For example, the child may be able to bring both hands to midline and to reach with the greatest elbow extension in sidelying. However, for functional use the child may need to be able to contact a switch on a surface while in an adapted sitting position. In an intervention session the therapist may initially work with the child in the sidelying position, then move to a supported sitting position to help the child generalize the skills to a functional position. Eventually the therapist may work with the child primarily in a supported sitting position. In any case the therapist almost always needs to specifically address carryover of skills across positions with the child, often through activities developed collaboratively with the parents or the teacher.

The therapist can use certain body positions to elicit specific hand skills. The supine position is effective for working with children on arm movements and visual regard of the hands during movement. The prone position on the forearms is appropriate for addressing shoulder stability and co-contraction in 90 degrees of elbow flexion, disassociation of the two sides of the body during weight bearing on one arm while manipulating with the other, gross bilateral manipulation of objects, and visual regard of the hands. Sidelying can be an effective position for encouraging unilateral arm movement to bat at an object and for hand-to-hand play. Visual regard of the hands and objects is difficult to address in the sidelying position.

Sitting at a table is often the position in which children are most likely to use fine motor skills. For optimal hand use, children need a stable chair with adequate foot support. The therapist should not expect a child who is not yet independent in sitting to work on sitting stability while working on hand skills. Such children need adaptations for sitting (e.g., lateral supports and chest straps) when working on hand skills. A tray or table surface should be a work surface rather than a support surface. The table or tray should be only slightly above elbow height because a lower table promotes use of body flexion and a higher surface promotes use of abduction and internal rotation of the arms. The therapist also may provide activities with the child in sitting on the floor or in a chair without a table, particularly when working on reaching skills or gross bilateral skills.

For children with mild-to-moderate motor involvement, standing may be an appropriate position for treatment of some hand skills. Many daily living skills that rely on hand skills are most commonly done while standing, such as brushing teeth, zipping and buttoning clothing, shaving and applying makeup, and cooking. For children who have substantial difficulties with standing, the therapist should use this position only after the child has mastered the skills in a sitting position.

Improving postural control

The child with increased tone throughout the body may need overall inhibition of tone before participating in hand skill activities. Use of slow rotary movements using small ranges of motion between internal and external shoulder rotation and between forearm pronation and supination can help inhibit tone (Finnie, 1975). Upper extremity weight bearing is particularly useful as a treatment technique for improving postural control and improving stability in the scapulohumeral area. The therapist can also use upper extremity weight bearing to encourage the child to maintain elbow cocontraction and some degree of wrist extension while engaging in slight weight shifting (Boehme, 1988; Danella & Vogtle, 1992). The therapist provides proprioceptive input during weight bearing. The primary focus for most children is on helping the child increase overall stability rather than concentrating on achieving full elbow, wrist, or finger extension. The therapist can carry out weight-bearing activities with the child in the prone position on the forearms, the prone position on extended arms, the side-sitting position, or the long-sitting position, depending on the child's skill level (Boehme, 1988).

For the child who has tightness in wrist flexion, a position of upper extremity weight bearing on hands with the arms extended is often difficult if not impossible to achieve. The most appropriate positions for these children to use for weight bearing include prone on the forearms and sidelying. The therapist can help the child position the wrists in neutral position, and some therapists use splints during weight bearing to assist with wrist and hand positioning (Kinghorn & Roberts, 1996).

Finger flexion is permitted during weight bearing as long as the thumb is not in an abnormal position. If the child's thumb is tightly adducted and flexed, the therapist should use handling techniques before weight bearing. The therapist can use his or her own hand to provide firm pressure over the first metacarpal joint and relax the child's hand through slow, small rotary and flexion-extension movements. Mildly and moderately involved children often can work toward maintaining full finger extension during weight bearing.

Using multiple-baseline single-subject design, Barnes (1986, 1989a, 1989b) found that children with cerebral palsy demonstrated increased use of wrist extension and finger extension after upper extremity weight bearing. The weight bearing, increased wrist extension during these activities, but did not affect grasp and voluntary release quality and skill. Chakarian and Larson's (1993) study of weight bearing with 10 children with cerebral palsy also found improvements in wrist and finger extension. Kinghorn and Roberts' (1996) single-subject study of weight bearing with splinting for a child with cerebral palsy did not show significant changes in objective measures of tone, positioning, or function. However, family members reported improved functioning.

■ HAND SKILL DEVELOPMENT

When addressing hand skill development in children, the therapist must select activities that are interesting and appropriately challenging to the child. To support skill development, the therapist must be able to repeat these activities. Therefore toys and games with many pieces and eating activities can be particularly useful and enjoyable. Engaging in play while addressing hand skills with the child can have important benefits for the child, including motivating the child to engage in activities repeatedly and building the child's play repertoire (Couch, Dietz & Kenny, 1998; Tobias & Goldkopf, 1995).

Promoting Isolated Arm and Hand Movements

The therapist may choose to address specific movements in the upper extremity in isolation of specific hand skills. For example, the therapist may assist the child in using elbow flexion-extension, supination-pronation, or wrist flexion-extension movements before integrating these movements into reaching, grasping, or releasing patterns. Helping children generalize the movement patterns that they have practiced and learned into a functional activity is an important aspect of motor learning theory. Such an approach is most successful with children who are able to follow verbal instructions and participate actively in working on specific hand skills. The therapist can use games or songs to practice the use of these movements. The therapist needs to emphasize specific movements and, in the same treatment session, use them in a functional context.

Supination control is one of the greatest areas of difficulty for children with disabilities, particularly for those with tone problems. Abnormal posturing at the trunk, shoulder, elbow, or wrist often compensate for difficulties with initiating or sustaining forearm supination. Supination is easiest to use when the elbow is fully flexed and most difficult to use with full elbow extension. Therefore

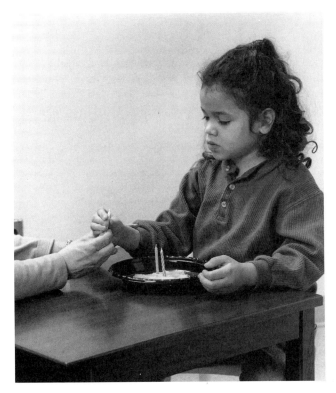

figure11-17 Arm support on the surface, elbow flexion, and vertical orientation of materials encourage this child's use of forearm supination in placing "candles" on a clay "birthday cake." *(Photo by Kanji Takeno.)*

the therapist can use activities that position the elbow in more than 90 degrees of flexion to facilitate supination. Examples of such activities include finger feeding, holding a kaleidoscope, and putting lotion on the face.

If the child can initiate supination but has poor control of this pattern, he or she can benefit from activities with the elbow held in 90 degrees, with the forearm stabilized on a surface and an object presented vertically (Figure 11-17). Gradually the therapist moves materials to encourage the child to use more elbow extension while maintaining the supinated position. Children with more severe involvement may only be able to achieve about 30 degrees of supination, the minimum amount needed to effectively handle materials on a table. The therapist should encourage children with less motor impairment to obtain and use at least 90 degrees of supination to accomplish functional activities such as drinking, eating with utensils, or turning a doorknob. It is also helpful to facilitate supination in the nonpreferred arm so that hand can stabilize materials more effectively.

Enhancing Reach Skills
Problems

Children with neuromotor disabilities exhibit typical problems in reach that limit range and control. Examples of problems in reach include the following:

- Use of abduction and internal rotation to initiate reach
- Use of shoulder elevation and lateral trunk flexion to increase the height of the arm for reaching
- Inability to coordinate the degree of hand opening or the hand position with the timing of the reach
- Difficulty maintaining an upright body posture when reaching forward or across midline

Goals

The following are examples of goals that the therapist can use for children with a variety of levels of disabilities. The goals are in approximate order of difficulty, although difficulty in using any one pattern can vary with individual children.

1. The child will maintain visual regard of the object while contacting the object with the hand.
2. The child will bring the hand into contact with objects in various planes.
3. The child will sustain some degree of finger extension while reaching for objects in various planes.
4. The child will reach with both hands together for an object presented at midline.
5. The child will orient the forearm appropriately for object contact during bilateral reaching.
6. The child will reach with 45 degrees of shoulder flexion, using neutral rotation of the humerus and elbow extension.

7. The child will reach with 90 degrees of shoulder flexion, using slight external rotation of the humerus, elbow extension, and forearm supination to midposition.
8. The child will use appropriate hand positioning for grasp with a mature reaching pattern.
9. The child will reach across midline with an erect trunk posture and humeral external rotation, elbow extension, and forearm supination to midposition.
10. The child will reach above the head with control.

Intervention strategies

When the child initiates little movement or is unable to open the hand during arm movement, the primary focus of intervention is on controlled initiation of arm movements. This includes using various types of arm movements and being able to place and hold the arm to allow for contact with objects. This type of reaching goal is a priority for children with extremely limited movement control or strength and those whose degenerative disease process results in skill regression. These movements are important for contact with others, and the child can use them to activate switches for toys and electronic equipment.

To facilitate arm movements and contact with objects, the therapist must identify the best position to promote postural stability and visual regard. The most commonly used position is sitting, with attention given to head and trunk control, visual regard, and visual tracking. However, the therapist can effectively use the supine and side-lying positions as well.

Children with severe motor involvement need toys and materials that are easy to activate and have no "failure" elements. Such toys include play foam, beans, rice, musical toys that are activated by light touch, and soap bubbles. The therapist can usually obtain the best results through proximal handling at the shoulders and upper arms while assisting the child with movements of either or both arms. Initial emphasis is on general arm movement, then on hand and arm placement, and finally on finger extension during arm movement as a precursor for reach with grasp.

When children are able to contact objects with some control, the therapist should introduce structured activities to assist the child with using elements of a more mature reaching pattern. Gradually these elements are combined to promote a smooth direct reach. The therapist needs to determine the placement of objects in relation to the child's body so the child can use the best reaching pattern possible. From that position the therapist can begin to vary object placement and orientation. For example, because presentation of objects at shoulder height often results in the child reaching with internal rotation and elbow flexion, initial presentation of objects at a level below the child's shoulder may facilitate the use of shoulder flexion and neutral rotation. Gradually the child can raise objects higher as he or she develops more control. The therapist can use activities that require lateral reaching with shoulder abduction and slight external rotation before encouraging reaching with shoulder flexion.

The therapist should also encourage the child to reach behind his or her body, combining humeral hyperextension with controlled internal rotation and various elbow positions. Many children have difficulty with this posterior reaching pattern, which is required in dressing and other daily living skills.

Some children can use neutral to slight external shoulder rotation in combination with humeral flexion if the therapist provides them with a minimal amount of handling at the humerus or elbow and appropriate object orientation. However, if such handling techniques are required for a child to use a mature reaching pattern, the therapist should present objects somewhat to the side or in front of the shoulder initially and then gradually toward midline. To encourage reaching that incorporates neutral to slight external rotation of the shoulder and forearm supination, the therapist should orient the objects vertically. Horizontal orientation of an object encourages use of forearm pronation.

Children with muscle weakness are better able to reach objects when they can use a table or tray surface that is at or slightly above elbow height. The therapist can use mobile arm suspension systems to support and assist the child who has muscle strength of fair-minus or less.

The therapist should provide objects that have high color contrasts or bright solid colors to children with visual impairment. In the presence of severe visual impairment, objects can combine both auditory stimuli and varied textures. If the child has not developed the ability to search for objects, the therapist should provide materials within a confined space or tied to strings so that the child can easily retrieve them after dropping.

Enhancing Grasp Skills
Problems

The following are problems in development of effective grasp:

- Fisting or finger flexion that prevents hand opening
- Wrist flexion (often with ulnar deviation) in combination with finger extension
- Excessive forearm pronation, which interferes with use of radial finger grasp patterns
- Thumb adduction, often with MCP or IP flexion
- Inability to use thumb abduction and adduction with MCP and IP extension
- Inability to initiate or sustain thumb opposition
- Inability to use grasp patterns that involve control of the intrinsic finger muscles
- Inability to vary grasp in accordance with object characteristics and activity demands

Goals

The following are examples of goals that the therapist can use for children with a variety of levels of disabilities. The goals are in approximate order of difficulty, although difficulty in using any one pattern can vary with individual children.

1. The child will demonstrate a sustained palmar grasp with the arm in a variety of positions.
2. The child will demonstrate finger surface grasp on a variety of objects.
3. The child will demonstrate a finger pad grasp with thumb opposition on objects that are small or have a small diameter.
4. The child will demonstrate an opposed grasp pattern varied in accordance with object shapes and characteristics.
5. The child will demonstrate an effective lateral pinch grasp pattern.
6. The child will demonstrate a controlled grasp with MCP flexion and IP extension to hold thin, flat objects.
7. The child will demonstrate a power grasp on a variety of tools in daily living tasks.

Intervention strategies

For children with delays and functional difficulties in grasp, the therapist needs to match preparation techniques, such as positioning, handling, or strengthening, to the child's problem.

Some children fist their hands or refuse to grasp objects because of tactile hypersensitivity, which also can influence the ability to maintain grasp. If this problem is present, grading tactile input from well tolerated to more difficult to tolerate is helpful. Initially, the child best tolerates firm objects with smooth surfaces and contours.

Tactile discrimination problems can contribute to grasp problems. Poor discrimination can affect dynamic use of grasp patterns and regulation of pressure in grasp. Problems with regulating pressure are seen in either holding objects with excessive force or dropping objects. Most children benefit from graded sensory input and attention to sensory discrimination as part of the intervention for grasp skills. Having the child actively explore the sizes, shapes, and textures of objects can precede emphasis on grasp in a treatment session.

In planning intervention that addresses grasp problems, the therapist should select objects with consideration of the child's interests, sensory needs, and motor skills. Properties to consider include the size, shape, color, weight, and texture of objects.

Children with severe disabilities. Children with severe disabilities need to develop an effective palmar grasp and, if possible, grasp patterns using the finger surface. If possible the therapist should stress abilities to initiate grasp and sustain grasp with the arm in a variety of positions. If the child is unable to open the hand readily for grasp, the therapist may explore whether changing the child's body position would be helpful. Sidelying may decrease stress on overall body posture and make it possible for the child to open the hand more easily. In supported sitting, the child may find opening the hand easier if the therapist places an object below the seat of the chair and lateral to the child's body. Boehme (1988) described other handling techniques that may assist the child with hand opening. The therapist should follow these techniques with movement of the open hand across objects and surfaces as a way of increasing the child's sustained hand opening and object interaction.

For the child who can independently open the hand but who shows wrist flexion with grasp, the therapist can emphasize wrist extension with grasp by positioning objects above the table surface or at chest height. Once the child can sustain wrist extension, the therapist can assist or encourage him or her to move the arm while maintaining grasp of an object. Sample activities using this skill include using a small stick to hit a suspended balloon or to break soap bubbles blown by the therapist, touching pictures on a wall or mirror with a stick, or holding onto clothing items while they are pulled up or down.

The child with a severe disability can wear a splint or other orthotic device during treatment and at other times of the day. Splinting techniques that may be useful in supporting hand function during treatment are described later in this chapter. Many of these children need adaptations to materials to support their performance of activities at home, school, and play. Use of standard materials may not be possible. Built-up handles that accommodate a palmar grasp pattern and larger objects, such as game pieces and blocks, may be used instead of smaller ones. Adapted page turners for books, switches for toys, and computer adaptations may be necessary to give the child some independence in play and school activities.

Children with moderate disabilities. Children with moderate disabilities are able to grasp but have difficulty in functional use of a variety of grasp patterns. They have problems in forearm control, wrist extension, thumb opposition, and control of the MCP and IP joints. Grasp may be initiated with wrist flexion. Grasp goals for these children usually are designed to address use of opposed grasp patterns and use of grasp patterns in which the hand effectively accommodates to objects.

Selection of objects for use in developing opposed grasp patterns is critical. The child must be able to use objects within the context of an activity that is interesting and meaningful to the child and that has elements that the child can repeat. Games and imaginary play materials can provide opportunities for repetitive presentation of objects to the child. The child can use opposed grasps with medium-sized, small, and tiny objects. Children often can demonstrate better thumb and finger control with small or medium-sized objects that have well-defined edges. Tiny objects require too much precision, such that the child often resorts to a more primitive grasping pattern. In fact, skill in using a pincer grasp usually is less critical for the child's functional performance of daily life tasks than skill in using and varying a three-point opposed grasp pattern. Once the child begins to acquire an opposed grasp pattern, the therapist can vary the objects by size, shape, texture, and weight.

The research findings of Case-Smith and others (1998) support these clinical observations that object characteristics are important in eliciting specific grasp patterns, particularly when these grasp patterns are emerging. To develop an opposed grasp pattern, the therapist can begin working on grasp alone rather than reach and grasp. The child's arm should be well stabilized when objects are presented. Having the wrist in a neutral or slightly extended position is critical; if appropriate, the therapist can stabilize the volar surface of the child's forearm on the table surface and give support over the dorsum of the forearm. The therapist should present objects in line with the shoulder and not at midline, because midline positioning has a tendency to encourage the use of pronation. With objects presented in line with the shoulder, neutral rotation of the humerus is encouraged (versus internal rotation), and slight forearm supination is likely to occur. The therapist holds the object with his or her fingers and presents the object directly to the child's fingers (Figure 11-18). After grasp, the child carries the object to a nearby container or surface. Practice of this strategy for grasp, carry, and release using a variety of objects is needed for the child to integrate this skill.

Once the child is able to use this pattern well, the therapist can move to the next skill level. At this level the therapist places the object in his or her cupped hand (just under the child's hand and in line with the child's shoulder) so that the object is stable and asks the child to grasp the object. When the therapist uses this strategy, the child needs to use more internal stability of the arm and some degree of prepositioning of the fingers before grasp.

As the child develops skill in grasping from the therapist's hand, the therapist can begin to place an object on the table surface. As at the prior two levels, the object is in line with the child's shoulder, not at midline. The therapist may need to stabilize the object or place it on a nonskid surface for the child who does not have sufficient arm stability to grasp without unintentionally moving the object.

After the child is able to grasp from the table surface with the object in line with the shoulder, the therapist can begin to move the object further away on the table surface, above the table surface, and closer to midline. In this way the therapist is structuring activities to combine reach with grasp (see Figure 11-18). This requires the child to stabilize the arm in space while controlling finger

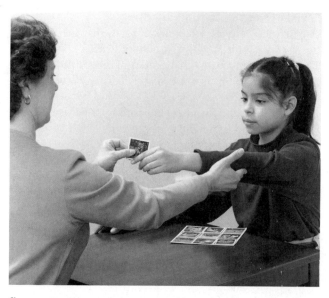

figure**11-18** Facilitation is provided to prompt use of slight humeral external rotation and forearm supination. The object is held vertically to assist this reaching pattern. A lotto card game is used to engage the child and allow for repetition of the pattern. *(Photo by Kanji Takeno.)*

movements. The therapist may use a variety of these object placements in a therapy session to elicit the child's best skills. Different object placements may be needed with various sizes and shapes of objects.

Children with mild disabilities. Children with mild disabilities typically have difficulties with small ranges of movements in supination and wrist extension. Sustained control with the intrinsic muscles of the hand may be difficult for these children to achieve. Fingertip control in grasp is often poor, as is the ability to control the palmar arches and to achieve radial-ulnar dissociation of movements within the hand. Goals for grasp skills for these children usually are focused on use of an effective pincer grasp and lateral pinch grasp pattern; use of a grasp with MCP flexion and IP extension to hold thin, flat objects; and/or use of a power grasp on a variety of tools in daily living tasks. The standard and lateral pinch patterns and the grasp for thin, flat objects require wrist stability and use of the intrinsic muscles.

The therapist can use a variety of treatment strategies, including verbal cueing and structuring of activities to elicit intrinsic muscle activity, with children who are working on these skills. Sample activities include holding all fingers in adduction and extension while rolling out clay, using finger abduction to stretch rubber bands placed around two or more fingers, playing finger games that require isolation and small ranges of finger movements, holding or hiding objects in a cupped hand, and squeezing clay or other objects between the pad of the thumb and the pads of one or more fingers.

Development of a power grasp relies on development of radial-ulnar disassociation and ability to extend the index finger and thumb during ulnar finger flexion. Emphasis on radial-ulnar dissociation in the hand and on grasp with MCP flexion and IP extension is helpful as a precursor to the power grasp pattern. To address radial-ulnar dissociation, the therapist structures activities in which the child holds two objects in one hand and releases one at a time, holds an object in the ulnar side of the hand with the ring and little fingers while grasping and releasing with the radial fingers and thumb, and engages in activities that develop finger-to-palm translation with stabilization skills. In addressing the power grasp within functional activities, the therapist carefully selects the type of tool that the child handles. Tools that have a narrow surface for index finger contact are particularly difficult for children to control. The therapist can use verbal cues, stickers, or dots on the handles of the tools to encourage appropriate finger placement. The child may need built-up handles to facilitate performance initially.

Carrying

The child must maintain grasp of an object during the carry phase. Therefore the therapist needs to attend to the child's ability to vary all joint positions in the arm while sustaining grasp and emphasize wrist extension with sustained finger flexion. The therapist should be especially attentive to the child's use of compensatory trunk movements and the child's difficulty dissociating arm and trunk movements. If these are present, the child may need intervention to improve sustained trunk control in midline and trunk rotation with arm movements. The use of adapted equipment to support the trunk in a symmetric, erect posture is helpful for many children. The therapist also may need to stabilize the shoulder to prevent scapular elevation.

The therapist can use facilitation of arm movements in a manner similar to that described for reaching to encourage carrying patterns of shoulder rotation, graded elbow movements, and forearm supination. Most children with increased tone or stability problems have more difficulty carrying small or thin objects. Use of objects that are larger in diameter, such as those adapted with built-up handles, can promote wrist extension and management of objects during carrying.

Voluntary Release
Problems

Therapists usually combine treatment for voluntary release problems with intervention for grasp. Children with difficulty in releasing objects may exhibit the following:
- Fisting and tight finger flexion
- Difficulty with sustained arm position during object placement and release
- Difficulty combining wrist extension with finger extension
- Inability to use slight forearm supination to allow for release in small areas or near other objects and with visual monitoring of the placement
- Overextension of the fingers in release, limiting control of specific object placement

Goals

The following are examples of goals that the therapist can use for children with a variety of levels of disabilities. These goals specifically define the size of an area in which the child can release the object (e.g., into a container with a 4-inch opening) or the height of a surface on which the child can release the object (e.g., a stack of six cubes). The following goals incorporate these commonly used measures of voluntary release skill. The goals are in approximate order of difficulty, although difficulty in using any one pattern can vary with individual children. The therapist should integrate these goals with the child's functional goals.
1. The child will demonstrate release of objects into a container placed on the floor.
2. The child will demonstrate release of objects into a container placed on a table surface with the container at arms' length from the child's body to encourage wrist extension with finger extension.
3. The child will demonstrate release of objects into a container at midline while using wrist extension.
4. The child will demonstrate release of tiny objects into a container with a small opening.
5. The child will demonstrate placement of objects within 1 inch of other objects without making other objects move or fall.
6. The child will demonstrate release of unstable, lightweight objects while keeping them in an upright position.
7. The child will demonstrate release of objects without visual monitoring.

Intervention strategies

Intervention focuses on one or more of the following areas, depending on the child's problems: hand opening for object release, arm placement and stability for release, and accuracy of object placement. Releasing patterns correlate with grasping patterns. A child who uses a palmar grasp will use full finger extension to release the object. A child who uses a pincer grasp can use voluntary release with good control of the intrinsic muscles as balanced with the extrinsics.

When the child shows excessive finger flexion (fisting), initial treatment for voluntary hand opening focuses on the child's ability to move the arm while maintaining some finger extension. Splinting may be helpful in supporting the child's wrist or facilitating increased wrist and finger extension. In children with fisting, asking the child to place the object into a container increases the child's fisting. Some children have success releasing to the side of their body because movement toward midline increases the pronation-flexion posturing, thus increasing the hand fisting.

If the child can accomplish this level of voluntary release, he or she can attempt release of large and medium-sized objects into a container with a large opening that is placed on the floor. For some children, transfer of objects from hand to hand is a reasonable strategy for encouraging release with object stabilization.

Children who can voluntarily open their hands but who use tenodesis patterns may benefit from intervention to increase voluntary finger extension while maintaining the wrist in a neutral position. For some children, structured activities and handling are effective; other children benefit from wearing a dorsal wrist splint. A therapist can have the child wear a splint during part of the therapy session and encourage finger extension through a variety of activities, including voluntary release. The therapist can use similar activities after splint removal.

Children who use wrist flexion with voluntary release may benefit from structured activities in which a container for objects is placed slightly laterally from the child's midline and at a sufficient distance from the child's body that the child needs to extend the elbow

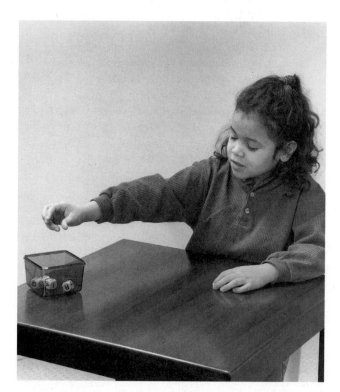

figure**11-19** Positioning materials to elicit elbow extension during release encourages the child's use of wrist extension. (*Photo by Kanji Takeno.*)

(Figure 11-19). This level of control is similar to that of an infant who releases objects with the arm held in a total extension pattern. Over time, the therapist can move the target containers closer to the child's body, requiring gradually increasing elbow flexion with wrist extension for release of objects. Sometimes the therapist can facilitate this pattern if he or she sets the containers at an angle. Once the child can release medium-sized objects into a container at midline while maintaining wrist extension to at least a neutral position, the therapist can decrease the size of the container opening.

Children with overextension of the fingers during voluntary release may benefit from activities described previously that address development of intrinsic muscle control. They also may need intervention to improve somatosensory awareness of their hands. Activities for these children often incorporate the use of lightweight materials and objects that vary in size and stability. Verbal cueing of the child to attend to object and hand placement and graded activities to facilitate increasing accuracy and visual monitoring of materials are often helpful.

In-Hand Manipulation
Problems

Children who have difficulty with in-hand manipulation skills drop objects, use surfaces for support during manipulation, or are slow in the execution of skills (Exner, 1990a). Case-Smith (1993) found empirical support for these problems in her study of children with and without fine motor delays. These problems are associated with tactile problems (Case-Smith, 1991). Praxis and motor control problems, particularly of the intrinsic muscles, also may be a major cause of limited in-hand manipulation skill development. Attentional and cognitive problems contribute to these problems in some children. Problems that limit in-hand manipulation include the following:

- Limited finger isolation and control
- Inability to effectively cup the hand to hold objects in the palm
- Inability to hold more than one object in the hand at the same time
- Insufficient stability for controlling object movement at the finger pads, resulting in objects being dropped frequently

Goals

The following are examples of goals that the therapist can use for children with a variety of levels of in-hand manipulation skill. The goals are in approximate order of difficulty, although difficulty in using any one pattern can vary with individual children.

1. The child will demonstrate finger-to-palm translation by moving a coin into the palm of the hand.

2. The child will demonstrate finger-to-palm translation with stabilization skills by holding several coins in one hand.
3. The child will demonstrate shift skills by adjusting a coin for placement into a slot in a bank.
4. The child will demonstrate simple rotation skills by adjusting utensils while eating or brushing teeth.
5. The child will demonstrate palm-to-finger translation (and palm-to-finger translation with stabilization) while eating small finger foods.
6. The child will demonstrate simple rotation with stabilization in handling pieces for a board game.
7. The child will demonstrate complex rotation skills by erasing with a pencil eraser.

Intervention strategies

The therapist's assessment of the causes of the child's problems and the therapist's determination of the child's potential for acquiring specific in-hand manipulation skills influence intervention goals and strategies. Many children with moderate and severe disabilities who lack the necessary prerequisite skills cannot develop in-hand manipulation skills. Children with mild disabilities usually can develop at least the lower-level in-hand manipulation skills.

Specific activity suggestions are given in Box 11-3. The following sections provide suggestions of strategies for therapists to use with children who differ in their level of skills. Exner (1995) provides additional information on treatment of in-hand manipulation skills.

Children with no in-hand manipulation skills. The therapist may encourage the child with no in-hand manipulation skills or only finger-to-palm translation to manipulate objects between the two hands and use support surfaces to assist in object manipulation. Use of these strategies can help the child begin to move the fingers actively over object surfaces. The therapist can use objects such as cubes that have pictures on all sides, kaleidoscopes, and textured toys. When the child can effectively move the fingers over objects, the therapist can introduce finger-to-palm translation activities in the context of "hiding object games" using various objects. Finger isolation games can be useful, and the therapist should incorporate the thumb into these activities. The child should be assisted in developing and functionally using a variety of grasp patterns, including those that combine flexion at the MCP joints with extension at the IP joints. The therapist can use tactile discrimination and proprioception activities to enhance awareness of fingers and areas of the palm of the hand.

Children with beginning in-hand manipulation skills. Children who can use finger-to-palm translation and beginning simple rotation, or shift, or palm-to-finger translation skills can work on refinement of these skills, expanding their repertoire of skills used without stabilization and beginning their ability to stabilize objects in the ulnar side of the hand while manipulating with the radial fingers.

Object selection for in-hand manipulation skills with these children is important. Objects that do not roll and that are small (not tiny) are often the easiest for the child to handle. Examples include dice-sized cubes, nickels, game pieces, and other small toys. With larger objects, the child must involve all fingers in the manipulation and use more hand expansion, so these are more difficult for the child to handle. With tiny objects, the child must have excellent tactile discrimination and fingertip control, so they are also more difficult to handle than small objects.

The therapist structures the presentation of objects to assist the child in using a particular in-hand manipulation skill and often cues the child in the use of the skill. In a study of preschool children without disabilities who had emerging in-hand manipulation skills, Exner (1990b) found that use of verbal cues or demonstration of skills had a positive effect on the children's scores (as a group). However, children with lower scores showed more improvement with cues than children with higher scores. These findings suggest that verbal cueing may be an important component of intervention for in-hand manipulation skills.

In addressing palm-to-finger translation, the therapist first places the object on the middle phalanx of the child's index finger. When the child is able to move the object from this position out to the pads of the fingers, the therapist places the object on the volar surface of the proximal phalanx of the index finger. Later the therapist places the object in the palm of the child's hand to promote thumb isolation and control to move the object.

The therapist can structure simple rotation skills by placing the object in the child's hand (in a radial grasp pattern) and asking the child to turn it upright. Pegs and peglike objects, such as candles and objects that look like little people, can be helpful in developing these skills.

Finger-to-palm translation with stabilization is the one skill with stabilization that is likely to be feasible for these children. This child often can facilitate this skill during finger-feeding activities and in play with coins. The therapist first encourages the child to hold one object in the hand while picking up and hiding another. After the child can manage two objects, the therapist can progress to using three or more objects.

Children with basic in-hand manipulation skills. For children with basic in-hand manipulation skills, the therapist emphasizes developing complex rotation skills and the use of stabilization with the other skills. The therapist introduces small- and medium-sized objects and emphasizes use of the skills in a variety of functional activities, such as dressing, hygiene, and school tasks. The child practices combinations of skills, such as finger-to-

box 11-3 *In-hand manipulation treatment activities*

Preparation activities

General tactile awareness activities
1. Using crazy foam
2. Using shaving cream
3. Applying hand lotion
4. Finger painting

Activities involving proprioceptive input
1. Weight bearing (wheelbarrow, activities on a small ball)
2. Pushing heavy objects (boxes, chairs, benches, etc.)
3. Pulling (tug-of-war)
4. Pressing different parts of the hand into clay
5. Pushing fingers into clay or therapy putty
6. Pushing shapes out of perforated cardboard
7. Tearing packages or boxes open
8. Playing clapping games

Activities involving regulation of pressure
1. Tearing edges off of computer paper
2. Rolling clay into a ball
3. Squeezing water out of a sponge or washcloth
4. Pushing snaps together

Activities involving tactile discrimination
1. Playing finger games and singing songs
2. Playing finger identification games
3. Discriminating among objects with the objects stabilized
4. Discriminating among shapes with the shapes stabilized
5. Writing on the body and identifying the shape, letter, or object drawn
6. Discriminating among textures

Specific in-hand manipulation activities

Translation (fingers to palm)
1. Getting a coin out of a change purse
2. Hiding a penny in the hand (magic trick)
3. Crumpling paper
4. Picking up and bringing a small piece of food into the palm

Translation (fingers to palm with stabilization)
1. Getting two or more coins out of a change purse, one at a time
2. Taking two or more chips off a magnetic wand, one at a time
3. Picking up pegs or paper clips one at a time and holding two or more in the hand at one time
4. Picking up several utensils one at a time and holding two or more in the hand at one time

Translation (palm to fingers)
1. Moving a penny from the palm to the fingers
2. Moving a chip to the fingers to put on a magnetic wand
3. Moving an object to put it into a container
4. Moving a food item to put it in the mouth

Translation (palm to fingers with stabilization)
1. Holding several chips to put on a wand, one at a time
2. Handling money to put it into a bank or soda machine
3. Putting one utensil down when holding several
4. Holding several game pieces (chips, pegs, or markers)

Shift
1. Turning pages in a book
2. Picking up sheets of paper, tissue paper, or dollar bills
3. Separating playing cards
4. Stringing beads (shifting string and bead as string goes through the bead)
5. Shifting a crayon, pencil, or pen for coloring or writing
6. Shifting paper in the nonpreferred hand while cutting
7. Playing with Tinker Toys (the long, thin pieces)
8. Moving a cookie while eating
9. Adjusting a spoon, fork, or knife for appropriate use
10. Rubbing paint, dirt, or tape off the pad of a finger

Shift with stabilization
1. Holding a pen and pushing the cap off with the same hand
2. Holding chips while flipping one out of the fingers
3. Holding fabric in the hand while attempting to button or snap
4. Holding a key ring with the keys in hand, shifting one for placement in a lock

Simple or complex rotation (depending on object orientation)
1. Removing or putting on a small jar lid
2. Putting on or removing bolts from nuts
3. Rotating a crayon or pencil with the tip oriented ulnarly (simple rotation)
4. Rotating a crayon or pencil with the tip oriented radially (complex rotation)
5. Removing a crayon from the box and preparing it for coloring
6. Rotating a pen or marker to put the top on
7. Rotating toy people to put them in chairs, a bus, or a boat
8. Rotating a puzzle piece for placement in the board
9. Feeling objects or shapes to identify them
10. Handling construction toy pieces
11. Turning cubes that have pictures on all six sides
12. Constructing twisted shapes with pipe cleaners
13. Rotating a toothbrush or eating utensils during use

Simple or complex rotation with stabilization
1. Handling parts of a small shape container while rotating the shape to put it into the container
2. Holding a key ring with keys, rotating the correct one for placement in the lock

palm translation, palm-to-finger translation, and simple rotation. The therapist also can stress speed of skill use by timing skills and reporting the speed to the child. Children who are working at this level of skill typically respond well to verbal cueing for strategies to use in performing skills and to feedback about the effectiveness and speed of their skills.

Bilateral Hand Use
Problems

Difficulties with bilateral hand use result from a combination of problems, of which motor factors are only one component. Some children with significant cognitive delays cannot attend to two objects simultaneously, thus reciprocal hand use or stabilization with one hand combined with object handling by the other hand is not possible. Deficits in integration of the two body sides may be present. Impaired sensation may contribute to a lack of attention to one body side. Lack of bilateral motor experience, as in children with hemiplegia or brachial plexus injuries, can cause children to approach all tasks in a one-handed manner. Other problems include the following:

- The child cannot effectively sustain both hands at midline.
- The child has difficulty using supination during bilateral activities.
- The child has overflow movements and associated reactions in one upper extremity when using the other.

Goals

The following are examples of goals that the therapist can use for children with a variety of levels of disabilities. These goals fit the categories of gross symmetric bilateral skills, stabilizing or manipulating with one hand while manipulating with the other hand, and bilateral simultaneous manipulation. The following goals show increasing levels of difficulty that are consistent with a developmental approach. This progression in skills may not be appropriate for children with significant weakness or motor problems on one body side.

1. The child will demonstrate the ability to bring both hands to midline for grasp of a large or medium-sized object.
2. The child will demonstrate the ability to use both hands together to push large objects.
3. The child will demonstrate the ability to use both hands together to lift and carry large objects.
4. The child will demonstrate the ability to stabilize materials on a table surface with one open hand while the other hand manipulates materials (e.g., coloring, writing, or holding a puzzle board while putting pieces in it).
5. The child will demonstrate the ability to stabilize materials using a palmar grasp while the other hand

manipulates materials (e.g., holding the handle of a small pan while pretending to cook).
6. The child will demonstrate the ability to stabilize materials using a variety of grasp patterns while the other hand manipulates materials (e.g., holding a cup while pouring liquid into it or holding a slice of bread while spreading butter on it).
7. The child will demonstrate the ability to manipulate objects with both hands simultaneously (e.g., buttoning, shoe tying, fixing hair, doing mechanical projects).

Treatment goals vary depending on the severity of the child's disability and the level of skills that the child is expected to acquire. The therapist must consider the child's need for and potential for gross symmetric hand use, stabilizing with one hand while manipulating with the other, and bilateral simultaneous manipulation.

Intervention strategies

Children with severe disabilities. Treatment of the child with significantly increased tone or marked asymmetry focuses on promoting the child's ability to stabilize materials with the more involved hand while manipulating with the more proficient hand. Activities that require stabilization with grasp are often easier for these children than are symmetric bilateral skills or stabilization without grasp. However, the child can accomplish stabilization without grasp as long as the child can use his or her hand in a fisted position with the wrist in neutral to slight extension. Symmetric bilateral hand use may receive some attention, particularly if these activities serve to increase awareness of one arm and to increase movement and/or control of that arm. Simultaneous bilateral manipulation skills usually are inappropriate for these children unless the therapist can use adaptations.

Special handling techniques can promote the child's ability to stabilize objects while manipulating them or to use gross bilateral skills. The therapist can sit behind the child and stabilize both shoulders to help the child bring and keep both hands at midline. The therapist should also encourage trunk rotation so that the child can cross midline effectively.

Toys and materials selected for bilateral activities must require both hands to be used, particularly in the early phases of treatment. Initially the child may be more successful with gross bilateral skills if he or she can sustain grasp and keep the forearms pronated, such as in holding a stick horizontally to hit a balloon. For the child who is working on stabilizing with one hand while manipulating with the other, presenting objects on a slippery surface may require the child to use one hand as a stabilizer. Objects that have handles are useful when the therapist is working on stabilization with grasp. Activities that are simple for the manipulating hand can allow the child to focus on the role of the stabilizing hand.

Usually the therapist places materials for bilateral skill development at midline. However, the therapist and the child should explore other positions if midline positioning is not optimal.

When a child cannot successfully stabilize materials and does not show potential for this skill in the near future, the therapist should consider adaptations. Nonskid surfaces and other devices can assist in stabilization of materials for table activities.

Children with moderate disabilities. Intervention for children with low tone or some degree of involuntary movement can approximate the normal sequence of bilateral hand skill development. Therapy initially focuses on improving symmetry and stability and proceeds through developing the child's skills in stabilizing with and without grasp. Children at this skill level may benefit from working on a slightly unstable surface to prompt spontaneous stabilization of materials during manipulation. The child may need adaptations for certain highly demanding activities in which one hand needs to be an effective stabilizer, such as in handwriting. Generally, simultaneous bilateral manipulation is not feasible for these children.

Children with mild disabilities. Children with mild disabilities may require further refinement of their gross symmetric bilateral skills and stabilizing with one hand while manipulating with the other. These children can also develop or improve their simultaneous bilateral manipulation skills. To enhance development of simultaneous bilateral manipulation skills, the therapist carefully selects, grades, and structures a variety of activities that elicit these skills. The therapist may also use functional activities of daily living to facilitate development of these skills.

Children with muscle weakness. Children with muscle weakness can often manage simultaneous manipulation activities well because little hand strength and movement of the arms against gravity is required. These children often need assistance or adaptations to develop the ability to stabilize materials with one hand because this demands more strength in the stabilizing arm. The child may be able to accomplish gross symmetric bilateral skills only on table surfaces that provide arm support.

■ GENERALIZATION OF SKILLS INTO FUNCTIONAL ACTIVITIES

Most children do not readily generalize skills from isolated activities to their everyday life activities without assistance. Therefore the therapist should present activities to the child with hand or arm function problems in a meaningful context, and he or she should seek ways in which the child can practice specific fine motor skills within everyday activities. For example, the child can carry out reaching program activities during dressing and

hygiene training or while playing with a toy that has many different parts. The therapist can incorporate grasp activities into independent eating and vocational readiness tasks. The child can facilitate in-hand manipulation by using materials from his or her pencil or crayon box or building with construction toys. The therapist can structure voluntary release into a game that uses moveable pieces. The child can develop bilateral hand use through meal preparation activities, play, and schoolwork. Many other combinations are possible to help the child develop mature function of hand or arm skills with increasing competence in daily life activities.

Research on Intervention for Hand Skill Problems

Studies on the efficacy of fine motor and hand skill intervention in children are beginning to be reported. Case-Smith (1996) conducted a study to assess outcomes of occupational therapy programs for 26 preschool-age children who were treated during one school year. The children showed significant change in several aspects of fine motor skills, including in-hand manipulation skills, motor accuracy, and tool use. In addition, the children showed significant improvement in their self-care skills.

In a follow-up study with a larger group of preschool-age children with problems and a group of children without problems, Case-Smith and others (1998) compared children who received services with those without problems. The children who received services made significant progress in the areas of in-hand manipulation skills and motor accuracy. The researchers also found that more consultation was significantly associated with the children's improvement in some fine motor skills.

■ SPLINTING FOR CHILDREN

Splinting is often a component of occupational therapy intervention for children with hand function problems. Children who have one or more of the following problems may benefit most:

- Sustained abnormal posturing
- Increased tone or markedly decreased tone
- Limitations in movement of the hand
- Limitations in functional skills secondary to problems with hand functions

Children with severe motor disability associated with CNS dysfunction may benefit from splints to reduce tone or improve mobility and functional skills. The child with minimal involvement secondary to CNS damage may have more difficulty with thumb use than with wrist or finger control. This child may need a thumb splint to decrease flexor muscle tone or provide thumb MCP stability so that function is enhanced.

Precautions and Indications for Splint Use

Precautions for splint use are always in order, particularly for nonverbal children who may have poor sensation. These factors make them vulnerable to skin irritations and pressure problems. Children may be unable to report sensory problems during or after splint application; therefore the therapist must carefully instruct the child's parents regarding the wearing schedule, possible problems, and postural changes to note.

Static splints generally are worn for shorter periods than splints that allow hand movement. Initially, children may tolerate wearing a splint for only 5 to 10 minutes. Usually the therapist can gradually increase these periods. If the child has increased tone, maximum wearing time for a static splint is usually 6 to 8 hours per day. However, if splints allow some hand movement and the therapist uses them to aid accomplishment of functional activities, the child may tolerate them for additional hours. Children generally wear night splints all night, but they should spend at least a portion of each 24-hour period without splints.

Not all children with increased tone need night resting splints. In many cases their hands are more relaxed during sleep, and their parents can position their arms and hands in neutral. Children who have neutral positioning at night generally are at less risk for development of contractures. However, the child who shows abnormal hand posturing during the day but not at night may require daytime splint application to increase function.

Boehme (1988) noted that some children have learned to use abnormal patterns of wrist flexion and ulnar deviation or thumb adduction to accomplish their daily activities. If a splint inhibits this pattern, the child may compensate by using another abnormal position of the hand or arm. Therefore before the therapist applies a splint, he or she must determine whether functional skill patterns that the child is using will be lost. Often the therapist needs to provide an increased frequency of intervention sessions when children are wearing splints so that they can develop better patterns of hand use.

The use of splinting rarely is questionable for children who have muscle weakness, traumatic injury of the hand or arm, or joint inflammation. However, splinting is more controversial in children with increased tone. Most of the related literature addresses problems of adults with abnormal tone; fewer studies (Exner & Bonder, 1983; MacKinnon, Sanderson, & Buchanan, 1975; McPherson, 1981) report the use of splints with children.

Types of Splints Used With Children

Splints are categorized into those that allow hand movement and those that do not. *Static splints* include resting pan splints, other volar and dorsal full hand and wrist splints, spasticity reduction splints, and thumb positioning splints. *Dynamic splints* assist the child with a particular wrist, finger, or thumb movement. A *neurophysiologically based* splint may provide stimulation to the hand or arm or assist with stabilization of one or more joints during hand or arm activities.

Doubilet and Polkow (1977) and Snook (1979) reported case studies suggesting that *spasticity reduction splints* help decrease tone in adults. McPherson (1981) examined the effectiveness of Snook's spasticity reduction splint in five adolescents with severe disabilities. Splint-wearing time was gradually increased from 15 minutes the first day to 2 hours daily by the fourth week. The outcome measure was passive muscle tone at the wrist, which was documented on a daily basis through use of a scale that measured pounds of force when the individual assumed wrist flexion. During the 4 weeks of splint application, the subjects' wrist tone decreased significantly. When they did not wear the splints for a week, their tone increased again.

When the therapist applies spasticity reduction splints, he or she should take care to control the thumb MCP joint. Distal force on the thumb can result in ". . . stretch or even rupture of the ulnar collateral ligament of the MCP joint of the thumb . . . " (Phelps & Weeks, 1976, p. 545) and subluxation of the MCP joint. Because children with spasticity usually demonstrate marked thumb adduction, distal control of the thumb moves the MCP and IP joints into hyperextension, thus control at the carpometacarpal (CMC) joint is needed to abduct and extend the first metacarpal CMC joint.

Resting pan splints may provide more support to and control of the thumb than some of the spasticity reduction devices. However, the therapist should plan and monitor splints carefully for reactions at the wrist and fingers. Children with increased tone may not tolerate the classic position for a resting hand splint in which the wrist is in 20 to 30 degrees of extension and fingers are in slight flexion. The child with moderately increased tone may have more tolerance for a resting splint that holds the wrist in neutral position and the fingers in slight flexion. However, if flexor spasticity is severe, splinting that begins with the wrist in marked flexion and emphasizes slightly increased finger extension (out of full fisting) may be most effective. Initially, the therapist should stabilize wrist position in just slightly more extension than the child normally achieves. The therapist then adjusts or reconstructs splints to position the wrist, thumb, and fingers. In general, the therapist increases extension at only the wrist *or* fingers at one time to prevent the occurrence of flexion or extension deformities in the fingers.

The therapist may use other *volar splints,* such as the wrist support splint, with children who respond to control of wrist flexion but who do not need or cannot tol-

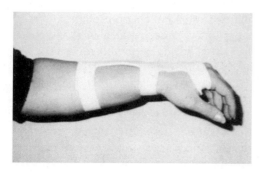

figure**11-20**   Dorsal splint to support the wrist in extension.

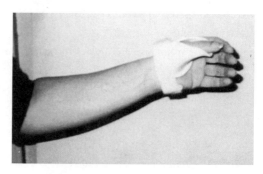

figure**11-21**   Short opponens thumb splint.

erate positioning of the fingers or thumb simultaneously. Wrist support splints allow the child to use the hand to perform functional activities, and the therapist may adjust them periodically to promote a progression of controlled finger extension during activities. The volar wrist splint should control ulnar deviation.

Controversy regarding the use of dorsal versus volar static splints is long standing and has yet to be resolved. From a functional perspective, dorsal splints are most effective with children who have muscle weakness and those with mild to moderately increased tone. The therapist uses the dorsal splint shown in Figure 11-20 on children with high tone and on those with low tone to hold their wrists in a neutral position. The splint provides support to the palmar arch. Although the child cannot use extreme wrist flexion, the therapist may use a small degree of wrist flexion in functional activities. Because no splint material contacts the volar surface of the hand and forearm, this splint interferes less with controlled arm use on a surface than a volar splint would; children have responded favorably to this splint. However, dorsal static splints have limited use in controlling abnormal finger position in children with CNS deficit.

The therapist uses thumb splints when a child has difficulty with thumb control but can adequately coordinate movements in other parts of the wrist and hand or when thumb control is the greatest problem. Exner and Bonder (1983) reported a study of short opponens thumb splint use with 12 children who had cerebral palsy with spastic hemiplegia. These splints controlled the thumb over the first metacarpal joint and extended onto the distal phalanx (Figure 11-21). The researchers used the splints 8 hours daily for 6 weeks. After this program, two children showed improvement in bilateral hand use and three children showed improved grasp. Some children found that wearing the splints on the nonpreferred hand interfered with stabilization of materials that could not be grasped. In clinical use, the splint is beneficial in improving children's functional use of their hands.

The therapist can use a soft splint to enhance thumb control in children with mildly increased tone. Neoprene

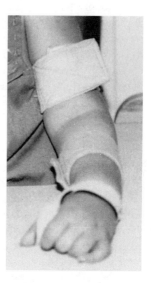

figure**11-22**   A neoplush thumb splint is worn with orthokinetic cuffs on the forearm and arm. Both orthokinetic cuffs are designed to promote extension and inhibit flexion.

or Neoplush is a commonly used material for soft splints. Use of the opponens splint pattern described previously is suitable when higher tone is present (Figure 11-22).

The therapist uses other orthotic devices that provide specific types of sensory stimulation to inhibit or facilitate muscle tone. MacKinnon and others (1975) introduced the *MacKinnon splint,* a device that uses a dowel in the child's hand to provide pressure against the metacarpal heads. The therapist attaches a piece of aquarium tubing to each end of the dowel and connects it to a small band that fastens around the child's wrist. Contact of the dowel with the metacarpal heads is believed to stretch and facilitate the intrinsic muscles of the hand and inhibit the long finger flexors. MacKinnon and others (1975) reported that children with spastic cerebral palsy improved in-hand awareness and bilateral hand use and showed a decrease in fisting.

Exner and Bonder (1983) modified the MacKinnon splint. They enlarged the forearm piece and used two

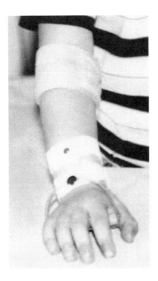

figure**11-23**   MacKinnon splint and forearm orthokinetic cuff.

straps to provide better stabilization (Figure 11-23). They found that the dowel contacted the palm of the child's hand rather than the metacarpal heads. They fitted the orthotic device with the child's hand in its most typical wrist position (in flexion, if necessary) so that they could maintain firm dowel contact with the palm. Wrist positioning is not a function of this splint. Children in their study wore the modified MacKinnon splints 8 hours daily for 6 weeks. Of the 12 children, 7 showed improvement secondary to use of this splint. Three children improved in both grasp and bilateral hand skills, two improved in grasp only, and two improved in bilateral hand skills only. The children with improved skills all had moderate to severe upper extremity motor involvement. All children tolerated the splint well and found that weight bearing could be accomplished comfortably during application periods.

There are several precautions regarding use of the MacKinnon splint. The splint is usually constructed by attaching aquarium tubing to the dowel with small nails. Even though these nails are covered with moleskin, the therapist should not use the splint if the child is likely to put objects in his or her mouth. An alternative is to roll thermoplastic material around the tubing in place of using a dowel. However, this alternative is not as readily adjustable. Hill (1988) noted that some children experience instability of the upper extremity with decreased tone secondary to MacKinnon splint use. Therefore careful monitoring, particularly in number of weeks for use, is recommended.

The therapist applies *orthokinetic devices* to facilitate tone in one muscle group and inhibit tone in the opposing muscles. These cuffs are made of elastic and nonelastic segments. The elastic portion may activate afferent fibers of skin exteroceptors and facilitate the motor neurons that innervate the muscles underlying the stimulated skin area (Blashy & Fuchs, 1959). Effectiveness of the device may be attributable to its inhibitory or facilitory functions or a combination of both. The authors noted that orthokinetic cuffs were more effective when tone imbalance between the muscle groups was pronounced.

Orthokinetic cuffs are made from three layers of elastic bandage material, with nonstretch fabric sewn into the areas that are to be inhibitory. The therapist should carefully fit the cuff before final sewing so that it is snug and the elastic portion does not extend onto the muscles to be inhibited. For facilitation of elbow extension, the therapist places the active (elastic) area of the cuff over the triceps and the inactive area over the biceps. The child can easily wear orthokinetic cuffs with other hand splints and during treatment activities.

The Exner and Bonder (1983) study of splint use with 12 children with cerebral palsy also tested application of orthokinetic cuffs. The researchers tested evaluation of effects over a 6-week period with 8 hours of daily use. They placed cuffs on the children's forearms, with the elastic (facilitory) portion over the muscle bellies of the fingers and wrist extensors. Four children demonstrated improvement in both functions. The study indicated that the device helped encourage wrist or finger extension when the child was able to use some active contraction of the muscles being facilitated.

Other orthotic devices are available for children with increased tone or contractures. Positioning children who have had head injuries to prevent loss of range is particularly important during extensive comatose, semicomatose, and recovery periods. The therapist uses inflatable air (pneumatic) splints (Hill, 1988) to decrease tone, maintain and increase joint range, and stimulate somatosensory function. Some therapists use casting with children who exhibit spasticity and contractures secondary to cerebral palsy or head injury (Hill, 1994; Yasukawa, 1992; Yasukawa & Hill, 1988). Tona and Schneck (1993) conducted a single-subject study using upper extremity casting. Their findings were positive regarding the effectiveness for that child.

■ SUMMARY

A description of the components of hand and arm function that are instrumental in the performance of play, self-maintenance, schoolwork, and vocational readiness activities were presented in this chapter. Factors that influence the development of hand function and types of problems in hand and arm use were discussed. The normal sequences of development for basic skills of reach, grasp, release, and carry, as well as advanced functions of in-hand manipulation and bilateral hand use, were presented. Intervention strategies for development of various hand skills were described, as well as the appropriate uses of splinting with children. The therapist should always frame assessment and intervention of hand and arm function problems within the context of the child's daily environments and his or her play, school, and self-care activities.

STUDY QUESTIONS

1. What are the major considerations for intervention with an adolescent who has spastic hemiplegia; demonstrates elbow flexion, forearm pronation, and fisting in the nonpreferred hand; and is having difficulty completing manual dexterity tasks in his or her vocational readiness program?

2. A 5-year-old girl with marked involuntary movements of her arms and poor postural stability would like to feed herself. What aspects of arm and hand function would the therapist assess to determine if she can do this with or without adaptive equipment? What intervention strategies would the therapist use to promote the most effective grasp of the spoon and cup and achievement of the plate-to-mouth pattern? What types of splinting could the therapist consider?

3. A 6-year-old boy has a diagnosis of autism. He does not sustain eye contact with objects and shows limited hand contact with objects. How would the therapist begin to determine treatment priorities for him? What strategies would the therapist use to assess his hand skills and factors contributing to the limited use? Are in-hand manipulation skills a priority to address in treatment? Why or why not?

4. An 8-year-old boy has illegible handwriting. How may problems with bilateral hand use and in-hand manipulation skills interact with short attention span and somatosensory problems to contribute to his handwriting difficulties?

5. What aspects of reach, grasp, release, and bilateral hand use should the therapist address with a 15-month-old infant who has Down syndrome and associated limited hand function and cognitive skills at the 8- to 10-month level?

6. A 10-year-old girl sustained a head injury 2 months ago. Before the accident she was left-hand dominant. She is now alert but has some memory deficits and motor planning problems. She has a left elbow contracture and shows moderately increased tone in wrist flexion, thumb adduction, and finger flexion. What types of splinting should the therapist consider? How can the therapist determine if the splinting devices are effective treatment?

References

Ager, C.L., Olivett, B.L., & Johnson, C.L. (1984). Grasp and pinch strength in children 5 to 12 years old. *The American Journal of Occupational Therapy, 38,* 107-113.

Ayres, A.J. (1958). Ontogenetic principles in the development of arm and hand function. *The American Journal of Occupational Therapy, 8,* 95-99.

Ayres, A.J. (1989). *Sensory Integration and Praxis Tests manual.* Los Angeles: Western Psychological Services.

Barnes, K.J. (1986). Improving prehension skills of children with cerebral palsy: A clinical study. *Occupational Therapy Journal of Research, 6* (4), 227-239.

Barnes, K.J. (1989a). Direct replication: Relationship of upper extremity weight bearing to hand skills of boys with cerebral palsy. *Occupational Therapy Journal of Research, 9,* 235-242.

Barnes, K.J. (1989b). Relationship of upper extremity weight bearing to hand skills of boys with cerebral palsy. *Occupational Therapy Journal of Research, 9,* 143-154.

Bertenthal, B., & von Hofsten, C. (1998). Eye, head and trunk control: The foundation for manual development. *Neuroscience and Biobehavioral Reviews, 22* (4), 515-520.

Blashy, M.R.M., & Fuchs, R.L. (1959). Orthokinetics: A new receptor facilitation method. *The American Journal of Occupational Therapy, 13,* 226-234.

Bobath, B. (1978). *Adult hemiplegia: Evaluation and treatment* (2nd ed.). London: Heinemann Educational Books.

Boehme, R.H. (1988). *Improving upper body control: An approach to assessment and treatment of tonal dysfunction.* Tucson: Therapy Skill Builders.

Bushnell E.W., & Boudreau, J.P. (1997). Exploring and exploiting objects with the hands during infancy. In K.J. Connolly (Ed.), *The psychobiology of the hand* (pp. 144-161). London: Cambridge University Press.

Case-Smith, J. (1991). The effects of tactile defensiveness and tactile discrimination on in-hand manipulation. *The American Journal of Occupational Therapy, 45,* 811-818.

Case-Smith, J. (1993). Comparison of in-hand manipulation skills in children with and without fine motor delays. *Occupational Therapy Journal of Research, 13,* 87-100.

Case-Smith, J. (1996). Fine motor outcomes in preschool children who receive occupational therapy services. *The American Journal of Occupational Therapy, 50,* 52-61.

Case-Smith, J., Bigsby, R., & Clutter, J. (1998). Perceptual-motor coupling in the development of grasp. *The American Journal of Occupational Therapy, 52,* 102-110.

Case-Smith, J., Fisher, A.G., & Bauer, D. (1989). An analysis of the relationship between proximal and distal motor control. *The American Journal of Occupational Therapy, 43,* 657-662.

Case-Smith, J., Heaphy, T., Marr, D., Galvin, B., Koch, V., Ellis, M.G., & Perez, I. (1998). Fine motor and functional outcomes in preschool children. *The American Journal of Occupational Therapy, 52,* 788-796.

Chakarian, D.L., & Larson, M. (1991, September). The effects of upper extremity weight bearing on hand function in children with cerebral palsy. *NDTA Newsletter,* 4-5.

Colangelo, C.A. (1999). Biomechanical frame of reference. In P. Kramer & J. Hinojosa (Eds.), *Frames of reference for pediatric occupational therapy* (pp. 233-305). Philadelphia: Lippincott.

Connolly, K., & Dalgleish, M. (1989). The emergence of a tool-using skill in infancy. *Developmental Psychology, 25,* 894-912.

Connor, F.P., Williamson, G.G., & Siepp, J.M. (1978). Movement. In *Program guide for infants and toddlers.* New York: College Press.

Corbetta, D., & Mounoud, P. (1990). Early development of grasping and manipulation. In C. Bard, M. Fleury, & L. Hay (Eds.), *Development of eye-hand coordination across the life span* (pp. 188-213). Columbia: University of South Carolina.

Couch, K.J., Dietz, J.C., & Kenny, E.M. (1998). The role of play in pediatric occupational therapy. *The American Journal of Occupational Therapy, 52,* 111-117.

Danella, E., & Vogtle, L. (1992). Neurodevelopmental treatment for the young child with cerebral palsy. In J. Case-Smith & C. Pehoski (Eds.), *Development of hand skills in the child* (pp. 91-110). Rockville, MD: AOTA.

Doubilet, L., & Polkow, L.S. (1977). Theory and design of a finger abduction splint for the spastic hand. *The American Journal of Occupational Therapy, 31* (5), 320-322.

Eliaason, A.C. (1995). Sensorimotor integration of normal and impaired development of precision movement of the hand. In A. Henderson & C. Pehoski (Eds.), *Hand function in the child* (pp. 40-54). St. Louis: Mosby.

Elliott, J.M., & Connolly, K.J. (1984). A classification of manipulative hand movements. *Developmental Medicine and Child Neurology, 26,* 283-296.

Erhardt, R.P. (1982). *Erhardt developmental prehension assessment.* Tucson: Therapy Skill Builders.

Exner, C.E. (1992). In-hand manipulation skills. In J. Case-Smith & C. Pehoski (Eds.), *Development of hand skills in the child* (pp. 35-45). Rockville, MD: AOTA.

Exner, C.E. (1990a). In-hand manipulation skills in normal young children: A pilot study. *Occupational Therapy Practice, 1* (4), 63-72.

Exner, C.E. (1990b). The zone of proximal development in in-hand manipulation skills of non-dysfunctional 3- and 4-year-old children. *The American Journal of Occupational Therapy, 44,* 884-891.

Exner, C.E. (1995). Remediation of hand skill problems in children. In A. Henderson & C. Pehoski (Eds.). *Hand function in the child: Foundations for remediation.* St. Louis: Mosby.

Exner, C.E., & Bonder, B.R. (1983). Comparative effects of three hand splints on the bilateral hand use, grasp, and arm-hand posture in hemiplegic children: A pilot study. *Occupational Therapy Journal of Research, 3,* 75-92.

Exner, C.E., & Henderson, A. (1995). Cognition and motor skill. In A. Henderson & C. Pehoski (Eds.), *Hand function in the child* (pp. 93-110). St. Louis: Mosby.

Fagard, J., & Jacquet, A.Y. (1989). Onset of bimanual coordination and symmetry versus asymmetry of movement. *Infant Behavior and Development, 12,* 229-236.

Finnie, N.R. (1975). *Handling the young cerebral palsied child at home* (2nd ed.). New York: E.P. Dutton.

Folio, R.M., & Fewell, R. (2000). *Peabody Developmental Motor Scales—Revised.* Chicago: Riverside.

Gesell, A., & Amatruda, C.S. (1947). *Developmental diagnosis.* New York: Harper & Row.

Gordon, A.M., & Forssberg, H. (1997). Development of neural mechanisms underlying grasping in children. In K.J. Connolly & H. Forssberg. (Eds.), *Neurophysiology and neuropsychology of motor development.* London: MacKeith Press.

Haron, M., & Henderson, A. (1985). Active and passive touch in developmentally dyspraxic and normal boys. *Occupational Therapy Journal of Research, 5,* 101-112.

Henderson, A. (1995). Self-care and hand skill. In A. Henderson & C. Pehoski (Eds.), *Hand function in the child* (pp. 164-183). St. Louis: Mosby.

Hill, J. (1994). The effects of casting on upper extremity motor disorders after brain injury. *The American Journal of Occupational Therapy, 48,* 219-224.

Hill, S.G. (1988). Current trends in upper extremity splinting. In R. Boehme (Ed.), *Improving upper body control* (pp. 131-164). Tucson: Therapy Skill Builders.

Hirschel, A., Pehoski, C., & Coryell, J. (1990). Environmental support and the development of grasp in infants. *The American Journal of Occupational Therapy, 44,* 721-727.

Humphry, R., Jewell, K., & Rosenberger, R.C. (1995). Development of in-hand manipulation and relationship with activities. *The American Journal of Occupational Therapy, 49,* 763-774.

Jeannerod, M. (1994). The hand and the object: The role of posterior parietal cortex in forming motor representations. *Canadian Journal of Physiology and Pharmacology, 72,* 535-541.

Johansson, R.S., & Westling, G. (1988). Coordinated isometric muscle commands adequately and erroneously programmed for the weight during lifting tasks with precision grip. *Experimental Brain Research, 71,* 59-71.

Kenney, W.E. (1963). Certain sensory defects in cerebral palsy. *Clinical Orthopedics, 27,* 193-195.

Kinghorn, J., & Roberts, G. (1996). The effect of an inhibitive weight-bearing splint on tone and function: A single-case study. *The American Journal of Occupational Therapy, 50,* 807-815.

Latch, C.M., Freeling, M.C., & Powell, N.J. (1993). A comparison of the grip strength of children with myelomeningocele to that of children without disability. *The American Journal of Occupational Therapy, 47,* 498-503.

Lawrence, D.G., & Kuypers, H.G. (1986). The functional organization of the motor system in monkey. Parts I & II. *Brain, 91,* 1-36.

Link, L., Lukens, S., & Bush, M.A. (1995). Spherical grip strength in children 3 to 6 years of age. *The American Journal of Occupational Therapy, 49,* 318-326.

Long, C., Conrad, P.W., Hall, E.A., & Furler, S.L. (1970). Intrinsic-extrinsic muscle control of the hand in power grip and precision handling. *Journal of Bone and Joint Surgery, 52A,* 853-913.

MacKinnon, J., Sanderson, E., & Buchanan, J. (1975). The MacKinnon splint: A functional hand splint. *Canadian Journal of Occupational Therapy, 42,* 157-158.

Mathiowetz, V., Rogers, S.L., Dowe-Keval, M., Donohoe, L., & Rennells, C. (1986). The Purdue Pegboard: Norms for 14-19 year olds. *The American Journal of Occupational Therapy, 40,* 174-179.

Mathiowetz, V., Weimer, D.M., & Federman, S.M. (1986). Grip and pinch strength: Norms for 6- to 19-year olds. *The American Journal of Occupational Therapy, 40,* 705-711.

McHale, K., & Cermak, S.A. (1992). Fine motor activities in elementary school: Preliminary findings and provisional implications for children with fine motor problems. *The American Journal of Occupational Therapy, 46,* 898-903.

McPherson, J.J. (1981). Objective evaluation of a splint designed to reduce hypertonicity. *The American Journal of Occupational Therapy, 35,* 189-194.

Monfraix, C., Tardieu, G., & Tardieu, C. (1961). Disturbances of manual perception in children with cerebral palsy. *Developmental Medicine and Child Neurology, 22,* 454-464.

Myers, C.A. (1992). Therapeutic fine-motor activities for preschoolers. In J. Case-Smith & C. Pehoski (Eds.), *Development of hand skills in the child* (pp. 47-59). Rockville, MD: AOTA.

Napier, J.R. (1956). The prehensile movements of the human hand. *Journal of Bone Joint Surgery, 38B,* 902-913.

Pehoski, C. (1992). Central nervous system control of precision movements of the hand. In J. Case-Smith & C. Pehoski (Eds.), *Development of hand skills in the child* (pp. 1-11). Rockville, MD: AOTA.

Pehoski, C. (1995). Cortical control of skilled movements of the hand. In A. Henderson, & C. Pehoski (Eds.), *Hand function in the child* (pp. 3-15). St Louis: Mosby.

Pehoski, C., Henderson, A., & Tickle-Degnen, L. (1997a). In-hand manipulation in young children: Rotation of an object in the fingers. *The American Journal of Occupational Therapy, 51,* 544-552.

Pehoski, C., Henderson, A., & Tickle-Degnen, L. (1997b). In-hand manipulation in young children: Translation movements. *The American Journal of Occupational Therapy, 51,* 719-728.

Phelps, R.E., & Weeks, P.M. (1976). Management of thumb-in-palm web space contracture. *The American Journal of Occupational Therapy, 30,* 543-556.

Ramsey, D.S., & Weber, S. (1986). Infant's hand preference in a task involving complementary roles for the two hands. *Child Development, 57,* 300-307.

Rosblad, B. (1995). Reaching and eye-hand coordination. In A. Henderson & C. Pehoski (Eds.), *Hand function in the child* (pp. 81-92). St. Louis: Mosby.

Ruff, H.A. (1980). The development of the perception and recognition of objects. *Child Development, 51,* 981-992.

Ruff, H.A., McCarton, C., Kurtzber, D., & Vaughan, Jr., H.G. (1984). Preterm infants' manipulative exploration of objects. *Child Development, 55,* 1166-1173.

Schneck, C., & Battaglia, C. (1992). Developing scissors skills in young children. In J. Case-Smith & C. Pehoski (Eds.), *Development of hand skills in the child* (pp. 79-89). Rockville, MD: AOTA.

Schoen, S., & Anderson, J. (1999). Neurodevelopmental treatment frame of reference. In P. Kramer & J. Hinojosa (Eds.), *Frames of reference for pediatric occupational therapy* (pp. 49-86). Williams & Wilkins.

Sheridan, M.D. (1975). *From birth to five years: Children's developmental progress.* Atlantic Highlands, NJ: Humanities Press.

Smith, R.O., & Benge, M.W. (1985). Pinch and grasp strength: Standardization of terminology and protocol. *The American Journal of Occupational Therapy, 39,* 531-535.

Snook, J.H. (1979). Spasticity reduction splint. *The American Journal of Occupational Therapy, 33,* 648-651.

Stillwell, J.M., & Cermak, S.A. (1995). Perceptual functions of the hand. In A. Henderson, & C. Pehoski (Eds.), *Hand function in the child* (pp. 55-80). St. Louis: Mosby.

Tachdjian, M.O., & Minear, W.I. (1958). Sensory disturbances in the hands of children with hemiplegia. *Journal of the American Medical Association, 155,* 628-632.

Tobias, M.V., & Goldkopf, I.M. (1995). Toys and games: Their role in hand development. In A. Henderson & C. Pehoski (Eds.), *Hand function in the child* (pp. 223-254). St. Louis: Mosby.

Tona, J.L., & Schneck, C.M. (1993). The efficacy of upper extremity inhibitive casting: A single-subject pilot study. *The American Journal of Occupational Therapy, 47,* 901-910.

Twitchell, T.E. (1965). The automatic grasping responses of infants. *Neuropsychologics, 3,* 247-259.

Verdonck, M.C., & Henneberg, M. (1997). Manual dexterity of South African children growing in contrasting socioeconomic conditions. *The American Journal of Occupational Therapy, 51,* 303-306.

von Hofsten, C. (1982). Eye-hand coordination in the newborn. *Developmental Psychology, 18* (3), 450-461.

von Hofsten, C. (1991). Structuring of early reaching movements: A longitudinal study. *Journal of Motor Behavior, 23* (4), 280-292.

Weiss, M.W., & Flatt, A.E. (1971). Functional evaluation of the congenitally anomalous hand. Part II. *The American Journal of Occupational Therapy, 25,* 139-143.

Wilson, B., & Trombly, C.A. (1984). Proximal and distal function in children with and without sensory integrative dysfunction: An EMG study. *Canadian Journal of Occupational Therapy, 51,* 11-17.

Yasukawa, A. (1992). Upper-extremity casting: Adjunct treatment for the child with cerebral palsy. In J. Case-Smith & C. Pehoski (Eds.), *Development of hand skills in the child* (pp. 111-123). Rockville, MD: AOTA.

Yasukawa, A., & Hill, J. (1988). Casting to improve upper extremity function. In R. Boehme (Ed.), *Improving upper body control* (pp. 165-188). Tucson: Therapy Skill Builders.

Suggested Readings

Duff, S.V. (1995). Prehension. In D. Cech & S. Martin (Eds.), *Functional movement development across the life span* (pp. 313-353). Philadelphia: W.B. Saunders.

Eliasson, A.C., Gordon, A.M., & Forssberg, H. (1991). Basic co-ordination of manipulative forces of children with cerebral palsy. *Developmental Medicine and Child Neurology, 33,* 661-670.

Gilfoyle, E.M., Grady, A.P., & Moore, J.C. (1990). *Children adapt* (2nd ed.). Thorofare, NJ: Slack.

Henderson, A., & Pehoski, C. (1995). *Hand function in the child.* St. Louis: Mosby.

Jensen, G.D., & Alderman, M.E. (1963). The prehensile grasp of spastic diplegia. *Pediatrics, 31,* 470-477.

Kopp, C.B. (1974). Fine motor abilities of infants. *Developmental Medicine and Child Neurology, 16,* 629-636.

Ruff, H.A. (1982). Role of manipulation in infants' responses to invariant properties of objects. *Developmental Psychology, 18,* 682-691.

Sugden, D.A., & Keogh, J.F. (1990). *Problems in movement skill development.* Columbia: University of South Carolina.

chapter **12**

Sensory Integration

L. Diane Parham
Zoe Mailloux

key terms

Sensory nourishment
Adaptive responses
Neural plasticity
Development of
    sensory integration
Sensory modulation
Sensory defensiveness
Sensory discrimination
Vestibular processing
    disorders

Dyspraxia
Classical sensory
    integration treatment
Compensatory skill
    development
Group therapy
    programs
Expected outcomes of
    sensory integration
    treatment

■ CHAPTER OBJECTIVES

1. Explain the neurobiologic concepts that are basic to an individual's sensory integrative function.
2. Explain the link between sensory input from the environment and the child's adaptive response.
3. Describe the development of sensory integration from prenatal life through childhood.
4. Explain the clinical picture and hypothesized basis for problems in sensory modulation, defensiveness, and discrimination.
5. Describe vestibular processing disorders and the types of behaviors that characterize children with vestibular processing problems.
6. Define developmental dyspraxia, and identify examples of behaviors that might be observed in a young child with dyspraxia.
7. Identify and describe tests, interviews, and instruments used in evaluation of sensory integration.
8. Define and explain classical sensory integrative treatment, and discuss limitations and benefits of using such an intervention approach.
9. Explain when individual therapy should focus on compensatory skill development.

10. Describe group therapy programs and consultative models, and explain the benefits of using these models in combination with classical treatment.
11. Identify the expected outcomes of an occupational therapy program using a sensory integrative approach.
12. Discuss the published research on the effectiveness of sensory integration.

The term *sensory integration* holds special meaning for occupational therapists. In some contexts it is used to refer to a particular way of viewing the neural organization of sensory information for functional behavior. In other situations this term refers to a clinical frame of reference for the assessment and treatment of persons who have functional disorders in sensory processing. Both of these meanings originated in the work of A. Jean Ayres, an occupational therapist and educational psychologist whose brilliant clinical insights and original research revolutionized occupational therapy practice with children.

Ayres' ideas ushered in a new way of looking at children and understanding many of the developmental, learning, and emotional problems that arise during childhood. Her innovative practice and groundbreaking research met a tremendous amount of resistance within the profession when introduced in the late 1960s and 1970s. Today the treatment methods that she pioneered continue to be questioned and investigated, but there is little doubt that her perspective has had a profound influence on occupational therapy practice. The presence of sensory integration concepts in nearly all of the chapters of this book attests to the extent to which these ideas have affected the thinking of pediatric occupational therapists. Furthermore, the research base of the sensory integration frame of reference is extensive. More research has been conducted in the area of sensory integration than in any other area of occupational therapy.

This chapter provides an in-depth orientation to this fascinating aspect of occupational therapy practice. The reader will gain a general sense of how sensory integration as a brain function is related to everyday occupations. Following is a description of how sensory integration is manifested in typically developing children and in relation to the daily-life problems of children who experience difficulty with sensory integration. The history of research on sensory integrative dysfunction is reviewed to give the reader a perspective on how this field came into being, what the major constructs are, and how they have changed—and continue to change—over time. Sensory integration, as a clinical frame of reference, is described by identifying types of sensory integrative dysfunction, reviewing approaches to clinical assessment, and outlining the characteristics of both direct and indirect modes of intervention. The issue of effectiveness research is addressed. Case examples of children who have been helped by occupational therapists using sensory integrative principles are presented.

■ SENSORY INTEGRATION IN CHILD DEVELOPMENT

One of the most distinctive contributions that Ayres made to understanding child development was her focus on sensory processing, particularly with respect to the proximal senses (vestibular, tactile, and proprioceptive). From the sensory integration viewpoint, these senses are emphasized because they are primitive and primary; they dominate the child's interactions with the world early in life. The distal senses of vision and hearing are critical and become increasingly more dominant as the child matures. Ayres believed, however, that the body-centered senses are a foundation on which complex occupations are scaffolded. Furthermore, when Ayres began her work, the vestibular, tactile, and proprioceptive senses were virtually ignored by scholars and clinicians who were interested in child development. She devoted her career to studying the roles that these forgotten senses play in development and in the genesis of developmental problems of children.

A basic assumption made by Ayres (1972b) was that brain function is a critical factor in human behavior. She reasoned, therefore, that knowledge of brain function and dysfunction would give her insight into child development and would help her understand the developmental problems of children. However, Ayres also had a pragmatic orientation that sprang from her professional background as an occupational therapist. She was concerned particularly with how brain functions affected the child's ability to participate successfully in daily occupations. Consequently, her work represents a fusion of neurobiologic insights with the practical, everyday concerns of human beings, particularly children and their families.

As Ayres developed her ideas about sensory integration, she used terms such as *sensory integration, adaptive response,* and *praxis* in ways that reflected her orientation. A glossary of terms that are commonly used within the framework of sensory integration theory is presented in Appendix 12-A. It may be helpful to the reader to refer to these definitions frequently while reading this chapter.

Ayres coined some of the terms in Appendix 12-A, whereas other terms were drawn from the literature of other fields. When Ayres borrowed a term from another field, however, she imparted a particular meaning to it. For example, Ayres did not use the term *sensory integration* to refer solely to intricate synaptic connections within the brain, as neuroscientists typically do. Rather, she applied it to neural processes as they relate to functional behavior. Hence her definition of sensory integration is the "organization of sensation for use" (Ayres, 1979, p. 5). It is the inclusion of the final clause "for use" that is a hallmark of Ayres because it ties sensory processing to the person's occupation.

Ayres introduced a new vocabulary of sensory integration theory and synthesized important concepts from the neurobiologic literature to organize her views of child development and dysfunction. Many of these ideas were first published in her classic book, *Sensory Integration and Learning Disorders* (Ayres, 1972b). Later she wrote a book for parents, *Sensory Integration and the Child* (Ayres, 1979), outlining the behavioral changes that can be observed in a child as sensory integration develops. Major points made in these books regarding neurobiologic concepts in relationship to development and the ontogeny of sensory integration are presented in the following sections.

■ NEUROBIOLOGICALLY BASED CONCEPTS

Sensory Nourishment

Sensory input is necessary for optimal brain function. The brain is designed to constantly take in sensory information, and it malfunctions if deprived of it. Sensory deprivation experiments conducted in the 1950s and

1960s make it clear that without an adequate inflow of sensation, the brain generates its own input in the form of hallucinations and subsequently distorts incoming sensory stimuli (Solomon et. al., 1961). If adequate sensory stimulation is not available at critical periods in development, brain abnormalities and resulting behavioral disorders result (Hubel & Wiesel, 1963; Kolb & Whishaw, 1985).

Ayres (1979) considered sensory input to be *sensory nourishment* for the brain, just as food is nourishment for the body. Wilbarger (1984), a colleague of Ayres, built on this concept with her notion of the *sensory diet* designed specially for the child with sensory integrative dysfunction. The therapeutic sensory diet provides the optimal combination of sensations at the appropriate intensities for an individual child. For most typically developing children, the sensory diet does not require conscious monitoring by caregivers. The environment continuously "feeds" the child a variety of nourishing sensations in the flow of everyday life.

As critical as input is to the developing brain, the mere provision of sensory stimulation is limited in value. Too much stimulation can generate stress that is detrimental to brain development and may reduce the person's subsequent ability to cope with stress (Gunnar & Barr, 1998). To have an optimal effect, the child must actively organize and *use* sensory input to act on the environment.

Adaptive Response

A child does not passively absorb whatever sensations come along. Rather the child actively selects those sensations that are most useful at the time and organizes them in a fashion that facilitates accomplishing goals. This is the process of *sensory integration*. When this process is going well, the child organizes a successful, goal-directed action on the environment, which is called an *adaptive response*. When a child makes an adaptive response, he or she successfully meets some challenge presented in the environment. The adaptive response is possible because the brain has been able to efficiently organize incoming sensory information, which then provides a basis for action (Figure 12-1).

Adaptive responses are powerful forces that drive development forward. When a child makes an adaptive response that is more complex than any previously accomplished response, the brain attains a more organized state and its capacity for sensory integration is enhanced. Thus sensory integration leads to adaptive responses, which in turn result in sensory integration that is more efficient.

Ayres (1979) provides the example of learning to ride a bicycle to illustrate this process. The child must integrate sensations, particularly from the vestibular and proprioceptive systems, to learn how to balance on the bicycle. The senses must accurately and quickly detect when the child begins to fall. Eventually, perhaps after many trials of falling, the child integrates sensory infor-

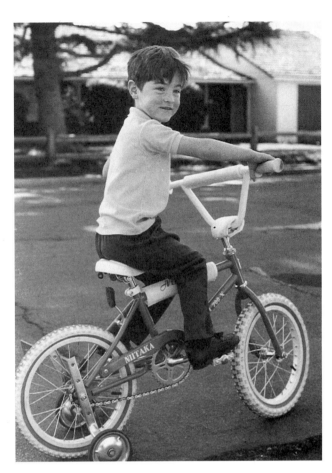

figure **12-1**   Adaptive responses help the child acquire skills such as riding a bicycle. Although training wheels reduce the challenge for this boy, his nervous system must integrate vestibular, proprioceptive, and visual information adequately to successfully steer the bicycle while it is moving. *(Courtesy of Shay McAtee.)*

mation efficiently enough to make the appropriate weight shifts over the bicycle to maintain balance. This is an adaptive response, and once made, the child is able to balance more effectively on the next attempt to ride the bike. The child's nervous system has changed and now is more adept at bicycle riding.

In making adaptive responses the child is an active doer, not a passive recipient. Adaptive responses come from within the child. No one can force a child to respond adaptively, although a situation may be set up that is likely to elicit adaptive responses from the child. For typically developing children and for most children with disabilities, there is an innate drive to develop sensory integration through adaptive responses. Ayres (1979) called this *inner drive* and speculated that it is generated primarily by the limbic system of the brain, a structure known to be critical in both motivation and memory. Ayres designed therapeutic activities and environments to engage the child's inner drive (elicit adaptive responses) and, in so doing, advance sensory integrative development and the child's occupational competence.

Neural Plasticity

It is thought that when a child makes an adaptive response, change occurs at a neuronal synaptic level. This change is a function of the brain's *neural plasticity*. Plasticity is the ability of a structure and concomitant function to be changed gradually by its own ongoing activity (Ayres, 1972b). It is well established in the neuroscientific literature that when organisms are permitted to explore interesting environments, significant increases in dendritic branching, synaptic connections, synaptic efficiency, and size of brain tissue result (Rosenzweig, Bennett, & Diamond, 1972). These changes are most dramatic in a young animal and probably represent a major mechanism of brain development, although it is clear that such manifestations of plasticity are characteristic of optimal brain functioning throughout the lifespan (Bach-Y-Rita, 1981).

Studies of the effects of enriched environments on animals indicate that the essential ingredient for positive brain changes is that the organism actively interacts with a challenging environment (Bennett, Diamond, Krech, & Rosenzweig, 1964). Passive exposure to sensory stimulation does not produce these same positive changes (Dru, Walker, & Walker, 1975). It can be hypothesized from these findings that adaptive responses activate the brain's neuroplastic capabilities. Furthermore, the brain's plasticity makes it possible for an adaptive response to increase the efficiency of sensory integration at a neuronal level.

Schaaf (1994) uses the activity of learning to ride a bicycle to illustrate how neuroplasticity may operate in development. She points out that a child first practices the basic skill of maintaining balance on the bicycle. Once this is mastered, the child uses it repeatedly in riding up and down the sidewalk for hours. After this is mastered, the child looks for greater challenges, such as riding up and down hills or jumping curbs. Schaaf (1994) interprets these behaviors using concepts of developmental plasticity. First the child solidifies the necessary neural pathways for bike riding and then later enhances or modifies these pathways by creating challenging environments. Schaaf (1994) further draws a parallel between this process and the opportunities that are afforded a child during sensory integrative treatment.

Central Nervous System Organization

Ayres (1972b) looked to the organization of the central nervous system (CNS) for clues as to how children organize and use sensory information and how sensory integration develops over time. At the time that she was developing her theory, *hierarchic* models of the CNS dominated thinking in the neurosciences.

Hierarchic models view the nervous system in terms of vertically arranged levels, with the spinal cord at the bottom, the cerebral hemispheres at the top, and the brainstem sandwiched in between. These levels are interdependent yet reflect a trend of ascending control and specialization. Thus the cerebral cortex at the top of the hierarchy is highly specialized and analyzes precise details of sensory information. Ordinarily the cortex assumes a directive role over lower levels of the hierarchy. For example, the cortex may command lower centers to "ignore" certain stimuli deemed unimportant. This process is called *descending inhibition* and is critical in enabling higher brain functions to work efficiently (Ayres, 1972b). The lower levels of the CNS, however, have functions that are more diffuse, primitive, less specialized, and yet potentially more pervasive in influence compared with those of the higher levels. One of the important responsibilities of the lower levels is to filter and refine sensory information before relaying organized sensory messages upward to the cerebral cortex. Thus cortical centers are dependent on lower centers for the receipt of essential, well-organized sensory information to analyze in preparation for the planning of action. According to hierarchic views, the higher levels of the CNS superimpose functions that are more sophisticated on the lower levels, but these do not replace the important lower-level functions (Ayres, 1972b).

Ayres (1972b) believed that critical aspects of sensory integration are seated in the lower levels of the CNS, particularly the brainstem and thalamus. Most of the CNS processing of vestibular information occurs in the brainstem, and much somatosensory processing takes place there and in the thalamus. One of the basic tenets of Ayres' theory is that, because of the dependence of higher CNS structures on lower structures, increased efficiency at the levels of the brainstem and thalamus enhance higher-order functioning (Ayres, 1972b). This view is in sharp contrast to mainstream neuropsychology and education, which tend to emphasize the direct study and remediation of high-level, cortically directed skills such as reading and writing.

In adopting a hierarchic view of the CNS, Ayres (1972b) also assumed that the CNS develops hierarchically from bottom to top, with spinal and brainstem structures maturing before higher-level centers. At the time that Ayres was developing her theory, this was somewhat speculative although generally accepted by neuroscientists. In research conducted in more recent years, the use of positron electron tomography (PET) scans on infants has provided direct support for the notion that brain development proceeds in a bottom-to-top direction (Chugani & Phelps, 1986).

The hierarchic approach to CNS functioning and development led Ayres to emphasize the more primitive vestibular and somatosensory systems in her work with young children. These systems mature early and are seated in the lower CNS centers (particularly the brainstem, cerebellum, and thalamus). Using the logic of hierarchy, Ayres reasoned that the refinement of primitive functions, such as postural control, balance, and tactile perception, provides a sensorimotor foundation for higher-order functions, such as academic ability, behavioral self-regulation, and complex motor skills (e.g., those required in sports). Thus she viewed the developmental process as one in which primitive body-centered functions serve as building blocks upon which complex cognitive and social skills can be scaffolded. This view undergirds a basic premise of the therapy approach that she developed: by enhancing lower-level functions related to the proximal senses, one might have a positive influence on higher-level functions.

On some points Ayres (1972b) departed from a strictly hierarchic view of the CNS. For example, she noted that each level of the CNS can function as a self-contained sensory integration system. Therefore the brainstem has the capacity to independently direct some sensorimotor patterns without being directed by the higher-level cortex. Furthermore, the sensory integrative process involves the brain working as a whole, not simply as a series of hierarchically controlled messages, as rigid hierarchic models might suggest. These ideas are more consistent with the view of some contemporary biologists that the brain is a *heterarchic* system. A heterarchy is a system in which different parts may assume the controlling role in different situations; control does not always flow in a top-down direction (Salthe, 1985). Ayres was ahead of her time in suggesting that the brain does not operate exclusively as a hierarchy but has holistic characteristics. These heterarchic notions strengthened her view that functions considered primitive were worthy of serious consideration in therapy.

■ SENSORY INTEGRATIVE DEVELOPMENT AND CHILDHOOD OCCUPATIONS

Ayres (1979) believed that the first 7 years of life is a period of rapid development in sensory integration. She drew this conclusion not only from her many years of observing children, but also from research in which she gathered normative data on tests of sensory integration (Ayres, 1972b). By the time most children reach 7 or 8 years of age, their scores on standardized tests of sensory integrative capabilities reflect almost as much maturity as an adult's.

Development, from a sensory integrative standpoint, occurs as the CNS organizes sensory information and adaptive responses with increasing degrees of complexity. Sensory integration, of course, enables adaptive responses to occur, which in turn promote the *development of sensory integration* and the emergence of occupational behaviors. As this process unfolds in infancy, the developing child begins to attach meaning to the stream of sensations experienced. The child becomes increasingly adept at shifting attention to what he or she perceives as meaningful, tuning out that which is irrelevant to current needs and interests. As a result the child can organize play behavior for increasing lengths of time and gains control in the regulation of emotions.

Inner drive leads the child to search for opportunities in the environment that are "just right challenges." These are challenges that are not so complex that they overwhelm or induce failure, nor so simple that they are routine or disinteresting. The just right challenge is one that requires effort but is accomplishable for the child. Because there is an element of challenge, a successful adaptive response engenders feelings of mastery and a sense of self as a competent being.

It is fascinating to watch this process unfold in typically developing children. They require no adult guidance or teaching to acquire basic developmental skills such as manipulating objects, sitting, walking, and climbing. Little if any step-by-step instruction is needed to learn daily occupations such as playing on playground equipment, dressing and feeding oneself, drawing and painting, and constructing with blocks. These achievements seem to just happen. They are the product of an active nervous system busily organizing sensory information and searching for challenges that bring forth behaviors that are more complex.

In the following sections, developmental hallmarks of sensory integration are identified and connected to the occupational achievements of childhood. The proximal senses dominate early infancy and continue to exert their influence in critical ways as the visual and auditory systems gain ascendancy. Also, because development is highly canalized (genetically programmed) in infancy, there is limited variation across children in the sequence in which developmental achievements unfold during the first year of life. Developmental variability becomes increasingly apparent after this first year. By kindergarten age, skills vary tremendously among children because of differences in environmental opportunities, familial and cultural influences, personal experiences, and genetic endowment.

Prenatal Period

The first known responses to sensory stimuli occur early in life, at approximately 5½ weeks after conception (Humphrey, 1969). These first responses are to tactile stimuli. Specifically, they involve reflexive avoidance reactions to a perioral stimulus (e.g., the embryo bends its head and upper trunk away from a light touch stimulus around the mouth). This is a primitive protective reaction. It is not until about 9 weeks' gestational age that an approach response (moving of the head toward the chest) occurs (Humphrey, 1969), probably as a function of proprioception.

The first known responses to vestibular input in the form of the Moro reflex also appear at about 9 weeks' postconception. The fetus continues to develop a repertoire of reflexes such as rooting, sucking, Babkin, grasp, flexor withdrawal, Galant, neck righting, Moro, and positive supporting in utero that are fairly well established by the time of birth. Thus when the time comes to leave the uterus, the newborn is well equipped with the capacity to form a strong bond with a caregiver and to actively participate in the critical occupation of nursing. These innate capacities require rudimentary aspects of sensory integration that are built into the nervous system.

Neonatal Period

Touch, smell, and movement sensations are particularly important to the newborn infant, who uses these to maintain contact with a caregiver through nursing, nuzzling, and cuddling. Tactile sensations, especially, are critical in establishing a mother-infant bond and thus play a key role in fostering feelings of security in the infant. This is just the beginning of the important role that the tactile system plays in a person's emotional life because it is directly involved in making physical contact with others (Figure 12-2). Proprioception is also critical in the mother-infant relationship, enabling the infant to mold to the adult caregiver's body in a cuddly manner. The phasic movements of the infant's limbs generate additional proprioceptive inputs. Together, all of these proprioceptive inputs set the stage for the eventual development of body scheme (the brain's map of the body and how its parts interrelate).

The vestibular system is fully functional at birth, although refinement of its sensory integrative functions, particularly its integration with visual and proprioceptive systems, continues through childhood. Of all the sensory systems, the vestibular system is the first to mature (Maurer & Maurer, 1988). Most caregivers, who use rocking and carrying to soothe and calm the infant, instinctively appreciate the influence of vestibular stimuli on the infant's arousal level. Ayres (1979) pointed out that sensations such as these, which make a child contented and organized, tend to be integrating for the child's nervous system.

Vestibular stimuli have other integrating effects on the infant as well. Being lifted into an upright position against the caregiver's shoulder is known to increase alertness and visual pursuit (Gregg, Hafner, & Korner, 1976). While being held in such a position, the young infant's vestibular system detects the pull of gravity and begins to stimulate the neck muscles to raise the head off the caregiver's shoulder. This adaptive response reaches full maturation within 6 months. In the first month of

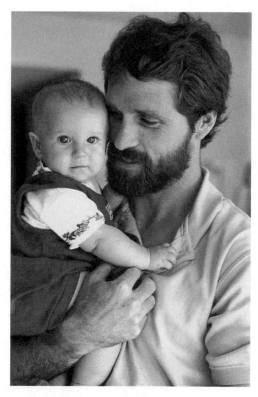

figure **12-2** Tactile sensations play a critical role in generating feelings of security and comfort in the infant and are influential in emotional development and social relationships throughout the life span. *(Courtesy of Shay McAtee.)*

life, head righting may be minimal and intermittent with much wobbling, but it will gradually stabilize and become firmly established as the baby assumes different positions (first when the baby lies in a prone position and later in the supine position).

The visual and auditory systems of the newborn are immature. The newborn orients to some visual and auditory inputs and is particularly interested in human faces and voices, although meaning is not yet attached to these sensations. Visually the infant is attracted to high-contrast stimuli, such as black and white designs, and the range of visual acuity for most stimuli is limited to approximately 10 inches. The infant's visual acuity and responsiveness to visual patterns expand dramatically over the first few months of life (Maurer & Maurer, 1988). During this time the infant begins to use eye contact to relate to the caregiver, further strengthening the bond between them.

First 6 Months

By 4 to 6 months of age a shift occurs in the infant's behavioral organization. The sensory systems have matured to the extent that the baby has much greater awareness and interest in the world, and developing vestibular-proprioceptive-visual connections provide the

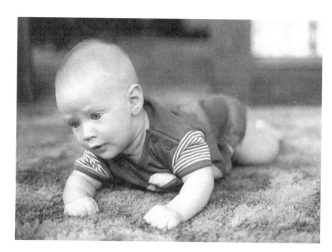

figure**12-3** Strong inner drive to master gravity is evident in this infant's efforts to lift his head and shoulders off the floor. This is an early form of the prone extension posture. *(Courtesy of Shay McAtee.)*

beginnings of postural control. During the first half of the first year the infant begins to show a strong inner drive to rise up against gravity (Figure 12-3), and this drive is evident in much of the baby's spontaneous play. Body positions during the first 6 months characteristically involve the prone position, with gradually increasing extension from the neck down through the trunk and arms gradually bearing more weight to help push the chest off the floor. By 6 months of age, many infants spend a great deal of time in the prone position with full active trunk extension, and most are able to sit independently, at least if propped with their own hands. These body positions usually are the infant's preferred positions for play and are reflective of the maturing lateral vestibulospinal tract. Head control is well established by 6 months of age and provides a stable base for control of eye muscles. This, of course, reflects the growing integration of vestibular, proprioceptive, and visual systems, which becomes increasingly important in providing a stable visual field as the baby becomes mobile.

Somatosensory achievements at this time are particularly evident in the infant's hands. The infant uses tactile and proprioceptive sensations to grasp objects, albeit with primitive grasps. Touch and visual information are integrated as the baby begins to reach for and wave or bang objects. The infant has a strong inner drive to play with the hands by bringing them to midline while watching and touching them. Connections between the tactile and visual systems pave the way for later hand-eye coordination skills. In addition, midline hand play is a significant milestone in the integration of sensations from the two sides of the body.

By now, neonatal reflexes no longer dominate behavior; the baby is beginning to exercise voluntary control over movements during play. The earliest episodes of motor planning occur as the infant works to produce novel actions. This becomes evident as the infant handles objects and begins to initiate transitions from one body position to another, as in rolling from prone position to supine. Although reflexes may play a role in such actions (such as grasp and neck righting reflexes), the infant's actions have a goal-directed, volitional quality and are not stereotypically reflex bound but are responsive to changing characteristics of the environment.

Second 6 Months

Another major transition occurs during the latter half of the first year. Infants become mobile in their environments, and by the first birthday they can willfully move from one place to another, many walking while others creep or crawl. These locomotor skills are the product of the many adaptive responses that have gone before, resulting in increasingly more sophisticated integration of somatosensory, vestibular, and visual inputs.

As the infant explores the environment, greater opportunities are generated for integrating a variety of complex sensations, particularly those responsible for developing body scheme and spatial perception. The child learns about environmental space and about the body's relationship to external space through sensorimotor experiences.

During the second 6 months of life, tactile perception becomes further refined and plays a critical role in the child's developing hand skills. The infant relies on precise tactile feedback in developing a fine pincer grasp, which is used to pick up small objects. Proprioceptive information is also an important influence in developing manipulative skills, and now the baby experiments with objects using a variety of actions. These somatosensory-based adaptive responses contribute to development of motor planning ability. Further development of midline skills is also apparent as the baby easily transfers objects from one hand to the other and may occasionally cross the midline while holding an object.

Through the first year, auditory processing plays a significant role in the infant's awareness of environment, especially the social environment. Auditory information is integrated with tactile and proprioceptive sensations in and around the mouth as the infant vocalizes. The fruits of this process begin to blossom in the latter half of this first year, when the infant begins to experiment with creating the sounds of the language used by caregivers. Vocalizations such as consonant-vowel repetitions ("baba" and "mamama") are common. Parents often attach meaning to these infant vocalizations and strongly encourage them, thus leading the infant also to attach meaning to these sounds. By their first birthday many infants have a small vocabulary of words or wordlike sounds that they use meaningfully to communicate desires to caregivers.

Another major landmark toward the end of the first year is beginning independence in self-feeding. This complex achievement requires refined somatosensory processing of information from the lips, the jaw, and inside the mouth to guide oral movements in the chewing and swallowing of food. Taste and smell sensations are also integral to this process, but self-feeding involves more than the mouth. All of the acquired sensory integrative milestones involving hand-eye coordination are important to self-feeding. The infant at this period of life uses the fingers directly to feed him or herself and to explore the textures of foods. At this stage, use of a utensil such as a spoon is not very functional and is messy because motor planning skills have not progressed to the point that the child can manipulate the utensil successfully. However, many infants begin to demonstrate a drive to use the spoon in self-feeding by the end of the first year. For many contemporary American infants, use of a spoon is the first real experience in using a tool (Figure 12-4).

The occupation of dining, then, begins to emerge in infancy as sensory integrative abilities mature, allowing the child to engage in self-feeding. As an occupation, dining in its fullest sense goes far beyond the physical, sensorimotor act of feeding. Dining usually takes place within a social context, whether at a family dinner at home or in a formal restaurant, so social standards for acceptable behavior and etiquette become increasingly important as the child develops. Furthermore, partaking in a meal and sharing certain types of food gradually come to take on powerful symbolic meanings. The sensory integrative underpinnings of the dining experience influence how the child experiences mealtimes and how others view the child as a dining partner, thus playing a role in shaping the social and symbolic aspects of this vitally important occupation.

Second Year

As the child moves into the second year of life, the basic vestibular-proprioceptive-visual connections that were laid down earlier continue to refine, resulting in growing finesse in balance and fluidity of dynamic postural control. Discrimination and localization of tactile sensations also become much more precise, allowing for further refinement of fine motor skills.

Increasingly complex somatosensory processing contributes to the continuing development of body scheme. Ayres (1972b) hypothesized that as body scheme becomes more sophisticated, so does motor planning ability. This is because the child draws on knowledge of how the body works to program novel actions (Figure 12-5).

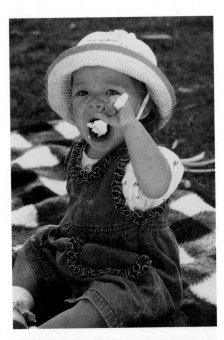

figure**12-4** Because somatosensory processing and visual-motor coordination strongly influence self-feeding skills, sensory integration is an important contributor to development of dining, a fundamental occupation. *(Courtesy of Shay McAtee.)*

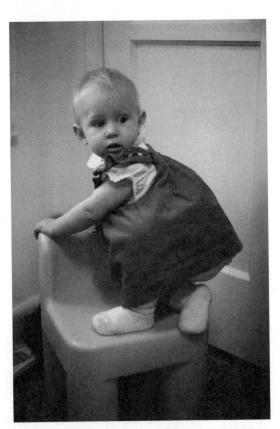

figure**12-5** As motor planning develops during the second year of life, the infant experiments with a variety of body movements and learns how to transition easily from one position to another. These experiences are thought to reflect development of body scheme. *(Courtesy of Shay McAtee.)*

Throughout the second year the typically developing toddler experiments with many variations in body movements. Imitation of the actions of others contributes further to the child's movement repertoire. In experiencing new actions, the child generates new sensory experiences, thus building an elaborate base of information from which to plan future actions.

While motor planning ability becomes increasingly more complex in the second year, another aspect of praxis, ideation, begins to emerge. Ideation is the ability to conceptualize what to do in a given situation. Ideation is made possible by the cognitive ability to use symbols, first expressed gesturally and then vocally during the second year of life (Bretherton et. al., 1981). Symbolic functioning enables the child to engage in pretend actions and to imagine doing actions, even actions that the child has never before done. By the end of the second year the toddler can join several pretend actions in a play sequence (McCune-Nicolich, 1981). Furthermore, the 2-year-old child demonstrates that he or she has a plan before performing an action sequence, either through a verbal announcement or through a search for a needed object (McCune-Nicolich, 1981). Thus a surge in practic development occurs in the second year as the child generates many new ideas for actions and begins to plan actions in a systematic sequence.

The burgeoning of praxis abilities plays an important role in the development of self-concept. Infant psychiatrist Daniel Stern (1985) suggests that the sense of an integrated core self begins in infancy as an outcome of the volition and the proprioceptive feedback involved in motor planning. The consequences of the child's voluntary, planned actions add to the developing sense of self as an active agent in the world. As praxis takes giant leaps during the second year, so does this sense of self as an agent of power. The child feels in command of his or her own life when sensory integration allows the child to move freely and effectively through the world (Ayres, 1979).

Third Through Seventh Years

The child's competencies in the sensorimotor realm mature in the third through seventh years of life, which Ayres (1979) considered a crucial period for sensory integration because of the brain's receptiveness to sensations and its capacity for organizing them at this time. This is the period when sensorimotor functions become consolidated as a foundation for higher intellectual abilities. Although further sensory integrative development can and usually does occur beyond the eighth birthday, the changes that take place are likely to be far more limited than those that occurred earlier.

In the third through seventh years, children have strong inner drives to produce adaptive responses that not only meet complicated sensorimotor demands but also sometimes require interfacing with peers. The chal-

lenges posed by children's games and play activities attest to this complexity. In the visual-motor realm, sophistication develops through involvement in crafts, drawing and painting, constructional play with blocks and other building toys, and video games (Figure 12-6). Children are driven to explore playground equipment by swinging, sliding, climbing, jumping, riding, pushing, pulling, and pumping. Toward the end of this period they enthusiastically grapple with the motor planning challenges posed by games such as jump rope, jacks, marbles, and hopscotch. It is also during this period that children become expert with cultural tools such as scissors, pencils, zippers, buttons, forks and knives, pails, shovels, brooms, and rakes (Figure 12-7). Many children begin to participate in occupations that present sensorimotor challenges for years to come, such as soccer, softball, karate, gymnastics, playing a musical instrument, and ballet. Furthermore, children develop the ability to organize their behavior into more complex sequences over longer timeframes. This makes it possible for them to become more autonomous in orchestrating daily routines, such as getting ready for school in the morning, completing homework and other school projects, and performing household chores.

As children participate in these occupations, they must frequently anticipate how to move in relation to changing environmental events by accurately timing and sequencing their actions (Fisher, Murray, & Bundy, 1991). This is particularly challenging in sports when peers, with their often unpredictable moves, are involved. Their bodies are challenged to maintain balance through

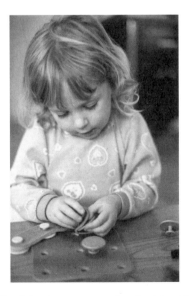

figure **12-6** Adaptive responses involved in this activity require precise tactile feedback and sophisticated praxis. During activities such as this one, the preschooler becomes adept at handling tools and objects that are encountered in daily occupations throughout life. (*Courtesy of Shay McAtee.*)

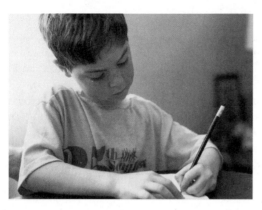

figure**12-7** By the time a child reaches school age, sensory integrative capacities are almost mature. The child now can devote full attention to demands of academic tasks because basic sensorimotor functions, such as maintaining an upright posture and guiding hand movements while holding a tool, have become automatic. *(Courtesy of Shay McAtee.)*

dynamic changes in body position. In fine motor tasks, children must efficiently coordinate visual with somatosensory information to guide eye and hand movements with accuracy and precision while maintaining a stable postural base.

Children meet these challenges with varying degrees of success. Some are more talented than others with respect to sensory integrative abilities, but most children eventually achieve a degree of competency that allows them to fully participate in the daily occupations that they are expected to do and wish to do at home, in school, and in the community. Furthermore, most children experience feelings of satisfaction and self-efficacy as they master those occupations that are heavily dependent on sensory integration.

■ WHEN PROBLEMS IN SENSORY INTEGRATION OCCUR

Unfortunately, not every child experiences competency in sensory integration. When some aspect of sensory integration does not function efficiently, the child may experience stress in the course of everyday occupations because processes that should be automatic or accurate are not. It may be stressful, for example, to simply maintain balance when sitting in a chair, to get dressed in the morning before school, to attempt to play jump rope, or to eat lunch in a socially acceptable manner. The child is aware of these difficulties and becomes frustrated by frequent failure when confronted with ordinary tasks that come easily for other children. Many children with sensory integrative problems develop a tendency to avoid or reject simple sensory or motor challenges, responding with refusals or tantrums when pushed to perform. If this

becomes a long-term pattern of behavior, the child may miss important experiences, such as playing games with peers, that are critical in building feelings of competency, mastering a wide repertoire of useful skills, and developing flexible social strategies. Thus the capacity to participate fully in the occupations that the child wants to do and needs to do is compromised.

Often behavioral, social, or motor coordination concerns are cited when a child with a sensory integrative dysfunction is referred to occupational therapy. The occupational therapist needs to evaluate whether a sensory processing problem may underlie these concerns. The therapist then must decide on a course of action to help the child move toward the goal of greater success and satisfaction in doing meaningful occupations. These challenges to the therapist—to identify a problem that may be hidden and to figure out how to best help the child— were the challenges to which Ayres devoted most of her career.

As mentioned previously, Ayres turned to the neurobiologic literature to give her insight into understanding children's learning and behavior problems. Ayres also took on the responsibility of conducting research to develop her theory of sensory integration. In doing so she produced a diagnostic system for clinical evaluation of children through the use of standardized tests. She also conducted research that was designed to evaluate the effectiveness of her treatment methods. After each study, Ayres always returned to her theory to revise and refine it in light of research findings. While she was doing this, she maintained a private practice; thus she had many years of firsthand, clinically based experience on which to ground her theoretic work.

The following sections examine the research that Ayres conducted to identify different types of sensory integrative dysfunction in children. The general categories of sensory integrative dysfunction that concern clinicians today, based on research findings and clinical experience, are discussed. The field of sensory integration continues to be a dynamic field that changes as future research generates new findings and as future experiences of clinicians generate new ways of interpreting those findings.

■ RESEARCH BASE FOR SENSORY INTEGRATIVE DYSFUNCTION

Throughout her professional career, Ayres was guided by her keen observation skills and her search to reach a deeper understanding of the clinical problems that she encountered in practice. To begin answering the questions that arose as she worked with children, Ayres initiated the process of developing standardized tests of sensory integration during the 1960s. She originally developed these tests solely as research tools to aid in theory development. At the time, she was working with children with learning disabilities, many of whom she suspected had covert difficulties processing sensory information, and she sought to uncover the nature of whatever sensory integrative difficulties might exist. It was after her initial efforts at research using her tests that other therapists asked to have access to the tests, instigating their publication by Western Psychological Services.

The first group of tests created by Ayres was published as the Southern California Sensory Integration Tests (SCSIT) (Ayres, 1972c). These were later revised and renamed the Sensory Integration and Praxis Tests (SIPT) (Ayres, 1989). Normative data were collected on a regional scale for the SCSIT and on a national scale for the SIPT. The tests were designed to measure aspects of visual, tactile, kinesthetic, and vestibular sensory processing as well as motor planning abilities.

Using first the SCSIT and later the SIPT with samples of children, Ayres used a statistic procedure called *factor analysis* to develop a typology of sensory integrative function and dysfunction. Tables 12-1 and 12-2 summarize results of her factor analytic studies, along with results of several studies conducted by other researchers. In factor analysis, sets of test scores are grouped according to their associations with one another. The resulting groups of associated test scores are called *factors*. Ayres interpreted the factors that emerged from her studies as representative of neural substrates underlying learning and behavior in children. For example, in her 1965 study, Ayres found that the tactile tests correlated highly with the motor planning tests, forming a factor. She hypothesized that there is an ability called *motor planning* that is dependent on somatosensory processing and influences one's interactions with the physical world. *Apraxia* is the term she used to identify a disorder in this ability. In her later work she subsumed the notion of motor planning under the construct of praxis and replaced the term *apraxia* with *dyspraxia* when referring to children.

In her last set of analyses with the SIPT, just before her death in 1988, Ayres used both factor analysis and another statistical technique called *cluster analysis,* which groups together children with similar SIPT profiles (see Table 12-1). This approach was used to further carve out diagnostic groupings of children that might be useful clinically. Today, consideration of both factor analysis and cluster groupings is a critical component in the interpretation of a child's SIPT scores.

Through the years as Ayres conducted her studies with different groups of children, she continually revisited her theory, bringing along new hypotheses based on new research results. Of particular interest were the patterns that recurred despite being generated from different samples of children. Among the most consistent findings was that children who had been identified as having learning or developmental problems often displayed difficulties in more than one sensory system. Ayres (1972b) interpreted this finding in light of the neurobiologic literature on intersensory integration, which indicates that the sensory systems tend to function synergistically with each other rather than in isolation. Thus the idea of intersensory integration as critical to human function became one of the major tenets of sensory integration theory.

Another finding, which emerged in early studies and in later SIPT studies, was that some patterns of scores were seen only in groups of children who had been identified as having disorders. In other words, some factors were not evident in typically developing children at any age. This led to the proposal that the sensory integrative disorders associated with these particular patterns were representative of neural dysfunction rather than developmental lag.

Yet another recurrent pattern was a relationship between tactile perception and praxis scores. This association appeared repeatedly in her studies and led Ayres to theorize that the tactile system contributes importantly to the development of efficient practic functions. The robustness of this finding across many studies influenced Ayres to emphasize the relationship between the tactile system and praxis, a relationship that has become a cornerstone of sensory integration theory.

Throughout her research, several patterns emerged that Ayres suspected were related to a discrete involvement of cortical rather than brainstem or intersensory dysfunction. Ayres came to view these types of problems as different than those classified as sensory integrative disorders and less likely to be responsive to the treatment techniques that she was developing. An example is the association of low Praxis on Verbal Command scores with high postrotary nystagmus scores. Praxis on Verbal Command is the only test on the SIPT with a strong language comprehension component. Postrotary nystagmus is a test that may reflect cortical dysfunction if scores are extremely high. In this example it is hypothesized that an underlying cortical dysfunction, possibly involving the left hemisphere (where language centers are located), is responsible for the pattern of scores. Ayres did not view this particular pattern as a sensory integrative dysfunction, although it could be detected by her tests.

As Fisher and Murray (1991) pointed out, some design flaws limit Ayres' factor analytic studies. Specifically, sample sizes were small in relation to the number of tests studied, and she repeated exploratory techniques with different groups of tests in her studies, rather than using confirmatory factor analysis to replicate results using the same group of tests. The presence of these flaws makes results vulnerable to instability because of associations that may occur by chance. It is important to note, however, that similar factors did recur across her studies despite these limitations (see Tables 12-1 and 12-2).

Text continues on p. 351

Year	Author	Purpose	Instruments	Hypothesis	Analysis	Subjects	Results	Contribution to Theory
1965	Ayres, A.J.	Identify relationships among sensory perception, motor performance, laterality in normal and children with perceptual problems Establish construct and discriminant validity	Early versions of the SCSIT, additional perceptual-motor and laterality tests, also freedom from hyperactivity and tactile defensiveness	Test results would identify factors for children with and without dysfunction Normal and dysfunctional children will demonstrate different factors	Thirty-three tests Two behavioral parameters Analysis of difference between group means Q- and R-technique factor analysis	n = 100 dysfunctional n = 50 normal Dysfunctional children had learning or behavioral disorders	Tests discriminated between normal and dysfunctional groups Five patterns detected: Apraxia Dysfunction form and space perception Deficit bilateral integration Visual figure-ground perception Tactile defensiveness	Established discriminant validity of early versions Most children demonstrated more than one factor, therefore factors related Sensory integration-clusters were not by sensory systems Praxis and tactile functions linked Tactile defensiveness, hyperactivity, distractibility linked Cognitive aspects deemphasized Eye-hand agreement not discriminative Empirical support for syndromes
1966a	Ayres, A.J.	Explore perceptual-motor relationships in a normal sample and compare with prior studies Establish construct validity	Frostig tests, early versions of the SCSIT Also freedom from hyperactivity and tactile defensiveness	That factors would emerge	Seventeen tests R-technique factor analysis (simplified matrix)	n = 92 Formed normal distribution, 10% abnormal, three with mild cerebral palsy	Praxis accounted for most variance Motor planning, kinesthesia, tactile functions, motor accuracy, bilateral coordination Visual perception factor: Ayres Space Test, Frostig	More support for praxis syndrome Visual component without motor element Perceptual-motor functions correlate as a whole in normative sample Kinesthesia closer to tactile than visual perception as in prior study

Year	Author	Purpose	Tests and Observations	Hypothesis	Sample	Method of Analysis	Findings	Implications
1966b	Ayres, A.J.	Provide an understanding of whether syndromes represent dysfunction or developmental lag; Establish construct validity	Nearly the same as 1966a	That variation in perceptual-motor abilities would be small in a group of typical children	n = 64; Adopted, all normal on Gesell	Sixteen tests; Two behavioral parameters; R-technique factor analysis	Visual motor ability accounted for most variation; Praxis and tactile perception were least variable; Hyperactivity, distractibility, tactile defensiveness factor; Factors weak because of lack of variance in performance of normal children	Suggested that low scores in praxis and tactile perception represent developmental deviation, not delay; Little systematic variation when tests given to normal children; Tactile defensiveness-hyperactivity may have a maturational component
1969	Ayres, A.J.	To provide an in-depth analysis of dysfunctional patterns in children with learning handicaps; Establish construct validity	Sixty-four tests and observations: SCSIT, psycholinguistic, intelligence, auditory, postural-ocular reactions, academic achievement	Brain functions involve several levels and will cluster accordingly	n = 36; Educationally handicapped children	Q-technique factor analysis	Five factors identified: ▪ Auditory language, sequencing ▪ Postural and bilateral integration ▪ Right hemisphere dysfunction ▪ Apraxia ▪ Tactile defensiveness	Hints to left hemisphere dysfunction
1971	Ayres, A.J.	To identify predictors of severity of sensory integrative syndromes	Forty-eight tests and observations: SCSIT, psycholinguistic, intelligence, eye-hand usage, postural responses	That predictive equations would emerge	n = 140; Educationally handicapped children	Ten-step regression equations for each syndrome calculated	Presence of more than one type of disorder was the norm; Prone extension best predictor of postural-bilateral integration; Imitation of postures best predictor of praxis	Somatosensory and praxis linked again; Elucidated best predictors of syndromes; As many children may have apraxia as have postural and bilateral coordination problems

SCSIT, Southern California Sensory Integration Test.

Continued

Year	Author	Purpose	Instruments	Hypothesis	Analysis	Subjects	Results	Contribution to Theory
1972	Ayres, A.J.	To further analyze and refine factors Establish construct validity	Same as above	That similar factors as previously would emerge	R-technique factor analysis	n = 148 Educationally handicapped children	Six factors identified: ▪ Form and space perception ▪ Auditory language ▪ Postural ocular ▪ Motor planning ▪ Reading-spelling and IQ ▪ Hyperactivity, tactile perception	Further confirmed left hemisphere dysfunction Reconfirmed syndromes found in other samples of learning-disabled children
1977	Ayres, A.J.	To further analyze interrelationships (add SCPNT) so that differential diagnosis can be further refined	SCSIT SCPNT, postural-ocular and lateralization measures, dichotic listening, ITPA, intelligence, academic achievement Flowers-Costello (auditory)	That clusters would continue to be refined	Series of R-technique factor analyses (not all measures entered each time)	n = 128 Learning disabled children	Five major domains identified: ▪ Somatosensory-motor planning ▪ Auditory-language ▪ Postural-ocular ▪ Eye-hand coordination ▪ Postrotary nystagmus	Further elucidated nature of interhemispheric integration Role of vestibular system clarified
1987	Ayres, A.J.	To continue to attempt to differentiate types of sensory integration dysfunction New praxis tests as well as many of the tests that had been used in past studies	SCSIT, SCPNT, selected ITPA test, sentence repetition Clinical observation of prone extension, supine flexion, ocular pursuits Preliminary versions of newly designed praxis tests: Sequencing Praxis, Praxis on Verbal Command, Oral Praxis, Block Building Test	Is praxis a unitary function? Would computer-generated clusters match those that had been identified clinically and through factor analysis?	Screen plot factor analyses, correlation coefficients Comparison of test profiles of children with diagnoses Use of computer generated clusters	n = 182 Learning or behavior disorders	Praxis tests were related with one another Visual tests correlated with tactile tests Somatovisual-practic factor identified Tactile scores and praxis related; short duration postrotary nystagmus; statistical association with praxis	Suggestion of a general somatopractic function Further verified close association of tactile score and praxis Computer-generated clusters were not meaningful

Year	Author	Purpose	Measure	Hypothesis	Analysis	Sample	Results	Conclusions
1989	Ayres, A.J.	Factor analyses: to clarify the nature of the constructs measured by the Sensory Integration and Praxis Tests (SIPT)	SIPT (17 tests)	That factors related to those of the SCSIT would emerge	Principal components analysis	Three analyses: n = 1750 Normative sample; n = 125 Learning or sensory integrative disorders; n = 293 Combined sample of learning or sensory integrative disorders and matched children from normative sample	Visuopraxis and somatopraxis factors emerged in all three analyses. Bilateral integration and sequencing factor and praxis on verbal command factor seen only in dysfunctional sample. Other factors related to vestibular and somatosensory processing identified	Expanded understanding of vestibular-bilateral disorders to include sequencing element. Somatopraxis factor reinforced previous findings linking tactile perception and praxis. Visuopraxis factor provided support for previous visual-motor linkages
1989	Ayres, A.J.	Cluster analyses: to assist in identifying children in need of different types of remediation or services	SIPT (17 tests)	That meaningful diagnostic groupings would emerge	Agglomerative cluster analysis, Ward method	n = 293 Same sample as above, combined dysfunctional and normative	Six cluster groups identified: ▪ Low average bilateral integration and sequencing ▪ Generalized sensory integrative dysfunction ▪ Visuo- and somatosensory dyspraxia ▪ Low average sensory integration and praxis ▪ Dyspraxia on verbal command ▪ High average sensory integration and praxis	Children with and without dysfunction can be differentiated on the basis of SIPT profiles. Identified specific SIPT profile that may be characteristic of left hemisphere dysfunction

ITPA, Illinois Test of Psycholinguistic Abilities; *SCPNT*, Southern California Postrotary Nystagmus Test; *SCSIT*, Southern California Sensory Integration Test; *SIPT*, Sensory Integration and Praxis Tests.

Continued

Year	Author	Purpose	Instruments	Hypothesis	Analysis	Subjects	Results	Contribution to Theory
1998	Mulligan, S.	To determine a plausible model for understanding sensory integrative dysfunction by evaluating a five factor model utilizing SIPT scores	SIPT	That sensory integrative dysfunction is a five-factor structure consisting of bilateral integration and sequencing, postural ocular movements, somatosensory processing, somatopraxis, and visuopraxis	CFA followed by SEM	n = 10,475 Children from the Western Psychological Services, primarily with mild disabilities such as learning, behavioral or motor problems. n = 995 Subset with learning disabilities	The CFA of the hypothesized five-factor model demonstrated a reasonably good fit. Correlations among the factors also supported the presence of a single, general dysfunction factor	Supported the idea of a generalized practic function. Suggested limited ability of the SIPT alone to identify problems related to postural ocular movement disorders. Replication of visual perception deficit, bilateral integration and sequencing deficit, dyspraxia, and somatosensory deficit factors with a large sample validated the existence of specific sensory integrative patterns of dysfunction. Proposed model that includes a general dysfunction as a second order factor, with four first order factors of visual perceptual deficit, bilateral and sequencing deficit, dyspraxia and somatosensory deficit

Year	Author	Purpose	Measures	Hypotheses	Analysis	Sample	Results	Conclusions
1998	Parham, L.D.	To examine whether sensory integrative measures are predictive of school achievement, when intelligence and other factors are taken into account, concurrently and over a 4-year period	SIPT, converted into 3 factor scores: Praxis, visual perception, & somatosensory; Intelligence reading & math achievement; Socioeconomic status	That sensory integrative performance at ages 6-8 years is related to achievement concurrently and predictively 4 years later; That sensory integrative performance at ages 10-12 is not related to achievement	Multiple regression analyses	n = 91, of whom 43 were identified as learning disabled; Children were 6-8 years old initially, 10-12 years old at follow-up	When controlling for IQ sensory integration: at ages 6-8 significantly correlated with math, but not reading; at ages 6-8 significantly predicted math and reading 4 years later; at ages 10-12 significantly predicted math and reading at same age. Strong relationships between praxis and math achievement identified	Supported the hypothesis that sensory integration, especially praxis, is related to achievement when taking IQ into account. Sensory integration continues to contribute to achievement at middle school age

CFA, Confirmatory factor analysis; *SIPT*, Sensory Integration and Praxis Tests; *SEM*, structural equation modeling.

Ayres, A.J. (1965). Patterns of perceptual-motor dysfunction in children: a factor analytic study. *Perceptual and Motor Skills, 20,* 335-368.
Ayres, A.J. (1966a). Interrelationships among perceptual-motor functions in children. *American Journal of Occupational Therapy, 20* (2), 68-71.
Ayres, A.J. (1966b). Interrelations among perceptual-motor abilities in a group of normal children. *American Journal of Occupational Therapy, 20* (6), 288-292.
Ayres, A.J. (1969). Deficits in sensory integration in educationally handicapped children. *Journal of Learning Disabilities, 2* (3), 44-52.
Ayres, A.J. (1971). Characteristics of types of sensory integrative dysfunction. *American Journal of Occupational Therapy, 25* (7), 329-334.
Ayres, A.J. (1972). Types of sensory integrative dysfunction among disabled learners. *American Journal of Occupational Therapy, 26* (1), 13-18.
Ayres, A.J. (1977). Cluster analyses of measures of sensory integration. *American Journal of Occupational Therapy, 31* (6), 362-366.
Ayres, A.J., Mailloux, Z., & Wendler, C.L.W. (1987). Development apraxia: is it a unitary function? *Occupational Therapy Research, 7* (2), 93-110.
Ayres, A.J. (1989). *Sensory Integration and Praxis Tests manual.* Los Angeles: Western Psychological Services.
Mulligan, S. (1998). Patterns of sensory integration dysfunction: A confirmatory factor analysis. *American Journal of Occupational Therapy, 52,* 819-828.
Parham, L.D. (1998). The relationship of sensory integrative development to achievement in elementary students: Four-year longitudinal patterns. *Occupational Therapy Journal of Research, 18,* 105-127.

table 12-2 Factors and Clusters Identified in Research

Date of Study	Author	Dyspraxia	Deficit in Visual Perception and Visual-Motor Functions	Deficit in Vestibular, Postural, and Bilateral Integration	Deficit in Auditory and Language Functions	Somatosensory	Miscellaneous
1965: 100 dysfunctional, 50 normal	Ayres, A.J.	Tactile tests Motor planning (Imitation of Posture, Motor Accuracy, Grommet) Eye pursuits	Frostig tests Kinesthesia Manual Form Perception Ayres' Space Test	Right-left discrimination Avoidance crossing midline Rhythmic activities	Not tested	Poor tactile perception Hyperactive-distractible behavior Tactile defensiveness	Figure-ground a separate factor Eye-hand agreement not related to perceptual-motor dysfunction
1966a: Normal distribution of Gesell developmental quotients	Ayres, A.J.	Accounted for most variance Motor planning Tactile and kinesthesia Motor accuracy Figure-ground Frostig tests	Figure-ground Frostig spatial relations Ayres' Space Test		Not tested	Low association of tactile defensiveness with praxis factor	Identified two main factors in normal sample: General perceptual-motor (somatosensory and motor) Visual perception
1966b: Only normal children	Ayres, A.J.		Frostig tests Ayres' Space Test Motor Accuracy Figure-ground	Integration two sides of body and tactile perception	Not tested	Tactile defensiveness and hyperactivity—may be a maturational factor involved	Visual-motor ability accounted for most variation in normal children Poor motor planning—tactile perception not seen in normal children
1969: Educationally handicapped children	Ayres, A.J.	Tactile Motor Planning	Most SCSIT; visual tests not included in analysis Possible right hemisphere dysfunction: eye movement deficits, better right-than left-sided function	Bilateral integration Postural reactions Reading and language problems	Possible left hemisphere dysfunction: Auditory-language Reading achievement Auditory and visual-motor sequencing	Tactile defensiveness and hyperactivity—loaded together but not a separate factor	

1972: Educationally handicapped children	Ayres, A.J.	Motor planning Hyperactivity Tactile defensiveness (more emphasis on motor than tactile)	Position in Space ITPA visual closure Space Visualization Design Copying Tactile tests	Poor ocular control Excessive residual primitive postural responses Relatively good left-hand coordination Bilateral integration symptom did not load	Auditory language Intelligence	Hyperactivity-distractibility Tactile perception	Reading-spelling load together Motor accuracy highly associated with all parameters
1977: Learning disabled children	Ayres, A.J.	*Analysis 5:* Imitation of Postures Composite tactile Kinesthesia	*Analysis 3:* Four SCSIT visual tests Manual Form Perception	*Analysis 5:* Prone extension Composite postural Flexion posture Composite tactile Kinesthesia Bilateral integration symptom did not load	*Analysis 5:* Composite language (ITPA) Dichotic listening Flowers-Costello (auditory)	Not measured	Visual tests have strong cognitive component (loaded with IQ on Analysis 2) SVCU associated with lateralization indices Motor accuracy loaded separately on all

ITPA, Illinois Test of Psycholinguistic Abilities; *SCSIT*, Southern California Sensory Integration Test; *SVCU*, Space Visualization Contralateral Use.

Continued

table 12-2 Factors and Clusters Identified in Research—cont'd

Date of Study	Author	Dyspraxia	Deficit in Visual Perception and Visual-Motor Functions	Deficit in Vestibular, Postural, and Bilateral Integration	Deficit in Auditory and Language Functions	Somatosensory	Miscellaneous
1989: Children with learning disorders and sensory integrative deficits and children from normative sample of SIPT	Ayres, A.J.	Somatopraxis (Oral Praxis, Postural Praxis, Graphesthesia) Visuo- and somatodyspraxia cluster	Visuopraxis (Constructional Praxis, Design Copying, Space Visualization, Figure-Ground)	Bilateral integration and sequencing (Sequencing Praxis, Bilateral Motor Coordination, Standing and Walking Balance) Low average bilateral integration and sequencing cluster	Praxis on Verbal Command Dyspraxia on verbal command cluster (high Postrotary Nystagmus with low Praxis on Verbal Command)	Not measured	High functioning group identified within normative sample Generalized dysfunction group identified within group with learning disorders and sensory integrative dysfunction
1998: 10,475 children primarily with mild learning, behavior, or motor problems.	Mulligan, S.	Dyspraxia (Oral Praxis, Postural Praxis, and Praxis on Verbal Command); Also suggests generalized practic function underlying all other factors.	Visual Perceptual Deficit (Design Copying, Constructional Praxis, Space Visualization, Manual Form Perception, Figure Ground Perception)	Bilateral Integration and Sequencing Deficit (Sequencing Praxis and bilateral Motor Coordination)	Not tested	Tactile tests and Kinesthesia	

Ayres, A.J. (1965). Patterns of perceptual-motor dysfunction in children: A factor analytic study. *Perceptual and Motor Skills, 20,* 335-368.
Ayres, A.J. (1966a). Interrelationships among perceptual-motor functions in children. *American Journal of Occupational Therapy, 20* (2), 68-71.
Ayres, A.J. (1966b). Interrelationships among perceptual-motor abilities in a group of normal children. *American Journal of Occupational Therapy, 20* (6), 288-292.
Ayres, A.J. (1969). Deficits in sensory integration in educationally handicapped children. *Journal of Learning Disabilities, 2* (3), 44-52.
Ayres, A.J. (1972). Types of sensory integrative dysfunction among disabled learners. *American Journal of Occupational Therapy, 26* (1), 13-18.
Ayres, A.J. (1977). Cluster analyses of measures of sensory integration. *American Journal of Occupational Therapy, 31* (6), 362-366.
Ayres, A.J. (1989). *Sensory Integration and Praxis Tests manual.* Los Angeles: Western Psychological Services.
Mulligan, S. (1998). Patterns of sensory integration dysfunction: A confirmatory factor analysis. *American Journal of Occupational Therapy, 52,* 819-828.

Furthermore, many of the factors were replicated recently by Mulligan (1998) in a study of over 10,000 children. The resilience of some of these factors across many studies strengthens the hypothesis that they reflect underlying patterns of function.

Ayres conducted her factor and cluster analyses to shed light on the types of sensory integrative dysfunctions that children experience, yet she did not view the resulting typologies as specific diagnostic labels to pin on individual children. Rather, the typologies were seen as general patterns exhibited time after time by groups of children who were struggling in school or with some other aspect of behavior or development. They provide the therapist with relevant information to consider when conducting clinical assessments. They do not provide prefabricated slots in which to fit children. Ultimately, the important job of interpreting an individual child's pattern of scores in relation to his or her unique life situation lies in the purview of the therapist's judgment.

■ SENSORY INTEGRATIVE DISORDERS

The results of research, combined with the experiences of clinicians and the work of scholars in the field, have generated many different ways of conceptualizing sensory integrative disorders over the past 30 years. The complexity of this domain can be initially confusing to the novice therapist, but it is also one of the most intriguing aspects of the field. The term *sensory integrative disorder* does not refer to one particular type of problem but to a heterogeneous group of disorders that are thought to reflect subtle, primarily subcortical, neural dysfunction involving multisensory systems. These disorders affect human behavior in ways that are often difficult to interpret unless seen through the eyes of someone with special training in sensory integration.

Most discussions of sensory integrative problems assume normal sensory receptor function. In other words, sensory integrative disorders involve central, rather than peripheral, sensory functions. This assumption has been supported in several well-designed studies. For instance, Parush, Sohmer, Steinberg, and Kaitz (1997) found that the somatosensory-evoked potentials of children with attention-deficit hyperactivity disorder (ADHD) differ from those of typically developing children with respect to indicators of central tactile processing but not in peripheral receptor responses. Many of the children with ADHD in this study were also identified as having tactile defensiveness, a sensory integrative problem. In another study, researchers found that children with learning disabilities, compared with nondisabled children, had impaired postural responses involving central integration of vestibular, proprioceptive, and visual inputs, whereas measures of peripheral receptor functions were normal (Shumway-Cook, Horak, & Black, 1987). Thus when sensory integrative disorders involving the vestibular system are discussed, these problems are generally thought to be based within brainstem structures and pathways (namely, the vestibular nuclei and its connections) rather than the vestibular receptor (i.e., the semicircular canals, utricle, or saccule). This has been a point of confusion in some studies in which measures of peripheral vestibular functioning were used to evaluate Ayres' concept of vestibular dysfunction (e.g., Polatajko, 1985). Wiss (1989) has provided an excellent discussion of this issue in relation to vestibular processing. The same point could apply to other sensory systems as well. In this chapter, the discussions of sensory integrative problems assume that peripheral function is normal.

As noted previously, different conceptualizations of sensory integrative disorders have been generated over the years. Recent categoric systems of sensory integrative dysfunction include, for example, those of Clark, Mailloux, and Parham (1989); Fisher et. al. (1991); and Kimball (1993). Although perfect consensus on how to categorize sensory integrative dysfunctions does not exist, clearly there are recurring themes across all authors. For the purposes of this chapter the following categories are used:
1. Sensory modulation problems
2. Sensory discrimination and perception problems
3. Vestibular processing disorders
4. Dyspraxia

The first two of these categories are observed in behavioral and social-emotional responses to sensory input; the latter two expressions involve motoric outcomes of sensory integration.

Sensory Modulation Problems

Sensory modulation refers to CNS regulation of its own activity (Ayres, 1979). With respect to sensory systems, this term is used to refer to the tendency to generate responses that are appropriately graded in relation to incoming sensory stimuli, rather than underreacting or overreacting to them. Cermak (1988) and Royeen (1989) have hypothesized that there is a continuum of sensory responsivity, with hyporesponsivity at one end and hyperresponsivity at the other. An optimal level of arousal and orientation lies in the center of the continuum (Figure 12-8).

Royeen and Lane (1991) point out that, ordinarily, individuals experience fluctuations across the continuum of sensory responsivity in the course of a day, with most activity falling in the midrange. Dysfunction is indicated when the fluctuations within an individual are extreme or when an individual tends to function primarily at one extreme of the continuum or the other.

Failure to orient   Optimal arousal   Overorientation

HYPORESPONSIVITY   **HYPERRESPONSIVITY**
Sensory registration   Sensory defensiveness
problem

figure**12-8** Continuum of sensory responsivity and orientation. (*Modified from Royeen, C.B., & Lane, S.J. [1991]. Tactile processing and sensory defensiveness. In A.G. Fisher, E.A. Murray, & A.C. Bundy [Eds.],* Sensory integration: Theory and practice. *Philadelphia: F.A. Davis.*)

An individual who tends to function at the extremely underresponsive end of the continuum may be said to have diminished sensory registration. This person fails to notice sensory stimuli that elicit the attention of most people. At the other extreme of the continuum is the individual with sensory defensiveness. This person is overwhelmed and overstressed by ordinary sensory stimuli. Because these problems tend to manifest themselves differently and are handled differently in treatment, they are discussed separately in this chapter.

Originally, Ayres (1979) thought of sensory registration problems as different in nature from sensory modulation problems such as tactile defensiveness. Soon after she introduced the concept of sensory registration, however, other experts in the field of sensory integration suggested that sensory registration and tactile defensiveness might be related through common underlying limbic system functions (Dunn & Fisher, 1983; Royeen & Lane, 1991). This idea contributed to the continuum model shown here. Recently, experts in the field have criticized the continuum model as overly simplistic, because the process of modulation probably involves complex processes and is influenced by the individual's history of personal experiences, interpretation of the situation, and multiple neural systems. It may also be that the neural mechanisms involved in sensory registration problems differ from those involved in sensory defensiveness. Miller, Reisman, McIntosh, and Simon (in press) differentiate between physiologic and behavioral elements of sensory modulation disorders (SMDs). They propose an ecologic model that includes both external and internal dimensions affecting sensory modulation. External dimensions identified are culture, environment, relationships, and tasks, and internal dimensions identified are sensory processing, emotion, and attention. The external dimensions highlight the importance of context, whereas the internal dimensions focus on enduring differences among individuals. In this model, external and internal dimensions are interlinked through multidirectional, rather than linear, relationships and must be viewed in total to design intervention for SMDs. This new model illustrates that modulation is not as simple as portrayed in the linear continuum model shown in Figure 12-8.

Sensory registration problems

As noted previously in this chapter, sensory integration is the "organization of sensory input for use" (Ayres, 1979, p. 184). However, before sensory information can be used functionally, it must be registered within the CNS. When the CNS is working well, it knows when to "pay attention" to a stimulus and when to "ignore it." Most of the time this process occurs automatically and efficiently. For example, a student may not be aware of the noise of traffic outside the window of a classroom while listening to a lecture, instead focusing his or her attention on the sound of the lecturer's words. In this situation the student registers the auditory stimuli generated by the lecturer but not the stimuli generated by the traffic. The process of sensory registration is critical in enabling efficient function so that people pay attention to those stimuli that enable them to accomplish desired goals. Simultaneously, if the process is working well, energy is not wasted attending to irrelevant sensory information.

Traditionally, occupational therapists, beginning with Ayres (1979), have used the term *sensory registration problem* to refer to the difficulties of the person who frequently fails to attend to or register relevant environmental stimuli. This kind of problem is often seen in individuals with autism, but it may also be seen in other individuals with developmental problems. When a sensory registration problem is present, the child often seems oblivious to touch, pain, movement, taste, smells, sights, or sounds. Usually more than one sensory system is involved, but for some children one system may be particularly affected. Sometimes the same child who does not register relevant stimuli may be over focused on irrelevant stimuli; this is commonly seen in children with autism. It is also common for children with severe developmental problems, such as autism, to lack sensory registration in some situations but react with extreme sensory defensiveness in other situations.

Safety concerns are frequently an important issue among children with sensory registration problems. For example, the child who does not register pain sensations has not learned that certain actions naturally lead to negative consequences, such as pain, and therefore may not withdraw adequately from dangerous situations. Instead of avoiding situations likely to result in pain, the child may repeatedly engage in activities that may be injurious, such as jumping from a dangerous height onto a hard surface or touching a hot object. Other children with sensory registration problems may not register noxious tastes and smells that warn of hazards. Similarly, sights and sounds such as sirens, flashing lights, firm voice commands, and hand signals or signs that are meant to warn of perils go unheeded if not registered.

This can be a life-endangering problem in some circumstances (e.g., when a child steps in front of a moving car).

A sensory registration problem interferes with the child's ability to attach meaning to an activity or situation. Consequently, in severe cases, the child lacks the inner drive that compels most children to master ordinary childhood occupations (e.g., the child who is generally unmotivated to engage in play activities or to practice skills). Therefore the long-term effects on the child's development can be profound.

It is thought that the lack of inner drive in children with autism and severe underresponsivity renders them among the most challenging children to treat using a sensory integrative approach. These children can benefit from individual occupational therapy, but gains may be slow to develop (Ayres & Tickle, 1980). Both clinical experience and research indicate that sensory registration can be enhanced in these children through vestibular stimulation, particularly linear stimulation, and proprioceptive input, particularly when it involves joint compression and traction (Ayres, 1979; Slavik, Kitsuwa-Lowe, Danner, Green, & Ayres, 1984).

Sensation-seeking behavior

Some children register sensations yet are underresponsive to the incoming stimuli. These children seem to seek intense stimulation in the sensory modalities that are affected. The child who is hyporesponsive to vestibular stimuli may seek large quantities of intense stimulation when introduced to suspended equipment in a clinic setting. This child registers the vestibular sensations and usually shows signs of pleasure from the sensations, but the input does not affect the nervous system to the extent that it does for most other children. The underresponsive child may not become dizzy or show any autonomic responses in response to intense stimulation that would be overwhelming for most peers. This is called *hyporesponsivity* because it refers to the underlying mode of sensory processing rather than to observable motor behavior. Although the child may appear to be active motorically, the child is not reacting to intense vestibular stimuli to the degree that most children do. In everyday settings these children often appear to be restless, motorically driven, and thrill seeking.

Some children seem to seek greater-than-average amounts of proprioceptive input. Typically these children often seek active resistance to muscles, deep touch pressure stimulation, or joint compression and traction (e.g., by stomping instead of walking; intentionally falling or bumping into objects, including other people; or pushing against large objects). They may tend to use strong ballistic movements such as throwing objects forcefully. Some of these children may not seem to register the positions of body parts unless intense proprioceptive stimulation is present.

The behaviors generated by sensation-seeking children may be disruptive or inappropriate in social situations. Safety issues frequently are of paramount concern, and often these children are labeled as having social or behavioral problems. A challenge for the occupational therapist working with these children may be to identify strategies by which they can receive the high levels of stimulation that they seek without being socially disruptive, inappropriate, or dangerous to self or others.

Sensory defensiveness

At the opposite end of the sensory modulation continuum are problems associated with hyperresponsivity, or *sensory defensiveness*. The child who has sensory defensiveness is overwhelmed by ordinary sensory input and reacts defensively to it, often with strong negative emotion and activation of the sympathetic nervous system. This condition may occur as a general response to all types of sensory input, or it may be specific to one or a few sensory systems.

The term *sensory defensiveness* was first introduced by Knickerbocker (1980) and later used by Wilbarger and Wilbarger (1991) to describe sensory modulation disorders involving multisensory systems. Wilbarger and Wilbarger suggest that more than one sensory system is typically involved when signs of hyperresponsivity are present. These include overreactions to touch, movement, sounds, odors, and tastes, any of which may create discomfort, avoidance, distractibility, and anxiety. Most knowledge regarding hyperresponsivity is related to the tactile and vestibular systems, on which occupational therapists have focused their research and clinical efforts.

Tactile defensiveness. Tactile defensiveness involves a tendency to overreact to ordinary touch sensations (Ayres, 1964; 1972b; 1979). It is one of the most commonly observed sensory integrative disorders involving sensory modulation. Individuals with tactile defensiveness experience irritation and discomfort from sensations that most people do not find bothersome. Light touch sensations are especially likely to be disturbing. Common irritants include certain textures of clothing, grass or sand against bare skin, glue or paint on the skin, the light brush of another person passing by, the sensations generated when having one's hair or teeth brushed, and certain textures of food. Common responses to such irritants include anxiety, distractibility, restlessness, anger, throwing a tantrum, aggression, fear, and emotional distress.

Common self-care activities such as dressing, bathing, grooming, and eating are often affected by tactile defensiveness. Classroom activities such as finger painting, sand and water play, and crafts may be avoided. Social situations involving close proximity to others, such as playing near other children or standing in line, tend to be uncomfortable and may be disturbing enough to lead to emotional outbursts. Thus ordinary daily routines can become traumatic for children with tactile defensiveness and for their parents. Teachers and friends are likely to misinterpret the child with tactile defensiveness as being rejecting, aggressive, or simply negative.

It is difficult for individuals with tactile defensiveness to cope with the fact that others do not share their discomforts and that situations they find so upsetting actually may be enjoyed by others. For a child with this disorder, who may not be able to verbalize or even recognize the problem, the accompanying feelings of anxiety and frustration can be overwhelming and the influence on functional behavior is likely to be significant.

An occupational therapist working with a child who is tactually defensive must become aware of the specific kinds of tactile input that are aversive and the kinds that are tolerated well by that particular child. Usually light touch stimuli are aversive, especially when they occur in the most sensitive body areas such as the face, abdomen, and palmar surfaces of the upper and lower extremities. Generally, tactile stimuli that are actively self-applied by the child are tolerated much better than stimuli that are passively received, as when being touched by another person. Tactile stimuli may be especially threatening if the child cannot see the source of the touch. Most individuals with tactile defensiveness feel comfortable with deep touch stimuli, and may experience relief from irritating stimuli when deep pressure is applied over the involved skin areas.

Knowledge of these characteristics of tactile defensiveness helps the occupational therapist identify strategies that help the child and others who interact with the child to cope with this condition. For example, the occupational therapist may recommend to the teacher that if the child needs to be touched, it should be done with firm pressure in the child's view, rather than with a light touch from behind the child.

Gravitational insecurity. Gravitational insecurity is a form of hyperresponsivity to vestibular sensations, particularly sensations from the otolith organs, which detect linear movement through space and the pull of gravity (Ayres, 1979). Children with this problem have an insecure relationship to gravity characterized by excessive fear during ordinary movement activities. The gravitationally insecure child is overwhelmed by changes in head position and movement, especially when moving backward or upward through space. Fear of heights, even those involving only slight distances from the ground, is a common problem associated with this condition.

Children who display gravitational insecurity often show signs of inordinate fear, anxiety, or avoidance in relation to stairs, escalators or elevators, moving or high pieces of playground equipment, and uneven or unpredictable surfaces. Some children are so insecure that only a small change from one surface to another, as when stepping off the curb or from the sidewalk to the grass, is enough to send them into a state of high anxiety or panic.

Common reactions of children with gravitational insecurity include extreme fearfulness during low-intensity movement or when anticipating movement and avoidance of tilting the head in different planes (especially backward). They tend to move slowly and carefully, and they may refuse to participate in many gross motor activities. When they do engage in movement activities such as swinging, many of these children refuse to lift their feet off the ground. When threatened by simple motor activities, they may try to gain as much contact with the ground as possible or they may tightly clutch a nearby adult for security. These children often have signs of poor proprioception in addition to the vestibular hyperresponsivity.

Playground and park activities are often difficult for children with gravitational insecurity, as are other common childhood activities such as bicycle riding, ice skating, roller skating, skateboarding, skiing, and hiking. Ability to play with peers and to explore the environment is therefore significantly affected. Functioning in the community may also be affected when the child needs to use escalators, stairs, and elevators.

A distinction can be made between gravitational insecurity and a similar condition called *postural insecurity*. Postural insecurity was the term originally used by Ayres to refer to all children with fears related to movement. Over the years, however, it became clear that some children moved slowly and displayed fears of movement not because of a hyperresponsivity to vestibular input but because they lacked adequate motor control to perform many activities without falling. The fears of these children, then, seemed to be based on a realistic appraisal of their motor limitations. The term *posturally insecure* is used to refer to these children.

Often it is difficult to discern whether a child's anxiety is based on sensory hyperresponsivity or limited motor control because these two conditions can, and often do, coexist in the same child. Sometimes, however, the distinction is clear. Children with mild spastic diplegia, for example, commonly have postural but not gravitational insecurity. These children typically (and appropriately) react with anxiety when faced with a minimal climbing task; however, they may show pleasure at receiving vestibular stimulation, including having the head radically tilted in different planes as long as they are securely held and do not have to rely on their own motor skills to maintain a safe position.

Defensiveness in other sensory modalities. Hyperresponsivities in other sensory systems can also have a significant influence on a person's life. For example, overreactions to sounds, odors, and tastes are often problematic for children with heightened sensitivities. These types of problems, like hyperresponsivity to touch and movement, may create discomfort, avoidance, distractibility, and anxiety. Most people interpret the raucous sounds found at birthday parties, parades, playgrounds, and carnivals as happy sounds, but these can be overwhelming to a child with auditory defensiveness. A visually busy and unfamiliar environment may evoke an unusual degree of anxiety in a child with visual defensiveness. Similarly, the variety of tastes and odors encountered in some environments may be disturbing to a child with hyperresponsivity in these systems.

Sensory Discrimination and Perception Problems

Sensory discrimination and perception allow for refined organization and interpretation of sensory stimuli. Some types of sensory integrative disorders involve inefficient or inaccurate organization of sensory information (e.g., difficulty differentiating one stimulus from another or difficulty perceiving the spatial or temporal relationships among stimuli). A classic example involving the visual system is the older child with a learning disability who persists in confusing a *b* with a *d*. A child with an auditory discrimination problem may be unable to distinguish between the sounds of the words *doll* and *tall*. A child with a tactile perception problem may not be able to distinguish between a square block and a hexagonal block using touch only, without visual cues.

Some children with perceptual problems have no difficulty with sensory modulation. However, modulation problems often coexist with perceptual problems. It makes sense that these two types of problems are associated. A child who often does not register stimuli probably has deficit perceptual skills because of a lack of experience interacting with sensory information. Conversely, the child who has sensory defensiveness may exert a lot of energy trying to avoid certain sensory experiences. Defensive reactions may make it difficult to attend to the detailed features of a stimulus and thereby may impede perception.

Discrimination or perception problems can occur in any sensory system. They are best detected by standardized tests, except in the case of proprioception, which is difficult to measure in a standardized manner. Professionals in many different fields, such as clinical psychology, special education, and speech pathology, are trained to evaluate perceptual problems, and their focus usually is on the visual and auditory systems. In contrast, occupational therapists are somewhat unique in their emphasis on somatosensory perception.

Tactile discrimination and perception problems

Poor tactile perception is one of the most common sensory integrative disorders. Children with this disorder have difficulty interpreting tactile stimuli in a precise and efficient manner. For example, they may have difficulty localizing precisely where an object has brushed against them or using stereognosis to manipulate an object that

is out of sight. Fine motor skills are likely to suffer when a tactile perception problem is present, especially if tactile defensiveness is also present (Case-Smith, 1991).

As discussed previously in this chapter, the tactile system is a critical modality for learning during infancy and early childhood. Tactile exploration using the hands and mouth is particularly important. If tactile perception is vague or inaccurate, the child is at a disadvantage in learning about the different properties of objects and substances. It may be difficult for a child with such problems to develop the manipulative skills needed to efficiently perform tasks such as connecting pieces of constructional toys, fastening buttons or snaps, braiding hair, or playing marbles. Inadequate tactile perception also interferes with the feedback that is normally used to precisely guide motor tasks such as writing with a pencil, manipulating a spoon, or holding a piece of paper with one hand while cutting with the other.

Tactile perception is associated with visual perception (Ayres, Mailloux, & Wendler, 1987); thus it is fairly common to see children with problems in both of these sensory systems. Not surprisingly, these children tend to have concomitant problems with hand-eye coordination. One of the most striking findings in Ayres' factor analytic studies is the link between tactile perception and motor planning, which recurred in different studies (Ayres, 1965, 1966a, 1966b, 1971, 1972a, 1977a; Ayres et. al., 1987). These findings led Ayres to hypothesize that tactile perception is an important contributor to the ability to plan actions. She speculated that the tactile system is responsible for the development of body scheme, which then becomes an important foundation for praxis.

Ordinarily, tactile perception operates at such an automatic level that, when it is impaired, compensation strategies take a great deal of energy. An example of this is the child who cannot make the subtle manipulations needed to fasten a button without looking at it. Because this child needs to use compensatory visual guidance, the task of buttoning, which is usually performed rapidly and automatically, becomes a tedious, tiring, and frustrating task. The necessity of using such compensatory strategies throughout the day tends to interrupt the child's ability to focus on the more complex conceptual and social elements of tasks and situations.

Proprioception problems

Another type of perceptual problem involves proprioception, which arises from the muscles and joints to inform the brain about the position of body parts. This is a difficult area to research because direct measures of proprioception are not available. However, the experience of many master clinicians indicates that many children have serious difficulties interpreting proprioceptive information.

Children who do not receive reliable information about body position often appear clumsy, distracted, and awkward. As with poor tactile perception, these children must often rely on visual cues or other cognitive strategies (e.g., use of verbalizations) to perform simple aspects of tasks, such as staying in a chair or using a fork correctly. Other common attributes of children with poor proprioception include using too much or too little force in activities such as writing, clapping, marching, or typing. Breaking toys, bumping into others, and misjudging personal space are other ramifications of poor proprioception, which have strong social implications.

Many children with proprioception problems seek firm pressure to their skin, or joint compression and traction. These sensation-seeking behaviors may be an attempt to gain additional feedback about body position, or they may reflect a concomitant hyporesponsiveness to proprioceptive sensations. In any case, if these behaviors are done in socially inappropriate ways or at inopportune times, such as leaning on another child during circle time or hanging from a doorway at school, the child's behavior may be misinterpreted as being willfully disruptive.

Visual perceptual problems

Visual perception is an important factor in the competent performance of many constructional play activities and fine motor tasks. Tests are available to measure figure-ground perception, spatial orientation, depth perception, and visual closure, to name just a few of the many aspects of visual perception that have been of concern to professionals in many disciplines.

Problems with visual perception are commonly seen in children with sensory integrative disorders, particularly when poor tactile perception or dyspraxia is present (Ayres, 1989; Ayres et. al., 1987). However, some children have only a specific visual perception problem without any other sign of a sensory integrative dysfunction. Generally, therapists do not consider that these children have a sensory integrative disorder. A classic sensory integrative treatment approach, as described later in this chapter, is inappropriate for these children, although an occupational therapist might choose to work with the child using another treatment approach, such as visual perception training, use of compensatory strategies, or skill training in specific occupations.

Other perceptual problems

Many other dimensions of perception and sensory discrimination exist. For example, perception of movement through space involves the integration of vestibular, proprioceptive, and visual integration and may be affected in children with vestibular-proprioceptive problems. Auditory perception is an important function that may be involved in some children with sensory integrative disorders. However, it often exists as a discrete problem in children with language disorders. A discrete auditory perception problem, therefore, usually would not be

considered a sensory integrative dysfunction but probably would be addressed by the speech pathologist. Many areas of perception are not well understood and warrant further research.

Vestibular Processing Disorders

Over the years the research of Ayres has identified a class of disorders thought to reflect a problem in central vestibular processing. The clinical signs related to this type of disorder involve the motor functions that are outcomes of vestibular processing, such as poor equilibrium reactions and low muscle tone, particularly of the extensor muscles, which are strongly influenced by the vestibular system. These disorders are assessed using informal and formal clinical observations and standardized test scores.

Different names have been applied to vestibular processing disorders at different points in time because of the changing patterns of research findings. In her early factor analytic studies, Ayres identified a linkage between postural-ocular mechanisms and integration of the two sides of the body. Clinically, she called the related dysfunction a disorder in "postural and bilateral integration," and she noted that it often occurred in children with learning disabilities, especially those with reading disorders (Ayres, 1972b). Additional problems commonly seen in this disorder include low muscle tone, immature righting and equilibrium reactions, poor right-left discrimination, and lack of clearly defined hand dominance.

Later in the 1970s Ayres included the Southern California Postrotary Nystagmus Test (SCPNT) (Ayres, 1975) in her research as a more specific measure of vestibular processing. This test continues to be used and is part of the SIPT. Based on analysis of SCPNT scores, Ayres (1978) identified a vestibular processing component to the postural and bilateral integration (PBI) disorder. At this point she replaced the old PBI concept with the term *vestibular-bilateral integration* (VBI) disorder. One of the main characteristics of this problem was depressed postrotary nystagmus scores, suggesting inefficient central processing of vestibular input. Also characteristic were other signs of vestibular-related dysfunction, such as low muscle tone, postural-ocular deficits, and diminished balance and equilibrium reactions. In addition, poor bilateral coordination was implicated in VBI.

Factor and cluster analyses using the SIPT led to further evolution of the concept of vestibular processing disorders. The SIPT studies identified a *bilateral integration and sequencing (BIS)* problem characterized by poor bilateral coordination and difficulty sequencing actions (Ayres, 1989). Ayres suggested that vestibular functioning was an important component of this set of dysfunctions, but she was only able to make preliminary conjectures about this before her death in 1988. Building on Ayres' ideas, Fisher (1991) also suggested that a vestibular-proprioceptive disorder is the basis for a bilateral and sequencing deficit, but she recommended that continued research is needed to investigate this putative relationship.

Fisher (1991) introduced an interesting new concept in relation to BIS: the notion of *projected action sequences.* A projected action sequence involves anticipating how to move as one's relationship to the environment changes, as when moving to kick a ball or catching a moving ball. Fisher suggested that difficulty with projected action sequences is related to poor vestibular-proprioceptive processing, and furthermore, that such deficits are a form of motor planning disorder. Thus Fisher has proposed a formal link between vestibular processing and praxis through the production of bilateral and sequenced movements.

Despite the variety of ways that have been used to describe vestibular processing disorders, certain classic clinical signs are common to all. In general, many children with vestibular processing disorders do not appear to have the level of dysfunction associated with other types of sensory integrative disorders, so the problem is easy to overlook. These children often exhibit poor equilibrium reactions, lower-than-average muscle tone, particularly in extensor muscles, poor postural stability, a tendency toward slouching, and difficulty in keeping the head upright. Impaired balance and equilibrium reactions are likely to affect function in activities such as bicycle riding, roller skating, skiing, and playing games such as hopscotch. Poor bilateral integration interferes with these activities as well. In addition, poor bilateral integration makes activities such as cutting with scissors, buttoning a shirt, or doing jumping jacks especially challenging. Vestibular processing problems that involve the vestibular-ocular pathways may adversely affect function when directing eye movements while moving, as when watching a rolling soccer ball while running to kick it. Neurologic connections between the reticular activating system and the limbic system also put children with vestibular processing disorders at risk for problems with attention, organization of behavior, communication, and modulation of arousal.

Dyspraxia

Praxis is the ability to conceptualize, plan, and execute a nonhabitual motor act (Ayres, 1979). *Dyspraxia* refers to a condition characterized by difficulty with praxis that cannot be explained by a medical diagnosis or developmental disability and that occurs despite ordinary environmental opportunities for motor experiences. When Ayres originally wrote about dyspraxia, she used the term *developmental apraxia* (Ayres, 1972b). However, because the term *apraxia* is often associated with brain damage in adults, she later replaced this term with *developmental dyspraxia* (Ayres, 1979, 1985). The prefix *developmental* implies that the condition emerges in early

childhood development and is not the result of traumatic injury.

As noted previously, Ayres was struck with the relationship between tactile perception and praxis that emerged in study after study. She hypothesized that good tactile perception contributes to development of an accurate and precise body scheme, which serves as a reservoir of knowledge to be drawn on when planning new actions. Her interest in praxis appeared to grow over time, as is evident in the number of praxis tests included in the SIPT as opposed to the older SCSIT. When Ayres (1989) discussed praxis in relation to her SIPT studies, she introduced the idea that praxis problems may be manifested in different forms, not all of which are sensory integrative in nature. She coined the term *somatopraxis* to refer to the aspect of praxis that is sensory integrative in origin and grounded in somatosensory processing. At the same time she introduced the term *somatodyspraxia* to refer to a sensory integrative deficit that involves poor praxis and impaired tactile and proprioceptive processing. By definition, somatodyspraxia involves a disorder in tactile discrimination and perception. Cermak (1991) noted that not all children with developmental dyspraxia demonstrate poor tactile perception; the term *somatodyspraxia* applies only to those who do.

The child with somatodyspraxia appears clumsy and awkward. Novel motor activities are performed with great difficulty and often result in failure. Transitioning from one body position to another and sequencing and timing the actions involved in a motor task may pose a great challenge. These children typically have difficulty relating their bodies to physical objects in environmental space. They often have difficulty accurately imitating actions of others. Directionality of movement may be disturbed, resulting in toys being broken unintentionally when the child forcefully pushes an object that should be pulled. Many of these children have difficulties with oral praxis, which may affect eating skills or speech articulation.

Some children with dyspraxia have problems with *ideation* (i.e., they have difficulty generating ideas of what to do in a novel situation). When asked to simply play, without being given specific directions, these children may not initiate any activity or they may initiate activity that is habitual and limited or seems to lack a goal. Typical responses, for example, are to wander aimlessly, to perform simple repetitive actions such as patting or pushing objects around; to randomly pile up objects with no apparent plan; or for the more sophisticated child, to wait to observe others doing an activity and then imitate them rather than initiating an activity independently.

For children with dyspraxia, skills that most children attain rather easily can be excessively challenging (e.g., donning a sweater, feeding self with utensils, writing the alphabet, jumping rope, and completing a puzzle). These skills can be mastered only with high motivation on the part of the child, coupled with a great deal of practice, far more than most children require. Participation in sports is often embarrassing and frustrating, and organization of schoolwork may be a problem of particular concern. Children who have somatodyspraxia and are aware of their deficits often avoid difficult motor challenges and may attempt to gain control over such situations by assuming a directing or controlling role over others.

Praxis is best evaluated using the SIPT, which is sensitive to difficulties in this area. However, parent interview and informal observations provide critical pieces in the assessment process. In fact, these are essential in evaluating ideation because standardized tests are extremely limited in their measurement of this aspect of praxis.

Secondary Problems Related to Sensory Integrative Dysfunction

In addition to the primary characteristics of sensory integrative dysfunctions, secondary problems may arise in the child's functioning at home, in school, and in the community. Following is an explanation of these indirect, but significant, influences on the child and family.

First, sensory integrative dysfunction is an "invisible" disability (i.e., not directly and easily seen by the casual observer) that is easily misinterpreted. Sensory integrative disorders can fluctuate in severity from one time to another within the same child. Moreover, the severity of dysfunction and the ways that dysfunction is expressed vary tremendously from one individual to another. This makes it difficult to predict which situations cause problems for a particular child, how much discomfort results, and when distress is likely to occur. Parents and teachers of children with these disorders often find the unpredictability of the child's behavior to be frustrating and difficult to understand. As a result, sensory integrative problems are frequently misinterpreted as purely behavioral or psychologic issues.

A second indirect effect of sensory integrative dysfunction on the child's life is its negative influence on skill development secondary to limited participation in childhood occupations. The child who avoids finger painting, because of tactile defensiveness, or rarely attempts climbing on the jungle gym, because of dyspraxia, misses more than these singular experiences. The child also misses experiences that hone underlying functions such as tactile discrimination, hand strength and dexterity, shoulder stability, balance and equilibrium, hand-eye coordination, bilateral coordination, ideation, and motor planning.

In addition to interference with the development of sensorimotor functions, interactions important to the development of communication and social skills do not occur. Thus some children with sensory integrative disorders may lack the ability to play successfully with peers partially because they have not been able to participate fully in the play occupations in which sensory, motor, cognitive, and social skills emerge and develop. The fear, anxiety, or discomfort that accompanies many everyday situations are also likely to work against the expression of the child's inner drive toward growth-inducing experiences. Therefore lack of experience and diminished drive to participate compound the direct effects of a sensory integrative disorder. Consequently, the development of competence in many domains of development may be seriously compromised.

A third indirect effect of sensory integrative dysfunction is the undermining of self-esteem and self-confidence over time. Children with sensory integrative dysfunction are often aware of their struggles with commonplace tasks, so it is natural for them to react with frustration. Frustration is likely to mount as the child observes peers mastering these same tasks effortlessly. Chronic frustration can negatively affect and detract from the child's feelings of self-efficacy. Instead, the child may develop feelings of helplessness. This leads to further limitations in the child's experiences because the child becomes less likely to attempt challenging activities.

■ ASSESSMENT OF SENSORY INTEGRATIVE FUNCTIONS

Assessment of sensory integration, like all other areas addressed in occupational therapy, requires a multifaceted approach because of the need to understand presenting problems, not only in relation to the individual who is being assessed, but also with respect to the family and environments in which that individual lives. Assessment by the occupational therapist begins with a general exploration of the occupations of the child and family, focusing on their concerns and hopes in relation to the child's participation in routine activities. A variety of tools are needed to help the therapist identify whether a sensory integrative disorder is a factor in the child's life and, if so, what the nature of the problem is and whether any intervention should be recommended. Assessment tools employed by occupational therapists using a sensory integration perspective include interviews and questionnaires, informal and formal observations, standardized tests, and consideration of services and resources available to and appropriate for the family.

Interviews and Questionnaires

The potential need for an occupational therapy assessment of sensory integration usually arises with a referral from someone who knows the child and something about the problems that the child is experiencing. Therefore the time of referral is often ideal for initiating the as-

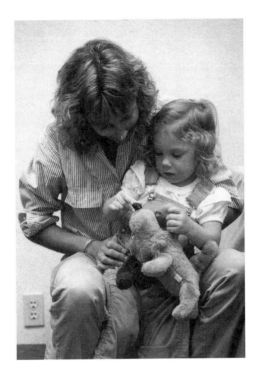

figure 12-9 Because parents know their child better than anyone else, they are invaluable sources of information to the therapist, especially in beginning phases of the assessment process. *(Courtesy of Shay McAtee.)*

sessment process. The referral source, family members, and others who work with the child may all be valuable sources of information through interview or questionnaire (Figure 12-9). This initial phase of evaluation serves to identify the presenting problems, or main concerns, about the child and begins the process of determining whether a sensory integrative dysfunction is a significant influence on the child's ability to function.

During the initial interview, as the parent, teacher, psychologist, physician, or other referral source describes the child's difficulties, the therapist may gather important information by probing to uncover hidden signs of sensory integrative dysfunction that may be present. For example, the teacher may report that the child is always fighting while standing in line and cannot seem to stay seated during reading circle time. Further questioning by the therapist may disclose signs of possible tactile defensiveness that might explain the child's behavior but were not considered important by the teacher who is unfamiliar with this condition. A parent may be able to provide critical information about the child's development, which may be helpful in identifying early signs of sensory integrative dysfunction. For instance, parents may have noticed that it always takes their child longer than others to learn new tasks, such as cutting with scissors or riding a tricycle; this is a possible sign of dyspraxia. Another important role of the interview is to uncover alternative ex-

planations of the child's difficulties that may rule out sensory integrative dysfunction, such as when a recent emotional crisis (e.g., a divorce or death) coincides with the onset of problems.

Questionnaires, checklists, and histories given by caregivers and other adults who know the child well are other means for gathering information that aid in identifying presenting problems, estimating how long they have been a concern, and clarifying the priorities of the family. One such instrument is a sensory history or similar questionnaire. Originally developed as an unpublished questionnaire by Ayres, this type of instrument asks parents questions regarding specific child behaviors indicative of sensory integrative dysfunction, and parents respond by rating the child using a Likert-style scale. In the past decade, the reliability and validity of these types of questionnaires have been evaluated with encouraging results. Currently, three such questionnaires are the most extensively researched: the Sensory Profile (Dunn, 1999), the Evaluation of Sensory Processing (ESP) (Johnson-Ecker & Parham, in press), and the Sensory Rating Scale (Provost, 1991).

Behavior checklists and other questionnaires that address classroom performance are often a convenient way to elicit information from teachers (Carrasco & Lee, 1993). An additional way to gather information in the initial phases of assessment is through clinical records, including reading previous reports from other professionals and reviewing medical histories.

It may be useful to talk with the child directly when possible. Royeen and Fortune (1990) developed a child questionnaire for the assessment of tactile defensiveness, called the *Touch Inventory for Elementary School-Aged Children (TIE)*. Children with enough verbal skills to discuss their own abilities, perceptions, and difficulties can sometimes provide invaluable insight into their condition through such a questionnaire-based interview. One 5-year-old girl, when asked, "Do fuzzy shirts bother you?" (an item on the TIE), responded with a 10-minute discussion regarding the types of clothes she could and could not wear. Even at this young age she had developed a clear awareness of her own tactile preferences and aversions. The Alert Program (Williams & Shellenberger, 1994), a group intervention program for older children and adults, includes a self-assessment of sensory preferences that can be adapted for assessment of younger children to help them identify and communicate their characteristic sensory responses.

The information garnered through the initial interview process is used to decide whether further assessment is warranted, and if so, which evaluation procedures are most appropriate. This information is also critical in interpreting the final pool of information gathered through assessment and in prioritizing goals for the child in light of the main concerns of the family.

Informal and Formal Observations of the Child

Direct observation of the child is essential to the evaluation of sensory integration. Informal observations, clinical observations, and standardized testing are commonly used.

Informal observations

Informal observation of the child in natural settings, such as a classroom, playground, or home, is informative and should be done whenever feasible. Informal observation will influence the conclusion as to whether a sensory integrative disorder is present and will, perhaps more importantly, indicate how the child's difficulties are interfering with daily occupations. For example, an experienced therapist can often detect signs of poor body awareness by observing the child at school. Such signs may include exerting too much pressure on a pencil, standing too close to classmates in line, misstepping when climbing on a jungle gym, and sitting in an ineffective position in a chair while doing class assignments. Teachers may not necessarily report these behaviors to the therapist if they perceive them as typical signs of inattentiveness or clumsiness.

Informal observation of the child in the clinical setting can also be useful in that it shows how the child responds to situations that are novel or unpredictable. A child with dyspraxia may have a great deal of difficulty figuring out how to mount an unfamiliar climbing structure in the clinic, even though performance is adequate on similar tasks at home or at school where the child has practiced them. The novelty of the clinical therapy room elicits responses from children that may be diagnostically relevant. For children with good ideation and sensory processing abilities, the endless opportunities afforded by sensory integration equipment in the clinic can be exhilarating. For the child with a disorder like dyspraxia, the same environment may be confusing, puzzling, or frustrating. A child with gravitational insecurity may be terrified by the prospect of equipment that moves, whereas a child with autism may be distressed by the clinic environment because of its unpredictability and discrepancy from familiar settings. Parham (1987) has provided some guidelines for organizing informal observations in the clinic, with special attention to issues related to praxis. Although her suggestions are focused on the assessment of preschoolers, they can also be applied to older children and may be particularly helpful in evaluating older children who are unable to cooperate with standardized testing.

Clinical observations

Formal observations that are highly structured and similar to test items are often used in an occupational therapy assessment of sensory integration. Usually referred to as *clinical observations*, these typically involve a

---

box 12-1 *Examples of commonly used clinical observations*

- *Crossing body midline:* A movement that has a tendency to occur when using the hand to reach for or manipulate an object in contralateral space. This tendency typically emerges during toddlerhood and early childhood and is related to the development of hand preference. Delays in midline crossing may be related to inadequate hand preference and bilateral integration.
- *Equilibrium reactions:* Automatic postural and limb adjustments that occur when the body's center of gravity shifts its base of support. These adjustments serve to restore the body's center of gravity over its base of support so that balance is maintained or restored. Difficulties with equilibrium reactions are associated with vestibular processing problems.
- *Muscle tone:* The readiness of a muscle to contract. Force with which a muscle resists being lengthened.
- *Prone extension:* Ability to assume and hold an "airplane" position (neck, upper body, and hips extended to lift head, arms, and legs off the floor) while lying prone. Difficulty maintaining this position for 30 seconds is related to inefficient vestibular processing in children 6 years of age and older.
- *Supine flexion:* Ability to assume and hold a curled position (neck, upper body, hips, and knees flexed so that knees are drawn close to the head) while lying supine. Difficulty maintaining this position for 30 seconds is related to poor praxis in children 6 years of age and older.

---

set of specific tasks, reflexes, and signs of nervous system integrity that are associated with sensory integrative functioning. Ayres (1965, 1966a, 1966b, 1969, 1971, 1972d, 1977a) included measures of such formal observations in her factor analytic studies, along with standardized tests. She also developed a set of clinical observations that she used in clinical practice. These unpublished, nonstandardized evaluation tools were intended to supplement standardized test scores and subsequently were revised and expanded upon by many other therapists over the years. Examples of some of the most commonly used clinical observations are described in Box 12-1.

One of the difficulties in using clinical observations as an assessment tool is that administration and scoring criteria have not been standardized. This means that they are administered using different procedures from one clinician to another. Furthermore, most of them lack any normative data to aid in interpretation of any scores that might be obtained. Some, but not all, clinical observations have research behind them to inform interpretation (e.g., Dunn, 1981; Gregory-Flock & Yerxa, 1984; Magalhaes, Koomar, & Cermak, 1989; Wilson, Pollock, Kaplan, & Law, 1994). Occupational therapists must rely on the information from these studies, as well as their personal expertise and judgment, to interpret the results of clinical observations. Without the requisite data in hand, occupational therapists are cautioned to avoid overinterpretation of clinical observations in light of the lack of standardized procedures and inadequate information regarding expected performance across age, gender, and other demographically related groups.

It is perhaps most problematic that most clinical observations address motor functions that may be strongly affected by conditions other than sensory integrative dysfunction. Therefore the therapist must master advanced knowledge of sensory integration theory before meaningful interpretations of these observations can be made.

Standardized Testing

Standardized tests are frequently used by occupational therapists in the evaluation of sensory integration. Although most relevant tests are not labeled as tests of sensory integration per se, they do include items or subtests from which inferences regarding sensory integration may be drawn. For example, the Miller Assessment for Preschoolers (Miller, 1988) includes tests of stereognosis, tactile perception, and some vestibular functions. Many tests, such as the Bruininks-Oseretsky Test of Motor Proficiency (Bruininks, 1978), measure aspects of fine and gross motor skills (such as bilateral coordination) that are related to sensory integrative functions. Other tests, such as the Developmental Test of Visual Motor Integration (Beery, 1997), provide specific information related to visual-perceptual and perceptual-motor skills.

Some tests geared toward the broader evaluation of occupation, such as the School Function Assessment (SFA) (Coster, Deeney, Haltwanger, Haley, 1998) are useful for identifying the extent to which sensory integrative disorders may be affecting the child's participation in occupations within specific settings. When the child being assessed is suspected of having a sensory integrative disorder, tests such as the SFA are most effectively used along with specific measures of sensory integration. When combined, these tests identify the functional problems to target in intervention and the reasons for the child's difficulties.

Although several tests are available that contribute incidental information regarding sensory integrative functions, the SIPT are the only set of standardized tests designed specifically for in-depth evaluation of sensory

integration. The SIPT evolved from a series of tests that Ayres developed in the 1960s (Ayres, 1963, 1964, 1966a, 1966b, 1969) and later published as the SCSIT (Ayres, 1972c) and the SCPNT (Ayres, 1975). The standardization process used in the development of the SIPT was rigorous, involving normative data on approximately 2000 children in North America and extensive reliability and validity studies (Ayres, 1989). Its 17 tests measure tactile, vestibular, and proprioceptive sensory processing; form and space perception and visuomotor coordination; bilateral integration and sequencing abilities; and praxis (Ayres & Marr, 1991). A list of the 17 tests and the functions measured by each is presented in Table 12-3.

The SIPT require about 2 hours to administer and another 30 to 45 minutes to score. Raw scores may be translated into standard scores by the therapist using a computer diskette available from the publisher. In addition, they may be sent to the publisher, Western Psychological Services, for an analysis using the normative data. After normative scores are obtained, the therapist critically examines them to determine if patterns of sensory integrative dysfunction are evident. Not only are patterns of test scores scrutinized, but also the observations that the therapist has made of child behavior during testing are considered in interpreting test scores. Finally, test scores and test behaviors are integrated with all other sources of information from the assessment in reaching a conclusion regarding the status of sensory integrative functioning.

Because it is a standardized test, the SIPT must be administered with strict adherence to standardized procedures (Figure 12-10). Specialized training is required to administer and interpret the SIPT. It is a complex set of tests and, unlike most published tests, cannot be self-taught by simply reading the manual. In addition to formal training for the SIPT, it is strongly recommended that therapists practice administration of the tests with children who do not have any known problems and with children who have recognized difficulties. With this experience and training, the therapist can administer the tests in a manner that produces reliable scores while allowing for observation of behaviors that provide additional information about the child's sensory integration and praxis abilities.

Consideration of Available Services and Resources

In addition to the information that is gathered about the child, an occupational therapy assessment of sensory integration should take into consideration the services and resources that are available to the child. Information regarding the type of services that the child is currently receiving, how he or she is responding to these services, and what services, programs, and resources are available to the child need careful consideration in light of the pur-

table 12-3	*Functions Measured by the Sensory Integration and Praxis Tests*
Function	**Description**
Space visualization	Motor-free visual space perception; mental manipulation of objects
Figure-ground perception	Motor-free visual perception of figures on a rival background
Manual form perception	Identification of block held in hand with visual counterpart or with block held in other hand
Kinesthesia	Somatic perception of hand and arm position and movement
Finger identification	Tactile perception of individual fingers
Graphesthesia	Tactile perception and practic replication of designs
Localization of tactile stimuli	Tactile perception of specific stimulus applied to arm or hand
Praxis on verbal command	Ability to motor-plan body postures on the basis of verbal directions without visual cures
Design copying	Visuopractic ability to copy simple and complex two-dimensional designs, and the manner or approach one uses to copy designs
Constructional praxis	Ability to relate objects to each other in three-dimensional space
Postural praxis	Ability to plan and execute body movements and positions
Oral praxis	Ability to plan and execute lip, tongue, and jaw movements
Sequencing praxis	Ability to repeat a series of hand and finger movements
Bilateral motor coordination	Ability to move both hands and both feet in a smooth and integrated pattern
Standing and walking balance	Static and dynamic balance on one or both feet with eyes opened and closed
Motor accuracy	Hand-eye coordination and control of movement
Postrotary nystagmus	Central nervous system processing of vestibular input assessed through observation of the duration and integrity of a vestibuloocular reflex

Reprinted from Mailloux, Z. (1990). An overview of the Sensory Integration and Praxis Tests. *American Journal of Occupational Therapy, 44,* 589-594.

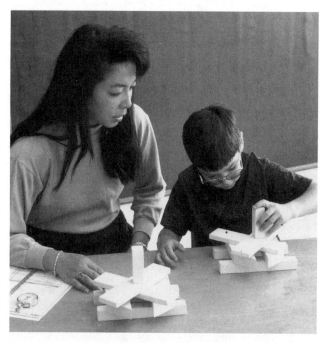

figure **12-10** The Constructional Praxis Test is one of 17 tests of the Sensory Integration and Praxis Tests (SIPT). The SIPT must be administered individually with strict adherence to standardized procedures. *(Courtesy of Shay McAtee.)*

pose and findings of the evaluation before recommendations can be formulated. For example, an occupational therapist may be asked to provide a reevaluation of a child who has been receiving occupational therapy for several years. If the child continues to demonstrate significant sensory integrative dysfunction and has shown a diminishing response to treatment using a classical sensory integration approach, the recommendations would be different than if the child no longer showed evidence of a significant sensory integrative dysfunction.

Similarly, a child who lives in an area in which there are no therapists qualified to provide occupational therapy using a classical sensory integration approach needs a different program recommendation than a child who has easy access to this type of service. Understanding family aspirations and values, as well as resources in terms of funding, transportation, time, and available caregivers, are also critical in identifying what kinds of services are most helpful to the child and family. These issues are just as important to the assessment process as the within-child factors that are addressed in a sensory integration evaluation.

Interpretation of Assessment Findings

Once all of the information from interviews, questionnaires, informal and formal observations, standardized tests, and consideration of available services and resources has been collected, the occupational therapist must integrate and interpret these data to reach meaningful conclusions and appropriate recommendations for the individual child. One of the first steps in this process is to evaluate whether a sensory integrative dysfunction is a contributor to the presenting problems of the child. To do this, data are classified into categories that either support or refute the presence of particular types of sensory integrative dysfunction. After a detailed analysis of the constellation of assessment findings, a hypothesis is generated as to whether a sensory integrative dysfunction appears to be present. If a sensory integrative dysfunction is thought to be present, the type of disorder is tentatively identified.

Whether a sensory integrative dysfunction is evident, it is critical to relate the findings to the presenting problems and initial concerns of the family or referral source. For example, an assessment may uncover signs of tactile defensiveness in a child described by the parents as destructive and impulsive. The evaluating therapist must explain how tactile defensiveness may be related to the child's behavior problems. Because sensory integrative problems are not commonly recognized, the therapist usually includes an educational component in the evaluation report to link assessment findings to the daily life experiences of the child and family.

If an assessment leads to a recommendation for intervention, it generally includes an estimate of the duration of time that the child should receive therapy, some indication of prognosis, and a statement regarding expected areas of change. The anticipated gains can be further clarified through the establishment of specific goals and objectives. The format in which goals are specified is often a function of the setting in which therapy is delivered. For example, a school district may tend to include certain types of goals as part of an individualized education plan, whereas a hospital setting may lean toward more medically related outcomes. Whatever the case, goals should be established in a manner that is culturally relevant for the family and considers the needs and wishes of the individual child.

■ SENSORY INTEGRATIVE DYSFUNCTION INTERVENTION

Planning an occupational therapy program for a child with a sensory integrative disorder requires the same careful analysis that is used when applying any theoretic framework in clinical practice. The constellation of child and family characteristics is analyzed in relation to the occupations of the individuals involved. In a sensory integration approach to intervention, the unique ways in which sensory integrative problems affect the occupa-

box 12-2 Guiding principles from sensory integration theory

1. Controlled sensory input can be used to elicit an adaptive response.
2. Registration of meaningful sensory input is necessary before an adaptive response can be made.
3. An adaptive response contributes to the development of sensory integration.
4. Better organization of adaptive responses enhances the child's general behavioral organization.
5. More mature and complex patterns of behavior are composed of consolidations of more primitive behaviors.
6. The more inner-directed a child's activities are, the greater the potential of the activities for improving neural organization.

tions of the particular child and his or her family provide the cornerstone upon which decisions regarding treatment are made.

The assessment process aids the therapist in deciding whether any intervention is recommended and, if so, in what format—individual therapy, group sessions, collaborative problem solving with parents and teachers, or consultation. Regardless of the form in which intervention is delivered, theory-based concepts regarding the nature of sensory integration are applied whenever a sensory integrative approach is selected. Six guiding principles from the work of Ayres (1972b, 1979, 1981) are summarized in Box 12-2. The key ideas behind these principles were introduced previously in this chapter in the sections on sensory integrative development and sensory integrative disorders.

Making decisions regarding the manner in which occupational therapy should be provided for children with sensory integrative disorders requires a great deal of expertise that is developed through advanced training and years of practice. The field of sensory integration is a complex, specialized area of occupational therapy practice that demands that the therapist synthesize information from many sources. Because it is a dynamically changing field of practice, it is important that the therapist stays abreast of new developments in sensory integration theory, practice, and research. These sources of information, in combination with the unique situation of the child and family being helped, all influence the decision of whether to intervene and, if so, how. In the following section, three of the primary methods of service delivery are described: individual therapy, group sessions, and consultation. Most of the time in clinical practice, these forms of intervention are used in combination rather than as the sole service delivery method. They may also be used with interventions based on other frames of reference, such as neurodevelopmental treatment or training of in-hand manipulation, as long as the underlying assumptions of the interventions are mutually compatible.

Individual Therapy

Individual occupational therapy for a sensory integrative disorder is the most intensive form of intervention. Individual therapy is usually recommended as the most effective way to initially help a child gain improved capabilities when sensory integrative problems are interfering with the child's occupations at home, in play, at school, or in the community. Individual occupational therapy for sensory integrative disorders can generally be classified into two categories: classical sensory integration treatment and compensatory skill development.

Classical sensory integrative treatment

In this section the term *classical sensory integration treatment* refers to the kind of individual occupational therapy that Ayres developed specifically to remediate sensory integrative dysfunction in children. Although she originally designed this therapy for children with learning disabilities (Ayres, 1972b), she and many other expert clinicians have used this kind of intervention to help children with other kinds of problems as well, including autism and other developmental disabilities.

In designing this specialized form of occupational therapy, Ayres was influenced by the neurobiologic literature, which shows that nervous systems have plasticity or changeability. Plasticity is particularly characteristic of the developing young child. This led Ayres to hypothesize that the neural systems that impair function may be remediable, especially in the young child. Accordingly, she set out to design a therapy that capitalized on the plasticity of the nervous system to remediate sensory integrative dysfunction. This is *not* to say that sensory integrative treatment cures conditions such as learning disability, autism, or developmental delays. Rather, the intent is to improve the efficiency with which the nervous system interprets and uses sensory information for functional use. Therefore in a classical sensory integration approach, therapy is aimed at promoting underlying capabilities and minimizing abnormal function to the greatest degree possible.

Classical sensory integrative treatment has several defining characteristics. It is virtually always applied on an *individual* basis because the therapist must adjust therapeutic activities moment by moment in relation to the individual child's interest in the activity or response to a specific challenge or sensory experience (Clark et. al., 1989; Kimball, 1999; Koomar & Bundy, 1991). This requires the therapist to continually focus attention on the child while being mindful of opportunities in the environment for eliciting adaptive responses. The therapist's decisions regarding how and when to intervene involve a delicate interplay between the therapist's judgment regarding the potential therapeutic value of an activity and the child's motivation to do the activity. The therapist does not use a "cookbook" approach in providing this therapy (e.g., by entering the therapy situation with a predetermined schedule of activities that the child is required to follow). Rather, the therapist enters into a relationship with the child that fosters the child's inner drive to actively explore the environment and to master challenges posed by the environment.

Treatment involves a *balance between structure and freedom* (Ayres, 1972b, 1979), and its effectiveness is contingent on the proficiency of the therapist in making judgments regarding when to step in to provide structure and when to step back and allow the child to choose activities. The therapist's job is to create an environment that evokes increasingly complex adaptive responses from the child. To accomplish this the child's needs and interests are respected, while taking opportunities to help the child successfully meet a challenge. An example is a child who needs to develop more efficient righting and equilibrium reactions and chooses to sit and swing on a platform swing. The therapist may allow the child to swing awhile to become accustomed to the vestibular sensations. Once the child seems comfortable, the therapist steps in to jiggle the swing to stimulate the desired responses. However, if the child responds to this challenge with signs of anxiety or fear, the therapist needs to intervene quickly to help the child feel safer. For example, the therapist might set an inner tube on the swing to provide a base to stabilize the lower part of the child's body and increase feelings of security while the child's upper body is free to make the required righting reactions. Therapeutic activities thus emerge from the interaction between therapist and child. Such individualized treatment can be fully realized only when there is a one-to-one ratio between therapist and child (Figure 12-11).

The emphasis on the *inner drive* of the child is another key characteristic of classical sensory integration therapy (Ayres, 1972b, 1979; Clark et. al., 1989; Koomar & Bundy, 1991). Self-direction on the part of the child is encouraged because therapeutic gains are maximized if the child is fully invested as an active participant. However, this is not to say that the child is permitted to engage in free play with no adult guidance. The optimal therapy situation is one in which a balance is struck between the structure provided by the therapist and some degree of freedom of choice on the part of the child (Ayres, 1972b, 1981). Drawing on the child's interests and imagination is often a key to encouraging a child to exert more effort on a difficult task or to stay with a challenging activity for a longer time. However, because chil-

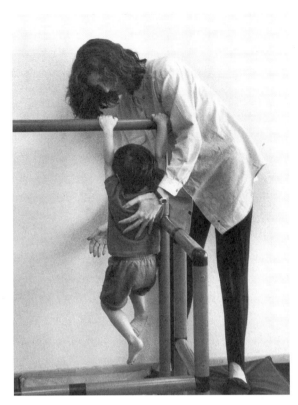

figure**12-11** Classical sensory integration treatment requires the therapist to attend closely to the child on a moment-by-moment basis to ensure that therapeutic activities are individually tailored to changing needs and interests of the child. *(Courtesy of Shay McAtee.)*

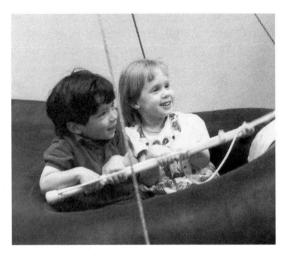

figure**12-12** Rather than passively imposing vestibular input on the child, classical sensory integration treatment emphasizes active participation and self-direction of the child. *(Courtesy of Shay McAtee.)*

dren with sensory integrative problems do not always demonstrate inner drive toward growth-inducing activities, it is often necessary to modify activities and to find ways to entice a child toward interaction. A high degree of directiveness often is needed when working with children with autism or other children whose inner drive is limited. Occasionally a therapist may use a high degree of directiveness within the context of a particular activity to show a child that the challenging activity is possible not only to achieve, but also to enjoy.

Related to inner drive is another key feature of sensory integration treatment—the valuing of *active participation,* rather than passive, on the part of the child. Because the brain responds differently and learns more effectively when an individual is actively involved in a task rather than merely receiving passive stimulation, it is considered optimal for a child to be an active participant to the greatest degree possible. For example, sensory integration theory posits that a child experiences a greater degree of integration from pumping a swing or pulling on a rope to make it go than from being swung passively.

Maximal active involvement generally takes place when therapeutic activities are at just the right level of complex-

ity, wherein the child not only feels comfortable and non-threatened but also experiences some challenge that requires effort. The course of therapy usually begins with activities in which the child feels comfortable and competent and then moves toward increasing challenges. For example, for children with gravitational insecurity, therapy usually begins with activities close to the ground and with close physical support from the therapist to help the child feel secure. Gradually, over weeks of therapy, activities that require stepping up on different surfaces and moving away from the floor are introduced as the therapist subtly withdraws physical support. Introducing just the right level of challenge, while respecting the child's need to feel secure and in control, is a key to maximizing the child's active involvement in therapy (Figure 12-12).

However, there are situations in which passive stimulation is needed to help prepare a child for more complex or challenging activities. For example, the child with autism may show improved sensory registration after receiving passive linear vestibular stimulation (Slavik et. al., 1984). The improved registration means that the child has greater awareness of the environment, and thus the passive stimulation is a stepping stone toward active involvement in an activity. Another example is the use of passive tactile stimulation as a means for reducing tactile defensiveness (Ayres, 1972b; Wilbarger & Wilbarger, 1991). However, this aspect of therapy is seen as only a limited component of a sensory integrative treatment program and then only as a step toward facilitating more active participation.

Another key characteristic of sensory integrative treatment is the *setting* in which it takes place. The provision of a special therapeutic environment is an important aspect of this kind of intervention and has been described in detail by other authors (Slavik & Chew, 1990; Walker, 1991). Based on the research that shows that brain structure and function are enhanced when animals are permitted to actively explore an interesting environment (Rosenzweig et. al., 1972), a sensory-enriched environment is designed to evoke active exploration on the part of the child. The clinic that is designed for classical sensory integrative treatment contains large activity areas with an array of specialized equipment. The availability of suspended equipment is a hallmark of this treatment approach (Clark et. al., 1989; Koomar & Bundy, 1991). Suspended equipment provides rich opportunities for stimulating and challenging the vestibular system. In addition, equipment and materials are available that provide a variety of somatosensory stimuli, including tactile, vibratory, and proprioceptive. Mats and large pillows are used for safety. Overall, this special environment provides the child with a safe and interesting place in which to explore his or her capabilities. At the same time it provides the therapist with a tool kit for creating sensory experiences that are enticing and for gently guiding the child toward activities that challenge perception, dynamic postural control, and motor planning (Figure 12-13).

Because of the prominence of vestibular stimulation in the classical sensory integration treatment environment, a few cautionary words are in order regarding this powerful tool. Vestibular stimulation, most often in the form of linear movement, is commonly introduced early in the course of treatment for many children because it is believed to have an organizing effect on other sensory systems (Ayres, 1972b, 1979, 1981). However, it can have a highly disturbing and disorganizing effect on the child if used carelessly. Vestibular stimulation may produce strong autonomic responses, such as blanching and nausea. It directly influences the arousal level and, if not regulated carefully, may produce hyperactive, distractible states or lethargic, drowsy states. Used in classical sensory integration treatment, vestibular stimulation is not passively imposed on the child. Rather, the child is allowed to initiate and actively control vestibular input as much as possible, with the therapist stepping in to help modulate it when indicated. For example, if a child is actively rotating while sitting in a tire swing and begins to exhibit mild signs of autonomic activation, the therapist may intervene. The therapist may reduce the intensity of the swinging by guiding the child to shift to slow linear swinging or by offering the child a trapeze to pull to increase the amount of proprioceptive input. Proprioceptive input is believed to have an inhibiting effect on vestibular input, based on results of animal research (Fredrickson, Schwartz, & Kornhuber, 1966). Therefore knowledge of the effects of vestibular stimulation and its interactions with other sensory systems is critical in this treatment approach. Responsible use of vestibular stimulation as a treatment modality absolutely requires advanced training in sensory integration.

To summarize the key features of classical sensory integrative treatment, therapeutic activities are neither predetermined nor are they simply free play. The flow of the treatment session results from a collaboration between the therapist and child in which the therapist encourages and supports the child in a way that moves the child toward therapeutic goals. This all takes place within a special environment that is safe yet challenging. The use of special equipment and powerful sensory modalities requires that the therapist have special training well beyond the entry level of practice in occupational therapy.

Classical sensory integration treatment is an intensive, long-term intervention. Although treatment schedules vary, a typical schedule involves two sessions per week, each lasting 45 minutes to 1 hour. A typical course of therapy lasts for about 2 years. Most experts agree that at least 6 months of therapy are needed to detect results.

After Ayres (1972b, 1979) developed the classical sensory integrative treatment approach, her colleagues and students continued to further develop and expand on her intervention concepts. Koomar and Bundy (1991) provided a particularly thorough description of the application of sensory integration procedures for specific types of sensory integrative disorders. Holloway (1993) has imported classical sensory integration treatment concepts into the neonatal intensive care unit (NICU), where the treatment principles are used to help young infants when their developing nervous systems are most plastic.

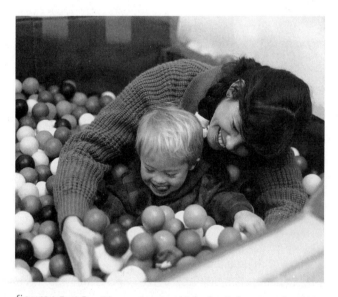

figure **12-13** The setting in which classical sensory integration treatment takes place provides a variety of sensory experiences. Immersion in a pool of balls presents challenges to sensory modulation. *(Courtesy of Shay McAtee.)*

Use of the classical sensory integration treatment approach requires advanced study and training. Koomar and Bundy (1991) advocated a mentorship process as the best preparation for learning how to clinically apply sensory integration principles. Ayres also advocated this and established a 4-month course in which therapists receive both didactic instruction and intensive hands-on experience treating children under close supervision. Ayres believed that this level of intensity was required to master the classical sensory integration approach. Because of the highly specialized and complex nature of the classical sensory integration approach, it is important that occupational therapists gain mentored experience in this area before independently engaging in this form of practice.

Compensatory skill development

In contrast to the classical sensory integrative treatment approach, the *compensatory skill development* approach does not attempt to remediate an underlying sensory integrative disorder. Instead it aims to help the child and family develop specific skills or coping strategies in the face of a sensory integrative disorder. This approach may be used to supplement or to replace classical sensory integrative treatment.

The compensatory approach may be appropriate when a therapist trained in classical sensory integrative treatment is not available. It may also be selected as the treatment of choice for a child who urgently needs to accomplish specific tasks or skills and cannot wait for the longer-range but more widely generalizable outcomes of classical sensory integrative treatment. It may also be a desirable alternative for the child who has reached an age at which expected gains from the classical treatment are minimal. The compensatory approach may also be introduced to a child who has been involved with classical sensory integrative treatment. Such cases include children who (1) have responded well to a classical sensory integrative treatment for some time but have reached a plateau in gains, (2) are approaching or have reached ages at which expected gains from the classical treatment are minimal, (3) do not appear motivated to participate or show waning interest in the classical approach, (4) do not demonstrate improvement in response to the classical sensory integrative approach after a reasonable amount of time (usually a 6-month trial), or (5) urgently need to accomplish specific tasks or skills that could be trained as a supplement or replacement for classical sensory integrative treatment.

When the compensatory skill approach is selected, therapy is aimed at training specific skills or using techniques that permit better performance on a given task. For example, a child with poor proprioceptive feedback may need to keep up with handwriting exercises assigned in his or her second grade class. The child is involved with classical sensory integrative treatment, which aims to help him or her develop better body awareness that eventually will help him or her not only with writing, but also with catching, throwing, cutting, buttoning, and many other proprioception-related difficulties. However, because of the everyday stress of the demands of handwriting, the child may not be able to afford to wait for these generalized capabilities to develop through sensory integrative treatment. For this child, specific handwriting training may be used to help him or her develop better handwriting skills, despite poor proprioceptive feedback. Adaptations may also be introduced to help the child compensate for the problem. For instance, a weighted pencil may provide augmented proprioceptive feedback regarding the position of the child's hand. Additionally, arrangements may be made with the child's teacher for the child to enter part of his or her schoolwork on a computer or to dictate it into a tape recorder to prevent poor writing skills from impeding other aspects of academic performance.

The therapist who chooses to use the compensatory skill development approach to individual therapy can do so while being mindful of the guiding principles of sensory integration theory (see Box 12-2). For example, it is optimal to involve self-direction and active participation as much as possible. This might be accomplished with the example child by having the child write his or her own stories related to his or her interests and experiences. Handwriting exercises that require active movement are expected to accomplish much more than any that are dependent on passive guidance of the child's hand. The therapist's ability to read the child's responses to writing activities helps ensure that the activities remain motivating and appropriately challenging. However, this approach generally tends to be much more therapist directed than the child-centered classical sensory integration approach.

Use of a compensatory skill approach for children with sensory integrative disorders requires that the therapist know enough about sensory integration to make sound judgments regarding when this approach is appropriate. Understanding the underlying sensory integrative disorder adequately is also essential so that the therapist does not interpret sensory-based problems as behavioral or neuromuscular in origin. Continuing education courses in specific training methods are available, particularly in the area of fine motor skills, and should be actively pursued by therapists desiring to use this approach.

Group Therapy Programs

Group rather than individual occupational therapy is sometimes recommended for children experiencing sensory integrative disorders. Sometimes *group therapy programs* are used as a transition from individual therapy so that the child can apply newly developed skills in a social peer context with less intensive support from a therapist

(Figure 12-14). The need to help a child learn to function in the context of school- and community-based groups, such as in classrooms or on sports teams, is another important reason to consider placing the child in a therapeutic group setting. Furthermore, sensory integrative disorders often create social problems for children, and treatment in groups can provide an opportunity to help the child develop important peer interaction skills.

The occupational therapist working with a group of children cannot provide the same level of vigilance to individual responses that takes place during individual therapy. Therefore some of the more intense applications of sensory stimulation or risk-taking behaviors that might be encouraged during classical sensory integrative treatment cannot be used within a group, nor can the therapist give the close guidance that is finely tuned to the individual child's needs every moment of the treatment session. Again, however, the principles of sensory integration theory outlined in Box 12-3 are important concepts to incorporate into the group format as much as possible.

Working with children in a group provides the opportunity to observe some of the ways in which sensory integrative disorders interrupt functional behavior in a social context. Some problematic child behaviors emerge only in a group situation and may not be evident during individual therapy. For example, tactile defensiveness may not be apparent in the safe constraints of individual therapy but may become obvious as a child tries to participate within a group of people who are brushing by in an unpredictable manner. Observing how the group dynamic affects the child can help the therapist know what aspects of the classroom, playground, park, or after-school activities are likely to pose a threat or challenge.

In some situations, external variables such as funding limitations, availability of staff, or organizational policies create the need for children to receive therapy in a group setting. It is important that occupational therapists make recommendations based primarily on the needs of the children being served, taking into consideration such outside factors, rather than allowing the external factors to dictate the type of intervention that is provided. It is also important to differentiate between what can be accomplished within a group versus an individual therapy session. Because group programs do not permit the same degree of intensive therapy as the classical sensory integration approach, they are not expected to lead to the same outcomes. Moreover, group programs usually resemble the compensatory skill approach more closely than classical sensory integrative treatment in aim and process, although some aim to facilitate and maintain sensory integrative functions.

Several resources are available to the therapist interested in developing group programs based on sensory integration concepts. Examples include group programs described by Bissell, Fisher, Owens, and Polcyn (1998), Inamura (1998), and Scheerer (1996). An especially innovative application of sensory integration concepts to groups is reflected in the work of Williams and Shellenberger (1994). Through a group format, their *Alert Program* helps children learn to recognize how alert they are

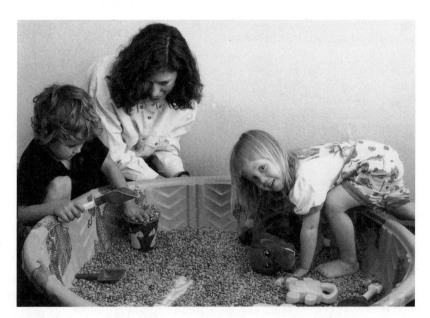

figure**12-14** Group programs provide opportunities for children with sensory integrative disorders to develop coping skills that help them function in social context with peers. *(Courtesy of Shay McAtee.)*

feeling, to identify the sensorimotor experiences that they can use to change their level of alertness, and to monitor their arousal levels in a variety of settings.

To apply sensory integration principles to a group program, an occupational therapist should be familiar enough with sensory integration theory to understand precautions and general effects of various sensory and motor activities. Experience and training in working with groups, including how to maintain the attention of children in a group, how to address varying skill and interest levels, and how to deal with behavioral issues, are also recommended for occupational therapists applying sensory integration in group programs.

Consultation

Sensory integrative disorders are complex and are often misinterpreted as behavioral, psychologic, or emotional in origin. Helping family members, teachers, and others who come into contact with the child to understand the nature of the problem can be a powerful means toward helping the child. The provision of information to those who are in ongoing contact with the child and the development of strategies through collaboration with them are important ways that the therapist can indirectly intervene to influence the child's life positively across a variety of settings. The term *consultation* broadly refers to this indirect form of intervention.

Although many of the concepts that make up sensory integration theory and practice are not usually familiar to family members, teachers, or other professionals, once they are explained in everyday terms, a newfound understanding of the child often ensues. Cermak (1991) aptly referred to this process as *demystification*. Parents commonly express relief at finally having a name for behaviors that they have observed, and they may experience release from feeling that they have caused these problems through a maladaptive parenting style. Teachers also may appreciate having an alternative way to view child behaviors, especially when this new perspective is coupled with the application of strategies that promote responses from the child that are more productive.

Helping those around the child understand their own sensory integrative processes is sometimes a good way to make these new concepts more meaningful. Williams and Shellenberger (1994) use this tactic when introducing their Alert Program to promote optimal arousal states. They encourage the adults who are involved with the program to develop awareness and insight into their own sensorimotor preferences. This first step of the consultation process, increasing an understanding of sensory integration, can be achieved through several avenues, including parent conferences, experiential sessions, lecture and discussion groups, professional in-services, and ongoing education programs. Whatever format is used, it is likely that the greater the understanding of the basic concepts of sensory integration, the greater the openness and willingness to address these problems (Figure 12-15).

Perhaps the most important component of any consultation program is providing guidance for how to cope with the problems that stem from the sensory integrative dysfunction. Sometimes specific activities can be suggested that will help a child to prepare for a challenging task. For example, a child who has tactile defensiveness may be better able to tolerate activities such as finger painting or sand play if some desensitization techniques, such as applying firm touch-pressure to the skin, are used just before the activity. Promoting success in activities can also be accomplished by suggesting individualized ways to help a child through difficult tasks. For example, some children with dyspraxia are likely to be more successful in completing a novel task when they receive verbal directions, whereas others respond optimally to visual demonstrations, and still others need physical assistance with the motion. Determining which method or combination of methods is most likely to help the individual child can assist adults in facilitating success.

Making adjustments in the environment can also be an important component of a consultation program for sensory integrative disorders. For example, children with autism often are highly affected by the sensory characteristics of their environments. Finding ways to manage sound, lighting, contact with other people, environmental odors, and visual distractions can make an important difference in attention, behavior, and ultimately, performance.

Consultation services may be provided before, during, or after direct occupational therapy intervention, or they may be recommended as the intervention of choice instead of direct individual or group therapy. Whichever

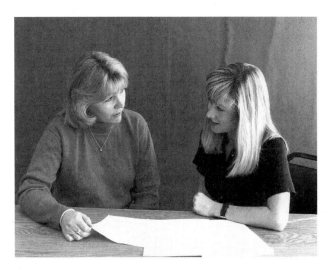

figure**12-15**   Consultation in school involves joint problem solving between the occupational therapist and the teacher. *(Courtesy of Shay McAtee.)*

the case, the consultation should not be used to take the place of direct intervention if this would be most beneficial to the child. As previously mentioned, external pressures should not influence the form of therapy that is provided to the child with sensory integrative disorders, nor should procedures or techniques that require advanced training of an occupational therapist be recommended to parents and other professionals. For example, an appropriate consultation program never attempts to train a parent or teacher to provide individual therapy using the classical sensory integration approach. Therapists should also be familiar enough with the child to be aware of any precautions that might apply before suggestions are made. For example, some children display delayed responses to vestibular stimulation and can become overstimulated or lethargic hours after such stimulation is received. Many aspects of sensory integrative techniques can lead to adverse reactions and must be used with care.

At its best, consultation as a form of intervention for sensory integrative disorders requires training and experience. However, therapists with lesser degrees of experience and training can use this approach successfully, albeit to a more limited extent, as long as they do not overstep the bounds of their knowledge. The same background and training that are needed to provide individual therapy for sensory integrative dysfunction are desirable for this approach because the therapist needs to be able to predict what the child's likely responses will be to various activities and situations, given the characteristics of the child's sensory integrative disorder. In addition, the therapist should be well enough versed in sensory integration concepts to be able to explain them in simple yet meaningful terms. Also, it is imperative that the therapist have excellent communication skills and respect for the various people and environments that are involved. Bundy (1991) provided an excellent description of the communication process involved in a good consultation program.

Expected Outcomes of Occupational Therapy

As discussed previously, occupational therapy is not expected to "cure" sensory integrative disorders. Rather, occupational therapy aims to improve the health and quality of life of a child through engagement in meaningful and important occupations. To accomplish this with a child who has sensory integrative problems, the occupational therapist may aim to improve sensory integrative functions through direct remediation or to minimize the effects of the problems by teaching compensatory skills and coping strategies to the child, parents, and teachers. Often, remediation and compensatory approaches are thoughtfully combined in an intervention plan that is tailored to the particular needs of the child and family.

The goals and objectives that are formulated as part of a child's treatment plan target specific occupations in which positive changes are expected. These goals and objectives can be conceptualized as falling under the traditional occupational categories of work, rest, play, and self-care. For example, a toddler who, because of severe sensory modulation difficulties, tends to be overstimulated much of the time, has difficulty falling asleep, and consequently is sleep deprived, a situation that aggravates his defensiveness and behavior problems. A goal addressing the occupational domain of rest may be for the child to acquire more predictable sleep patterns with adequate amounts of sleep. A corresponding behavioral objective might be that the child will take a midday nap of at least 1 hour for 3 days per week. The intervention could involve both direct remediation to reduce the sensory defensiveness generally and parent consultation to teach strategies such as calming activities, a very predictable activity schedule including a specific rest time ritual, and creation of an arousal-reducing environment after lunch (e.g., lights dimmed and noise reduced and screened with rhythmic sounds or "white noise").

Sometimes specific behavioral objectives that address performance components are appropriate as a way to monitor progress toward the desired changes in daily occupations. Goals can be conceptualized as falling into seven general categories of expected outcomes that address component and occupational performance. These are summarized in Box 12-3 and discussed further in the following sections.

---

box **12-3** *Expected outcomes of occupational therapy using sensory integration principles*

1. Increase in the frequency or duration of adaptive responses
2. Development of increasingly more complex adaptive responses
3. Improvement in gross and fine motor skills
4. Improvement in cognitive, language, and academic performance
5. Increase in self-confidence and self-esteem
6. Enhancement of occupational engagement and social participation
7. Enhancement of family life

Increase in the frequency or duration of adaptive responses

As discussed in the introduction of this chapter, adaptive responses occur when an individual responds to environmental challenges with success. Application of sensory integration principles helps the therapist envision how to create opportunities for the child to make adaptive responses. This may be accomplished through controlled sensory input that promotes organization within the child's nervous system. Ensuring that the sensory inputs inherent in activities are organizing rather than disorganizing and integrating rather than overwhelming requires careful monitoring on the part of the therapist, who must be sensitive to the child's response to each aspect of an activity and to each type of sensory input involved. The classical sensory integrative treatment approach intensively focuses on the child's demonstration of higher-level adaptive responses. However, compensatory skill approaches, group programs, and consultation services may also boost the frequency and duration of adaptive responses by changing the child's everyday environments in ways that enable the child to make adaptive responses more easily.

Increasing the duration and frequency of adaptive responses is an important outcome of sensory integration because it is on simple adaptive responses that functional behavior and skills are developed. For example, a child who has difficulty staying with an activity for more than a few seconds tends to shift from one activity to another. A desirable outcome for that child might be to stay for a longer time with a simple activity, such as swinging, in a therapy environment. Achievement of this simple adaptive response may eventually contribute to the functional behavior of staying with the reading circle in the school classroom for the required amount of time, despite the many distractions and cognitive challenges imposed by this occupation.

Development of increasingly more complex adaptive responses

Adaptive responses can vary in complexity, quality, and effectiveness (Ayres, 1981). A simple adaptive response might be simply holding onto a moving swing. A more complex adaptive response involving timing of action might be releasing grasp on a trapeze at just the right moment to land on a pillow. Over time, effective intervention is expected to enable the child to make adaptive responses that are more complex. This outcome is based on the assumption that sensory integrative procedures promote more efficient brainstem organization of multisensory input. Better neural organization of primitive functions is expected to enhance functions that are more complex. Put into functional terms, the result is an improvement in the child's ability to make judgments

about the environment, what can be done with objects, and what specific actions need to be taken to accomplish a goal (Ayres, 1981).

Although repetition of a familiar activity may be important while a child is assimilating a new skill and may be useful in helping a child get ready for another more challenging activity, development of increasingly more complex abilities occurs only when tasks become slightly more challenging than the child's prior accomplishments. This is one of the main tenets of classical sensory integrative treatment. Because of the high degree of personal attention continuously given to the child during this kind of therapy, a fine gradient of complexity can be built into therapeutic activities while simultaneously ensuring that the child experiences success and a growing sense of "I can do it!"

Group program activities, compared with individual therapy, tend to place greater demands on children for several reasons, including limited opportunity for individualization of activities, the presence of other children with their unpredictable behaviors, and reduced opportunity for direct assistance from the therapist. Thus a limitation posed by group programs is that challenges imposed on the group may at times be too great for an individual child, leading to frustration and failure. The therapist who provides a group program needs to be alert to the potential for this undesirable effect and strive to avoid it as much as possible. Whatever format for intervention is used, the therapist uses activity analysis, assessment information, ongoing observations, and knowledge of child development to ensure that the program engages the child's inner drive as much as possible to draw forth increasingly more complex interactions within the clinical, home, or community environments.

Improvement in gross and fine motor skills

The child who makes consistent and more complex adaptive responses shows evidence of improved sensory integration. Moreover, this child meets new challenges with greater self-confidence. A net result of these gains frequently is greater mastery in the motor domain. An example is the child with a vestibular processing disorder who exhibits greater competency and interest in playground activities and sports after classical sensory integrative treatment, even though these activities were not practiced during therapy. Motor skills may be among the earliest complex skills to show measurable change in response to a classical sensory integrative approach, probably because of the extent of the motor activity that is inherent in this treatment approach. Compensatory skill treatment, group intervention, or consultation for children with sensory integrative disorders should result in improvement of specific motor skills if these are targeted by the intervention. For example, if a compensatory approach to handwriting is used to help a child with poor somatosensory perception, specific gains in handwriting performance should follow if the intervention is successful.

Improvement in cognitive, language, or academic performance

Although cognitive, language, and academic skills are not specific objectives of occupational therapy for sensory integrative disorders, improvement in these domains has been detected in some intervention studies involving the provision of classical sensory integration treatment (Ayres, 1972a, 1976, 1978; Ayres & Mailloux, 1981; Cabay, 1988; Magrun, Ottenbacher, McCue, & Keefe, 1981; Ray, King, & Grandin, 1988; White, 1979). Application of classical sensory integration procedures is thought to generate broad-based changes in these areas secondary to enhancement of sensory modulation, perception, postural control, or praxis (Ayres, 1979, 1981; Cabay & King, 1989). For example, a child with autism may be helped through a sensory integrative approach to respond in a more adaptive way to sights, sounds, touch, and movement experiences that initially were disturbing. This improvement in sensory modulation may lead to a better ability to attend to language and academic tasks; thus improvement in these areas may follow. A child who has a vestibular processing disorder may improve in postural control and equilibrium, freeing the child to more efficiently concentrate on academic material without the distraction of frequent loss of sitting balance or loss of place while copying from the blackboard. This child's vestibular-related improvements are also likely to have a positive effect on playground and sports activities because effects of classical sensory integration treatment are expected to generalize to a wide range of outcome areas.

Occupational therapy aimed at developing compensatory skills such as improved handwriting also may free the child to focus on the conceptual aspects of academic tasks rather than the perceptual-motor details of how to write letters on a page or how to keep a sentence on a printed line. In such compensatory programs, effects on outcome skills tend to be limited to the specific task of concern. Similarly, consultation programs may enhance language, cognitive, or academic skills by providing strategies for reducing the effect of sensory integrative disorders on these functions. For instance, helping a teacher understand how best to seat a child in class (such as in a bean bag chair versus a firm wooden chair or in the front corner of the room near the teacher's desk) may assist in reducing the effects of a sensory integrative disorder by making it easier for the child to attend to instruction in the classroom.

Increase in self-confidence and self-esteem

Ayres (1979) asserted that enhanced ability to make adaptive responses promotes self-actualization by allowing the child to experience the joy of accomplishing a task that previously could not be done. The outcome of therapy that encourages successful, self-directed experiences is a child who perceives the self as a competent actor in the world. Individual and group programs and direct and indirect services all can be geared to helping the child master the activities that are personally meaningful and essential to success in the world of everyday occupations. Mastery of such activities is expected to result in feelings of personal control that, in turn, lead to increased willingness to take risks and to try new things (Ayres, 1979). For example, a child with gravitational insecurity may experience not only fear responses to climbing and movement activities, but also feelings of failure and frustration at not being able to participate in the play of peers. In such a case, an increase in self-confidence and comfort in one's physical body is often accompanied by a general boost in feelings of self-efficacy and worth.

Enhanced occupational engagement and social participation

Occupational therapy programs that address sensory integrative dysfunction encourage the child to organize his or her own activity, particularly in the classical sensory integration approach. As the child develops general sensory integrative capabilities and improved strategies for planning action, gains are seen in relation to ability to master self-care tasks, to cope with daily routines, and to organize behavior more generally (Ayres, 1979). As a result, the child often is able to participate more fully in the occupations that are typical for his or her peers, a broad but critically important outcome of social participation. For example, intervention may help the child who is overly sensitive to touch or movement to deal with sensations in a more adaptive manner. As a result, the child approaches and engages in the challenges of everyday occupations, such as getting himself or herself ready for school in the morning, sharing a table with others in the school cafeteria, behaving appropriately in the classroom, and playing with friends on the playground with greater security and confidence. Not only is participation in daily occupations performed with greater competency and satisfaction, but also relationships with others are likely to become more comfortable and less threatening. Group therapy programs are ideal arenas in which the increases in self-confidence made in individual therapy can be tried out in the more challenging context of a social setting. Gains in occupational engagement and social participation are among the most significant of intervention outcomes.

Enhanced family life

When children with sensory integrative problems experience positive changes during intervention, their lives and the lives of other family members may be enhanced. One possible by-product of intervention based on sensory integrative principles is that parents gain a better understanding of their children's behavior and begin to generate their own strategies for organizing family routines in a way that is supportive of the entire family system. This kind of change can be particularly powerful for parents of children with autism, whose perceptions of child behaviors may be reframed as the parents become familiar with the sensory integrative perspective. For example, behavior that is interpreted as bizarre, such as insisting on wearing rubber bands on the arms, may be reframed as a meaningful strategy that the child uses to obtain deep pressure input for self-calming (Anderson, 1993). Instead of viewing the behavior as a frustrating, pathologic sign that should be eliminated, such reframing may lead the parents to explore other ways that they could provide the child with the deep pressure experiences that he or she seeks. Thus changes in parents' understanding of the child may generate new coping strategies and alleviate parental stress. As Cohn and Cermak (1998) have suggested, reduction in parental stress may be an important outcome of sensory integrative intervention.

Research on Effectiveness of Intervention

Therapists who wish to use a sensory integration approach in practice need to keep themselves up to date on research in this field to ensure that intervention is informed by the growing knowledge base. With respect to effectiveness research, more exists in the area of sensory integration than in any other practice area of occupational therapy. In one compendium of published research in sensory integration (Daems, 1994), a total of 57 efficacy and effectiveness studies were reviewed. Most of this research is oriented toward the individualized classical sensory integration approach, although there is great variability in how this approach has been operationalized. Some studies have examined group intervention programs, but little research has focused on compensatory skill training or consultation programs that are guided specifically by sensory integration principles.

In general, effectiveness studies indicate that classical sensory integration treatment produces gains in participants' motor, language, or academic skills. Early studies were particularly encouraging in this regard (e.g., Ayres, 1972a, 1976, 1978; Ayres & Mailloux, 1981; Cabay, 1988; Magrun et al., 1981; Ottenbacher, 1982; White, 1979). However, more recent experimental design studies have found that, although children receiving sensory integration treatment tend to make gains after inter-

vention, they do not significantly outperform other children receiving an alternative treatment such as tutoring (Wilson, Kaplan, Fellowes, Gruchy, & Faris, 1992) or perceptual-motor training (Humphries, Wright, Snider, & McDougall, 1992; Polatajko, Law, Miller, Schaffer, & Macnab, 1991).

In a recent meta-analysis of experimental research on sensory integrative treatment, Vargas and Camilli (1999) analyzed 16 studies comparing sensory integrative treatment with no treatment and 16 studies comparing sensory integrative treatment with alternative treatments. A significant overall average effect size of 0.29 was found for sensory integrative treatment compared with no treatment, indicating an advantage for children receiving the treatment. The largest effect sizes were found for psychoeducational and motor outcome measures. However, older studies had a significantly higher effect size than more recent studies, which did not have a significant effect size when considered by themselves. The average effect size for sensory integrative treatment compared with alternative treatments was 0.09, and the sensory integrative treatments did not differ significantly from alternative treatments in effect size. This latter finding indicates that sensory integrative treatment methods are as effective as other treatment methods, such as tutoring or perceptual-motor training.

The chronologic-related decline in effect size of sensory integrative treatment studies is puzzling. The authors of the meta-analysis (Vargas & Camilli, 1999) suggest that the reason for this finding may lie in some unidentified difference in treatment implementation or with selection and assignment of participants to experimental and control groups in the older studies versus the more recent ones. They point out that, in general, the studies examined sensory integration intervention in isolation and therefore do not represent the ways that sensory integration is implemented clinically, which usually involves incorporation of treatment methods that do not strictly adhere to classical sensory integration principles. It may also be that the sensory integration interventions delivered in the more recent studies were overly restrictive with respect to what therapists were permitted to do and not do in comparison with the original concept of classical sensory integration treatment, which allows for a great deal of flexibility in activity choice. This probably was related to efforts by the researchers to increase rigor by ensuring that therapists followed a designated treatment protocol.

In examining the experimental group design studies of sensory integration intervention, it is important to remember that every study is imperfect in design and that limitations must be considered when interpreting results. For example, many studies use unclear or unsound methods to identify who is to receive sensory integration treatment; this creates the possibility that some children who do not have sensory integrative dysfunction are assigned to this treatment inappropriately. Another common flaw is that researchers attempt to use a standard treatment protocol to ensure that the sensory integration treatment is well defined and adheres to strict criteria. The problem associated with this is that the highly individualized, child-centered, fluid nature of classical sensory integration treatment may be diminished; therefore results of the study do not fully represent the effects of the classical treatment. This may especially be an issue in studies contrasting sensory integration treatment with similar interventions, such as perceptual-motor treatment. In classical sensory integration treatment, if a child is motivated to practice specific motor skills, this may be permitted even though this activity may make the intervention temporarily indistinguishable from perceptual-motor treatment. Such blurring of boundaries between treatment approaches would not be allowable in a research study that aims to compare effectiveness of these treatments. In such a study, it would be necessary to make "perceptual-motor-like" activities off-limits for the sensory integration intervention, thus artificially limiting the range of therapeutic activities that may be done within sensory integration treatment.

Another potential problem is related to selection of outcome measures. Often children's responses to classical sensory integration treatment are as individualized as the methods used with them in intervention, making it difficult, perhaps impossible, for the researcher to select tests and other measurements that target the precise areas of gain for individual children. Moreover, it is likely that children with different types of sensory integrative dysfunction respond to this treatment with different kinds of gains. For example, children with tactile defensiveness are likely to show gains in different outcome domains than children with vestibular processing disorders; yet, almost all of the research studies lump children together with sensory integrative dysfunction as if they should have similar responses to a standard treatment. This certainly was not Ayres' view, because she spent considerable effort attempting to identify subgroups of children with sensory integrative dysfunction who might differ from one another with respect to degree and type of responsiveness to intervention (Ayres, 1972a, 1978; Ayres & Tickle, 1980). Hopefully, researchers who conduct future effectiveness studies will become more sensitive to this important issue.

Despite the methodologic problems and conflicting results that characterize experimental group effectiveness studies, it is encouraging that these studies generally indicate that children who participate in classical sensory integration treatment are likely to benefit. Another encouraging finding reported by Wilson and Kaplan (1994) suggests that children receiving sensory integration intervention may receive long-term benefits that are not shared by children receiving other interventions. These researchers re-tested children who had participated in an earlier study comparing sensory integration intervention with tutoring. Although no significant differences in outcomes were found between the two intervention groups in the original study (Wilson et. al., 1992), at follow-up 2 years later, only the children who had received the sensory integration treatment maintained the gross motor gains that they had made after intervention. Maintenance of intervention gains is a critical issue that has an influence on cost-effectiveness questions. Replication of Wilson and Kaplan's findings (1994) would make an important contribution to understanding the extent to which gains after sensory integration treatment can be maintained.

Although group experimental treatment designs are considered to be the "gold standard" of effectiveness studies, other research designs examining treatment outcomes also make valuable contributions to an understanding of the potential effects of sensory integration intervention. Single system research has been particularly useful in revealing individual differences in responses to sensory integrative treatment (see reviews in Daems, 1993). In this kind of research, a child serves as his or her own control and is monitored repeatedly before intervention (the baseline phase) and during intervention. An advantage to this approach is that treatment and behavioral outcomes can be highly individualized. A recent example of this type of research is the study conducted by Linderman and Stewart (1999) on two preschoolers with pervasive developmental disorders. The researchers measured three behavioral outcomes for each child. Each outcome was observed in the child's home and was tailored to address functional issues for each child (e.g., response to holding and hugging for one child and functional communication during mealtime for the other). Results indicate significant improvements between baseline and intervention phases for five of the six outcomes measured.

A great deal of investigation remains to be done to explore questions regarding effectiveness of sensory integration treatment. It would be particularly beneficial to be able to better predict who will be the best responders to the classical sensory integration approach and who may be better served by other interventions. The effectiveness of combining classical sensory integration treatment with compensatory skill treatment, group programs, consultation, or other intervention methods is another area in need of research, particularly because such intervention combinations are what is typically done in clinical practice. The kinds of outcomes likely to proceed from various treatment approaches and the time-frames in which those outcomes can be expected to emerge deserve close examination in effectiveness studies. Long-term maintenance of gains, particularly of those related to outcomes that are more global, such as social participation, is a particularly important question that should be addressed in research. Finally, studies need to explore which intervention outcomes are most meaningful to the families of children with sensory integrative dysfunction to ensure that intervention programs are responsive to the needs of the people served.

Case Study 1
History

Drew was diagnosed with autism (high functioning) when he was 7 years of age. His mother is Korean, and his father is American. All of Drew's early developmental milestones were attained within normal limits, except for language acquisition. He did not speak any words until 2 years of age, and by 3 years of age his family was concerned about his development because of delayed language skills. Drew attended an English language preschool at 3 years of age and then a Korean language preschool. (His family speaks both Korean and English at home.) He was asked to leave the second preschool because of aggressive behavior. At 4 years of age Drew attended a private special education school where he received speech therapy and participated in a language-intensive playgroup. When Drew reached kindergarten age, he was enrolled in public special education programs where he attended specialized classrooms for speech and language disorders, autism, and multiple handicaps.

Reason for referral

Drew initially was referred by the state regional center for developmental disabilities to an occupational therapy private practice for evaluation when he was nearly 8 years of age. His regional center counselor thought that Drew had signs of a sensory integrative disorder, and he believed that Drew might benefit from occupational therapy. Drew's mother reported that her main concerns for Drew were related to his poor socialization skills, his limited ability to play with games and toys, and his tendency to become easily frustrated.

Evaluation procedure

Although the Sensory Integration and Praxis Tests (SIPT) were attempted during the initial occupational therapy assessment, Drew was unable to follow the directions or attend to the tests sufficiently to obtain reliable scores. Therefore his occupational therapy evaluation consisted of a parent interview, including completion of a developmental and sensory history, and observation of Drew in a clinical therapy setting. At the time of assessment it was not possible to interview Drew's teacher. However, information about Drew's performance at school was obtained from his mother, who often observed him in the classroom.

Evaluation results

Drew demonstrated inefficiencies in sensory processing in a number of sensory systems. During the assessment, signs of inconsistent responses to tactile input were evident. For example, Drew demonstrated a complete lack of response to some stimuli such as a puff of air on the back of his neck or the light touch of a cotton ball applied to his feet when he was not visually attending. However, he withdrew in an agitated fashion when the therapist attempted to position him. His mother reported that he showed extreme dislike for certain textures of food and clothing and that he disliked being touched. She also stated that he seemed to become irritated by being near other children at school and sometimes pinched or pushed peers who came close to him. Drew also appeared easily overstimulated by extraneous visual and auditory stimuli. His mother stated that he often covered his ears at home when loud noises were present and that at school he sometimes seemed confused as to the direction of sounds. He was observed to pick up objects and look at them very closely, and he appeared to rely on his vision a great deal to complete tasks. In response to movement, he enjoyed swinging slowly but became fearful with an increase in velocity. His mother stated that he often became fearful at the park when climbing.

Drew's balance was observed to be poor, and his equilibrium reactions were inconsistent. He also had trouble positioning himself on various pieces of equipment, showing poor body awareness. During the assessment he appeared to seek touch-pressure stimuli, including total body compression. He was reported to jump a great deal at home and at school. These types of proprioception-generating actions appeared to have a calming effect on Drew.

In the areas of praxis, Drew was able to imitate positions and follow verbal directions to complete motor actions, but he had a great deal of difficulty initiating activities on his own or attempting something that was unfamiliar to him. He also had difficulty timing and sequencing his actions. His mother reported that he tended not to participate in sports or in park activities and that he had trouble throwing, catching, and kicking balls. Drew was able to complete puzzles, string beads, and write his name; however, bilateral activities such as cutting and pasting were difficult for him.

Socially, Drew demonstrated poor eye contact and tended to use repetitive phrases that he had heard in the past. His mother stated that he wanted to play with peers but found it hard to make friends. Drew was independent in all self-care skills, except for tying shoes and managing some fasteners.

Based on an interview and questionnaire with Drew's mother, as well as observation of Drew in a clinical therapy setting, it was determined that he displayed irregularities in sensory processing, including hypersensitivity to some aspects of touch, movement, visual, and auditory stimuli. He also demonstrated difficulty with position sense, balance, bilateral integration, and the ideation, timing, and sequencing aspects of praxis. These difficulties were thought to interfere with Drew's ability to play purposefully with toys and to participate in age-appropriate games and sports. These problems, in combination with his language delays, were interfering significantly with his social skills, ability to make friends, and tendency to become frustrated, which were the major concerns of his parents.

Recommendation

Individual occupational therapy was recommended to address Drew's sensory integrative dysfunction and the development of specific fine and gross motor skills. Because socialization issues were such a major concern for Drew's family and were interfering with his performance at school, the evaluating therapist also recommended that Drew participate in an after-school group occupational therapy program to facilitate the acquisition of social skills.

Occupational therapy program

Drew received individual occupational therapy in a therapy clinic for 1 year. This individual therapy involved a combination of classical sensory integration and a compensatory skill development approach. During this time, Drew demonstrated significant gains in sensory processing with no further significant signs of tactile defensiveness or fear of movement activities. Motor planning of novel actions improved but continued to be of some concern for Drew. He did make notable gains in being able to catch and throw a ball and in writing and scissors skills. Through the group occupational therapy program, Drew became able to initiate and maintain interaction with peers, share objects, and play cooperatively with some assistance and structure from adults.

After this year of clinically based individual and group occupational therapy, it was recommended that individual therapy be continued at school. The focus of this occupational therapy program was to help Drew apply his improved sensorimotor and social skills in the natural context of school. Through a combination of direct service and consultation, several activities and adaptations were made to facilitate his performance at school. Because the initial year of intensive therapy using a classical sensory integrative approach had helped Drew tolerate and respond appropriately to sensory information and because he had developed many of the specific skills that he needed in the classroom during individual therapy, he was much better able to focus on the demands expected of him at school at that time. By the end of the school year, Drew's occupational therapist recommended that

occupational therapy be discontinued because she believed that his teacher would be able to continue to help him in the areas that had been addressed through the consultation program.

However, when the individualized educational program (IEP) team met to discuss Drew's transition to a new school, there was significant concern about the possibility of Drew regressing in a new setting where he would need to adjust to many different routines. The IEP team requested that occupational therapy continue to ensure a smooth transition for Drew and to put in place a plan that would continue to help him develop socially.

When school resumed in the fall, the occupational therapist had arranged a "big buddy" program with a local high school. Two high school seniors worked with Drew as part of a social service assignment during recess for the fall semester. The occupational therapist trained the high school students to carry out a socialization program aimed at helping Drew feel comfortable with a new set of peers. Drew seemed to look up to the high school students and responded well to the "big buddy" program.

By the end of the fall semester in the new school, Drew played cooperatively with peers, interacting independently and communicating appropriately. His occupational therapy program was formally discontinued at this time, although the occupational therapist continued to check in with Drew's teacher when at his school site to work with other children. No additional intervention has been needed, but the option for further consultation or direct intervention is available should the need arise.

Case Study 2
History

Karen was born after a full-term pregnancy complicated by gestational diabetes. Labor, which was induced at 40 weeks, was long, and it was believed that Karen broke her right collar bone during delivery. Karen achieved her early motor and language milestones within average age ranges. However, she was described as an irritable baby who had difficulty breastfeeding, startled easily, and could only be calmed by swinging. Karen attended a parent cooperative child development program as a toddler, and at 4 years of age she was found eligible for a special education preschool program through her school district. She has not been given any specific medical or educational diagnosis.

Reason for referral

Karen's mother expressed concern about Karen's fine and gross motor skills to a neurologist, who referred Karen for an occupational therapy assessment when she was 4 years of age. When asked why she was seeking an evaluation for Karen, her mother wrote, "Up until recently I had been very patiently waiting for normal development to occur (for example, handedness, fine motor). The school psychologist feels that this still may occur, but I am convinced that something isn't right. Karen's increasing frustration and decreasing belief in herself prompted me to seek evaluations. While a part of me wishes to have a 'normal child,' the other part will be relieved to find that the child I have had so many doubts about since infancy does indeed have some behaviors and actions that are unusual."

Evaluation procedures

The Sensory Integration and Praxis Tests (SIPT) were administered in one testing session. Karen was also observed in a clinical therapy setting and at home. In addition, Karen's mother was interviewed, and she completed a developmental and sensory history on which she provided detailed accounts of Karen's early and current sensorimotor, language, cognitive, social, and self-care development.

Evaluation results

On the SIPT, Karen scored below average for age expectations on 7 of 17 tests. Her profile of SIPT scores is shown in Figure 12-16. This profile was generated through computer scoring by the test publisher. The unit of measure represented by the scores is a statistic measure called a *standard deviation*, which represents how different the child's score is from that of an average child of the same age. The closer a child's score is to 0 on the horizontal axis, the closer to average is the child's performance on that test. Karen's scores are plotted as solid squares that are connected by a dark line on the computer-generated profile. Scores falling below −1.0 on the horizontal axis are considered to be possibly indicative of dysfunction.

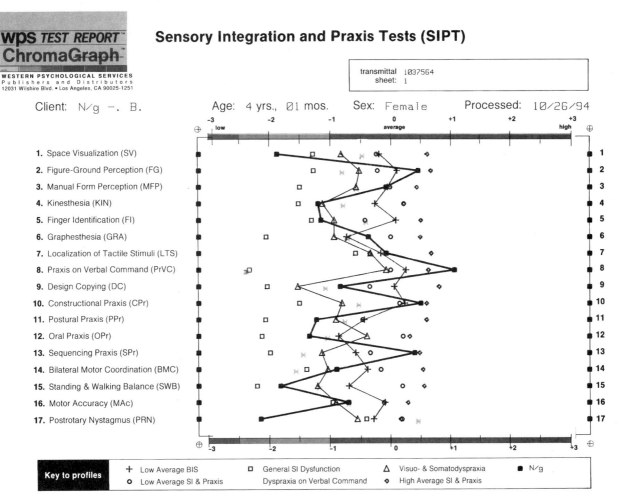

figure **12-16**   Karen's Sensory Integration and Praxis Tests profile. *(Used with permission of Western Psychological Services. [1989]. Los Angeles.)*

One of Karen's scores was low on a motor-free visual perception test (space visualization), and it was noted that she had difficulty fitting a geometric form into a puzzle board during this test. Her mother reported that she knew colors at 18 months of age but had trouble learning shapes. However, she was reported to have a strong visual memory for roads, signs, and faces. These findings suggested difficulty with spatial orientation of objects but relative strengths in visual memory.

Karen had several low scores and showed signs of difficulty performing on several of the tests of somatosensory and vestibular processing. A low score on finger identification suggested inefficient tactile feedback involving the hands. This was corroborated by observations of poor manipulative skills during activities such as buttoning and using utensils. She was also observed to have signs of tactile defensiveness, also corroborated by her mother's report. Her low score on kinesthesia, as well as her difficulty in exerting the appropriate amount of pressure on a pencil and in positioning her body for dressing, suggested problems with proprioceptive feedback. Karen's lowest score on the SIPT was on the post-rotary nystagmus test (-2.2 standard deviations). This low score, as well as below average scores on standing and walking balance, observations of poor functional balance in dressing and playground activities, a tendency not to cross her body midline, poor bilateral coordination in activities such as cutting, and reports that she never appeared to get dizzy, all pointed to the probability of vestibular processing problems.

Karen showed above-average performance on a praxis test on which she could rely on verbal directions. However, tests of motor planning that were more somatosensory dependent (oral praxis and postural praxis) were substantially more difficult for her. Karen was unable to ride a tricycle, pump a swing, or skip. She had extreme difficulty planning her movements to dress herself or even to let someone else dress her. She also had a great deal of difficulty using utensils during eating and often choked on food and drinks. Writing skills have been particularly difficult for Karen, and her lack of hand preference, immature grasp, and hesitancy to cross her midline have hampered her attempts at drawing or writing.

Karen was reported to be a social child who was liked by adults and younger peers. However, her mother worried that she did not seem able to "pick up on the hints and unwritten rules of her peers" and was "definitely starting to march to her own beat." She noticed increasing signs of frustration that she thought were beginning to impinge on Karen's willingness to participate with peers.

Overall, the evaluation results suggested deficits in sensory processing of some aspects of visual, tactile, proprioceptive, and vestibular sensory information. These difficulties were seen as related to somatodyspraxia, poor balance and bilateral integration, difficulties with specific gross and fine motor skills, and emerging concerns around socialization. Karen's strengths included age-appropriate cognitive and language skills, good ability to motor plan actions using verbal directions, and an exceptionally supportive and involved family.

Recommendations

Based on the evaluation results and a meeting of Karen's IEP team, who met shortly after the assessment, it was recommended that Karen receive individual occupational therapy using a sensory integration approach to enhance foundational sensory and motor processes. This program was funded by the school district as part of her special education program, but because of her significant sensory integrative problems and need for a specialized approach, the therapy was recommended to initially occur in a therapy clinic equipped for classical sensory integrative treatment.

Occupational Therapy Program

In the first 6 months of individual occupational therapy a classical sensory integration approach was used. In addition to the classical treatment, a brushing program (Wilbarger & Wilbarger, 1991) and a series of oral motor activities were initiated to attempt to reduce Karen's tactile defensiveness and her habit of frequently sucking in her cheeks. These aspects of her individual occupational therapy, although not part of the classical sensory integration treatment per se, used principles of sensory integration theory to help Karen overcome specific difficulties related to her sensory integration problems.

After 6 months of therapy, Karen has shown decreasing tactile defensiveness, a reduced tendency to choke on food, acquisition of the ability to ride a tricycle, and an improved ability to plan new or unusual motor actions. Although these are significant gains for Karen, she continues to exhibit substantial difficulties with many aspects of sensory processing, general motor planning ability, and many age-appropriate fine and gross motor skills. If she continues to respond to occupational therapy using a classical sensory integration approach, it is expected that by the beginning of the next school year (in about 6 months) she will have improved in basic sensory and motor functions to the extent that some specific skill training will become more appropriate. It is likely that at that time some therapy will occur at school with the introduction of a consultation program for her teacher. Her parents have already begun a home program, which appears to support the gains she is making through direct services. Karen's young age and initial positive response to therapy make her an optimal candidate for application of the sensory integration approach, and her long-term outlook is excellent.

STUDY QUESTIONS

1. How did A. Jean Ayres use the term *sensory integration?*

2. Describe how sensory integration plays a role in normal development. Provide specific examples of behaviors seen in infancy and early childhood, and explain how they relate to the development of sensory integration.

3. Identify the four main types of sensory integrative dysfunction, and describe some of the ways that each can influence daily function.

4. Imagine that you are explaining sensory modulation to a teacher who has never heard of this concept before. How would you communicate to this person that sensory modulation disorders affect classroom functioning?

5. What types of analyses did Ayres conduct to develop sensory integrative theory? What were some of the main tenets of sensory integration theory that emanated from these research studies?

6. Discuss the different methods that can be used as part of an occupational therapy assessment using a sensory integration approach.

7. Describe the Sensory Integration and Praxis Tests and the general domains that they assess.

8. Contrast the application of the classical sensory integration treatment approach with the compensatory skill approach. What would be the rationale for using one versus the other?

9. Under what circumstances would a group occupational therapy program or a consultation program be the intervention of choice for a child with a sensory integrative disorder?

10. How might expected outcomes of treatment differ for classical sensory integrative treatment versus compensatory skill, group, or consultation approaches?

References

Anderson, E.L. (1993). *Parental perceptions of the influence of occupational therapy utilizing sensory integrative techniques on the daily living skills of children with autism.* Unpublished Master's thesis. Los Angeles: University of Southern California.

Ayres, A.J. (1963). The Eleanor Clark Slagle Lecture. The development of perceptual-motor abilities: A theoretical basis for treatment of dysfunction. *American Journal of Occupational Therapy, 17* (6), 221-225.

Ayres, A.J. (1964). Tactile functions: Their relation to hyperactive and perceptual motor behavior. *American Journal of Occupational Therapy, 18* (1), 6-11.

Ayres, A.J. (1965). Patterns of perceptual-motor dysfunction in children: A factor analytic study. *Perceptual and Motor Skills, 20,* 335-368.

Ayres, A.J. (1966a). Interrelationships among perceptual-motor functions in children. *American Journal of Occupational Therapy, 20* (2), 68-71.

Ayres, A.J. (1966b). Interrelations among perceptual-motor abilities in a group of normal children. *American Journal of Occupational Therapy, 20* (6), 288-292.

Ayres, A.J. (1969). Deficits in sensory integration in educationally handicapped children. *Journal of Learning Disabilities, 2* (3), 44-52.

Ayres, A.J. (1971). Characteristics of types of sensory integrative dysfunction. *American Journal of Occupational Therapy, 25* (7), 329-334.

Ayres, A.J. (1972a). Improving academic scores through sensory integration. *Journal of Learning Disabilities, 5,* 338-343.

Ayres, A.J. (1972b). *Sensory integration and learning disorders.* Los Angeles: Western Psychological Services.

Ayres, A.J. (1972c). *Southern California Sensory Integration Tests.* Los Angeles: Western Psychological Services.

Ayres, A.J. (1972d). Types of sensory integrative dysfunction among disabled learners. *American Journal of Occupational Therapy, 26* (1), 13-18.

Ayres, A.J. (1975). *Southern California Postrotary Nystagmus Test.* Los Angeles: Western Psychological Services.

Ayres, A.J. (1976). *The effect of sensory integrative therapy on learning disabled children: The final report of a research project.* Los Angeles: Center for the Study of Sensory Integrative Dysfunction.

Ayres, A.J. (1977). Cluster analyses of measures of sensory integration. *American Journal of Occupational Therapy, 31* (6), 362-366.

Ayres, A.J. (1978). Learning disabilities and the vestibular system. *Journal of Learning Disabilities, 11* (1), 30-41.

Ayres, A.J. (1979). *Sensory integration and the child.* Los Angeles: Western Psychological Services.

Ayres, A.J. (1981). *Aspects of the somatomotor adaptive response and praxis.* (Audiotape). Pasadena, CA: Center for the Study of Sensory Integrative Dysfunction.

Ayres, A.J. (1985). *Developmental dyspraxia and adult-onset apraxia.* Torrance, CA: Sensory Integration International.

Ayres, A.J. (1989). *Sensory Integration and Praxis Tests manual.* Los Angeles: Western Psychological Services.

Ayres, A.J., & Mailloux, Z. (1981). Influence of sensory integration procedures on language development. *American Journal of Occupational Therapy, 35* (6), 383.

Ayres, A.J., Mailloux, Z., & Wendler, C.L.W. (1987). Developmental apraxia: Is it a unitary function? *Occupational Therapy Research, 7* (2), 93-110.

Ayres, A.J., & Marr, D. (1991). Sensory Integration and Praxis Tests. In A.G. Fisher, E.A. Murray, & A.C. Bundy (Eds.), *Sensory integration: Theory and practice* (pp. 203-250). Philadelphia: F.A. Davis.

Ayres, A.J., & Tickle, L. (1980). Hyperresponsivity to touch and vestibular stimuli as a predictor of positive response to sensory integration procedures in autistic children. *American Journal of Occupational Therapy, 34,* 375-381.

Bach-Y-Rita, P. (1981). Brain plasticity. In J. Goodgold (Ed.), *Brain plasticity.* St. Louis: Mosby.

Beery, KE. (1997). *The Developmental Test of Visual-Motor Integration* (4th ed.). San Antonio: Psychological Corporation.

Bennett, E.L., Diamond, M.C., Krech, D., & Rosenzweig, M.R. (1964). Chemical and anatomical plasticity of brain. *Science, 146,* 610-619.

Bissell, J., Fisher, J., Owen, C., & Polcyn, P. (1998). *Sensory motor handbook: A guide for implementing and modifying activities in the classroom.* San Antonio, TX: Therapy Skill Builders.

Bretherton, I., Bates, E., McNew, S., Shore, C., Williamson, C., & Beeghly-Smith, M. (1981). Comprehension and production of symbols in infancy: An experimental study. *Developmental Psychology, 17,* 728-736.

Bruininks, R.H. (1978). *Bruininks-Oseretsky Test of Motor Proficiency examiner's manual.* Circle Pines, MN: American Guidance Service.

Bundy, A.C. (1991). Consultation and sensory integration theory. In A.G. Fisher, E.A. Murray, & A.C. Bundy (Eds.), *Sensory integration: Theory and practice* (pp. 318-332). Philadelphia: F.A. Davis.

Cabay, M. (1988). *The effect of sensory integration–based treatment on academic readiness of young, "at risk" school children.* Annual conference of the American Occupational Therapy Association, Phoenix, AZ.

Cabay, M., & King, L.J. (1989). Sensory integration and perception: The foundation for concept formation. *Occupational Therapy in Practice, 1,* 18-27.

Carrasco, R.C., & Lee, C.E. (1993). Development of a teacher questionnaire on sensorimotor behavior. *Sensory Integration Special Interest Section Newsletter, 16* (3), 5-6.

Case-Smith, J. (1991). The effects of tactile defensiveness and tactile discrimination on in-hand manipulation. *American Journal of Occupational Therapy, 45,* 811-818.

Cermak, S.A. (1988). The relationship between attention deficits and sensory integration disorders (Part I). *Sensory Integration Special Interest Section Newsletter, 11* (2), 1-4.

Cermak, S.A. (1991). Somatodyspraxia. In A.G. Fisher, E.A. Murray, & A.C. Bundy (Eds.), *Sensory integration: Theory and practice* (pp. 137-170). Philadelphia: F.A. Davis.

Chugani, H.T., & Phelps, M.E. (1986). Maturational changes in cerebral function in infants determined by 18FDG positron emission tomography. *Science, 231,* 840-843.

Clark, F.A., Mailloux, Z., & Parham, D. (1989). Sensory integration and children with learning disorders. In P.N. Pratt & A.S. Allen (Eds.), *Occupational therapy for children* (2nd ed.). (pp. 457-509). St. Louis: Mosby.

Cohn, E.S., & Cermak, S.A. (1998). Including the family perspective in sensory integration outcomes research. *American Journal of Occupational Therapy, 52,* 540-546.

Coster, W. (1998a). Occupation-centered assessment of children. *American Journal of Occupational Therapy, 52,* 337-344.

Coster, W., Deeney, T., Haltwanger, J., & Haley, S. (1998). *School Function Assessment.* San Antonio, TX: Therapy Skill Builders.

Daems, J. (Ed.). (1994). *Reviews of research in sensory integration.* Torrance, CA: Sensory Integration International.

Dru, D., Walker, J.P., & Walker, J.B. (1975). Self-produced locomotion restores visual capacity after striate lesion. *Science, 187,* 265-266.

Dunn, W.W. (1981). *A guide to testing clinical observations in kindergartners.* Rockville, MD: American Occupational Therapy Association.

Dunn, W.W. (1999). *Sensory Profile.* San Antonio, TX: Psychological Corporation.

Dunn, W., & Fisher, A.G. (1983). Sensory registration, autism, and tactile defensiveness. In J. Melvin (Ed.), *Occupational therapy in practice* (Vol. 1). (pp. 181-182). Rockville, MD: American Occupational Therapy Association.

Fisher, A.G. (1991). Vestibular-proprioceptive processing and bilateral integration and sequencing deficits. In A.G. Fisher, E.A. Murray, & A.C. Bundy (Eds.), *Sensory integration: Theory and practice* (pp. 69-107). Philadelphia: F.A. Davis.

Fisher, A.G., & Murray, E.A. (1991). Introduction to sensory integration theory. In A.G. Fisher, E.A. Murray, & A.C. Bundy (Eds.), *Sensory integration: Theory and practice* (pp. 3-26). Philadelphia: F.A. Davis.

Fisher, A.G., Murray, E.A., & Bundy, A.C. (Eds.). (1991). *Sensory integration: Theory and practice.* Philadelphia: F.A. Davis.

Fredrickson, J.M., Schwartz, D.W., & Kornhuber, H.H. (1966). Convergence and interaction of vestibular and deep somatic afferents upon neurons in the vestibular nuclei of the cat. *Acta Otolaryngologica, 61,* 168-188.

Gregg, C.L., Hafner, M.E., & Korner, A. (1976). The relative efficacy of vestibular-proprioceptive stimulation and the upright position in enhancing visual pursuit in neonates. *Child Development, 47,* 309-314.

Gregory-Flock, J.L., & Yerxa, E.J. (1984). Standardization of the prone extension postural test on children ages 4 through 8. *American Journal of Occupational Therapy, 38,* 187-194.

Gunnar, M.R., & Barr, R.G. (1998). Stress, early brain development, and behavior. *Infants and Young Children, 11* (1), 1-14.

Holloway, E. (1997). Early emotional development and sensory processing. In J. Case-Smith (Ed.), *Pediatric occupational therapy and early intervention* (pp. 163-197). Boston: Andover Medical Publishers.

Hubel, D.H., & Wiesel, T.N. (1963). Receptive fields of cells in striate cortex of very young, visually inexperienced kittens. *Journal of Neurophysiology, 26,* 994-1002.

Humphrey, T. (1969). Postnatal repetition of human prenatal activity sequences with some suggestions of their neuroanatomical basis. In R.J. Robinson (Ed.), *Brain and early behavior.* New York: Academic Press.

Humphries, T., Wright, M., Snider, L., & McDougall, B. (1992). A comparison of the effectiveness of sensory integrative therapy and perceptual-motor training in treating children with learning disabilities. *Journal of Developmental and Behavioral Pediatrics, 13,* 31-40.

Inamura, K.N. (1998). *Sensory integration for early intervention: A team approach.* San Antonio, TX: Therapy Skill Builders.

Johnson-Ecker, C.J., & Parham, L.D. (in press). The Evaluation of Sensory Processing: A validity study using contrasting groups. *American Journal of Occupational Therapy.*

Kimball, J.G. (1999). Sensory integrative frame of reference. In P. Kramer & J. Hinojosa (Eds.), *Frames of reference for pediatric occupational therapy.* Baltimore: Williams & Wilkins.

Knickerbocker, B.M. (1980). *A holistic approach to learning disabilities.* Thorofare, NJ: C.B. Slack.

Kolb, B., & Whishaw, I.Q. (1985). *Fundamentals of human neuropsychology* (2nd ed.). New York: W.H. Freeman.

Koomar, J.A., & Bundy, A.C. (1991). The art and science of creating direct intervention from theory. In A.G. Fisher, E.A. Murray, & A.C. Bundy (Eds.), *Sensory integration: Theory and practice* (pp. 251-317). Philadelphia: F.A. Davis.

Linderman, T.M., & Stewart, K.B. (1999). Sensory integrative-based occupational therapy and functional outcomes in young children with pervasive developmental disorders: A single-subject study. *American Journal of Occupational Therapy, 53,* 207-213.

Magalhaes, L.C., Koomar, J., & Cermak, S.A. (1989). Bilateral motor coordination in 5- to 9-year-old children. *American Journal of Occupational Therapy, 43,* 437-443.

Magrun, W.M., Ottenbacher, K., McCue, S., & Keefe, R. (1981). Effects of vestibular stimulation on spontaneous use of verbal language in developmentally delayed children. *American Journal of Occupational Therapy, 35,* 101-104.

Maurer, D., & Maurer, C. (1988). *The world of the newborn.* New York: Basic Books.

McCune-Nicolich, L. (1981). Toward symbolic functioning: Structure of early pretend games and potential parallels with language. *Child Development, 52,* 785-797.

Miller, L.J. (1988). *Miller Assessment for Preschoolers manual* (Rev. ed). San Antonio, TX: Psychological Corporation.

Miller, L.J., Reisman, J., McIntosh, D.N., & Simon, J. (in press). An ecological model of sensory modulation: Performance of children with Fragile X Syndrome. In E. Blanche, S. Roley, & R. Schaaf (Eds.), *Sensory integration and developmental disabilities*. San Antonio, TX: Therapy Skill Builders.

Mulligan, S. (1998). Patterns of sensory integration dysfunction: A confirmatory factor analysis. *American Journal of Occupational Therapy, 52,* 819-828.

Ottenbacher, K. (1982). Sensory integration therapy: affect or effect. *American Journal of Occupational Therapy, 36,* 571-578.

Parham, L.D. (1987). Evaluation of praxis in preschoolers. *Occupational Therapy in Heaalth Care, 4* (2), 23-36.

Parush, S., Sohmer, H., Steinberg, A., & Kaitz, M. (1997). Somatosensory functioning in children with attention deficit hyperactivity disorder. *Developmental Medicine and Child Neurology, 39,* 464-468.

Polatajko, H.J. (1985). A critical look at vestibular dysfunction in learning-disabled children. *Developmental Medicine and Child Neurology, 27,* 283-291.

Polatajko, H.J., Law, M., Miller, J., Schaffer, R., & Macnab, J. (1991). The effect of a sensory integration program on academic achievement, motor performance, and self-esteem in children identified as learning disabled: Results of a clinical trial. *Occupational Therapy Journal of Research, 11,* 155-176.

Provost, E.M. (1991). *Measurement of sensory behaviors in infants and young children.* Doctoral dissertation. Albuquerque, NM: University of New Mexico.

Ray, T., King, L.J., & Grandin, T. (1988). The effectiveness of self-initiated vestibular stimulation in producing speech sounds in an autistic child. *Occupational Therapy Journal of Research, 8,* 186-190.

Rosenzweig, M.R., Bennett, E.L., & Diamond, M.C. (1972). Brain changes in response to experience. *Scientific American, 226* (2), 22-29.

Royeen, C.B. (1989). Commentary on "Tactile functions in learning-disabled and normal children: Reliability and validity considerations." *Occupational Therapy Journal of Research, 9,* 16-23.

Royeen, C.B., & Fortune, J.C. (1990). TIE: Touch Inventory for Elementary School-Aged Children. *American Journal of Occupational Therapy, 44,* 165-170.

Royeen, C.B., & Lane, S.J. (1991). Tactile processing and sensory defensiveness. In A.G. Fisher, E.A. Murray, & A.C. Bundy (Eds.), *Sensory integration: Theory and practice* (pp. 108-136). Philadelphia: F.A. Davis.

Salthe, S.N. (1985). *Evolving hierarchical systems.* New York: Columbia University.

Schaaf, R. (1994). Neuroplasticity and sensory integration. Part 2. *Sensory Integration Quarterly, 22* (2), 1-7.

Scheerer, C. (1996). *Sensorimotor groups: Activities for school and home.* San Antonio, TX: Therapy Skill Builders.

Short-DeGraff, M.A. (1988). *Human development for occupational and physical therapists.* Baltimore: Williams & Wilkins.

Shumway-Cook, A., Horak, F., & Black, F.O. (1987). A critical examination of vestibular function in motor-impaired learning-disabled children. *International Journal of Pediatric Otolaryngology, 14,* 21-30.

Slavik, B.A., & Chew, T. (1990). The design of a sensory integration treatment facility: The Ayres Clinic as a model. In S.C. Merrill (Ed.), *Environment: Implications for occupational therapy practice* (pp. 85-101). Rockville, MD: American Occupational Therapy Association.

Slavik, B.A., Kitsuwa-Lowe, J., Danner, P.T., Green, J., & Ayres, A.J. (1984). Vestibular stimulation and eye contact in autistic children. *Neuropediatrics, 15,* 333-336.

Solomon, P., Kubzansky, P.E., Leiderman, P.H., Mendelson, J.H., Trumball, R., & Wexler, D. (Eds.). (1961). *Sensory deprivation.* Cambridge: Harvard University.

Stern, D.N. (1985). *The interpersonal world of the infant.* New York: Basic Books.

Todd, V.R. (1999). Visual perceptual frame of reference: An information processing approach. In P. Kramer & J. Hinojosa (Eds.), *Frames of reference for pediatric occupational therapy* (pp. 177-232). Baltimore: Williams & Wilkins.

Vargas, S., & Camilli, G. (1999). A meta-analysis of research on sensory integration treatment. *American Journal of Occupational Therapy, 53,* 189-198.

Walker, K.F. (1991). Sensory integrative therapy in a limited space: An adaptation of the Ayres Clinic design. *Sensory Integration Special Interest Section Newsletter, 14* (3), 1, 2, 4.

White, M. (1979). A first-grade intervention program for children at risk for reading failure. *Journal of Learning Disabilities, 12,* 26-32.

Wilbarger, P. (1984). Planning an adequate "sensory diet": Application of sensory processing theory during the first year of life. *Zero to Three,* pp. 7-12.

Wilbarger, P., & Wilbarger, J.L. (1991). *Sensory defensiveness in children aged 2-12.* Denver, CO: Avanti Educational Programs.

Williams, M.S., & Shellenberger, S. (1994). *"How does your engine run?" A leader's guide to the Alert Program for Self-regulation.* Albuquerque, NM: TherapyWorks.

Wilson, B.N., & Kaplan, B.J. (1994). Follow-up assessment of children receiving sensory integration treatment. *Occupational Therapy Journal of Research, 14,* 244-266.

Wilson, B.N., Kaplan, B.J., Fellowes, S., Gruchy, C., & Faris, P. (1992). The efficacy of sensory integration treatment compared to tutoring. *Physical and Occupational Therapy in Pediatrics, 12,* 1-36.

Wilson, B.N., Pollock, N., Kaplan, B.J., & Law, M. (1994). *Clinical Observations of Motor and Postural Skills (COMPS).* Tucson: Therapy Skill Builders.

Wiss, T. (1989). Vestibular dysfunction in learning disabilities: Differences in definitions lead to different conclusions. *Journal of Learning Disabilities, 22,* 100-101.

Definitions of Terms

Adaptive response. A successful response to an environmental challenge (Ayres, 1979). The adaptive response is an important mechanism of sensory integrative development and is a central concept in classical sensory integration treatment.

Bilateral coordination. The ability of the two sides of the body to work together motorically.

Bilateral integration. The brain function that enables coordination of functions of the two sides of the body.

Body scheme. An internal representation of the body; the brain's "map" of body parts and how they interrelate.

Dyspraxia. A condition in which the individual has difficulty with praxis. In children, this term is usually used to refer to praxis problems that cannot be accounted for by a medical condition, developmental disability, or lack of environmental opportunity.

Gravitational insecurity. A condition in which there is a tendency to react negatively and fearfully to movement experiences, particularly those involving a change in head position and movement backward or upward through space.

Hyperresponsivity. A disorder of sensory modulation in which the individual is overwhelmed by ordinary sensory input and reacts defensively to it, often with strong negative emotion and activation of the sympathetic nervous system.

Hyporesponsivity. A disorder of sensory modulation in which the individual tends to ignore or be relatively unaffected by sensory stimuli to which most people respond. In some cases the person may have an excessive craving for intense stimuli.

Ideation. The ability to conceptualize a new action to be performed in a given situation (Ayres, 1981, 1985). This aspect of praxis involves generating an idea of what to do. It precedes motor planning, which addresses the plan for how to perform the action.

Motor planning. The process of organizing a plan for action. This aspect of praxis is a cognitive process that precedes the performance of a new action.

Perception. The organization of sensory data into meaningful units. For example, stereognosis, a type of tactile perception, involves the organization of tactile details so that an object can be recognized by touch.

Praxis. The ability to conceptualize, organize, and execute nonhabitual motor tasks (Ayres, 1979, 1981).

Sensory defensiveness. A condition characterized by hyperresponsivity in one or more sensory systems.

Sensory discrimination. The ability to distinguish between different sensory stimuli. This term is usually used to refer to the ability to make fine distinctions between stimuli of one sensory modality, such as discriminating between two points of tactile contact or differentiating between similar sounds.

Sensory integration. The organization of sensation for use (Ayres, 1979); a complex set of processes in the central nervous system that include modulation, perceptual, and praxic functions. This term is also used to refer to a frame of reference for treatment of children who have difficulty with these neural functions.

Sensory modulation. The tendency to generate responses that are appropriately graded in relation to incoming sensations, neither underreacting nor overreacting to them.

Sensory processing. A term referring generally to the handling of sensory information by neural systems, including the functions of receptor organs, peripheral, and central nervous systems.

Sensory registration. The process by which the central nervous system attends to stimuli; this usually involves an orienting response.

Sequencing. The ability to appropriately order a series of actions, an important element of motor planning. This term also is sometimes used to refer to the ability to replicate a series of sensory stimuli in the correct order.

Somatopraxis. An aspect of praxis that is heavily dependent on somatosensory processing (Ayres, 1989).

An impairment of this aspect of praxis is termed *somatodyspraxia* (Cermak, 1991) and is characterized by poor tactile and proprioceptive processing as well as poor praxis.

Somatosensory. Pertaining to the tactile and proprioceptive systems.

Tactile defensiveness. A condition in which there is a tendency to react negatively and emotionally to touch sensations (Ayres, 1979).

Vestibular. Pertaining to the inner ear receptors, the semicircular canals and otolith organs, that detect head position and movement as well as gravity.

chapter 13

Visual Perception

Colleen M. Schneck

Visual-receptive component
Visual-cognitive component
Attention
Visual memory
Visual discrimination
Object (form) perception
Spatial perception

■ CHAPTER OBJECTIVES

1. Define *visual perception*.
2. Describe typical development of visual perceptual skills.
3. Identify factors that contribute to typical or atypical development of visual perception.
4. Explain the implications of visual perceptual problems for performance of play, self-care, and school performance.
5. Describe models and theories that may be used in structuring intervention plans for children who have problems with visual perceptual skills.
6. Identify assessments and methods useful in evaluation of visual perceptual skills in children.
7. Describe intervention strategies for assisting children in improving or compensating for problems with visual perceptual skills.
8. Illustrate principles of evaluation and intervention with case examples of children.

Although one may question which of the senses is the most important for performance, some consider vision to be the most influential sense in humans (Bouska, Kauffman, & Marcus, 1990; Hellerstein & Fishman, 1987;

Nolte, 1988). There is little argument that vision is the dominant sense in human perception of the external world; it helps to monitor what is happening in the environment outside of the body. Because of the complexity of the visual system, it is difficult to imagine the influence of a visual perceptual deficit on daily living. Functional problems that may result from a visual perceptual deficit include difficulties with eating, dressing, reading, writing, locating objects, driving, and many more activities necessary for functional independence.

Given that occupational therapists' focus on functional independence in the performance of activities of daily living, work and productive activities, and play and leisure activities, the focus on the performance component of visual perception is critically important. Although visual perception is a major intervention emphasis of occupational therapists working with children, it is one of the least understood areas of evaluation and treatment (Warren, 1993a). The information presented in this chapter describes current information on visual perception that relates to evaluation and intervention with children. The information in this area of visual perception continues to evolve as research in this area confirms or disproves explanatory models of the visual perceptual system.

■ DEFINITIONS

Visual perception is defined as the total process responsible for the reception and cognition of visual stimuli (Zaba, 1984). The *visual-receptive component* is the process of extracting and organizing information from the environment (Solan & Ciner, 1986), and the *visual-cognitive component* is the ability to interpret and use what is seen. These two components allow a person to understand what he or she sees, and they are both necessary for functional vision. Visual perceptual skills include the recognition and identification of shapes, objects, colors, and other qualities. Visual perception allows a person to make accurate judgments of the size, configuration, and spatial relationships of objects.

Kwatney and Bouska (1980) defined the following as functions of the mature visual system. These functions demonstrate the interaction of the visual-receptive and visual-cognitive components:

1. Respond and adjust to retinal stimuli (anatomic and physiologic integrity)
2. Move both the head and eyes to collect raw data (oculomotor and vestibuloocular control)
3. Effectively interpret visual information (visuoperceptual ability)
4. Respond to visual cues through efficient limb movements (visuomotor ability)
5. Accomplish integration of all of these abilities

The term *visual information analysis* has been used recently to define this ability to extract and organize information from the visual environment and to integrate this information with other sensory information, previous experience, and higher cognitive functions (Tsurumi & Todd, 1998). Therefore integration of the visual-receptive and visual-cognitive systems is essential for functional vision.

■ PERFORMANCE COMPONENTS

Visual-Receptive Components

Hearing and vision are the distant senses that allow people to understand what is happening in the environment outside of his or her body or in extrapersonal space. These sense organs transmit information to the brain, whose primary function is to receive information from the world for processing and coding. The visual sensory stimuli are then integrated with other sensory input and associated with past experiences. The eye, oculomotor muscles and pathways, optic nerve, optic tract, occipital cortex, and associative areas of the cerebral cortex (parietal and temporal lobes) are all included in this process. Approximately 70% of the sensory receptors in the human are allocated to vision.

As an occupational therapist, it is imperative to understand the neurophysiologic interactions in the central nervous system (CNS) to effectively evaluate and treat children with problems in the visual system. This discussion begins with the sensory receptor, the eye.

Anatomy of the eye

A basic understanding of the anatomy and physiology of the eye aids in understanding its influence on perception (Figure 13-1). The eye functions to transmit light to the retina. It focuses images of the environment onto the retina. The eye is shaped to refract the rays of light so that the most sensitive part of the retina receives rays at one convergent point. The cornea covers the front of the eye and is part of the outermost layer of the eyeball. It plays a large part in focusing or bending the rays of light entering the eye. Behind the cornea is the aqueous humor, which is a clear fluid. The pressure of this fluid helps maintain the shape of the cornea and helps in focusing the rays. The colored part of the eye, or iris, with its center hole, the pupil, is directly behind the cornea. The iris governs the amount of light entering the eye by increasing or decreasing the size of the pupil. The light then progresses through the crystalline lens, which does the fine focusing for near or far vision, and through the jellylike substance called the *vitreous humor*. The eye has three layers: the sclera is fibrous and elastic, helping to hold the rest of the eye structure in place; the choroid is primarily blood vessels that nourish the eye; and the retina is the innermost layer. The retinal layer is composed of receptor nerve cells that contain a chemical that is activated by light. The retina has three types of receptor cells:

1. *Cones.* Used for color perception and visual acuity
2. *Rods.* Used for night and peripheral vision
3. *Pupillary cells.* Controls opening (dilation) and closing (constriction) of the pupil

The fovea centralis (located in the retina) is the point of sharpest and clearest vision. It is most responsive to daylight and must receive a certain quantity of light before it transmits the signal to the optic nerve. The retina responds to spatial differences in intensity of light stimulation, especially at contrasting border areas, and it provides basic information about light and dark areas. Light stimulates the visual receptor cells in the retina, causing electrochemical changes that trigger an electrical impulse to flow to the optic nerve. The optic nerve (cranial nerve II) transmits the visual sensory messages to the brain for processing. This information travels to the brain in a special way. Fibers from the nasal half of each retina divide, and half of these fibers cross to the contralateral side of the brain. Fibers from the outer half of each retina do not divide, and so they carry visual information ipsilaterally. Therefore visual information from either the left or right visual field enters the opposite portion of each retina and then travels to the same hemisphere of the brain. This organization means that even with the loss of vision in one eye, information is transmitted to both hemispheres of

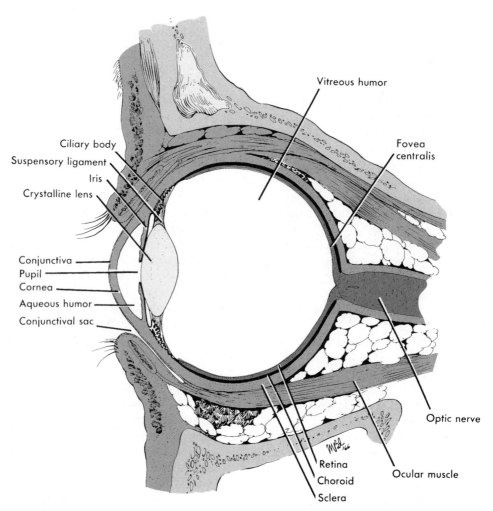

figure**13-1**   Cross-section of the eye. *(From Ingalls, A.J., & Salerno, M.C. [1983]. Maternal and child health nursing [5th ed.]. St. Louis: Mosby.)*

the brain. This also means that damage in the region of the left or right occipital cortex can cause a loss of vision that is referred to as a *field cut* in the opposite visual field.

The optic nerve leads from the back of the eye to the lateral geniculate nucleus in the optic thalamus. It is here that binocular information is received and integrated at a basic level, which may contribute to crude depth perception. Information then passes from the two lateral geniculate bodies of the thalamus to the visual cortex in the occipital lobe (area 17). From the occipital cortex the refined visual information is sent in two directions via visual areas 18 or 19 (Rafal & Posner, 1987; Ratcliff, 1987). Some impulses flow upward to the posterior parietal lobe where visual spatial processing occurs, focusing on the location of objects and their relationships to objects in space. Other impulses flow downward to the temporal lobe where visual object processing takes place. Information sent here is analyzed for the specific details of color, form, and size needed for accurate object identification; the focus is on pattern recognition and detail and remembering the qualities of objects.

Oculomotor system

The oculomotor system makes possible the reception of visual stimuli (visual-receptive). The visual-receptive components include *fixation, pursuit and saccadic eye movements, acuity, accommodation, binocular vision and stereopsis,* and *convergence and divergence. Visual fixation* on a stationary object is a prerequisite skill for other ocular-motor responses such as shifting gaze between objects (scanning) or tracking. Each eye is moved by the coordinated actions of the six extraocular muscles. These are innervated by the third, fourth, and sixth cranial nerves: oculomotor, trochlear, and abducens. The oculomotor nuclei are responsible for automatic conjugate eye movements: lateral, vertical, and convergence. They also help regulate the position of the eyes in relation to the position of the head. The nuclei receive most of their information from the superior colliculus.

Two types of eye movements are used to gather information from the environment: pursuit eye movements, or tracking, and saccadic eye movements, or scanning. *Visual pursuit,* or *tracking,* involves the continued fixation on a moving object so that the image is maintained continuously on the fovea. The smooth pursuit system is characterized by slow, smooth movements. Tracking may occur with eyes and head together or with eyes moving independently from the head. *Saccadic eye movements,* or *scanning,* are defined as a rapid change of fixation from one point in the visual field to another. A saccade may be voluntary, as when localizing a quickly displaced stimulus or when reading, or it may be involuntary, as during the fast phases of vestibular nystagmus. A saccadic movement is precise, although the presence of a slight overshoot or undershoot is normal.

In addition to voluntary control of eye movements, the vestibular-ocular pathways control conjugate eye movements reflexively in response to head movement and position in space. These pathways enable the eyes to remain fixed on a stationary object while the head and body move.

In addition to the tasks of visual fixation, pursuit movements, and saccadic movements, other visual-receptive components include the following:

- *Acuity.* The capacity to discriminate the fine details of objects in the visual field. 20/20 means that a person can perceive as small an object as an average person can perceive at 20 feet.
- *Accommodation.* The ability of each eye to compensate for a blurred image. Accommodation refers to the process used to obtain clear vision (i.e., to focus on an object at varying distances). This occurs when the internal ocular muscle (the ciliary muscle) contracts and causes a change in the crystalline lens of the eye to adjust for objects at different distances. Focusing must take place efficiently at all distances, and the eyes must be able to make the transition from focusing at nearpoint (a book or a paper) to farpoint (the teacher and the blackboard) and vice versa. It should take only a split second for this process of accommodation to occur.
- *Binocular fusion.* The ability to mentally combine the images from the two eyes into a single percept. There are two prerequisites for binocular fusion to occur. The first is that the two eyes must be aligned on the object of regard. This is termed *motor fusion;* it requires coordination of the six extraocular muscles on each eye and precision between the two eyes. *Sensory fusion* is the second aspect. This requires that the size and clarity of the two images be compatible. Only when these two aspects have occurred can the brain combine what the two eyes see into a single percept; binocular fusion has taken place.
- *Convergence and divergence.* The ability of both eyes to turn inward toward the medial plane and outward from the medial plane.
- *Stereopsis.* Binocular depth perception or three-dimensional vision.

For further description of these components' functions, see Gentile (1997).

Visual-Cognitive Components

Interpretation of the visual stimulus is a mental process involving cognition, which gives meaning to the visual stimulus (visual-cognitive). The visual-cognitive components include *visual attention, visual memory, discrimination,* and *integration of the visual stimulus* with other sense modalities.

Visual attention

Visual attention involves the selection of visual input. It also provides an appropriate time frame through which visual information is passed by the eye to the primary visual cortex of the brain, where visual perceptual processing can occur. Voluntary eye movements of localization, fixation, ocular pursuit, and gaze shift lay the foundation for optimal functioning of visual attention (Erhardt, 1989).

The four components of visual attention are as follows:
1. *Alertness* is reflective of the child's natural state of arousal. Alerting is the transition from an awake to an attentive and ready state needed for active learning and adaptive behavior.
2. *Selective attention* the ability to choose relevant visual information while ignoring the less relevant information; it is conscious, focused attention.
3. *Visual vigilance* is the conscious mental effort to concentrate and persist at a visual task. This skill is exhibited when a child plays diligently with a toy or when writing a letter.
4. *Divided, or shared, attention* is the ability to respond to two or more simultaneous tasks. This skill is exhibited when a child is engaged in one task that is automatic while visually monitoring another task.

Visual memory

Visual memory involves the integration of visual information with previous experiences. Long-term memory is the permanent storehouse, which has expansive capacity. In contrast, short-term memory can hold a limited number of unrelated bits of information for approximately 30 seconds.

Visual discrimination

Visual discrimination is the ability to detect features of stimuli for recognition, matching, and categorization. The specific visual discrimination abilities require the ability to note similarities and differences among forms and symbols with increasing complexity and then relate these back to information previously stored in long-term memory. These three abilities are described as follows:
1. *Recognition.* The ability to note key features of a stimulus and relate them to memory

2. *Matching.* The ability to note the similarities among visual stimuli
3. *Categorization.* The ability to mentally determine a quality or category on which similarities or differences can be noted

Visual perceptual abilities aid in the manipulation of a visual stimulus for visual discrimination (Todd, 1999). Visual perception has not been consistently defined. In addition, resources on visual perception use different terms and categories to define the same visual perceptual skills. This contributes to confusion because each discipline may define the same terms differently.

It is also important to note that a distinction exists between object (form) vision and spatial vision (Mishkin, Ungerleider, & Macko, 1983). Object vision is implicated in the visual identification of objects by color, texture, shape, and size (i.e., what things are). Spatial vision is concerned with the visual location of objects in space (i.e., where things are). These two classes of function are mediated by separate neural systems. The cortical tracts for both object vision and spatial vision are projected to the primary visual area, but the object vision pathway goes to the temporal lobe and the spatial vision pathway goes to the parietal lobe.

Based on studies after brain damage, these two functions have been shown to be independent (Necombe & Ratcliff, 1989). That is, disturbances of object recognition can occur without spatial disability, and spatial disability can occur with normal object perception. The following are definitions of the object (form) and spatial perceptual skills. Although they may not be separate entities, these groups of abilities or skills are labeled as follows:

1. Object (form) perception
    a. *Form constancy.* The recognition of forms and objects as the same in various environments, positions, and sizes. Form constancy helps a person develop stability and consistency in the visual world. It enables the person to recognize objects even when there are differences in orientation or detail. Form constancy enables a person to make assumptions regarding the size of an object even though visual stimuli may vary under different circumstances. The visual image of an object in the distance is much smaller than the image of the same object at close range, yet the person knows that the actual sizes are equivalent. An example of form constancy is that a school-age child can identify the letter *A* whether it is typed, written in manuscript, written in cursive, written in upper- or lower-case letters, or italicized.
    b. *Visual closure.* The identification of forms or objects from incomplete presentations. This enables the person to quickly recognize objects, shapes, and forms by mentally completing the image or by matching it to information previously stored in

memory. This allows the person to make assumptions regarding what the object is without having to see the complete presentation. For example, a child working at his or her desk is able to distinguish a pencil from a pen, even though both are partially hidden under some papers.
    c. *Figure-ground.* The differentiation between foreground or background forms and objects. It is the ability to separate essential important data from distracting surrounding information and the ability to attend to one aspect of a visual field while perceiving it in relation to the rest of the field. It is the ability to visually attend to what is important. For example, a child is able to visually find a favorite toy in a box filled with toys.

2. Spatial perception
    a. *Position in space.* The determination of the spatial relationship of figures and objects to oneself or other forms and objects. This provides the awareness of an object's position in relation to the observer or the perception of the direction in which it is turned. This perceptual ability is important in understanding directional language concepts such as in, out, up, down, in front of, behind, between, left, and right. In addition, position in space perception provides the ability to differentiate among letters and sequences of letters in a word or in a sentence (Frostig, Lefever, & Whittlesey, 1966). For example, the child knows how to place letters equal spaces apart, touching the line; he or she is able to recognize letters that extend below the line, such as *p, g, q,* or *y.*
    b. *Depth perception.* The determination of the relative distance between objects, figures, or landmarks and the observer and changes in planes of surfaces. This provides an awareness of how far away something is. This perceptual ability also helps us move in space (e.g., walking down stairs).
    c. *Topographic orientation.* The determination of the location of objects and settings and the route to the location. *Wayfinding* is dependent on a cognitive map of the environment. These maps include information about the destination, spatial information, instructions for execution of travel plans, recognizing places, keeping track of where one is while moving about, and anticipating features. These are important means of monitoring one's movement from place to place (Garling, Book, & Lindberg, 1984). For example, the child is able to leave the classroom for a drink of water from the water fountain down the hall and then return to his or her desk.

Visual imagery

Another important component in visual cognition is visual imagery, or visualization. Visual imagery refers to the ability to "picture" people, ideas, and objects in the mind's eye, even when the objects are not physically present. Developmentally, the child is first able to picture objects that make certain sounds and those that are familiar by taste or smell. The ability to picture what words say is the next step. This level of visual-verbal matching provides the foundation for reading comprehension and spelling.

Developmental Framework for Intervention

Warren (1993a) presented a developmental framework based on a bottom-up approach to evaluation and treatment. Using the work of Moore (Gilfoyle, Grady, & Moore, 1990), Warren suggested that with knowledge of where the deficit is located in the visual system, the therapist could design appropriate evaluation and treatment strategies to remediate basic problems and improve perceptual function. To apply this approach, it is necessary for the occupational therapist to have an understanding of the visual system, including both the visual-receptive and visual-cognitive components. Although Warren's model was presented as a developmental framework for evaluation and treatment of visual perceptual dysfunction in adults with acquired brain injuries, it is useful as a model for children with visual perceptual deficits. A hierarchy of visual perceptual skill development in the CNS is presented in Figure 13-2. The definitions of components of each level are provided in the following list and are used in later descriptions of intervention.

1. Three primary visual skills form the foundation for all visual functions.
   a. *Oculomotor control.* The efficient eye movements that ensure that the scan path is accomplished.

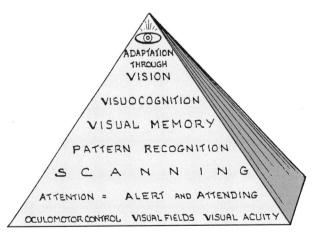

figure**13-2** Hierarchy of visual perceptual skill development. *(From Warren, M. [1993]. A hierarchial model for evaluation and treatment of visual perceptual dysfunction in adult acquired brain injury. Part 1.* American Journal of Occupational Therapy, 47, *42-54.)*

b. *Visual fields.* Register the complete visual scene.
   c. *Visual acuity.* Ensures that the visual information sent to the CNS is accurate.
2. *Visual attention.* The thoroughness of the scan path depends on visual attention.
3. *Scanning.* Pattern recognition is dependent on organized, thorough scanning of the visual environment. The retina must record all of the detail of the scene systematically through the use of a scan path.
4. *Pattern recognition.* The ability to store information in memory requires pattern detection and recognition. This is the identification of the salient features of an object.
   a. Configural aspects (shape, contour, and general features).
   b. Specific features of an object (details of color, shading, and texture).
5. *Visual memory.* The mental manipulation of visual information needed for visual cognition requires the ability to retain the information in memory for immediate recall or to store for later retrieval.
6. *Visual cognition.* The ability to mentally manipulate visual information and integrate it with other sensory information to solve problems, formulate plans, and make decisions.

Warren's model provides a framework for assessing vision alone without consideration of the other sensory systems. When visual perceptual problems relate to sensory integration (SI) dysfunction, models based on SI theories guide evaluation and intervention (Burpee, 1997). These models consider organization of multisensory systems and the influence of vision as it integrates with other sensory systems.

Skeffington (1963) recognized that vision was more than light coming from the physical environment, entering the eye, and then becoming transformed into an external phenomenon. He believed that vision cannot be separated from the total individual nor from any of the sensory systems because it is integrated into all human performance. He proposed a model that describes the visual process as the meshing of audition, proprioception, kinesthesia, and body sense with vision. This interaction is presented by four connecting circles, each denoting one important subsystem (Figure 13-3). The core, where each circle connects with the others, is vision. It should be clear from the model that visual perception is not obtained by vision alone. It comes from combining visual skills with all other sensory modalities, including the proprioceptive and vestibular systems.

Through extension of Skeffington's model, vision can be viewed as a dynamic blending of sensory information in which new visual and motor input are combined with previously stored data and then used to guide a reaction. Research demonstrates an expansive interconnectivity of

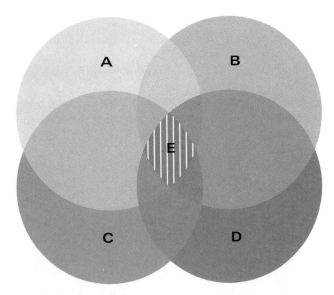

figure **13-3**   Skeffington model of vision. **A,** Antigravity: coming to terms with gravity to move. **B,** Centering: ability to locate objects in space. **C,** Identification: ability to focus on information, to refine and discriminate detail, and to save that information in the brain. **D,** Speech audition: ability to communicate through speech and gesture and to use hearing. **E,** Vision: interweaving of all these modalities (**A** through **D**). *(From Skeffington, A.N. [1963].* The Skeffington Papers, *Series 36, No. 2 [p. 11]. Santa Ana, CA: Optometric Extension Program.)*

sensory systems (Damasio, 1989; Thelen & Smith, 1994). Studies of brain activity confirm that when an individual is using the visual system, many areas of the brain are activated. Evidence of full brain activity when visualizing supports the concept that vision should be viewed within the totality of all sensory systems.

■ DEVELOPMENTAL SEQUENCE

Visual-Receptive Components

Like other areas of development, the development of visual-receptive components takes place according to a prescribed timetable, which begins in the womb. By gestational week 24, gross anatomic structures are in place, and the visual pathway is complete. Between gestational weeks 24 and 40, the visual system, particularly the retina and visual cortex, undergo extensive maturation, differentiation, and remodeling (Glass, 1993). As early as the fifth gestational month, eye movements are produced by vestibular influences (DeQuiros & Schranger, 1979). At birth the infant has rudimentary visual fixation ability and brief reflexive tracking ability. The visual system at this age is relatively immature compared with other sensory systems, with considerable development occurring over the next 6 months (Glass, 1993).

Toward the end of the second month, accommodation, convergence, and oculomotor subsystems are established (Bouska et. al., 1990). Maximum accommodation is reached at 5 years of age, and the child should be able to sustain this skill effort for protracted periods at a fixed distance.

Controlled tracking skills progress in a developmental pattern from horizontal eye movements to eye movements in vertical, diagonal, and circular directions. By kindergarten a child should be able to move his or her eyes with smooth control and coordination in all directions. This can be demonstrated by asking the child to follow a moving object at 8 to 12 inches. If the child moves his or her head along with the eyes, this skill is still developing. Visual acuity is best at 18 years of age and tends to decline thereafter.

Visual-Cognitive Components

Some visual-cognitive capacities are present at birth, and other higher-level visual-cognitive tasks are not fully developed until adolescence. This development occurs through perceptual learning, the process of extracting information from the environment. This increases with experience and practice and through stimulation from the environment.

Object (form) vision

Long before infants can manipulate objects or move around space, they have well-developed visual perceptual abilities, including pattern recognition, form constancy, and depth perception. Infants as young as 1 week of age show a differential response to patterns, with complex designs and human faces receiving more attention than simple circles and triangles. The infant learns to attend to relevant aspects of visual stimuli, to make discriminations, and to interpret available cues according to experiences.

Visual perception develops as the child matures, with most developmental changes taking place by 9 years of age. However, children vary in the rate at which they acquire perceptual abilities, in their effective use of these capacities, and in the versatility and comfort with which they apply these functions (Levine, 1987).

These abilities to perceptually analyze and discriminate objects systematically increase throughout childhood. It is generally believed that visual perception develops in the following ways:

- General to specific
- Whole to parts
- Concrete to abstract
- Familiar to novel

However, these sequences have not been proven, and in certain instances the opposite may occur. For example, visual development may follow specific to general. The child first learns to recognize an object

table 13-1 Developmental Ages for Emergence of Visual Perceptual Skills

Perception	Developmental Age
OBJECT (FORM)	
Figure-ground perception	Improves between 3 and 5 years of age; stabilized growth at 6 to 7 years of age
Form constancy	Dramatic improvement between 6 and 7 years of age, with less improvement from 8 to 9 years of age
SPATIAL	
Position in space	Development complete at 7 to 9 years of age
Spatial relationships	Improves to approximately 10 years of age

Modified from Williams, H. (1983). *Perceptual and motor development.* Englewood Cliffs, NJ: Prentice Hall.

based on its general appearance and not by specific details. As the child learns to classify objects into categories and types, it becomes apparent that the child is able to extract the features that make the object part of that category (Mussen, Conger, & Kagan, 1979). For example, the child learns to categorize cars as certain types or classify animals according to their species. Further study is needed in this area. Williams (1983) estimated the developmental ages when primary visual perceptual skills develop (Table 13-1).

Bouska and others (1990) described three areas in which a child demonstrates increasing ability to visually discriminate. These include the ability to (1) recognize and distinguish specific distinctive features (e.g., that *b* and *d* are different because of one feature), (2) observe invariant relationships in events that occur repeatedly over time (e.g., a favorite toy is the same even when distance makes it appear smaller), and (3) find a hierarchy of pattern or structure, allowing the processing of the largest unit possible for adaptive use during a particular task (e.g., a map is scanned globally for the shape of a country, but subordinate features are scanned for the route of a river) (Gibson & Levin, 1975).

The child's first perceptions of the world develop primarily from tactile, kinesthetic, and vestibular input. As these three basic senses become integrated with the higher-level senses, vision and audition gradually take over. Young children or beginning readers tend to prefer learning through their tactile and kinesthetic senses and have lower preferences for visual and auditory learning (Carbo, 1983). At 6 or 7 years of age, most children appear to prefer kinesthetic, tactile, visual, and auditory learning, in that order. They learn easily through their sense of touch and whole-body movement and have difficulty learning through listening activities. Generally, boys are less auditory and verbal and remain kinesthetic longer than girls (Restak, 1979). Around third grade most children become highly visual, and not until fifth grade do many children learn well through their auditory sense.

In the young child, visual discrimination of forms precedes the visual motor ability of copying forms by years. Throughout elementary school the child is able to handle more internal detail of figures and to understand, recall, and recreate such configurations (Levine, 1987). Children begin to use simultaneous and sequential data to develop strategies, and cognitive or learning styles begin to emerge. In addition, children learn best through their dominant sensory input channel. About 40% of school-age children remember visually presented information, whereas only 20% to 30% recall what is heard (Carbo, Dunn, & Dunn, 1986).

Information processing in the visual perceptual–motor domain has been identified as one of the major factors that can predict readiness for the first grade. There is evidence that the child who enters school with delayed perceptual development may not catch up with his or her peers in academic achievement (Morency & Wepman, 1973). Adequate perceptual discrimination is considered necessary for the development of reading and writing skills (Moore, 1979).

Children gradually develop the abilities to attend to, integrate, sort, and retrieve increasingly larger chunks of visual data. These stimuli from the environment usually arrive for processing either in a simultaneous array or in a specific serial order (Levine, 1987). An example of simultaneous processing involves observing and later trying to recall what someone wore.

Sequential processing involves the integration of separate elements into groups whose essential nature is temporal where each element leads only to one another. It enables the child to perceive an ordered series of events (Kirby & Das, 1978). An example of sequential processing is the visual information provided in the written instructions for assembling a plastic model. An effective learner in the classroom needs to be able to evaluate, retain, process, and produce both simultaneous and sequential packages of information or action. In addition, children must learn to analyze and synthesize material containing more detail at a faster rate.

In adolescence, perceptual skills are enhanced by their interrelationship with expanding cognitive skill. Thus the adolescent can imagine, create, and construct complex visual forms. The adolescent is able to mentally manipulate visual information to solve increasingly complex problems, formulate plans, and make decisions.

Spatial vision

In the developmental process of organizing space, the child first acquires a concept of vertical dimensions, followed by a concept of horizontal dimensions. Oblique and diagonal dimensions are more complex, and perception of these spatial coordinates matures later. The 3- to 4-year-old child can discriminate vertical lines from horizontal ones but is unable to distinguish vertical, horizontal, and oblique lines until about 6 years of age (Cratty, 1970). The ability to discriminate between mirror or reversed-imaged numbers and letters, such as *b* and *d*, and *p* and *q*, does not mature until around 7 years of age (Ilg & Ames, 1981).

The child develops an understanding of left and right from the internal awareness that his or her body has two sides (Suchoff, 1987). This understanding of left and right is called *laterality* and proceeds in stages, according to Cratty (1970). A child's awareness of his or her own body is generally established by 6 or 7 years of age. Before 7 years of age, a child is not yet ready to handle spatial concepts on a strictly visual basis. The child must relate them back to his or her own body.

Around the eighth year the child begins to project the laterality concepts outside himself or herself. The child then develops *directionality*, or the understanding of an external object's position in space in relationship to himself or herself. This allows the child to handle spatial phenomena almost exclusively in a visual manner. By sensing a difference between body sides, the child becomes aware that figures and objects also have a right and a left. The child "feels" this visually.

Directionality is thought to be important in the visual discrimination of letters and numbers for both reading and writing. First a child learns these concepts in relation to himself or herself and then transfers them to symbols and words.

■ SPECIFIC VISUAL PERCEPTUAL PROBLEMS

Visual-Receptive Components

The importance of good vision for classroom work cannot be emphasized enough. More than 50% of a student's time is spent working at near-point visual tasks such as reading and writing. Another 20% is spent on tasks that require the student to shift focus from distance to near and near to distance, such as copying from the board. Thus for more than 70% of the day, tremendous stress is being put on the visual system (Ritty, Solan, & Cool, 1992). Many students with vision dysfunctions can have difficulty meeting the behavioral demands of sitting still, sustaining attention, and completing their work.

Figure 13-4 presents a sample list of behaviors noted in children with specific visual problems (Optometric Ex-

tension Program Foundation, 1985). In addition to these behaviors noted in the list, Seiderman (1984) suggested that individuals with functional vision problems may use any of the following compensatory techniques:

- Avoidance of reading work
- Asthenopic symptoms (visual fatigue)
- Adaptation through the development of a refractive error to perform near-centered visual task demands

Disruption of oculomotor control can occur through disruption of cranial nerve function or disruption of central neural control. The pattern of oculomotor dysfunction depends on the areas of the brain that have been injured and the nature of the injury (Leigh & Zee, 1983). Oculomotor problems can limit ability to control and direct gaze. In addition, when large amounts of energy must be used on the motor components of vision, little energy may be left for visual-cognitive processing (Hyvarinen, 1988). See Warren (1993a) for a detailed description of oculomotor deficits and other deficits seen in visual-receptive components.

Refractive errors

The child who is nearsighted has blurred distant vision but generally experiences clarity at near point. The child who is farsighted frequently has clear distant and near vision but has to exert extra effort to maintain clear vision at near point. The child with astigmatism experiences blurred vision at distance and near, with the degree of loss of clarity depending on the amount of astigmatism. Measures of visual acuity alone do not predict how well children interpret visual information (Hyvarinen, 1988). Other determinants include the ability to see objects in low-contrast lighting conditions, the ability of the eye to adapt to different lighting conditions, visual field problems, accommodation, and other oculomotor functions (Hyvarinen, 1988).

If accommodation takes longer than previously described, words appear blurry and the child tends to lose his or her place, missing important information and understanding. When accommodation for near objects is poor, presbyopia exists; this individual is described as farsighted.

When the conditions of motor fusion and sensory fusion have not been met for binocular fusion to occur (this process was described previously), single binocular vision is at best difficult and at worst impossible. If one eye overtly turns in, out, up, or down because of muscular imbalance, the condition is known as *strabismus*, sometimes referred to as a *crossed* or *wandering eye*. This can result in double vision or a mental suppression of one of the images. This, in turn, can have effects on the development of visual perception. Some children have surgery to correct an eye turn. Although this intervention can correct the eye cosmetically, it does not always result in binocular vision.

1. **Appearance of eyes**
   One eye turns in or out at any time _____
   Reddened eyes or lids _____
   Eyes tear excessively _____
   Encrusted eyelids _____
   Frequent styes on lids _____
2. **Complaints when using eyes at desk**
   Headaches in forehead or temples _____
   Burning or itching after reading or
     desk work _____
   Nausea or dizziness _____
   Print blurs after reading a short time _____
3. **Behavioral signs of visual problems**
   a. Eye movement abilities (ocular motility)
      Head turns as reads across pages _____
      Loses place often during reading _____
      Needs finger or marker to keep place _____
      Displays short attention span in
        reading or copying _____
      Too frequently omits words _____
      Repeatedly omits "small" words _____
      Writes up or down hill on paper _____
      Rereads or skips lines unknowingly _____
      Orients drawings poorly on page _____
   b. Eye teaming abilities (binocularity)
      Complains of seeing double (diplopia) _____
      Repeats letters within words _____
      Omits letters, numbers, or phrases _____
      Misaligns digits in number columns _____
      Squints, closes, or covers one eye _____
      Tilts head extremely while working
        at desk _____
      Consistently shows gross postural
        deviations at all desk activities _____
   c. Eye-hand coordination abilities
      Must feel things to assist in any
        interpretation required _____
      Eyes not used to "steer" hand
        movement (extreme lack of
        orientation, placement of words
        or drawings on page) _____
      Writes crookedly, poorly spaced:
        cannot stay on ruled lines _____
      Misaligns both horizontal and vertical
        series of numbers _____
      Uses hand or fingers to keep place
        on the page _____
      Uses other hand as "spacer" to control
        spacing and alignment on page _____
      Repeatedly confuses left-right directions _____

   d. Visual-form perception (visual compar-
      ison, visual imagery, visualization) _____
      Mistakes words with same or similar
        beginnings _____
      Fails to recognize same word in next
        sentence _____
      Reverses letters and/or words in
        writing and copying _____
      Confuses likenesses and minor
        differences _____
      Confuses same word in same sentence _____
      Repeatedly confuses similar beginnings
        and endings of words _____
      Fails to visualize what is read either
        silently or orally _____
      Whispers to self for reinforcement
        while reading silently _____
      Returns to "drawing with fingers" to
        decide likes and differences _____
   e. Refractive status (e.g., nearsightedness,
      farsightedness, focus problems) _____
      Comprehension reduces as reading
        continued; loses interest too quickly _____
      Mispronounces similar words as
        continues reading _____
      Blinks excessively at desk tasks and/or
        reading; not elsewhere _____
      Holds book too closely; face too close
        to desk surface _____
      Avoids all possible near-centered tasks _____
      Complains of discomfort in tasks that
        demand visual interpretation _____
      Closes or covers one eye when reading
        or doing desk work _____
      Makes errors in copying from chalk-
        board to paper on desk _____
      Makes errors in copying from reference
        book to notebook _____
      Squints to see chalkboard, or requests
        to move nearer _____
      Rubs eyes during or after short periods
        of visual activity _____
      Fatigues easily; blinks to make chalk-
        board clear up after desk task _____

   NOTE: Students found to have any of the visual or eye problems on the checklist should be referred to a behavioral optometrist. Referral lists of behavioral optometrists are available from Optometric Extension Program Foundation, 2912 S. Daimler, Santa Ana, CA 92705.

figure**13-4**   Checklist of observable clues to classroom vision problems.

Another type of binocular dysfunction is termed *phoria*. Phoria refers to a tendency for one eye to go slightly in, out, up, or down but with the absence of overt misalignment of the two eyes. A phoria requires that the child expend additional mechanical effort to maintain motor fusion of the two eyes, whether focusing near or far. The extra effort frequently detracts from the child's ability to process and interpret the meaning of what he or she sees.

Visual-Cognitive Components
Attention

To review, visual attention is composed of alertness, selective attention, vigilance, and shared attention. If the child's state of alertness or arousal is impaired, the child may demonstrate behaviors of overattentiveness, underattentiveness, or poor sustained attention (Todd, 1999). Children who are overattentive may be compelled to respond to visual stimuli around them rather than attend to the task at hand, may be easily distracted by visual stimuli, and may demonstrate continual visual searching behaviors. Children who are underattentive may have difficulty orienting to visual stimuli, may habituate quickly to a visual stimulus, and may fatigue easily. At this level a child may refrain from attending to a familiar stimulus. A child with poor sustained attention may demonstrate a high activity level and be easily distracted.

Selective attention is the next level of visual attention, and a child with difficulty in this area demonstrates a reduced ability to focus on a visual target. The child may have difficulty screening out unimportant or irrelevant information, focus on irrelevant stimuli, and be distracted by irrelevant stimuli. A child with difficulty in selective attention is easily confused. The child may focus on unnecessary tasks or information and therefore not obtain the specific information needed for the task.

A child with reduced vigilance skills shows reduced persistence on a visual task and poor or cursory examination of visual stimuli. The child cannot maintain visual attention. The more complex the visual structure of an object, the lengthier the process of visual analysis and the greater vigilance skills are needed. A child with deficits in shared attention can only focus well on one task at a time. He may be easily confused or distracted if required to share visual attention between two tasks.

Enns and Cameron (1987) suggested that visual inattention is the result of an inability to select the features that differentiate objects in a visual array. The child cannot see, recognize, or isolate the salient features and therefore does not know where to focus visual attention. Luria (1966) suggested that problems of visual recognition represent a breakdown of active feature-by-feature analysis necessary for interpreting a visual image.

Memory

The child with visual memory deficits has poor or reduced ability to recognize or retrieve visual information and to store visual information in short- or long-term memory. The child may fail to adequately attend, fail to allow for storage of visual information, or show a prolonged response time. The child may demonstrate the inability to recognize or match visual stimuli presented previously because he or she has not stored this information in memory or he or she may not be able to retrieve it from memory (Todd, 1999). The child may have good memory for life experiences but not for factual material and may fail to relate information to prior knowledge. The child may demonstrate inconsistent recall abilities, and the child may demonstrate poor ability to use mnemonic strategies for storage.

Visual discrimination

The child with poor discrimination abilities may demonstrate an inadequate ability to recognize, match, and categorize. Ulman (1986) proposed that a finite set of visual operations, or "routines," are performed to extract shape properties and spatial relations. Usually an individual recognizes an object by orienting to its top or bottom. A child with poor matching skills may demonstrate difficulty matching the same shape presented in a different spatial orientation or may confuse similar shapes. A child with poor matching skills may have difficulty in recognizing form within a complex field.

Object (form) vision. Children with form constancy problems may have difficulty recognizing forms and objects presented in different sizes or different orientations in space, or when there are differences in detail. This interferes with the child's ability to organize and classify perceptual experiences for meaningful cognitive operations (Piaget, 1964). This may result in difficulty recognizing letters or words in different styles of print or in making the transition from printed to cursive letters.

A child with a visual closure deficit may be unable to identify a form or object if an incomplete presentation is made. Therefore the child would always need to see the complete object to identify it. For example, a child would have difficulty reading a sign whose letters were partially occluded by tree branches.

The child with figure-ground problems may not be able to pick out a specific toy from a shelf. The child may have difficulty with sorting and organizing personal belongings. The child may overattend to details and miss the big picture or may overlook details and miss the important information. Children with figure-ground problems may have difficulty attending to a word on a printed page because they cannot block out other words around it. The child with figure-ground difficulties may not have good visual search strategies. Marr (1982) suggested that control of the direction of gaze is a prerequisite for efficiency of visual search. Cohen (1981) described these visual search strategies:

1. The reviewer looks for specific visual information and makes crude distinctions between figure and ground by isolating one figure from another.
2. The viewer determines which figures are most meaningful (the process stops here when recognition is immediate).
3. When recognition is not immediate, the viewer makes a hypothesis about the visual information received and directs attention to selected items to test the hypothesis.

Rogow and Rathwill (1989) found that good readers more frequently proceeded from the left to the right and from the top down to find "hidden figures" than did poor readers. Good readers were also more flexible in their approach; they rotated the page as needed and were not content until they found as many hidden figures as possible. The good readers also were less distressed by ambiguity, and they understood that pictures could be viewed in different ways.

Spatial vision. A child with position-in-space difficulty has trouble discriminating among objects because of their placement in space. These children also have difficulty planning their actions in relation to objects around them. They may show letter reversals past 8 years of age and may show confusion regarding the sequence of letters or numbers in a word or math problem (e.g., was/saw). Writing and spacing letters and words on paper may be a problem. The children may show difficulty in understanding directional language such as in, out, on, under, next to, up, down, and in front of.

Decreased depth perception can affect the child's ability to walk through spaces and to catch a ball. The child may be unable to visually determine when the surface plane has changed and may have difficulty with steps and curbs. Transference of visual spatial notations across two visual planes can make copying from the blackboard difficult. Faulty interpretation of the spatial relationships can contribute to a problem with sorting and organizing personal belongings.

A child who has diminished topographic orientation may be easily lost and unable to find his or her way from one location to the next. The child may also demonstrate difficulty determining the location of objects and settings.

Diagnoses With Problems in Visual Perception

When children with disabling conditions have visual problems, the effects of the visual impairments can be tremendous. Numerous studies have found a high frequency of vision problems among individuals with disabilities (Ciner, Macks, & Schanel-Klitsch, 1991; Duckman, 1979; Fanning, 1971; Scheiman, 1984). Severe

refractive errors are common among children with developmental problems (Rogow, 1992). Impaired visual attention can have a pervasive negative influence on the functional behavior of these children. Often considered distractible, these children may be able to locate objects but have difficulty sustaining eye contact or recognizing objects visually (Rogow, 1992).

Retinopathy of prematurity is the single most often cited cause of blindness in preterm infants. Cortical visual impairment also occurs in preterm infants and is generally associated with severe CNS damage, such as periventricular leukomalacia. Other visual disorders common in preterm children include lenses that are too thick, poor visual acuity, astigmatism, extreme myopia, strabismus, amblyopia, and anisometropia (unequal refraction of the eyes) (Fledelius, 1976). These children also have difficulty processing visual information. Measures of visual attention, pattern discrimination, visual recognition, memory, and visual motor integration are lower than those for full-term infants (Caron & Caron, 1981; Rose, 1980; Sigman & Parmelee, 1974). Studies of older children suggest that these problems often persist (Siegel, 1983).

Children with developmental disabilities commonly have a coexisting diagnosis of blindness or other visual impairment. In addition, these children may have sensory integrative deficits that further complicate their functional abilities (Roley-Smith & Schneck, in press).

Children with cerebral palsy (CP) have frequently been identified as a group with visual perception deficits (Abercrombie, 1963; Breakey, Wilson, & Wilson, 1994). Children with CP often have a strabismus, ocular motor problems, convergence insufficiencies, or nystagmus. These problems may also limit ability to control and direct visual gaze (Rogow, 1992).

Early research indicated that the degree of perceptual impairment in persons with CP was related to the type and severity of the motor impairment (Birch, 1964). Children with athetosis have been found to have fewer visual perceptual disorders than children with spasticity (Abercrombie, 1963). In a comparison study, children with CP scored significantly lower scores on a motor-free test of visual perception (Menken, Cermak, & Fisher, 1987) than typical children. These findings supported earlier studies showing that the group with spastic quadriplegia demonstrated the greatest problems in visual perception.

In children with language delay, poorly developed visual perception may contribute to their language difficulties. For example, language moves from the general to the specific. Young children call every animal with four legs a dog. Eventually they are able to visually discriminate between dogs and lions, and the vocabulary follows the visual perceptual lead. Next, they can tell dalmatians from dachshunds, but they are unable to recognize that they are both dogs. Finally, the ability to categorize and generalize emerges somewhere between 7 and 9 years of age. In addition, the child who has visual spatial perception deficits may show difficulty in understanding directional language such as *in, on, under,* and *next to.*

Not all children with learning disabilities have visual perception problems (Hung, Fisher, & Cermak, 1987). However, visual perceptual problems are found more frequently in persons who show significantly higher verbal scores than performance scores on intelligence testing.

Children with learning disabilities may have difficulty filtering out irrelevant environmental stimuli and therefore present with erratic visual attention skills. Children who have difficulty interpreting and using visual information effectively are described as having visual perceptual problems because they have not acquired adequate visual perceptual skills in spite of normal vision (Todd, 1999).

Daniels and Ryley (1991) studied the incidence of visual perceptual and visual motor deficits in children with psychiatric disorders. In this study, visual-motor skills deficits occurred far more frequently than visual perception skills deficits. When visual perception problems did occur, they were in conjunction with visual-motor skill problems. Some children with autism have demonstrated poor oculomotor function (Rosenhall, Johansson, & Gilberg, 1988). Children with autism often do not appear to focus their vision directly on what they are doing (Osterling & Dawson, 1994). A possible explanation is that they are using peripheral vision to the exclusion of focal vision.

Effects of Visual Perceptual Problems on Performance Areas

The effects of visual perceptual problems may be subtle in nature, with no obvious disabilities. However, when the child is asked to perform a visual perceptual task, he or she may be slow or unable to perform the task. Visual perception dysfunction affects the child's ability to use tools and relate materials to one another (Ayres, 1979); thus bilateral manipulative skills are affected to a greater degree than the child's basic prehension patterns indicate. The child with visual perceptual deficits may show problems with cutting, coloring, constructing with blocks or other construction toys, doing puzzles, using fasteners, and tying shoes. Visual perception deficits can influence children's self-care, work, and play and leisure performance.

Children with visual perception problems may demonstrate difficulty with activities of daily living (ADLs). In grooming, the child may have difficulty obtaining the necessary supplies and using a mirror to comb and style hair. Applying toothpaste to the brush may be difficult for the child. Fasteners; donning and doffing clothing, prostheses, and orthoses; tying shoes; and matching clothes may present problems. The skilled use of hand-

writing, telephones, computers, and communication devices may all present difficulty for the child with visual-cognitive problems. Community mobility may be difficult because the child is unable to locate objects and find his or her way. In play, the child may demonstrate difficulty with playing games and sports, drawing and coloring, cutting with scissors, pasting, constructing, and doing puzzles.

Work and productive activities such as home management and classroom assignments may present problems for the child with visual perceptual problems. For example, the child may have trouble sorting and folding clothes as a home management task. Educational activities such as reading, spelling, writing, and math may be difficult for the child. The following section elaborates on the educational problems seen in the school-age child.

Problems in reading

Gibson (1971) has delineated different characteristics of printed (written) information necessary for reading. These include a word's graphic configuration, orthography (order of letters), phonology (sounds represented), and semantics (meaning). The child benefits from these multiple simultaneous clues in reading. If the child has difficulty with one characteristic, he or she can rely on his or her perception of the other characteristics to extract the meaning. In early reading, children first encounter the visual configuration (graphics) and orthographics in a printed word. The child then must break the written word into its component phonemes (phonology), hold them in active working memory, and then synthesize and blend the phonemes to form recognizable words (semantics). After practice, this step is accomplished and the word can then be dealt with as a gestalt and added to the child's growing sight vocabulary. Sight vocabulary consists of words that are instantly recognized as gestalts. As a child's reliance on sight vocabulary increases, decoding takes less time and the child develops automaticity, which allows the child to begin to concentrate on comprehension and retention.

Understanding sentences requires adding two more variables, context (word order) and syntax (grammatic construction), to the skills previously discussed (Levine, 1987). To read paragraphs, chapters, and texts, it is assumed that decoding is well automatized. A hierarchy can be assumed here in that any developmental dysfunctions that impair decoding or sentence comprehension impede text reading.

The segmenting of written words in early reading calls for a variety of skills. First, children must be able to recognize individual letter symbols. This requires visual attention, visual memory, and visual discrimination. In the presence of severe dysfunction, recognition of words may be impaired (Levine, 1987) and thus interfere with the acquisition of sight vocabulary. Problems with visual perception might be suspected in a child who appears to be better at understanding what was read than at actually decoding the words. This child has good language abilities but some trouble processing written words.

Visual perceptual attributes are different from the capacity to assimilate visual detail. The child may be diagnosed as having visual perceptual problems when he or she is limited in attending to or extracting data presented simultaneously. In this instance the child does not have difficulty with the specific perceptual content but with the amount of information that must be simultaneously perceived to understand the whole.

Memory deficiencies also present reading problems (Levine, 1987). Children with visual memory problems may be unable to remember the visual shape of letters and words. Such children may also demonstrate the inability to associate these shapes with letters, sounds, and words (Greene, 1987). Children with weaknesses of visual-verbal associative memory have difficulty establishing easily retrievable or recognizable sound-symbol associations. They are unable to associate the sound, visual configuration, or meaning of the word with what is seen or heard.

Children with difficulty with active working memory cannot hold one aspect of the reading process in suspension while pursuing another component. It is closely related to perceptual span, or the ability to recall the beginning of the sentence while reading the end of it. The child must take a second look at the beginning of a sentence after reading the end of it.

Children with visual discrimination deficits may not be able to recognize symbols and therefore may be slow to master the alphabet and numbers. Their relatively weak grasp of constancy of forms may make visual discrimination an inefficient process. Some children, therefore, cannot readily discern the differences between visually similar symbols. Confusion between the letters *p, q,* and *g* and between *a* and *o,* as well as letter reversals, may ensue, such as the notorious differentiation between *b* and *d.* Visual discrimination abilities (form perception and spatial perception) are somewhat less important at advanced stages of the learning-to-read process than they are during the initial stages of reading acquisition (deHirsch, Jansky, & Langford, 1966; Jansky & deHirsh, 1972; Lyle, 1969).

Confusion over the directionality and other spatial characteristics of a word may result in weak registration in visual memory, again possibly creating significant delays in the consolidation of a sight vocabulary. Thus even frequently encountered words need to be analyzed anew each time they appear. A child with visual spatial deficits has difficulty with map reading and interpretation of instructional graphics such as charts and diagrams. Graphic representations require the child to integrate, extract the most salient elements from, condense, and organize

the large amount of stimuli presented at once. Again, the child may not have difficulty with the perceptual content, but the amount of information to be simultaneously assimilated is more than the child can integrate and remember (Levine, 1987).

Problems in spelling

Children with impaired processing of simultaneous visual stimuli may have difficulty with spelling (Boder, 1973). Their inability to visualize words may result from indistinct or distorted initial visual registration. Such children who have a strong sense of sound-symbol association may make what Boder calls *dyseidetic errors*— spelling words phonetically (e.g., lite for light), yet incorrectly. They exhibit spelling inaccuracies that reflect good phonetic approximations but are inaccurate. Visual sequential memory is necessary for remembering the sequence of letters in a word. The child may exhibit poor spelling and be unaware of letters omitted.

Problems in handwriting

Pilot studies have begun to explore the relationship between visual-cognitive skills and handwriting (Chapman & Wedell, 1972; Yost & Lesiak, 1980; Ziviani, Hayes, & Chant, 1990). Tseng and Cermak (1993) suggested that the role of visual perception shows little relationship to handwriting, whereas kinesthesia, visual motor integration, and motor planning appear to be more closely related to handwriting. However, further research is necessary to provide information concerning the role of visual perception in handwriting.

Visual-cognitive abilities may affect writing in any one or any combination of the following. Children with problems in attention may have difficulty with the correct letter formation, spelling, mechanics of grammar, punctuation, and capitalization and the formulation of a sequential flow of ideas necessary for written communication. For the child to write spontaneously, he or she must be able to revisualize letters and words without visual cues. Therefore if the child has visual memory problems, he or she may have difficulty recalling the shape and formation of letters and numbers. Other problems seen in the child with poor visual memory would be the child mixing small and capital letters within a sentence, the same letter written many ways on the same page, and the inability to print the alphabet from memory. In addition, legibility may be poor, and the child may need a model to write.

Visual discrimination problems may affect the child's handwriting. The child with poor form constancy does not recognize errors in his or her own handwriting. The child may be unable to recognize letters or words in different prints and therefore have difficulty in copying from a different type of print to handwriting. The child may also show poor recognition of letters or numbers in different environments, positions, or sizes. If the child is unable to discriminate a letter, he or she may show poor letter formation. A child with visual-closure difficulty always needs to see the complete presentation of what he or she is to copy. If the child has figure-ground problems, he or she may have difficulty in copying because he or she is unable to determine what is to be written. Therefore the child may omit important segments.

Visual spatial problems can affect the child's handwriting in many ways. The child may show reversals of letters such as *m, w, b, d, s, c,* and *z* and of numbers *2, 3, 5, 6, 7,* and *9*. If the child is unable to discriminate left from right, he or she may have difficulty with the left-to-right progression of writing words and sentences. The child may demonstrate overspacing or underspacing and have trouble keeping within the margins. He or she may be unable to relate one part of the letter to another part of the letter and therefore show inconsistency in letter size. The child may have difficulty with the placement of letters on a line and the ability to adapt the letter sizes to the space provided on the paper or worksheet.

Visual-motor integration

In handwriting, the ability to integrate the visual image of letters or shapes with the appropriate motor response is necessary. Visual-motor integration is not well understood because it is not a unitary process and consequently can be disrupted for a variety of reasons. Failure on visual-motor tests may be caused by underlying visual-cognitive deficits, including visual discrimination, poor fine motor ability, inability to integrate visual-cognitive and motor processes, or a combination of these abilities. Therefore careful analysis is necessary to determine the underlying problem. Tseng and Murray (1994) examined the relationship of perceptual motor measures to legibility of handwriting in Chinese school-age children, and visual-motor integration was found to be the best predictor of handwriting.

Mathematics

The child with visual perceptual problems has difficulty correctly aligning columns for calculation, and therefore the answers are incorrect because of alignment and not because of calculation skills. Worksheets with many rows and columns of math problems may be disorganizing to children with figure-ground problems. Children with poor visual memory may have difficulty using a calculator. Visual memory may also present problems for students when addition and subtraction problems require multiple steps. Geometry, because of its spatial characteristics, presents much difficulty for the child with visual spatial perception problems. Problem solving often involves recognizing, discriminating, and comparing object form and space as a foundation for higher-level mathematic skills. Visual imagery required to match and compare forms and shapes is difficult for students with

visual perceptual problems and interferes with learning these underlying skills.

■ EVALUATION METHODS

In evaluation of visual perceptual function, the therapist considers the entire process of vision and examines the relationship of visual function to behavior and performance (Seiderman, 1984). Visual-receptive and visual-cognitive components may represent different issues in a child's school performance. Problems can and do exist in either area, with differing effects on the learning process. However, visual-receptive components can influence the information obtained for visual-cognitive analysis. Because receptive and cognitive components are important in the visual processing of information, individual assessment of the child should be conducted within a multidisciplinary approach, realizing that the interplay between visual-receptive, visual-cognitive, and school success is different for each child (Flax, 1984).

Reports generated by other educational or medical specialists often provide standardized measures of performance. Securing this information will often eliminate the need for the occupational therapist to spend time administering additional visuomotor or visual perceptual tests that yield the same information. This information may also assist the occupational therapist in selecting alternative measures that yield different data that could further help in understanding a child's problem. An interview with the teacher or classroom observation should be a major component in the assessment process. For example, information on the visual stimulation in the classroom, which could affect the students' attention and focus, should be determined. Another example is to determine whether most visual work is done at near point or far point for copying.

Thus the occupational therapist's findings can be integrated with those of the reading specialist, psychologist, speech-language pathologist, and classroom teacher as a part of the multidisciplinary team. By combining test results and analysis of the child's performance, the team ascertains the nature of the interaction of the disability with the activity. A vision specialist, such as an opthalmologist or an optometrist, may be needed to assess visual-receptive dysfunction and to remediate the condition.

Visual-Receptive Assessment

Evaluation should begin by focusing on the integrity of the visual-receptive components, including visual fields, visual acuity, and oculomotor control (Warren, 1993b). If deficits occur in these foundation skills, then insufficient or inaccurate information regarding the location and features of objects is sent to the CNS. Therefore the quality of learning through the visual sense is severely affected. Warren (1990) suggested that what sometimes appear to be visual-cognitive deficits are actually visual-receptive problems, which may include oculomotor disturbances. Therefore visual-receptive and visual-cognitive deficits may be misdiagnosed. The occupational therapist should be familiar with visual screening because the assessment of vision and oculomotor skills assists in assessing and analyzing their influence on visual perception and functional performance (Todd, 1999).

Visual screening consists of basic tests administered to select those children who are at risk for inadequate visual functions (Bouska et. al., 1990). The purpose of the screening is to determine those children who should be referred for a complete diagnostic visual evaluation. Therefore the purpose of the screening of the visual-receptive system is to determine how efficient the eyes are in acquiring visual information for further visual-cognitive interpretation. The observational checklist in Figure 13-4 assists in alerting the therapist to visual symptoms commonly found in those who demonstrate poor visual performance.

Perimetry, confrontation, and careful observation of the child as he or she performs daily activities gives useful information regarding field integrity in measuring visual fields (Warren, 1993a). Missing or misreading the beginning or ends of words or numbers may indicate the presence of a central field deficit.

The child's refractive status, which is the clinical measurement of the eye, should be measured. A school nurse or vision specialist usually conducts the measurement. A student's refractive status determines whether there is nearsightedness (myopia), farsightedness (hyperopia), or astigmatism. There are several methods used to measure the child's refractive status. One method, the Snellen Test, is used to screen children at school or in the physician's office. However, this test measures only eyesight (visual acuity) at 20 feet. This figure, expressed commonly as x/20, has little predictive value for how well a child uses his or her vision. It is estimated that this measurement shows less than 5% of visual problems (Seiderman & Marcus, 1990). When a child passes this screening, he or she may be told that the existing vision is fine. However, it is only the eyesight at 20 feet that is fine.

Some schools and clinics use a Telebinocular or other similar instrument in vision screening. This provides information on clarity or visual acuity at both near and far distances, as well as information on depth perception and binocularity (two-eyed coordination). Warren (1993b) suggested that the Contrast Sensitivity Test is best for measuring acuity. A pediatric version is available (Vistech Consultants Inc., Dayton, OH).

The occupational therapist may observe oculomotor dysfunction in the child. The screening test should answer several questions (Warren, 1993b):
1. Do the eyes work together? How well?
2. Where is visual control the most efficient? The least efficient?

3. What types of eye movements are the most efficient? The least efficient?

Screening tools that can be used by occupational therapists are presented in Table 13-2.

In addition, the child's ocular health should be ascertained. The presence of a disease or other pathologic condition such as glaucoma, cataracts, or a deterioration of the nerves or any part of the eye, for instance, must be ruled out. An interview with the family regarding significant visual history helps identify any conditions that may be associated with visual limitations. A record review can also help obtain this information, as can a consultation with other professionals involved in direct care of the child (e.g., teacher or physician).

When visual problems are detected in screening, the child may be referred to a vision specialist such as an optometrist. The specialist can help determine if the child has a visual problem that might be causing or contributing to school difficulties. The therapist will then be able to understand what effect those deficits have on function and the strategies needed for intervention. With this information the therapist can design and select appropriate activities that are within the visual capacity of the child (Bouska et. al., 1990).

Visual-Cognitive Assessment

Clinical evaluation and observation may be the occupational therapist's most useful assessment methods. The therapist should observe for difficulty in selecting, storing, retrieving, or classifying visual information. Observations could include visual search strategies used during visual perceptual tasks (e.g., outside borders to inside), how the child approaches the task, how the child processes and interprets visual information, the child's flexibility in analyzing visual information, methods used for storage and retrieval of visual information, and amount of stress associated with visual activities. The therapist should carefully analyze the tasks observed to determine what visual skills are needed and to identify where the child has difficulty.

Visual-cognitive evaluations that are typically administered by occupational therapists and those typically administered by other professionals are presented in Tables 13-3 to 13-6. Tsurumi and Todd (1998) have applied task analysis to the nonmotor tests of visual perception. This information greatly assists the therapist in analyzing the results of these tests. Currently, the best evaluation method of visual attention in children is informal observation during occupational performance tasks. Further description of assessments that may be used follows:
- *Bruininks-Oseretsky Test of Motor Proficiency* (Bruininks, 1978)
- *The Reversals Frequency Test* (Gardner, 1978). A norm-referenced test for children between 5 and 15 years of age. This test measures reversals in a recognition and execution mode and includes a questionnaire for the

table 13-2 *Vision Screening Tests*

Test	Author (Date)	Description
Functional Visual Screening	Langley (1980)	Screening developed for the severely or profoundly handicapped, which consists of 12 items, including pupillary reactions, blinking, peripheral orientation, fixation, gaze shift, tracking, and convergence.
Visual Screening	Bouska, Kauffman, & Marcus (1990)	Comprehensive screening of distance and near vision, convergence near point, horizontal pursuits, distant and near fixations, and stereoscopic visual skills to select those children who should be referred to a qualified vision specialist for a complete diagnostic visual evaluation.
Erhardt Developmental Vision Assessment	Erhardt (1989)	Assessment that measures motor components of vision from fetal and natal periods to 6 months of age; the 6-month age level is considered to be a significant stage of maturity, and this is appropriate for older children. The motor components of vision measured include both reflexive visual patterns and voluntary eye movements of localization, fixation, ocular pursuit, and gaze shift.
Sensorimotor Performance Analysis	Richter & Montgomery (1991)	Assessment of visual tracking, visual avoidance, visual processing, and hand-eye coordination during gross and fine motor tasks.
Crane-Wick Test	Crane & Wick (1987)	A norm-references test that can be administered individually or in a group, for children in kindergarten through grade 12; a sustained near-point visual skills test that is used to identify children with vision problems that interfere with learning and work activities. Subtests included are accommodation, saccadic eye movement, near point of convergence, eye teaming, pursuit of movement, visual processing, and functional hearing.
Visual Skills Appraisal	Richards & Oppenheim (1984)	An individually administered, norm-referenced test for children 5 to 9 years of age. Six subtests include pursuit, scanning, alignment, locating movements, hand-eye coordination, and fixation unity. Resulting subtest scores are converted to a scale, and a specialist provides cutoff points to indicate whether a student requires further examination.
OK Vision Kit	Williamson (1994)	A test that measures visual acuity using observable reflexive optokinetic nystagmus.
Pediatric Clinical Vision Screening for Occupational Therapists	Scheiman (1991)	A test that screens accommodation, binocular vision, and ocular motility.
Clinical Observations of Infants	Ciner, Macks, & Schanel-Klitsch (1991)	Description methods for testing vision in early intervention programs.
Clinical Observation for Adults	Warren (1993b)	Detailed description of visual screening is outlined for adults, but many items may be applied to children.

teacher to complete that indicates the type and frequency of a child's reversals in both reading and writing.

■ *Test of Pictures, Forms, Letters, Numbers, Spatial Orientation, and Sequencing Skills* (Gardner, 1992). This test measures the ability to visually perceive forms, letters, and numbers in the correct direction and to visually perceive words with letters in the correct sequence. There are seven subtests in this norm-referenced test for children 5 to 9 years of age; it can be administered individually or in a group.

■ *Concepts of Left and Right Test* (Laurendau & Pinard, 1970). This instrument evaluates the child's understanding of left and right, from total lack of understanding to full internalization.

■ *Test of Visual Perceptual Skills (Non-Motor), revised (TVPS)* (Gardner, 1997).

■ *Test of Visual Analysis Skills.* This is an individually administered criterion-referenced test for children 5 to 8 years of age. The child taking this untimed test is asked to copy simple to complex geometric patterns. The purpose

table 13-3　Assessments of Visual Attention

Description	Test	Author (Date)
SCANNING Saccadic eye movements: rapid change of fixation from one point in the visual field to another.	• Line Bisection* • Letter Cancellation*	Warren (1993a)
VISUAL VIGILANCE Ability to handle substantial simultaneous detail. The task requires the child to sustain attention and emphasizes visual attention to detail by having the child find a particular rarely occurring design embedded in many others.	• Matching Familiar Figures Test* • Visual Vigilance task on the Pediatric Early Elementary Examination • Visual Vigilance task on the Pediatric Examination of Educational Readiness at Middle Childhood (PEERAMID) (PEEX)	Cairns & Cammock (1978) Levine & Rapport (1983) Levine (1985)
VISUAL SEQUENCING Registration and immediate recall of visual sequences.	• Picture Arrangement subtest of Wechester Intelligence Scale for Children (WISC-III) • Visual Sequential memory subtest of the Test of Visual Perception Skills (Nonmotor)*	Wechsler (1991) Gardner (1997)

*Tests administered by occupational therapists.

table 13-4　Assessments of Visual Memory

Description	Test	Author (Date)
VISUAL RETRIEVAL MEMORY TESTS Visualization and recall of entire configurations. In these tests a child studies a geometric form and then is asked to reproduce it from memory.	• Benton Visual Retention Test* • Visual Memory Scale* • Spatial Memory subtest from the Kaufman Assessment Battery for Children	Benton (1974) Carroll (1975) Kaufman & Kaufman (1983)
VISUAL RECOGNITION MEMORY Short-term visual memory. The child is shown a design and later asked to select it from among similar sets of stimuli.	• Visual recognition subtests of Pediatric Early Elementary Examination (PEEX) • Visual recognition subtests of Pediatric Examination of Education Readiness at Middle Childhood (PEERAMID) • Visual Memory subtest of the Test of Visual Perception Skills (Nonmotor)*	Levine & Rapport (1983) Levine (1985) Gardner (1997)

*Tests administered by occupational therapists.

of the assessment is to determine if the child is competent or in need of remediation in perceiving the visual relationships necessary for integrating letter and word shapes.

■ *Developmental Test of Visual Perception (DTVP) (2nd ed.)* (Hammill, Pearson, & Voress, 1993). This test is unbiased relative to race, gender, and handedness. It is a norm-referenced test for children 4 to 10 years of age.

There are eight subtests, which include hand-eye coordination, copying, spatial relations, position in space, figure-ground, visual closure, visual-motor speed, and form constancy.

■ *Jordon Left-Right Reversal Test—Revised* (Jordon, 1980). This is a standardized test for children 5 to 12 years of age that can be administered individually or in a

table 13-5 *Assessments of Visual Discrimination*

Description	Test	Author (Date)
OBJECT (FORM) PERCEPTION Matching one design with another or finding a specific stimulus embedded within a complex background (usually administered as a motor-free assessment).	• Motor Free Visual Perception Test*	Colarusso & Hammill (1996)
	• Test of Pictures, Forms, Letters, Numbers, and Spatial Orientation*	Gardner (1997)
	• Developmental Test of Visual Perception (2nd ed.)*	Hammill, Pearson, & Voress (1993)
	• Subtests of the Test of Visual-Perception Skills (Nonmotor)*	Gardner (1997)
SPATIAL PERCEPTION Match a design to one that has experienced some transformation but retains its identity (mirror image or rotation).	• Visual Form Constancy subtest of the Test of Visual-Perception Skills (Nonmotor)*	Gardner (1997)
	• Matrix Analogies subtest of the Kaufman Assessment Battery of Children (ABC)	Kaufman & Kaufman (1983)
	• The Reversals Frequency Test*	Gardner (1978)
	• Jordon Left-Right Reversal Test—Revised*	Jordon (1980)
	• Concepts of Left and Right Test*	Laurendau & Pinard (1970)
	• Block Design and Object Assembly subtest of Wechsler Intelligence Scale for Children (WISC-III)	Wechsler (1991)

*Tests administered by occupational therapists.

table 13-6 *Assessment of Visual Motor Integration*

Description	Test	Author (Date)
Integration of spatial input with fine motor production. The child is shown a geometric form and asked to copy it.	• Bender Visual Motor Gestalt*	Bender (1963); see Koppitz scoring, 5-10 years of age Koppitz (1963)
	• Benton Visual Retention Test	Benton (1974)
	• Developmental Test of Visual Motor Integration (VMI)*	Beery (1997)

*Test administered by occupational therapists.

group. It is an untimed test and takes about 20 minutes to administer and score. The test is used to detect visual reversals of letters, numbers, and words. The manual includes remediation exercises for reversal problems.

These tests can be used to evaluate how the child is processing, organizing, and using visual-cognitive information. Care in interpreting and reporting test results should be taken because it is not always clear what visual perceptual tests are measuring. Because of the complexity of the tests, it is certain that they tap different kinds and levels of function, including language abilities. The effectiveness of any treatment method is largely determined by how the child is diagnosed; therefore careful analysis of test results and observations is important.

∎ INTERVENTION

Theoretic Approaches

The theoretic approaches that guide evaluation and treatment of visual perceptual skills can be categorized as *developmental* or *compensatory.* Warren's (1993a, 1993b) developmental model, described in a previous section, is based on the concept that higher-level skills evolve from integration of lower-level skills and are subsequently affected by disruption of lower-level skills. Skill levels within the hierarchy function as a single entity and provide a unified structure for visual perception. As pictured in Figure 13-2, oculomotor control, visual field, and acuity form the foundation skills, followed by visual attention, scanning, pattern recognition or detection, memory, and visual cognition. The identification and remediation of deficits in lower-level skills permit integration of higher-level skills. Occupational therapists who follow this model need to evaluate lower-level skills before proceeding to higher-level skills to identify where the deficit is in the visual hierarchy and to design appropriate evaluation and intervention. Following this model, vision deficits should be addressed by the vision professional and compensatory strategies should be addressed by the occupational therapy practitioner (Tsurumi & Todd, 1998).

The *neurophysiologic* approaches aim to address the maturation of the human nervous system and the link to human performance. These approaches help create environmental accommodations to sensory hypersensitivity, and visual distractibility. They also promote organization of movement around a goal, reinforcing the sensory feedback from that movement. Neurophysiologic approaches emphasize the importance of postural stability for oculomotor efficiency. The role of visual perception as part of sensory integration and how the child perceives his envioronment are discussed in Chapter 12. The neurophysiologic approaches focus on improving visual-receptive and visual-cognitive components to enhance a child's occupational performance. Learning theories and behavioral approaches emphasize a child's development of visual analysis skills. The therapist provides the child with a systematic method for identifying the pertinent, concrete features of spatially organized patterns, thereby enabling the child to recognize how new information relates to previously acquired knowledge on the basis of similar and different attributes. The child learns to generalize to dissimilar tasks so that improvement in visual perceptual skills leads to increased levels of occupational performance.

Perceptual training programs use learning theories to remediate deficit or prerequisite skills and have been implemented in the public schools for more than two decades. Occupational therapists generally use activities from these approaches in combination with neurophysiologic and compensatory approaches.

In *compensatory approaches,* classroom materials or instructional methods are modified to accommodate the child's limitations. The environment can also be altered or adapted. Adaptation and compensation techniques can include decreasing the classroom visual distractions, providing visual stimuli to direct attention and guide response, and modifying the input and output of computer programs. In daily living skills, adaptations to increase grooming, dressing, eating, and communication skills can be made. In play situations, toys can be made more accessible, and in work activities, adaptations to promote copying, writing, and organizational skills can be made. Box 13-1 outlines compensatory instruction guidelines.

---

box 13-1 *Compensatory instruction guidelines*

1. Limit the amount of new material presented in any single lesson.
2. Present new information in a simple, organized way that highlights what is especially pertinent.
3. Ensure that the child has factual knowledge.
4. Link up the new information with the information that the child already knows.
5. Use all senses.
6. Provide repeated experiences to establish the information securely in long-term memory; practice until the child knows it and does not need to figure it out.
7. Group children with similar learning styles together.

Optometry

Optometry and occupational therapy have common goals related to the effects of vision on performance (Hellerstein & Fishman, 1987; Kalb & Warshowsky, 1991; Scheiman, 1997). Collaboration is frequent and has been successful (Downing-Baum & Maino, 1996). When a visual dysfunction is identified, sometimes only environmental modifications, such as changes in lighting, desk height, or surface tilt, may alleviate the problem. In many cases, glasses (lens therapy) are prescribed to reduce the stress of close work or to correct refractive errors. Other times optometric vision therapy may be prescribed by an optometrist and carried out by an occupational therapy practitioner (Downing-Baum, 1995). Through vision therapy, optometrists provide structured visual experiences to enhance basic skills and perception.

Intervention Strategies

For any age child, one important treatment strategy is education (Tsurumi & Todd, 1998). The occupational therapy practitioner can help to interpret the functional implications of the vision problem for the parents, caregivers, teachers, and the child. At times this can be the most helpful intervention for the child. The following sections give intervention suggestions according to age groups. However, activities should be analyzed and then selected according to the child's needs rather than according to his or her age group. These activities illustrate both the developmental and compensatory approaches. Often activities combine approaches. For example, when classroom materials are adapted so that the print is larger and less visual information is presented (compensatory approach), the child might be better able to use visual perceptual skills with resulting improvement in those skills (developmental approach).

Infants

Glass (1993) presented a protocol for working with preterm infants in a neonatal intensive care unit (NICU). Dim lighting allows the newborn to spontaneously open his or her eyes. Stimulating the body senses (i.e., tactile-vestibular) can influence the development of distance sense (e.g., visual), which matures later (Rose, 1980; Turkewitz & Kenny, 1985). Based on research of neonatal vision, Glass suggested ways to use the human face as the infant's first source of visual stimulation. The intensity, amplitude, and distance of the stimulus are dependent on whether the intent is to arouse or quiet the infant. Glass also recommended beginning with softer, simpler forms and three-dimensional objects and to vary the stimuli on the intent to soothe or arouse the infant. Mobiles hung over cribs should be placed approximately 2 feet above the infant and slightly to one side. This allows for selective attention by the infant. In addition, Glass suggested that black and white patterns be reserved for full-term infants who are visually impaired and unable to attend to a face or toy. Once a visual response is elicited with the high-contrast pattern, a shift to a pattern with less contrast should be made.

Preschool and kindergarten

Occupational therapists can help preschool and kindergarten teachers organize the classroom activities to help children develop the readiness skills needed for visual perception. Teachers should understand the increased need for a multisensory approach with young children who are struggling with shape, letter, and number recognition. For example, the child might benefit from tactile input to help learn shapes, letters, and numbers. By using letters with textures the child has additional sensory experiences on which he or she can rely when visual skills are diminished. Children should be encouraged to feel shapes, letters, and words through their hands and bodies. Letters can be formed with clay, sandpaper, beads, or chocolate pudding (Figure 13-5).

All preschool, kindergarten, and primary classes should include frequent activities that develop body-in-space concepts. Even with a range of levels of understanding among young students, group activities, such as Statue, shadow dancing, and Simon Says, can reinforce body-in-space comprehension. Children benefit from watching and imitating one another. The therapist may pair children so that one can model for the other in an obstacle course or other gross motor activity. In the occupational therapy literature, several publications detail activities for both classroom teachers and therapists (see Appendix 13-A).

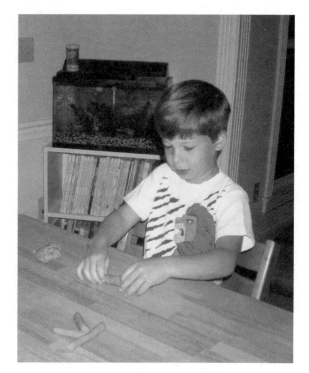

figure**13-5**   Kyle making letters with clay.

Elementary school

Therapy should begin at the level of the visual hierarchy where the child is experiencing difficulty. If the child is experiencing difficulty with visual-receptive skills, the cooperative efforts between the occupational therapist and the optometrist may be helpful.

Organizing the environment. Visual perception affects a child's view of the entire learning environment. Visually distracting and competing information can be problematic to the child who has not yet fully developed his or her skills. The child may require that the classroom be less "busy" visually to be successful. Limiting a distractible child's peripheral vision by using a carrel is often helpful (Figure 13-6). In addition, levels of illumination and the control of glare needs to be monitored.

The child needs a stable postural base that allows his or her eyes to work together. Children often sit at ill-fitting furniture, which can compound their problems. The occupational therapist can assist the teacher in properly positioning children. The therapist could add bolsters to seat backs, put blocks under a child's feet, or provide the child with a slant-board if any of these materials will help the child use vision more efficiently or increase productivity. The therapist could also stress the importance of encouraging different positions for visual activity. Figure 13-7 illustrates such alternative positions as prone, the TV sit position, and side lying for visual perceptual activities such as reading. Each position should

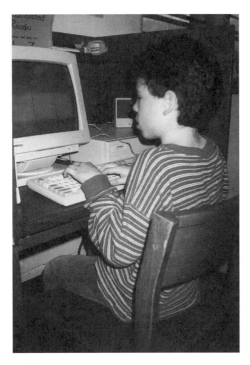

figure**13-6**   Todd in a study carrel.

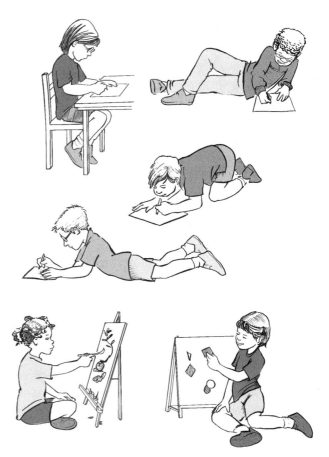

figure**13-7**   Alternate positions for visual perceptual activities.

place the child in good alignment and should offer adequate postural support.

Children may benefit from color-coded worksheets to assist them in attending to what visually goes together. However, children with color vision problems may have difficulty with educational materials that are color-coded, particularly when the colors are pastel or muddy. Therefore it is important to differentiate an actual visual color deficit from a problem with either color naming or color identification (Ciner et. al., 1991).

Christenson and Rascho (1989) proposed strategies to assist the elderly in topographic orientation, which can also be adapted for children. These authors found that use of landmarks and signage can enhance way-finding skills and topographic orientation. They recommended the use of pictures or signs that are realistic, simple, and of high color contrast. For example, a simple, graphic depiction of a lunch tray with food could be used for the cafeteria door.

Visual attention. Following a neurophysiologic frame of reference, general sensory stimulation or inhibition may be done during or before visually oriented activities to improve visual attending skills. If the child is overaroused, the therapist can diminish sensory input to calm him or her; if the child is underaroused the therapist selects alerting activities to increase the level of arousal.

For the child with impaired visual attention, the therapist addresses goals using varied activities and time segments that are achievable. The therapist identifies activities that are intrinsically motivating to the child because these will help maintain the child's attention. The therapist should plan activities together with the child and use as many novel activities as possible. Most challenging to the therapist is the ability to adapt or modify task activities while maintaining a playful learning environment for the child. Elimination of extraneous environmental stimuli is helpful at each level of visual attention.

Developmentally appropriate and visually and tactilely stimulating activities enhance visual attention skills. Manual activities of drawing or manipulating play dough or clay encourage the eyes to view the movements involved (Rogow, 1992). In addition, the hand helps educate the eye about object qualities such as weight, volume, and texture and helps direct the eye to the object (Rogow, 1987). Simultaneous hand and eye movements construct internal representations of objects and serve the function of object recognition.

Activities to compensate for limitations in attention include (1) placing a black mat that is larger than the worksheet under it to increase high contrast to assist in visual attention to the worksheet, (2) drawing lines to group materials, and (3) reorganizing worksheets (Todd, 1999). Visual stimuli on a worksheet or in a book can be reduced by covering the entire page except the activity on which the student is working or by using a mask that uncovers one line at a time (Figure 13-8). Reducing competing sensory input in both the auditory and visual modalities can be helpful for some students with poor visual attention. For example, headphones can be worn when working on a visual task. Good lighting and use of pastel-colored paper helps reduce the glare. Additionally, encouraging children to search for high-interest photographs or pictures can help increase visual attention skills (Rogow, 1992). *Where's Waldo* and other similar books are highly motivating and encourage children to develop search strategies and visual attention. Other suggestions include cuing the child to important visual information by using a finger to point, a marker to underline, or therapist verbalization to help the child maintain visual attention. Cooper (1975) found that subjects tended to look at a picture when it was named. The therapist can use large colorful pictures combined with rhyming chants to encourage attention to the pictures (Rogow, 1992). Visual work should be presented when the student's energy is highest and not when he or she is fatigued (Rogow, 1992).

Visual memory. Children with visual memory problems need repeated consistent experiences; therefore the therapist should consult with the parents and teachers so that these activities can be done at home and in the classroom. Grouping information in ways that provide retrieval cues can help a child remember interrelated data (Schneck, 1998). Several strategies may be helpful. "Chunking" is organizing information into smaller units, or chunks. This can be done by cutting up worksheets and presenting one unit or task at a time. "Maintenance rehearsal" (repetition) helps the child hold information in his or her short-term memory but seems to have no effect on long-term storage. An example of this strategy would be repeating a phone number until the number is dialed. "Elaborative rehearsal" is a strategy in which new information is consciously related to knowledge already stored in long-term memory. By the time a child is 8 years of age, he or she can rehearse more than one item at a time and can rehearse information together as a set to remember. Children can also relate ideas to more than one other idea. Mnemonic devices are memory-directed tactics that help transform or organize information to enhance its retrievability through use of language cues such as songs, rhymes, and acronyms. Gibson (1971) suggested that memory is composed primarily of distinctive features (what makes something different). Occupational therapists can help the child determine differences in visual stimuli to promote storage into memory. Games such as concentration, copying a sequence after viewing it for a few seconds, or remembering what was removed from a tray of several items can be enjoyable ways to increase visual memory. The therapist first provides the student with short, simple tasks that the child can complete quickly and with success; then gradually, as the student accomplishes tasks, the therapist increases the length and complexity of the tasks.

Visual discrimination. The therapist must use task analysis to design an intervention program. By analyzing the continuum of a task, the therapist can grade the activity from simple to complex to allow success while challenging the child's visual abilities (Blanksby, 1992). Remediation therefore should follow an orderly design (Bouska et. al., 1990) so that the child can make sense of each performance. Intervention strategies should aim to help children recognize and attend to the identifying features by teaching them to use their vision to locate objects and then to use object features as well as other cues to form identification hypotheses (Schneck, 1998). Teaching children to visually scan or search pictures instructs the child on the value of looking and finding meaning. With high-interest materials the therapist can teach the child to look from top to bottom and left to right (Rogow, 1992). Using pictures from magazines, the therapist removes an important part of a picture and asks the student to identify what part is missing. Drawing, painting, and other art and craft activities encourage exploration and manipulation of visual forms. As the

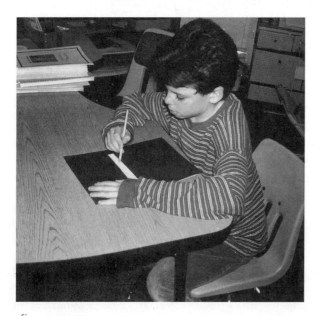

figure**13-8** Todd's mask uncovers one line at a time.

child moves from awareness to attention and then to selection, he or she becomes better able to discriminate between the important and unimportant features of the environment.

Occupational therapists can assist teachers in reorganizing the child's worksheets. Color coding different problems may assist the child in visually attending to the correct section. Worksheets can also be cut up and reorganized to match the child's visual needs. It is important to gradually fade out the restructuring of the worksheets so the child can eventually use the sheets as they are presented in the workbooks.

When a child has problems copying from the chalkboard, an occupational therapist might recommend that the chalkboard be regularly cleaned in an effort to reduce clutter and provide high contrast for chalk marks. Notations on chalkboards, bulletin boards, or overhead transparencies should be color coded, well spaced, and uncluttered. These practices may reduce figure-ground problems. The therapist may also suggest that a teacher reduce use of the chalkboard by having the children copy from one paper to another with both papers in the same plane. A teacher may be encouraged to try bean bag games in which the targets are placed at approximately the same distance from the child's eyes as the chalkboard so that a student can practice focusing and fixating eyes near and far in play.

Reducing the amount of print on a page (less print, fewer math problems) and providing mathematical problems on graph paper with numbers in columns in the ones, tens, and hundreds places help students with figure-ground difficulties. Masking the part of the worksheet that is not being worked on can help the child focus on one problem at a time. Cooper (1985) proposed a theoretic model for the implementation of color contrast to enhance visual ability in the older adult. Principles of color contrast and the ways in which color contrast can be achieved by varying hue, brightness, or color saturation of an object in relation to its environment are the foundation of the method of intervention. This helps a child identify the relevant information, such as the classroom materials and supplies.

Decoding problems in reading. Children with difficulty distinguishing between similar visual symbols may benefit from a multisensory approach. This includes tracing the shapes and letters, hearing them, saying them, and then feeling them. This permits a number of routes of processing to help supplement weak visual perceptual processing. Thus the child sees it, hears it, traces it, and writes it. Eating letters is an activity loved by children; alphabet cereal, gelatin jigglers, cookies, and french fries in the shape of letters can be served for snack. The children can trace the letters with frosting from tubes onto cookies and catsup from packets for french fries.

For children with word recognition difficulty, the initial emphasis should be on recognition rather than retrieval. The child can be given a choice of visually similar words to complete sentences that have single words missing. In addition, using word families (ball, call, and tall) to increase sight vocabulary enhances word recognition skills. Phonic approaches may also be the best reading instruction method for children with poor word recognition. Textbooks recorded on audiotape cassettes can be ordered from local and state libraries from the American Printing House for the Blind (Louisville, Kentucky). The student can hear and read the textbook at the same time.

If the child has strong verbal skills, verbal mediation (talking through printed words) should be stressed, and the child could be encouraged to describe what he or she sees to retain the information. A strategy that may assist a child who reverses letters in words is to follow along the printed lines with a finger. This technique helps stress reading the letters in the correct sequence. Reading material rich in pictorial content such as comic books, pictures with captions and cartoons, and computer software designed to enhance sight vocabulary can strengthen these associations.

Visualization. The development of visualization techniques, or visual imagery, may be delayed. Like all skills, this proceeds from the concrete to the abstract. Therapists can start by helping students picture something that they can touch or feel. Using a grab bag with toys or objects inside that the child identifies without vision is a good way to do this.

As material becomes less concrete, more visual skills are drawn into play. A student might be asked to visualize something that he or she has done. The occupational therapist can facilitate the child's thinking by reminding him or her to consider various factors such as color, brightness, size, sounds, temperature, space, movement, smells, and tastes. Hopefully, once the child practices orally, he or she will generalize the visualization process to reading (Bell, 1991).

Children with poor visualization may have difficulty spelling and may need to learn spelling rules thoroughly. They may also demonstrate reading comprehension problems. In addition, they may have difficulty forming letters because they are unable to visualize them. This would become evident when children write from dictation. Sometimes the child can visualize a letter from the sound but it is reversed or missing parts.

Learning styles. All students have a preferred learning style (Carbo, et. al., 1986). When a student is taught through his or her preferred style, the child can learn with less effort and remember better. Figure 13-9 illus-

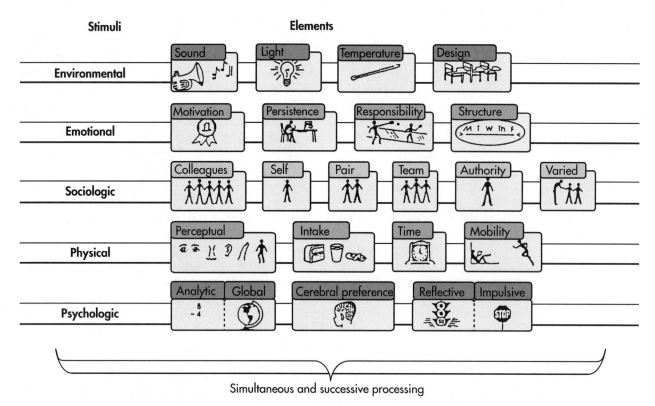

figure**13-9**   Diagnostic learning styles. *(Courtesy of Rita Dunn, Ed.D. Director, Learning Styles Network, The Center for the Study of Learning and Teaching Styles, School of Education & Human Services, St. John's University, Jamaica, NY.)*

table 13-7 *Matching Reading Methods to Perceptual Strengths*

Reading Method	Description	Reading-Style Requirements
Phonics	Isolated letter sounds or letter clusters are taught sequentially and blended to form words.	Auditory and analytic strengths
Linguistic	Patterns of letters are taught and combined to form words.	Auditory and analytic strengths
Orton-Gillingham	Consists of phonics and tactile stimulation in the form of writing and tracing activities.	Auditory and analytic strengths combined with visual weaknesses
Whole-word	Before reading a story, new words are presented on flash cards and in sentences, with accompanying pictures.	Visual and global strengths
Language-experience	Students read stories that they write.	Visual, tactile, and global strengths
Fernald	Language-experience method and student traces over new words with index finger of writing hand.	Tactile and global strengths combined with visual weaknesses
Choral reading	Groups read a text in unison.	Visual and global strengths
Recorded book	Students listen two or three times to brief recordings of books, visually track the words, then read the selection aloud.	Visual and global strengths

From Carbo, M. (1987). Deprogramming reading failure: Giving unequal learners an equal chance. *Phi Delta Kappa, Nov.,* 35.

trates diagnostic learning styles. All students need to be taught through their strongest senses and then reinforced through their next strongest sense.

Auditory learners are those who recall at least 75% of what is discussed or heard in a normal 40- to 45-minute period (Carbo et. al., 1986). Visual learners remember what they see and can retrieve details and events by concentrating on the things that they have seen. Tactual and kinesthetic learners assimilate best by touching, manipulating, and handling objects. They remember more easily

13-2 *Suggestions for tactile and kinesthetic learners*

- At story time, give the child a prop that relates to the story. The child can act out something that they just heard using the prop.
- Provide letter cubes to make words.
- Provide simple written and recorded directions (see and hear written directions simultaneously, which increases their understanding and retention) to enable the student to build models and projects.
- Use games such as bingo, dominoes, or card games to teach or review reading skills. These activities allow movement, as well as peer and adult interaction.
- Use writing activity cards. Paste colorful, high-interest pictures on index cards and add stimulating questions.
- Encourage the child to participate actively while they read. For example, children can write while they read, underline or circle key words or place an asterisk in the margin next to an important section as they read, and inscribe comments when appropriate.
- Use glue letters.
- Use blocks from a Boggle game.
- Play Scrabble (Carbo et. al., 1986).

when they write, doodle, draw, or move their fingers. It is best to introduce material to them through art activities, baking, cooking, building, making, interviewing, and acting experiences. If a child has weaknesses in visual processing, it is more difficult for him or her to learn through the visual sense. This child may learn more effectively through the kinesthetic and tactile senses. See Box 13-2 for suggestions for kinesthetic learning.

Occupational therapists can greatly assist teachers by helping to determine a child's perceptual strengths and weaknesses so that an appropriate reading program can be matched to the child's preferred perceptual modality. Once the child is in first grade, it is important to determine what reading program the teacher is using. Table 13-7 matches reading methods to perceptual strengths and weaknesses and global and analytic styles. For example, the Orton-Gillingham method (Gillingham & Stillman, 1968; Orton, 1937) teaches decoding through a multisensory approach.

In addition to perceptual strengths, the therapist must also keep in mind the child's preferred manner of approaching new material. For instance, global learners require an overall comprehension first and then can at-

tend to the details. Analytic learners piece details together to form an understanding.

Visual-motor integration

To review, the therapist should first focus on the underlying visual-receptive functions and then focus on the visual-cognitive functions. This should precede in the sequence of visual attention, visual memory, visual discrimination, and specific visual discrimination skills. A multisensory approach to handwriting may be helpful to a child with visual-cognitive problems. Working with eyes closed can be effective in reducing the influence of increased effort that vision can create and in lessening the visual distractions. Keeping the eyes closed can also improve the awareness of the kinesthetic feedback from letter formation.

Use of a vibrating pen provides augmented tactile and proprioceptive input to the child's hand during handwriting and can reinforce learning of correct letter formation. The child whose preferred learning style is through the auditory system can be assisted in learning handwriting through use of a talking pen. Handwriting programs that are easier for children with visual-cognitive problems include Loops and Other Groups (Benbow, 1990) and Handwriting without Tears (Olsen, 1996). Olsen described strategies to help children correct or avoid reversals. During handwriting lessons the child should proofread his or her own work and circle the best-formed letters. Chapter 18 has comprehensive information on developing handwriting skills.

Children with visual spatial problems often choose random starting points, which can confuse the writing task from the onset. Concrete cues must be used to teach abstract handwriting concepts. For example, colored lines on the paper or paper with raised lines can be helpful for the child who is having trouble knowing where to place the letters on the page. In addition, green lines drawn to symbolize *go* on the left side of the paper and red lines to symbolize *stop* on the right side may help a child know which direction to write his or her letters and words. Upright orientation of the writing surface may also lessen directional confusion of letter formation (up means up and down means down) versus at a desk on a horizontal surface, where up means away from oneself and down means toward oneself (Schneck, 1998).

Directional cues can be paired with verbal cues for the child who commonly reverses letters and numbers. These cognitive cues rely on visual images for distinguishing letters and include the following:

1. With palms facing the chest and thumbs up, the student makes two fists. The left hand will form a *b* and the right hand will form a *d*.
2. Lower-case *b* is like *B*, only without the top loop.

3. To make a lower-case *d*, remember that *c* comes first, then add a line to make a *d*.

The therapist can develop cue cards for the student to keep at his or her desk with common reversals.

Children with visual-cognitive problems often overspace or underspace words. The correct space should be slightly more than the width of a single lower-case letter. When a child has handwriting spacing problems, the occupational therapist may recommend using a decorated tongue depressor to use for spacing words, using a pencil, or simply having the child use his or her finger as a guide. The child can also imagine a letter in the space to aid in judging the distance.

When students need additional help to stop at lines, templates with windows can be used in teaching handwriting. These templates can be made out of cardboard with three windows; one for one-line letters (*a, c, e, i, m,* and *n*), one for two-line letters (*b, d, k, l,* and *t*), and another window for three-line letters (*f, g, j, p, q, z,* and *y*). It is important to consider that visual memory is used to recognize the letters or words to be written, and motor memory starts the engram for producing the written product. Therefore it may be that motor memory, not visual memory, is the basis for the problem.

Computers

Many excellent educational computer programs for young children are already on the market that the occupational therapist can use. Software programs are available that are highly motivating for children of all ages. Living books on the computer reinforce the written word with the spoken word and assist in developing a sight word vocabulary.

The computer can be used as a motivational device to assist in increasing the child's attention to the task. The computer also provides a way to practice skills in an independent manner. Drill and practice software record data on accuracy and time taken to complete the drills, thus allowing the therapist to record the child's progress. The therapist can adapt the computer program by changing the background colors to those that enhance the child's visual perceptual skills. The therapist can also enlarge the written information so that there is less information on the screen.

■ SUMMARY

Children with visual perceptual problems often receive the services of occupational therapists. This chapter described a developmental approach that emphasizes methods for identifying the underlying components of visual-receptive and visual-cognitive skills. The relationship of these components to various performance areas was described. Using the developmental approach, the occupational therapist helps the child increase his or her visual perceptual skills by improving his or her underlying components of performance. By adapting classroom materials and instruction methods, the therapist also helps the child compensate for visual perception problems. Intervention often includes a combination of developmental and compensatory activities. This holistic approach enables the child with visual perceptual problems to achieve optimal function and learning.

Case Study 1

When Todd was a 9-year-old student in the third grade, a majority of his day was spent in the regular third-grade classroom, where he functioned at grade level in all areas of academics except in reading. Todd received daily resource room instruction in this area. His resource instruction consisted of copying, worksheet completion, and drill and repetition techniques and did not include opportunities for manipulative activities.

An occupational therapy evaluation indicated that Todd's perceptual skills were about 2 years delayed, with weaknesses noted in visual-spatial relations, figure-ground perception, and visual sequential memory. From interviewing the teacher, the therapist learned that Todd was not moving from learning to read to reading to learn. His decoding was not automatic, and therefore he was spending considerable time figuring out what the words were rather than comprehending what he was reading. He also reported that his eyes tired easily while reading. Good eye movements were needed to sustain reading for longer periods. Because of poor spatial abilities, Todd had difficulty discerning differences in visually similar symbols and had difficulty with words that only differed by sequence (*three* and *there*) or spatial orientation (*dad* and *bad*). The third-grade reading books had more print per page and fewer illustrations to give cues. Too many words on the page made it difficult for Todd because of his poor figure-ground abilities. He demonstrated an inability to recall exact order of words, poor sight vocabulary, and poor spelling caused by poor visual sequential memory.

The therapist referred Todd for optometric evaluation because of his reported visual fatigue during reading tasks. Planning together with Todd, the therapist developed strategies to assist him in increasing his visual memory. Initially, short visual memory tasks were used, and then gradually the length of tasks was increased. This was done using visual memory games and activities on the computer. In addition, visual discrimination tasks were started, beginning with simple forms and moving to forms that were more complex.

In consultation with the teacher, the therapist recommends decreasing the amount of print per page and masking what is not immediately needed when this could not be done. Phonics approaches to word recognition are recommended (see Table 13-7), as is using verbal mediation to decode words.

STUDY QUESTIONS

1. Describe the relationship of the visual-receptive and the visual-cognitive components.

2. What are the differences between object (form) vision and spatial vision? Describe different forms of each.

3. Define three occupational therapy recommendations for a second-grade teacher who has a child with difficulties in visual attention?

References

Abercrombie, M.L.J. (1963). Eye movements, perception, learning. In *Visual disorders and cerebral palsy*. London: William Heinemann.

Ayres, A.J. (1979). *Sensory integration and the child*. Los Angeles: Western Psychological Services.

Beery, K.E. (1997). *Developmental Test of Visual-Motor Integration*. (4th ed.). Los Angeles: Western Psychological Corporation.

Bell, N. (1991). *Visualizing and verbalizing for language comprehension and thinking*. Paso Robles, CA: Academy of Reading Publishers.

Benbow, M. (1990). *Loops and other groups*. Tucson: Therapy Skill Builders.

Bender, C.L. (1963). *Bender Visual-Motor Gestalt Test*. Cleveland: The Psychological Corporation.

Benton, A.L. (1974). *Benton Visual Retention Test*. Chicago: The Psychological Corporation.

Birch, H.G. (1964). *Brain damage in children: The biological and social aspects*. New York: Williams & Wilkins.

Blanksby, B.S. (1992). Visual therapy: A theoretically based intervention program. *Journal of Visual Impairment and Blindness, 86*, 291-294.

Boder, E. (1973). Developmental dyslexia: A diagnostic approach based on three atypical reading-spelling patterns. *Developmental Medicine and Child Neurology, 15*, 661.

Bouska, M.J., Kauffman, N.A., & Marcus, S.E. (1990). Disorders of the visual perception system. In D. Umphred (Ed.), *Neurological rehabilitation* (2nd ed.). (pp. 522-585) St. Louis: Mosby.

Breakey, A.S., Wilson, J.J., & Wilson, B.C. (1994). Sensory and perceptual functions in the cerebral palsied. *Journal of Nervous and Mental Diseases, 158*, 70-77.

Bruininks, R.H. (1978). *Bruininks-Oseretsky Test of Motor Proficiency*. Circle Pines, MN: American Guidance Service.

Burpee, J.D. (1997). Sensory integration and visual functions. In M. Gentile (Ed.), *Functional visual behavior: A therapist's guide to evaluation and treatment options*. Bethesda, MD: The American Occupational Therapy Association.

Cairns, E., & Cammock, T. (1978). Development of a more reliable version of the matching familiar figures test. *Developmental Psychology, 14*, 555.

Carbo, M. (1983). Reading styles change from second to eighth grade. *Education Leadership, 40*, 56-59.

Carbo, M. (Nov. 1987). Deprogramming reading failure: Giving unequal learners an equal chance. *Phi Delta Kappa, 35*.

Carbo, M., Dunn, R., & Dunn, K. (1986). *Teaching students to read through their individual learning styles*. Englewood Cliffs, NJ: Prentice-Hall.

Caron, A., & Caron, R. (1981). Processing of relational information as an index of infant risk. In S. Friedman & M. Sigman (Eds.), *Preterm birth and psychological development*. New York: Academic Press.

Carroll, J.L. (1975). *Visual memory scale*. Mt Pleasant, MI: Carroll Publications.

Chapman, L.J., & Wedell, K. (1972). Perceptual-motor abilities and reversal errors in children's handwriting. *Journal of Learning Disabilities, 5*, 321-325.

Christenson, M.A., & Rascho, B. (1989). Environmental cognition and age-related sensory change. *Occupational Therapy Practice, 1*, 28-35.

Ciner, E.B., Macks, B., & Schanel-Klitsch, E. (1991). A cooperative demonstration project for early intervention vision services. *Occupational Therapy Practice, 3* (1), 42-56.

Cohen, K.M. (1981). The development of strategies of visual search. In D.F. Fisher, R.A. Monty, & J.W. Senders (Eds.), *Eye movements: Cognition and visual perception*. Hillsdale, NJ: Lawrence Erlbaum.

Colarusso, R.P., & Hammill, D.D. (1996). *Motor-Free Visual Perception Test, revised*. Novato, CA: Academic Therapy Publications.

Cooper, B.A. (1985). A model for implementing color contrast in the environment of the elderly, *American Journal of Occupational Therapy, 39*, 253-258.

Cooper, L.A. (1975). Mental rotation of random two-dimensional shapes. *Cognitive Psychology, 7* (2), 20-43.

Crane, A., & Wick, B. (1987). *Crane-Wick Test*. Houston: Rapid Research Corporation.

Cratty, B.J. (1970). *Perceptual and motor development in infants and children*, New York: Macmillan.

Damasio, A.R. (1989). Time-locked multiregional retroactivation: A systems' level proposal for the neural substrates of recall and recognition. *Cognition, 33*, 25-62.

Daniels, L.E., & Ryley, C. (1991). Visual perceptual and visual motor performance in children with psychiatric disorders. *Canadian Journal of Occupational Therapy, 58* (30), 137-141.

deHirsch, K., Jansky, J., & Lanford, W. (1966). *Predicting reading failure*. New York: Harper & Row.

DeQuiros, J.B., & Schranger, O.L. (1979). *Neuropsychological fundamentals in learning disabilities*. Novato, CA: Academic Therapy Publications.

Downing-Baum, S. (1995, June, 15). Exercises in pediatric vision therapy. *OT Week, 9*, 20-22.

Downing-Baum, S., & Maino, D. (1996, November 4). Case studies show success in OT-OD treatment plans. *ADVANCE for Occupational Therapists*, 18.

Duckman, R. (1979). The incidence of anomalies in a population of cerebral palsied children. *Journal of the American Optometric Association, 50*, 1013.

Enns, J.T., & Cameron, S. (1987). Selective attention in young children: The relation between visual search, filtering, and priming. *Journal of Experimental Child Psychology, 44*, 38-63.

Erhardt, R.P. (1989). *Erhardt Developmental Vision Assessment (EDVA)* (Rev. ed.). Tucson: Therapy Skill Builders.

Fanning, G.S. (1971). Vision in children with Down's syndrome. *Australian Journal of Optometry, 54*, 74.

Flax, N. (1984). Visual perception versus visual function. *Journal of Learning Disabilities, 17*, 182-185.

Fledelius, T. (1976). Prematurity and the eye. *Acta Ophthalmology*, 128-134.

Frostig, M., Lefever, W., & Whittlesey, J.R.B. (1966). *Administration and scoring manual for the Marianne Frostig Developmental Test of Visual Perception*. Palo Alto, CA: Consulting Psychologists Press.

Gardner, M.F. (1992). *Test of Pictures-Forms-Letters-Numbers-Spatial Orientation & Sequencing Skills*. Burlington, CA: Psychological and Educational Publications.

Gardner, M.F. (1997). *Test of Visual-Perceptual Skills (Non-Motor), revised (TVPS)*. Burlington, CA: Psychological & Educational Publications.

Gardner, R.A. (1978). *Reversals frequency test*. Cresskill, NJ: Creative Therapeutics.

Garling, R., Book, A., & Lindberg, E. (1984). Cognitive mapping of large-scale environments: The interrelationship of action plans, acquisition and orientation. *Environment and Behavior, 16,* 3-34.

Gentile, M. (1997). *Functional visual behavior: A therapist's guide to evaluation and treatment options.* Bethesda, MD: The American Occupational Therapy Association.

Gibson, E.J. (1971). Perceptual learning and the theory of word perception. *Cognitive Psychology, 2,* 351.

Gibson, E.J., & Levin, H. (1975). *The psychology of reading.* Cambridge, MA: The MIT Press.

Gilfoyle, E., Grady, A., & Moore, J. (1990). *Children adapt* (2nd ed.). Thorofare, NJ: Slack.

Gillingham, A., & Stillman, B. (1968). *Remedial teaching for children with specific disability in reading, spelling and penmanship.* Cambridge, MA: Educator's Publishing Service.

Glass, P. (1993). Development of visual function in preterm infants: Implications for early intervention. *Infants and Young Children, 6* (1), 11-20.

Greene, L.J. (1987). *Learning disabled and your child: a survival handbook.* New York: Ballantine Books.

Hammill, D.D., Pearson, N.A., & Voress J.K. (1993). *Developmental Test of Visual Perception* (2nd ed.). Austin, TX: Pro Ed.

Hellerstein, L., & Fishman, B. (1987). Vision therapy and occupational therapy: An integrated approach. *American Occupational Therapy Sensory Integration Special Interest Section Newsletter, 10* (3), 4-5.

Hung, S.S., Fisher, A.G., & Cermak, S.A. (1987). The performance of learning-disabled and normal young men on the test of visual-perceptual skills. *American Journal of Occupational Therapy, 41,* 790-797.

Hyvarinen, L. (1988). *Vision in children: Normal and abnormal.* Medford, Ontario: Canadian Deaf, Blind and Rubella Association.

Ilg, F.L., & Ames, L.B. (1981). *School readiness.* New York: Harper & Row.

Jansky, J., & deHirsh, K. (1972). *Preventing reading failure: Prediction, diagnosis, and intervention.* New York: Harper & Row.

Jordon, B.A. (1980). *Jordon Left-Right Reversal Test* (2nd ed.). Los Angeles: Western Psychological Services.

Kalb, L., & Warshowsky, J.H. (1991). Occupational therapy and optometry: Principles of diagnosis and collaborative treatment of learning disabilities in children. *Occupational Therapy Practice, 3* (1), 77-87.

Kaufman, A.S., & Kaufman, N.L. (1983). *Kaufman Assessment Battery for Children.* Circle Pines, MN: American Guidance Service.

Kirby, J., & Das, J.P. (1978). Information processing and human abilities. *Journal of Educational Psychology, 70.*

Koppitz, E.M. (1963). *The Bender Visual-Motor Gestalt Test for Young Children.* New York: Grune & Stratton.

Kwatney, E., & Bouska, M.J. (1980). *Visual system disorders and functional correlates: Final report.* Philadelphia: Temple University Rehabilitation and Training Center No. 8.

Langley, M.B. (1980). *Functional vision inventory for the severely/profoundly handicapped.* Chicago: Stoelting.

Laurendau, M., & Pinard, A. (1970). *Development of the concept of space in the child.* New York: International University Press.

Leigh, R.J., & Zee, D.S. (1983). *Neurology of eye movements.* Philadelphia: F.A. Davis.

Levine, M. (1985). *The ANSER system.* Cambridge, MA: Educator's Publishing Service.

Levine, M. (1987). *Developmental variation and learning disorders.* Cambridge, MA: Educators Publishing Service.

Levine, M., & Rapport, L. (1983). *The ANSER system.* Cambridge, MA: Educator's Publishing Service.

Luria, A. (1966). *Higher cortical functions in man.* New York: Basic Books.

Lyle, J.G. (1969). Reading retardation and reversal tendency: A factorial study. *Child Development, 40,* 833-843.

Marr, D. (1982). *Vision.* San Francisco: Freeman.

Menken, C., Cermak, S.A., & Fisher, A.G. (1987). Evaluating the visual-perceptual skills of children with cerebral palsy. *American Journal of Occupational Therapy, 41* (10), 646-651.

Mishkin, M., Ungerleider, L., & Macko, K. (1983). Object vision and spatial vision: Two cortical pathways. *Trends in Neuroscience, 6,* 414-417.

Moore, R.S. (1979). *School can wait.* Provo, UT: Bigham Young University Press.

Morency, A., & Wepman, J. (1973). Early perceptual ability and later school achievement. *Elementary School Journal, 73,* 323.

Mussen, P.H., Conger, J.J., Kagan, J. (1979). *Child development and personality* (5th ed.). New York: Harper & Row.

Necombe, F., & Ratcliff, G. (1989). Disorders of spatial analysis. In E. Boller & J. Grafman (Eds.), *Handbook of neuropsychology* (Vol. 2). New York: Elsevier Science.

Nolte, J. (1988). *The human brain* (2nd ed.). St. Louis: Mosby.

Olsen, J.Z. (1998). *Handwriting without tears.* Potomac, MD: Olsen.

Optometric Extension Program Foundation. (1985). Santa Ana, CA: The Foundation.

Orton, S.T. (1937). *Reading, writing, and speech problems in children.* New York: W.W. Norton.

Osterling, J., & Dawson, G. (1994). Early recognition of children with autism: A study of first birthday video tapes. *Journal of Autism and Developmental Disorders, 24,* 247-257.

Piaget, J. (1964). *Development and learning.* Ithaca, NY: Cornell University Press.

Rafal, R.D., & Posner, M.I. (1987). Cognitive theories of attention and the rehabilitation of attentional deficits. In M.J. Meier, A.L. Benton, & L. Diller (Eds.), *Neuropsychological rehabilitation.* New York: Guilford.

Ratcliff, G. (1987). Perception and complex visual processes. In M.J. Meier, A.L. Benton, & L. Diller (Eds.), *Neuropsychological rehabilitation* (pp. 182-201). New York: Guilford.

Restak, R. (1979). *The brain: The last frontier.* New York: Doubleday.

Richards, R.G., & Oppenheim, G.S. (1984). *Visual skills appraisal.* Novato, CA: Academic Therapy Publications.

Richter, E., & Montgomery, P. (1991). *The sensorimotor performance analysis.* Hugo, MN: PDP Products.

Ritty, J.M., Solan, H., & Cool, S.J. (1993). Visual and sensory-motor functioning in the classroom: A preliminary report of ergonomic demands. *Journal of the American Optometric Association 64* (4), 238-244.

Rogow, S.M. (1987). The ways of the hand: hand function in blind, visually impaired, and visually impaired multiple handicapped children. *British Journal of Visual Impairment, 5* (2), 58-63.

Rogow, S.M. (1992). Visual perceptual problems of visually impaired children with developmental disabilities. *Review, 24* (2), 57-64.

Rogow, S.M., & Rathwill, D. (1989). Seeing and knowing: An investigation of visual perception among children with severe visual impairments. *Journal of Vision Rehabilitation, 3* (3), 55-66.

Roley Smith, S., & Schneck, C. (In press). Sensory integration and the child with visual impairment and blindness. In S. Roley Smith, E. Blanche, & R. Schaff (Eds.), *Sensory integration and developmental disabilities.* Tuscan: Therapy Skill Builders.

Rose, S.A. (1980). Enhancing visual recognition memory in preterm infants. *Developmental Psychology, 16,* 85.

Rosenhall, J., Johansson, E., & Gilberg, C. (1988). Oculomotor findings in autistic children. *Journal of Laryngeal Otology, 102,* 435-439.

Scheiman, M. (1984). Optometric findings in children with cerebral palsy. *American Journal of Optometric Physiology Opt., 61,* 321-323.

Scheiman, M. (1991). *Pediatric clinical vision screening for occupational therapists.* Philadelphia: Pennsylvania College of Optometry.

Scheiman, M. (1997). *Understanding and managing vision deficits: A guide for occupational therapists.* Thorofare, NJ: Slack, Inc.

Schneck, C.M. (1998). Intervention for visual perceptual problems. In J. Case-Smith (Ed.), *Occupational therapy: Making a difference in the school system*. Bethesda, MD: American Occupational Therapy Association.

Seiderman, A.S. (1984). Visual perception versus visual function. *Journal of Learning Disabilities, 17,* 182-185.

Seiderman, A.S., & Marcus, S.E. (1990). *20/20 is not enough: The new world of vision.* New York: Alfred B. Knopf.

Siegel, L. (1983). The prediction of possible learning disabilities in pre-term and fullterm children. In T. Field & A. Sostek (Eds.), *Infants born at risk: Physiological, perceptual, and cognitive processes.* New York: Grune & Stratton.

Sigman, M., & Parmelee, A. (1974). Visual preferences of four month old premature and fullterm infants. *Child Development, 45,* 969-965.

Skeffington, A.N. (1963). *The Skeffington Papers,* Series 36, No. 2 (p. 11). Santa Ana, CA: Optometric Extension Program.

Solan, H.A., & Ciner, E.B. (1986). *Visual perception and learning: Issues and answers.* New York: SUNY College of Optometry.

Suchoff, I.B. (1987). *Visual-spatial development in the child* (2nd ed.). New York: State University of New York, State College of Optometry.

Thelan, D., & Smith, L.B. (1994). *A dynamic systems approach to the development of cognitions and action.* Cambridge, MA: MIT Press.

Todd, V.R. (1999). Visual perceptual frame of reference: An information processing approach. In P. Kramer & J. Hinojosa (Eds.), *Frames of reference for pediatric occupational therapy* (2nd ed.). Baltimore: Williams & Wilkins.

Tseng, M.H., & Cermak, S.A. (1993). The influence of ergonomic factors and perceptual-motor abilities on handwriting performance. *The American Journal of Occupational Therapy, 47* (10), 919-926.

Tseng, M.H., & Murray, E.A. (1994). Differences in perceptual-motor measures in children with good and poor handwriting. *The Occupational Therapy Journal of Research, 14* (1), 19-36.

Tsurumi, K., & Todd, V. (1998). Tests of visual perception: What do they tell us? *School System Special Interest Section Quarterly, 5* (4), 1-4.

Turkewitz, G., & Kenny, P.A. (1985). The role of developmental limitations of sensory input on sensory/perceptual organization. *Developmental Behavioral Pediatrics, 6,* 302.

Ulman, S. (1986). Visual routines. In S. Pinker (Ed.), *Visual cognition.* Cambridge: MIT Press.

Warren, M. (1990). Identification of visual scanning deficits in adults after CVA. *American Journal of Occupational Therapy, 44,* 391-399.

Warren, M. (1993a). A hierarchical model for evaluation and treatment of visual perceptual dysfunction in adult acquired brain injury. Part 1. *American Journal of Occupational Therapy, 47* (1), 42-54.

Warren, M. (1993b). A hierarchical model for evaluation and treatment of visual perceptual dysfunction in adult acquired brain injury. Part 2. *American Journal of Occupation Therapy, 47* (1), 55-66.

Wechsler, D. (1991). *Wechsler Intelligence Scale for Children-III.* New York: Psychological Corporation.

Williams, H. (1983). *Perceptual and motor development.* Englewood Cliffs, NJ: Prentice-Hall.

Williamson, T. (1994). *OK Vision Test.* Farmersville, OH: Vision Lyceum.

Yost, L.W., & Lesiak, J. (1980). The relationship between performance on the developmental test of visual perception and handwriting ability. *Education, 101,* 75-77.

Zaba, J. (1984). Visual perception versus visual function. *Journal of Learning Disabilities, 17,* 182-185.

Ziviani, J., Hayes, A., & Chant, D. (1990). Handwriting: A perceptual motor disturbance in children with myelomeningocele. *Occupational Therapy Journal of Research, 10,* 12-26.

Publications on Classroom Activities

1. *Sensory Motor Handbook* (Bissell et. al., 1988). A wonderful guide for implementing and modifying activities in the classroom. Both visual perceptual and spatial concerns are addressed. Exercises are indexed according to the skill that they are designed to remediate.
2. *Little Kim's Left and Right Book* (McMonnies, 1992a). A picture book for preschoolers that is very appealing.
3. *A Practical Guide for Remedial Approaches to Left/Right Confusion and Reversals* (McMonnies, 1991).
4. *Overcoming Left/Right Confusion and Reversals: A Classroom Approach* (McMonnies, 1992b). Includes group and individual remediation exercises for older children. These 18 remedial procedures outlined by McMonnies follow a developmental sequence, starting with body awareness of oneself, which is used as a basis for acquiring an ability to project that internal awareness into space (directionality). The aim is to provide variety to activities that will establish an internal/automatic/reflex/somatesthetic awareness of right and left that does not depend on external cues such as identifying the writing hand, watch-wearing hand, or ring-wearing hand. Specific activities are used to help children overcome difficulty with left-to-right reading. All of McMonnies' materials are being distributed in the United States through the Optometric Extension Program (OEP), Santa Ana, CA.
5. *Reversal Errors: Theories and Therapy Procedures* (Lane, 1988) and *Developing Your Child for Success* (Lane, 1991). For use by school-based practitioners, teachers, and parents.
6. *Classroom Visual Activities (CVA)* (Richards, 1988). More than two dozen exercises are provided to remediate underlying laterality, directionality, and midline problems, as well as activities focused on the underlying visual skills necessary to achieve efficient visual perception. The exercises are categorized by the areas addressed, which include muscle movement, oculomotor skills, accommodation, and visualization.
7. *Songs for Sensory Integration: The Calming Tape and the Vision Tape* (Hickman, 1992). Auditory tapes. Optometrist Lynn Hellerstein is the narrator of the latter. Included is a clear, simple explanation of vision and exercises that can be used to supplement optometric vision therapy.
8. For children who are having trouble remembering letters, and their sounds, Pavlak (1985) presents 41 letter- and letter-sound recognition activities and 52 consonant- and vowel-recognition activities.

References

Bissell, J., Fisher, J., Owens, C., & Polcyn, P. (1988). *Sensory motor handbook*. Torrance, CA: Sensory Integration International.

Hickman, L. (1992). *Songs for sensory integration: The calming tape and the vision tape*. Boulder, CO: Belle Curve Records.

Lane, K.A. (1988). *Reversal errors theories and therapy procedures*. Santa Ana, CA: Vision Extension.

Lane, K.A. (1991). *Developing your child for success*. Santa Ana, CA: Vision Extension.

McMonnies, C.W. (1991). *A practical guide for remedial approaches to left/right confusion and reversals*. Sydney, Australia: Superior Educational Publication.

McMonnies, C.W. (1992a). *Little Kim's left and right book*. Sydney, Australia: Superior Educational Publications.

McMonnies, C.W. (1992b). *Overcoming left/right confusion and reversals: A classroom approach*. Sydney, Australia: Superior Educational Publications.

Pavlak, S.A. (1985). *Classroom activities for correcting specific reading problems*. West Nyack, NY: Parker Publishing.

Richards, R.G. (1988). *Classroom visual activities (CVA)*. Novato, CA: Academic Therapy Publications.

chapter 14

Psychosocial and Emotional Domains

Anne F. Cronin

key terms

Temperament
Social competence
Mastery motivation
Self-efficacy
Learned helplessness
Social referencing
Anxiety disorders
Disruptive behavior
 disorders
Affective disorders

Child abuse
Pediatric pain
Social learning and
 behavioral
 approaches
Occupational behavior
 perspective
Self-management and
 values clarification
Behavior management

■ CHAPTER OBJECTIVES

1. Understand the typical stages of psychosocial and emotional development and their influence on occupational performance.
2. Introduce the complex innate and environmental pressures on the individual that influence personality and behavior.
3. Identify and describe some features of atypical psychosocial and emotional development and their influence on occupational performance.
4. Specifically describe features of common psychosocial and behavioral problems that occur in childhood and adolescence.
5. Explain how child abuse and family mental illness influence psychosocial development.
6. Describe secondary emotional and behavioral problems associated with physical disabilities, long-term health problems, or pain.
7. Apply occupational therapy frames of reference for the prevention of psychosocial dysfunction in children and adolescents.
8. Describe evaluation of psychosocial function through interviews, inventories, and observation.

9. Discuss methods to enhance psychosocial development and to establish a positive therapy environment.
10. Describe behavioral management strategies.

As scientific and social research becomes more sophisticated, occupational therapists have become increasingly aware that all human functions and performance skills are intimately interrelated. Research suggests that a large part of what is called *personality* is inborn. Social and emotional responses develop as a product of these inborn characteristics (the child's human and nonhuman environments and sum of experience). Children with atypical development, including problems such as attention-deficit hyperactivity disorder (ADHD), spina bifida, and Down syndrome, are likely to have difficulties in psychosocial and emotional development.

Occupational therapists can serve an important role in enhancing and supporting the social and emotional health of the children with whom they work. Occupational therapists can help families identify risk factors and distinguish between the normal emotional turmoil of childhood and problems requiring professional intervention.

In both theory and research, therapists have identified links between cognition, self-esteem, volition, motivation, and personal choice of activity to functional performance and health (Henry & Coster, 1997; Kielhofner, 1995). Although most occupational therapy referrals focus on sensorimotor delays, the therapist should always consider social and emotional development in assessment and intervention. Without considering these aspects of development in a sensorimotor assessment, the therapist greatly reduces the chances of establishing an intervention plan that will result in lasting functional change.

Certain developmental transitions that stress children (e.g., starting school and puberty) challenge a child's ability to adapt. Most children need social and emotional support during childhood transitions. The sensitive therapist can ease these normal transitions as a part of meeting his or her client's developmental needs.

In all pediatric, school, or early intervention settings, occupational therapists need to recognize each child's social and emotional skills and assess how well these match the demands of the child's environment. Because the children served by occupational therapists are generally at risk for psychosocial problems, it is crucial that the therapist understands and incorporates the psychosocial and emotional domains of behavior in interventions. The challenge to the therapist is to develop both the cultural and ethnic sensitivities to support children and their families without being prescriptive about social values (Dillard et. al., 1992). An objective understanding of social behavior and emotional development is one goal of this chapter.

This chapter is organized into four sections. The first section presents typical developmental issues in the psychosocial and emotional domains of behavior. Discussions of temperament and social learning as the building blocks of psychosocial and emotional behavior offer the occupational therapist a neutral and objective basis for analyzing child behavior. This section also discusses the role of the environment in the development of social and emotional skills. Clinical examples offer insights into the environmental influences and cultural contexts of social and emotional behavior.

The second section includes an overview of atypical development that can influence occupational performance, including a discussion of maladaptive learned behaviors such as learned helplessness and behavior common to children who have experienced abuse. This section describes tools that the therapist can use to enhance psychosocial function.

The third section presents occupational therapy theories, evaluation, and intervention. The fourth section focuses on the everyday clinical setting and the promotion of psychosocial function in children. This section focuses on ways that the therapist can establish and maintain a positive therapy environment. It reviews behavior management strategies for use in the clinical, home, and classroom settings. This section ends with a discussion of issues surrounding the transition to adult life that are common to persons at risk for psychosocial and emotional difficulties.

■ DEVELOPMENT OF EMOTIONAL AND SOCIAL FUNCTIONS

Temperament Defined

Occupational therapists have long considered personality to be composite of nature and nurture. In this conception nature represents those characteristics, both genetic and congenital, that are innate to the individual. Nurture consists of environmental influences, such as social expectation, opportunity, and mastery experiences, and the social and interpersonal behaviors that the individual uses to respond to the environment. This section discusses the importance of nature.

For about 30 years the pioneering work of Chess and Thomas (1983, 1984, 1987) proposed that the child's nature strongly influences the role of nurture. A genetic predisposition, described by Chess and Thomas (1987) as *temperament*, exists in personality and behavioral style.

All standardized pediatric tests reveal variations in the rate of skill acquisition. Children also vary in the development of interests, habits, talents, and social competence. Therapists previously paid little attention to the range of differences in social and emotional development. These differences in behavior were the focus of Chess and Thomas' research. They considered information on caregivers' behavior and expectations and on the child's specific environmental experience. Their research focused on children's style of responding to various experiences, such as individual differences in carrying out activities such as sleeping, eating, and exploring objects (Chess & Thomas, 1987).

Although some authors have expanded the concept of temperament, research suggests nine characteristics of temperament. Box 14-1 provides the nine categories with their definitions. Temperament characteristics are neutral, and behaviors are not inherently good or bad. No child or parent is at fault for a child's activity level, intensity, or mood. Temperament is an individual's genetic predisposition to certain types of behavior in each category.

All of the characteristics listed in Box 14-1 are important in describing a child's behavioral style. Many of these attributes are not obvious in a therapy setting. Figure 14-1 provides typical examples of a high and low rating for each category. Children who are not at extremes in any direction may have the easiest time negotiating the social and emotional demands of childhood, but the determination of function or dysfunction has much to do with *goodness of fit*.

Categories of temperament

1. *Activity level.* Motor activity and the proportion of active and inactive periods
2. *Rhythmicity.* The predictability or unpredictability of the timing of biologic functions, such as hunger, sleep-wake cycle, and bowel elimination
3. *Approach or withdrawal.* The nature of the initial response to a new situation or stimulus (e.g., a new food, toy, person, or place); approaches are more positive, and the child may display them by mood expression (smiling, speech, or facial expression) or motor activity (swallowing a new food or reaching for a new toy); withdrawal reactions are negative, and the child may display them by mood expression (crying, fussing, speech, or facial expression) or motor activity (moving away, spitting new food out, or pushing new toy away)
4. *Adaptability.* Long-term responses to new or altered situations; the concern is not the nature of the initial responses but the ease with which the child modifies them in desired directions
5. *Sensory threshold.* The intensity level of stimulation necessary to evoke a discernible response, regardless of the specific form that the response may take
6. *Quality of mood.* The amount of pleasant, joyful, friendly mood expression as contrasted with the amount of crying, unfriendly behavior, and mood expression
7. *Intensity of reactions.* The energy level of response (positive or negative)
8. *Distractibility.* The effectiveness of an outside stimulus in interfering with or changing the direction of the child's ongoing behavior
9. *Persistence and attention span.* Persistence is the continuation of an activity in the face of obstacles or difficulties; attention span concerns the length of time that an activity is pursued without interruption

Modified from Chess, S., & Thomas, A. (1987). *Know your child* (pp. 28-31). New York: Basic Books.

Temperament Types

Chess and Thomas (1983) described three patterns of temperament that occurred commonly and resulted in patterns of behavior. They gave these combinations the labels *easy child, difficult child,* and *slow-to-warm-up child* (see Figure 14-1).

The *easy child* is positive in mood and approach to new stimuli. This child is calm, expressive, malleable, and has a low to moderate activity level. Children characterized as easy may vary greatly. They may vary in activity level (high activity is generally considered difficult), distractibility, and attention span. The *difficult* child is at the opposite end of the temperament spectrum. Characteristics that make a child difficult are a negative mood and approach, slow adaptability, a high activity level, and high emotional intensity. Extremes of sensory threshold often occur among children with a difficult temperament pattern. A *slow-to-warm-up* child demonstrates mild-intensity negative reactions to new stimuli in combination with slow adaptation. These children require several therapy sessions to become comfortable with the therapy environment and do not change therapists easily. Once a slow-to-warm-up child has established a routine, this child functions well. Transitions are problematic for children of this temperament type.

In an attempt to increase the usefulness of temperament in clinical settings, Turecki and Wernick (1994) elaborated on the original temperament categories. For greater clarity, they expanded the original 9 categories to 18. They also equated *high* and *low* levels of the categories with easy (potential asset) and difficult (potential liability) behaviors.

Turecki and Wernick (1994) described behavior characteristics that place the child at risk for developing positive relationships with others. These categories apply when the described behaviors are persistent. Occasional gloominess or impulsive behavior is normal and not a risk. Box 14-2 provides the temperament characteristics that Turecki and Wernick identified as potential liabilities.

Recent research has linked parental stress in child-rearing (Honjo et. al., 1998), school performance (Balck & Glass, 1998), developmental psychopathology (Kagan and Zentner, 1996; Nigg & Goldsmith, 1998), adolescent substance abuse (Weinberg et. al., 1998), and disruptive behavioral disorders (Harden & Zoccolillo, 1997) to temperament characteristics.

Occupational therapists usually see children at risk for delays in social and emotional development secondary to disability or physical injury. With the added stress of disability and illness, difficult personality traits have an exaggerated influence on the child.

Although innate temperament characteristics influence many aspects of development and behavior, the therapist must not underplay the role of the environment. The environment, or the "nurture" part of the formula, greatly influences the manifestations and interpretation of temperament (Chess & Thomas, 1987; Goldsmith, Buss, & Lemery, 1997). The economic level of the family often affects the child's social and emotional development. If the family does not meet basic needs of nourishment and shelter, the child can have difficulty in forming social relationships and establishing a healthy self-concept. The child's cultural background

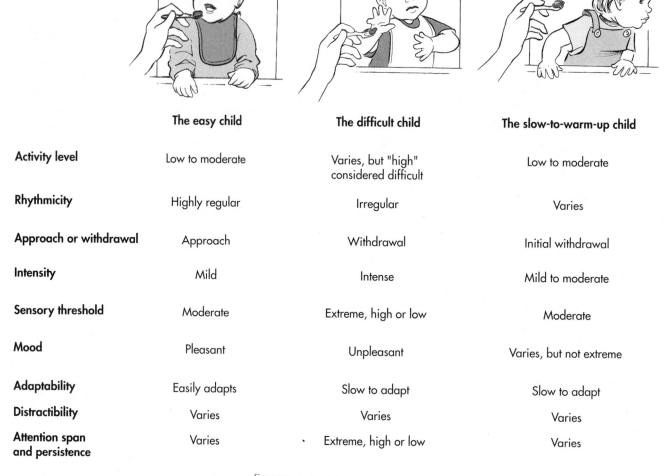

	The easy child	The difficult child	The slow-to-warm-up child
Activity level	Low to moderate	Varies, but "high" considered difficult	Low to moderate
Rhythmicity	Highly regular	Irregular	Varies
Approach or withdrawal	Approach	Withdrawal	Initial withdrawal
Intensity	Mild	Intense	Mild to moderate
Sensory threshold	Moderate	Extreme, high or low	Moderate
Mood	Pleasant	Unpleasant	Varies, but not extreme
Adaptability	Easily adapts	Slow to adapt	Slow to adapt
Distractibility	Varies	Varies	Varies
Attention span and persistence	Varies	Extreme, high or low	Varies

figure **14-1**   Temperament types.

may influence the development of certain temperamental characteristics.

Chess and Thomas (1987) were interested in learning about the influence of personality characteristics on the parent-child relationship and the child's development. They took the statistic concept, *goodness of fit,* and applied it to interpersonal relationships. When the demands and expectations of persons important to the child are compatible with the child's temperament, there is a good fit. Although Chess and Thomas focused on parent-child fit, other research has supported the findings in teacher and peer relationships (Keogh, 1986; Keogh & Burstein, 1988). Temperament and fit can be valuable teaching tools for therapists working to improve parent-child dynamics.

Social Competence

The child is not a passive recipient of social and environmental experiences. Even in infancy the therapist can observe active social patterns. Therapists have demonstrated active synchrony between infant movement and the structure of adult speech (Condon & Sander, 1974). Young infants imitate simple adult facial expressions (Meltzoff & Moore, 1983) and are socially aware and socially active. Research on the social and cognitive behavior of newborns affirms that infants identify with other human beings and respond with some self-awareness (Field & Fox, 1985).

Social competence is the result of the diverse skills and behaviors that allow individuals to learn, care for their daily needs, and maintain satisfactory human relationships within their cultural context. It provides the foundation from which an individual can successfully negotiate social and emotional challenges. Children develop skills for the environments in which they must function. Social competence in an infant includes sensory and perceptual skills, such as orienting to smiles and imitating facial expressions.

box 14-2 *Potential liability temperament characteristics*

Predominant mood: gloomy
Disposition: high-strung
Consistency of mood: changeable
Emotional sensitivity: high
Sociability: shy, timid
Expressiveness: reserved, taciturn
Initial response: withdrawal
Expression of anger: hot-tempered
Self-control: impulsive
Intensity: loud, forceful
Activity level: very high
Concentration: distractible
Regularity: irregular
Adaptability: poor; upset by transitions
Sensory threshold: low
Preferences: particular, strong
Negative persistence: stubborn, resistant
Positive persistence: gives up easily

Modified from Turecki, S., & Wernick, S. (1994). *The emotional problems of normal children* (pp. 102-105). New York: Bantam Books.

A socially competent 3-year-old child demonstrates a variety of complex skills. He or she reads the nonverbal cues of adults in the environment to learn about the desirable or dangerous aspects of unfamiliar situations. The 3-year-old child has mastered the nonverbal and gestural communication appropriate to his or her culture and imitates expected social behaviors well. Although the child may not understand the meaning or intent of certain learned behaviors, he or she understands that the performance of the behavior is expected. An example of this understanding is the child who folds his or her hands in prayer before meals. The child is imitating the behavior but is unlikely to understand prayer.

Social competence requires communication, motor, cognitive, emotional, and sensory perceptual skills. It usually involves interpersonal communication. Initially, communications are simple and nonverbal, like the infant's expression of distress or pleasure. Communication becomes more complex as children develop language. The communication skills of a preschooler indicate his or her understanding of the intangible meaning of words for emotions and thoughts. Although the child may not be able to define words, such as *happy, angry, understand, scared, feel, sad,* and *sorry,* a 3-year-old child correctly uses them (Bretherton & Beeghly, 1982; Wellman & Estes, 1987). By 3 years of age, social competence has become dynamical and interactive.

Problems in other performance areas can negatively affect social competence. Visual impairment is an example of a sensory processing impairment that influences social competence development. Vision helps the child identify distant features in his or her environment. Distant features are important in interpersonal activity and in recognizing context-specific behavior. Recognition of facial, gestural, and other behavioral cues that encourage a child to engage socially is limited in children with visual impairment. When visual or other sensory deficits limit the child, the occupational therapist can help provide an enriched environment and consistent social information to enhance the child's awareness and the development of compensatory behaviors to provide the needed social information.

Social competence implies that the child can appropriately adjust social behaviors according to location and audience. For example, most children play differently with peers versus with adults or in church versus on the playground. The therapist should consider the child's ability to adjust social interactions according to differing environments and situations when evaluating social competence. The therapist should also consider cultural and social aspects of the environment when evaluating the child's competence because the child's cultural experience and environmental pressures shape his or her social behavior.

Social behavior is difficult for the therapist to measure objectively in children who are not members of the predominant social group. For example, a 5-year-old child raised in a Vietnamese community may fail to prepare cereal and play board or card games when given the Denver Developmental Screening Test—Revised (Frankenburg, et. al., 1990). This indicates that the child may have some social difficulties with middle-class suburban playmates in the United States. However, such test item failures are not a delay in the absence of further indicators of social problems in the child's home, play, or school environments.

Competence is the ability to interact effectively with the environment while maintaining individuality and growth (Matheson & Bohr, 1997; White, 1971). For the child to achieve task competence, he or she must understand the function of any objects involved, the sensorimotor skill needed to act on that object in an effective manner, and the mastery motivation needed to accept the task challenge. Parent-child interactions may help or hinder a child's ability to organize and master developmental tasks. Most toddlers form selective attachments to certain adults in their world. This social attachment emotionally grounds the child and facilitates the child's ability to form new attachments. A lack of security in early social relationships influences peer relationships several years later. Children without secure adult relationships in early life often have difficulty making and sustaining friendships (Rutter, 1987).

Social competence in the preschool child requires an ability to imitate and learn the family's social rules. Over time children increasingly participate in larger social arenas, such as school. As their experience expands, the socially successful child modifies and expands his or her repertoire of social skills. The child's intrinsic motivation for social interaction enhances this process of social learning. Therefore social competence is "rooted in a sense of oneself, *both* as an individual and as a participant in a social world" (Holly & Schuster, 1992, p. 470).

Mastery Motivation

Mastery motivation is an "innate drive to find solutions" (Holly & Schuster, 1992, p. 462). Mastery motivation challenges people and drives them to practice and learn new skills.

Theories of mastery motivation emphasize the child's active role in his or her own learning. At around 9 months of age, children begin to engage in task-directed behavior. At this time, the child repeats successful cause-and-effect tasks like operating a pop-up box or ringing a toy telephone. Gentle praise of the child's play, especially focusing on what he or she does independently, reinforces the child's pleasure in the achievement.

Critical to the growth of mastery motivation is the freedom to initiate and learn from activity (Linder, 1990). Play is one of the earliest and most important arenas for learning social competence. Children who do not imitate or initiate play are likely to have difficulty in many areas of childhood performance. Competent play strengthens the child's motivation and encourages a positive sense of self. Parents or therapists who are too invested in the child's performance may not allow the child the freedom to experiment in play. Often a child can get frustrated when working toward a goal, and occupational therapists and parents are often too quick to rescue the struggling child. While relieving the child's frustration, this "help" may also reduce the child's sense of competence. The following is an example of a child experiencing mastery motivation:

> Two-year-old Bronwyn declares her need for independence by pushing her mother away, announcing, "No Mommy! Me do it myself!" as she shoves both legs into the same leg of her pajamas. Bronwyn is an intense and persistent child. She has begun to understand the function of objects and to connect that new understanding with her own growing skills.

To enhance the development of competence, Bronwyn's parents should allow her to persist at this task as long as she is interested. Her mother can participate and gently guide her explorations through social interactions like "You are working very hard at that. Look at your silly feet in the same hole; can you think of a way to fix that?" When Bronwyn is ready for help, she will let her mother know.

Parents and therapists need to encourage independence without giving the child insurmountable tasks. Bronwyn's mother can help her daughter gain skill and a sense of mastery by selecting clothing items appropriate to her daughter's developmental level. Slightly oversized elastic-waist shorts may make Bronwyn's explorations more positive than a pair of tights.

Self-Efficacy

Mastery motivation and the degree to which it is nurtured provide the basis for self-efficacy, a sense of self as individual and vital. Self-efficacy is a sense of personal value. The intrinsic awareness that one can accept challenges and potentially master them is the core of self-esteem (Chess & Thomas, 1983).

Average, or typical, children begin creating ideas about themselves and about their emotions between 18 months and 3 years of age (Greenspan & Greenspan, 1985). As young children begin to understand and remember the emotional aspects of their interactions, they begin to form ideas about their own value and the value of others. They play with language labels. They may offer the statements "You are my very best friend" and "I love you" indiscriminately to toys, family members, and strangers. Through the fourth year, children distinguish between *me* and *you* and develop an understanding of social expectations and standards. The therapist can enhance this developmental process by providing an emotionally supportive environment and modeling appropriate means of expressing difficult emotions like anger, fear, and sadness.

In older children and in children with atypical development, the nurturing adult often must contend with a social environment that frustrates the child's abilities and must combat the social learning associated with failures.

Children with atypical development may not be fully aware of their differences until about 7 years of age (Butler, 1989). At this time these children are likely to be more emotionally and socially vulnerable than the average child. Even typical school-age children sometimes assume that they are responsible for major negative events in their lives, such as the death of a sibling or their parents' divorce (Rothbaum & Weisz, 1989).

Children who need a great deal of adult direction and support are less likely to demonstrate initiative in learning and play. In the example of Bronwyn, if her parents consistently squelch her independence in the interest of efficiency, Bronwyn may begin to lose her motivation to initiate self-care independently. In therapy sessions, children with atypical aspects to their development are more likely to look externally for direction of their activity. The following are observations of personal causation as children react to the therapy environment.

> When he enters the therapy room, 6½-year-old Andre explodes with activity. He finds the large balls irre-

sistible. He rolls forward onto the mat and makes an ob-stacle course before the therapist begins his intervention. He shows good internal motivation in his attempts to or-ganize and stay with his undertaking. He quickly responds to verbal prompts and needs a minimum of adult reinforcement in exploratory play.

Seven-year-old Michael bounces into the therapy room and flits from one piece of equipment to another. He pulls a large ball out of the box and then abandons it to investigate the rope ladder. He spreads toys all over the floor but does not stay with any undertaking. He has little internal motivation to persist. With suggestions of-fered by the therapist, Michael is a little more organized but continues to need verbal praise and extravagant ges-tures of encouragement to persist.

Learned Helplessness

A child learns to expect a certain outcome based on ex-perience. Mastery motivation and self-efficacy are central for the child to establish the perspective that he or she can control outcomes and events. When a child believes that he or she has no control, helpless feelings result. When a child does not experience success, he or she loses motiva-tion to act. With repeated failures the child learns that his or her actions will not have an effect on the environment. As this occurs the child is less likely to initiate or persist at the behavior in question. This pattern of behavior is called *learned helplessness*. Learned helplessness occurs when an individual is exposed to unsolvable problems. Children who have learned that they fail in school no matter how hard they try soon quit trying. Learned helplessness is the actualization of the individual's perception of hopeless-ness: "Nothing that I do matters; why try?"

Learned helplessness is present in all areas of occupa-tional performance. It is most typically characterized by cognitive and affective disturbances (Schuster, 1992b). Schuster notes that "if the child learns early in life that outcomes are independent of responses, cause-effect re-lationships are not learned. It becomes more difficult to learn later in life that response can produce an outcome" (p. 284). Kashani, Soltys, Dandoy, Vaidya, and Reid (1991) investigated patterns of hopelessness in children with psychiatric problems. These researchers noted that children with high hopelessness demonstrated lower cog-nitive performance; had difficult temperament character-istics, more anxiety, and lower self-esteem than children with low hopelessness.

The therapist can avoid the development of learned helplessness through interactions that support and en-courage the child's initiation of action and persistence in tasks. Children who have experienced many failures lose the intrinsic motivation to master tasks. The therapist should notice whether the child is performing an activity to please adults or solely for external reinforcement (praise or rewards). If a child is not strongly motivated internally, the therapist needs to build support and en-couragement into all interventions and home programs. As the child begins to succeed and a sense of mastery de-velops, the therapist's reinforcement should become more subtle and less frequent.

■ DEVELOPMENT OF INTERPERSONAL RELATIONSHIPS IN CHILDREN AT RISK

Interpersonal reciprocity occurs naturally between human infants and their mothers (Brazelton, Tronick, Adamson, Als, & Wise, 1975). This reciprocity relies on both parties reading and interpreting the other's nonver-bal cues. The social interactions of the child with a dis-ability or with atypical development also are atypical. Low muscle tone results in minimal to absent facial ex-pression (Goldberg, 1977). A difficulty in reading adult or infant cues can strain this crucial relationship.

Children with low muscle tone or multiple sensory impairments are also likely to be less active and less inter-active than other children (Field, 1983; Linder, 1990). Although families often learn to read and respond to their atypical children, communication with others re-mains a problem. These children often become increas-ingly socially isolated at the developmental period when their peers have mastered language and begin to ex-pand their social horizons. In addition, the unusual physical appearance and stigma associated with disabili-ties may further impede social development (Bracegirdle, 1990).

Clearly the growth of social competence has an im-portant developmental influence on the child. Poor social skills may affect self-esteem and self-efficacy throughout the life span. Social awareness and sensitivity to the child's needs can reduce family stress and allow the fam-ily to focus on more positive interactions. In many cases the child's immature social behavior, rather than specific cognitive or physical limitations, restricts the child's community contact. Particularly in older children and adolescents, social difficulties exaggerate other difficul-ties that the child has and may isolate them from normal friendships and opportunities for peer support. The fol-lowing is an example of a child with social difficulties:

According to his family and teachers, 9-year-old Der-rick is an intense, emotional child. Derrick sometimes gets overexcited in play, but he is not an aggressive child. He is always in trouble on the playground, is frequently suspended for hitting and fighting on the playground, and his teacher is considering him for special placement with a "behavior disorder" because of these playground fights. When questioned, Derrick seems confused. He does not know why the other kids do not like him. He feels singled out and picked on by his classmates and teachers.

After observing Derrick during social interactions, his teacher notices that some of the other children are taunting him. Derrick cannot distinguish sarcasm or teasing from direct insults. He responds intensely and physically to these perceived insults, striking out and yelling. His classmates have recognized and played with this weakness. With discussion and role-playing, Derrick is able to develop responses to his peers that are more appropriate, and all of the adults in his life work to help him sort out the subtle cues that distinguish playful teasing from true insult.

Derrick has ADHD. His high activity level seems to be associated with a low sensory threshold. His difficulty with perception of nonverbal social cues suggests some difficulty with right-hemisphere processing. Derrick needs special coaching, demonstration, and language cues to respond in a socially appropriate way.

Communication

Communication is critical to the development of interpersonal skills. Children's earliest forms of communication are nonverbal, consisting of gestures, movements, facial expressions, taking turns, vocal pitch, and loudness. In the developmental process, children understand language (receptive language) long before they are able to talk (expressive language).

For the typical child, spoken language serves many social functions, including the ability to control other people's behavior, share feelings or information, and sustain social exchanges (Smolak, 1992).

Developmental issues involving language can affect the child's occupational performance. The pragmatics of language (i.e., the social rules governing the use of language) are especially important for the occupational therapist to understand because of their influence on interpersonal relationships.

Many interpersonal skills are based on language pragmatics. Pragmatics are context and audience specific. Pragmatics also involve active listening and respect for the communication of others. Highly verbal children may still have difficulty with pragmatics. The following is an example of a child with pragmatics difficulty:

"Hello, my name is Clariece Parker. I live at 1114 Long Street, Lake City, Florida, 66602. My subdivision is Pine Knoll, and I have a dog named Skip." This may seem to be an impressive greeting from a 4-year-old child, but when Clariece presents it in its entirety every time she faces a new person or a new situation, it is socially inappropriate.

In play with peers and in the therapy session Clariece seldom responds to conversations around her. When she wants to interact with another person, she interjects, into whatever conversation had been going on, a long discourse on one of her "topics." Clariece has monologues on listing the full addresses of everyone she

knows, the eating habits and life cycle of hermit crabs, and her bedtime routine. Although this impresses some adults, it alienates her in peer interactions and significantly limits her social experience.

Clariece's speech is often attention seeking. Her intended meaning in requesting and protesting things is appropriate. Other aspects of implied meaning (that her greetings are stereotypic and not tailored to the environment and that Clariece often does not acknowledge the speech of others) causes social problems for her. In addition, Clariece has significant difficulties with discourse skills. She gives fleeting attention to a conversation partner. She does not appropriately take turns, maintain a topic, or change the topic. Attempts to verbally direct her in therapy or in the classroom are frustrating. Clariece's peers dislike and avoid her in preschool and at church.

The therapist can appropriately prompt and reinforce these language skills as a part of the occupational therapy intervention. In particular the therapist needs to educate Clariece's family about her social language difficulties. Family members often grow so familiar with their child and his or her behavior that they have difficulty seeing how it may interfere outside of the home. This is particularly true of Clariece because her performance is better with adults than with children. Adults notice her memory and vocabulary more than the inappropriate timing and poor conversational relevance of her speech. Peers, however, are put off by her interruptions and self-centered focus. Unless the therapist identifies and explains the problem to Clariece's family, they will not understand why their articulate daughter has so much difficulty making friends.

Goodness of Fit

Two children with identical temperament types adapt differently based on the parents' temperament and style of caregiving. The interaction of child and adult temperaments on a day-to-day basis is called *goodness of fit* (Chess & Thomas, 1987). With a healthy parent-child fit, "the demands and expectations of the parents and other people important to the child's life are compatible with the child temperament, abilities, and other characteristics" (Chess & Thomas, 1987, p. 56). Teachers, therapists, and any other adult who has behavioral expectations for the child must balance their own expectations against the child's own behavioral set.

Goodness of fit includes a child's social context, behavior expectations, and family and social values. Figure 14-2 outlines the continuum from biologic impairment to behavioral outcome. *Social fit* is the heart of the interaction. The fit of the child's performance with social demands, both at home and in the community, determines whether a child must deal with the stress and frustration of social failure. The occupational therapist must consider the fit in establishing therapy goals. For example, the therapist can ask the following questions when considering a child's social fit:

- Will intensive therapy for increasing tongue lateralization improve the occupational performance of a 9-year-old child with athetoid cerebral palsy?
- What are the concerns and interests of this child?
- What are his or her family, school, and community demands?

Although remediation for tongue lateralization may be an appropriate intervention, such a focus is unlikely to address this child's difficulties with social fit.

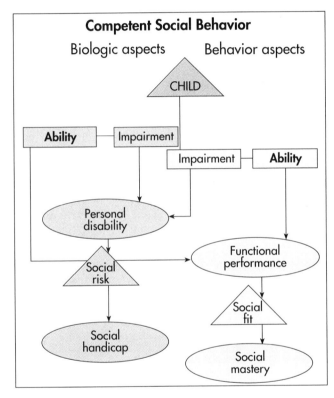

figure14-2   Social mastery.

Social Referencing

As noted previously, the child begins to compare himself or herself with peers around 7 years of age (third grade). Throughout the toddler and preschool years the child gradually becomes aware that he or she is different than other people. At this time the child is usually unaware of the long-term effect that his or her disability will have on social life (Schuster, 1992a). As the child begins *social referencing,* he or she confronts the reality of being different. Schuster (1992a) described the process of adaptation associated with growing up "different" in a series of stages (Table 14-1).

During the early elementary school years, the typical child struggles with normal peer influences and the need to fit in. The child often is rebellious and acts out during this period as he or she tries to take control and "defy" the disability. As many as 50% of chronically impaired children experience some form of depression by 10 years of age (Rodgers, Hilemeier, O'Neill, & Slonim, 1981; Russell, 1985; Schuster, 1992a). During this time it is common for the child to blame all of his or her problems on the disability. Over time children may assume that because the disability is "no good" they are "no good." In the elementary school years, children with a physical disability often report feeling that they are rejected, less popular, and more often victimized (Dudgeon, Massagli, & Ross, 1997; Yude, Goodman, & McConachie, 1998). The occupational therapist must learn to support and enhance the child's self-efficacy and provide opportunities for success. In addition the occupational therapist should help identify the child's unique needs, educate others, and be sensitive to the warning signs of depression.

As adolescence approaches, the child is more likely to act out, be noncompliant with medication or treatment regimens, and engage in high-risk behaviors. By late adolescence the successful child values himself or herself and accepts the disability. The risk for these individuals is that they will overfocus on the disability and maintain a negative outlook on the future. Although depression becomes

table 14-1 *Process of Adaptation When Growing Up "Different"*

Stage	Cognitive	Affective	Manifestations
Infancy	Naïveté	Naïveté	Unawareness of difference
Early childhood	Awareness	Naïveté	Curiosity
Middle childhood	Rebellion	Awareness	Uncooperativeness
Early adolescence	Adaptation	Rebellion	Socially acting out
Late adolescence	Acceptance	Adaptation	Prominent disability

Adapted from Schuster, C. (1992a). Adaptation to Uniqueness. In C. Schuster & S. Ashburn. *The process of human development: A holistic life-span approach* (3rd ed.). (pp. 351-375). Philadelphia: Lippincott.

less of a risk, these teens often need help making realistic life plans.

Summary

This section focused on issues in the typical development of emotional and social functions that are consistent in children. In children with disabilities, psychosocial stress may be great and social competence may be delayed. The therapist must understand these issues and value the principle of goodness-of-fit for successful interventions with children in all practice settings.

■ PSYCHOSOCIAL DYSFUNCTION IN CHILDREN

Occupational therapists typically see children who are at risk for difficulties in social and emotional functioning. Although about 2% of children and adolescents receive intervention for psychosocial problems (Cohen, Cohen, & Brook, 1993; National Advisory Mental Health Council, 1990), epidemiologic studies of the general population of children suggest that about 20% of children have psychosocial behavior that meets psychiatric diagnostic standards. The behavior of children and adolescents in home and school environments most commonly provides the basis for identifying and treating psychosocial dysfunction.

Recognizing Psychosocial and Behavioral Disorders

Parents are usually the first to notice atypical or worrisome behaviors in their child (American Academy of Child and Adolescent Psychiatry, [AACAP] 1995a), and teacher often is the first to notice these behaviors in the school environment. Most children occasionally behave in unusual or undesirable ways. For this reason it is sometimes difficult to discriminate ordinary behavior from dysfunctional behavior. Many emotional problems in children are a combination of problems in the child, family, and environment. There are four general categories of children's behavior patterns:

1. *Ordinary behavior.* The child occasionally does unusual or destructive things, but the behavior is well within expectations for his or her developmental age and situation.
2. *Problem behavior in response to extraordinary circumstances.* This occurs when the ordinary child faces a specific personal, health, or family crisis. When the child's crisis is resolved, the child functions adequately.
3. *Problem behavior in response to home environment.* This occurs when the ordinary child faces chronic

upheaval or dysfunction in the home environment. If the problems with the family or the physical environment are removed, the child functions normally.

4. *Troubled behavior.* This occurs in the child who carries his or her own pathologic condition. The problems are persistent and impair the child's ability to function and learn.

The degree and persistence of the problem are critical considerations in identifying mental health problems in children. The first approach to the first three types of behavior is to provide emotional support and promote self-awareness, self-efficacy, problem solving, and interpersonal skills. When a child's problematic behavior persists and the behavior is unusual for the child's developmental level, the therapist should consult a specialist.

The following signs in young children, particularly when observed in combination, are indications to refer him or her for psychosocial interventions (AACAP, 1995a):

- Marked fall in school performance; poor grades
- High levels of worry or anxiety, as shown by regular refusal to go to school, sleep, or take part in activities that are normal for the child's age
- Hyperactivity; fidgeting; constant movement beyond regular playing
- Persistent nightmares
- Persistent disobedience or aggression (longer than 6 months) and provocative opposition to authority figures
- Frequent, unexplainable temper tantrums

In older children, preadolescents, and adolescents, the following are some additional considerations (AACAP, 1995a; AACAP 1997a):

- Abuse of alcohol and/or drugs
- Inability to cope with problems and daily activities
- Marked changes in sleeping and/or eating habits
- Many complaints of physical ailments
- Aggressive or nonaggressive consistent violation of rights of others
- Opposition to authority, truancy, thefts, vandalism
- Intense fear of becoming obese with no relationship to actual body weight
- Depression shown by sustained, prolonged negative mood and attitude, often accompanied by poor appetite, difficulty sleeping, or thoughts of death
- Frequent outbursts of anger

When children exhibit these affective changes or problem behaviors, teachers and family members may seek the occupational therapist's advice regarding professional intervention. The therapist should be able to determine whether the family can handle the problem at home, the family may benefit from support in occupational therapy, and the child needs a referral to a specialist.

Major Classification of Psychosocial Dysfunction Used With Pediatric Populations

A summary of common pediatric psychosocial classifications follows. It is not comprehensive, and the practitioner specializing in this area should review this topic in greater depth.

Anxiety disorders

Anxiety is a normal response to stress and challenge. All children experience anxiety at some time. Typically, preschool children have intense but short-lived fears of things in their environment, such as animals, storms, or the dark. Therapists do not consider anxiety atypical in childhood until it persists and begins to interfere with occupational performance. The only form of anxiety disorder that is unique to childhood is separation anxiety disorder (Kaplan & Sadock, 1996). When therapists diagnose older children and adolescents with *anxiety disorders,* they base the diagnosis on the adult categories of the fourth edition of the *Diagnostic and Statistical Manual of Mental Disorders (DSM-IV)* (APA, 1994).

Generalized anxiety disorder refers to excessive anxiety and worry about events or activities such as school. The child or adolescent has difficulty controlling worries. Symptoms include restlessness, fatigue, difficulty concentrating, irritability, muscle tension, and sleep difficulties (AACAP, 1997c).

Separation anxiety usually centers on separation from a major attachment figure or place. The child with separation anxiety disorder experiences excessive anxiety, sometimes to the point of panic, when leaving a parent, the home, or some other secure fixture. Degrees of separation anxiety are normal in the preschool years. This disorder reaches clinical proportions when the behavior extends beyond the expected developmental level (as in a middle-school child) or when it occurs to such a degree that it interferes with normal activities. Separation anxiety occurs in approximately 3% to 4% of school-age children and 1% of adolescents (Kaplan & Sadock, 1996). A child or adolescent with severe separation anxiety may show the following (AACAP, 1995b):

- Constant thoughts and fears about safety of self and parents
- Refusal to go to school
- Frequent stomachaches and other physical complaints
- Overly clingy behavior at home
- Panic or tantrums at times of separation from parents

In a typical school or clinical setting the types of behaviors common to children with anxiety difficulties include fear of meeting new people and a tendency to have few friends. The therapist suspecting an anxiety disorder should immediately refer the child for further assessment. To assist the child's ability to function, the therapist can respect and help the child function when faced with feared events and offer reassurance in activities. The American Academy of Child and Adolescent Psychiatry (1995b) warns that because anxious children may also be quiet, compliant, and eager to please, their difficulties may be missed. Parents should be alert to the signs of severe anxiety so that they can intervene early to prevent future difficulties, such as loss of friendships, failure to reach social and academic potential, and feelings of low self-esteem.

Posttraumatic stress disorder (PTSD) is an intense, chronic anxiety reaction to traumatic emotional or physical stress. Research suggests that this diagnosis is appropriate for some victims of child abuse (APA, 1994; Famularo, Kinscherff, & Fenton, 1990; Rowan & Foy, 1993). The most notable effects of childhood PTSD are poor emotional bonding to children or adults, difficulty making friends, apathy, and depression. Children may demonstrate an acute form of PTSD with a relative increase in spontaneously acting as though the trauma were recurring, difficulty falling asleep, hypervigilance, nightmares, and generalized anxiety and agitation. A more chronic form of PTSD, and the form that therapists most likely observe, includes detachment, restricted range of affect, dissociative episodes, and sadness (Famularo et. al., 1990).

Disruptive behavior disorders

This category of atypical psychosocial behavior is characterized by actions directed externally. The *disruptive behavior disorders* described in *DSM-IV* are conduct disorders and oppositional defiant disorder.

The child with conduct disorder exhibits repetitive and persistent patterns of behavior that violate social expectations. Many children occasionally behave in ways that violate the rights of others or offend social sensibilities. Therapists reserve this diagnosis for serious and persistent infractions of social rules. Conduct disorder includes aggression toward people or animals, destruction of property, deceitfulness or theft, and serious violations of rules. Overall, conduct disorder is about twice as common in boys as in girls. The peak incidence in boys is 10 years, with a steady rate decline throughout adolescence. In girls the rate begins increasing between 10 and 16 years of age. Incidence is similar across genders by 16 years of age, and the rate for girls abruptly decreases after 16 years of age. These statistics suggest developmental periods of increased risk for conduct disorder. The most common explanation for these findings is the role transitions that the child experiences (Cohen et. al., 1993). The ages and the incidence of this disorder are likely to vary within cultural groups because the disorder is defined by cultural expectations.

Oppositional defiant disorder includes negative, hostile, and defiant behaviors often directed toward authority figures. Oppositional defiant disorder differs from conduct disorder primarily in that the disruptive behavior does not violate the rights of others. Behaviors common to this disorder include exhibiting temper tantrums, actively defying adult direction, and blaming others for their own actions. The individual is often angry and resentful (APA, 1994). This disorder shows similar prevalence and age patterns for boys and girls. The incidence increases in adolescents between 13 and 16 years of age and then becomes much less common (Cohen et. al., 1993). Like conduct disorder, the incidence of oppositional defiant disorder is likely to vary within different ethnic groups based on cultural expectations.

The presence of one or more of the following increases the risk of violent or dangerous behavior (AACAP, 1998a):

- Past violent or aggressive behavior or threats directed toward self or others
- Access to guns or other weapons
- Family history of violent behavior or suicide attempts
- Unwillingness to accept responsibility for one's own actions
- Recent experience of humiliation, shame, loss, or rejection
- Bullying or intimidating peers or younger children
- Being a victim of abuse or neglect (physical, sexual, or emotional)
- Abuse or violence in the home
- Themes of death or depression evident in conversation, written expressions, reading selections, or artwork
- Preoccupation with themes and acts of violence in television shows, movies, music, magazines, comics, books, video games, and Internet sites
- Use of alcohol or illicit drugs
- Poor peer relationships and/or social isolation
- Involvement with cults or gangs
- Little or no supervision or support from parents or other caring adult

Attention-deficit hyperactivity disorder

ADHD is the most common behavioral disorder in childhood and occurs in approximately 3% to 5% of school-age children. This disorder occurs three to five times more often in boys than in girls (Kaplan & Sadock, 1996). ADHD includes a cluster of behavioral limitations that include a short attention span, poor impulse control (including poor safety awareness), difficulty completing tasks, high levels of motor activity, emotional lability, and poor interpersonal awareness. ADHD is especially difficult to diagnose objectively because the age and gender of the client likely modify the clinical manifestations of the disorder. Although many children have high activity levels, the "hyperactivity" associated with ADHD is characterized by ". . . haphazard, poorly organized

and not goal-directed" behavior (APA, 1994). Children with ADHD may exhibit several of the following school and classroom behaviors (AACAP, 1995c; Kaplan & Sadock, 1996):

- Has difficulty organizing work
- Is easily distracted; gives the impression that he or she has not heard instructions
- Makes careless, impulsive errors
- Frequently calls out in class
- Has difficulty waiting his or her turn in group situations
- Fails to follow through on teachers' and therapists' requests
- Is unable to play games for the same amount of time as peers

Children with *task impersistence* have difficulty completing tasks, particularly challenging ones, without being prompted. This problem critically limits the social and emotional development and school performance of the child. Children with task impersistence have difficulty sustaining participation in games and often cooperate poorly. They have little sense of the overall task, or the "whole picture," in terms of organized games. These children are often avoided, or even ostracized, in middle childhood because their behaviors disrupt organized group activities.

ADHD can contribute to school failure, difficulties making and keeping friends, learned helplessness, and poor self-efficacy. Children with ADHD have cognitive deficits that impair social learning and affect the child's innate ability to mediate behavior. Many children with ADHD have secondary psychosocial diagnoses. Secondary labels like conduct disorder or overanxious disorder can result as the child attempts to compensate for the hyperactivity and limited ability to attend (Friedman & Doyal, 1992). In many cases the ADHD symptoms begin to diminish in late adolescence, although social impairments may persist.

Mood disorders

Mood disorders may be present in individuals throughout the lifespan and are characterized by the sustained internal state of the person. Mood disorders, or *affective disorders*, are relatively common, occurring in about 5% of children and adolescents in the general population. "Children under stress, who experience loss, or who have attentional, learning, conduct or anxiety disorders are at a higher risk for depression" (AACAP, 1998a). Although the *DSM-IV* does not separate mood disorders of childhood and adolescence from those of adults, the behavior of children and teenagers with mood disorders often differs from that of adults. The primary signs of depression in childhood include the following (AACAP, 1997c):

- Frequent sadness, crying, and hopelessness
- Decreased interest in activities or inability to enjoy previously favorite activities

- Social isolation, poor communication, or difficulty with relationships
- Increased irritability, anger, or hostility
- Low self-esteem and guilt
- Extreme sensitivity to rejection or failure
- Frequent complaints of physical illnesses such as headaches and stomachaches
- Frequent absences from school or poor performance in school
- Poor concentration
- A major change in eating and/or sleeping patterns
- Talk of or efforts to run away from home
- Thoughts or expressions of suicide or self-destructive behavior

Children and adolescents who cause trouble at home or school may actually be depressed but do not know it. Because the child may not always seem sad, parents and teachers may not realize that troublesome behavior is a sign of depression. Although they may not appear sad, when asked directly, these children may state that they are unhappy or sad (AACAP, 1998a).

Major depressive disorder

In children and adolescents the prevailing mood can be either depression or irritability. Depressed children may fail to gain weight as expected with normal growth. They often have little interest in daily activities and often fall behind in their schoolwork. Excessive fatigue and sleep disorders are common. All areas of development are likely to be impaired during a depressive episode, and the child may be misdiagnosed with a learning disability (Kaplan & Sadock, 1996). These disorders tend to be insidious, and in adolescents they often are associated with substance abuse. Other symptoms include suicidal thoughts or actions or psychotic symptoms (APA, 1994). In childhood and late adolescence, rates for major depression are low with no significant gender differences. Cohen and others (1993) observed a sharp increase in the incidence of major depression in girls around the age of puberty. This finding suggests that the biologic changes of puberty predispose young women to this problem. Another hypothesis is that changing social expectations play a role. Depression is 1.5 to 3 times more common among children with a depressed parent than in the general population (APA, 1994).

Bipolar disorders, such as manic-depressive illness, usually appear in adolescents and adults before 35 years of age. People with manic-depressive illness have a combination of extremely high (manic) and low (depressed) moods (Kaplan & Sadock, 1996). Some of the behaviors associated with manic-depressive illness "are similar to those that occur in teenagers with other problems such as drug abuse, delinquency, ADHD, or even schizophrenia. The diagnosis can only be made with careful observation over an extended period of time. . . ." (AACAP, 1995d).

Teenagers with manic-depressive illness can be treated with psychiatric care effectively. The occupational therapist needs to be aware of this disorder to make appropriate referrals for evaluation and treatment. Therapists also monitor adolescents with diagnoses of bipolar disorder for signs of exacerbation or treatment side effects such as drug toxicity. Occupational therapists in mental health settings may be involved in increasing occupational function, rebuilding self-esteem, and improving relationships while the teen is hospitalized.

Obsessive-compulsive disorder

Obsessive-compulsive disorder (OCD) is relatively common, occurring in 2% to 3% of the general population (Kaplan & Sadock, 1996). OCD usually begins in adolescence or young adulthood and is characterized by recurrent obsessions and/or compulsions that are intense enough to cause severe distress. To be diagnosed with OCD, the obsessions must be recurrent and persistent thoughts, impulses, or images that the child does not want and that cause marked anxiety or distress. These obsessions are often unrealistic or irrational. Compulsions are repetitive behaviors (e.g., hand washing, hoarding, and keeping things in order) or mental acts (e.g., counting and avoiding) (Kaplan & Sadock, 1996).

OCD is associated with some childhood disorders, including Prader-Willi syndrome and Tourette's syndrome. Obsessive-compulsive behavior patterns interfere with the child's normal routine, academic functioning, social activities, or relationships (AACAP, 1997d). Children and adolescents often feel shame and embarrassment about their OCD, and many fear that it means that they are crazy. Communication between parents and the child with OCD is critical. Understanding of the problem helps parents appropriately support their child (AACAP, 1997d).

Eating disorders

Eating disorders is common during adolescence. The incidence of the two primary psychiatric eating disorders, anorexia nervosa and bulimia nervosa, is increasing in the United States. As many as 10 in 100 young women suffer from an eating disorder (AACAP, 1998b). The therapist should be aware that these disorders also occur in boys but much less often.

Anorexia nervosa is an eating disorder that generally occurs in females between 10 and 30 years of age. It is characterized by secret, self-imposed dietary limitations that result in a body weight less than 85% of that expected for height and build (APA, 1994). Although its incidence is relatively small, anorexia is life threatening and usually results in hospitalization. Persons who are admitted to university hospitals for treatment have a mortality rate of 10%, usually caused by starvation, suicide, or electrolyte imbalance (APA, 1994). Individuals with anorexia have highly distorted body images and experience intense fear of gaining weight despite being emaciated. Because teenage girls often have distorted body images, they are developmentally more vulnerable to this problem. The mean age of onset is 17 years. Atkins and Silber (1993) suggested that the development of anorexia in children relates to a complex combination of factors, including physical maturation, entry into junior high, loss of friendships, or some combination of these factors.

Early warning signs of anorexia include the following (APA, 1994; Kaplan & Sadock, 1996):
- The person is typically a perfectionist and a high achiever.
- The person often suffers from low self-esteem, irrationally believing that he or she is fat regardless of how thin he or she becomes.
- The teenager desperately needs a feeling of mastery over life.

Some common medications, such as the stimulants commonly used to treat attention problems (e.g., dexedrine or methylphenidate), can cause medicine-induced anorexias in some children. Therapists who suspect anorexia should refer the child or adolescent for careful evaluation and possible intervention. In extreme cases, this condition can be life threatening.

Bulimia nervosa is like anorexia nervosa in that it is a response to a distorted body image and occurs most frequently in young women. Bulimia is less destructive and life threatening than anorexia and is less likely to require hospitalization. Bulimia involves recurrent episodes of binge eating followed by a self-induced purging. Although anorexia is often episodic, bulimia is more likely to be chronic for many years. Mental disorders often seen with bulimia include depression, anxiety, and substance abuse of alcohol or stimulants (APA, 1994).

Warning signs of bulimia are as follows (AACAP, 1998b; APA, 1994):
- The person binges on large quantities of high-caloric food and purges his or her body of dreaded calories by self-induced vomiting and use of laxatives.
- These binges may alternate with severe diets, resulting in dramatic weight fluctuations.
- Teenagers may try to hide the signs of throwing up by running water while spending long periods of time in the bathroom.

Although the purging of bulimia is not likely to be life threatening, it presents a threat to the individual's physical health, including dehydration, hormonal imbalance, and damage to vital organs.

Developmental issues in psychiatric diagnosis

Many children who have psychosocial problems, particularly disruptive behaviors, receive multiple diagnoses (Cohen et. al., 1993). In particular, ADHD creates greater-than-average social and emotional stress. In addition, many psychosocial diagnoses follow a typical developmental course as the child matures. Table 14-2 shows that boys with ADHD have a steady decline in all disruptive behavior disorders throughout their teenage years. Where incidence rates decline steadily, the gradual growth in skills, self-control, social maturity, and conformity to gender role expectations probably accounts for the improvement (Cohen et. al., 1993). These typical progressions suggest that intervention emphasizing developmental social skills may alleviate some problems in the younger child and help speed the resolution of the disorder.

As mentioned previously, the pattern for disruptive behavior disorders in girls is initially low, peaks in the 14- to 16-year-old age group, and then diminishes. Therapists can give support and specific social skill intervention to help provide the teenage girl with positive behavior to help her through this biologically and socially stressful time.

Cultural and social environment

Culture is a complex interaction of ethnicity, formal belief systems, social experience, and language. Families, schools, classrooms, and playgroups have their own "cul-

table 14-2	*Disruptive Behavior Disorders (Prevalence in Percentage)*					
	Attention Deficit Disorder		Conduct Disorder		Oppositional Disorder	
Age (yr)	Girls	Boys	Girls	Boys	Girls	Boys
To 13	8.5	17.1	3.8	16.0	10.4	14.2
14-16	6.5	11.4	9.2	15.8	15.6	15.4
17-20	6.2	5.8	7.1	9.5	12.5	12.2

Modified from Cohen, P., Cohen, J., Kasen, S., Velez, C., Hartmark, C., Johnson, J., Rojas, M., Brook, J., & Streuning, E. (1993). An epidemiological study of disorders in late childhood and adolescence: I. Age- and gender-specific prevalence. *Journal of Child Psychology and Psychiatry, 34,* 851-867.

ture" for insiders. The cultural environment is in some ways similar to the physical environment in that it influences the individual's behavior in a particular setting. This occurs in the spontaneous change of affect seen when the child transitions from the playground to the classroom or from home to school.

Illustrating an American cultural ideal in their study of adolescents with cerebral palsy, Magill and Hurlbut (1986) found that the subgroup of teenage girls with cerebral palsy had low self-esteem:

> [These girls] scored significantly lower than the boys with (cerebral palsy), the nondisabled boys, and nondisabled girls on physical self-esteem. . . . The scores of the boys with (cerebral palsy) were similar to those of the nondisabled groups (p. 402).

This study probably reflects a cultural view of beauty. Abnormal movements and poor control of facial musculature, which are common to cerebral palsy, place girls with these problems at odds with cultural values. These young women are likely to stand out among their peers and have fewer opportunities for social and emotional growth because of the societal valuation of women's beauty. Children with disabilities of all types encounter social constraints that limit their active participation in the daily life of the community, sometimes in subtle ways.

A white, middle-class, American child with Prader-Willi syndrome inevitably fails to live up to cultural expectations. Society considers compulsive eating to be a character flaw, even when it is based in a biologic condition. Compulsive eating in Prader-Willi syndrome does not respond to behavior modification or other social learning strategies. The child with Prader-Willi syndrome is likely to be unfashionably over weight and will never be able to live without another person controlling and limiting his or her food intake. Although persons with other mental retardation syndromes like Down syndrome or fragile X syndrome have the possibility of functioning semi-independently in a group home situation, the person with Prader-Willi syndrome is limited to more restrictive living arrangements because of compulsive eating. Therefore the individual with this diagnosis exemplifies a poor person-culture fit. His or her compulsive eating negatively influences the acceptance and perceived competence of this individual.

Family and mental illness

Children are better able to adapt to stress when there is a positive parent-child relationship. Specific relationship assets include positive parental attitudes, involvement, and guidance (Gribble et. al., 1993). The positive parent-child relationship mediates childhood stress, and children from this type of family function with greater resilience. Children can adjust more effectively to physical

disorders when the parent-child relationship is strong and positive (Lavigne & Faier-Routman, 1993).

In general, positive family interactions optimize the child's health and functional performance. When family relations are strained, the child is at increased risk for dysfunction (Vessey & Caserza, 1992). Mental illness in parents is a definitive risk for children in the family (i.e., these children have a higher risk for developing mental illnesses than other children). The risk is greatest when the parent's illness is manic-depressive illness, schizophrenia, alcoholism or other drug abuse, or major depression (AACAP, 1995e). Intervention for a child whose parents have mental illness should include the following:
- Convincing the child that he or she is not to blame for the parent's illness
- Supporting self-esteem and good coping skills in the child
- Facilitating a strong relationship with a healthy adult
- Supporting the child's friendships
- Promoting interest in and success at school
- Helping the child develop healthy, social interests and activities

Child abuse

The same children who are at risk for psychosocial and emotional difficulties are at risk for *child abuse*. The therapist needs to support the child and the family and has the responsibility to objectively consider parents' current ability to adequately care for their child. Because occupational therapists work with children at high risk for abuse, they should understand and evaluate the abuse risk factors as a component of any child assessment.

Three factors associated with abuse are (1) the characteristics of the child, (2) environmental stress, and (3) the parents' personality and background. Abuse is most prevalent in preschoolers, particularly those whose cognitive, social, or physical developmental delays extend the child's dependency and demands on their caregivers. Therapists associate physical abuse with difficult temperament characteristics and neurologic impairments. The school-based occupational therapist commonly treats children who are survivors of child abuse. In these cases it is important for the therapist to know that the emotional trauma remains long after the abusive incident. The therapist can address these emotional "hidden bruises" with early recognition and treatment to minimize the long-term effects of physical abuse. Children who have been abused may display the following (AACAP, 1998c):
- Poor self-image
- Sexual acting out
- Aggressive, disruptive, and sometimes illegal behavior
- Anger and rage
- Self-destructive or self-abusive behavior; suicidal thoughts
- Passive or withdrawn behavior

- Anxiety and fears; lack of trust in others
- School problems or failure
- Feelings of sadness or other symptoms of depression
- Flashbacks, nightmares
- Drug and alcohol abuse

The severe emotional damage to abused children often remains hidden until adolescence or later. Whether or not the emotional effects of abuse are evident, the therapist needs to implement social and emotional support strategies for the child or adolescent with a history of child abuse.

Assessment of the child at risk should include observations of the child's physical appearance and affective and social behavior. Observations documented over time are more reliable and court admissible than those documented only once. The therapist should use norm-referenced evaluation tools whenever possible because these also provide the most reliable evidence should the case go to court (Davidson, 1995).

Assessment of the home environment and the parent teaching style is valuable in planning all interventions but vital when the child is at risk for abuse. The *Developmental Interview for Parents of Young Children at Risk* (Davidson, 1995) offers an interview format designed to identify problems in the child's home environment. The *Nursing Child Assessment Teaching Scale (NCATS)* (Barnard, 1980) also focuses on the family and home environment. This assessment includes the observation of a parent teaching the child a play activity. By comparing the parent's report of their teaching style with direct observation, the therapist can identify discrepancies and potential problem areas.

The following example, drawn from the work of Davidson (1995), illustrates some of the issues important for the occupational therapist working with children and parents:

> Four-year-old Monique is new in the early intervention program. During developmental assessment she maintains a flat affect and has no spontaneous exploratory play. She is compliant and waits quietly for the therapist to direct her. Monique's mother arrives late to pick her up. She appears stressed and disorganized.
>
> Monique does not acknowledge her mother's presence. Monique's mother abruptly demands, "Has she been bad again?" After the therapist explains that Monique worked well, her mother replies, "I've had a headache all day and nothing to eat. Come on, Monique, you can't sit there all day." The family leaves without further comment.

When working with children at risk for abuse, prevention is best (i.e., identifying and supporting families at risk, thus heading off the potential for abuse). If the therapist believes that a family is at risk for abuse, he or she needs to carefully observe the child's behaviors and physical appearance. The therapist following Monique documented the exchange described previously, along with other worrisome incidents as they occurred:

> In a parent-child teaching activity, Monique's mother is asked to help her daughter string beads for a necklace. Both mother and daughter are enthusiastic about the idea. Given the beads, Monique's mother worries about the aesthetics of the necklace, correcting Monique's choices and undoing her daughter's work. As the interaction progresses, Monique becomes apathetic and passive.

This type of interaction exemplifies behavioral indicators of risk for child abuse. Monique relates poorly to adults in general and shows limited attachment behaviors toward her mother. Monique's mother appears overwhelmed and socially limited. She does not interact with her daughter in a nurturing manner. Monique's mother is preoccupied with her own needs and excludes those of Monique. The therapist should continue to evaluate the child and parent, followed by preventive intervention or referral to Child Protective Services.

The therapist has a responsibility to refer the family to the state Child Protective Services agency if he or she suspects abuse or neglect. Referrals involve a telephone call, followed by a letter that outlines the client's name, age, address, and a summary of the reasons for concern. The Child Protective Services agency categorizes the reports according to severity and type and schedules investigations accordingly. The therapist should make repeated reports if continued observations of the problem behavior occur. The case sometimes requires multiple referrals before it qualifies for an in-depth Child Protective Services evaluation or legal intervention.

The therapist can initiate preventive intervention for the family at risk for abuse at any point in the therapy relationship. The therapist can assist parents by facilitating the establishment of a social support network and educating them regarding child development and parenting skills. The development of a support system begins with the parent-therapist relationship. Parent groups and parenting classes also provide valuable information and social contacts. The therapist should not limit these groups to abusive or "at-risk" families. Some facilities routinely offer parenting seminars presented by members of the interdisciplinary team. This approach offers nonjudgmental support that may alleviate the pressure at home and reduce the likelihood of abuse (Davidson, 1995).

Children with chronic health problems

In some cases, children are referred to occupational therapy services for the treatment of emotional problems that are secondary to medical illness and long-term hospitalization (Frank et. al., 1991; Stowell, 1987). Disorders in interests, motivation, and play behavior are common in hospitalized children. Emotional and behavioral problems are often associated with children who have incurred traumatic brain injury or other neurologic (cognitive) impairment. The first noticeable signs of cognitive impairment are often social affective deficits (Table 14-3).

Emotional lability in children with traumatic brain injury means that moods change abruptly. Emotional response may be inappropriate to the situation or may be more intense than the situation seems to warrant. In particular, the child is easily upset when challenged. Perhaps in response to their perception of having little control, children with cognitive problems sometimes become bossy and negative. These children perform poorly in directive environments, such as most classroom and therapy situations.

Chronic conditions in childhood affect the child's overall development. The pediatric therapist sees a scope of chronic conditions that changes with alterations in health care delivery and health technology. Stowell (1987) presented a model of psychosocial intervention with pediatric bone marrow transplantation patients. This article outlined the social and emotional challenges

table 14-3 *Early Signs of Emotional Distress*

Problem	Signs
Emotional lability	Has abrupt mood changes
	Is sensitive to criticism
	Exaggerates emotional outbursts in response to ordinary events
Negativity	Finds fault with every suggestion or activity
	Refuses to participate in activity or participates without making any effort to succeed
Social withdrawal	"Shuts down" and does not talk to the therapist even in response to direct questions
	Relates poorly to others (even parents)
Low frustration tolerance	Throws toys and objects rather than persisting at challenging tasks
	Quits working abruptly and does not complete activities
Poor task initiation	Does not mentally organize tasks and has difficulty knowing where to begin
	Requires an external prompt to begin a task
Oppositional	May become bossy and negative
	Argues with the therapist's ideas and plans
	Denies that personal behavior is relevant to problems with completing tasks

secondary to a disease process that was once fatal and a treatment process that impairs the child's development.

Another condition that therapists see in early intervention programs is perinatal human immunodeficiency virus (HIV) infection (Anderson, Hinojosa, Bedell, & Kaplan, 1990). Children with perinatal HIV infection have difficulties in neuromotor, developmental, and psychosocial performance. Interventions should be sensitive to the overall developmental needs of the child and the needs of the caregivers.

With HIV, cancer, and many other childhood conditions, the prognosis affects therapist and caregiver decisions. Children who are expected to have little chance of survival into the adult years are treated differently than other children. Establishing future goals, long-term plans, and skill building for competence help shape developing cognitive skills. A child who is therefore sheltered because of his or her potentially limited life span may lose important developmental learning experiences (Vessey & Caserza, 1992).

Atypical development in any performance area places the child at risk for inappropriate expectations (Turecki & Wernick, 1994). Children who have chronic health problems in addition to problems with cognition or depression are the likely to have secondary difficulties with psychosocial development (Pollock, 1986; Youssef, 1988). These problems occur more typically in elementary or middle-schoolage children (Barkley, Anastopoulos, Guevremont, & Fletcher, 1991; Simmons et. al., 1987). Important considerations when treating children and adolescents with chronic health problems include the child's temperament, medication side effects, and the influence of the disease process on the child and on his or her family. A look at the varied environments in which a child needs to function may help by anticipating problems, especially peer problems that affect the child's social and emotional development (Creer, Stein, Rappaport, & Weiss, 1992; Pollock, 1986).

Pediatric pain

Many pediatric conditions are associated with chronic or recurrent pain. Notable among these forms of *pediatric pain* are juvenile rheumatoid arthritis, postsurgical rehabilitation, and burn rehabilitation. Chronic and recurrent experiences with pain are associated with depression and delayed return of functional status (Solomon, Walco, Robinson, & Dampier, 1998). There has been much recent research in the area of children's pain experiences. Some of the findings of importance to the occupational therapist are as follows:

- Song and others (1998) found that of 73 children followed for chronic musculoskeletal pain, 36 had no identifiable organic etiology for their pain. The researchers recommend the increased use of psychosocially based pain management techniques for these children.

- Researchers have documented a pattern of inconsistent use of prescribed pain medications in children, and 25% of children in their study said that the pain management available was ineffective (Boughton et. al., 1998).
- The child achieves an understanding of pain with the development of cognition, and pain measures must correspond with the child's level of cognitive development to be useful (Lederhaas, 1997).
- Cultural and parental beliefs about pain and pain medications strongly influence a child's expression of pain (McGrath & Frager, 1996).
- Adults vary in their abilities to recognize signs of pain in children.
- Perceived lack of personal control exaggerates children's perception of pain (McGrath & Frager, 1996).

Any disorder that causes pain, limits the child's activity, or causes increased dependence on adults has the potential to influence the child's development and psychosocial function. Pain is a complex interaction of biologic, psychologic, and sociologic phenomena. Turnquist and Engel (1994) reported that children with prolonged pain experience a sense of loss of control. This sense may result in a decrease in courage, motivation, and constructive activity. These children often develop a sense of learned helplessness.

A child's cognition, coping strategies, ability to communicate feelings, and temperament affect the pain experience. Schechter, Bernstein, Beck, Hart, and Scherzer (1991) found that parental anticipation of their child's distress greatly influenced the distress level manifested by the child.

The therapist can teach the child strategies to self-manage chronic pain, and the child may benefit from pain management protocols similar to those used with adult clients. Therapists recommend relaxation training and the use of visualization for the psychologic management of children's pain.

Pain clearly affects children's functional performance, and prolonged pain can leave the child at risk for other emotional and social problems. In children with arthritis, disease severity and disease activity are associated with behavioral problems and poor social competence (Daltroy et. al., 1992). Although therapists focus on functional outcomes, those who evaluate pain and provide pain management interventions can better meet the needs of children with painful conditions.

Summary

Children's development is a dynamical and multifaceted process. The child's neurologic and genetic makeup, experience, and environment influence his or her psychosocial development. Many children with atypical development, physical impairment, and chronic illness are at risk for emotional problems. Occupational therapists in all pediatric settings must address the child's social and behavioral competencies as a routine part of clinical assessment and intervention.

■ THEORETIC APPROACHES AND FRAMES OF REFERENCE APPLIED TO OCCUPATIONAL THERAPY INTERVENTION

The theoretic models of occupational therapy for children with psychosocial problems can be categorized as (1) developmental theories, including sensory integration (SI); (2) social learning and behavioral approaches; and (3) occupational behavioral models. This section presents each model briefly and gives specific examples of occupational therapy interventions incorporating these models.

Developmental Theories

Developmental theories provide much of the foundation for pediatric occupational therapy practice. The first developmental approaches (e.g., Gesell) assumed that children follow orderly, predictable patterns of development with successively higher levels of nervous system control. These models, focusing on "top down" control, are called *hierarchic theories of development.* Therapists widely use this type of theoretic model in screening instruments because it offers general developmental guidelines for normative performance. Hierarchic models of development posit that atypical development is the result of an unusual occurrence, such as a disabling condition or severe social stress. Therapists can use this approach to determine stage- and age-appropriate behavior expectations and as a guide to direct intervention. Hierarchic models of development are less useful in explaining behavior and development with an atypical nervous system (as in cerebral palsy or autism) or with atypical sensory systems (as in vision or hearing impairment).

More recent approaches to developmental theory have integrated systems theory and dynamical action theory (Shumway-Cook & Woollacott, 1995). Systems theories consider the child as a whole, subject to internal and external forces that effect change. Systems theory offers a dynamic and integrated look at the child within the context of home and school pressures. This model is limited in that there are few assessment instruments, and those that exist do not answer the question of how one child's development compares with that of his or her peers. Dynamical action theory emphasizes the development of patterns and self-organization. This model has been used in recent research of cognitive and social development. The dynamical action approach to theory is widely reflected in the occupational performance theories.

Therapists often use the SI frame of reference with children who have social and emotional problems (see Chapter 12). In addition to a focus on motor development, SI theory also addresses sensory-affective development. Children with disorders in sensory modulation often have difficulty behaving in school. In addition, individuals with sensory modulation problems may experience anxiety related to hypersensitivity that limits interest in and enjoyment of social contact (Wilbarger & Wilbarger, 1991). The Wilbargers (1991) described this pattern of atypical social and emotional development as a "disorder of sensory modulation." These children seem to perform better in a child-centered atmosphere, where they can have some control of the activity and suspend the pressures of the social world. The observable changes are reinforcing for many families and often influence social-emotional function (e.g., in self-esteem and confidence).

When using an SI approach, the therapist establishes a child-centered environment that the child perceives as a safe environment to first try challenging social and emotional skills. Helping parents and teachers understand SI dysfunction, accommodation, and remediation can promote appropriate adaptations at home and school.

Social Learning and Behavioral Approaches

Social learning and behavioral approaches include a group of theories based on the premise that all behavior is a consequence of learning. Whether a behavior is adaptive or maladaptive depends on the social context. Adaptive and maladaptive behaviors result from the same basic principles of behavior acquisition and maintenance. A pattern of maladaptive behavior may result when a child fails to learn an important behavior (Kaplan & Sadock, 1996). If Javan, whose mother is hearing impaired, fails to learn to modulate the volume of his voice, he will have difficulty in the structured environment of school. In this case he has not received normal social feedback and needs to learn it to meet social expectations. If Javan is hearing impaired, the same problem may occur; he may not be able to modulate his voice, but in this case learning to meet expectations is a more difficult process.

Maladaptive behavior also occurs as a consequence of inappropriate learning (Kaplan & Sadock, 1996). As noted previously, children with a parent who has a depressive disorder are likely to demonstrate poor social competence. The following is an example of a child with maladaptive behavior:

> Six-year-old Nikki is the middle child of three children living with her alcoholic mother. Nikki's mother withdraws for days at a time, leaving the children to fend for themselves. Nikki seldom attends school, has poor hygiene, steals, is physically aggressive, and uses inappropriate language at school.

Nikki has learned extreme behaviors, perhaps to earn the attention of her nonresponsive mother. Nikki can learn more appropriate behavior, but ideally her parents should be involved in changing her environment. The therapist can influence the child's inappropriate learning by guiding him or her through successive approximations of the difficult skills and modeling the appropriate behavior. Reality testing activities help the older child sort out her personal situation. Another approach is to reinforce a positive behavior inconsistent with the inappropriate one. Behavior management techniques are common in school and clinical settings. Among the techniques that therapists most often use are time out, performance contracts, self-management and personal responsibility training, and values clarification.

Theories Reflecting the Occupational Behavior Perspective

As the science of studying occupation matures, therapists extend and adapt theories to better reflect the unique nature of human occupation. Four practice-oriented theoretic approaches used in occupational therapy that are derived from an *occupational behavior perspective* are described. These are (1) the model of human occupation, (2) occupational adaptation, (3) the ecology of human performance, and (4) the model of social interaction.

The *model of human occupation* presents adaptive functioning and social competence as the result of efficient, organized occupational behaviors (i.e., play activities, self-care activities, and work). Optimally, these behaviors are organized into patterns or routines that become habit. By relegating everyday behaviors to habit, the child is free to direct more energy to explore, learn, and challenge the environment. Therapists conceptualize the individual as an open system consisting of layers of subsystems. This model addresses the motivation for occupation and the influence of the environment on occupation.

Assessment and treatment planning using the model of human occupation require consideration of the child's volition (personal causation, values, goals, interests, and personal performance standards), habituation (child's perceived roles, behavior habits, and routines), performance (sensorimotor and cognitive skills), and environment (object, task, interpersonal, and cultural). The therapist notes patterns of function and dysfunction in each area and plans treatment to interrupt dysfunctional cycles and replace them with the performance skills

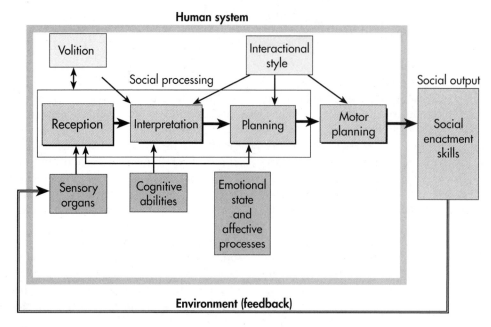

figure**14-3**   Model of social interaction. *(From Doble, S.E., & Magill-Evans, J. [1992]. A model of social interaction to guide occupational therapy practice.* Canadian Journal of Occupational Therapy, 59 *[3], 143).*

needed to enhance the child's development and adaptive behavior.

Occupational adaptation is an integrated model based on analysis of the internal adaptation process that occurs through occupation. This approach emphasizes the life-long process of adapting to internal and external performance demands. In this model the focus of intervention is on the individual's internal adaptation process. This model prescribes no specific type of assessment but rather mandates that the therapist use assessment data to facilitate occupational adaptation. This model does not focus on performance skills but on the internal processes that organize and direct performance skills. This approach is more client focused and is well suited to the needs of the adolescent populations described in this chapter.

In the *ecology of human performance,* the contexts of performance are a focus in this intervention model. This approach describes human performance as a transactional process through which the person, context, and task performance affect one another (Neistadt & Crepeau, 1998). Therapeutic intervention in this model improves performance through alteration of the person, context, task, or transaction among them. This approach with its emphasis on context offers important insight for school-based therapists in inclusive classrooms.

The model of social interaction (Doble & Magill-Evans, 1992) is a useful addition to occupational therapy theory. Drawing from the model of human occupation and other sources, this model views the individual as an open system whose output is socially oriented occupational be-

havior. Figure 14-3 illustrates the components of this model. The *social processing* component consists of three separate processes: reception, interpretation, and planning. Through social processing the individual makes sense of social information and develops a cognitive plan for response.

The first component, social processing, is the focus of social interaction problems for children with right-hemisphere dysfunction syndrome who cannot make sense of social information. Impulsive children, such as those with ADHD or closed-head injury, are likely to have difficulty making a plan.

The next component, motor planning, is the action after the cognitive plan. Children with SI dysfunction or other motor disorders are likely to be limited in motor planning. The observable output of this step is called *social enactment skills.*

As a part of a dynamic open system, the social enactment skills of the individual result in a change in the environment that provides feedback to the individual. Social enactment skills "enable us to communicate our needs and intentions to others and to respond to the messages of others in a competent manner" (Doble & Magill-Evans, 1992, p. 146). Social enactment skills may be verbal or nonverbal. They include the following major categories of interaction: acknowledging skills, sending skills, timing skills, and coordinating skills (Box 14-3). This model provides a structured analysis of the social process and grounds intervention in occupational therapy theory.

box **14-3** *Examples of social enactment skills*

1. Acknowledging skills
   Looks and gazes
   Touches
   Positions
   Gestures (e.g., nods head)
   Says "yes"
2. Sending skills
   Greets
   Initiates
   Asks and inquires
   Accepts
   Encourages
   Refuses
   Reveals
   Disengages and terminates
3. Timing skills
   Initiates without hesitation
   Speaks without unnecessary interruption
   Speaks without repeating information unnecessarily
   Maintains a reasonable pace when speaking
   Ends message without perseverating
   Ends message without stopping prematurely
   Ends message after reasonable period (does not go
      on and on)
4. Coordinating skills
   Sends message compatible with social partner's
      abilities (e.g., language comprehension)
   Sends message compatible with social partner's
      interests
   Sends message compatible with social partner's
      affective tone
   Sends message variations in message styles
      (alternates questions with disclosure and
      information provision)

From Doble, S.E., & Magill-Evans, J. (1992). A model of social interaction to guide occupational therapy practice. *Canadian Journal of Occupational Therapy, 59* (3), 147.

■ EVALUATION

In all areas of occupational therapy practice, assessment must include insight into the client's social and behavioral function. Although health care professionals tend to focus on limitations in physical performance, they must recognize and acknowledge the crucial role that psychosocial skills play in organizing and adapting behavior for everyday function. Children with sensorimotor and developmental delays are at risk for delays in the development of social, emotional, and adaptive behaviors.

In selecting assessments for children, the therapist must remember that a child's function in a particular environment may differ from the skill demonstrated in a controlled testing situation. For instance, a child may be independent in eating when tested in the clinic, but the same child may be so distracted and overstimulated in the school lunchroom that he or she does not persist at the activity. His or her distractibility may lead to excessive spillage and inadequate food intake. Besides causing social problems, being hungry all afternoon does not improve the child's mood or ability to learn. Assessments that consider parent and teacher reports are especially useful in singling out daily function from abilities that they may have in controlled settings.

Another important consideration is that children diagnosed with psychosocial or emotional conditions may be taking medications to influence their behavior. The therapist must ask whether the child takes medications and whether he or she is taking medications at the time of testing. This is particularly important when children are taking methylphenidate (Ritalin). Methylphenidate has a short active period in the body. This medication can greatly influence the child's performance. Some well-coordinated children with attention deficits appear clumsy because of impulsiveness and inattention to tasks when they have not taken their medication. These children may exhibit delays in motor coordination and poor concentration when they are tested without their medications; however, their performance is normal when medicated.

Medications are frequently prescribed for psychosis and affective and anxiety disorders. In acute settings, children with these problems are often medicated in the manner of adults with the same problem. Controversy about the long-term use of these medications exists, and medications alone do not remediate the difficulties in social behavior that are so disabling in school and community situations. The occupational therapist needs to know the intended effects and side effects of all medications to help monitor the drug's effectiveness and safety.

Naturalistic Observation

A naturalistic assessment may be as simple as a systematic series of lunchroom observations to determine aspects of the environment that are problematic for a particular child. In interventions designed to help the child function in his or her everyday environment, test scores showing how many standard deviations that a child is from the mean are not helpful to planning. Naturalistic observation is most useful when the therapist conducts it in a systematic, organized manner. Table 14-4 provides three examples of this approach.

Children with social or behavioral difficulties often perform better in nondirective environments. Allowing 10 or 15 minutes of child-directed play before formal

table 14-4	*Naturalistic Assessments*			
Test	**Author/Date**	**Comments**		**Age (yr)**
Transdisciplinary Play-Based Assessment (TPBA)	Linder (1990)	Provides information on all areas of functional performance		0-4
Preschool Play Scale	Knox (1997)	Provides information on many areas of functional performance; simpler but less comprehensive than TPBA		0-4
Ethnographic Classroom Analysis	Griswold (1994)	Provides information about social and environmental demands in the classroom		5-18

Linder T.W. (1990). *Transdisciplinary play-based assessment: A functional approach to working with young children.* Baltimore: Brookes.
Knox, S. (1997). Development and current use of the Knox Preschool Play Scale. In L.D. Parham & L. Fazio (Eds.), *Play in occupational therapy for children.* St. Louis: Mosby.
Griswold, L.A. (1994). Ethnographic analysis: A study of classroom environments. *The American Journal of Occupational Therapy, 48* (5), 397-402.

testing provides valuable clinical observations and may greatly improve the child's compliance on structured test items.

Informal Scales and Structured Observation

Informal scales provide information about a child's self-awareness and social roles. Interviews, such as *The University of Texas Medical Branch Initial Interview* (Figure 14-4), are an example of an informal scale. These scales provide an organized format but allow therapists to expand the questions at their own discretion. Although researchers have published several excellent role assessments, it is difficult to get reliable responses from an unhappy 13-year-old child in the test environment. Open-ended questions that the therapist can expand based on the child's answers are the best type of question with children and young adolescents.

Observational checklist

Another common use for informal scales is to document the quality of a child's performance. *The University of Texas Medical Branch Task Performance Scale* is an example of this type of scale (Figure 14-5). Another example of this type of tool is a group behavior survey that identifies the specific social behaviors in a group situation. This type of tool is especially useful when the child has difficulties with peer relations and social interaction.

The *Developmental Interview for Parents of Young Children at Risk* (Davidson, 1995) offers an interview structure to identify problems between the parent, child, and environment. This tool provides valuable information about the family environment, daily routines, and the parent's expectations of the child. Therapists designed this instrument to help identify families at risk for child abuse. Because many of the risk factors for child abuse parallel those for children's social and emotional problems, this instrument provides useful insights for all pediatric therapists.

Interest and role checklists

Therapists often use Interest checklists in clinical settings. Neville and Kielhofner (1983) developed a modification of the checklist format that includes current interests and historic and current reporting of participation in activities. This gives a clearer idea of how the child uses his or her time. It identifies discrepancies between interests and activities and helps the therapist review how the child's leisure behavior has changed.

Therapists have developed role checklists that are appropriate for older adolescents (Florey & Michelman, 1978). Role assessment is an important tool in assessing childhood performance, but children's roles are less discrete than those of adults. Therapists can interpret roles from the information collected on many other tests, including play assessments and developmental assessments. The therapist can use this information to add informal questions directed at the child and caregiver to clarify the child's current role function.

Sensory reactivity histories

Sensory responsiveness histories are important when a child has social or emotional problems because children often have sensorimotor difficulties as well. Therapists often link sensory processing and sensory modulation problems to social problems and often associate these disorders with inappropriate social behavior, social avoidance, and sometimes aggression. Children with either extremely high or extremely low sensory thresholds are likely to have difficulties similar to those associated with sensory modulation disorders. The Sensory Profile (Dunn, 1999) helps the therapist interpret a child's sensory processing based on the caregivers' report.

INITIAL INTERVIEW

Biographic Information

How old are you? _____   When is your birthday? _____

Where do you live (city)? _____   What is the street address? _____

Home

Who lives in your house? What are the ages of siblings?

Do you have any pets?

What is your room like?

What chores do you do at home?

Does your mother/father work?   What does your mother/father do at work?

What do you do at home that gets you in trouble?

Who gets mad at you when you get in trouble?   What do they do?

What does your mother/father do that gets you mad?   What do you do?

School

What grade are you in school?

What do you like most about school?

What do you like least about school?

Peers

Who is your best friend?   What activities do you like to do with him or her?

Who are some of your other friends?

Is there anyone around your house or at school that you do not like?

Why don't you like him or her?

figure**14-4**   Child psychiatric initial interview at the University of Texas Medical Branch.

Continued

Work/Play/Leisure

What do you do after school?   What kinds of games do you like to play?

What do you do on weekends?

Do you have any hobbies?

Personal Here and Now Status

Why are you in the hospital?

What do you want to change while you are in the hospital?

Tell me something good about yourself.

If you could change anything about yourself by wishing, what would it be?

Length of Interview _____

Observations

Good/poor eye contact
Cooperative/uncooperative
Appeared comfortable/uncomfortable
Easy/difficult to obtain responses to questions
Direct/rambling responses
Information reliable/unreliable

Additional Comments/Observations

Interviewer _____

figure **14-4, cont'd**   For legend see page 437.

Psychosocial assessments

Many broad-spectrum developmental tests include social and emotional development items. This type of test is often a primary measurement tool for occupational therapists working with preschool children. Therapists have an important role in determining the underlying cause of a child's difficulties in meeting performance expectations. Although some social and emotional screening tools are presented in this section, the occupational therapist must refer children quickly and appropriately when he or she suspects an emotional problem. For the therapist in a mental health program, some standardized tests that are specifically useful in assessing psychosocial issues in school-age children are as follows:

- *Kinetic family drawings and Draw-a-Person Tests* (Welsh, 1992) are used by professionals of various *disciplines* as a quick screen of the child's emotional well-being. An advantage to these tests is the ease with which the therapist can administer and score them.

- The *Piers-Harris Children's Self-Concept Scale* (Piers, 1984) is appropriate for children between 8 and 18 years of age. This test provides information about the child's perception of his or her own behavior, intelligence, school performance, physical appearance, anxiety, popularity, and happiness.

- The *Vineland Adaptive Behavior Scales* (Sparrow, Balla, & Cicchetti, 1987) is an interview-based survey that therapists administer to parents and caregivers. This provides a general assessment of strengths and weaknesses and an overall measure of social behaviors compared with developmental norms.

- The *Gardener Social Developmental Scale* (Gardener, 1994) compares parent reports of a child's behavior with a normative sample of behaviors reported by parents. The parent completes this test questionnaire, which provides standard information on the child's social behavior.

Project _____

Structure   None   Minimal   Moderate   High

Completed in _____ sessions

TASK COMPONENTS

Type of Directions Used
___ Written
___ Verbal
___ Demonstrated

Ability to Follow Directions
___ Unable
___ Needed directions at each step
___ Needed directions at the beginning of the project with few reminders during process

Organization
___ No organization; trial and error approach
___ Developed a plan with assistance; needed help in breaking task into sequential steps
___ Organized task with little or no assistance

Problem Solving
___ Unable to recognize problems or suggest solutions
___ Able to recognize problems but not suggest solutions
___ Able to recognize problems and suggest realistic solutions

Attention Span
___ Less than 15 minutes
___ 15 to 30 minutes with few interruptions
___ 30 to 45 minutes with few interruptions

Concentration
___ Worked only when environmental distractions were at a minimum (outside the group)
___ Worked when environmental distractions were at a moderate level (in clinic, others doing quiet tasks)
___ No problems noticed (in clinic, others doing loud tasks)

figure **14-5**   Task Performance Scale. The University of Texas Medical Branch.
Continued

Work Quality
___ Poor, messy
___ Average
___ Above average

Safety
___ Did not recognize or was careless with potentially dangerous tools or situations
___ Was aware of potentially dangerous tools or situations, but required frequent supervision
___ Adhered to safety precautions when working with potentially dangerous tools or situations, required minimal supervision

Work Satisfaction
___ Indifferent towards work
___ Not satisfied with work
___ Satisfied with work

Frustration Tolerance
___ Easily frustrated with simple tasks
___ Easily frustrated with more difficult tasks
___ Seldom frustrated with more difficult tasks

INTERACTIONS

Response to adults
___ Opposed adult supervision; frequently argues with adult; refuses to cooperate
___ Occasionally opposed adult supervision, argues and/or refuses to cooperate
___ Accepted adult supervision, seldom argues or refuses to cooperate

Response to peers
___ Minimum to no interaction with peers in a positive or negative way
___ Interacted with peers but in a negative, non-productive manner
___ Interacted with peers in a positive, productive manner

figure**14-5, cont'd** For legend see page 439.

■ The *Social Adjustment Inventory for Children and Adolescents (SAICA)* (John, Gammon, Prusoff, & Warner, 1987) is a semistructured interview schedule that assesses patterns of social function in children and adolescents in school, in leisure activities, and with peers, siblings, and parents.

■ PRIMARY INTERVENTION STRATEGIES

Environmental Adaptation

Many of the occupational therapy approaches described in this chapter use environmental adaptation as a primary strategy. The therapist adapts the child's environment to alter the sensory input, help the child organize materials, affect the child's mood and affect, and encourage specific behaviors. Environmental adaptation requires analysis of the cognitive and psychosocial functions of the individual and then alteration of the environments in which he or she must function to maximize those abilities. Environmental adaptation provides an external device (or place) to organize behaviors. This device may be a notebook with reminders of work and school routines or a quiet place where the student can sit when stressed. Other examples of environmental adaptation include organizing a child's work space at school with labeled compartments so that he or she knows where to locate and store the tool needed in school, or programming a telephone with frequently called numbers. Environmental adaptation can involve assistive technology, such as electronic reminders to take medicines, do homework, or walk the dog.

Adapting the sensory environment is a component of SI interventions. Children who have low sensory thresholds or a sensory modulation disorder may need clothes of only natural fibers or oversized clothes to be comfortable enough to attend to other things. A machine that emits white noise may help some easily aroused children go to sleep. Each of these environmental adaptations compensates for the lack of a particular skill that the child needs.

The functional goal in children with task impersistence is independence in task completion. Attention is an important aspect of persistence. To improve the child's success with tasks, the therapist needs to structure the tasks and provide clear cues to help the child orient him or herself as needed. The therapist's job is to organize the task and then teach the child to use cues and self-monitoring strategies. The therapist can teach older children to organize tasks and cues for themselves.

The therapist should also adapt the child's social environment when necessary. The therapist must consider the number of individuals in the room with the child and who those individuals are. Do the adults in the room give the child nonverbal or verbal cues to help him or her self-correct? Are they consistently reinforcing the child for positive interactions?

Social Behavioral Interventions

The focus of social and behavioral intervention is learning positive, functional-oriented skills. This type of intervention is well suited to occupational therapy, and therapists use it often. Some specific examples of social behavior interventions follow.

Self-management and values clarification

Therapists use *self-management and values clarification* discussion groups as intervention strategies with adults. The same types of groups have worked well with adolescents, with attention paid to normal developmental issues in adolescence. Self-management remains an important goal with younger children. In children with a neurobiologic basis to their behavior problems (e.g., ADHD or closed-head injury), improvement in self-management may have a positive effect on the development of social skills.

Self-management interventions with preschool children include modeling and teaching productive peer relations, making the child aware of the behaviors expected in specific environments, and organizing or altering the environment to enable positive performances. By school age, children are often able to articulate concerns, complaints, and fears in a manner specific enough to engage in discussions about hypothetical situations and solutions. Performance contracts are a step toward self-management that the child can carry out in all environments. A successful performance contract must be a collaborative effort. The child and supervising adult (therapist, parent, or teacher) review an area of problem performance, and the child describes behaviors that impede progress. The child negotiates the performance standards and consequences of the contract (rewards and punishments). The following example describes the use of self-management intervention:

Ten-year-old Travis is worried about an upcoming class field trip. The principal suspended him from school after the last field trip because of aggressive and disruptive behavior on the school bus. This upcoming trip will involve 5 hours on the bus. He wants to see the museum but is considering skipping the field trip to stay out of trouble. The occupational therapist encourages Travis to describe specifically what happened before and why he thinks it is so difficult to ride the bus.

Travis has an intense temperament, a high activity level, and a low sensory threshold. The therapist observes tactile defensiveness. Travis says that the bus is "too loud," he gets a headache, and he feels "edgy" when riding for even short periods. Travis has difficulty remaining seated for long periods and experiences a low frustration tolerance and high distractibility.

Travis also dislikes being bumped and stepped on by other kids. Travis is polite and cooperative at home and in occupational therapy sessions. At school he is rude and disruptive. He says that he feels "out-of-control" and that the teacher "sets him up" for problems. Travis struggles with the important roles of student, team member, and friend. His intensity and poor impulse control leave him at risk for continuing problems in cooperative activity. He and the therapist consult with his family and the teacher as they develop their strategy. Travis will bring his tape player and headphones to eliminate some of the bus noise. He will arrive or come early so that he can pick a good seat near the front of the bus (he is sure less jostling happens here) and by the window where he is less likely to be stepped on.

Travis has a successful field trip. He also learns that he can think through difficult situations and gain control of them. He gains the respect of his teacher for trying to constructively change his behavior, and his teacher becomes more sensitive to his needs. Travis and his family are excited to have found a way to anticipate and negotiate difficult situations.

Values clarification groups, in their traditional format, are above the developmental levels of most pediatric clients. Therapists can apply the idea of using social and personal values in concrete, functional terms with school-age children. This is done much in the same way as self-management. The therapist presents specific places and activities, with leading questions about appropriate and inappropriate behavior. For example, questions such as "Do you like going to the grocery store?" "Why?" "What happens when you get in trouble?" "Why did you want to do that?" "Who had to pick up all the cans?" "Did anyone get hurt?" "Could anyone have gotten hurt?" lead to a discussion regarding responsibility for the safety of others and personal behavior in public places. The therapist can follow this up with a trip to the grocery store to help the child remember and apply the discussion.

The therapist can use noncompetitive board games in a group situation to demonstrate cooperation and turn taking. For younger children the therapist can adapt a variety of noncompetitive games for clinical use. The game *Funny Face* (Deacove, 1987) promotes noncompetitive interaction. This game has playing cards requesting specific facial expressions and gestures as the game progresses. It helps children be aware of nonverbal communication in a lighthearted style.

The structure and format of these games make them accessible to young adolescents. This provides a forum for values clarification with younger clients. Therapeutic board games that therapists often use are *The Ungame* (Zakich, 1989), which offers a noncompetitive format that prompts the child to express likes, dislikes, and emotions in a group setting, and *Stop, Relax, & Think* (Bridges, 1990), which promotes cognitive strategies to overcome impulsivity and increase prosocial behavior in a variety of situations.

Interest groups

A child's social environment dramatically expands soon after he or she begins school. Middle childhood is when children understand that they have different roles in different social environments. As children seek to identify a sense of self, they begin to develop interests or habits. Most school-age children in North America can explain what they like about school, sports, and music. The acquisition of social and personal values is a precursor to adult decision making. Interest groups for children can better be called self-awareness groups because the focus is on questions such as "Who am I?" "What do I do well?" "What frustrates me?" and "What makes a game fun?" Children begin to distill personal and social interests from these questions. Many children with social and emotional problems have limited social interests, and they focus much of their time on things that frustrate them. This adds to their sense of helplessness and isolation. The child can identify and develop interests to interrupt a negative cycle.

During adolescence, interest groups can evolve into vocational interest groups. Children with a history of school failure may not be able to picture themselves in a competent adult role. Children with severe physical disabilities may have a sense of physical helplessness that limits the possibilities that they consider. Exploring vocational interests while supporting the development of community skills is an appropriate direction for adolescent interventions.

Socratic questioning

Socratic questioning (SQ) is a familiar technique in education and cognitive therapy and is well suited to occupational therapy interventions. The therapist structures and directs SQ, yet he or she gives power and responsibility to the child. SQ involves facing a task or activity as a problem. The therapist asks the child questions such as "What do you need to do first?" and guides each of the child's responses by further questions, such as "Why did you choose that?" or "Is there another way to do it?" The therapist leads the child through skillful questioning to organize the problem and come to an answer.

This approach helps the child sort out and learn to organize his or her thoughts. As the child learns foundation skills (e.g., basic social rules), these skills can serve as prompting questions when he or she must learn new behaviors. With this approach, children have a growing sense of accomplishment that results from coming to the answers themselves. A strength of this approach is that the learning seems to be more readily internalized so that the child can solve problems independently in new situations. The following is an example of a child who the therapist leads through SQ:

James loves sports, but his teacher and parents do not allow him to participate in after-school programs because of his disruptive behaviors. James has a personal goal of playing basketball on the playground in the after-school program. The occupational therapist encourages a dialogue with James about this issue, asking the following question sequence:

- "Why won't the teachers let you play?"
- "Why do you think the teachers don't like you?"
- "Do all the kids think that the teachers are mean, or just you?"
- "Why do you think the teachers single you out?"
- "Do you like getting into all those fights?"
- "Why do you get into so many fights?"

This process continues until James states that his behavior is the reason that his teachers and peers exclude him. At this point the therapist asks, "What happened before you felt like hitting Bobby?"

In time the therapist directs James to acknowledge his responsibility in the problem and some of the precipitating factors and potential solutions that will allow him to play basketball. As James gains skill in the SQ process, the therapist can use it as a problem-solving tool for accomplishing difficult school tasks, solving social problems, and working things out with his parents.

SQ is a powerful therapy tool and is relatively easy to learn. The difficult part of SQ for the therapist is persisting with the resistive child long enough to elicit productive responses. The SQ approach is useful in task-focused applications, and is more easily accepted when used in the context of a specific task.

Social skills instruction

Occupational therapists have developed commercial social skills training programs for teachers to enhance social behavior in children (e.g., Borba & Borba, 1978; Korb-Khalsa, Azok, & Leutenberg, 1992; Pincus, 1994). Therapists generally develop these programs for a classroom activity but may individualize and use them successfully in the therapy setting. Therapists should use these programs with theory-guided assessment and intervention planning. With a theory-based and developmentally delineated understanding of social behaviors to guide decisions, the therapist may successfully teach social and interpersonal skills without a commercial program. The following description of a young girl exemplifies the critical nature of social skills to all functional areas and roles:

Sophia is 8 years old when she is referred to occupational therapy at school for sensorimotor delays. A social worker removed Sophia from an abusive home, where her parents confined her to a small room, when she was 5 years of age. Before the social worker placed her in a foster home, Sophia had never been around other children, had seldom been out in public, and had habitually spent 10 to 12 hours alone daily with the television on. Her medical record indicated a suspicion of fetal alcohol syndrome, and both biological parents had a history of polysubstance abuse.

After her foster parents adopted her, Sophia participated in intense psychotherapy and was home-schooled for 2 years. Sophia is now entering school as a first grader. She is quiet and withdrawn in the classroom. She can do the academic work but does not interact with the teacher or peers in the classroom. She does not consistently speak when spoken to, and she resists cooperative activities. Sophia has good language comprehension but difficulty in all other cognitive areas associated with interpretation of social information. She has poor awareness of social rules and difficulty inferring the meaning of social behaviors based on contextual cues. For example, on the playground several children are playing "freeze tag." Sophia has never seen any sort of tag game before. When a boy runs by her and tags her roughly, Sophia runs away crying hysterically. She later says that she was afraid that he was going to hurt her because she was in the way. Sophia is unaware that her self-imposed isolation punctuated by dramatic outbursts makes her classmates uncomfortable. She is fearful and has a highly externalized sense of control. Sophia's usual first response to social overtures is a failure to acknowledge or respond.

Her occupational therapy program goals focus on sensorimotor delays and teaching basic social rules in therapy (and later playground) situations. Sophia's motor skills improve rapidly, and her behavior in occupational therapy begins to change. From a quiet withdrawn child, she becomes physically boisterous and impulsive. Her social interactions are extreme and unpredictable. The intervention team speculates that as Sophia gains skill and confidence in motor skills, she feels secure enough to explore and try new behaviors.

The therapist initiates an activity program based on art and handwriting skill training to capitalize on Sophia's growing social awareness. As Sophia draws, she becomes involved in a story-telling game. She and the therapist take turns adding to the story and drawing new aspects to the mural that they make. The focus of this intervention is solving problems in social situations. Sophia quickly understands and begins to use appropriate sending and timing skills. When the therapist includes her in a handwriting skills group, Sophia begins to demonstrate appropriate acknowledging behaviors and to learn how to negotiate and coordinate with her peers.

Child-Centered Intervention

Child-centered intervention (CCI) activity was first developed as a form of psychotherapy (Guerney, 1983). With this approach, interventions have a flexible sequence, involve exploration and creativity, and are centered in the child's choices and interests. In CCI the child is the initiator of activity and the adult is the facilitator. The therapist must organize the therapy environment for CCI to make activities available that promote development. Part of the art of this approach is creating an appealing environment that limits inappropriate play choices without adult intervention. CCI is useful in all types of pediatric interventions. Therapists have used it successfully for improvement of sensorimotor problems and for enhancing social and behavioral skills (DeGangi, Wietlisbach, Goodin, & Scheiner, 1993).

The CCI approach to the child emphasizes interpersonal interaction by relying on negotiation and flexibility rather than structure and verbal praise. CCI is useful in initial therapy sessions for establishing rapport and a positive environment. As the child recognizes that he or she has some control and that his or her opinion is solicited, antisocial behaviors tend to decrease. CCI often works well with children who have difficult temperaments because it seems to disarm their struggle to take control. CCI gives the child some control, so he or she accepts the therapist and therapy environment more readily. Even in situations better suited to structured interventions, CCI is useful as a transition technique. It can be a gentle introduction to therapy, and the therapist can use it later when inappropriate behavior interferes with therapy progress. CCI is a positive, supportive intervention that helps when the child appears stressed.

Sophia is withdrawn and passive in her first contact, so the occupational therapist decides to use CCI to establish rapport. In the first session the therapist gives Sophia a choice of toys and activities and warmly invites her to play. She sits quietly and does not explore the room. The therapist then walks around the room pointing out the equipment, toys, and art supplies. Shyly, Sophia takes a piece of paper and some markers to the table. The therapist mirrors her activity. As Sophia draws, the therapist remarks, "I'm drawing too. I want to make a picture like yours"; "That is a very pretty cat. I want to try and draw a cat too"; or "Your picture has a lot of yellow in it. I will put some yellow on my picture." During the entire session, Sophia verbalizes very little, but her affect brightens, she makes eye contact more often, and she does not demonstrate the avoidance gestures that she demonstrates in the classroom.

Soon Sophia has ideas about what she wants to do in therapy and requests them. By retaining the CCI approach the therapist can support social and sensorimotor skill development. When the relationship seems secure, the therapist begins making activity suggestions, although Sophia continues to have veto power. Sophia comes to trust that the therapist will choose activities that are fun and not too hard for her. As she speaks more, the therapist begins simple negotiations of play activities, allowing the presentation of social play rules and allowing Sophia to practice skills that she needs in peer interactions.

The CCI approach may allow the child to exert autonomy and control over the environment, to organize attention and play schemes, and to seek out environmental stimuli that are more self-organizing. Child-centered activity is also useful in eliciting imaginative play and storytelling. For children with difficulty in appropriately expressing emotions and with poor social skills, CCI provides a safe, stimulating therapy environment in which the therapist can explore these skills.

Expressive Interventions

Expressive interventions include diverse activities such as role-playing, art and craft projects, and drama. Fraenkel and Tallant (1987) presented a structured drawing program as a projective media for school-age children. The program uses a structured drawing workbook with captions such as "This is me" and "Things that bug me." The following are suggested occupational therapy treatment objectives:
1. To encourage the expression of feelings and conflicts
2. To facilitate the expression of fantasies and wishes
3. To help the child gain insight and self-awareness
4. To encourage the child to become aware of and relinquish his or her maladaptive defense mechanisms
5. To enhance the development of decision-making skills

Other examples of occupational therapy interventions incorporating expressive aspects in pediatric interventions are Bracegirdle's (1990) analysis of uses of play and Fazio's (1992) application of the therapeutic metaphor. In both of these examples the psychodynamical aspect is only a part of the intervention. These approaches focus on acquisition of skills and improved daily function. Expressive interventions are also appropriate to the model of human occupation and the model of social interaction.

Therapy Considerations to Promote Psychosocial Development in All Children with Disabilities
Social values reasoning

Culture is the social background that children learn and use to evaluate things and behaviors. Culture influences all aspects of human life. Different cultures value possessions, formal education, food, and time in different ways. The occupational therapist needs to be sensitive to the possibility that certain behaviors, including a family's failure to follow through with the therapist's recommendations, may be a result of differing cultural values. The occupational therapist should identify those cultural issues that create conflict. In the case of the uncooperative family, the conflict may be between the goals that the therapist establishes and those that the family values. Conflict may also exist between the values of the family and the values of the community.

When the conflict is between family cultural values and the community's values system, the occupational therapist acts as mediator. The reason that the situation requires a mediator is that most children must deal with the culture of their family and that of the community. A warm, supportive home environment that embraces the child's physical disability as a unique aspect of the child is an ideal that is offered in many homes. The home environment may also pair this loving nurturance with a tendency to exclude the child from social responsibility as he or she reaches adolescence. The rude 3-year-old child with cerebral palsy is cute, but the rude 15-year-old child is disabled physically and socially. There is a fine line between preparing a child to face the adult world and imposing middle-class values on persons from differing cultural backgrounds.

Establishing a positive therapy environment

The first step that the therapist takes in managing the child's behavior is establishing a positive and supportive therapy environment. Affirmation and positive reinforcement of behavior help establish appropriate responses. Praising specific appropriate behavior causes that behavior to increase and informs the child about the therapist's expectations. It is important to praise specific behaviors. For example, the therapist informs the child, "You are aiming those beanbags very carefully" rather than "Good boy" and "I like the careful way you are listening" rather than "Nice work."

Another important strategy that therapists employ is intermittent echoing of appropriate speech. Repeating and paraphrasing the child's speech shows respect for the child and his or her ideas and indicates to the child that the therapist is listening. This approach has the advantage of improving and increasing the child's verbal communication while modeling appropriate turn taking in conversation. If the child says, "This is going to be a picture of a spider," the therapist replies, "It is fun to draw interesting things like spiders." When the child says, "I like to go fast on the swing," the therapist replies, "It's really fun to go fast on that swing."

A final and often overlooked part of the therapy environment is the therapist's affect. The therapist should clearly demonstrate that he or she has enjoyed the time with the child. Laughter and clowning convey this impression, as does seriously and respectfully listening to the child's ideas or concerns. The therapist's delight in the interaction helps the child feel valued, and over time it helps him or her develop positive feelings about the therapy experience.

Behavior management interventions

Behavior management is based on behavior modification methods and is an effective tool for improving both social and academic behaviors. Behavior management includes the use of external controls (such as time out) and techniques to teach individuals to control their own behavior (such as performance contracts). The management of behavior is important with all occupational therapy interventions. Inappropriate behavior can limit the child's function and the child's progress on therapy goals.

The therapist expects to manage the behavior of a child who is labeled "emotionally handicapped," but most children seen for therapy need some degree of external behavior control during the course of therapy. Children with disabilities do not always learn basic manners and social behaviors. These physically disabled, or "ill," children who have no psychosocial disorders, often develop dysfunctional interpersonal behaviors that exaggerate their disability. Their behaviors often limit social interactions more dramatically than their disability ever would.

Rude behaviors gain attention even though they isolate the individual. Children with disabilities need to be respected as individuals with feelings, ideas, and emotional needs. Likewise, children with disabilities need to respect other individuals. Manners are a social tool reflecting respect. The occupational therapist needs to model and expect developmentally appropriate social interactions in the therapy session. The theory and intervention models presented in this chapter provide specific approaches to this type of intervention.

Society does not deal well with long-term disability, often allowing the individual who has a disability to break social rules. Society may inadvertently foster overdependency and passivity. Parents are often caught up in day-to-day matters and do not see how their child's social behavior will affect them as adults. The occupational therapist needs to discuss these concerns with the parents and include the family in any plan to introduce social skills training. This is a sensitive area because families often interpret it as a poor reflection on their parenting. Therapists need to be sensitive to this possibility in describing the problem and soliciting family input for remediation.

Routine behavioral strategies for managing problems in therapy. Therapists should establish behavior rules early in the therapy relationship and repeat them before "at-risk" activities. The therapist can post rules when appropriate. A sign stating "Ask before using the swings" is neutral and lets the child know that the rule is for everyone. Rules for intervention groups should be more extensive than those for individual behaviors. Group rules should reflect respect for the rights of others. Obvious rules may be "No physical contact without permission" or "Each person is allowed 2 minutes to talk in circle time." School-age children can help develop their own group rules and consequences. If the therapist includes children in the rule-making process, they are more likely to accept the rules. When the therapist negotiates group rules with the children, the rules need to apply to both children and adults.

The therapist should carefully grade behavior interventions based on their consequences for others (e.g., which ones are irritating or rude and which ones are dangerous or destructive). Many irritating behaviors are attempts at gaining attention, and withholding attention keeps the behavior from increasing. Children can exhibit extremely inappropriate behaviors to disconcert adults.

Ignoring means being silent about the behavior; it is important for the therapist to not use nonverbal or verbal cues that reveal feelings about the behavior. Although this approach ultimately decreases some behaviors, the behaviors usually get worse before they get better. With a child like Sophia, whose sudden unexpected outbursts disrupt activity, the therapist must keep interactions task focused. If the outburst disrupts the task, the therapist should casually change the task or the child should deal with the natural consequences of the resultant disarray. The therapist makes this transition without comments or offers to clean up the destroyed activity. The therapist should not allow the child to control the flow of therapy with this behavior. Once the child believes that he or she cannot gain the attention of the therapist, the behavior will discontinue.

As the therapist initiates these difficult early stages in the therapy relationship, he or she should use the power of praise and imitation. The therapist must give praise for positive behaviors, especially those that are incompatible with the problem behavior. The therapist should mirror the child's positive behaviors with his or her own. For example, if the child draws a spider, the therapist compliments the good idea and then proceeds to draw another spider, not competing artistically with the child. If the therapist has decided to ignore spitting, he or she ignores it when the child spits on the floor and instead praises the spider drawing. If the child spits at the therapist, the game stops without discussion or bargaining. Spitting is so socially offensive that the therapist cannot ignore it, so he or she must move to a more serious level of behavior control.

Sequence of behavioral controls. Therapists should alternate liked and disliked activities whenever possible. This rewards the child with a liked activity as he or she completes a difficult one. In addition, it reminds the child that the difficult task has an end and it will not fill the whole session once he or she completes it. The therapist can combine this alternation with a rule that any activity started must be completed. The therapist can shorten or simplify an activity if it appears too challenging for the child. If a child procrastinates on a disliked activity once the therapist establishes the rule, he or she can remind the child that time is being lost for the reward activity.

Establishing simple rules such as those described in the previous paragraph can lead to establishing performance contingencies. The therapist needs to give children control in the therapy session, and the child needs to understand what that control means. At first the therapist rewards any approximation of the desired behavior, then he or she increases the standards as the child makes progress. The therapist should replace criticism or commands with reminders about rewards and repercussions.

Organization. Many attention-getting and avoidance behaviors are subtle. The child may leave therapy having accomplished little for no apparent reason. The therapist should develop a behavior recording system to establish or document maladaptive behaviors and should look for antecedent behaviors, such as tapping the pencil on the table, that can indicate the imminence of offensive behavior. Ideally the therapist can change the activity or redirect the child before the offensive behavior occurs.

Recording the child's behavior helps identify behaviors that are not negative in isolation (e.g., telling stories) but that the child uses as an effective stalling technique. Before the therapist can effectively manage behaviors, he or she needs to target the specific problems and deal with them one at a time.

The therapist then organizes a reward system. The therapist should record what the child seems to particularly enjoy. The activities or objects may be found in or out of the therapy environment. Questions that the therapist can ask the child include "If you had fifty cents, how would you spend it?" and "If you could do something special in occupational therapy, what would it be?" The therapist can enlist parents and teachers to identify a "menu" of reinforcers. A choice of reinforcing activities is important so that the therapist can verify the rewards. The child who earns a sticker for each completed activity will soon tire of stickers. The therapist must frequently update the menu because the interests of children frequently change.

Coordinated strategies between family and team. Behavior management works best if it is consistently applied. If Joey is spitting in occupational therapy, he is probably spitting in the classroom and at home. All of the adults working to help Joey need to make a team decision as to what is and is not acceptable. Maybe Joey's occupational therapist can ignore the spitting, but his teacher cannot. If the teacher ignores Joey's spitting in the classroom, other children will begin to imitate the behavior. Behavior management is most efficient when it occurs in all aspects of a child's day. The same is true of reinforcers. Young children need to be quickly reinforced, even for small successes. One method to reinforce an older child is to award points. For example, 10 points may earn the child 10 minutes on the playground after school or 30 seconds with a can of silly string chasing the therapist. If the family is involved, points may earn the child a favorite meal, a movie, or cash.

Behavior-recording charts. Well-designed charts make the behavior goals and progress clear to even a young child. They serve as a tool to remind others to praise positive behaviors and to give the child assurance that he or she can succeed. Behavior change is an abstract idea to young children, but stickers on a chart are concrete. The therapist can individualize behavior-recording charts to the child's level of understanding. As the therapist begins a behavior management program, he or she should reward progress immediately. A coloring chart, such as the ice cream cone in Figure 14-6, is a good reinforcer for short-term goals. Every 5 minutes that pass without the child whining entitles him or her to color a section. The therapist draws the chart to ensure that the child can earn the "big" reward in a short time. For example, the ice cream cone in Figure 14-6 has six parts so that a 30-minute session with no whining may earn the child a trip to the ice cream parlor. Once the therapist established the program, the child can color sections every 10 minutes.

A spider chart for 9-year-old Joey may look something like Figure 14-7. For every 10 minutes without spitting, Joey gets to put a bug sticker on his chart. In this case the therapist and the child can negotiate the level of compliance that earns a reward. The chart records 2 weeks of therapy behavior. If Joey earns 10 of 18 possible stickers, he may earn 30 minutes of playing video games. The therapist can adjust this to 12 then 15 stickers as Joey begins to control his behavior. With the older child, behavior-recording charts should focus on self-control of behaviors. When feasible, the child should be in charge of keeping his or her behavior records in therapy.

Older children and teenagers can keep and carry their behavior-recording charts between classes at school and at home. If the child is responsible for keeping a chart and recording his or her performance at regular intervals, he or she is more likely to think about his or her behavior. In this type of self-recording system, the child records posi-

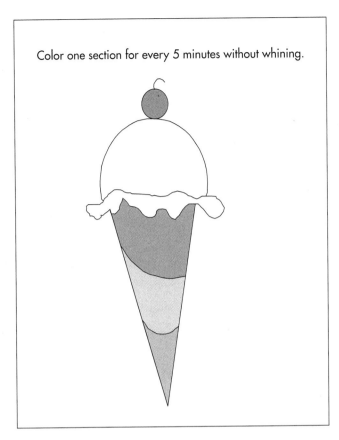

Color one section for every 5 minutes without whining.

figure**14-6**   Coloring project for behavior reinforcement.

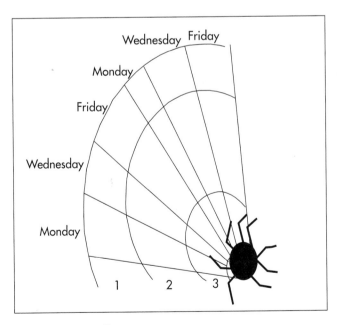

figure**14-7**   Joey's spider.

tive and negative behaviors. Children are less likely to misuse the system if they are documenting progress and problems. The therapist can follow the self-recording with self-evaluation and then self-reinforcement, moving the child toward behavior self-management.

Time-out process. Time-out is a process that is widely used for punishment in schools and clinical settings because it is often effective and typically reduces the need for physical management. The purpose of time-out is to exclude the child from attention and preferred activity. The first step to using time-out effectively is choosing the time-out location. It should be a neutral place, boring maybe but not unpleasant, providing a quiet space for the child to regroup. Time-out also provides an opportunity for the child to practice compliance to adult directives. A chair or carpet square should define the "quiet" or "thinking" place. The use of a timer is important. When the therapist keeps the time, staying in time-out may continue to be a power struggle. The neutral timer takes some of the emotion and control issues out of the situation. Many experts advocate requiring 1 minute of quiet time-out for each year of age (up to 5 minutes). The child should receive time-out in a firm and gentle manner with minimal discussion.

The timer runs while the child is quiet and cooperative. If the child is uncooperative, the timer does not start until he or she is quiet. Young children may not have a developed sense of time or numbers. Stopping and resetting the timer is more concrete than adding minutes. Time-out "quiet" times should not exceed 5 minutes. The time-out process may take much longer, with warnings and resetting the timer until a 5-minute quiet time results. Figure 14-8 presents a flow sheet of the time-out process. This model shows how to make time-out a learning time for the child.

It is important to teach children when time-out will be implemented. This can be done informally at first, with appropriate behavior modeled. Praising and allowing the child more control in the therapy setting are good rewards for appropriate behavior. When behavior is not appropriate, the therapist must be certain that the child knows that the behavior is wrong. Before initiating any punishment, the therapist explains to the child why the behavior is not acceptable and establishes rules to guide future behavior.

When a behavior is not dangerous or highly offensive, the child should receive one verbal warning. If the verbal cue results in improved behavior, the therapist should focus on the positive behavior. The therapist does not need to qualify the praise by referencing the unacceptable behavior. For some children, any reaction or response to the negative behavior is enough reinforcement to continue the behavior. If the child does not change his or her behavior with the warning, he or she receives the time-out.

The time-out process becomes complicated when the child who refuses to go to or stay in time-out. Because the purpose of the time-out is to *withdraw* attention, the therapist must maintain a calm, flat affect. If the therapist must carry the child to time-out, he or she should do it silently. The therapist must remove the

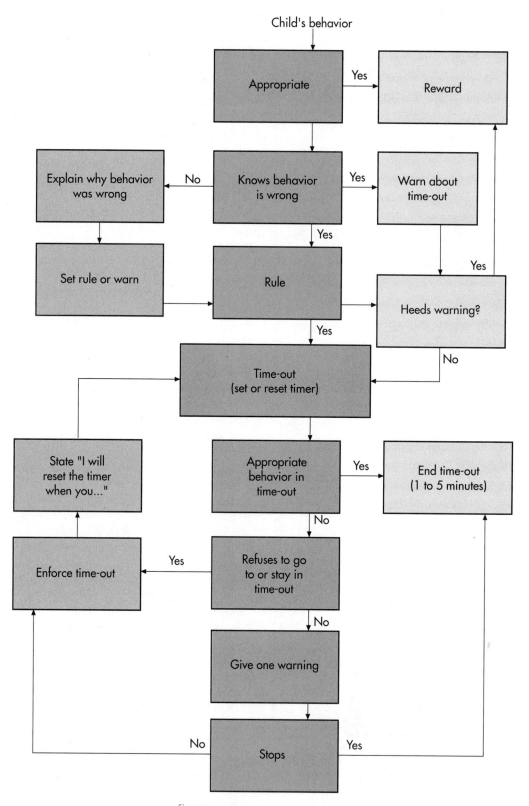

figure **14-8**   Time-out process.

child's power to control the situation, at least in appearance. When the therapist is unable to keep the child in time-out, he or she should involve the family and interdisciplinary team. Children can lose television time or another favorite activity for a short time if they resist time-out. Physically holding the child in time-out can be effective, but the therapist should only do this as a last resort and with the parents' support. Most child mental health settings have policies and training opportunities to ensure appropriate physical management of children and adolescents.

The therapist should inform the child's parents about difficult behavior and strategies for changing that behavior. The therapist should encourage the family to praise and reward the positive behaviors. Behavior change takes a long time, and the therapist may devote several therapy periods to time-out before the child begins to work appropriately. The child's behavior should not excuse him or her from therapy, nor should the therapist make the parents feel responsible for behavior in the therapy session.

For children around 8 years of age, the therapist often needs to use other forms of time-out, such as withdrawal of television privileges. With older children the therapist needs to negotiate the behavioral consequences with the family. There are other behavior management techniques that the therapist may use. Performance contracts (discussed previously) signed by the child and therapist work well with school-age children. The therapist should make the terms of the contract public either by posting or presenting copies to the child's parents (Davidson & LaVesser, 1998).

■ TRANSITION TO ADULTHOOD

Developmental Issues

The therapist needs to understand the normal social and emotional changes associated with adolescence. In the middle school and early high school years, children begin the transition to adulthood and toward dealing with complex adult issues. The individual's movement toward personal independence characterizes this age. Common themes associated with adolescence include the following:

- Struggle with sense of identity
- Awkward or strange feeling about one's self and one's body
- Focus on self, alternating between high expectations and poor self-concept
- Moodiness
- Improved ability to use speech for self-expression
- Tendency to return to childish behavior, particularly when stressed

In the early adolescent period teenagers focus primarily on the present. This may pose some problems for the therapist trying to ensure compliance with medical regimens or promote healthy behavior relative to the adolescent's physical condition. Early adolescence is also when issues of sexuality (e.g., sexual interests and sexual advances) typically emerge. Students often question therapists in public schools about sexual issues or concerns. At the same time, adolescence is a period when teenagers view adult concern as interference and peers have greater influence than adults (e.g., therapists). Adolescence is the most typical age range for experimentation with sex and drugs, and some teenagers become either destructive or self-destructive. These behaviors can be serious, and the therapist should refer adolescents with these behaviors for further evaluation.

The early and middle adolescent years are challenging; often the adolescent is more oriented to the present than the future. The late high school years typically bring the following changes:

- Increased independent functioning
- Firmer and more cohesive sense of identity
- Decreased conflict with parents
- Increased ability for delayed gratification and compromise
- Increased emotional stability
- Increased self-reliance
- Improved work habits
- Increased concern for the future

Although planning ideally begins in the early teen years, the occupational therapist should focus on easing the transition to adulthood for those in the middle of adolescence. By this stage the adolescent with a disability may reap criticism for not meeting societal expectations. Common problems in disabled adults are social isolation, lack of occupation, frustrated sexual feelings, and limited recreational and leisure opportunities (Schuster, 1992a).

The transition to adult lifestyles and adult responsibilities is an important aspect of psychosocial and emotional development. In the child with atypical development, poorly developed personal causation, learned helplessness, and difficult interpersonal skills can contribute to a difficult transition to adulthood. Although successful neuromuscular interventions and technologic aids, such as power wheelchairs, may make the young adult with cerebral palsy or spinal cord injury eligible for placement in community living, poor interpersonal skills can make such a placement impossible. Common problems include the inability to negotiate and cooperate with peers, passive dependence in money management and personal hygiene, inability to relate effectively with personal care assistants, and lack of respect for social rules.

A critical responsibility of the occupational therapist is to prepare children and adolescents to be a part of the community. This is not a responsibility limited to those therapists who treat adolescents. Long-term considerations of a child's psychosocial and emotional needs are critical. What types of outcomes can be expected? How will the child's behavior change in 5 or 15 years? The bear hug of a young boy with Down syndrome quickly becomes socially inappropriate as he becomes a young adult. The boy hospitalized for a conduct disorder needs more than a hierarchy of privileges in the hospital setting to develop a sense of control and responsibility for the effects of his or her behavior. Even in the hospital, goals should incorporate skills that the child or adolescent needs to gain acceptance in the society to which he or she will return. Another important role for occupational therapists is as an advocate for the development of community resources, such as independent living apartments, accessible public recreation facilities, and school-based supported work environments.

Interests and Roles In Adolescence

Adolescence is a time of acquiring social and personal values and a time when many people begin to work outside of the home. Adolescents in North America are aware of money and the acquisition of things. Money becomes a critical factor in the leisure and work roles of adolescents. Planning for and budgeting money often interests adolescents and are important for the adolescent to establish self-reliance. Adolescents can direct their interests toward careers and consider leisure time as time to earn money. Adolescents want to be in control of their lives. By helping them understand how they can channel their time-use decisions and interests to increase their control, caregivers can lead adolescents toward self-reliance.

Before developing true vocational skills, the adolescent needs to develop good interpersonal skills, some form of reliable communication, self-direction in activities of daily living (ADLs), task orientation, task persistence, and task organization abilities. The occupational therapist should assess each of these areas and plan appropriate interventions.

For interests and roles to mature into an adult pattern, the individual needs experience. Most young adolescents have ideas about careers and interests that are based on fantasy rather than experience. The adolescent seen in occupational therapy is likely to have even less experience and less awareness of his or her own abilities than the average adolescent. Most public schools offer career awareness programs, but it may be difficult for a child with an atypical history to see how those potential careers relate to him or her. The following are major goals toward an adolescent's career development (Jordan & Heyde, 1979):

- Crystallization of interests
- Realistic self-appraisal of strengths and deficits in relation to vocational choice
- Development of work experience
- Acceptance of responsibility in acquiring skills
- Self-direction in the development and implementation of a vocational or career plan
- Self-reliance in transportation and mobility in the community

The occupational therapist should work with the school or vocational counseling personnel to help the adolescent apply interests and career information to their own future planning. The adolescent client may benefit from help appraising work abilities and work demands. The management of personal self-care extends beyond acquiring skills to an awareness of proper grooming and social rules about grooming behavior. Transition services and supported employment programs are presented at length in Chapter 31.

■ SUMMARY

Occupational therapy with children requires an understanding of and sensitivity to the domains of psychosocial and emotional development. Nearly all clients of pediatric occupational therapists are at risk for disruptions in these areas of development. Overlooking critical dimensions of development, such as the development of interpersonal relations, can greatly affect the individual's function and resources as he or she faces adulthood.

Routine assessment should include an overview of the child or adolescent's function in social performance areas. Play with family members and peers is an important part of the child's ability to learn and assimilate social behaviors. In addition to measures of the individual's performance, this chapter includes several approaches to family and environmental assessment. These assessments help develop meaningful goals for the child in his or her own situation. These assessments also can help identify children at risk for abuse, and the therapist can use them to structure programs that include support of family members.

Decisions about specific theoretic approaches and interventions should reflect the intervention setting, the team's values and theoretic orientations, and the family's concerns. Occupational therapists use psychosocial interventions and follow theories on occupational performance, development, neurophysiologic function, and behavior. Occupational therapists use a variety of holistic approaches and strategies that include consultation with family and teachers to optimize psychosocial function in the children whom they serve.

STUDY QUESTIONS

1. Review the case study of Derrick (p. 419). Using the examples in the text, consider how Derrick's temperament characteristics are likely to affect his academic performance. What kind of classroom adaptations may make it easier for him to succeed?

2. Robert has difficulty with a sense of mastery in academic work. When asked what their biggest concern was about their child, Robert's parents responded, "His inability to make friends and his lack of concern with his schoolwork. He has a lack of self-esteem." Explain mastery motivation in a way that may help Robert's parents understand his behavior and the relationship between mastery, self-esteem, and personal causation.

3. Four-year-old Rex has Down syndrome. He has difficulty imitating sequential behaviors and organizing his play. Consider your early intervention goals for Rex and his family. How do the issues of learned helplessness and locus of control influence your intervention decisions?

4. Review the characteristics of temperament. Do you think your temperament is extreme in any aspect? How do you think your temperament affects your study style, your friendships, or your behavior when you are ill? Answer these questions again while considering a sibling or peer. How does the "fit" between you work or not work?

5. Review the case study of Travis (p. 439). Using the examples in the text, what sort of an activity group would you suggest for Travis? Defend your answer with examples of his behavior and the need for specific skill development.

6. Fourteen-year-old Bryce arrives for sensorimotor testing. He is rude, offensive, and uncooperative throughout testing. The only way you can finish testing is by threatening to end the test session and return him to the classroom. Bryce has some sensorimotor delays, but his behavior is so extreme that it exaggerates his problems and makes him a poor candidate for traditional sensorimotor intervention. What are some additional tests that may be appropriate to understand Bryce's problems? What information will let you know if Bryce needs to be referred for specific psychosocial intervention?

7. Review the characteristics of disruptive behavior disorders. How would your approach to these behaviors change in an early intervention, public school, or acute psychiatric clinic setting? Choose a theoretic model and a therapy format for treatment of a 10-year-old child with conduct disorder in a setting of your choice.

8. Review the case example of 14-year-old Bryce from study question 6. Bryce continues to be rude, offensive, and uncooperative in therapy sessions. His interests are tennis, video games, and skateboarding. He says that he hates school and does not want to do well in any school-related task. Bryce has some sensorimotor delays, but because of his age he should be looking beyond his school days. He needs to develop work and interpersonal skills to make a successful transition to adult life. Consider the strategies listed in this chapter for maintaining a positive therapy environment and making the transition to adult life. Organize a behavior management program for Bryce that is appropriate for his age and that you can grade toward increasing self-control.

9. Review the case study of Sophia (p. 441). Sophia has a history of fetal alcohol syndrome and physical abuse. Her current home environment is warm and supportive, but she still retains many of the behaviors common to an abused child. The therapist following Sophia has given her a diagnosis of posttraumatic stress disorder (PTSD). The therapist continues to use child-centered intervention (CCI) to support social skill development. However, as Sophia gains skill, her behavior becomes more difficult to manage. She is impulsive and sometimes explosive emotionally. She will be playing on a swing and then throw herself to the ground, screaming, "I hate her! I hate her!" and pounding her fists. Review the discussions of child abuse, PTSD, and behavior management to develop a strategy to help Sophia and her family.

10. Review the behavioral indicators of risk for child abuse presented in the case of Monique (p. 428). How may these behaviors look in a school-age child? How is a history of abuse likely to affect development and the transition to adulthood? What type of performance skills would you emphasize in a 15-year-old child with a history of abuse?

References

American Academy of Child and Adolescent Psychiatry. (1995a). *Facts for families: Being prepared: Know when to seek help for your child.* Washington, DC. Available at www.aacap.org/factsfam/whenhelp.htm.

American Academy of Child and Adolescent Psychiatry. (1995b). *Facts for families: The anxious child.* Washington, D.C. Available at www.aacap.org/factsfam/anxious.html.

American Academy of Child and Adolescent Psychiatry. (1995c). *Facts for families: Children who can't pay attention.* Washington, D.C. Available at www.aacap.org/factsfam/noattent.html.

American Academy of Child and Adolescent Psychiatry. (1995d). *Facts for families: Manic-depressive illness in teens.* Washington, D.C. Available at www.aacap.org/factsfam/bipolar.html.

American Academy of Child and Adolescent Psychiatry. (1995e). *Facts for families: Children of parents with mental illness.* Washington, D.C. Available at www.aacap.org/factsfam/parentmi.html.

American Academy of Child and Adolescent Psychiatry. (1997a). *Facts for families: Normal adolescent development: middle and early high school years.* Washington, D.C. Available at www.aacap.org/factsfam/develop.html.

American Academy of Child and Adolescent Psychiatry. (1997b). *Facts for families: Normal adolescent development: late high school years.* Washington, D.C. Available at www.aacap.org/factsfam/develop2.html.

American Academy of Child and Adolescent Psychiatry. (1997c). *Glossary: Anxiety.* Washington, D.C. Available at www.aacap.org/aacap/glossary/anxiety.html.

American Academy of Child and Adolescent Psychiatry. (1997d). *Facts for families: Obsessive-compulsive disorder in children and adolescents.* Washington, D.C. Available at www.aacap.org/factsfam/ocd.html.

American Academy of Child and Adolescent Psychiatry. (1998a). *Facts for families: Children's threats: When are they serious* [Fact sheet number 65 released on the World Wide Web]. Washington, D.C. Available at www.aacap.org/factsfam/65.html.

American Academy of Child and Adolescent Psychiatry. (1998b). *Facts for families: Teenagers with eating disorders.* Washington, D.C. Available at www.aacap.org/factsfam/eating.html.

American Academy of Child and Adolescent Psychiatry. (1998c). *Facts for families: Child abuse: The hidden bruises.* Washington, D.C. Available at www.aacap.org/factsfam/chldabus.html.

American Psychiatric Association. (1994). *Diagnostic and statistical manual of mental disorders* (4th ed.). Washington, DC: American Psychiatric Association.

Anderson, J., Hinojosa, J., Bedell, G., & Kaplan, M.T. (1990). Occupational therapy for children with perinatal HIV infection. *The American Journal of Occupational Therapy, 44* (3), 249-255.

Atkins, D.M., & Silber, T.J. (1993). Clinical spectrum of anorexia nervosa in children. *Journal of Developmental and Behavioral Pediatrics, 14* (4), 211-216.

Balck, R., & Glass, P. (1998). Temperament and school performance. *Pediatrics Review, 19* (5), 177.

Barkley, R.A., Anastopoulos, A.D., Guevremont, D.C., & Fletcher, K.E. (1991). Adolescents with ADD: Patterns of behavioral adjustment, academic functioning, and treatment utilization. *Journal of the American Academy of Child and Adolescent Psychiatry, 30* (5), 752-761.

Barnard, K.E. (1980). *Nursing Child Assessment Teaching Scale.* Seattle, WA: NCAST Publications.

Bledsoe, N., & Sheperd, J. (1982). A study of reliability and validity of a preschool play scale. *The American Journal of Occupational Therapy, 36* (12), 783-788.

Borda, M., & Borba, C. (1978). *Self-esteem: A classroom affair.* San Francisco: Harper Publications.

Boughton, K., Blower, C., Chartrand, C., Dircks, P., Stone, T., Youwe, G., & Hagen, B. (1998). Impact of research on pediatric pain assessment and outcomes. *Pediatric Nursing 24,* (1), 31-35, 62.

Bracegirdle, H. (1990). The acquisition of social skills by children with special needs. *British Journal of Occupational Therapy, 53* (3), 107-108.

Brazelton, T.B., Tronick, E., Adamson, L., Als, H., & Wise, S. (1975). Early mother-infant reciprocity. In *Parent-infant interaction: Ciba Foundation Symposium 33.* Amsterdam: Associated Scientific Publishers.

Bretherton, I., & Beeghly, M. (1982). Talking about internal states: The acquisition of an explicit theory of the mind. *Developmental Psychology, 18,* 906-921.

Bridges, B. (1990). *Stop, relax, and think: A game to help impulsive children think before they act.* Childsplay Childswork: The Center for Applied Psychology.

Butler, R. (1989). Mastery versus ability appraisal: A developmental study of children's observations of peers' work. *Child Development, 60,* 1350-1361.

Chess, S., & Thomas, A. (1983). Dynamics of individual behavioral development. In M.D. Levine, W.B. Carey, A.C. Crocker, & R.T. Gross (Eds.), *Developmental-behavioral pediatrics* (pp. 158-175). Philadelphia: W.B. Saunders.

Chess, S., & Thomas, A. (1984). *Origins and evolution of behavior disorders: Infancy to adult life.* New York: Brunner/Mazel.

Chess, S., & Thomas, A. (1987). *Know your child.* New York: Basic Books.

Cohen, P., Cohen, J., & Brook, J. (1993). An epidemiological study of disorders in late childhood and adolescence: II. Persistence of disorders. *Journal of Child Psychology and Psychiatry, 34* (6), 869-877.

Cohen, P., Cohen, J., Kasen, S., Velez, C., Hartmark, C., Johnson, J., Rojas, M., Brook, J., & Streuning, E. (1993). An epidemiological study of disorders in late childhood and adolescence: I. Age- and gender-specific prevalence. *Journal of Child Psychology and Psychiatry, 34* (6), 851-867.

Condon, W.S., & Sander, L.W. (1974). Neonatal movement is synchronized with adult speech: Interactional participation and language requisition. *Science, 183,* 99-101.

Creer, T.L., Stein, R.E., Rappaport, L., & Lewis, C. (1992). Behavioral consequences of illness: Childhood asthma as a model. *Pediatrics, 90* (5 Pt 2), 808-815.

Daltroy, L.H., Larson, M.G., Eaton, H.M., Partridge, A.J., Pless, I.B., Rogers, M.P., & Liang, M.H. (1992). Psychosocial adjustment in juvenile arthritis. *Journal of Pediatric Psychology, 17* (3), 277-289.

Davidson, D. (1995). Physical abuse of preschoolers: Identification and intervention through occupational therapy. *The American Journal of Occupational Therapy, 49* (1), 235-243.

Davidson, D., & LaVesser, P. (1998). Facilitating adaptive behaviors in elementary school-aged children. In J. Case-Smith (Ed.), *Occupational therapy: Making a difference in school based practice.* Bethesda, MD: AOTA, Inc.

Deacove, J. (1987). *Funny face.* Perth, Ontario: Family Pastimes.

DeGangi, G., Wietlisbach, S., Goodin, M., & Scheiner, N. (1993). A comparison of structured sensorimotor therapy and child-centered activity in the treatment of preschool children with sensorimotor problems. *The American Journal of Occupational Therapy, 47* (9), 777-786.

Dillard, M., Andonian, L., Flores, O., Lai, L., MacRae, A., & Shakir, M. (1992). Culturally competent occupational therapy in a diversely populated mental health setting. *The American Journal of Occupational Therapy, 46* (8), 721-726.

Doble, S.E., & Magill-Evans, J. (1992). A model of social interaction to guide occupational therapy practice. *Canadian Journal of Occupational Therapy, 59* (3), 141-150.

Dudgeon, B., Massagli, T., & Ross, B. (1997). Educational participation of children with spinal cord injury. *The American Journal of Occupational Therapy, 51* (7), 553-561.

Dunn, W. (1999). The Sensory Profile. San Antonio, TX: Psychological Corporation.

Famularo, R., Kinscherff, R., & Fenton, T. (1990). Symptom differences in acute and chronic presentation of childhood post-traumatic stress disorder. *Child Abuse and Neglect, 14* (3), 439-444.

Fazio, L. (1992). Tell me a story: The therapeutic metaphor in the practice of pediatric occupational therapy. *The American Journal of Occupational Therapy, 46* (2), 112-119.

Field, T.M. (1983). High-risk infants "have less fun" during early interactions. *Topics in Early Childhood Special Education, 3,* 77-87.

Field, T.M., & Fox, N.A. (Eds.). (1985). *Social perception in infants.* Norwood, NJ: Ablex.

Florey, L., & Michelman, S. (1978). Occupational role history: A screening tool for psychiatric occupational therapy. *The American Journal of Occupational Therapy, 32,* 301.

Fraenkel, L., & Tallant, B. (1987). Mostly me: A treatment approach for emotionally disturbed children. *Canadian Journal of Occupational Therapy, 54* (2), 59-64.

Frank, G., Huecker, E., Segal, R., Forwell, S., & Bagatell, N. (1991). Assessment and treatment of a pediatric patient in chronic care. *The American Journal of Occupational Therapy, 45* (3), 252-263.

Frankenburg, W.K., Dodds, J.B., Archer, P., Bresnick, B., Maschka, P., Edelman, N., & Sapiro, H. (1990). *Denver II Developmental Screening Test.* Denver: Denver Developmental Materials.

Friedman, R., & Doyal, G. (1992). *Management of children and adolescents with attention deficit-hyperactivity disorder* (3rd ed.). Austin, TX: Pro-Ed.

Gardener, M. (1994). *Gardener Social Developmental Scale.* Burlingame, CA: Psychological and Educational Publications.

Goldberg, S. (1977). Social competency in infancy: A model of parent-child interaction. *Merrill-Palmer Quarterly, 23,* 163-177.

Goldsmith, H., Buss, K., & Lemery, K. (1997). Toddler and childhood temperament: Expanded content, stronger genetic evidence, new evidence for the importance of environment. *Developmental Psychology, 33* (6), 891-905.

Greenspan, S., & Greenspan, N.T. (1985). *First feelings: Milestones in the emotional development of your baby and child.* New York: Penguin Books.

Gribble, P.A., Cowen, E.L., Wyman, P.A., Work, W.C., Wannon, M., & Raof, A. (1993). Parent and child views of parent-child relationship qualities and resilient outcomes among urban children. *Journal of Child Psychology and Psychiatry, 34* (4), 507-519.

Griswold, L.A. (1994). Ethnographic analysis: A study of classroom environments. *American Journal of Occupational Therapy, 48* (5), 397-402.

Guerney, L.F. (1983). Client-centered (nondirective) play therapy. In C.E. Schaefer & K.J. O'Connor (Eds.), *Handbook of play therapy* (pp. 21-64). New York: John Wiley & Sons.

Harden, P.W., & Zoccolillo, M. (1997). Disruptive behavior disorders. *Current Opinions in Pediatrics, 9* (4), 339-345.

Henry, A.D., & Coster, W. (1997). Competency beliefs and occupational role behavior among adolescents: Explication of the personal causation construct. *The American Journal of Occupational Therapy, 51* (4), 267-276.

Holly, K., & Schuster, C. (1992). Cognitive development during the school-age years. In C. Schuster & S. Ashburn. *The process of human development: A holistic life-span approach* (3rd ed.). (pp. 444-466). Philadelphia: Lippincott.

Honjo, S., Mizuno, R., Ajiki, M., Suzuki, A., Nagata, M., Goto, Y., & Nishide, T. (1998). Infant temperament and child-rearing stress: Birth order influences. *Early Human Development, 51* (2), 123-135.

Jackson, P., & Vessey, J. (1992). *Primary care of the child with a chronic condition.* St. Louis: Mosby.

John, K., Gammon, G.D., Prusoff, B.A., & Warner, V. (1987). The Social Adjustment Inventory for Children and Adolescents (SAICA): Testing of a new semi-structured interview. *Journal of the American Academy of Child and Adolescent Psychiatry, 26,* 898-911.

Jordan, J.P., & Heyde, M.B. (1979). *Vocational maturity during the high school years.* New York: Teachers College Press.

Kagan, J., & Zentner, M. (1996). Early childhood predictors of adult psychopathology. *Harvard Review of Psychiatry, 3* (6), 341-350.

Kaplan, H., & Sadock, B. (1996). *Concise textbook of clinical psychiatry* (7th ed.). Baltimore: Williams and Wilkins.

Kashani, J.H., Soltys, S.M., Dandoy, A.C., Vaidya, A.F., & Reid, J.C. (1991). Correlates of hopelessness in psychiatrically hospitalized children. *Comprehensive Psychiatry, 32* (4), 330-337.

Keogh, B.K. (1986). Temperament and schooling: Meaning of "goodness of fit"? *New Directions in Child Development, Mar* (31), 89-108.

Keogh, B.K., & Burstein, N.D. (1988). Relationship of temperament to preschoolers' interactions with peers and teachers. *Exceptional Child, 54* (5), 456-461.

Kielhofner, G. (Ed.). (1995). *A model of human occupation: Theory and application.* Baltimore: Williams & Wilkins.

Knox, S. (1997). Development and current use of the Knox Preschool Play Scale. In L.D. Parham & L. Fazio (Eds.), *Play in occupational therapy for children.* St. Louis: Mosby.

Korb-Khalsa, K., Azok, S., & Leutenberg, E. (1992). *SEALS+Plus: Self-esteem and life skills.* Beachwood, OH: Wellness Reproductions.

Lavigne, J.V., & Faier-Routman, J. (1993). Correlates of psychological adjustment to pediatric physical disorders: A meta-analytic review and comparison with existing models. *Journal of Developmental and Behavioral Pediatrics, 14* (2), 117-123.

Lederhaas, G. (1997). Pediatric pain management. *Journal of the Florida Medical Association, 84* (1), 37-40.

Linder, T.W. (1990). *Transdisciplinary play-based assessment: A functional approach to working with young children.* Baltimore: Brookes.

Magill, J., & Hurlbut, N. (1986). The self-esteem of adolescents with cerebral palsy. *The American Journal of Occupational Therapy, 40*(6), 402-407.

Matheson, L., & Bohr, P. (1997). Occupational competence across the life span. In C. Christiansen & C. Baum. *Occupational therapy: Enabling function and well-being* (pp. 429-457). Thorofare, NJ: Slack.

McGrath, P., & Frager, G. (1996). Psychological barriers to optimal pain management in infants and children. *Clinical Journal of Pain Management, 12* (2), 135-141.

Meltzoff, A.N., & Moore, M.K. (1983). Newborn infants imitate adult facial gestures. *Child Development, 54,* 702-709.

National Advisory Mental Health Council. (1990). *National plan for research on child and adolescent mental disorders.* Washington, DC: National Institute of Mental Health.

Neistadt, M., & Crepeau, E. (1998). *Willard and Spackman's occupational therapy* (9th ed.). Philadelphia: J.B. Lippincott.

Neville, A., & Kielhofner, G. (1983). *The modified interest checklist.* Unpublished workbook. Washington, DC: National Institutes of Health.

Nigg, J., & Goldsmith, H. (1998). Developmental psychopathology, personality, and temperament: Reflections on recent behavioral genetics research. *Human Biology, 70* (2), 387-412.

Piers, E.V. (1984). *Piers-Harris Children's Self-Concept Scale* (Revised manual). Los Angeles: Western Psychological Services.

Pincus, D. (1994). *Feeling good about others.* Carthage, IL: Good Apple.

Pollock, S. (1986). Human responses to chronic illness: Physiologic and psychosocial adaptation. *Nursing Research, 32,* 4-9.

Rodgers, B., Hilemeier, M., O'Neill, E., & Slonim, M. (1981). Depression in the chronically ill or handicapped school aged child. *The American Journal of Maternal and Child Nursing, 6,* 266-273.

Rothbaum, F., & Weisz, J. (1989). *Child psychopathology and the quest for control.* Beverly Hills, CA: Sage.

Rowan, A.B., & Foy, D.W. (1993). Post-traumatic stress disorder in child sexual abuse survivors: A literature review. *Journal of Traumatic Stress, 6* (1), 3-20.

Russell, P. (1985). *The wheelchair child: How handicapped children can enjoy life to its fullest.* Englewood Cliffs, NJ: Prentice-Hall.

Rutter, M. (1987). The role of cognition in child development and disorder. *British Journal of Medical Psychology, 60,* 1-16.

Schechter, N.L., Bernstein, B.A., Beck, A., Hart, L., & Scherzer, L. (1991). Individual differences in children's response to pain: Role of temperament and parental characteristics. *Pediatrics, 87* (2), 171-177.

Schultz, S. (1992). School-based occupational therapy for students with behavioral disorders. *Occupational Therapy in Health Care, 8,* 173-196.

Schuster, C. (1992a). Adaptation to Uniqueness. In C. Schuster & S. Ashburn. *The process of human development: A holistic life-span approach* (3rd ed.). (pp. 351-375). Philadelphia: Lippincott.

Schuster, C. (1992b). Preparation for school. In C. Schuster & S. Ashburn. *The process of human development: A holistic life-span approach* (3rd ed.). (pp. 277-294). Philadelphia: Lippincott.

Shumway-Cook, A., & Woollacott, M. (1995). *Motor control: Theory and practical applications.* Williams and Wilkins: Baltimore.

Simmons, R.J., Corey, M., Cowen, L., Keenan, N., Robertson, J., & Levison, H. (1987). Behavioral adjustment of latency age children with cystic fibrosis. *Psychosomatic Medicine, 49* (3), 291-301.

Smolak, L. (1992). Development of communication and language. In C. Schuster & S. Ashburn. *The process of human development: A holistic life-span approach* (3rd ed.). (pp. 254-276). Lippincott: Philadelphia.

Solomon, R., Walco, G., Robinson, M. & Dampier, C. (1998). Pediatric pain management: program description and preliminary evaluation results of a professional course. *Journal of Developmental and Behavioral Pediatrics 19* (3), 193-195.

Song, K., Morton, A., Koch, K., Herring, J., Browne, R., & Hanway, J. (1998). Chronic musculoskeletal pain in childhood. *Journal of Pediatric Orthopedics, 18*(5), 576-581.

Sparrow, S., Balla, D., & Cicchetti, D. (1987). *The Vineland Adaptive Behavior Scales.* Circle Pines, MN: American Guidance Service.

Stowell, M. (1987). Psychosocial role of the occupational therapist with pediatric bone marrow transplant patients. *Occupational Therapy in Mental Health, 7* (2), 39-50.

Turecki, S., & Wernick, S. (1994). *The emotional problems of normal children.* New York: Bantam Books.

Turnquist, K., & Engel, J. (1994). Occupational therapists' experiences and knowledge of pain in children. *Physical and Occupational Therapy in Pediatrics, 14* (1), 35-51.

Vessey, J.A., & Caserza, C.L. (1992). Chronic conditions and child development. In P.L. Jackson & J.A. Vessey (Eds.), *Primary care of the child with a chronic condition* (pp. 26-44). St. Louis: Mosby.

Weinberg, N., Rahdert, E., Colliver, J., & Glantz, M. (1998). Adolescent substance abuse: A review of the past 10 years. *Journal of the American Academy of Child and Adolescent Psychiatry, 37* (3), 252-261.

Wellman, H.M., & Estes, D. (1987). Children's early use of mental verbs and what they mean. *Discourse Processes, 10,* 141-156.

Welsh, J. (1992). The use of drawings in the pediatric office. In S. Dixon & M. Stein (Eds.), *Encounters with children: Pediatric behavior and development* (2nd ed.). (pp.425-435). St. Louis: Mosby

White, R. (1971). The urge toward competence. *The American Journal of Occupational Therapy, 25,* 271-274.

Wilbarger, P., & Wilbarger, J. (1991). *Sensory affective disorders: Beyond tactile defensiveness.* Santa Barbara, CA

Youssef, N.M. (1988). School adjustment of children with congenital heart disease. *Maternal and Child Nursing Journal, 17*(4), 217-30.

Yude, C., Goodman, R., & McConachie, H. (1998). Peer problems of children with hemiplegia in mainstream primary schools. *Journal of Child and Adolescent Psychiatry, 39* (4), 533-541.

Zakich, R. (1989). *The ungame.* Anaheim, CA: Talicor.

chapter 15

Feeding Intervention

Jane Case-Smith
Ruth Humphry

key terms

Co-occupation of feeding
Social interactions during feeding
Self-feeding
Sucking and drinking
Suck-swallow-breathe sequence
Biting and chewing
Feeding evaluation
Videofluoroscopic swallow studies

Oral hypersensitivity
Oral motor problems
Swallowing disorders
Transition from nonoral to oral feeding
Oral structural problems
Interactional and social issues
Nutrition and nutritional issues

■ CHAPTER OBJECTIVES

1. Analyze problems in feeding, eating, and mealtime occupations.
2. Articulate the importance of social contexts in feeding and feeding dysfunction.
3. Understand the sequence of typical feeding and self-feeding skills.
4. Apply a systems model to relate performance components to changes in feeding.
5. Define feeding as a co-occupation and a critical element of the parent-child relationship.
6. Analyze how a disability can interfere with feeding interactions and strategies to support optimal parent-child interaction during feeding.
7. Comprehend the influence of developmental problems and the potential influence of experience on acquisition of age-appropriate feeding skills.
8. Explain evaluation of and intervention for impairments, including oral sensory, oral motor, cognitive, and psychosocial problems, as they affect feeding skills of children.
9. Define and describe swallowing disorders and intervention for swallowing problems.

10. Describe common oral structural problems and explain interventions to promote early feeding in children with these problems.
11. Describe interventions that enhance the child's ability to self-feed and to drink from a cup.
12. Identify and explain nutritional aspects of feeding and the nature of collaboration with nutritionists.
13. Explain behavioral issues that interfere with feeding and intervention strategies to improve mealtime behaviors.

Eating meals is an essential occupation that occurs several times a day and provides children with nutritional intake and learning and interactional experiences that affect every aspect of the young child's life. Mealtimes create a temporal organization to the day and give the child opportunities to practice object manipulation, experience new sensations, and learn how to communicate needs and desires. The nurturing that the child receives during feeding helps the parent bond with the child and helps the child trust in and rely on the parent to meet his or her needs. For children, eating food occurs as a co-occupation with caregiving adults who select the types of food, amount presented, time of eating, and method of feeding. The caregiver bases these carefully made selections on what he or she believes is age-appropriate performance, what is nutritional sound, and what he or she values as cultural tradition.

Children experience problems in feeding for various reasons. Premature infants and those born with congenital problems such as heart defects may lack the ability to organize behavior or the energy to suck effectively. Other children born with oral anomalies, such as cleft palate, require parents and health care professionals to implement compensation strategies so that he or she can ingest food. Children who have underlying problems with motor control (e.g., cerebral palsy) or difficulty learning everyday skills (e.g., mental retardation) can experience associated problems with eating or mastering utensil use. Other children have delayed feeding skills secondary to problems that the parent experiences in presenting food or understanding what to expect of young children at mealtime. To plan effective interventions for a child's problem in feeding, the therapist synthesizes information about the mealtime environment, performance of the child and caregivers, and relationship of the child's performance to an eating task. Given the complexity of performing this occupation and the interactive effect of the occupation, person, and environment described in Chapters 3 and 4, the occupational therapist works at many levels in helping a child with feeding problems.

The first section of this chapter focuses on the child's occupational performance and related elements. It first describes developmental changes in the acquisition of feeding skills, or the ability to bring food to the mouth. Occupational performance of feeding for typically developing children goes through major transformations in the first 3 years, starting with total dependency to independence in using spoons and forks and consuming various foods. The first section also presents a general framework for evaluation of feeding problems and examines specific considerations and interventions for feeding problems. Because interventions place priority on maintaining the child's health, the section describes nutritional concerns and modifications in intervention strategies.

The next section of this chapter focuses on issues related to the parent or other caregiver who engages the child in this co-occupation. Typically, when the child has feeding problems, the therapist needs to collaborate with the parent or adult caregivers about how or what they feed the child. Part of this section also addresses the implications for parent-child interactions and other aspects of the child's development if there are feeding difficulties.

The final section illustrates to the importance of family characteristics that determine the environment for feeding. At all times the therapist must provide services that are appropriate to social context and consistent with the family's priorities and strategies.

■ FEEDING AS CO-OCCUPATION OF PARENT AND CHILD

The parent orchestrates the child's occupations during the day and provides support and assistance to enable the child's successful participation in activities. The parent or other caregiver who engages in co-feeding with the child prepares and presents food in a manner consistent with the child's developmental abilities. The adult uses the child's cues regarding speed, taste preferences, and comfort to adjust the feeding process. Parents vary in eating expectations and routines. Appreciating parents' decisions regarding how to support the child's mealtime occupations is an important aspect of parent-therapist collaboration.

Since developmental changes in the child's eating and self-feeding skills require new mealtime challenges, the parent's expectations of his or her child are important. Parents receive guidelines about child development and feeding in books and through informal resources such as advice of family or friends. However, parents express varied and poorly formulated expectations of when they think their children should reach developmental milestones in eating (Humphry & Thigpen-Beck, 1997). Parents integrate many perspectives when dealing with day-to-day family life. Mealtime selections involve a parent's unique perspective of the child and what he or she ate previously and beliefs about child development. The following is an example of a child whose behavior indicates a need for change in mealtime challenges:

> When asked how she knew that it was time to give her 7-month-old daughter soft table food, Julie responds, "She grabbed at my french fries one day. I said, 'OK, but you might not like them.' She liked it and only coughed once. The pediatrician told me at the 6-month check-up that something like a teething cracker would be OK, and my sister told me that I was starving her by not giving her more than baby food. I didn't think she was ready until she asked for it." This parent considers her daughter's readiness to change food texture because she was given formal and informal advice, but she ultimately bases her decision on the infant's behaviors.

Parents make decisions about how to feed their children and the appropriate amount of flexibility based on what they believe the child should learn from the situation. For example, in a descriptive study, researchers asked parents whether they approve of flexibility with a child when he or she refuses to eat a dish (Humphry & Thigpen-Beck, 1997). The results of this study reveal the multidimensional nature of feeding. Social contexts are important in understanding how different parents responded. Older, more educated parents were more inclined to be flexible and change what they fed the child. Parents who believed that good behavior and obedience are important were less likely to accept flexibility. A larger agenda often influences the type of feeding strategy that the parents use and how parents interpret the child's behaviors at mealtime (Humphry & Thigpen-Beck, 1998).

Occupational science demonstrates that observable caregiving behaviors involve reasoning and attitudes and that the meaning of each occupation is important. Preparing meals and feeding family members communicate symbolic and emotional meanings while meeting a need for nourishment (DeVault, 1991). Many adults believe that to nourish the child is to nurture. Parents view the weight gain of an infant as success in the caregiver role. Feeding an infant can be a warm, positive experience for the caregiver and enhances the bond between adult and child. When the caregiver does not take pleasure in feeding a child, the task can lose much of its meaning and becomes a job (Brazelton, 1993), changing the experience of the co-occupation for the adult and child. The parent or teacher who approaches interactions with a sense of duty decreases the effectiveness of his or her efforts and teaches the child that eating is work rather than pleasure.

■ TYPICAL SEQUENCE OF CHANGES IN FEEDING

As with other developing occupations, a child's eating and self-feeding skills emerge from physical maturation, changing performance components, new challenging tasks that the caregiver presents, and feedback about success in performance. Eating, although almost automatic for adults, requires that the child have considerable skill and does not develop automatically with maturation. At times the therapist needs to consider maturity of the child's performance components, such as motor control of the tongue, but the relationship of motor performance to quality of feeding is not hierarchic (i.e., the maturation of the performance component does not always come first with a subsequent change in occupational performance). Rather there is an interaction between occupation and performance components in the developmental process. For example, underlying control of the lips to remove food from the spoon depends to some extent on maturation of nerves controlling oral motor actions. Understanding a spoon's function in self-feeding requires cognitive abilities in recognition and classification of objects. The child's motivation to self-feed may improve the quality of oral motor control and promote learning of form and space. Practice with a spoon enables discovery of new patterns of lip movement, which contributes to the child's self-feeding skills. Concurrently, through ma-

nipulation of the spoon into the mouth, the child alters his or her understanding of the nature of tools. A child challenged to change patterns of feeding before he or she is ready to apply new sensorimotor or cognitive abilities will become distressed and uncooperative with meals. Thus therapists must consider the child's readiness to learn new eating skills before introducing new tasks.

The occupation of feeding consists of different phases as the child progresses from breast-feeding to self-feeding a complete meal of table foods with utensils. During early infancy, changes occur in the method of the infant's sucking from a nipple. Health care professionals usually encourage parents to give the infant breast milk or formula in the first few months. Typically, changes in eating and self-feeding demonstrate a sequence of new behaviors as parents present new feeding challenges. Because the timing to introduce new eating experiences varies from one family to the next and typically developing children mature at varying rates, the range in the ages when new skills in feeding are demonstrated is great.

The child's occupational performance in feeding depends on his or her dynamical integration of sensorimotor, cognitive, and social components, which are also developing. Specific oral sensorimotor changes for drinking and eating are presented in detail later in this chapter; however, *the occupation organizes behavior and motivates the child* (i.e., consuming food in the context of a social experience). The changing quality of the child's occupational performance is gradual, and emerging skills to eat and drink require practice before the child shows consistent mastery. Therapists have gained insight into development of sensorimotor components as related to feeding and documented their findings. In designing intervention, the occupational therapist considers occupational performance (feeding) and underlying systems that contribute to performance (oral motor, sensorimotor, cognitive, and psychosocial abilities).

■ TYPICAL DEVELOPMENT OF ORAL STRUCTURES

Intact oral structures and cranial nerves are prerequisites for eating and drinking. Different actions of the mouth develop concurrently as the child gains control of jaw, tongue, cheek, and lip movement. The anatomic structures of the mouth and throat change significantly in the first 12 months. The growth and maturation of the oral structures allow for development of more mature feeding patterns. Table 15-1 lists the oral structures involved in feeding.

The newborn has a small oral cavity filled with fatty cheeks and the tongue. When the nipple is placed inside the mouth, the tight fit enables the infant to easily compress the nipple and achieve automatic suction. The nega-

table 15-1　*Functions of Oral Structures in Feeding*

Structure	Parts	Function During Feeding
Oral cavity	Hard and soft palate, tongue, fat pads of cheeks, upper and lower jaws, and teeth	Contains the food during drinking and chewing and provides for initial mastication before swallowing
Pharynx	Base of tongue, buccinator, oropharynx, tendons, and hyoid bone	Funnels food into the esophagus and allows food and air to share space; the pharynx is a space common to both functions
Larynx	Epiglottis and false and true vocal folds	Valve to the trachea that closes during swallowing
Trachea	Tube below the larynx and cartilaginous rings	Allows air to flow into bronchi and lungs
Esophagus	Thin and muscular esophagus	Carries food from the pharynx, through the diaphragm, and into the stomach; at rest it is collapsed and distends as food passes through it

Modified from Wolf, L.S., & Glass, R.P. (1992). *Feeding and swallowing disorders in infancy: Assessment and management.* Tucson: Therapy Skill Builders.

tive pressure that automatically occurs during sucking movements of the jaw expresses liquid from the nipple (Morris & Klein, 1987). Therefore the full-term, healthy newborn is successful in sucking from a breast or bottle nipple.

The structures in the infant's throat are also in close proximity to one another. The infant's epiglottis and soft palate are in direct approximation. As a result, the liquid from the nipple safely passes from the base of the tongue to the esophagus. During swallowing, the larynx elevates and the epiglottis falls over it to protect the trachea. Therefore aspiration is unlikely before 4 months of age, and the infant can safely feed in a reclined position.

As the infant grows, the neck elongates and the relationship of the oral and throat structures changes. The oral cavity becomes larger and more open. The fatty tongue becomes thin and muscular, and the cheeks lose much of their fatty padding. With the increase in oral cavity space, the tongue, lips, and cheeks must provide greater control of liquid or food within the mouth. New sucking patterns emerge to enable the infant to handle liquid without the structural advantages of early infancy. These include up-and-down movements of the tongue to express liquids from the nipple. The increasing oral space also provides room to masticate food and to move the tongue in the rolling pattern required during chewing.

As the infant approaches 12 months of age, the hyoid, epiglottis, and larynx descend, creating space between these structures and the base of the tongue. The hyoid and larynx become more mobile during swallowing, elevating with each swallow. The infant requires greater coordination of these structures during the suck-swallow-breathe sequence. With the elongation of the pharynx, feeding in a reclined position creates a greater possibility of aspiration. The pull of gravity in a reclined position can interfere with the control needed by the infant to move the liquid to the entrance of the esophagus. Figure 15-1 shows the structures of the mouth and pharynx of the infant.

■ TYPICAL ORAL MOTOR DEVELOPMENT ASSOCIATED WITH FEEDING SKILLS

The development of sucking, drinking, biting, and chewing is highly related to the overall sensorimotor development of the child. The development of more mature oral patterns occurs as the child has changing nutritional needs, demonstrates interest in self-feedings, and expands communication efforts. The changes in jaw, tongue, lip, and cheek movements are associated with the development of skills in (1) sucking and drinking, (2) coordinating sucking, swallowing, and breathing; and (3) biting and chewing.

Sucking and Drinking Skills

The sucking reflex is present in the fetus and predominates as the method of oral feeding through the first 8 to 10 months of life. Sucking patterns differ when the child is sucking on a pacifier (nonnutritive) compared with sucking on a bottle nipple (nutritive). The nonnutritive pattern is rapid and rhythmic, usually about two sucks per second. The nutritive pattern is rhythmic but is characterized by a burst-and-pause pattern. This pattern allows the infant to breathe and rest between sucking bursts.

Premature infants typically are fed by nonoral means through 33 weeks' gestational age. Before this age the infant demonstrates a rhythmic nonnutritive sucking pattern, but sucking strength and endurance limit oral feeding. In a healthy premature infant of 35 weeks' gestational age, the jaw and tongue movements are sufficiently strong to allow for oral feeding at least part of the time. The rate of sucking, the force of suction or compression, and the length of time that the infant eats determines the amount of liquid taken in. Two characteristics that are important to feeding efficiency are the rhythm of sucking and the type of suction (i.e., negative pressure for expression of liquid) that the infant is able to achieve and sustain over

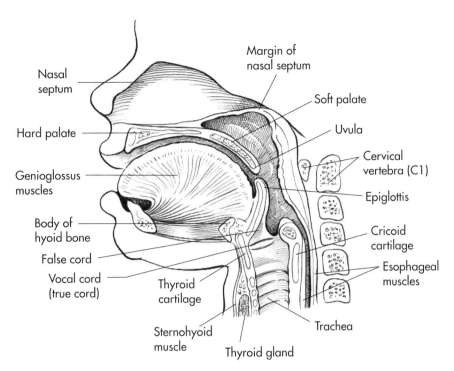

Nasal
septum

Margin of
nasal septum

Soft palate

Hard palate

Uvula

Cervical
vertebra (C1)

Genioglossus
muscles

Epiglottis

figure**15-1** Anatomic structures of
the mouth and throat.

Body of
hyoid bone

Cricoid
cartilage

False cord

Esophageal
muscles

Vocal cord
(true cord)

Thyroid
cartilage

Sternohyoid
muscle

Trachea

Thyroid gland

time (Daniels, Devlieger, Casaer, & Eggermont, 1986). Wolf and Glass (1992) explained that both compression and suction are needed to express liquid. The infant achieves these aspects of feeding through sucking patterns that include sealing the lips around the nipple and moving the tongue in a simultaneous extension and retraction and up-and-down movements. By 36 weeks' gestational age, the typical premature infant takes all food by mouth and uses a sucking pattern similar to that of the full-term infant.

The full-term infant (born at 40 weeks' gestation) has strong oral reflexes that enable him or her to take in liquid nutrition without difficulty. Given tactile stimulation near the mouth, the hungry infant's rooting reflex induces the infant to turn his or her head, thereby allowing him or her to latch onto any potential nutritional source. The infant also exhibits a gag and cough reflex to protect the airway from the intake of liquid.

The sucking pattern of the full-term infant is rhythmic, sustained, and efficient, diminishing appropriately with satiation. The pattern of each infant is unique and varies in efficiency of sucking according to the infant's level of fatigue and hunger. Most infants complete an oral feeding in 20 to 25 minutes.

The infant's first sucking pattern is termed *suckling* (Morris & Klein, 1987). A forward-backward movement of the tongue characterizes this pattern. Jaw opening and closing accompany this rhythmic back-and-forth tongue movement (Yokochi, 1997). The tongue typically extends to but not beyond the border of the lips.

Suckling predominates in the first 4 months. The pattern may cause slight liquid loss and intake of air and is

primarily observed in the second and third months of life, after the infant's physiologic flexion has disappeared and before the infant has established mature oral motor control. At 4 months of age the tongue begins to move in an up-and-down direction that characterizes a true sucking pattern. The wide jaw excursions of the young infant are reduced. Less liquid is lost, and suction on the nipple increases.

The 6-month-old infant demonstrates strong up-and-down tongue movement with minimal jaw excursion during sucking. Jaw stability increases and allows for better control of tongue movement. The lip seal is good, such that the infant does not lose liquid during sucking on a nipple. Many cultures in the United States introduce the cup to the infant at 6 months of age (usually a sipper cup with a spout). When first presented a cup, the infant will try to continue to use a suckling pattern so the jaw continues to move up and down and the tongue moves forward and backward in the mouth. The wide jaw excursions result in liquid loss. Some coughing may occur as the infant first attempts this skill.

By 9 months of age the infant continues to feed from the bottle, using strong sucking patterns. Long sequences of continuous sucks occur when the infant drinks from the cup. The jaw is not consistently stable on the rim of the cup, so the infant is messy drinking from a cup.

At 12 months of age many infants make the transition from the bottle to the cup for drinking during mealtime but continue to bottle-feed at other times. Jaw stability for supporting the cup's rim remains incomplete. The tongue may protrude slightly beneath the cup to provide additional stability (Morris & Klein,

1987). For the first time, tongue tip elevation occurs during swallowing.

With practice the infant uses an up-and-down sucking pattern to obtain liquids from a cup. He or she bites on the rim of the cup to obtain external jaw stabilization. The upper lip closes on the edge of the cup to provide a seal for drinking. The tongue elevates to bring the liquid into the mouth.

At 24 months of age the child can efficiently drink from a cup. He or she uses up-and-down tongue movements and tip elevation. Internal jaw stabilization emerges so that the jaw appears still. Therefore the rim of the cup rests on the stable jaw, and biting on the cup's rim is no longer necessary. The child swallows with easy lip closure and does not lose liquids from the cup. Lengthy suck-swallow sequences occur.

Coordination of Sucking, Swallowing, and Breathing

As the infant demonstrates increasing control of jaw, tongue, and lip movement, he or she also learns to coordinate and sequence oral movements into rhythmic patterns of sucking, swallowing, and breathing. The coordination of the oral structures as they work together to prepare and swallow food are perhaps more important to the feeding process than development of control of any one oral structure.

The 1-month-old infant demonstrates one suck to one swallow at the beginning of the feeding. He or she can sequence two to three sucks per swallow after his or her initial hunger has been satiated. By 3 or 4 months of age the infant sequences 20 or more sucks from the breast or bottle before pausing. Swallowing occurs intermittently (after four to five sucks) and without pausing. Breathing slows during sucking and occurs within and between sucking sequences. Occasionally the infant may cough or choke when he or she momentarily loses coordination of sucking, swallowing, and breathing.

As the infant approaches 12 months of age, these long sequences continue in bottle- or breast-feeding. When the infant begins to drink from the cup, he or she loses this coordination. At 9 months of age the infant stops to swallow or breathe after one to three sucks from the cup. By 12 months of age, swallowing follows sucking without pausing and the infant takes three continuous swallows before pausing. Swallowing is efficient (without coughing) when liquid flow presents at an appropriate rate.

By 15 to 18 months of age the infant has excellent coordination of sucking, swallowing, and breathing. When drinking from a cup, the infant's swallowing follows sucking without pauses. The infant performs at least three suck-swallow sequences before pausing, and the amount of liquid swallowed each time increases to at least 1 ounce. Coughing or choking rarely occurs.

Biting and Chewing

The first *biting or chewing* movements of the infant are reflexive. At 4 to 5 months of age the infant uses a rhythmic, stereotypic, phasic bite-and-release pattern on almost any substance placed in the mouth (e.g., a soft cookie, cracker, or toy). Jaw movements are up and down rather than diagonal. When the phasic bite-and-release pattern is used in a repeated rhythm, it is termed a *munching pattern*. The munch is characterized by jaw movement in the vertical direction and tongue movement in extension and retraction (lateralization has not yet developed). Therefore the munching pattern appears as an effective solution when the infant receives pureed foods or soft foods that quickly dissolve.

By 7 to 8 months of age the infant demonstrates some variability in the up-and-down munching pattern. He or she begins to use some diagonal jaw movement when the texture of the food requires variation in jaw movement. The infant continues to use the phasic bite-and-release pattern when he or she receives a cookie, thus the jaw closes abruptly on the cookie and then the infant sucks on it. The jaw holds the cookie but the infant cannot yet successfully bite through it. A bite is obtained by breaking off the piece while the jaw is held closed on the cookie. When the infant receives food on a spoon, the upper lip actively cleans it from the spoon. The lips become more active during sucking and maintaining the food within the mouth.

By 9 months of age the infant handles pureed and soft food well. He or she continues to use a munching pattern; however, the vertical up-and-down jaw movements now include diagonal movements. The infant transfers the food from the center of the mouth to the side using lateral tongue movements. These same lateral movements keep the food on the side during munching, making that process effective in mastication of soft or mashed table food. The lips are active during chewing, so they make contact as the jaw moves up and down.

Rotary chewing movements begin at approximately 12 months of age, made possible as the child gains jaw stability and controlled mobility. This control is also exhibited when the child demonstrates sustained, well-graded bite on soft cookies. The tongue is active in chewing by moving food from the center of the mouth to the sides, licking food from the lips, and demonstrating tip elevation on occasion. The infant is able to retrieve food on the lower lip by drawing it inward into the mouth.

The infant at 18 months of age demonstrates well-coordinated rotary chewing. He or she is able to chew soft meat and various table foods. The child can control and sustain bite and can bite off a piece of a hard cookie or pretzel. The tongue becomes increasingly mobile and efficiently moves food within the mouth.

At 24 months of age the child can eat most meats and raw vegetables. The child can grade and sustain the bite and can bite on hard foods with ease. Circular rotary jaw movements that characterize mature chewing are present. The tongue transfers food from one side of the mouth to the other using a rolling movement. The tongue moves skillfully to clear the lips and gums. Lip closure during chewing prevents food loss.

Self-Feeding Skills

Motivation to eat and the social meaning of eating can be equally important for the therapist to develop interventions for *self-feeding skills*. To consider cognitive and psychosocial development relative to activities of daily living (ADLs), Humphry and Morrow (1998) provide insights into how children play with and master toys (Barrett & Morgan, 1995; Piaget, 1952) to suggest how these components influence performance of occupations. The caregiver can introduce new challenges in mealtimes even before the child shows full mastery in an earlier area of performance. Table 15-2 outlines the developmental sequence of self-feeding. The ages are approximate and overlapping.

The infant displays his or her active nature of "discovering" new forms of feeding when given baby cereal for the first time on a spoon. Initially, the infant tries to use a suckling action, so the tongue pushes forward and pushes the food out of the mouth. With repeated challenge across several meals, the child applies alternative motor patterns of the lips and tongue to manage the new food texture. Learning to move the baby cereal to the back of the mouth takes time, sometimes several weeks. The infant elicits active learning by experience, and regardless of whether baby food is introduced at 5 or 7 months of age, the infant's first response is to use the original suckling pattern used with the nipple. Older infants master the action quicker than younger ones.

Children are often eager to feed themselves. As early as 6 months of age the infant may bring his or her hands up to the bottle and try to hold it. The caregiver should not prop the bottle because the infant lacks motor skills necessary to remove the bottle if choking occurs. Also the infant typically lacks the cognitive understanding that if the bottle is dropped it can be retrieved and put back into the mouth. Infants over 8 months of age actively hold the bottle, but the caregiver should monitor their self-feeding to ensure adequate intake because infants are easily distracted once they satisfy their initial hunger.

Typically, finger feeding develops quickly and naturally as the infant receives soft cookies or crackers to hold by about 8 months of age. At this age infants typically exhibit a radial digital grasp, which positions the cookie well for entry into the mouth. From 9 to 13 months of age the infant develops several skills that contribute to his or her ability to self-feed. Control of sitting posture and improved sitting balance, development of refined pincer grasp with controlled release, and refinement of isolated forearm and wrist movements result in efficient finger-feeding. By 12 months of age, finger-feeding is generally a preferred and enjoyed activity and matches changes in psychosocial components as the infant wishes to have increased independence and may refuse to be fed. The selection of finger foods should match the child's oral motor skills (e.g., cooked vegetables are easily grasped and mashed with the tongue and gums). The infant should not be given nuts, hard candy, chunks of hot dog, and grapes because these can occlude the airway if they are aspirated.

Infants under 1 year of age will grab, wave, and bang spoons when being fed. Around 12 months of age the infant demonstrates an understanding of the spoon by poking at a bowl of food with a spoon and bringing it to the mouth. The infant is easily frustrated as visual monitoring of the spoon's position is poor and he or she has difficulty sequencing movements to scoop or adjusting the forearm and wrist. The food frequently slips from the spoon before it reaches the mouth. Attending to the whole activity and recognizing when the spoon is empty (sufficient cognitive changes to use feedback) is necessary before the infant starts to control the wrist and forearm sufficiently for spoon-feeding. Infants, despite marginal ability, will frequently insist on self-feeding even though independence means less success at satisfying hunger.

Proficiency in spoon feeding emerges between 15 and 18 months of age when the infant brings the spoon with sticky food, such as yogurt, into the mouth with minimal spillage. The infant holds the spoon in a pronated gross grasp and uses primarily shoulder movement to bring it to the mouth. By 24 months of age the child spoon-feeds without spillage (with more solid foods). He or she holds the spoon in the radial fingers with the forearm supinated and is able to obtain the food and efficiently place the spoon into the mouth. Between 30 and 36 months of age the child may begin to prefer a fork for "stabbing" foods and may learn to eat foods that are more difficult to maintain on a spoon (e.g., cold cereal and rice with gravy).

Drinking

The infant may demonstrate interest in drinking from a cup as early as 6 months of age. However, skills in drinking from a cup do not emerge until about 12 months of age. At that time the infant is better able to correctly orient the cup to the mouth and to tip it to a degree that spillage is not inevitable. Several types of cups are available that make learning to drink from a cup an easy transition for the child. The first cup that the infant uses has a lid and a spout. It may have handles or may be a small cup that the infant can hold in one hand. Initially, the parent places only a small amount in the cup to decrease spillage and promote the child's success in directing the flow of liquid. The child may begin to use a small (4- to 6-ounce) cup without a lid at 24 months of age;

table 15-2 *Developmental Continuum in Self-Feeding and Associated Component Areas*

Age (mo)	Eating and Feeding Performance	Concurrent Changes in Performance Components		
		Sensorimotor	Cognition	Psychosocial
5-7	Takes cereal or pureed baby food from spoon	Has good head stability and emerging sitting abilities; reaches and grasps toys; explores and tolerates various textures (e.g., fingers, rattles); puts objects in mouth	Attends to effect produced by actions, such as hitting or shaking	Plays with caregiver during meals and engages in interactive routines
6-8	Attempts to hold bottle but may not retrieve it if it falls; needs to be monitored for safety reasons		Object permanence is emerging and infant anticipates spoon or bottle	Easily distracted by stimuli (especially siblings) in the environment
6-9	Holds and tries to eat cracker but sucks on it more than bites it; consumes soft foods that dissolve in the mouth; grabs at spoon but bangs it or sucks on either end of it	Good sitting stability emerges; able to use hands to manipulate smaller parts of rattle; guided reach and palmar grasp applied to hand-to-mouth actions with objects	Uses familiar actions initially with haphazard variations; seeks novelty and is anxious to explore objects (may grab at food on adult's plate)	Recognizes strangers; emerging sense of self
9-13	Finger feeds self a portion of meals consisting of soft table foods (e.g., macaroni, peas, dry cereal) and objects if fed by an adult	Uses various grasps on objects of different sizes; able to isolate radial fingers on smaller objects	Has increased organization and sequencing of schemas to do desired activity; may have difficulty attending to events outside visual space (e.g., position of spoon close to mouth)	Prefers to act on objects than be passive observer
12-14	Dips spoon in food, brings spoonful of food to mouth, but spills food by inverting spoon before it goes into mouth	Beginning to place and release objects; likely to use pronated grasp on objects like crayon or spoon	Recognizes that objects have function and uses tools appropriately; relates objects together, shifting attention among them	Interest in watching family routines
15-18	Scoops food with spoon and brings it to mouth	Shoulder and wrist stability demonstrate precise movements	Experiments to learn rules of how objects work; actively solves problems by creating new action solutions	Internalizes standards imposed by others for how to play with objects
24-30	Demonstrates interest in using fork; may stab at food such as pieces of canned fruit; proficient at spoon use and eats cereal with milk or rice with gravy with utensil	Tolerates various food textures in mouth; adjusts movements to be efficient (e.g., forearm supinated to scoop and lift spoon)	Expresses wants verbally; demonstrates imitation of short sequence of occupation (e.g., putting food on plate and eating it)	Has increasing desire to copy peers; looks to adults to see if they appreciate success in an occupation; interested in household routines

however, spillage is inevitable at that time. The child continues to use a small cup.

Straw drinking emerges at about 2 years of age. It may become a skill before that time if the caregiver exposes the child to straw drinking. Use of a straw requires good lip seal and strong suction to bring the liquid into the mouth. In addition to the oral motor skills required to draw the liquid into the mouth, cognitive skills are needed to problem-solve how to use the straw. The infant often bites or blows on the straw before learning how to suck through it. This framework of typical development helps the therapist identify problems and establish realistic intervention goals and expected outcomes.

■ EVALUATION

Once the therapist identifies a concern about feeding, he or she must examine this self-care occupation and determine if the child's performance presents issues in the following areas: health and safety, adequate skill for age, efficiency related to the time required to eat a meal, the child's endurance, types of foods the child eats, and the satisfaction of parent and child in the occupation. If the therapist identifies issues in any of these parameters, then he or she collects additional information to determine what contributes to the problem. By understanding the emerging nature of occupations, the therapist examines the types of challenges that the parent presents and the meaning attributed to feeding routines. The following is an example of a child with performance issues:

> Emanuel, a 2½ year old, is referred to an interdisciplinary feeding clinic. His pediatrician is concerned because Emanuel, who is developing normally in other ways, is not feeding himself with a spoon. The occupational therapist interviews Emanuel's parents. They explain that nurturance is demonstrated in their family by feeding young children, and Emanuel's grandmother feeds him to demonstrate that she cares for him. The therapist does not indicate an intervention in this case because the family does not see independence in spoon feeding as desired despite the fact that Emanuel has not reached the expected milestone. The therapist needs comprehensive information, generally obtained from multiple team members, to plan feeding interventions.

Parent Interviews

A discussion regarding the feeding problem from the perspective of the parents is critical for determining its basis and for developing an intervention plan. The parents' primary concerns should become the priorities of the feeding team that works with the child. Are the parents most concerned about weight gain? Is the length of time required for feeding dominating the parent's daily activities? Does the child seem to lose most of the food consumed during feeding (e.g., through vomiting or re-

flux)? Is the child's behavior during feeding creating havoc for the entire family during mealtime? Although the parents' expressed concerns become the focus of intervention, the therapist should consider concerns of the professionals in developing the feeding plan when they differ from the concerns of the parents.

The parents also provide the team with information about the child's developmental history and feeding history. Obtaining this history helps the therapist identify the basis of the feeding problem (e.g., if long-standing sensory or behavioral issues have influenced feeding performance). By asking about the feeding history, the therapist also obtains a sense of the parents' frustration and ability to cope with the child's feeding issues. The techniques that the parents use and their experiences in feeding the infant are helpful in identifying appropriate intervention strategies. Parents whose children have received therapy services in the past probably have important information to share regarding interventions that worked and those that did not.

The therapist must obtain information about the current feeding methods. He or she can often gather detailed information by simply asking the parents to describe feeding over the course of a typical day. This open-ended request allows the parents to bring forward their concerns. After this the therapist can guide the discussion to obtain comprehensive information. Box 15-1 provides a list of guiding questions.

Medical and Development History

Several medical conditions found in children can lead to feeding problems or poor weight gain. The therapist should obtain and review all medical records. Reports of metabolic or neurologic evaluations, including results of computerized tomography (CT) scans or brain imaging scans, may help the therapist understand systemic problems. Instances of pneumonia and frequent and prolonged upper respiratory infection suggest a problem with swallowing. The therapist should carefully read results of barium swallow and *videofluoroscopic swallow studies* (VFSSs) if they have been done.

Recorded developmental histories supplement the parents' report. The written reports of other occupational and physical therapists, early childhood specialists, and teachers provide foundational knowledge about the child. For example, a child with sustained hospitalization for another condition may not have been given the same opportunities to progress, or an early history of restricted upper extremity movement may lead to restricted oral play, influencing sensory system and secondarily the ability to eat. Understanding the child's developmental course and rate of change in other occupational performance areas such as object play and social interactions is important for the therapist to make realistic goals for what will change in the next few months, prioritize objectives, and select appropriate intervention strategies.

box 15-1 *Questions regarding feeding at home*

1. Who feeds your child at home?
   a. Do different caregivers feed your child in different ways (e.g., different positions)?
   b. Does your child seem to respond differently to various feeders?
   c. If only one caregiver feeds your child, what is the effect of this total responsibility on this caregiver?
2. Describe your child's problems with feeding.
   a. Does your child have difficulty sucking or drinking?
   b. Does your child have problems biting or chewing?
   c. Does your child cough or choke? When? How often?
   d. What do you think is causing your child's problems with eating?
3. How much help does your child need with feeding?
   a. Do you manually assist your child in chewing and drinking?
   b. Does your child self-feed or do you assist him or her in self-feeding?
   c. Is your child independent in using a cup or do you have to assist him or her?
4. How do you know when your child is hungry?
5. How do you know when your child has had enough to eat or drink?
   a. Does your child stop eating when satiated?
   b. Can your child's endurance cause him or her to stop eating before he or she is full?
6. When and how often is your child fed, and how long does a meal take?
7. How much formula, milk, baby food, or other food does your child consume? Each meal? Each day?
8. If your child gets something other than formula, milk, and baby food, do you do anything special to prepare the food (e.g., mash it or cut it into small bites)?
9. When your child is fed at home, where does he or she sit (e.g., in a regular chair at the table, in a high chair, or in a wheelchair)?
   a. How do you position your child?
   b. Is there anything special that you do to adapt the seating?
10. What bottles, nipples, or spoons are used in feeding? (Explore specific types or shapes).
    a. If adapted equipment is used for feeding, what is it and how is it used?
    b. Have you tried special equipment before and decided that it was not working for you and your child?
11. Describe your child's response to feeding. When does your child most enjoy feeding?
12. How does your child react to foods that are new or that have different textures, tastes, or temperatures?
13. Does your child's performance and behavior during feeding differ in the morning, midday, or night?
14. Who is around during most meals, and what else is going on in the room?
15. Has anyone given you suggestions on how to feed your child? How did these work for you?

Feeding Observation

The feeding observation should be as naturalistic as possible. Ideally the therapist has an opportunity to play with the child before feeding. During play the therapist can observe overall exploration and play performance and can analyze which systems (e.g., cognitive, motor) constrain performance. The therapist should focus on cognitive ability and interest in imitation, response to sensory input, communication style, postural control, ability to manipulate objects, and if age appropriate, use toys in a functional manner. This information helps the therapist plan the *feeding evaluation* (e.g., how to position the child, whether to offer opportunities to use a utensil, and how to communicate with the child during the feeding observation). This play session also helps build rapport between the therapist and the child. The relaxed and positive interaction can influence the nature of the interaction during feeding, given that feeding experiences may have a history of being stressful and uncomfortable for the child.

If the evaluation takes place in a clinic or school, the child should receive foods that he or she typically eats. Parents should help the team select the menu, or the team may ask them to bring preferred foods from home. The therapist should place the child in his or her typical feeding position and provide feeding utensils and methods familiar to the child. The therapist initially asks one parent to feed the child a portion of the meal.

The observation of the parent-child interaction helps the therapist understand factors that may promote or inhibit the child's intake. During this time the therapist reflects on the potential meaning of the occupation to the child and his or her interest in participating. Observations of parent-child interaction also give the therapist insights into the everyday context for feeding from which to make recommendations. Does the parent talk to the child? Does the parent respond to his or her nonverbal cues?

Communication with the child during eating can facilitate the child's participation and foster eating independence. Many children with severe motor problems have difficulty sending clear cues and have limited communication. Parents of children with severe disabilities develop a high level of sensitivity and responsivity to successfully foster communication during feeding. The therapist should discuss with the parents their interpretation of the child's cues and alternative communication strategies when verbal responses are limited.

After observing feeding by the caregiver, the therapist should also feed the child. This gives the therapist additional information about the child's responses to new positions and different foods. This part of the evaluation helps the therapist determine the potential effectiveness of compensation techniques that will improve the child's ability to eat or self-feed. Therefore the therapist obtains assessment information regarding what intervention strategies seem to promote skills and the child's responsiveness to different intervention methods.

The focus of the observational assessment is to explore hypothesized impairments that may relate to the health, safety, endurance, interactional issues identified through interview and record review. Throughout the evaluation, the therapist considers the child's ability to communicate, respond, and interact during eating. Component level analysis includes the child's oral sensitivity; postural control; jaw, lip, cheek, and tongue movements; coordination of those movements; and overall strength and endurance during feeding. A speech pathologist may assist in analysis of oral motor skills.

Videofluoroscopic Swallow Study

VFSS is an important tool in analyzing feeding disorders and is particularly important for children who aspirate or are at high risk for aspiration because of severe motor problems (Gisel, Applegate-Ferrante, Benson, & Bosma, 1995). Factors that suggest swallowing problems include gagging or choking, repeated ineffective swallows, and reflux. Many times the aspiration may be silent, so the only indications are wet, noisy respiration after feeding and the occurrence of repeated respiratory infections (Benson & Lefton-Greif, 1994). The therapist should distinguish aspiration from penetration. *Penetration* describes the flow of food into the airway immediately before or during the apneic period of swallowing, and *aspiration* refers to food entering the airway after a swallow, assisted by inhalation during the resumption of respiration (Gisel et al., 1995). The feeding team can identify and distinguish these problems with a VFSS.

The VFSS is also referred to as a *modified barium swallow*. The therapist or technician saturates a food substance with barium and videotapes ingestion of the barium to show how the food passes from the mouth

through the pharynx. The therapist consults with the radiologist so that he or she can place the infant or child in typical feeding positions or potentially therapeutic positions. The therapist also selects the types of food textures based on knowledge of the child's current diet and feeding goals (Schuberth, 1994).

In a typical VFSS, the therapist mixes liquid barium with other liquids or pureed foods and spreads barium paste on crackers or cookies. The therapist can give the food using a bottle, cup, or spoon. The purpose of the VFSS is to identify whether the child aspirates and how the child handles different textures in different positions. Because the video record shows how the food travels through the mouth and pharynx, the therapist receives detailed information about the swallowing problem. After the therapist has imaged and studied typical feeding procedures, he or she should attempt and videotape therapeutic methods (Logeman, 1983; Wolf & Glass, 1992). For example, the therapist can feed the child thickened liquids or feed the child in new positions. The therapist can observe swallowing when the child is fatigued after he or she consumes various foods and liquids.

The results of the VFSS indicate the safety and appropriateness of oral feeding and guide the therapist's recommendations (Zerilli, Stefans, & DiPietro, 1990). For example, the therapist may recommend positions and textures for the parents to use during feeding that seem to result in optimal swallowing patterns without aspiration. Often a speech pathologist contributes to interpretation of the results (Benson & Lefton-Greif, 1994). Although the VFSS gives the therapist important information and insight regarding the swallowing problem, it may not be representative of the child's typical feeding in a more natural environment.

Having completed the assessment process, which ideally includes several opportunities to interact with the child and family, the therapist designs an intervention plan. Intervention for feeding problems considers the whole child, involves the family, and includes collaboration with professionals of other disciplines. The following sections identify key issues that affect feeding in infants and children. Although the issues are discussed separately, feeding problems are seldom attributable to a singular cause and usually are the result of delays or impairment in multiple performance areas. For example, children with severe sensory problems generally have oral motor skill delays, and children with swallowing disorders often have motor deficits.

■ INTERVENTION FOR SENSORY ISSUES

Young children with feeding problems often exhibit hypersensitivity in and around the mouth. They demonstrate aversive responses to touch in the mouth and demonstrate extreme responses to textured food within the mouth. Behaviors observed when pureed food on a spoon is placed in the mouth include spitting, coughing, or gagging. These behaviors are typical when a new texture is introduced to most children. However, the child with oral tactile defensiveness persists beyond the time usually required to develop tolerance. Infants with sensory problems may hold the food in their mouths to avoid moving it through the mouth. Sensory defensiveness is a critical problem for the child because it often limits the amount of nutritional intake, restricts variety of foods, and creates a negative interaction that is disruptive to the co-occupation of feeding. Adding textured food to the infant's meal is important to facilitating higher levels of oral motor skill (i.e., chewing and diagonal tongue movements are elicited when the texture of the food requires those movements). Knowing the basis of the child's defensiveness is important for the therapist to plan an intervention program that helps resolve the problem. Oral hypersensitivity can relate to any one of three causative factors (Wolf & Glass, 1992):

1. Oral hypersensitivity is often associated with the early experiences of the child (i.e., as a newborn and young infant). Newborns with medical problems at birth often endure procedures that are noxious to the oropharyngeal area. Examples of nursing and medical procedures associated with oral tactile defensiveness are mouth and lung suctioning, intubation, and nasal gastric feeding. In each of these procedures, hard plastic tubes are entered into the mouth and throat, almost always causing gagging and coughing. Over time, when such experiences are repeated, the infant develops defensive responses to all oral-sensory input, perhaps in an attempt to protect that highly sensitive area.

2. Sensory defensiveness also may result in the child who is not fed by mouth for an extended period. When the child does not receive oral feedings and compensatory oral stimulation, he or she develops hypersensitivity of the oral area. Oral stimulation is critical at certain developmental periods for establishing sensory processing around and inside the mouth. Lack of oral experiences may be the easiest type of sensory defensiveness to overcome.

3. A neurologic impairment that directly affects the sensory tracts can also cause oral-sensory defensiveness. Infants with neurologic immaturity often have difficulty with sensory modulation and are hypersensitive to tactile input. Children with cerebral palsy or other disorders may demonstrate oral defensiveness as a manifestation of neurologic impairment. Children with autism or attention-deficit hyperactivity disorder (ADHD) may exhibit general sensory defensiveness and may require a program that addresses overall sensory integration (SI). In children with general sensory defensiveness, hypersensitivity of the oral area may be a long-standing problem.

Oral hypersensitivity often is the result of a combination of these three causative factors. Infants with neurologic impairment with associated hypersensitivity often are recipients of nonoral feedings and invasive oral procedures. Feeding intervention is particularly challenging for children whose defensiveness seems to be related to both offensive oral experiences and general sensory impairment.

Evaluation

The therapist should assess the child's ability to accept various sensory stimuli in his or her mouth through a parent or caregiver interview and observation. In the interview the therapist explores the questions outlined in Box 15-1. The child with sensory defensiveness may accept only one or two food textures, may swallow food without mastication or preparation, may spit out foods on a regular basis, or may exhibit a hyperactive gag that seems unrelated to the amount of food placed into the mouth.

The therapist should precede trial of different textures with relaxed play with the child so that he or she becomes comfortable and to establish rapport. To observe the child's sensory responses, the therapist should use various textures and attempt placement of food in different parts of the mouth. When the child exhibits aversive responses to food inside the mouth, the therapist asks the parent if the responses are typical or exaggerated because of discomfort with an unfamiliar environment or a different feeder.

Intervention

Sensory defensiveness can seriously interfere with the nutritional intake and oral motor skills of the child. It is often a problem that can improve significantly with intervention. At first the therapist should implement intervention activities at times other than during meals. Because intervention activities are often uncomfortable and challenging for the child, the therapist may best perform them between feedings to avoid disruption of mealtimes and the child's nutritional intake.

The therapist must first establish a relationship of trust with the child. The child may distrust anyone who attempts to place food in his or her mouth; therefore good rapport and positive interactions are critical. The therapist should place activities to desensitize in the context of play, the activities should be as self-guided as possible, and the therapist should introduce the activities gradually. Once the therapist begins oral desensitization, he or she can maintain the trust relationship if he or she always acknowledges the child's physical cues of discomfort (by at least a verbal response and when appropriate by withdrawal of the oral stimulus). The therapist should also allow turn taking, decision making, and as much active participation by the child as possible. Children will tolerate greater sensory input if the activity is under the child's control and provided in the context of a motivating, developmentally appropriate activity.

The therapist should begin oral desensitization by encouraging the infant to explore his or her mouth with his or her own hands. The infant can begin to suck on his or her hands and fingers with the guidance of the therapist's hand. The therapist can introduce rubber toys into the oral play. The therapist may use the NUK toothbrush or a regular toothbrush to brush and massage the gums (Morris & Klein, 1987). The therapist can engage in turn-taking games with the infant using a rubber toy or toothbrush in a hide-and-seek game to stimulate different areas of the mouth using different degrees of pressure. The parent can rub the infant's gums with a warm washcloth, applying firm sustained pressure and allowing the child to chew or suck on the cloth. The texture of the washcloth is easily accepted by children and is helpful in improving sensory tolerance of other textures. For older children with higher-level oral motor skills, the therapist can use blow toys to desensitize the oral area. Blowing bubbles and making sounds are particularly motivating activities that help the child become more aware of his or her mouth and oral movements.

Desensitization activities between meals should include small amounts of food. The therapist can dip rubber toys in pureed food and toothbrushes in fruit juice before entry into the infant's mouth. The therapist should introduce the taste and texture of different foods into the oral play as much as possible. Once the child is in preschool, snack time is an excellent time to focus on oral desensitization because it may not be as important to eat a certain amount of food. Turn-taking games and sharing with peers can encourage oral intake and improve the child's willingness to try new textures.

Oral desensitization is also important immediately before the child's mealtime. The therapist should develop a program that prepares the child for oral intake and requires only a brief amount of time and energy by the caregiver and child. Using a warm washcloth around and inside of the mouth can desensitize this area before feeding. The child may tolerate the washcloth better than the therapist's finger. The child generally accepts the therapist's finger inside a nipple or inside an infa-dent toothbrush, which can offer some protection to the therapist's fingers as he or she rubs the gums, tongue, and palate (Klein & Delaney, 1994). When applying any method of direct oral stimulation, the therapist should wear gloves and follow Occupational Safety and Health Administration (OSHA) guidelines for exposure to body fluids such as saliva (Federal Register, 1991). These regulations require that "gloves be worn when it can be reasonably anticipated that the employee may have hand contact with blood, other potentially infectious materials, mucous membranes, and nonintact skin" (pp. 64133-64134). The therapist should systematically apply sensory preparation, beginning with stroking in body areas where

it is tolerated. Firm rubbing and deep pressure are stimuli that desensitize and increase tolerance to touch (Klein & Delaney, 1994). Gradually, and based on the child's response, the therapist applies the tactile stimulation to the cheeks, outer lips, inside of the mouth, gums, and tongue (Glass & Wolf, 1998). Sustained firm pressure to the upper palate desensitizes the entire mouth, enabling the child to accept touch in other parts of his or her mouth. This pressure can produce calming and more organized responses. Certain children (e.g., those with autism) seem to benefit from vibration applied to the lower jaw and around the mouth. The therapist should allow the child to guide this strong proprioceptive input, and the child may request vibration to the gums and inside the mouth. The therapist should monitor responses to vibration; the proximity to the vestibular receptor may cause vestibular system reactions. If tolerated by the child, vibration can decrease sensitivity and increase oral motor responses.

In addition to these preparatory activities, the therapist should consider adaptations to the child's position and the texture of the food. The therapist should support the child's trunk and head so that the child feels secure and stable but not confined. Children who have generalized sensory defensiveness may be more comfortable in a chair than in the arms of the caregiver because human touch is a very powerful stimulus. The therapist should position children with concomitant respiratory problems to allow for maximum thoracic expansion and optimal respiration during feeding.

Adjusting the texture of the child's food is perhaps the most important intervention that the therapist can offer to the child with tactile defensiveness. Box 15-2 provides guidelines for adapting food texture to accommodate and decrease the child's sensory defensiveness.

The therapist should introduce new textures gradually and in a way that makes them palatable to the child and easily consumed. For example, the therapist can mix mashed potatoes with other vegetables and soft meats to help hold those foods together. The child may accept this sensory experience better than the new food alone, which may become a collection of discrete bits after chewing. The therapist should encourage parents to add the right amount of moisture to food to make it easily manageable in the mouth. Thickening foods becomes important for the child with poor oral motor control because the thicker substance moves more slowly within the mouth and provides more sensory input, making it easy for the child to control.

When the therapist recommends changes in the types of food (e.g., more fruits and vegetables), consultation with a nutritionist regarding the effect of the dietary change is important. Children with disabilities are often on high-caloric and high-protein intake, making the balance of nutrients more difficult to achieve.

In addition to adjusting the food texture, the therapist should assess the utensils used and the placement of the

---

box 15-2 *Guidelines for adapting food texture for children with sensory defensiveness*

1. The therapist should ensure adequate nutritional intake by attending to the nutrient value and amount of food intake when changing the texture of foods consumed.
2. Pureed, smooth foods are the first solid foods that the therapist should attempt with a child with severe oral-sensory defensiveness. The therapist can gradually increase the texture of pureed foods by adding food with lumps or of more coarse texture.
3. The therapist should vary the textures within any one meal from those least tolerated to those most tolerated. When the child successfully eats a food with strong sensory input, the therapist can reward him or her with a spoonful of a favorite food.
4. Soft foods that have cohesion when masticated offer increased sensory experiences. Cheese, chicken, and well-cooked vegetables with no skins increase chewing when placed between the teeth.
5. Graham crackers, butter cookies, and some cereals (e.g., Cheerios) provide discrete bits of food in the mouth that promote desensitization. Soft crackers and cookies promote chewing and dissolve quickly

once inside the mouth, presenting less danger of choking.
6. For children who need altered food texture over time, a food grinder to puree the child's food is a useful tool. The therapist can progressively alter the food texture by changing the food grinder setting.
7. Grainy breads provide more texture than soft white breads, which tend to form a ball and adhere to the upper palate.
8. It may be helpful to introduce textured foods that require some chewing by mixing them in with foods that are familiar to the child and that add cohesion to the food bolus.
9. The therapist should maintain a pleasant, fun atmosphere during feeding and, when appropriate, use play and verbal interaction to distract the child from focusing attention on the food within his or her mouth. Verbal encouragement and looks of delight are rewarding to the child who has eaten a new food. Offering another bite can be frustrating rather than rewarding.

Modified from Case-Smith, J. (1999). Self care strategies for children with developmental deficits. In C. Christiansen (Ed.), *Ways of living: Self-care strategies for special needs* (pp. 83-122). Bethesda, MD: AOTA.

---

spoon in the child's mouth relative to the child's tolerance. The child better tolerates food placed in the anterior part of the mouth as opposed to food placed on the posterior tongue. He or she may better tolerate food on the center of the tongue than on the sides. However, food placement on the side is often desirable for increasing chewing and tongue lateralization.

Table 15-3 is a chart of food progression from smooth, pureed foods to coarse and chewy foods. The chart lists foods in different nutrient groups in the sequence that a typical child learns to tolerate and handle solid foods. The food groups also follow the progression of oral motor skills achievement.

■ INTERVENTION FOR MOTOR IMPAIRMENTS

Children with significant motor impairments often exhibit oral motor delays. Examples of children with motor dysfunctions that can affect feeding are those with cerebral palsy, traumatic brain injury, prematurity, or genetic syndromes such as trisomy 21. Problems in oral motor control in infants are often different from those of older children. Delays in feeding skills caused by oral motor dysfunction may not occur until the child progresses to

solid food and he or she requires more sophisticated oral motor responses.

Often the muscle tone of children with cerebral palsy in the proximal areas of the face, neck, and trunk is hypotonic, resulting in poor head and trunk stability. The child's jaw tends to move in wide excursions, completely open or clamped shut. The child often demonstrates inability to grade the jaw's movement in the midranges typically observed in sucking and chewing. When the child has low facial muscle tone, the mouth is often open, resulting in excessive drooling and loss of food from the mouth during feeding. An open mouth during feeding also makes swallowing difficult. In a recent study of 58 children with severe physical disabilities, more than half exhibited an up-and-down pattern of jaw movement to take in food. Protrusion of their tongues often occurred with mouth open, making movement of the food for swallowing difficult. In more than a third of the children, their mouths were open some or all of the time during feeding (Yokochi, 1997).

In the child with hypotonia, the tongue may be inactive, moving primarily with the lower jaw. The tongue may move only in extension and retraction, or it may move into extreme ranges (e.g., completely retracted into the back of the mouth) (Yokochi, 1997). The tongue's extreme ranges or lack of movement may be as-

table 15-3 *Food Progression Based on Texture Consistency**

Food Group	Food and Food Forms from Easier to More Difficult Textures to Eat
Meats and meat substitutes	Strained meats and egg yolk
	Commercial junior meats; soft meats ground fine in baby food grinder with liquid added; mashed egg yolk
	Ground meats with gravy or other liquid added; soft-cooked eggs
	Ground meats without liquid added; scrambled eggs; smooth peanut butter
	Well-cooked and soft meats, fish, and poultry; hard-cooked eggs
	Cut up meats of increased texture (roast beef and ham)
Dairy products	Strained cottage cheese; thinned puddings; plain yogurt; thinned, strained cream soups
	Fork mashed cottage cheese; pudding; custard; thickened cream soups
	Cottage cheese
	Yogurt with soft fruits; ice cream; some soft cheeses (muenster and American)
	Harder cheeses (Swiss and cheddar)
Breads and cereals	Infant cereal thinned with milk
	Thicker infant cereals; Cream of Wheat; farina
	Cooked cereals such as oatmeal or Malto-meal; crackers; toast; plain cookies; bread without crust
	Cooked cereals with soft fruits added; bread with crust; well-cooked pasta (noodles and spaghetti)
	Dry cereals with milk; sandwiches with smooth filling and cut in small pieces; rice; firmer texture pasta
	Sandwiches with various fillings
Fruits and vegetables	Strained fruits and vegetables
	Junior fruits; applesauce; ripe, mashed bananas; junior vegetables; mashed potatoes
	Fork-mashed, soft canned fruits without skins; soft, ripe, mashed fresh fruits (peeled); fork-mashed, well-cooked vegetables without skins; boiled or baked potatoes without skins
	Canned fruits (peaches and pears); soft, ripe fresh fruits (peeled); well-cooked vegetables cut in small pieces
	Canned fruits of increased texture (fruit cocktail and pineapple); vegetables of increased texture (steamed carrots and broccoli); soups with well-cooked vegetables
	Raw or dried fruits; raw vegetables; vegetables with skins (corn, peas and lima beans); chunky soup

*The therapist should use these suggestions for texture progression as part of a treatment plan for children with oral sensory or motor problems. These suggestions identify foods and food forms in each category that may be appropriate in progressing toward a regular diet.

sociated with poor jaw stability such that the jaw does not function as a base for tongue movement. These patterns also may relate to the primitive movement patterns exhibited by children with cerebral palsy.

The lips of children with cerebral palsy are often inactive and hypotonic. Lip seal on the bottle's nipple, the cup rim, or a spoon is inadequate and results in food loss or air intake. Hypotonic cheeks result in less suction of the nipple and difficulty maintaining food in the tongue's center.

Children with hypotonic oral musculature often have overall postural instability. Postural instability results in poor postural alignment and increased difficulty with oral motor skills. When upright, the child may fall into trunk and cervical flexion. When slightly reclined, his or her head may fall into extension. The child may also elevate the shoulders and retract the arms in an attempt to stabilize the head. When the child's neck is in hyperextension, neck alignment is not appropriate for safe and efficient swallow.

When a child demonstrates hypertonicity in the face and mouth, usually he or she has spastic cerebral palsy.

Sometimes a child who initially exhibits low tone may exhibit spasticity as he or she matures and attempts to assume positions more upright against gravity. Children with hypertonicity tend to exhibit hyperextension of the trunk and neck without reciprocal flexion. They may exhibit tonic oral reflexes or abnormal oral motor patterns that are never observed in a typically developing child. Children with hypertonicity differ from children with low muscle tone who exhibit delayed oral motor patterns that are observed in children who are younger. The following are examples of oral motor patterns observed in children with hypertonicity:

- *Tonic bite.* The gums or teeth close or clamp together in a forceful motion. Once closed, the jaw remains clamped and the therapist may need to reposition the child to open the mouth. The tonic bite occurs more often when the child is inappropriately positioned in some neck extension or when he or she has extreme tactile defensiveness.
- *Tongue thrust.* In tongue thrust the child completely extends his or her tongue outside the border of the lips. The tongue's movement is forceful and is often main-

tained in the extended position. Tongue thrust also occurs more often when the child is positioned in trunk and neck extension. This forceful tongue movement results in loss of food or liquid from the mouth and does not initiate a swallow. Children with severe tongue thrust may lose much of the food presented to them and may be diagnosed as failure-to-thrive. Without knowledge of how much of the food that enters into the mouth is swallowed, it is difficult to estimate the amount of food consumed. The therapist may observe jaw thrust (a strong, forceful, downward movement of the lower jaw) with tongue thrust. The therapist observes this movement when the child is in a position of extension.

- *Lip retraction and lip pursing.* Some children with high muscle tone associated with cerebral palsy exhibit lip retraction. The lips pull away from the midline and stay fixed in the retracted position when utensils and food or a cup and drink are entered into the mouth. This stiffening replaces the soft seal of the lips typically observed. Lip pursing is a response in which the lips draw tightly together at midline. Both movement patterns result in food loss and difficulty obtaining the food from the spoon or the drink from the cup. These movement patterns occur most frequently when the neck is extended and appropriate head and trunk alignment is not achieved. They also occur when the child experiences an emotional reaction to a situation.

Evaluation

Specific assessment of the child's motor control as it affects feeding includes the following:
- Overall evaluation of motor patterns, strength, and muscle tone
- Assessment of postural alignment and postural control, including asymmetries, with a focus on head and trunk stability
- Evaluation of jaw, tongue, cheek, and lip movement patterns (note typical delayed and atypical patterns)
- Evaluation of the coordination and sequencing of jaw, tongue, and lip movements during feeding (i.e., coordination of suck-swallow-breathe)
- Observation of how oral movement patterns are affected by the child's posture using different external sources of postural support (e.g., in the caregiver's lap versus in a feeder chair or small child's chair)
- Observation of changes in oral motor patterns when the jaw or cheeks are supported and observation of child's responses to handling around the mouth before and during feeding

The goal of the evaluation is to assess oral motor skills with the child in typical positioning, with optimal positioning and environmental conditions, and during application of intervention strategies. The resulting information provides the therapist with guidance as to the nature of the child's oral motor strengths and problems and the types of intervention that seem to promote improved oral motor control.

Intervention
Postural alignment

Improving the child's postural alignment and stability through good positioning is often helpful in promoting oral motor function. Some oral motor problems immediately resolve when the child is well positioned in good postural alignment. Appropriate alignment for feeding consists of the following:
- Neutral pelvic alignment of the trunk. Pelvic alignment is promoted when the child sits well supported against a flat back, on a flat seat, and square on the buttocks with 90 degrees of hip flexion and 90 degrees of knee flexion
- Good head, neck, and shoulder alignment with the head in slight flexion or at neutral
- Chin tuck with the neck in an elongated position

The child can achieve correct postural alignment in various positions, depending on the size of the child and his or her postural stability. One guideline for the therapist is to provide the child with more external postural stability than he or she needs. The therapist positions the child with oral motor deficits associated with a motor delay in a slightly reclined position with head and trunk fully supported. Feeding requires high-level, intricate oral movement and focused concentration; therefore complete postural stability, excellent alignment, and comfort are critical to successful eating.

Characteristics of feeding positions and positioning devices

- *Infant held sideways in the caregiver's arms.* This position allows for full body contact. It is appropriate for infants; however, it may be difficult for the caregiver to maintain alignment. This position is fatiguing and is inappropriate for the older infant or the infant who has poor postural control.
- *Infant held on caregiver's thighs facing caregiver* (Figure 15-2). This position provides excellent stability and good alignment and promotes midline. It frees both of the caregiver's hands. This intimate position allows for eye contact and therefore promotes communication. It does not work with older, larger children.
- *Infant placed in an infant seat.* The infant seat works well for infants with fair head control who are not yet independent in sitting. The caregiver can adapt the infant seat with small rolls on the side to maintain a symmetric posture. When the infant is placed in the infant seat, the caregiver can free his or her hands and use them for support at the chin or chest during feeding. Straps are available with this seat, and the cost is low.

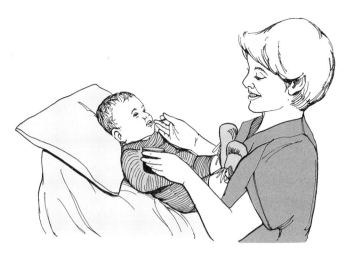

figure**15-2**   Face-to-face position for feeding.

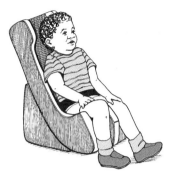

figure**15-3**   Tumble Forms Feeder Chair offers support and an adjustable feeding angle.

The infant seat is not an appropriate device for an infant with established sitting balance or for the infant who weighs more than 25 pounds.

- *Infant placed in a cradle bouncer.* This seat is similar to an infant seat. It holds the infant in more extension and is inappropriate for an infant with increased extensor muscle tone. The bouncing motion of the seat can promote rhythmic movement during feeding but is a distraction to the infant who has difficulty tolerating vestibular system input.
- *Infant placed in a foam-filled (Tumble Forms) feeder seat.* This positioner offers full head and trunk support and promotes good alignment. The feeder seat comes with a strapping system, and the caregiver can order different chest straps. The curved sides of the chair promote midline and decrease shoulder retraction. The caregiver can recline the infant seat to the angle desired for feeding (i.e., the angle at which the head is in an optimal position). The Tumble Forms chair is available in two sizes and is easily cleaned, easily transported, and safe when used on the floor. It is more expensive than an infant seat and is inappropriate for infants who sit independently (Figure 15-3).
- *Infant placed in a regular car seat.* The car seat has features similar to the Tumble Forms seat. Most car seats provide good alignment and postural stability for the infant. Usually adjusting the seat's degree of tilt is more difficult and small adjustments are not possible.
- *Child placed in a transport chair or wheelchair.* A transport chair or pediatric wheelchair may be the optimal seating device for feeding a child with severe motor limitations. It is typically the most supportive seating arrangement for the child. Transport chair offers individualized seating with customized head support, lateral supports, and trunk straps. Therefore the chair offers optimal external stability of the child's posture.

The tray provides an additional truncal support and a surface for weight bearing on arms. A key feature beneficial to children with poor head control is that the chair tilts into various positions while maintaining optimal postural alignment for feeding (neutral pelvis and 90 degrees hip and knee flexion). This tilt-in-space feature allows the child to recline in small increments. The transport chair places the child at a height that makes feeding convenient for the adult. A disadvantage of feeding in the transport chair is that its height can create a barrier to peer interaction, as in a preschool setting where the children eat snacks seated in small chairs at a low-level table.

- *Child placed in a beanbag chair.* The beanbag chair is a comfortable seating option for the child who otherwise may be in a wheelchair or on the floor. It brings the child into a semi-upright position for visualization of the environment and for eye contact with peer or adults. The beanbag chair is not the best option for feeding because postural alignment is difficult to control and the infant tends to be primarily in extension. The beanbag is particularly inappropriate for children with extensor posturing because it does not successfully inhibit these postures.
- *Infant placed in a high chair.* A high chair is standard furniture for many families with infants learning to eat solid foods. It is the positioner of choice if the infant has adequate postural stability and motor control. Minimally, the infant should be able to independently maintain a propped sitting position for several seconds. The high chair provides back support, side supports, pelvic strapping, and a tray. The caregiver can easily adapt it to give additional foot support and lateral support. The high chair places the infant at a height that allows him or her to participate in the family's mealtime. This height is convenient for the caregiver who is

feeding. The high chair is desirable because it is readily available and economical; it is particularly appropriate for the infant who will soon be sitting independently.

Summary. Caregivers should have a range of options for positions; however, the therapist should discourage certain positioning choices. For example, although holding the infant in the caregiver's lap is a comforting position, it does not give the caregiver optimal control when the infant has poor control of movement. Infants with postural instability benefit from placement in a stable seating device that helps the infant focus on oral movements and frees the caregiver's hands for providing manual assistance to the infant's oral movements.

Handling techniques in support of oral movement

The therapist applies all of the techniques after positioning the child in good postural alignment with optimal postural stability. The techniques involve touch in and around the mouth; therefore desensitization of the oral area is often a required prerequisite to handling.

Occupational therapists often collaborate with speech pathologists in developing an intervention program to address oral motor issues. Occupational and speech therapists have described handling techniques to either compensate for motor impairments or support the development of oral motor abilities associated with eating (Klein & Delaney, 1994; Morris & Klein, 1987; Wolf & Glass, 1992). These handling techniques have evolved over years of applied experience, but therapists have only recently subjected them to systematic study. The reflective clinician recognizes that certain handling techniques are more effective with some types of oral movement problems than with other conditions affecting children's oral motor abilities. The therapist also needs to consider pragmatic issues, such as the immediate need to help families incorporate safe and effective feeding methods and the frequency and duration of direct therapy services, in selecting treatment techniques and describing expected outcomes.

Some handling techniques can provide mechanical assistance when the child does not have the muscle strength or oral motor control to do the occupation independently. Compensation strategies, such as good positioning, immediately influence quality of occupational performance. Researchers have investigated the effectiveness of oral support using the therapist's fingers on the infant's cheeks and under the chin in a study of premature infants (Einarsson-Backes, Deitz, Price, Glass, & Hays, 1994). Preterm infants have the potential but lack the neurologic maturation to perform sucking movements in an organized manner. The therapist's hands provide necessary stability and control and may provide the bridge until the infant matures sufficiently to acquire his or her own control.

Handling before feeding. The therapist can best address certain neuromotor problems both before and during feeding. Children with hypotonicity of the oral musculature often benefit from techniques to at least temporarily improve muscle tone. Glass and Wolf (1998) described techniques that improve muscle tone and therefore muscle responsivity during feeding. Tapping or quick stretch of cheeks and lips provides sensory input that increases muscle tone around the mouth. The therapist should apply the tapping or stretch symmetrically and rhythmically, repeating the stimulation several times within a brief period immediately before feeding. Vibration is a stronger stimulus that can increase tone and ready muscles for movement. Children with low muscle tone and sensory defensiveness often benefit from vibration around the mouth.

Preparation for children with hypertonicity. When the child has high muscle tone of the lips, cheeks, and tongue, the therapist can apply deep and firm pressure using a downward stroking motion symmetrically to the cheeks and around the lips. The therapist can apply firm rhythmic sustained pressure through the lower jaw (chin), facilitating a chin tuck position. He or she can also apply touch pressure to the child's cheeks to inhibit or decrease lip retraction.

In the child with oral hypertonicity, often the tongue retracts to the back of the mouth or extends beyond the lips. Good postural alignment often helps inhibit these extreme tongue positions. Facilitation techniques can temporarily change movements of the tongue. The therapist can place his or her finger (or the bowl of the spoon) in the middle of the tongue and apply rhythmic, downward pressure. The pressure should be forward for the retracted tongue and backward for the extended tongue. Rhythmic pressure using a downward motion of one beat per second can promote a sucking pattern (Morris & Klein, 1987). Jiggling or lateral movement of the spoon or finger on the tongue can be inhibitory and should be used based on the child's response. Once feeding begins, the therapist should continue downward pressure with the use of the bowl of the spoon.

Techniques during feeding. The therapist's fingers can provide external support of the jaw under and around the lower jaw. The therapist can apply his or her hand to the child's chin either from the front or from the side (Figure 15-4). One finger places pressure through the front of the chin to promote chin tuck, and another provides support under the jaw. The finger under the jaw provides a source of stability, inhibits wide jaw excursions, and provides a support base for tongue movement. Important aspects of successfully using jaw support include use of the flat side of the finger (rather than the fingertip) and use of the finger as a source of support to the child's jaw movement, not to direct the child's movement. Forcefully moving the child's jaw is inappropriate.

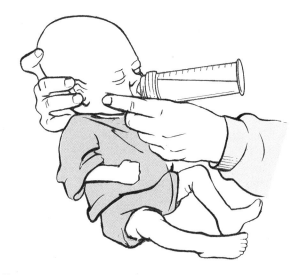

figure**15-5** Jaw and cheek support of the infant during bottle-feeding.

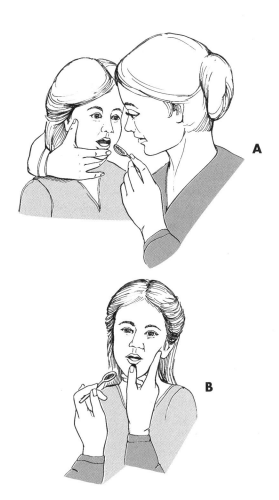

figure**15-4** Jaw control and oral support. **A,** From the side. **B,** From the front.

The therapist should maintain his or her hand under and around the jaw during the entire feeding rather than removing and reapplying it with each bite. The therapist should place the finger under the chin midway between the tip of the jaw and the throat and be careful not to move the hand's pressure into the throat. This support to the jaw may be particularly critical when the child is drinking from a cup, at which time the jaw's movement may increase. The goal of this activity is for the child to gain adequate internal jaw stability for independent mouth closure during eating and drinking.

Cheek support. In infants the therapist may apply touch pressure to the cheeks using the thumb and index finger (with the third finger under the jaw). This pressure is appropriate only during bottle-feeding as a method to increase negative pressure within the mouth and therefore improve suction on the nipple (Einarsson-Backes et. al., 1994). The pressure to the cheeks can improve the lip's seal and sucking patterns (Figure 15-5).

Spoon placement. A small spoon with a swallow bowl allows for easy food removal. The placement of the spoon can influence the child's oral motor responses.

Downward pressure of the spoon on the center of the tongue can facilitate a sucking response. This can be effective for moving the food to the back of the tongue for swallowing.

Downward and inward pressure with the spoon (or nipple) can promote the up-and-down tongue movement observed in mature sucking. This pressure can also inhibit tongue thrust during feeding. Central placement of the spoon is appropriate when the child has only a sucking pattern and the tongue moves in extension and retraction. To encourage tongue lateralization and the beginning of chewing patterns, the therapist should place the spoon to the side. Food placement between the gums and teeth directly promotes chewing. The therapist should consider placing the food on alternating sides to prevent development of skills on one side only and maintaining food in the central to anterior part of the mouth. Placement of the spoon or food on the posterior portion of the tongue results in gagging and does not allow the child to move, chew, and control the food before swallowing.

Head position. A chin tuck position with the head well aligned on the shoulders is generally best for feeding. This head position may require the support of the caregiver or therapist's arm in back of the neck or under the occipital lobe.

Although complete upright posture allows for correct swallowing and helps reduce the possibility of aspiration, certain children may need a position of slight neck flexion to help them swallow. Positioning the head slightly forward in neck flexion reduces the possibility of aspiration because it reduces the distance that the larynx must move upward to initiate the swallow.

The therapist should use a position of neck flexion with caution because it may interfere with breathing. Some children posture in neck hyperextension despite efforts to hold them in a position of neutral neck alignment. This is the case with children who have difficulty breathing and are seeking a completely open air passageway. A VFSS may help elucidate if aspiration occurs in this position, giving guidance to the therapist as to how important neutral neck alignment is to the child's feeding. The therapist should avoid pushing the neck into extension during feeding by handling the neck at key points to improve neck alignment (e.g., manual pressure on the upper chest).

Altering the sensory quality of foods. The progression of the food textures listed in Table 15-3 provides examples of food consistencies that require progressively higher-level oral motor skills. Although the therapist and parent use strategies to help the child develop improved oral motor skills, foods selected for the child's diet should accommodate the child's current skill level and should challenge the child to develop higher-level skills. Thin liquids are the most difficult consistency to control in the mouth and should be thickened when the child has poor tongue control and an inefficient suck-swallow pattern.

Eating pureed foods requires no more than a suck-swallow response; therefore giving the child pureed foods elicits sucking. To elicit munching and chewing patterns, the child must receive soft foods. Increasing the sensory input using highly textured foods facilitates tongue lateralization and tip elevation, active lip movements, and increased chewing responses.

The therapist can hold a long piece of vegetable or soft meat between the child's side teeth to promote graded biting. He or she may initially use strips of soft cheese, chicken, or a long green bean. Soft cookies and crackers placed to the side can also promote controlled biting. Pretzels and apple slices require more jaw strength and can be tried as a next step in promoting biting skills.

Certain foods can increase muscle tone and chewing. Fruit Rollups promote rotary chewing and graded jaw movements but at the same time dissolve fairly quickly to minimize the risk of choking. Some dried fruits (e.g., apricots and apples) can help increase chewing. Tough or fibrous meats are contraindicated. Box 15-3 provides a list of foods that are indicated and contraindicated for children with immature oral motor skills.

Efficacy of techniques. Therapists have guided traditional treatment for children with cerebral palsy through handling techniques designed to provide sensorimotor experiences that replicated normal movements (Adams & Snyder, 1998). Therapists, over time, found that higher parts of the motor system would learn and be able to replicate the experienced movement as part of an action during an occupation. Therapists have questioned the effectiveness of techniques that emphasize practicing movements if there is significant motor impairment (Heriza, 1991; Mathiowetz & Haugen, 1994). Gisel and others (1995) examined the efficacy of sensorimotor treatments for 27 children with cerebral palsy over 10- to

---

> **box 15-3** *Foods indicated and contraindicated for children with immature oral motor skills*
>
> **Properties of indicated foods**
> Even consistency
> Increased density and volume
> Thick (liquids)
> Uniform texture
> Stays together (will not break up in the mouth)
> Easy to remove and suck
>
> **Properties of contraindicated foods**
> Multiple textures and consistencies (tacos, vegetable soup, stews, and salads)
> Sticky (peanut butter)
> Greasy (fried foods)
> Tough (red meat, processed meats, and diced fruit)
> Fibrous and stringy (celery, citrus fruits, and raw vegetables)
> Skins (raw fruits and peanuts)
> Spicy (pepper and horseradish)
> Seeds and nuts (plain or in breads and cakes)
> Thin (liquids such as water, carbonated drinks, broth, coffee, tea, and apple juice)
> Quickly liquefying (jello and watermelon)
> Foods that break up in the mouth (some cookies and flaky pastries)
> Crunchy (chips and carrots)

20-week periods. They individualized treatment to the child, which lasted 5 to 7 minutes, 5 days a week. The children practiced components of oral motor skills, including tongue lateralization, lip control, and vigor of chewing. The researchers used food to elicit specific oral movements. Treatment included monitoring progress to introduce more food texture during snack or lunch as new oral motor skills were observed. The researchers found some significant changes in the children's ability to eat. After intervention, the researchers decreased the duration of meals slightly and the children progressed to eating increased texture. These gains were modest but suggested that the intervention may produce greater change if implemented over a longer period of time.

In selecting handling techniques to promote oral motor skills, therapists continually monitor the effects of their strategies on the child's eating skill. If the handling technique does not change how effectively the child eats, then the therapist may question a sustained effort to improve that performance component (e.g., lip closure or increased tongue lateralization). Working at the level of components is likely to be a long-term process and can be worthwhile if the functional goal is kept in mind (Rogers & Holms, 1998). The therapist should maintain eating food and drinking liquids as the source of motivation and the goal that organizes movement (Humphry & Morrow, 1998). Handling techniques will be most effective if the strategy feels natural and can be incorporated into daily routines by caregivers and parents.

■ INTERVENTION FOR SWALLOWING PROBLEMS

Swallowing and Coordinating the Suck-Swallow-Breathe Sequence

Children with *swallowing disorders* tend to have severe sensorimotor impairments or physiologic immaturity that interferes with the coordination of the *suck-swallow-breathe sequence*. To understand swallowing disorders related to neuromotor dysfunction or physiologic immaturity, this section briefly describes the normal phases of swallow.

Oral phase

In the first phase of swallow, the oral phase, the food enters into the mouth, where it is processed. This phase consists of biting, sucking, chewing, or munching. The food is moved side to side for chewing and comes to the center as a bolus for transit to the back of the tongue. In the oral transit phase, the masticated food or liquid is moved to the back of the tongue, where swallowing is initiated. Therefore swallowing is essentially a reflexive response to the sensory input of the food on the posterior portion of the tongue.

Pharyngeal phase

In the pharyngeal phase the bolus moves from the back of the tongue through the pharynx to the opening of the esophagus. The propulsion of the bolus is based on negative pressure; therefore closure of the nasal, laryngeal, and oral openings is important for efficient bolus transit. The larynx is protected by the closure of the epiglottis over the trachea and the contraction of the true and false vocal cords. At the same time that the esophagus opens, the negative pressure propels the bolus through the pharynx to the esophagus opening.

Esophageal phase

In the esophageal phase the food or liquid moves through the esophagus using peristalsis. The swallow itself and the sensation of the food involuntarily initiate peristalsis (Tuchman, 1994). The oral and oral transit phases are the only swallow phases that the child controls. These phases establish the timing and coordination of the swallow and are therefore critical to efficient swallowing. Therapeutic input to influence swallowing improves the child's control of the initial oral phases.

Problems

The following problems can affect the child's ability to coordinate sequential swallows without aspiration. When sensorimotor problems are severe, the tongue moves primarily in extension or demonstrates minimal movement and tone. Children with severe oral motor dysfunction are often unable to gather the food into a bolus for swallowing. The food may trickle over the sides of the tongue and the pharynx without eliciting a swallow. Foods that break apart can scatter in the mouth, and bits may fall into the pharynx. When a swallow is not triggered, the protective closure of the epiglottis does not occur, leaving the trachea open, and aspiration becomes highly probable. When liquids and food pool in the pharynx, the child is at high risk for aspiration. When the oral transit phase is slow or is without a rhythmic sequence, the swallow either appears delayed or seems to occur at random. The primary problem created by delayed swallowing is that food enters the pharynx before or after the swallow, where it pools or where it may enter the larynx.

The child with a respiratory disorder is also at high risk for swallow dysfunction. Although the child typically demonstrates adequate oral motor skills and swallowing, the suck-swallow-breathe sequence is poorly coordinated. Typically the infant with respiratory distress syndrome demonstrates rapid and shallow breathing patterns. The infant's oxygen level may plummet when breathing momentarily pauses to allow for swallowing. Rapid breathing in an irregular pattern prevents development of a regular, rhythmic pattern of swallowing. The infant who struggles to breathe has increased respiratory difficulty when feeding. He or she may attempt to breathe and swallow at the same time.

Evaluation

Assessment of swallowing disorders or the possibility of a swallowing disorder includes all of the strategies described previously in the chapter, including obtaining the following:
- History of feeding from the caregiver
- Medical history by written or parental report
- Clinical observation of feeding
- VFSS

Parental report

As described previously, the therapist requests a detailed description of typical feeding from the parent. From the parent's description, the therapist needs to ask the following questions regarding feeding at home. He or she can ask these questions during or after the parent's narrative description of mealtime.
1. How, where, and when is the child fed?
2. What kinds of foods are given to the child?
3. How does the child respond during feeding? Does he or she demonstrate aversive responses and, if so,

to what types of food? Does the child choke, gag, or cough? Is food lost during feeding?

4. Does the child sound raspy during feeding? Does his or her breathing sound noisy (wet) during or after feeding?

5. Does the child have frequent upper respiratory infections?

For the child who is underweight or is eating a restricted diet because of problems swallowing some types of food, a detailed record of the amount of food eaten over a 3-day period is important for the therapist to identify nutritional intake (Crist, Napier-Phillips, McDonnel, Dedwidge & Beck, 1998. The nutritionist analyzes this record to develop a comprehensive intervention plan for increased nutritional intake and a balanced diet.

Medical history

The therapist should obtain all medical records, including records of neurologic examination and results of CT scans and brain imaging scans. Frequently occurring pneumonia and upper respiratory infections are typical in the child who regularly aspirates. The therapist should carefully read past records of the results of VFSS and consider them in the intervention plan. Consultation with a speech pathologist who has completed an evaluation of the child can also help the therapist gain understanding of the child's oral motor function.

Clinical observation

The therapist should observe in the child's natural environment when possible. If the evaluation takes place in a clinic or school, the therapist should use foods that the child typically eats. The therapist should place the child in his or her typical feeding position and use feeding utensils and methods familiar to the child. After observing typical feeding, the therapist should attempt new positions and different foods as appropriate. The foods and methods tried during the evaluation are techniques that the therapist postulates will improve oral motor skill and swallow. Therefore the therapist obtains assessment information regarding what intervention strategies seem to promote skills and the child's responsiveness to different intervention methods. As discussed previously, the therapist should ask the parent if the child's behaviors are typical or unique to the stress of the evaluation situation (i.e., interacting with strangers in an unfamiliar setting).

Videofluoroscopic swallow study

The VFSS is an important component of the evaluation process. Often the VFSS provides the most conclusive evidence of the swallowing problem and results in specific recommendations for food consistencies and feeding positions that seem to promote oral motor skill and reduce the possibility of aspiration (Zerilli et. al., 1990).

Intervention

Intervention for swallowing dysfunction relates specifically to the child's unique strengths and limitations as shown in the evaluation. The following techniques were outlined by Glass and Wolf (1998) and address components of eating. At all times the first concern of the therapist is safety, so his or her first consideration is compensation strategies to ensure safe intake of nutrition.

Increase rhythmic initiation of swallowing

The therapist can activate the muscles involved in swallowing by applying cold stimulation to the tongue and soft palate using a frozen pacifier. When the muscles are readied for action, the swallow reflex is initiated more quickly. Wolf and Glass (1992) also recommend the use of chilled formula to quicken the swallow reflex. In an older child, the therapist can use a popsicle or piece of ice before feeding or intermittently during feeding. As with any technique, the therapist should carefully evaluate and adjust the effect of using cold stimulation as needed.

Improve oral transit

Many children have swallowing dysfunction associated with poor oral motor control. The food is not efficiently masticated, gathered into a bolus, and moved to the back of the tongue, where the swallow reflex is triggered. This child may benefit from head and jaw support. The jaw support should include facilitation of mouth closure and tongue movement. Jaw support allows the child to focus on moving the tongue within the mouth. Improving mouth closure can increase pressure gradients in the mouth, thereby improving the efficiency of swallowing. Thickening liquids is often extremely helpful in improving swallowing. The thickened liquid moves more slowly within the mouth, allowing the child to better control it; it also has greater adhesion and therefore tends to remain a bolus. Thickened liquid also is heavier and therefore gives more proprioceptive input to the tongue during oral transit.

Position can improve the child's ability to swallow. When the child is positioned in extension, he or she has less control of the food's movement because of the effects of gravity. With the neck extended the child has difficulty with mouth closure and efficient tongue movements. Positioning the child's head in neck flexion can improve closure of the larynx during swallowing, therefore decreasing the possibility of aspiration. Good neck alignment increases the child's ability to control the food's movement.

Handling and intervention during feeding

When children have respiratory disorders, swallowing is problematic as it relates to breathing and the child's coordination of the suck-swallow-breathe sequence. In therapy with the infant who remains on some oxygen support, use of a nasal cannula or another source of oxygen during feeding is important. With oxygen support, rapid breathing is slowed to a pace that better allows for intermittent swallowing. Slowing of respiration encourages better control of the suck-swallow-breathe sequence.

Placing the child in a full upright position can also improve respiration during feeding and can facilitate coordination of swallowing. Often the infant with a respiratory disorder struggles during feeding because he or she initiates a rapid sequence of sucking and is unable to establish an appropriate suck-swallow-breathe sequence. As a result the infant coughs or chokes when the breathing becomes an absolute, immediate necessity. Glass and Wolf (1998) recommended a technique termed *external pacing*. To pace the infant's sucking pattern, the therapist breaks the infant sucking sequence by gently removing the nipple from the mouth. By interrupting an otherwise long sucking sequence, the therapist gives the child an opportunity to breathe and relax. This method gives the child an externally imposed pace and suck-swallow-breathe sequence.

Modify the infant's food

Children with respiratory or cardiac disorders typically have poor endurance and less oral intake than other children. One way to improve their nutrient and caloric intake is to increase the caloric density of their food. Formula is available in different caloric densities, and Karo syrup can be added. For older children the caregiver can add peanut butter, butter, gravies, and powdered milk to foods. These diet changes require consultation and direction by a nutritionist. The therapist should discuss any diet change with a nutritionist or the physician to ensure that the child's overall nutritional intake is positively affected.

Nonoral Feeding

Several methods of nonoral feeding are available to infants with persistent swallowing disorders that result in aspiration, with poor feeding endurance that results in failure to thrive or with limitations in oral motor function that prevent adequate food intake. Nonoral methods include nasogastric tubes, oral gastric tubes, gastrostomy tubes, and feeding tubes that extend into the intestines. In any infant or child whose food intake is inadequate for growth or whose lack of oral motor skills and swallow efficiency make feeding unsafe, the therapist should consider nonoral feedings. The therapist should view nonoral feeding as a method to improve the health and developmental status of the child. It should not result in complete removal of oral stimulation or complete removal of the feeding interaction. In many instances the placement of a gastrostomy or the use of other nonoral feeding methods is a temporary measure to promote the child's nutritional status and growth.

Hyperalimentation, also termed *parenteral nutrition,* involves a medical procedure in which a central line introduces highly nutritional solutions directly into the bloodstream. It provides protein and calorie intake sufficient to sustain life and to promote growth in the absence of adequate gastrointestinal tract function. Hyperalimentation is used for children with congenital bowel anomalies or in severe medical crises (Coley & Procter, 1989).

A surgical procedure is required to insert the catheter into a large vein, typically a vein near the heart. The surgeon may use the brachial artery. The surgeon pumps the fluid into the blood stream, requiring that the child be connected to an intravenous pump at all times (Coley & Procter, 1989). A complication of this form of nutritional intake is yeast and bacterial infection, which can result in death. Although long-term use of hyperalimentation is possible, generally children who cannot make the transition to another form of nutritional intake do not survive beyond infancy.

Use of nonoral feeding should not end the child's oral experiences and the enjoyment of interaction during feeding. When the therapist gives bolus feedings, he or she can also give the child oral stimulation. The therapist can give the child small amounts of food before the nonoral feeding or during the feeding. He or she can implement simple tastes and sucking experiences during gastrostomy feeding if the child has routine aspiration. The goal is to link a pleasurable oral experience with the satiation of hunger. This type of oral stimulation during nonoral feeding is particularly critical for the child who is expected to return to oral feeding.

Transition from Nonoral to Oral Feeding

The therapist initiates the *transition from nonoral to oral feeding* with a physician's recommendation, based on the child's medical status and an evaluation of the child's oral motor skills by an occupational or speech therapist. After considering the health care team's recommendations, the family decides whether a transition to oral feeding is desirable and, if so, when and how they would like to approach this process. Occupational therapists often are instrumental in each phase of the transition.

The first step in a program to transition a child from nonoral to oral feeding is *oral motor intervention.* The child must demonstrate that he or she is capable of oral feeding. The therapist works with the child to desensitize the areas around the mouth and the structures within the mouth. The therapist facilitates specific oral motor skills during sensory play. Activities to desensitize include chewing and sucking of rubber toys, a NUK toothbrush, and a textured cloth (described in the section on sensory defensiveness). The therapist gradually offers small amounts of food textures to the child, usually while feeding the child through the gastrostomy tube (Schauster & Dwyer, 1996).

Other activities that encourage oral motor skill development are making sounds, blowing bubbles, and giving kisses. The therapist emphasizes brushing teeth and oral play with toys. The therapist can point out the small successes that the child makes and can help the parent and child maintain an appropriate perspective on the goals (e.g., enjoyment of oral-sensory experiences). The therapist praises and encourages whatever the child chooses to do with food.

Often the child vies for control of the oral sensory experiences, perhaps because of the discomfort involved and the associated lack of meaning of the occupations around meals. The parent, who has anxiety about the child's achieving oral feeding and successfully making the transition without weight loss or health problems, often awards the child's avoidance or manipulative behaviors during feeding with increased attention. Approaches to behavior issues are described in later sections of this chapter.

Another component of the transition from nonoral to oral feeding is *manipulation of the gastrostomy feedings* so that bolus feedings are given rather than continuous feeding (e.g., feeding overnight). The therapist gives bolus feedings four to five times per day to emulate a meal schedule. Once the child's digestive tract adjusts to the bolus feedings, health and weight are evaluated to determine if feedings can be reduced. If the child is expected to accept food by mouth, he or she needs to experience hunger; therefore the child must receive a reduced amount of food. Schauster and Dwyer (1996) suggested that a reduction of 25% of the tube feeding is necessary to stimulate hunger. Often children who require gastrostomy feedings are not medically and nutritionally stable enough to reduce their caloric intake; therefore the transition to oral feeding requires a lengthy time. Some weight loss almost always results from this process; therefore children who cannot tolerate any weight loss are not candidates for making the transition.

The therapist's support and encouragement are important to the child's and the parents' success in this process. The longer the child has been on nonoral feeding, the more difficult the transition. *Continual support* to the family is needed, and regular communication with the family is critical. The parents need encouragement for the small increments of progress and the loss of progress that occurs at times. The therapist's encouragement helps the parents maintain the energy and positive attitude needed to successfully reach the goal of oral feeding. Parents who experience feeding problems with their child can provide mutual support and assist each other in problem solving. Parent-to-parent support can strengthen their abilities to cope with stressful problems on a day-to-day basis (Chamberlin, Henry, Roberts, Sapsford, & Courtney, 1991). Parent

groups are particularly appropriate when children have difficult feeding problems that include behavioral issues that need to be managed over lengthy periods.

■ INTERVENTION FOR ORAL STRUCTURAL PROBLEMS

Children with *oral structural problems* at birth may have feeding problems that directly relate to the structural deficits, and a compensation strategy is indicated. Two structural problems that can occur are *cleft lip and palate* and *micrognathia*. Cleft lip and palate is the fourth most common disability in children, affecting almost 1 in 700 children in the United States. These problems often create feeding difficulties, particularly in the perinatal period (Emondson & Reinhartsen, 1998). The role of the occupational therapist is to make recommendations for feeding equipment, adapted methods, and positions to be used until the child undergoes plastic surgery or outgrows the structural problem. Because oral structural problems rarely occur with neurologic impairment, the child with cleft lip and palate or micrognathia typically demonstrates intact oral movement and effective suck-swallow coordination once the structural problems are resolved.

Cleft Lip and Palate

A cleft is a separation of parts of the mouth usually joined together during the early weeks of fetal development. A cleft lip is separation of the upper lip and often the upper dental ridge. A cleft palate is a separation of the hard or soft palate and occurs with or without a cleft lip. Because of the lack of closure between the oral and nasal cavities, newborns have difficulty maintaining sufficient negative pressure to express liquid from a nipple. The infant's tongue does not have an upper surface to express milk from the breast or bottle.

Cleft lips and palates are closed through surgery. Surgeons can repair cleft lips in the first few months of life. Repair of a cleft palate is more extensive, and the surgeon generally waits until the infant reaches a certain weight, usually by 12 months of age. Generally, surgeons perform multiple procedures to correct the abnormalities. These surgeries include bone grafting, orthodontic repair, and placement of ear tubes.

Micrognathia

Micrognathia refers to a small, receded lower jaw. The mouth and tongue may be of normal size but are posteriorly positioned in relation to the upper jaw and the airway. Children with Pierre Robin syndrome have both micrognathia and cleft palate.

Evaluation

Evaluation involves inspection of the oral structures and assessment of how the defects limit the feeding process. Evaluation should include observation of feeding to assess how the food travels through the mouth and how well the infant can express liquids from the nipple.

During the evaluation process the therapist should try several different feeding devices, methods, and positions to identify methods that overcome the structural defects and allow safe oral intake. The therapist may need a VFSS to identify if aspiration occurs or if liquids move into the nasal passageway.

Intervention

A variety of nipples are designed for use with children who have structural problems. These nipples compensate for lack of negative pressure and for limitations in tongue position and movement. Adaptive nipples that deliver flow without requiring suction include the Haberman feeder and the Ross cleft palate nipple. The therapist sometimes uses a prosthetic device (i.e., an obturator) to lengthen the palate to prevent liquid from escaping into the nasal cavity (Edmondson & Reinhartsen, 1998).

The therapist can use squeeze bottles with care to express liquids into the infant's mouth when suction is limited. Some nipples adjust the flow of the liquid during feeding by turning the nipple's rim. The therapist can use long thin nipples to carry the liquid to the back of the mouth past the cleft palate to avoid liquid flow into the nasal passageway. Wolf and Glass (1992) suggested that therapists avoid cross-cut nipples because they create an uneven flow that is more difficult for the infant to control. The therapist must work carefully with the parent so that the liquid flows easily from the bottle but is not excessive, resulting in a flow that the child cannot control. The therapist should consider the nipple characteristics in Table 15-4 when making recommendations to parents or nurses.

The infant with cleft lip and palate or micrognathia benefits from upright positioning. By holding the infant in a vertical position, the risk of aspiration is reduced. Upright positioning can promote forward movement of a recessed jaw and can prevent nasal and pharyngeal aspiration in the infant with cleft palate.

When micrognathia is severe the tongue may occlude the airway. When the condition compromises respiration, the child may need placement of a tracheostomy and gastrostomy. These procedures provide temporary support of respiration and nutrition until the surgeon can repair the structural problems.

The following example illustrates the role of the occupational therapist with the infant with Pierre Robin syndrome.

Sarah was born with Pierre Robin syndrome and presented with a small recessed chin and retracted tongue. She also had a deep cleft in her hard and soft palates. She struggled with her first feedings. On the third day of life her retracted tongue fell into her airway, completely occluding it. Because Sarah was connected to a monitor,

table 15-4 Nipple Characteristics Related to Use with Children Who Have Oral Structural Defects

Nipple Type	Characteristics
Long, thin nipples	Work well when the tongue is recessed; can bring the tongue forward
Single nipple hole	Results in a steady liquid stream, which can be easier to handle than bursts of liquid
Wide nipple	Can be compressed for liquid expression for the child with a cleft palate
Broad-based nipple	Can help the infant with a cleft lip gain suction
Nipple with cross-cut hole	Can create an uneven liquid flow or a burst of fluid that is difficult for the infant to control
Nipple with enlarged hole	Should be used with great care; when the caregiver enlarges the hole, it is difficult to predict what type of liquid flow will result
Soft, pliable nipple	Appropriate for infants with cleft palates who are unable to achieve suction
NUK nipple	Has the hole on top of the nipple and should not be used with children with cleft palates; this nipple may be functional if its position on the tongue is reversed

the medical team immediately intubated her. She then received a tracheostomy and gastrostomy to avoid further complications caused by the position of her tongue. She was discharged home on continuous feedings and moist air to her tracheostomy. She required respiratory treatment and frequent suctioning to keep her lungs clear. In the first few months she had frequent pneumonia but became healthy by 3 months of age. Her growth was adequate, although she remained in the fifth percentile of weight for height.

An occupational therapist initiated home-based therapy to develop an oral motor program that would promote development of her oral motor skills while she received gastrostomy feedings and awaited surgery, which was anticipated to occur at 18 months. The therapist initiated and recommended that the family implement a program of graded oral input. Because Sarah did not exhibit mouthing of her hands or objects, the therapist's first efforts were to initiate a hand-to-mouth movement pattern and to rub her gums with the pacifier. Sarah used the pacifier for brief periods, but she was unable to maintain suction on it to independently hold it in her mouth. Her preferred oral stimulus was her mother's finger.

The therapist applied slow, rhythmic stroking to Sarah's tongue to bring it forward. By 5 months of age Sarah could hold the pacifier in her mouth. At that time the therapist dipped her pacifier in fruit juice to introduce tastes. She frequently mouthed her fingers. Sarah's mother began using the NUK toothbrush for additional stimulation, and Sarah enjoyed chewing on it. Sarah demonstrated increased tolerance of a warm washcloth on her face.

By 7 months of age, Sarah learned to sit upright when supported at the pelvis and to sit at midline in an infant seat. Her increased stability of neck and trunk allowed for more oral motor experiences. The therapist introduced pureed foods, first on the nipple and NUK toothbrush. The therapist applied desensitization, using stroking with a washcloth to increase her sensory tolerance. She then began to take two to five spoonfuls of pureed fruits. The therapist applied downward and forward pressure with the bowl of the spoon. Sarah tolerated this procedure and seemed to enjoy it after several weeks. She developed good suction on the pacifier. The physician recommended that the therapist give feedings in boluses to emulate oral feedings. When the therapist began bolus feedings, she performed oral stimulation immediately before the gastrostomy feeding with the hope that Sarah would be hungry and more receptive to oral stimulation. She was receptive but did not consume more than five spoonfuls. She was not hungry because she received total nutrition through the gastrostomy. At that time her suck-swallow sequence was well coordinated, and her tongue was in a forward position.

At 9 months of age, Sarah tolerated various food textures in her mouth. Oral motor skills rapidly progressed and were only slightly behind those of her typically developing peers. Her tongue and mandible had moved into a forward position, and the physician recommended that she transition to oral feedings without waiting for repair of the cleft palate, which was 9 months in the future. The therapist and nutritionist met with Sarah's mother to design a diet that would increase oral intake and simultaneously reduce gastrostomy feedings. Because oral sensory issues had been addressed in the occupational therapy program and because Sarah's oral motor skills were almost age appropriate, the team thought that the transition would proceed quickly. As the therapist reduced gastrostomy feedings, she carefully monitored Sarah's weight to ensure that her oral intake maintained the nutritional intake required for growth. Although children almost always lose weight in the transition from nonoral to oral feedings, Sarah did not. She and her mother were ready for oral feedings to begin, and Sarah successfully made the transition in 2 weeks.

■ INTERACTIONAL ASPECTS OF THE CO-OCCUPATION OF FEEDING.

As described in Chapter 5, a parent and child form a subsystem within the dynamical family system. Children engage in the occupation of eating and feeding when adults initiate it while enacting the occupation of caregiving. The shared nature of the *co-occupation of feeding* re-

sults in reciprocal influences between the occupational performances of the child and adult. Therefore any intervention that targets how the child eats affects the parent who is responsible for feeding. When therapeutic activities occur without participation of the child's usual feeders and out of context of mealtimes, the meaning of the occupation for the child is diminished. Fisher (1998) describes activities in which the therapist, rather than the natural flow of the individual's occupational pattern, creates the meaning as more a contrived activity than a true occupation. When intervention targets impairments or performance components (e.g., practice of lip closure or tolerance of textures by sucking on a toy), the therapist should make a plan for incorporating the newly emerging components into mealtime tasks. Naturally this generalization of skill needs to involve the child's feeders.

A systems model of the feeding process suggests that one cannot isolate the cause from the consequences of feeding dysfunction in understanding the parent's and child's behaviors around meals (Humphry, 1995). Except in situations where structural oral problems such as cleft lip make immediate identification possible, frequently the therapist does not identify feeding dysfunction until after the parent and child have had weeks, sometimes months, of frustrating experiences in the co-occupation of feeding. The insights into occupations that therapists bring enable them to work with adult caregivers such as parents and teachers in a collaborative manner.

This section first uses the lens of occupational science (Clark, Wood, & Lawson, 1998) to articulate factors influencing the parent's occupational performance around feeding children and the meaning that feeding carries for most adults. Understanding factors that influence a parenting process such as feeding is important since the parent responds at an intuitive, emotional level, which makes problems difficult for the parent to articulate (Papousek & Papousek, 1995). Many of the therapeutic skills that all occupational therapists use in supporting adults in the modification or reconstruction of their occupations are needed to provide services around feeding problems of children.

Adult's Occupational Challenge: Child With Feeding Problems

Parents of children with feeding problems frequently report that their difficulties begin when the child is 6 months of age (Ramsay, Gisel, & Boutry, 1993). Some parents show great perseverance and creativity in trying to accommodate their child's special needs (Bakker & Woody, 1995). However, these early experiences can have a negative effect on parents and subsequent caregiving behaviors. Mothers of infants with eating problems feed their infants more frequently, feed them for longer periods, worry more about the infant's health, and experience more isolation from social support systems than mothers of infants with no feeding problems (Hagekull & Dahl, 1987). Among infants and preschool-age children with a history of mealtime problems, the parent is more likely to be coercive and have behaviors that can contribute to or sustain feeding problems in the child (Sanders, Patel, LeGrice, & Shepherd, 1993).

Statements made by parents about their choices at mealtimes help the therapist understand how meanings of feeding as an occupation influence adult's choices. In a qualitative study, Bakker and Woody (1995) interviewed parents of children with developmental disabilities who had feeding problems. They found one common theme—*the importance of nutrition*—suggesting that parents understand the implications of the child's problems for general health. However, sometimes the importance of nutrition is in conflict with another theme—*what is best for the child*. Parents' ideas about what their children experienced during meals helps them define what is best. At times the parent has to decide which theme will guide caregiving decisions. The following is an example of a parent who determines what will guide her decisions:

> Joan, the mother of a 5 year old with athetoid cerebral palsy, worried that her son would not feel that he was part of the family if he sat in his chair and used a tray rather than sit at the table to eat. In spite of the fact he had better control of the spoon in supported seating with a tray and dropped food onto himself and the floor when he was sitting at the table, Joan wanted the family to be together.

As described previously, part of parenting is integrating advice with what the parent thinks about that child and the meaning of the occupation. In the Bakker and Woody interviews (1995), Sarah said the following while looking at her daughter:

> In the chair there she'll do all this stuff, but in my lap, she relaxes. Of course now she sees people at the evaluation center and they all have hissy fits that I do this. Honest. It's more relaxing just to feed her like this than to put her in that chair or to fight her, and it's just me as a mom.

This parent understands the desired therapeutic actions for feeding her daughter with severe motor problems. However, the occupational therapist needs to address how positioning alters the meaning of the occupation for the parent before the parent can expect any substantial changes in the child's seating during meals.

Occupational therapy intervention for feeding problems facilitates behavioral change in both the child and the parent or other adult caregiver. The therapist first considers how to establish a working relationship with the parent and communicate intervention strategies in a way that supports adaptive and effective strategies that the parent already uses and respects the feelings that the parent expresses about what is important about feeding the child. The therapist recognizes that the parent may experience a sense of failure as a caregiver if nutritional status and growth are poor. Acknowledging the legitimate basis for the parent's stress is a first step in the parent being able to articulate his or her needs. As adults who think about their occupations, parents also have their own theories about why the child is not eating well (Humphry, 1995). Once the therapist and parent establish a collaborative relationship, the therapist can suggest alternative strategies to achieve a feeding goal and ask the parent to select those that he or she feels comfortable implementing. Two important strategies to promote success are to recommend ways that feeding techniques can be incorporated into daily routines and to allow the parent to decide when and how frequently he or she will implement the techniques. A parent may determine that working on drinking from a cup is only realistic at night, just before he or she changes the child's clothes for bed. Another parent may decide that giving the child time to practice self-feeding is only possible on weekends.

Using a systems model enables the occupational therapist to address the complex issue of feeding and to focus on more than one part of the system at a time. Using this model helps the therapist understand how a busy, overstimulating environment and a mother pressed for time can negatively influence the child's ability to use lip closure in taking food from the spoon. Conversely, a child who has difficulty feeding and requires continual caregiver assistance may be disruptive to the family's mealtime, and the therapist can recognize that the family's first priority is social aspects of dinner. In this situation it may be necessary to address nutritional needs in another context.

A focus on the child or parent and their feeding interaction is important when working with children who are diagnosed with failure to thrive. In the past when children did not gain weight, therapists categorized failure to thrive as either organic (a medical problem that led to poor nutrition) or nonorganic (a problem related to parenting and factors in the environment). The interactive systems model offers a more complete picture of feeding (Humphry, 1995). Children who are diagnosed with nonorganic failure to thrive, where parental neglect and inappropriate feeding practices are identified problems, may also demonstrate oral motor delays that affect their amount of nutritional intake and compound the other issues, such as limited time allotted by the parent for the meal. Regardless of the source of feeding problems, the multilevel systems model helps the therapist consider the quality of fit between the parent and child and suggests intervention that will enhance feeding skill acquisition in the child, parenting practices, and interaction of the feeding dyad.

Consequences of Co-Occupation Changes When a Child Has a Feeding Problem

Because children eat several times a day, meals represent frequent learning opportunities that can influence sensorimotor, cognitive, and psychosocial components of function. The perception of hunger, signaling need, and receiving adult response are the first contingency-response experiences of many infants. Children, especially infants, create opportunities to interact with adults. Once the immediate feelings of hunger are satiated, infants use feeding time to engage and interact with their caregivers (Brazelton, 1993). The reciprocity developed during feeding experiences may be a foundation for subsequent communication. The close physical contact during breast-feeding or bottle-feeding also provides various sensorimotor experiences. As the infant gets older, self-feeding is one of the first experiences to negotiate the issue of autonomy between the child and parent. For preschool- and school-age children, verbal interactions of families during meals provide learning experiences that promote language and concepts about the world (Beals, 1993).

When a child has feeding problems, the occupational therapist and other team members need to consider how to help the family compensate for the secondary effects on parent-child interaction and play. Collaboration with nurses and speech language pathologists who are also interested in parent-child interaction helps the therapist consider how the feeding program assists or at least does not diminish opportunities for general development. Clinicians, teachers, and parents also can work together to understand the child's typical communicative acts. If the child signals preferences by making faces or looking toward a desired drink, caregivers should recognize and honor these communications. The following is an example of an interaction between a teacher and a child:

> Megan is a 3-year-old girl with spastic cerebral palsy. When feeding Megan, the teacher implemented the occupational therapist's suggestions to promote jaw stabilization by placing her fingers under Megan's jaw as she offered a bite of ground food. The teacher noted that Megan looked at the chocolate pudding on the side of the tray. The teacher could acknowledge Megan's interest in the pudding by naming it and talking about how she could have the pudding after her meal. If Megan's feeders only concentrated on head position and jaw stability, Megan would learn that her efforts at making her needs known were not worth the effort.

■ INTERVENTION FOR SELF-FEEDING ISSUES

Delays in self-feeding skills result when the child has cognitive, behavioral, or sensorimotor problems or delays. The respondents of a survey of occupational therapists who were interested in developmental disability reported that the largest proportion of children with feeding delays were experiencing problems primarily associated with motor deficits (41%). The second most common issues influencing feeding were sensory problems (30%) and general developmental delays or behavioral problems (22%) (Thigpen-Beck & Dovenitz, 1995). In planning intervention, the first consideration of the therapist is to determine that the child can safely eat daily and with reasonable efficiency for his or her parents and teachers. After ensuring that safety and daily nutritional needs are met, the therapist will work to promote development in the performance area.

Intervention

Occupational therapists propose compensation strategies to improve the fit between the child's abilities and the occupation of self-feeding. Strategies during mealtime include position of the child, handling techniques, adaptation of the tasks, and use of adapted equipment. Behavior issues in self-feeding require a comprehensive team approach. Many general issues about behaviors are discussed in Chapter 14. Interventions at the impairment level to improve arm and hand strength and control are described in Chapter 11.

Positioning

Correct postural alignment and stability are critical to the child's success in self-feeding. Control of the arm in space while bringing the spoon to the mouth requires a stable postural base. Children with cerebral palsy often lack adequate postural stability for a base of arm control, moving the arm toward midline. The child must feel secure and relaxed during self-feeding so that his or her endurance is adequate to feed the entire meal. Various seating arrangements are available to stabilize the child for self-feeding.

Wheelchair. The child's wheelchair may offer ideal positioning and comfort for feeding and often has a tray to support the plate and cup. Positioning with the head, neck, and trunk in upright alignment is similar to the positioning described previously for feeding the child. Correct posture for self-feeding includes a tucked chin, depressed shoulders, and a neutral pelvis. The child can maintain an upright position for feeding if the wheelchair has a firm seat and is an appropriate size. Pelvic and hip abductor straps and lateral trunk support help support the position of a neutral pelvis and a symmetric, upright trunk. When the child tends to retract his or her shoulders, padded humeral "wings" on the back of the chair or on the wheelchair tray can maintain the arms in a forward protracted position. These "wings" help increase arm stability and maintain the child's hands at midline for self-feeding.

Rifton child's chair. Once the child has fair to good sitting stability, the Rifton chair is an excellent choice for feeding. The Rifton chair places the child in a completely upright position and requires good head control. This chair has a firm seat and back, adjustable foot rests, arm supports, and pelvic strapping. A pelvic abductor pad can be added to the system. A tray is desirable for weight bearing on arms during feeding and for additional sitting stability. The tray provides a surface for play with food or for self-feeding if the child has those skills.

Child's high chair. The advantages of using a high chair are discussed in the previous section and apply to self-feeding as well.

Tray adaptations. Regardless of the chair selected, the tray fitted for the chair offers opportunities for modification of positioning. A tray adaptation that helps increase arm stability and improve the arm's position for feeding is a small (short) bolster that can be placed under the arm. By separating the elbow from the trunk, the shoulder is abducted and the elbow is stabilized at a height that enables the child to scoop food onto the spoon and reach the mouth using a pattern of elbow flexion. The bolster serves as a lever from which the child can efficiently reach the tray (and food) and his or her mouth.

Another effective compensation strategy to improve control of the hand-to-mouth pattern is to raise the tray or feeding surface. Raising the tray brings it higher on the child's trunk, thereby assisting with trunk stability. A higher tray also holds the arms in greater humeral abduction, which decreases the distance that the hand travels to reach the mouth and can improve control of the hand-to-mouth movement. By stabilizing the elbow on the tray, the child can move in a simple pattern of elbow flexion and extension to self-feed.

Handling strategies during self-feeding

Self-feeding is a particular challenge for children with poor arm and hand control, such as those with athetoid cerebral palsy. These individuals may benefit from handling during feeding to improve control and to enhance the movement patterns used during feeding. The techniques that therapists use often involve facilitation of shoulder depression and protraction and scapular stability to increase the child's control of distal arm movement. The therapist may place his or her hand on top of the child's shoulders or scapula. Support or guidance of the humerus may be necessary to establish a smooth hand-to-mouth pattern. The therapist helps stabilize and support the arm as it moves through space rather than forcefully moving it through the range. Arm support should be intermittent and as needed based on the responses of the child.

Other children have poor control of free movement in space and rely on vision to guide movements. This is especially challenging since self-feeding involves moving the hand through space toward a target that the child cannot visualize (the mouth). The child lacks feedback about wrist position and when the food spills, and he or she has difficulty understanding what to change. In one recommended technique the therapist holds the spoon handle between the extended index and third fingers. The therapist slips these fingers into the child's palm with a thumb on the dorsum of the child's hand. The child holds onto the fingers and spoon using a palmar grasp, and the therapist facilitates a self-feeding pattern using subtle and natural facilitation from within the child's hand. Klein and Delaney (1994) recommended that the therapist hold the spoon in the child's palm by placing one finger in the palm and the thumb on the back of the wrist. Using this handling technique the therapist can facilitate wrist extension and apply pressure in the palm to encourage sustained grasp. These techniques are particularly successful with a child who has developed a basic hand-to-mouth pattern but has difficulty placing the spoon into his or her mouth (Case-Smith, 1999).

One disadvantage of these handling techniques is that they require the therapist, teacher, or parent to be seated behind or to the side of the child. This positioning limits eye-to-eye interaction with the child during feeding and can create a barrier to communication. This limitation is not as important in a group situation, such as the family mealtime or the school's snack time. Practice of self-feeding using these techniques on an intermittent basis can improve the movement pattern when the caregiver provides consistent feedback and reinforcement to the child regarding his or her self-feeding efforts. In applying these techniques, the therapist's goal is to facilitate the child's success and gradually decrease the amount of physical assistance and adaptive equipment required in self-feeding.

Adaptive equipment

A variety of adaptive equipment has been specifically designed to accommodate the needs of children who experience difficulty in self-feeding. Often the equipment provides simple, yet critical, adaptations to the feeding experience that enable the child to be independent in self-feeding. Examples of adapted feeding equipment include utensils, plates, bowls, cups, and straws. Utensils with built-up handles that are easier to grasp or straps on the handle to secure it to the hand can compensate for limited grasp. Children with orthopedic impairments that influence the upper extremity may be more successful with spoon handles that are longer or shorter or that are curved or bent. Children need sturdy spoons with short handles and small, shallow bowls. Various spoons are available for children and may cost less than special equipment ordered through catalogs. To scoop food onto the spoon, the child may need a dish with a raised edge. These "scoop dishes" often have suction cups underneath to stabilize them on the tray or table. The high curved side of the dish makes scooping the food easier when the child is unable to use an assisting hand to obtain the food. The fork is generally introduced after the spoon. A short fork with blunt prongs can work well even when the child uses a palmar grasp. Cups with lids reduce spillage by controlling the flow of liquid into the mouth. Lids without spouts are recommended when the child exhibits suckling tongue movement. Straws can promote the child's ability to suck and can allow the child to drink without lifting the cup from the table surface. Straw drinking can also promote a chin tuck position because the child must move forward using active neck flexion to obtain the straw. More sophisticated adapted equipment, such as the electric feeder, may enable a child to self-feed without using the arms. Criteria for selecting adaptive equipment to improve the child's independence in self-feeding include durability, ease of cleaning and use, and developmental appropriateness.

Task modifications

Children who have problems controlling the spoon because of abnormal muscle tone can also benefit from modification of the self-feeding activity itself. For example, children with ataxic cerebral palsy who exhibit tremor in the upper extremity during purposeful activities often have difficulty having enough control to self feed. Without the experience needed for feedback, the child does not learn more refined modifications of the arm and wrist. If children struggle when attempting to eat spillable foods on a spoon, stabbing food with a blunt fork may be a more effective self-feeding method.

In addition to learning how to control the utensil, the child learns to perform self-feeding occupations in a manner consistent with his or her social context. The adult usually sets the performance criteria and provides feedback regarding what is or is not finger food. Another powerful force in providing information about adequate self-feeding is observations of peers. Siblings and classmates eating the meal at the same time act as models for adequate occupational performance or will challenge the child to learn a new skill. Therefore part of intervention planning includes strategies to ensure that the child engages in self-feeding as a part of the social context of the family or classroom.

■ NUTRITION

Adequate nutrition is necessary for a healthy life. Malnutrition is of particular concern for children with development disabilities who demonstrate the feeding problems described in this chapter. This compromised feeding and nutritional status results from a combination of factors, including exceptional nutritive requirements, limited feeding skills, and drug- or disease-induced food intolerance. In addition, the parent's emotional, physical, and social stresses associated with caring for a child with special health care needs can disrupt the feeding interac-

tion (Baroni & Sondel, 1995; Brizee, Sophos, & McLaughlin, 1990).

Malnutrition or a failure-to-thrive condition can exacerbate or worsen the developmental condition. Accordingly, the therapist needs to adjust diets with higher or lower daily requirements of certain nutrients to provide optimal nutrition and prevent detrimental side effects of the medications. Unfortunately, early interventionists, including occupational therapists, often do not make appropriate referrals to nutritionists (Clark, Oakland, & Brotherson, 1998). Clinicians sometimes assume that if the family receives assistance through programs such as Women, Infants, and Children (WIC), a nutritionist is involved with the family and will provide sufficient guidance. Because children with special needs have exceptionally complex problems the WIC nutritionist does not have sufficient time or knowledge to address these issues.

The occupational therapist can perform nutritional screening with guidance by the nutritionist. Therapists will also see children for eating problems. The following require a referral to a nutritionist and incorporation of recommendations (Clark et. al., 1998):
- The child consumes less than the desired 16 to 32 ounces of milk or formula.
- The child has constipation.
- The parent expresses concerns.
- The child's diet is not consistent with his or her chronologic age.
- The child has problems with eating and self-feeding.
  A nutritional screening consists of the following:
1. Interviewing the caregivers regarding amounts and types of foods consumed daily
2. Collecting data on height, weight, and weight for height
3. Observing general appearance of skin, hair, and gums
4. Reviewing medical records

The following are problems identified in the screening that indicate the need for a more in-depth nutritional assessment and services (Brizee et. al., 1990):
- Weight for height below the tenth percentile
- Weight for height above the ninetieth percentile
- Height and weight below the fifth percentile
- Parents' concern about nutrition
- Behavioral or oral motor problems that result in severe limitations in the types or amounts of food ingested

The following is an example of a child who required in-depth nutritional assessment:

When Joey was 5 years old, the preschool interdisciplinary team in the Powell school district followed his development. His home-based teacher asked for additional input from the rest of the team because she suspected that Joey had autism. His parents wanted Joey to start in a kindergarten program but were worried about meals. Although he fed himself, Joey refused to eat anything but Cheerios and drink milk. His weight was at the twentieth percentile. The preschool interdisciplinary team referred Joey to the nutritionist because of his restricted diet. His analysis revealed adequate caloric intake but a diet that was missing many nutrients typically found in fruits and vegetables. The team began vitamin supplements immediately and agreed that one of the first priorities was for the occupational therapist to work with the teacher on expanding Joey's tolerance of different types of foods.

With the close link between nutrition and health, priorities in intervention are to promote nutrition by adjusting occupational therapy strategies. The following principles apply to the occupational therapist's intervention and its potential effect on the child's nutritional status.

When oral intervention for sensory or motor problems is stressful for the child, the intervention activities should occur at times other than mealtime. Mealtime should be the time for the child to receive an optimal amount of nutrition and experience the satisfaction of satiation. Challenging oral interventions, particularly those that strongly influence the sensory system, may upset or frustrate the child and result in food refusal. Mealtime can then evolve into a battle of the child who exerts control of a situation that creates discomfort or stress by refusing food. When the therapist addresses oral desensitization and new oral motor skills at times other than mealtime, the child and the parent or therapist can approach these activities in a more relaxed, playful manner.

The therapist should always consider the consequences of food intake and nutrition when developing therapeutic strategies to improve oral motor abilities. Strategies that prolong a meal beyond 40 minutes may make unreasonable demands on the caregivers' time or may exhaust the child before he or she has consumed a sufficient amount of food (Gisel et. al., 1995).

Often therapists recommend changes in food texture. To overcome an aversive response to sensory challenges, they may select sweet food, like cookies or pudding, to increase motivation. When the therapist attempts new textures, he or she should consider the nutritional value. Acceptance does not translate into good nutrition, especially if the snack for therapy translates into less hunger for the next meal. When attempting new textures of food, the therapist should reinforce the importance of nutrition by selecting foods with high nutritional value. The therapist should use cheese and fruits to work on chewing rather than cookies and monitor intake at other meals.

A nutritionist should assess all major changes in the child's diet. For example, blanket recommendations to use high-caloric foods can be inappropriate, even when the goal for the child is weight gain. Sometimes high-caloric food supplements actually decrease the child's overall appetite and food intake. The therapist needs to balance increases in the caloric density of foods with increases in fluid intake. The therapist should consider the long-term effects of artificially increasing caloric density.

Collaboration with the nutritionist is essential for children who are underweight, and frequent consultation with the nutritionist is critical for the therapist to avoid malnutrition and improve the child's overall health and development. Often the therapist interacts with the failure-to-thrive child and his or her family more frequently than the nutritionist and is privy to information regarding the child's eating. Food refusal and loss of appetite can be particularly detrimental to these children. The therapist can share insight into the interactional components of the problem. Issues other than failure to thrive warrant referral to the nutritionist. The therapist may recommend that the family consult with a nutritionist in the following instances:

- When certain medications have been used for long periods
- When changes in the child's health suggest concern for drug and nutrient interaction
- When the child gains or loses weight suddenly
- When major changes in diet occur
- When conditions such as constipation are long-standing problems

Although these problems do not always require direct intervention and changes in diet, it is important that the nutritionist monitor them and follow recommendations to improve the child's nutrition.

■ IMPLICATIONS OF SOCIAL CONTEXTS IN FEEDING

All aspects of the environment—cultural, physical, and interpersonal—influence feeding. Meals also have a temporal context in other life routines, so feeding must occur within the demands of time for other family or classroom occupations. Direct observation is an ideal strategy for the therapist to understand contextual factors in feeding. When this is unrealistic, the therapist should ask the parent to describe a typical meal and request specific details of the child's behaviors and the environment to appreciate variations in the elements of the social context.

As discussed at the beginning of the chapter, the family's cultural background can determine selection and preparation of food and the interactive rituals during mealtimes. The first component of social context is the ethnicity of and implications for feeding practices. For example, despite common recommendation that children not be given products with cow's milk, a mother from the Middle East may feel that yogurt, a common food in a family's diet, is an ideal first food for an infant. Asking parents about the different foods in their culture helps build rapport because it shows the therapist's interest in the family's traditions.

The family's interactive routines may also determine physical features of mealtime. For example, some families strive to always eat together watching a television show or sitting in a special dining area. In addition, the family's background may determine how the child is seated during feeding; therefore therapists must consider whether changing positions is essential.

Another component of the social context of feeding is the generally shared assumptions about good parenting and feeding. Confusion exists about the amount of food that children typically eat at different ages even among parents of typically developing children. Occupational therapists are just one of many sources of information on feeding. Caregivers acquire information about how and what to feed an infant from family members, neighbors, texts on child development, and other health professionals. The occupational therapist who asks about the feeding techniques that the parent has tried should specifically explore suggestions that have come from relatives and neighbors (see Box 15-1). If the family structure is hierarchic, the therapist may need to discuss feeding alternatives with the family member who has the authority to make decisions rather than the primary caregiver who is feeding the child. The therapist often needs to meet with several family members to come to a consensus. The occupational therapist may see the child in a clinic or special part of the classroom where the social and physical context of feeding cannot be directly observed. Questions about meals (see Box 15-1) are important for the therapist to make effective suggestions.

■ SUMMARY

Intervention to promote co-occupation in feeding and the child's eating skills is an important role of the occupational therapist. For the child, ability to participate in mealtime is influenced by performance components such as oral sensory and motor function, physiologic parameters, cognitive understanding of the occupation, and psychosocial abilities to appreciate meaning and standards of performance that are consistent with those of his or her family. For the parent or caregiver other factors influence his or her occupational performance as the feeder, including informal ideas about feeding a child and the adult's social context brought to the occupation.

The quality of interaction during meals is a product of occupational performance of child and adult. Although these aspects of feeding are addressed separately in the chapter, they are interrelated. Therefore, feeding interventions require a holistic approach in which multiple aspects of the child's behaviors and the environment are considered. Because of the complexity and critical importance of feeding interaction and nutritional intake, a collaborative interdisciplinary approach is recommended, with the family's concerns and priorities central to the intervention plan. This chapter provides a foundation for

occupational therapists to help children develop eating skills that allow for good nutritional intake and thus for growth and development. The occupational therapist emphasizes interventions that support positive interactions during feeding and helps caregivers gain confidence, skill, and enjoyment in feeding their children.

Case Study 1

Carol was born prematurely at 30 weeks' estimated gestational age and had hyperbilirubinemia, respiratory distress, and a grade III intraventricular hemorrhage. A developmental assessment at 12 months of age indicated mild delays in gross and fine motor skills. Her parents fondly called her their "lazy baby." She was alert and pleasant and had recently begun to babble in long sequences. She learned to sit independently at 11 months of age. She rolled from place to place and did not creep or cruise. She could hold two objects, one in each hand, waving and banging them. She did not yet combine objects and had limited control of release.

The therapist interviewed Carol's mother at the 12-month assessment. She reported that Carol fed completely from the bottle. Her mother had tried pureed foods on several occasions; however, Carol spit them from her mouth and became upset. These behaviors prevented Carol's mother from continuing to try pureed foods and cereals. Carol demonstrated a strong sucking pattern, but she did not demonstrate tongue lateralization or graded bite. Her jaw was unstable when she attempted cup drinking. Although her weight was appropriate for her age, her mother wanted to introduce new foods and progress to feeding with a spoon and cup.

Feeding evaluation

The therapist's evaluation indicated that Carol was hypersensitive in and around her mouth. Although she exhibited an effective sucking pattern, her tongue and jaw movement were unorganized when she was introduced to pureed foods. She coughed and choked on pureed food, losing most of the food placed on her tongue. Carol's parents were anxious to progress to a variety of foods and a more balanced diet. The failed attempts to introduce new foods into Carol's diet discouraged her parents.

Intervention

The therapist first addressed Carol's oral sensory defensiveness at times other than feeding. Using a warm, wet washcloth, the therapist began by stroking her face around the mouth and then in the mouth, rubbing the gums and palate. The therapist used the NUK toothbrush to rub her gums. Carol seemed to like this; therefore the therapist used the NUK toothbrush to introduce food tastes and textures. The therapist dipped the toothbrush into fruit baby food before oral stimulation. The therapist then dipped a nipple with her finger inside into the baby food and pressed it onto the anterior tongue, lateral tongue, and gums.

As Carol's tolerance of the baby food presented on the nipple and toothbrush increased, the therapist introduced a latex-covered spoon with pureed food. The therapist used smooth pureed food at first, and then introduced foods with greater texture. The therapist provided jaw support to inhibit her jaw's excessive movement and to promote the tongue's movements. The therapist removed this support as Carol's suck-swallow sequence of pureed foods became efficient.

By 15 months of age, Carol's diet included a variety of pureed foods. At this time the therapist introduced coarse foods and the therapist and parent initiated placement of the food on the side of her tongue and between her gums. The therapist reintroduced jaw support as a support of tongue lateralization. When the therapist observed tongue lateralization, she placed the food completely to the side between the gums.

The therapist introduced cup drinking at this time because Carol's jaw stability had increased. The therapist used a small, transparent plastic cup. Its transparency helped the parents and therapist regulate the flow of liquid into Carol's mouth. The therapist gave small, single sips at first and then facilitated a sequence of suck-swallow movements.

By 18 months of age, Carol was eating soft foods. Because she was unable and unsuccessful in self-feeding with a spoon, she preferred finger foods, such as strips of soft cheese or processed meats such as turkey. Cup drinking remained difficult, although she was learning to bite on the cup for stability. Her mother used thickened liquids, such as milk with yogurt and juice with baby food, to slow the movement of the liquid and to give her a better opportunity to control its flow. At that time oral sensitivity was no longer a primary issue, although she exhibited mild discomfort when new foods were introduced. Carol's mother was pleased with the variety of foods that Carol consumed and with her continued weight gain and growth.

Case Study 2

Jonathan was diagnosed with spastic quadriparesis when he was 6 months old. His lower extremities exhibited high muscle tone, particularly in hip adductors and hamstrings. As a result he demonstrated a scissoring pattern when standing or when held in his mother's arms. At 2½ years of age he had many assets: a ready smile, good social skills and responsivity to social interaction, beginning language (about 20 words), and a pleasant affect. He sat with minimal assistance, had begun to crawl on his belly, and rolled segmentally about the room. He required external postural support to play with toys; however, once he had postural stability, he brought his hands to midline, grasped using a radial palmar grasp, released toys in a container, transferred objects, and began to fit an object into a precise space. Although hand-eye coordination was emerging, he continued to have difficulty with integrating visual skills with arm and hand movements.

Evaluation

Parent interview. Jonathan ate soft foods and had begun to try some harder foods such as pretzels, ham, and apples. He took the food from a cup or spoon using active lip movements. Lip closure while chewing was fair, but not perfect, as he continued to have some food loss. He used both a munching pattern and some rotary chewing. He reverted to a vertical up-and-down munching pattern with more difficult foods (e.g., those that were hard or tough). He used a sucking pattern with pureed foods and a diagonal rotary pattern with soft foods. Jonathan demonstrated a variety of patterns of tongue movement, including tip elevation, lateralization, and beginning rolling. Jaw control was emerging; he exhibited a sustained bite pattern, and jaw stabilization increased on the cup rim. He continued to bite on the cup during drinking. The occupational therapist and Jonathan's parent implemented a program to upgrade the texture of his foods, and he made continual progress in feeding skills. Drinking thin liquids remained difficult, and his mother managed his drinking by providing some manual head and jaw support and by thickening his liquids to a nectar quality. Jonathan handled liquids better when using a straw and when taking small sips of liquid at a time. As his appetite increased and he continued to demonstrate improvements in oral skills, he showed increasing interest in self-feeding. He began to finger feed bites of sandwiches, crackers, cheese, and strips of ham or chicken.

Jonathan's mother gave him a spoon on several occasions; his first attempts at self-feeding resulted in much more food going on his face and clothes than in his mouth. His mother tried to have Jonathan self-feed in his high chair using an adult spoon and a bowl of yogurt. In spite of his lack of success, Jonathan seemed eager to try to use the spoon and often grabbed it from his mouth during feeding. The occupational therapist evaluated his feeding to help his mother develop a system for self-feeding that was efficient and began to address self-feeding as a goal in the intervention program.

Feeding observation. In the high chair, Jonathan was without foot support and had minimal trunk support. He frequently fell to one side. The therapist evaluated the self-feeding movements; he successfully scooped the yogurt, then fully abducted his shoulder and flexed his elbow to bring the spoon to his mouth. Although this motion brought the food to his mouth, Jonathan was unable to turn the spoon for entry into his mouth. His efforts to

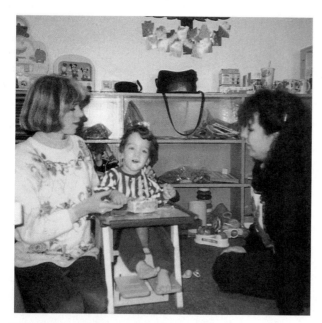

figure **15-6** Rifton chair provides a firm base of support to trunk and feet during self-feeding.

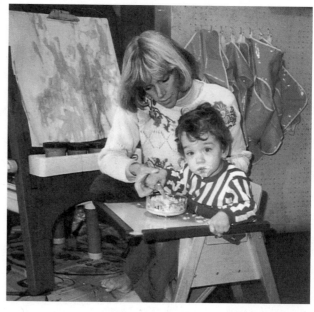

figure **15-7** Therapist supports and guides the child's hand during self-feeding using thumb on hand dorsum and finger in his palm.

get the food resulted in spillage. Although he failed to get food into his mouth, he remained highly motivated and seemed to enjoy the activity.

Intervention

The therapist adjusted Jonathan's position for self-feeding and recommended simple equipment to enhance the quality of fit between Jonathan and the desired occupation, self-feeding. Instead of feeding in the high chair, the occupational therapist suggested that he sit in the Rifton chair for self-feeding. He was stable in the Rifton chair, which had lateral supports, foot supports, and a tray that could be positioned close to his body at a height that enabled solid weight-bearing on elbows. He demonstrated his best hand and arm control in this chair (Figure 15-6). The therapist used a scoop dish with suction cups on the bottom. This bowl allowed him to obtain food without holding the bowl with his other hand. The therapist also used a small child's adapted spoon. The spoon selected was short; had a bent angle at the bowl; and had a flat, small bowl and a thick handle. Jonathan could easily handle the spoon with a radial palmar grasp and could enter it into his mouth without wrist rotation or radial deviation. Initially the therapist provided some support at his hand by entering her index finger into his hand and placing her thumb on the hand's dorsum as he grasped the spoon. The therapist's hand supported his arm and wrist movements, and she only exerted pressure when his arm movement appeared inadequate for entry into his mouth (Figure 15-7). The therapist soon eliminated this assistance. The therapist used a small padded block under his elbow, which proved to be helpful as an extra source of

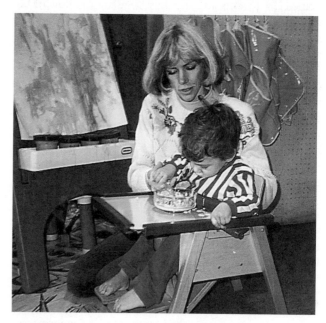

figure **15-8** Foods that are successful when first attempting self-feeding are those that stick together, are easily scooped, hold to the spoon, and taste good.

stability. Jonathan maintained his elbow on the pad and used elbow flexion to bring food to his mouth.

The therapist suggested that pudding be the first food used in feeding practice because of its cohesive, sticky texture. The therapist soon added yogurt and ice cream, which quickly became Jonathan's favorite treats (Figure 15-8).

The therapist and Jonathan's mother developed a plan to increase the fine motor skills that Jonathan needed to improve self-feeding. Activities to enhance self-feeding with the spoon included games that required forearm supination with objects held in a radial digital grasp. Examples included placing pegs vertically into a pegboard, placing peg people into a school bus or airplane, and using a toy accordion with vertically oriented handles. Jonathan performed these activities in the Rifton chair or corner chair with a tray, where he was well supported and posturally stable with feet flat. With this equipment and position, Jonathan regularly practiced self-feeding.

STUDY QUESTIONS

1. You receive a referral for a 9-month-old infant who refuses all attempts to be fed pureed baby foods. She currently takes six bottles of formula per day. Your initial evaluation indicates that she has severe tactile defensiveness of the oral area. Describe the first three activities that your would implement in intervention. Identify two recommendations that you would give to her parents.

2. You are working with a 12-year-old child who has severe motor delays and difficulty feeding. He has fair head control and poor trunk control, and he is not a candidate for self-feeding at this time. He demonstrates primitive oral movements; his jaw is unstable and moves in wide excursions, and his tongue moves in extension and retraction. He often loses food from his mouth and frequently chokes and coughs during feeding. Coughing is most frequent during drinking. Describe in detail how you would position him for feeding and what positioning devices you may use. What types of food and drink would you recommend?

3. You are the occupational therapist for a 6-year-old child with feeding difficulties. When you feed her at school, you suspect that she is aspirating some of her food and drink. List two ways that you would pursue investigating this possibility. What are two questions that you would ask her parents? What may you ask of the physician to further investigate the possibility of aspiration?

4. One of the children with whom you are working on oral feeding is demonstrating a keen interest in feeding himself. He has poor control of his upper extremities. His shoulder stability is poor, and he exhibits only a gross grasp and involuntary release. He does not yet have the ability to maintain grasp of a utensil while guiding it to his mouth. What activities may you implement to improve his ability to self-feed? What would be the first foods and eating activities that would allow him to succeed in self-feeding?

5. When a child has significant oral motor problems, often drinking is a more difficult skill to achieve than eating solid foods. Given the importance of maintaining hydration, what are three recommendations that you would make for children whose oral motor skills suggest the possibility of aspiration when drinking liquids?

References

Adams, R.C., & Snyder, P. (1998). Treatments of cerebral palsy: Making choices of intervention from an expanding menu of options. *Infants and Young Children, 10* (4), 1-22.

Bakker, T., & Woody, A. (1995). *Primary caregivers' experiences with children with feeding issues.* Unpublished research project, University of North Carolina at Chapel Hill.

Baroni, M., & Sondel, S. (1995). A collaborative model for identifying feeding and nutrition needs in early intervention. *Infants and Young Children, 8* (2), 26-36.

Barrett, K.C., & Morgan, G.A. (1995). Continuities and discontinuities in mastery motivation during infancy and toddlerhood: A conceptualization and review. In R.H. MacTurk & G.A. Morgan (Eds.), *Mastery motivation: Origins, conceptualization, and applications* (pp. 57-93). Norwood, NJ: Ablex.

Beals, D.E. (1993). Explanatory talk in low-income families' mealtime conversations. *Applied Psycholinguistics, 14,* 489-513.

Benson, J.E., & Lefton-Greif, M.A. (1994). Videofluoroscopy of swallowing in pediatric patients: A component of the total feeding evaluation. In D.N. Tuchman & R. Walter (Eds.), *Disorders of feeding and swallowing in infants and children* (pp. 187-200). San Diego: Singular Publishing Group.

Blackman, J.A., & Nelson, C.L.A. (1987). Rapid introduction or oral feeding to tube-fed patients. *Journal of Developmental and Behavioral Pediatrics, 8,* 63-66.

Brazelton, T.B. (1993). Why children and parents must play while they eat: An interview with T. Berry Brazelton. *Journal of the American Dietetic Association, 93,* 1485-1487.

Brizee, L.S., Sophos, C.M., & McLaughlin, J.F. (1990). Nutrition issues in developmental disabilities. *Infants and Young Children, 2* (3), 10-21.

Case-Smith, J. (1999). Self care strategies for children with developmental deficits. In C. Christiansen (Ed.), *Ways of living: Self-care strategies for special needs (2nd ed.)* (pp. 83-122). Bethesda, MD: AOTA.

Chamberlin, J., Henry, M.M., Roberts, J.D., Sapsford, A.L., & Courtney, S.E. (1991). An infant and toddler feeding group program. *The American Journal of Occupational Therapy, 45,* 907-911.

Clark, F., Wood, W., & Lawson, E.A. (1998). Occupational science: Occupational therapy's legacy for the 21st century. In M.E. Neisdtadt & E.B. Crepeau (Eds.), *Willard & Spackman's occupational therapy* (pp. 13-21). Philadelphia: J.B. Lippincott.

Clark, M.P., Oakland, M.J., & Brotherson, M.J. (1998). Nutrition screening for children with special health care needs. *Children's Health Care, 27,* 231-245.

Coley, I.L., & Procter, S.A. (1989). Self-maintenance activities. In P. Pratt & A. Allen (Eds.), *Occupational therapy for children* (pp. 442-456). St. Louis: Mosby.

Crist, W., Napier-Phyillips, A., McDonnell, P.,Ledwidge, J., & Beck, M. (1998). Assessing restricted diet in young children *Children's Health Care, 27* (4), 247-257.

Daniels, H., Devlieger, H., Casaer, P., & Eggermont, E. (1986). Nutritive and non-nutritive sucking in preterm infants. *Journal of Developmental Physiology, 8,* 117-121.

DeVault, M.L. (1991). *Feeding the family: The social organization of caring as gendered work.* Chicago: Chicago Press.

Edmondson, R., & Reinhartsen, D. (1998). The young child with cleft lip and palate: Intervention needs in the first three years. *Infants and Young Children, 11* (2), 12-20.

Einarsson-Backes, L., Deitz, J., Price, R., Glass, R., & Hays, R. (1994). The effect of oral support on sucking efficiency in preterm infants. *The American Journal of Occupational Therapy, 48,* 490-498.

Federal Register, 56 (235), December 6, 1991.

Fisher, A.G. (1998). Uniting practice and theory in an occupational framework. *The American Journal of Occupational Therapy, 52,* 490-498.

Gisel, E.G., Applegate-Ferrante, T., Benson, J.E., & Bosma, J.F. (1995). Effect of oral sensorimotor treatment on measures of growth, eating efficiency and aspiration in the dysphagic child with cerebral palsy. *Developmental Medicine and Child Neurology, 37,* 528-543.

Glass, R., & Wolf, L. (1998). Feeding and oral motor skills. In J. Case-Smith (Ed.), *Pediatric occupational therapy and early intervention* (pp. 225-288). Boston: Butterworth-Heineman.

Hagekull, B., & Dahl, M. (1987). Infants with and without feeding difficulties: Maternal experiences. *International Journal of Eating Disorders, 6,* 83-98.

Heriza, C. (1991). Motor development: Traditional and contemporary theories. In *Contemporary management of motor control problems.* Fredericksburg, VA: APTA.

Humphry, R. (1995). The nature and diversity of problems leading to failure to thrive. *Occupational Therapy in Health Care, 9,* 73-90.

Humphry, R., & Morrow, J. (1998). *Developmental processes behind the acquisition of occupations in self care.* Unpublished manuscript. University of North Carolina at Chapel Hill.

Humphry, R., & Thigpen-Beck, B. (1997). Caregiver role: Ideas about feeding infants and toddlers. *Occupational Therapy Journal of Research, 17,* 237-263.

Humphry, R., & Thigpen-Beck, B. (1998). Parenting values and attitudes: Views of therapists and parents. *The American Journal of Occupational Therapy, 52,* 835-843.

Klein, M.D., & Delaney, T.A. (1994). *Feeding and nutrition for the child with special needs.* Tuscon: Therapy Skill Builders.

Logemann, J.A. (1983). *Evaluation and treatment of swallowing disorders.* San Diego: College Hill Press.

Mathiowetz, V., & Haugen, J.B. (1994). Motor behavior research: Implications for therapeutic approaches to central nervous system dysfunction. *The American Journal of Occupational Therapy, 48,* 733-745.

Morris, S.E., & Klein, M.D. (1987). *Pre-feeding skills.* Tucson: Therapy Skill Builders.

Papousek, H., & Papousek, M. (1995). Intuitive parenting. In M.H. Bornsteing (Ed.), *Handbook of parenting* (Vol. 2). (pp. 117-136). Mahwah, NJ: Lawrence Erlbaum Associates.

Ramsay, M., Gisel, E.G., & Boutry, M. (1993). Non-organic failure to thrive: Growth failure secondary to feeding-skills disorder. *Developmental Medicine and Child Neurology, 35,* 285-297.

Rogers, J.C., & Holm, M.B. (1998). Evaluation of occupational performance areas. In M.E. Neistadt & E.B. Crepeau (Eds.), *Willard & Spackman's occupational therapy* (9th ed.). (pp. 185-208). Philadelphia: J.B. Lippincott.

Sanders, M.R., Patel, R.K., LeGrice, B., & Shepherd, R.W. (1993). Children with persistent feeding difficulties: An observational analysis of the feeding interactions of problem and non-problem eaters. *Health Psychology, 12,* 64-73.

Schuberth, L.M. (1994). The role of occupational therapy in diagnosis and management. In D.N. Tuchman & R. Walter (Eds.), *Disorders of feeding and swallowing in infants and children* (pp. 115-130). San Diego: Singular Publishing Group.

Shauster, H., & Dwyer, J. (1996). Transition for tube feedings to feedings by mouth in children: Preventing eating dysfunction. *The Journal of the American Dietetic Association, 96* (3), 277-281.

Thigpen-Beck, B., & Dovenitz, S. (1995). *The values, beliefs, and attitudes of occupational therapists regarding selected baby behaviors associated with eating.* Unpublished research project. University of North Carolina at Chapel Hill.

Tuchman, D.B. (1994). Physiology of the swallowing apparatus. In D.N. Tuchman & R. Walter (Eds.), *Disorders of feeding and swallowing in infants and children* (pp. 1-25). San Diego: Singular Publishing Group.

Wolf, L.S., & Glass, R.P. (1992). *Feeding and swallowing disorders in infancy: Assessment and management.* Tucson: Therapy Skills Builders.

Yokochi, K. (1997). Oral motor patterns during feeding in severely physically disabled children. *Brain & Development, 19* (8), 552-555.

Zerilli, K.S., Stefans, V.A., & DiPietro, M.A. (1990). Protocol for the use of videofluoroscopy in pediatric swallowing dysfunction. *The American Journal of Occupational Therapy, 44* (5), 441-446.

chapter **16**

Self-Care and Adaptations for Independent Living

Jayne Shepherd

Instrumental activities
  of daily living
Performance context
Compensatory
  approach
Grading techniques
Backward chaining
Forward chaining
Cues
Prompts

Assistive devices
Environmental
  adaptations
Adaptive positioning

■ CHAPTER OBJECTIVES

1. Heighten awareness of the effect of temporal, cultural, social, and physical contexts on a child's performance and parental expectations for self-care occupations.
2. Identify the intrinsic variables and performance components that may affect a child's self-care performance.
3. Identify evaluation procedures and methods in self-care and independent living occupations that target child and family preferences for intervention.
4. Describe general and specific intervention strategies and approaches.
5. Describe the selection and modification of equipment, techniques, and environments for selected occupations in self-care and instrumental activities of daily living (IADLs).

Self-care tasks and *instrumental activities of daily living* (IADLs) encompass some of the most important tasks that children learn as they mature. Basic self-care tasks include grooming, bathing, toileting, dressing, feeding, achieving functional mobility and communicating. As a child matures, he or she learns to perform these tasks in socially appropriate ways. Other self-care tasks may be assumed, such as taking his or her own medications, maintaining health (e.g., exercise, nutrition, and visiting health care professionals), taking care of personal devices, responding to emergencies, and expressing sexual needs (AOTA, 1994).

IADLs are more complex ADLs needed to function independently in home, school, community, and work environments (Brown et. al., 1991; Spencer, Murphy, Bean, & Schelly, 1991). IADLs include home management skills such as caring for clothing, cleaning, preparing meals, shopping, managing money, maintaining the household, and following safety procedures. Independence in IADLs determines an individual's ability to live independently in the community.

This chapter discusses the dynamic interaction between child characteristics and the temporal and environmental contexts in which a child performs self-care tasks and IADLs. Assessment methods, approaches, and strategies for improving performance in self-care tasks and IADLs are described. Typical development, problems, and adaptations for toileting, dressing, bathing, grooming, and performing other related self-care tasks are given (feeding is discussed in Chapter 15). IADL occupations are discussed in relation to performance in home, community, and school environments. Examples of adaptations to physical and social environments are given while considering cultural influences.

■ IMPORTANCE OF DEVELOPING SELF-CARE AND IADL SKILLS

The foundations for self-care begin in infancy and are refined throughout the various stages of development. As unique individuals living within certain contexts, children develop these skills at varying rates and have occasional regression and unpredictable behaviors. Cultural values, social routines, and the physical environment influence the timing of when children assume self-care and IADL skills. Overall, society and families assume that children develop increasing levels of competence and self-reliance to meet their own self-care and IADL needs. Growth and maturity allow the child to participate within various roles and environments with decreasing levels of adult supervision.

When a child is born with a disability or acquires a disability, parental and child expectations for self-care and daily living independence are modified. Occupational therapists are instrumental in helping parents and children learn how to modify tasks and routines so that children use self-care and IADL occupations daily. Active participation in a child's self-care has several benefits, including improving sensorimotor skills (e.g., strength, endurance, range of motion, and coordination) and cognitive skills (e.g., sequencing, concept formation, and memory) and mastery of tasks that are meaningful to the child. As the child learns new tasks, he or she develops a sense of accomplishment and pride in his or her abilities. The child becomes responsible for developing and maintaining routines that prevent further illness (e.g., checking skin conditions, maintaining cleanliness of self and environment, and cooking nutritious meals) and meeting role expectations for community living. This increasing independence also gives parents, teachers, siblings, and other caregivers more time and energy for other tasks.

■ FACTORS AFFECTING PERFORMANCE

Child characteristics and the performance context influence the child's opportunity and ability to successfully participate in self-care occupations. Child characteristics include sensorimotor, cognitive, and psychosocial performance components. The performance context consists of two areas that are interwoven with each other: the temporal context and the environment context (Dunn,

Brown & McGuigan, 1994). The temporal context relates to the time period in which the occupation occurs. Temporal context variables include the child's chronologic age, developmental stage, disability status, and place in the life cycle within the family. The environment context includes the physical, social, and cultural variables within the environment.

Child Characteristics and Performance Components

Occupational therapy intervention to increase self-care and IADL function considers what the child and family value and the context in which the tasks occur. The level of independence, safety, and adequacy of skill performance to the child and family determine if the child's sensorimotor, cognitive, and psychosocial abilities are adequate to perform self-care occupations.

The child has specific skills and limitations that affect self-care and IADL performance. For example, children with tactile defensiveness may cry during dressing and refuse to dress despite being cognitively and motorically able to dress themselves. They may dislike the textures, or they have learned to cry for their mother's attention (psychosocial). Children with visual impairments may use the sensations in their hands (tactile and proprioceptive) in brushing their hair even though they cannot see it. A child with cerebral palsy may not have the postural control to sit up during dressing but may have the cognitive skills (e.g., problem solving and sequencing), perceptual skills (e.g., right-left discrimination and figure-ground), and gross motor skills to dress in a side-lying position.

Interest level, self-confidence, and motivation are strong forces that help children attain levels of performance that are either above or below expectations. Children with mental retardation, traumatic brain injury, or multiple disabilities experience difficulties in coordination, initiative, attention span, sequencing, memory, safety, and the ability to learn and generalize skills across environments. However, with the proper instruction and opportunity (Kellegrew, 1998), self-care tasks and IADLs are sometimes the tasks that these children can perform most competently (Orelove & Sobsey, 1996). Adaptations to the activities, equipment, and the environment assist students in participating in self-care occupations. In general, children can improve their abilities in self-care occupations if they are highly motivated and are given the opportunity to practice self-care within their every day environments.

Developmental and chronologic age

Children typically develop self-care and IADL skills in a sequence, achieving specific skills as overall competency increases. The sequence of self-care development helps therapists and families form realistic expectations for children; and it helps determine the appropriate timing for teaching tasks. For example, in the Western culture, if a 2-year-old child cannot dress independently, intervention is not appropriate because most children are not independent in dressing until 5 or 6 years of age. By the same token, if a 14-year-old child has never crossed the street alone, the therapist may focus on this community mobility skill as an essential objective.

By considering the child's age, therapists can also determine when it is time to stop working on specific skills. For example, 6-year-old Tilly had occupational therapy for 5 years to increase lip closure and develop a more efficient suck-swallow pattern. If she did not learn this skill in the past 5 years, what are her chances of learning it this year? It may be time for the therapist to work on self-feeding strategies or an IADL skill, such as operating an appliance with a switch for meal preparation.

Therapists need to be aware of the developmental stage of maturation when choosing an activity. Planning self-care and IADL intervention for an adolescent is different than planning for a 2-year-old child. The therapist needs to give both children choices, but the adolescent needs more privacy and autonomy, and self-care and IADL needs have a different focus. The therapist may intervene for skills in personal grooming skills, functional graphic communication, community mobility, medication routine, emergency responses, sexual expression, homemaking skills, money management (allowance), and community skills. The therapist may focus the intervention for the 2-year-old child on feeding, bathing, dressing, and playing.

Disability status

The disability or health status of the child can affect his or her opportunity and ability to perform self-care tasks and IADLs (Brown & Gordon, 1987). Disability status includes when the onset of disability occurred, the acute or chronic effects of the disability, and the prognosis for recovery. The therapist considers the child's capacity for learning and ability to complete difficult tasks safely. Pain, fatigue, the amount of time it takes the child to complete the task, and the child's satisfaction with his or her performance influence choice of self-care occupations (Holm, Rogers, & James, 1998).

Children who are acutely ill or who have multiple disabilities with numerous procedures done throughout the day (e.g., tube feeding, tracheostomy care, and bowel and bladder care) may not have time or energy to work on self-care tasks and IADLs. For example: Jenna, a 10-year-old child with a C6 spinal cord injury and quadriplegia, can dress herself independently within a 45-minute period, but she and her family prefer that someone else dress her so that she has more energy for school tasks.

Children with progressive or terminal diseases may complete self-care tasks with modifications or complete assistance (e.g., later stages of acquired immunodeficiency syndrome [AIDS] or Duchenne's muscular dystrophy). These children and children with multiple disabilities may physically be unable to do all or any part of self-care tasks, but they can direct others on how to care for them. Children with psychosocial problems may cease doing normal self-care and IADL routines because of depression or anxiety or as an effort to have control over their environment. Occupational therapists use their medical knowledge and the preferences of the child and family to clinically judge when and what type of intervention is appropriate.

Placement in the family life cycle

The family is influential in establishing the role expectations and the routines for the child. Parents or other family members are typically the primary caregivers who are responsible for the child's daily living needs and who are with the child most consistently. Families vary in their ability and availability to assist and encourage the child to perform self-care tasks and IADLs. This ability often depends on where the family and child are in the family life cycle and their ability to be flexible in everyday routines (Turnbull & Turnbull, 1997).

Occupational therapists need to be aware of the child's and family's place in the life cycle because self-care and IADL issues change accordingly (Turnbull & Turnbull, 1997). In early childhood (birth to 3 years of age), feeding is usually of utmost importance because infants depend completely on their parents for nutrition. Parents often seek instruction on how to dress and bathe the infant at this stage. By 3 years of age the child's self-feeding, dressing, and toileting skills may become issues for parents.

When the child enters school by 6 years of age, self-care occupations (e.g., functional mobility within the school environment), dressing (especially outerwear), toileting, socialization with peers, grooming (e.g., washing hands and face), and functional communication (e.g., writing, drawing, and expressing needs) become increasingly important. Simple household tasks, such as taking out the trash, setting and clearing the table, making a simple sandwich, washing or dusting countertops, and following safety precautions, are appropriate goals. Older siblings may become more aware of and sensitive to their brother's or sister's disability, and the therapist may ask them to help their sibling learn self-care tasks and perform more household tasks.

During adolescence (13 to 21 years of age), increasing independence in self-care tasks and IADLs often determines if a child will "fit in" with peers or be successful in obtaining a job outside of the school environment. The child takes on increased responsibility for personal device care, medication routines, and health maintenance routines. During this stage, families further investigate current community resources as they think about future living arrangements, vocational opportunities, and the availability of other recreational activities for their child (Turnbull & Turnbull, 1997). Parent issues may focus on the child's ability to express sexual needs, be safe within many environments, and respond to emergency situations appropriately. The therapist may address additional skills during this stage, including caring for clothing, preparing meals, shopping, managing money, and maintaining a household.

During adolescence, concerns and goals for therapy may differ between parents and their children. Both may be concerned about the adolescent's independence in self-care tasks and IADLs; however, adolescents may have more concerns about fitting in with a social group (McGavin, 1998). Children with severe disabilities who require maximum physical assistance in ADLs become a great concern to parents as they approach adulthood. For the first time, parents may not have the physical strength to handle the daily care needs of their child.

Performance Context

Within the context of performing self-care occupations, the social, cultural, and physical environments influence the initiation and completion of tasks. Children in early and middle childhood often perform self-care tasks and IADLs in different settings. The four primary settings that children experience are home, school, community, and work. Once the occupational therapist understands the contexts in which occupation occurs, he or she may choose intervention strategies to be congruent with the environment or to change the aspects of the environment that are barriers to the child's performance of self-care tasks and IADLs.

The social environment, family, other caregivers, and peers provide encouragement and support self-care independence. They also hold certain expectations regarding the child's self-care occupations.

Family

The number of members in the family and the family expectations, roles, and routines for managing daily living needs (Turnbull & Turnbull, 1997) influence the child's development of self-care and IADL skills. Large families may assign different members to perform or help with specific self-care tasks for a child with a disability, whereas in other families the parent may be the sole person responsible for the daily living needs of their child. For example, parents living on a farm may expect their child to get up at dawn, put on overalls and boots, complete chores like feeding the animals, receive home schooling, and help sell eggs to augment the family in-

come. The parents and therapist must discuss these role expectations, personal preferences, and routines so that they can choose appropriate and meaningful assessment and intervention strategies.

The therapist considers personal characteristics of family members, such as temperament, coping skills, flexibility, and health status, when planning treatment (Turnbull & Turnbull, 1997) (see Chapter 5). Family members' abilities influence the kind of routines and assistance they provide, and the therapist needs to choose activities, techniques, equipment, and assistive devices carefully and collaboratively. Parents may have different expectations for children who have a disability. For example, the mother may place her child in the "mothering" role if she is depressed and unable to get out of bed to cook dinner. Another child may not learn how to complete yard chores if his or her father is disorganized and has not structured the tasks for the child. Parents with mental retardation or mental health problems may need to see a therapist modeling to learn how to cue and structure tasks for their children (Turnbull & Turnbull, 1997). Parents with physical problems may need instructions and practice in using specific techniques and assistive devices safely.

Other caregivers

Children grow up with assistance, support, and guidance of many caregivers. Other caregivers such as teachers, aides, nurses, attendants, and child care providers are part of the social environment. They have short-term involvement, and their role is determined by the nature of the program. The number of caregivers available in a particular environment and the child-adult ratio affect the relationship between the caregiver and the child. Interventions should be simple in situations where time is at a premium and multiple caregivers are involved.

Therapists, parents, teachers, and other professionals may vary in their expectations for the child because each has a different viewpoint. For example, in a rehabilitation program, the nurses' expectations for self-dressing may not include the child picking out his or her own clothes and getting them from the closet before dressing. Therefore the therapist collaborates with the family and other caregivers to discuss expectations, bring them into perspective, and establish them on a consistent basis. As a consultant, the therapist demonstrates specific methods for promoting self-care occupations and makes broad suggestions that allow caregivers to use their own ideas to incorporate self-care into everyday routines (Kellegrew, 1998).

Peers

Peers can positively or negatively influence a child's ability and willingness to perform tasks. For example, peers at school are often fascinated with assistive devices, such as adapted spoons, augmentative communication devices, wheelchairs, or computers, used by the child with a physical disability. This interest may encourage the child to use the device and may begin friendships. Peers also can make fun of a child's method of dressing or use of an adaptive button hook. This may discourage the child from using adaptive methods and interacting with peers. Social interactions and networks of peers or friends in school, home, recreational, and community environments can be extremely powerful in the success of an intervention strategy.

Social routines

An analysis of social routines helps determine when and how self-care tasks and IADLs are taught. Within home, school, community, and recreational environments, routines may differ significantly, and children need to adapt to these differences. The variation in routine may confuse or disorganize children with mental retardation, autism, or attention deficit disorders but may be motivating to children without attention, sensory, or cognitive problems. School-based and early intervention therapists need to be aware of the social routines so that they can choose appropriate times to teach tasks. When tasks are taught or practiced at times and places where they naturally occur, they more quickly become part of the child's behavior repertoire (Brown et. al., 1991). For example, school-based therapists may meet children at the bus to work on functional mobility skills and as the child removes his or her coat to work on dressing skills. When tasks are embedded throughout all environments, children receive multiple opportunities to practice skills and learn how to use the natural cues within the environment to modify their behavior. The therapist considers social routines and norms within a community when planning individual or group therapy. Children usually practice toileting, dressing, and bathing skills individually, but they may be able to cook or clean together as a cooperative effort within the school environment.

Cultural environment

As therapists work with children and families in an array of service provision models, they need to be aware of their own and of others' cultural beliefs, customs, activity patterns, and expectations for performance in self-care tasks and IADLs (Lynch & Hanson, 1998). Occupational therapists usually become involved with a family because someone else believed that their services were needed. The family may not welcome these services as the therapist asks personal questions about a child's and family's self-maintenance occupations and routines. Lynch and Hanson (1998) edited a useful guide to help interventionists develop skills in working with families and chil-

dren from different cultures. Therapists need to ask parents questions and use community resources to better understand the cultural backgrounds of their clients.

Cultural expectations of the family, caregivers, and social group as a whole may determine behavior standards. Family beliefs, values, and attitudes about child rearing, autonomy, and self-reliance influence how parents perceive self-care tasks and IADLs. In Anglo-European cultures, parents are usually concerned about children meeting developmental milestones (Hanson, 1998), yet other cultures (e.g., Hispanic) may be more relaxed about milestone attainment (Zuniga, 1998). This basic difference may determine whether parents see the importance of intervention. In some adult-centered Indian cultures, parents expect children to be independent at an early age. The parents and society reward the children for taking the initiative to do chores around the house or community. In other cultures, parents may give children more time to be childlike and not push them to do adult-like skills and chores until a later age (Willis, 1998).

Social role expectations and routines are influenced by culture. Many Anglo-European parents encourage children to become independent and self-reliant (Hanson, 1998). In contrast, many Hispanic (Zuniga, 1998) and Asian (Chan, 1998) families may encourage dependency or interdependency within the family. Routines for dressing, feeding, bathing, going to bed, and carrying out household tasks vary among cultural groups.

Culture also influences the type and availability of activities, tools, equipment, and materials that a child uses to perform self-care tasks or IADLs. Customs and beliefs may determine how parents dress their children, what they feed their children, what utensils they use in the kitchen, how they prepare and store food, what type of bed they use, or how they meet health care needs. Economic conditions, geographic location, and opportunities for education and employment can influence the resources and supports that are available to families.

Physical environment

Several barriers within the physical environment can hinder the child's development of self-care and IADL skills, including building construction, terrain, furniture, and objects within the environment. Inaccessible buildings and rooms crowded with furniture limit how children in wheelchairs move throughout the environment. Differences in the terrain or room surface also affect mobility. For example, a child who can run outdoors on an asphalt playground may trip and fall inside when walking on a rug. Other physical characteristics that the therapist assesses relate to the type of furniture, objects, or assistive devices in the environment and whether they are usable and accessible. This includes the type of equipment, household items, clothing, or toys. Sensory aspects of the physical environment often influence performance (e.g., the type of lighting, noise level, visual stimulation, and tactile or vestibular input of tasks). In particular, children with autism or attention-deficit hyperactivity disorder (ADHD) can be overly sensitive to and distracted by the sensory aspects of an environment.

■ EVALUATION OF SELF-CARE AND IADL SKILLS

Families and their children have key roles in determining which evaluation procedures to use. By collaboratively working with families, therapists learn about the characteristics of the child, the contexts in which task performance occurs, and the expectations and concerns of the family. When children get older and are able to communicate, the therapist includes them in determining what areas of self-care and IADL skills are important to them. When the therapist gives the parents and children a chance to select or refuse evaluations and choose where the evaluation is done, by whom, and when, the family is often more vested in the results (Giangreco, Cloninger, & Iverson, 1997). Therapists also have a better understanding of the contexts in which the child performs occupations.

Evaluation Methods

Interviews, inventories, and structured and naturalistic observations are evaluation methods that therapists typically use to measure self-care and IADL performance in occupational therapy. The therapist can use these methods alone or in combination to develop intervention strategies and measure outcomes of treatment (Snell & Brown, 1993). Table 16-1 lists instruments that assess children's self-care and IADL skills.

Self-care and IADL independence involves the child obtaining (setting up) and using supplies to complete a particular task. The therapist generally rates performance according to the child's ability to set up and complete a task and may assess performance by grading the child's level of independence. Table 16-2 gives one example of how the therapist may rate a child's independence in bathing. The therapist can use a system for grading the child's level of independence with any of the methods or purposes discussed in the following section.

Interviews and inventories

Interviews in which the therapist asks the interviewee (e.g., parents, children, teachers, and other significant caregivers) questions about the child's abilities, environmental characteristics, or goals and dreams can be informal or unstructured. Inventories are questionnaires or interviews that ask the rater to answer questions about

the child's ability to perform self-care tasks and IADLs and perhaps about future goals and concerns for the child. The therapist may use interviewing methods and inventory methods together to obtain useful information about how the child performs within different contexts. These assessments depend on the ability of the person to accurately answer the questions.

Structured and naturalistic observation

Structured observation occurs when the therapist gives the child a task to do and then rates the child's performance. The therapist can perform this testing in any environment with various materials. For example, while a child with a traumatic brain injury is receiving occupational therapy as an outpatient, the therapist may take the child to the occupational therapy kitchen and ask him or her to make a sandwich. The child's performance on this evaluation may vary significantly because of unfamiliarity of materials and equipment in the occupational therapy kitchen. Structured observation provides information regarding how well the child performs the task in a structured situation, but it does not determine if the child will begin the task at the appropriate time or perform the task in different environments (e.g., will the child make a sandwich for lunch when left alone?).

In *naturalistic* or *ecological observation,* the therapist gathers information in the typical or natural setting in which the activity occurs. Usually the therapist completes a task analysis to identify the component processes and subskills of an activity. In a naturalistic task analysis, the therapist evaluates the child's ability to do the task itself and the physical, social, and cultural characteristics of the environment. For example, when observing a child's ability to use the toilet at school, the therapist notes accessibility barriers, the sensory characteristics of the environment, typical classroom routines and expectations for toileting, and any cultural aspects of the toileting process (e.g., type of clothing the child is wearing). By understanding these contexts the therapist can choose intervention strategies more appropriately. Environmental observations can be time consuming, but they provide an abundance of information when used in a team effort. The therapist also examines each component or subskill of the task and notes steps that the child takes to complete the task. Snell and Vogtle (2000) suggested that task analyses are best if steps are sequenced logically and the size of each step is similar in size to the other steps. In addition to performance, the therapist identifies the necessary amount of assistance and modifications.

Ecological or environmentally referenced assessments are appropriate for all children and are particularly useful for children with moderate to severe disabilities who have difficulty generalizing tasks from one environment to another (Orelove & Sobsey, 1996; Sailor et. al., 1986; York-Barr, Rainforth, & Locke, 1996). A *top-down ap-*

| table 16-1 | *Self-Care and Instrumental Activities of Daily Living (IADL) Assessments for Children and Adolescents* | | | |

Instrument, Author, Publisher	Interview/ Inventory	Observation	Age Range	Description
AAMR Adaptive Behavior Scales (ABS) (Lambert, Windmiller, Cole, & Figueroa, 1975) American Association on Mental Deficiency 5201 Connecticut Avenue, NW Washington, DC 20015	X	X	4 years and up	• ABS is a standardized, criterion-referenced measure for adaptive behaviors in 10 domains, with 7 domains related to IADLs (independent functioning, economic activity, numbers and time, domestic self-direction, responsibility, socialization, and vocational and recreational). • Maladaptive behaviors are measured in 14 domains. • ABS is useful for children with moderate to severe disabilities.
Assessment of Motor Processing Skills (AMPS) (Fisher, 1994) Unpublished manual Dr. Anne Fisher Department of Occupational Therapy Colorado State University 100 Humanities Building Fort Collins, CO 80523	X	X	Child to adult	• AMPS is a criterion-referenced test for IADL tasks that assesses the underlying motor and process skills used to perform the task. • Clients can choose five to six IADL tasks that they want to perform (56 possible) as they are videotaped. • Examiners need to be trained; examiner ratings are calibrated. • AMPS appears to be useful for all ages and disabilities. • AMPS for performing school tasks is in research phase.
Battelle Developmental Inventory (BDI) (Newborg, Stock, Wnek, Guidubaldi, & Szinicki, 1988) Riverside Publishing 425 Spring Lake Drive Itasca, IL 60143-2079	X	X	Birth to 8 years	• The ADL domain includes grooming, toilet hygiene, dressing, and eating. • The evaluator can use an in-depth assessment or a screening format.
Carolina Curriculum for Preschoolers with Special Needs (Johnson-Martin, Attermeier, & Hacker, 1990) Paul Brookes Publishing Co. P.O. Box 10624 Baltimore, MD 21285	X	X	3-6 years	• Self-care is one of five domains measured. • The Carolina Curriculum includes sequences in responsibility, self-concept, interpersonal skills, and self-help. • The Carolina Curriculum does not include psychometric testing.

Continued

table 16-1   Self-Care and Instrumental Activities of Daily Living (IADL) Assessments for Children and Adolescents—cont'd

Instrument, Author, Publisher	Interview/ Inventory	Observation	Age Range	Description
Choosing Options and Accomodations for Children (2nd ed.). (Giangreco, Cloninger, & Iverson, 1998) Paul Brookes Publishing Co. P.O. Box 10624 Baltimore, MD 21285	X	X	3 to 21 years	• This is a curriculum-referenced, transdisciplinary team assessment and curriculum with four domains: personal management, community, home, and vocational. • Each evaluator scores skills and gives a potential priority and rank. • This is for children with moderate, severe, or profound disabilities but has been used with younger children with mild disabilities.
Functional Independence Measure (FIM) (Uniform Data System for Medical Rehabilitation, 1993) The State University of New York University at Buffalo Buffalo, NY 14214	X	X	8 years to adult	• FIM is a functional outcome measure for clients with physical disabilities. • Six domains are assessed (self-care, mobility, locomotion, sphincter control, communication, and social cognition), and there are 18 subdomains. • FIM uses a 7-point ordinal scale to measure the level of independence. • FIM is norm-referenced.
Functional Skills Screening Inventory (FSSI) (Becker, Schur, Paoletti-Schelp, & Hammer, 1986) Functional Resources Enterprises, Inc. 2743 Trail of the Madrones Austin, TX 78746	X	X	6 years and above	• FSSI is a criterion-referenced test of adaptive behavior. • The evaluator assesses self-care, independent living, vocational, recreational, and social emotional domains with five other domains. • FSSI includes optional computer scoring, visual profiles, and identification of priorities. • FSSI is appropriate for children with moderate to severe disabilities.
Hawaii Early Learning Profile (HELP) (Furuno et. al., 1984) VORT Corporation P.O. Box 11132 Palo Alto, CA 94306	X	X	Birth to 3 years	• HELP is a curriculum-referenced assessment. • Self-care is one of six domains. • HELP includes an inventory of developmental skills, an activity guide, and other materials related to parents with disabilities. • HELP does not include psychometric testing.

table 16-1	Self-Care and Instrumental Activities of Daily Living (IADL) Assessments for Children and Adolescents—cont'd				

Instrument, Author, Publisher	Interview/ Inventory	Observation	Age Range	Description
Klein-Bell Activities of Daily Living Scale (Klein & Bell, 1979) Educational Resources University of Washington Seattle, Washington Results with children: Law & Usher. (1988). Validation of the Klein-Bell Activities of Daily Living Scale with children. *Canadian Journal of Occupational Therapy, 55,* 63-68.		X	1 year to adult	• This scale is a criterion-referenced assessment that evaluates six domains: dressing, mobility, elimination, bathing and hygiene, eating, and emergency communication. • The evaluator scores 170 items as achieved or not achieved and rates according to difficulty of task. • The final score yields a percentage for overall independence. • Limited-reliability and predictive-validity studies have been completed.
Pediatric Evaluation of Disability Inventory (PEDI) (Haley, Coster, Ludlow, Haltiwanger, & Andrellos, 1992) Psychological Corporation Therapy Skill Builders 555 Academic Court San Antonio, TX 78204-2498	X		6 months to 7 years	• PEDI is a normative, judgment-based (parent interview) outcome measurement • Three domains (self-care, mobility, and social function) are assessed using two subscales: functional skills (197 tasks) and caregiver assistance (20 tasks).
Vineland Adaptive Behavior Scales (Sparrow, Balla, & Cicchetti, 1984) American Guidance Service Circle Pines, MN 55014	X		Birth to adult	• These scales involve norm-referenced evaluation. • These scales assess social competency with behavioral observations in ADL, communication, socialization, and motor domains. • These scales assess an optional maladaptive behavior domain for children 5 years of age and older.

Continued

table 16-1	**Self-Care and Instrumental Activities of Daily Living (IADL) Assessments for Children and Adolescents—cont'd**			
Instrument, Author, Publisher	**Interview/ Inventory**	**Observation**	**Age Range**	**Description**
				• Three versions are available: interview/ survey form, interview/expanded form, and classroom/teacher form (3 years to 12 years, 11 months of age). • These scales are appropriate for students with or without disabilities.
WeeFIM (Functional Independence Measure for Children) (Hamilton & Granger, 1991) WeeFIM Research Foundation of the State University of New York University at Buffalo Buffalo, NY 14214	X	X	6 months to 6 years	• WeeFIM is a functional evaluation for children with physical disabilities. • Six domains (self-care [grooming, dressing, and feeding], mobility, locomotion, sphincter control, communication, and social cognition) and 18 subdomains are assessed. • WeeFIM is a direct adaptation of the Functional Independence Measure (FIM) for adults. • WeeFIM is undergoing standardization procedures.

proach considers the contexts in which the child performs valued occupations, in addition to what skills the child can or cannot perform (Bryze & Curtin, 1993; Coster, 1998; Trombly, 1995). The therapist asks the parent and child what they want or need to do. Then the therapist considers the environments where the task occurs, the task components, and the child's skills. The therapist then identifies specific areas within the environment and determines the components of the task. The therapist compares the requirements of an identified task with the child's actual performance of the components of the task. The therapist identifies and prioritizes the discrepancies between the child's current abilities and those skills needed to perform in the environment.

Evaluation for Program Planning

Team members who share the responsibility for the assessment process typically use curriculum-referenced or guided assessments in settings like early intervention or school system practice. Self-care is often one area of the assessment. Therapists may use interview, inventories, direct testing, or environmental observation methods for these assessments. The Carolina Curriculum for Preschoolers with Special Needs (Johnson-Martin, Jens, Attermeier, & Hacker, 1991) and the Hawaii Early Learning

Profile (Furuno, O'Reilly, Hosaka, Zeisloft, & Allman, 1994) are typical curriculum-referenced assessments used in early intervention. Others are listed in Table 16-1.

Giangreco, Cloninger, and Iverson (1997) developed a useful transdisciplinary, curriculum-based assessment and guide, *Choosing Options and Accommodations for Children (COACH)*. Therapists use COACH to assess school-age children with moderate to severe disabilities and to help plan inclusive educational goals with a family prioritization interview and environmental observations. The therapist identifies priorities, outcomes, and needed supports for specific environments and across environments in the areas of communication, socialization, personal management, leisure and recreation, and applied academics. Team members plan goals together and write interdisciplinary goals on the child's educational plan.

Measurement of Outcome

Within the past decade, professionals in the fields of rehabilitation and occupational therapy have developed universal assessments to measure the outcomes of self-care tasks and IADLs. In rehabilitation there are few functional outcome measures appropriate for use with children and adolescents. The Functional Independence Measure (FIM) is a universal assessment tool developed

table 16-2 *Example of Rating Self-Care Skill Independence when Using a Task Analysis*

Levels of Independence	Definition	Bathing Example
Independent	Child does all of tasks, including setup	Child gets out needed supplies and equipment; bathes, rinses and dries self without assistance
Independent with setup	After someone sets up task, child does all of task	Caregiver places bathtub seat in tub and organizes bathing supplies; child bathes, rinses, and dries self without assistance
Supervision	Child performs task by self but is unsafe to be left alone; may need verbal cueing or physical prompts for 1% to 24% of task	Child bathes, rinses, and dries self without assistance but needs monitoring when getting in and out of tub and reaching lower extremities because of poor balance and judgment
Minimal assistance or skillful	Child does 51% to 75% of task independently but needs physical assistance or other cueing for at least 25% of task	Child bathes and rinses body parts independently; needs physical assistance getting in and out of tub and is cued to monitor water temperature and dry body parts
Moderate assistance or 26% to 50% partial participation	Child does 26% to 50% of task independently but needs physical assistance or other cueing for at least 50% of task	Child adjusts water temperature and washes and rinses face, torso, and upper extremities independently; needs physical assistance getting in and out of tub and washing and rinsing lower extremities and back
Maximal assistance or 1% to 25% partial participation	Child does 1% to 25% of task independently but needs physical assistance or other cueing for 75% of task	Child independently washes, rinses, and dries face but needs verbal cues to wash torso; needs physical assistance getting in and out of tub and washing other body parts
Dependent	Child is unable to do any of task	Caregvier physically picks up child, places in tub, and washes, rinses, and dries child's body parts; child does not lift body parts to be washed or dried

Adapted from Trombly, C.A., & Quintana, L.A. (1989). Activities of daily living. In C.A. Trombly (Ed.), *Occupational therapy for physical dysfunction* (3rd ed.). (p. 387). Baltimore: Williams and Wilkins.

for adolescents and adults. Therapists use the FIM for Children (WeeFIM) (Hamilton & Granger, 1991) and the Pediatric Evaluation of Disabilities Inventory (Haley, Coster, Ludlow, Haltiwanger, & Andrellos, 1992) with children 6 years of age and younger (see Table 16-1). The FIM and WeeFIM are limited in their sensitivity to children's progress because the rehabilitation team rates the 18 tasks.

The Assessment of Motor Processing Skills (AMPS) (Fisher, 1994) is an assessment tool that considers occupational performance within various environments. Therapists can use it with adolescents and adults with different cultural backgrounds and an array of disabilities (Bryze & Curtin, 1993; Fisher, 1994). In the AMPS, the therapist gives the adolescent a list of approximately 56 ADLs and chooses five to six tasks for the adolescent to perform. The therapist assesses process and motor skills, and results help the therapist predict what other ADLs the adolescent may or may not be able to perform. The AMPS tasks use a top-down approach to evaluating skills (Bryze & Curtin, 1993) and give a comprehensive view of how the child is functioning within performance contexts.

The Canadian Occupational Performance Measure (COPM) (Law et. al., 1994) assesses a client's perception of his or her self-care, productivity, and leisure occupations. The COPM provides a framework for children and families to identify how they are performing in everyday occupations and environments and how satisfied they are with their performance. Personal care, functional mobility, and community management are the areas discussed in self-care performance. The child identifies his or her most important concern and rates his or her performance and satisfaction with the task of concern, helping him or her prioritize intervention goals (McGavin, 1998).

■ INTERVENTION STRATEGIES AND APPROACHES

Intervention procedures consider the child's characteristics and performance skills in relation to temporal and environmental contexts. Therapists need to be sensitive to parents' and other caregivers' needs and concerns. Therapists must listen, give reassurance, involve parents in making observations, and engage them in problem solving. When planning treatment for children with performance problems in self-care tasks and IADLs, the therapist needs to answer the following questions (Brollier, Shepherd, & Markley, 1994; Snell, 1994).

1. What self-care tasks and IADLs are *useful* in current and future contexts?
2. What are the *preferences* of the child or the family?
3. Are the tasks *age appropriate* (used by peers without disabilities)?
4. Is it *realistic* to expect the child to perform or master this task? Can he or she learn it and, if so, how quickly?
5. What *alternative way* can the child use to perform tasks (e.g., methods or assistive technology)?
6. Does learning this task *improve the child's health and safety?*
7. Do *cultural issues* influence how tasks are taught?
8. Can the task be assessed, taught, and *practiced in a variety of environments?*

Therapists can use various approaches to improve self-care and IADL skills in children, including (1) developmental, (2) remedial, (3) compensatory, and (4) educational approaches. Therapists often use a combination of these approaches and various theoretic orientations to help children participate in self-care occupations. Table 16-3 gives examples of these four approaches and possible theoretic orientations for the therapist to use when teaching a child to button his or her shirt. These approaches are discussed throughout each area of self-care tasks and IADLs in later sections of the chapter.

Developmental Approach

The therapist may use a developmental approach to teach self-care tasks to children. Therapists consider the child's developmental and chronologic age and plan treatment according to a typical developmental sequence. In this approach the therapist teaches underlying performance components (e.g., fine motor coordination and tactile discrimination). This approach helps therapists select skills to target in intervention and gives parents some expectations for skill development (Kramer & Hinojosa, 1999), but it rarely considers the contexts in which self-care occupations occur. A developmental approach is useful for the therapist when working with infants and preschoolers with mild disabilities, but therapists use it cautiously because it assumes that children learn skills in a developmental sequence and that certain skills are necessary precursors to higher-level skills.

Many children with developmental disabilities do not learn or acquire tasks the same way that their peers do, nor do they learn tasks in the same typical developmental sequence (Orelove & Sobsey, 1996; Snell & Vogtle, 2000). Their developmental age may be significantly below their chronologic age, yet they are able to perform higher-level skills when taught skills in everyday environments (Sailor et. al., 1986). For example, 15-year-old Jimmy is functioning at a 3-year-old level in sensorimotor and cognitive skills. However, with adaptive aids and techniques and practice in his home environment, he is independent in bathing, dressing, grooming, toileting, and achieving functional mobility.

Remedial Approach

In a remedial approach, therapists identify gaps in skills and intervene to remediate the underlying problem that is interfering with a child's ADL performance. This approach focuses on the child's deficits in sensorimotor, cognitive, or psychosocial components. Therapists often use biomechanical, neurodevelopmental, sensory integration (SI), or perceptual motor approaches to restore skills. For example, before dressing a child with spastic cerebral palsy and tight extensors, the therapist may use handling techniques to inhibit the child's tone. The therapist places the child in a supine position and slowly rolls the child's hips from one side to the other to reduce the tone, increase range of motion, and encourage trunk rotation (Boehme, 1988). After this preparation, the child's task performance improves and the therapist may then facilitate movement patterns by stabilizing body parts while the child performs the task. While using this approach, therapists provide parents and children ideas on how to practice these movement patterns in various tasks. Besides dressing, this increased range of motion may improve the child's mobility skills to crawl to the changing table or to reach his or her foot and pull off a sock.

Compensatory Approach

In the *compensatory approach,* when the therapist does not expect a performance component skill to be remediated, he or she uses alternative physical techniques, substitute movement patterns, or other adaptive skills to complete a task. Compensatory strategies may include modification of the task or task method, use of assistive technology, or adaptation of the environment (Geyer, Kurtz, & Byram, 1998; Geyer, Okinom, & Kurtz, 1996). Therapists often use a combination of these strategies to improve a child's performance while considering the performance context. Table 16-4 gives examples of typical compensatory approaches used with different functional problems.

table 16-3   *Approaches to Improving Self-Care Performance*

Approach	Problem: Buttoning Without Use of Right Hand
Developmental	This approach uses shape-sorting boxes, pegboards, and coins in a piggy bank to help the child work on fine motor skills before beginning with buttons.
Remediation	This approach improves the range of motion of the child's hand and uses dexterity activities to improve fine motor control. This approach decreases tone in the upper extremities and hands. The child plays with foam or playdough to give the hands sensory input. The therapist provides rewards after each attempt to button.
Compensatory • Modify the task method	The child uses a one-handed buttoning technique. The child uses a pullover shirt so that buttoning is not an issue or uses an extra-large shirt with buttons already buttoned. The child wears buttoned shirts over a pullover (e.g., an open jacket).
• Adapt the object or use assistive technology	The therapist replaces buttons with other buttons with long shanks or buttons according to the child's tactile preference. The child uses a button hook, elastic sewn on buttons, or pressure-sensitive tape. The therapist positions the child and devices for stability during the activity (e.g., in a chair with arms to button).
• Adapt the task environment	The child practices buttoning in a bedroom away from distracting toys or siblings. The child asks a parent, sibling, or peer to button his or her shirt. The child uses a shirt with buttons since it is culturally important to the teen not to wear a pullover.
Education	The therapist educates children and parents according to their identified goals for treatment. The therapist models to the child and parent how to use previous approaches. The therapist gives home ideas to develop opportunities to practice tasks within everyday routines. The therapist gives written, pictorial, verbal, or video instructions.

Adapted from Holm, M.B., Rogers, J.C., & James, A.B. (1998). Treatment of occupational performance areas: Section 1, treatment of activities of daily living. In M.E. Neistadt & E.B. Crepeau (Eds.), *Willard and Spackman's occupational therapy* (9th ed.). (pp. 323-364). Philadelphia: J.B. Lippincott.
Smith, R., Benge, M., & Hall, M. (1994). Technology for self-care. In C. Christiansen (Ed.), *Ways of living: Self-care strategies for special needs* (pp. 379-422). Rockville, MD: American Occupational Therapy Association.

table 16-4 *Typical Compensatory Principles Used With Children and Adolescents With Disabilities*

Behavior/Disability	Compensatory Principles
Low vision or hearing or both	• Use intact or residual senses • Amplify sensory characteristics (e.g., color, size, tactile, and auditory) of objects • Give cues consistently to determine whether activity is beginning or ending • Use tactile, verbal, visual, or object cues (e.g., put hand on washcloth or say, "it's time to wash your face") • Use gestures (e.g., point to arm that is put in sleeve first) • Decrease auditory and visual distractions
Dislike for being touched (tactile defensive)	• Prepare for touch by giving deep pressure and organized, rhythmic touch • Give child choices for tactile preferences (e.g., clothes, washcloths, and brushes) • Let child perform touching on himself or herself (e.g., use tooth brush or wash face or body) • Let child wear snug clothes (e.g., turtleneck) or loose clothes (e.g., child's preference)
Inability to find clothes or understand top, front, or bottom	• Amplify characteristics • Reduce distracters (e.g., only one utensil on countertop for cooking activity) • Use visual or gestural cues (e.g., mark medial border of shoes with happy faces to keep shoes on correct feet) • Use systematic scanning when searching for objects (e.g., clothes in closet)
Inability to sit up or maintain balance	• Provide support externally (e.g., positioning device) • Change position of child (e.g., sit to put on shoes or dress in sidelying) • Change position of activity (e.g., keep grooming items together in bucket on top of sink)
Limited reach	• Reduce amount of reach needed • Change position of activity • Lengthen handles (e.g., long-handled bath sponge or reacher)
Difficulty grasping objects	• Build up handles to objects (e.g., brushes and spoons) • Substitute assistive devices so grasping is not necessary (e.g., universal cuffs or straps) • Stabilize objects with other body parts (e.g., in teeth or between legs)
Weakness with little endurance	• Eliminate gravity (e.g., prop elbow or dress in sidelyling) • Use lightweight objects • Use power equipment
Difficulty controlling movement	• Provide stable base of support (e.g., sit on floor with wide base) • Eliminate need for fine control (e.g., use an enlarged zipper pull) • Use weighted devices to give proprioceptive feedback (e.g., weighted tooth brushes and cups)
Poor memory; inability to remember sequences or directions	• Establish and practice set routines and sequences • Use partial participation, grading techniques, and backward and forward chaining • Use visual cues (e.g., pictures, labels, checklists, or color code) • Substitute assistive technology (e.g., alarm on watch or timers) • Use verbal cues (e.g., "first, then second", jingles, rhymes, or songs) • Use real life materials in the setting in which the occupation occurs
Tendency to become easily frustrated; outbursts	• Identify purpose of "problem behavior" (e.g., escape, avoid, attention, obtain, transition, or stimulate) by analyzing antecedents and consequences • Limit exposure to context associated with misbehavior • Use preferred tasks and give choices • Reinforce, coach, and expand appropriate alternate behaviors • Provide personal assistance and coaching (use partial participation) • Use grading, prompting, fading prompts, and generalization

Developed from Geyer, L.A., Kurtz, L.A., & Byram, L.E. (1998). Promoting function in daily living skills. In J.P. Dormans & L. Peliegrino (Eds.), *Caring for children with cerebral palsy: A team approach* (pp. 323-346). Baltimore: Brookes; and Koegel, L.K., Koegel, R.L., Kellegrew, D., & Mullen, K. (1996). Parent education for prevention and reduction of severe problem behaviors. In L.K. Koegel, R.L. Koegel & G. Dunlap (Eds.), *Positive behavioral support: Including people with difficult behavior in the community* (pp. 3-30). Baltimore: Brookes.

Therapists practice compensatory strategies in various contexts and modify them until they become functional. For example, a child with a bilateral upper-extremity amputation can have several compensatory strategies to use for self-care tasks. As an adapted method, the child can use his or her feet or mouth to write or dress, or he or she can learn new movement patterns to operate a prosthetic arm (assistive device) for manipulating objects. Another compensatory strategy may include using personal assistance within the home or school environment. A child's mother can place clothes in the drawers that the child can reach while sitting in a wheelchair.

Modifying task methods

By modifying tasks or the methods for teaching the task, children can participate in self-care occupations. The search for these methods involves creative teamwork between the therapist, child, and caregivers. A prompt from the therapist (e.g., "How can you do this?") often taps the child's motivation to find his or her own solution to the problem. The therapist observes and analyzes the child's attempts and then guides and adapts the most promising effort toward success.

The therapist often modifies tasks by using *grading techniques.* Grading is the adaptation of a task or portions of a task to fit the child's capabilities. By using a task analysis, the therapist rates subtasks of the activity and varies them according to their degree of ease or difficulty for the child. The child independently practices those skills that he or she is capable of performing. The therapist may modify the task for other difficult skills. The therapist may grade the tasks according to qualities, including gross to fine, light to heavy, and simple to complex. Grading of a task may include gradually increasing the number of steps for which the child is responsible, fading the amount of personal assistance that the child receives, or decreasing the amount of time that the child uses to complete an activity. The therapist also grades the sensory qualities of the environment to meet the specific sensory processing problems of the child. Developmental and remedial approaches also use grading techniques.

Each self-care task and IADL involves a series of steps that are performed together in a specific sequence. Through *task analysis,* the therapist gains an understanding of the sequence of steps involved in each self-care task. The therapist uses *personal assistance* when a child cannot complete a task independently or when completion of the task takes too much of the child's energy for other more important task (Smith, Benge, & Hall, 1994). The therapist uses *partial participation* when a child cannot complete a task independently and the child performs some steps of the task and a caregiver completes the remainder of the task. This helps the child be part of the activity and use current skills (Ferguson & Baumgart, 1991) and is often used when children are first learning a task or when they have severe limitations in their abilities.

Therapists use backward or forward chaining to teach the task and to involve the child in the task. In *backward chaining,* the therapist performs most of the task and the child performs the last step of a sequence to receive positive reinforcement for completing the task. Practice continues with the therapist performing fewer steps and the child completing additional steps. This method is particularly helpful for children with a low frustration tolerance or poor self-esteem because it gives immediate success. In *forward chaining,* the child begins with the first step of the task sequence, then the second step, and continues learning steps of the task in a sequential order until he or she can perform all steps in the task. Forward chaining can be helpful for children who have difficulties with sequencing and generalizing skills.

The therapist can give varying amounts of *cues,* or *prompts,* before or during an activity. Therapist or person cues and environment or task cues can occur naturally or artificially within an environment. Therapists use verbal, gestural, or physical cues or a combination of all three (Snell & Vogtle, 2000). Environmental or task cues may include picture sequences or checklists, color coding, positioning, or adapting the sensory properties of the environment or materials used in a task. Reese and Snell (1991) described a hierarchic approach to presenting artificial cues from being least intrusive to most intrusive: verbal cues, verbal and gestural cues, and verbal and physical cues. In tooth brushing, Reese and Snell (1991) described a hierarchy of physical cues: shadowing the child's movements, using two fingers to guide the child, and using a hand-over-hand approach to guide movement. The therapist or parent uses the least amount of cues possible and fades cues to promote independence.

Adapting the task object or using assistive technology

Several *assistive devices* are available through equipment vendors, catalogs, and specialty department stores and are changing constantly. These aids vary in complexity, price, and quality. Assistive devices are commercially available or custom-made by the therapist, skilled craftsmen, orthotists, or rehabilitation engineers. By using local and national databases and publications on product comparison (e.g., Abledata, HyperAbledata) therapists can keep informed of new assistive devices to find equipment for unique or specific problems (Smith et. al., 1994).

The choice of an assistive device is a cooperative decision made by the child, parents, therapists, and other persons who work with the child. Together they systematically evaluate what the child needs to do, his or her performance contexts, the child's abilities and limitations, and the capabilities of the ■ device itself. They choose the device that has the best "environmental fit." Adolescents who are striving to identify with their peers tend to reject devices that call attention to their disabilities. Children are easily frustrated if using the device exceeds their coordination abilities, attention spans, or gadget tolerances. To be worthwhile, an assistive device should have the following qualities:

- *Assists in the task* that the child is trying to complete without being cumbersome
- Is *acceptable* to the child, family, and contextual environments in which it is used (e.g., appearance, functions, upkeep, and storage)
- Is *practical and flexible* for the environments in which it is used (e.g., dimensions, portability, positioning, and use with other assistive devices)
- Is *durable* and easy to clean
- Is *expandable* (e.g., will meet the needs for the child now and when the child has grown and has more sophisticated skills)
- Is *safe* for the child to use (e.g., cognitive, behavioral, or physical characteristics such as drooling, throwing, or difficulty with sequencing will not interfere with using the device)
- Has a *system of maintenance or replacement* with continued use
- *Meets the cost constraints* of the family or purchasing agency

Overall, the child should complete tasks at a higher level of efficiency using this device than without using it. Trial use of a device is highly recommended. This helps determine the feasibility of using the device and demonstrates its value to the child and primary caregivers.

Adaptations to the environment

In all of the approaches discussed, the therapist uses the interaction between the child and the environmental contexts to improve performance. The therapist can adapt physical environments by recommending modifications of architectural and other physical barriers or sensory characteristics. To facilitate wheelchair access, the child's caregivers can install ramps or move furniture. For example, the family can place their computer on a more usable work surface in a more accessible location so that the child who is wheelchair dependent can use it for doing homework and communicating with his brother at college. For some children, therapists minimize sensory stimuli and eliminate visual and auditory distractions. Other children may require increased environmental stimulation to cue their performance (e.g., color or music). Table 16-5 gives examples of how physical and social environments can be adapted.

The physical environment is filled with useful tools, materials, and equipment that the therapist can adapt to enhance a child's occupational performance. Children

learn to eat with utensils; sit in chairs; read books, magazines, and newspapers; and write with a pen and pencil. Typical adaptations include enlarging the object, adding pieces to the object or elongating pieces for better mechanical advantage to make handling easier. Physical, social and cultural environments provide *natural prompts,* or *cues,* to improve self-care performance. For example, if a child observes other family members washing their hands for dinner, he or she is given the natural cue to wash his or her hands. This cue is repeated in other environments (e.g., before eating a snack at school or eating out at a restaurant, almost all persons wash their hands). Peers at school can prompt children in eating and dressing activities.

The therapist can adapt social routines and roles to improve the child's performance. The following is an example of such a situation:

> Pam can dress independently but does not dress on the rehabilitation unit. Assessment reveals that social routines and roles are interfering with Pam's performance. When the therapist asks the nurses to change the social routine so that patients have to dress before eating and Pam is given the role to set trays out (cultural expectation within rehabilitation hospital dining room) for selected patients, Pam independently dresses herself.

Work surface. The work surface supports the child, materials, tools, and assistive devices in an activity (Eriksson et. al., 1987). Boundaries of the work space help children keep within usable or safe environments. For example, a cutout surface on a table or a lip on a wheelchair tray or a sink countertop makes boundaries for children. The therapist adds various textures, colors, and pictures to the work surface area to give sensory cues about boundaries and to motivate children. Even with these adaptations, some children (e.g., those with weakness in one side of the body) need assistance in stabilizing objects. Table 16-6 gives suggestions for stabilizing objects placed on the work surface or when held by the child.

Characteristics of the work surface that are amenable to adaptation include height, angle of incline (Figure 16-1), size, distance from the body, distance from other work areas, and general accessibility of a work surface. Changes in these characteristics enhance the child's function in various ways, including improving arm support, increasing the visual orientation of a task, adapting seat height for transfers, and improving table height for wheelchair access.

Positioning options. Therapists consider the position of the child and the position of the materials or activity when planning intervention. Children who have problems with posture and movement often lack sufficient control to assume or maintain stable postures during activity performance and benefit from positioning adap-

Architectural Barrier	Structural Changes	Possible Assistive Devices	Task Modification
Entrances and exits	Hand rails Hand stairs Ramp Built-up terrain to door height Stair lift In-home elevator Increase door width (33-36″ minimum) Step back hinges Door rehinged to open in or out Pocket door Folding door Electric door openers	Strapping or loop on door handle Lever handles Portable door knob Built-up key holders Combination locks Environmental control unit	Use different entrance Remove inside doors Use curtains for privacy Use hip or wheelchair to open doors
Bathrooms	Increase door width (33-36″ minimum); French doors or accordion door Enlarge room Sink mounted low Open space under cabinet Showers with a built-in seat Change placement of tub faucets Ramped shower stall Toilet bidet installed Linen closet shelves with no door	Safety rails Seat reducer Raised commode seat Step placed in front of commode Wheelchair commode Insulated pipes Single lever faucets Tub seats Wheelchair shower chair Hydraulic lifts Toilet paper tongs Toilet paper mounting Angled mirrors Wall-mounted hairdryer with switch Suction-cupped bucket to hold supplies	Free standing commode in secluded area Use a urinal Bed bath Sponge bath Use liquid soap Soap on a string Shampoo pump Dry shampoo
Bedroom	Downstairs bedroom Enlarged space Enlarged closet doors Low closet pole Closet storage system with shelves Built-in bookshelves at low and medium heights Cut holes in work surfaces for holding objects and electrical cords Built-in dressers or dressers bolted to the wall Special glides for wall drawers	Leg extenders Bed rails Firm mattress Straps or rope ladders Mounted shoe rack Environmental control units or switches for TV, radio, and light access Enlarge or add loop to drawer handles Positioning devices Adaptive chairs	Place bed on floor Keep most used clothes in accessible drawers Use shelves instead of dresser drawers for clothes Toys stored in shoe bag
Kitchen	Enlarge space Lowered countertops Lowered cabinets Sink with no cabinets under it Built-in rangetop Sliding drawers and organizes in cabinet Wall-mounted, side-by-side oven Dishwasher mounted higher Front-opening washer	Adapted utensils Nonslip matting Automated learning devices for appliances turned on by switches Adapted seats Wheelchair laptray Use barstool	Items most used in low cupboards Bowls and pans hang on wall instead of in cabinet Eat on wheelchair laptray instead of table Water kept in insulated bottle with pump on table Most used items kept on accessible surfaces Stool for washing dishes

table 16-6 *Stabilization Materials and Application Procedures*

Materials	Application Procedures
Tape	Applies quickly but often is a temporary solution; includes cellophane, masking, electrical, and duct tapes (duct tape is sturdy with holding power)
Nonslip pressure-sensitive matting	Fits under objects or around them; can be glued to objects; friction between materials minimizes slipping and sliding of objects; available in rolls or pads
Suction cup holders	Hold lightweight materials; single-faced suction cups applied permanently to object (e.g., nail, screw, or glue); double-faced suction cups moved from object to object; maintain suction between the object and work surface
C-clamps	Secure flat objects to lap trays, table edges, and other surfaces
Tacking putty	Sticks posters onto a wall; holds lightweight objects on tables, lap trays, angle boards, walls, etc.
Pressure-sensitive hook and loop tapes (Velcro)	Sewn to cloth or glued to the base of objects and work surfaces; soft loop tape used on areas that will contact the child's skin or clothing
Wing nuts and bolts	Secure objects to a table surface or lapboard when holes are drilled through the object and holding surface; sturdy and more permanent
Magnets	Affix to an object; stabilize objects on metallic surfaces such as refrigerator doors, metal tables, and magnetic message boards
L-brackets	Hold objects in an upright plane; holes drilled in both the work surface and the object to correspond with the L-bracket holes; objects secured with nuts and bolts
Soldering clamps	Hold small items for intricate work (e.g., mending a shirt, sewing on a button, or putting on a bracelet); mounted to free-standing base; bases weighted, suction-cupped, or held to surface with a C-clamp
Elastic or webbing straps	Attach to or around objects or positioning devices to hold them down; secure flat objects onto a work surface; straps secured by tying, pressure-sensitive hook and loop tape, D-rings and buckles, grommets, or screws

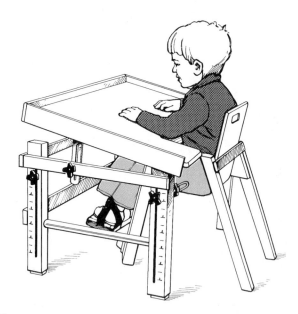

figure **16-1** Commercially available chair with positioning components and a desk with an adjustable height and adjustable inclined work surface.

tations. There are various body positions for self-care tasks, and no one position is best. Lying down, sitting, and standing are the positions most often used, with numerous options in each. When possible, the therapist uses the most typical position for a given activity and the lowest number of restrictions or adaptations to stabilize the body for function (Bergen, Presperin, & Tallman, 1990).

Alternative body positions are extremely helpful to children with disabilities. These changes help compensate for physical limitations in strength, joint movement, control, or endurance and provide relief to skin areas and bony prominences. They also allow children to experience different spatial relationships and thus develop a perceptual set for spatial orientation (Bergen & Colangelo, 1985; Ward, 1983).

A therapist considers positions that maximize independent task performance. Key points for stability that enable the child to use available voluntary movement are the pelvis and trunk, head, and extremities. When muscle weakness occurs, the therapist determines where support is needed or, for the child with muscle tightness, whether a preferred and comfortable position is contraindicated.

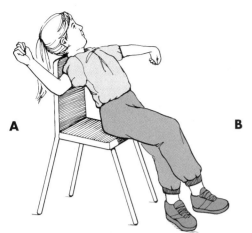
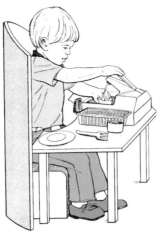

figure16-2 Sitting postures. **A,** Incorrect sitting resulting from a massive extension pattern and an asymmetric tonic reflex posture. **B,** Correct sitting posture. Weight equally distributed on the sitting base and feet and elbows supported.

Looking carefully at the entire body of the child, the therapist asks the following questions:

- Is the child *aligned properly?* Where are the hips, shoulders, and head in relation to the trunk? (Figure 16-2)
- What positions or devices increase *trunk stability?* Inserting lateral supports? A surface for supporting the feet? Widening the sitting base by abducting the legs?
- Does positioning in the *sidelying* or *sitting* position allow the child to use balanced flexion and extension? Does it inhibit flexion patterns that are dominant in the prone position and the extension patterns seen in the supine position? Is adequate anterior, posterior, and lateral support provided?

Seating. Sitting and sometimes standing are the most appropriate positions for the child to perform self-care tasks. In addition to postural alignment, the therapist recommends positions that provide the child with (1) good orientation of his or her body to the work surface and the materials being used, (2) good body and visual orientation to the therapist (if instruction is being given), and (3) the ability to independently get to and leave the place where self-care occurs. The therapist modifies chair heights so that the child's feet are touching the floor to support postural stability and facilitate transfers. If the therapist raises the seat height, he or she provides a foot rest. The therapist shortens or lengthens chair legs with blocks or leg extenders.

Kangas (1998) advocates a "task ready position" for children with moderate to severe motor disabilities. Instead of positioning the child's hips, knees, and ankles at 90-degree angles, Kangas positions them so that they are ready to move. In the task ready position the pelvis is secure, the trunk and head are slightly forward so that the shoulders are in front of the pelvis, the arms and hands are in front of the body, and the feet are flat on the floor or behind the knees. The therapist removes or loosens

as many restraints or chair adaptations as are safely possible so that the child has maximal potential for movement. The movement, even when subtle, provides visual, vestibular, proprioceptive, and kinesthetic feedback. A carved or molded seat and a seat belt across the thighs gives additional sensory feedback and are used for positioning of the pelvis and safety.

Education

Child and caregiver education is essential in all therapy for children. This education helps children perform self-care occupations within their environments and helps caregivers and children learn safety information and coping strategies. When providing information, occupational therapy practitioners consider the learning capacity and the temporal and environmental contexts of children and their families (Holm et. al., 1998).

A young child or a child with moderate developmental delays may not be ready to assume health maintenance tasks independently, so parents, caregivers, and occasionally siblings are responsible for learning appropriate methods and adaptations to perform self-care tasks and IADLs. Instructional methods depend on individual preferences, family life cycle needs, and the physical, learning, and psychosocial capacities of children, families, and caregivers.

Therapists present child or caregiver education in various ways. Therapists often demonstrate how to do the task (e.g., tub transfers) when instructing. In addition the therapist may use visual aids, written instructions, audiotapes, videotapes, and checklists. The method chosen often depends on the comfort level and preferences of the parents and therapists and the contextual demands.

Children require multiple opportunities to practice new tasks, and families may need help assessing routines and identifying when children can practice self-care occupations (Koegel, Koegel, Kellegrew, & Mullen, 1996). In a study by Kellegrew (1998), parents used self-monitoring forms to record the number of opportunities that the child could perform a self-care task and the amount of assistance that they gave the child during the task. The parents did not receive specific instructional methods; they received only broad concepts telling parents that self-care skills are important, their children are ready and able to learn, and their children require many opportunities to practice the tasks. Families were creative in finding ways and opportunities to help their children practice tasks, and self-care skills increased only when children were given more opportunities to engage in self-care as an occupation. These results suggest that it is important for the therapist to assess a child's opportunities to practice tasks before developing complex methods for home programs.

An educational approach provides parents and children the chance to make informed choices about the services, methods, assistive technology, and *environmental adaptations* that they will use (Bayzak, 1989). Grading, forward and backward chaining, partial participation, and modeling help train caregivers. Unfortunately, parent education and information given may not receive adequate emphasis in some programs (King, Law, King, & Rosenbaum, 1998). In this chapter, education of caregivers and children is discussed as an integral part of the intervention approaches for self-care tasks and IADLs.

■ SPECIFIC INTERVENTION TECHNIQUES FOR SELECTED SELF-CARE TASKS

Specific intervention strategies for toilet hygiene, dressing, bathing, oral hygiene, grooming, functional communication, and expressing sexuality are described in the following sections. Interrelationships between performance components, occupational performance, and contextual demands are considered. A combination of approaches and strategies described previously are employed to help children become as independent as possible in self-care occupations.

Toilet Hygiene
Typical developmental sequence

Independent toileting is an important self-maintenance milestone with wide variation among individual children. It carries considerable sociologic and cultural significance. Self-sufficiency may determine participation in day care centers, school programs, recreational and community opportunities, and secondary school vocational choices. Like other self-care tasks, toileting is a complex task requiring a set of subskills. To begin to learn this task, a child must be physically and psychologically ready. Also, parents or caregivers need to be ready to devote the time and effort to toilet training the child. A communication system between caregivers and the child is essential.

At birth a newborn voids reflexively and involuntarily. Changes in position, handling by others, and other stimuli can trigger micturition. As the child matures, the spinal tract is myelinated to a level for bowel and bladder control at the lumbar and sacral areas and the child learns to control sphincter reflexes for the volitional holding of urine and feces. Children are often physiologically ready for toileting if they have a pattern of urine and feces elimination.

Bowel control precedes bladder control, and studies indicate that girls are trained an average of 2.50 months earlier than boys (Erickson, 1976). Independence in toileting includes getting on and off the toilet, managing fasteners and clothing, cleansing after toileting, and washing and drying hands efficiently without supervision. Children progress in sequence, according to each child's unique pace of development. Table 16-7 gives the typical developmental sequence for toileting.

Typical problems interfering with toileting independence

Children with spinal cord injury, spina bifida, or other conditions that produce full or partial paralysis require special management for bowel and bladder activities. Loss of control over these bodily functions can produce embarrassment and decreased feelings of self-esteem. School-age children are characteristically modest about their bodies, and adolescents are struggling with identity issues and the need to be like their peers.

The type of bladder problem depends on the level and type of neurologic impairment. When the lesion is in the lumbar region or below, the bladder is flaccid (lower motor neuron bladder). The reflex arc is not intact, and the bladder has lost all tone. When the lesion is above the level of bladder innervation, an automatic bladder, or an upper motor neuron bladder, results. The child undertakes training programs for the upper motor neuron bladder to develop an automatic response. Children with a flaccid bladder cannot be trained because the bladder has no tone to empty (Shepherd, Proctor, & Coley, 1996).

The therapist determines bladder training and management programs after medical testing and collaborative discussions with children and their parents. Depending on medical test results, there are four main methods to manage urine: (1) condom catheterization (for males), (2) indwelling catheters, (3) intermittent catheterizations (every 4 to 6 hours), and (4) ileal conduits. The therapist restricts the child's fluid intake to prevent bladder distention. When girls have partial control of bladder function, they wear disposable diapers or incontinence pants.

table 16-7	*Typical Developmental Sequence of Toileting Skills*

Approximate Age (yr)	Toileting Skill
1	• Indicates discomfort when wet or soiled • Has regular bowel movements
1½	• Sits on toilet when placed there and supervised (short time)
2	• Urinates regularly
2½	• Achieves regulated toileting with occasional daytime accidents • Rarely has bowel accidents • Tells someone that he or she needs to go to the bathroom • May need reminders to go to the bathroom • May need help with getting on the toilet
3	• Goes to bathroom independently; seats self on toilet • May need help with wiping • May need help with fasteners or difficult clothing
4-5	• Is independent in toileting (e.g., tearing toilet paper, flushing, washing hands, managing clothing)

Modified from Coley, I. (1978). *Pediatric assessment of self care assessment* (p. 145, 149). St. Louis: Mosby; Orelove, F., & Sobsey, D. (1996). Self-care skills. In F. Orelove & D. Sobsey (Eds.), *Educating children with multiple disabilities* (2nd ed.). (p. 342). Baltimore: Brookes.

A basic principle for success in bowel reeducation is to have a regular, consistent evacuation of the bowel. The time for this is a matter of choice, but there should be a schedule that remains constant. In some cases the child receives suppositories and a warm drink before evacuation. This stimulates contraction and relaxation of muscle fibers within the walls of the intestine that move the contents onward. Other techniques include digital stimulation, massage around the anal sphincter, or manual pressure using the Credé's method on the abdomen. Occasionally, removal of the stool by hand or a colostomy is recommended. Similar to an ileostomy, colostomy collection bags are emptied and cleansed on a regular basis.

Although nurses are often the professionals who teach bowel and bladder control methods, the occupational therapist may be involved to provide assistive devices or to help design adapted methods. Children performing catheterizations or bowel programs may have difficulty in any of the following areas: maintaining a stable yet practical position, hand dexterity, perceptual awareness, strength, range of motion, and stability and accuracy when emptying collection devices. Memory, safety, and sensory awareness are needed to use any of these procedures.

Closely associated with bowel and bladder care is care of the skin in the perineal area. Skin should be cleansed thoroughly to protect the tissue against contact with waste matter and to eliminate odor. All children with decreased sensation are susceptible to decubiti, which are pressure sores that occur fairly rapidly when blood vessels are compressed (e.g., around a bony prominence such as the ischial tuberosity). This can result in ischemia, or lack of tissue nourishment.

Children with limited motor skills

Diapering becomes a difficult task when infants or children have strong extensor and adduction patterns in their legs. Therapists teach the mother remedial methods to decrease extensor patterns before diapering and incorporate these methods into the diapering routine. For example, the mother may first place a pillow under the child's hips, flex the hips, and slowly rock the hips back and forth before she helps the child abduct the legs for diapering.

Toileting independence may be delayed in children with limitations in strength, endurance, range of motion, postural stability, and manipulation or dexterity. With unstable sitting posture, the child has difficulty relaxing and maintaining a position for pressing down and emptying the bowels. With weakness and limited range of motion, the child may be unable to manage fastenings because of hand involvement or may have problems in sitting down or getting up from the toilet seat because of hip-knee contractions or quadriceps weakness.

Cleansing after a bowel movement may be difficult if the child cannot supinate the hand, flex the wrist, or internally rotate and extend the arm to cleanse after a bowel movement. An anterior approach may work. The therapist must caution girls against contamination from feces, which can cause vaginitis. If at all possible, girls should wipe the anus from the rear. Solutions to cleansing problems are difficult and often discouraging. These children may require remediation, strategies to improve performance components (e.g., active range of motion), or compensatory strategies (e.g., assistive technology and environmental adaptations) to perform the toileting task.

Children with cognitive limitations

Children with mental retardation take a longer period to learn toileting skills, but they often become independent (Orelove & Sobsey, 1996). Problems with awareness, initiation, sequencing, memory, and dexterity in managing their clothes are typical. As with all children, physiologic readiness for toileting is a prerequisite before beginning training programs. The therapist uses task analysis to determine which steps of the process are a problem. He or she then determines what cues and prompts are needed to achieve the child's best performance. Finally the therapist evaluates which methods work as successful reinforcement (Snell & Vogtle, 2000).

Compensatory Strategies for Improving Toileting Independence

Compensatory strategies include remodeling or restructuring the environment, selecting assistive devices, or devising alternative methods to enhance independence. Adaptations to provide privacy are particularly important for the older child and adolescent. The therapist also addresses caregiver needs as the child becomes heavier and more difficult to assist with toileting.

Characteristics of physical and social environments at home or school influence how a child manages toileting hygiene. Assisting children in determining where to perform the procedure and how to manage it within their home, school, and recreational environments is often a challenge. Social routines and expectations are also important variables for the therapist to consider when making recommendations for managing toileting. These expectations depend on the child's age and abilities and how the family perceives the child's ability to manage this part of his or her self-care.

Social environment

Of all self-care tasks, toileting requires the most sensitive approach on the part of those who work with the child on a self-maintenance program. Children may purposely restrict their fluid intake at school in an effort to avoid the need for elimination. Unfortunately, limited fluid intake promotes infections, which increases the difficulty of regulating the bowel and bladder. Families, teachers, nurses, and paraprofessionals work with therapists to evaluate the social environment and find the "best" place, time, and routine for the child. When self-catheterization occurs in the school or community environment, the child can ensure privacy by using the health room, a private bathroom stall, or a time when children are usually not taking bathroom breaks. Carrying catheterization supplies in a fanny pack or a small nylon (nontransparent) bag also protects the child's privacy.

Therapists help children who lack bowel and bladder control develop routines and health habits that eliminate possible odors. The therapist needs to reinforce and incorporate regular cleaning and changing of appliances (collection bags for ileal conduits and colostomies) and urine collection bags into schedules. Also a good fluid intake is recommended to prevent odors and bacteria growth.

Physical environment

The bathroom is often the most inaccessible room in the house, yet it is essential that every family member has access to it. The floor space inside is rarely sufficient to allow the child to turn a wheelchair for a toilet transfer. Sensory aspects of the objects in the environment may hinder performance. Children with hypersensitivity may have difficulty tolerating sensory features such as a padded toilet seat, air freshener, or rug by the toilet.

Toileting adaptations

Numerous adaptations for toileting are available to assist the child in positioning and maintaining cleanliness after toileting. Urinals, catheters, leg bag clamps, long-handled mirrors, positioning devices to provide postural stability or to hold legs open, and universal cuffs with a catheter or digital stimulator attached are some examples of assistive devices that therapists may provide.

For children with good postural control but limited range of motion or grasp, simple, inexpensive aids include various types of toilet paper tongs and toilet paper holding devices.

A combined bidet and toilet offers a means for total independence. Several models are available that attach to a standard toilet bowl. A self-contained mechanism spray-washes the perineal area with thermostatically controlled warm water and dries it with a flow of warm air. The child can operate controls with the hand or foot (Figure 16-3). Self-care of skin for children who are catheterized or have a flaccid bladder includes inspecting of the skin daily by mirror and avoiding sitting in wet garments or one position for long periods. Various special cushions designed to prevent tissue trauma are commercially available.

The type of clothing worn during toileting can often hinder the child's independence or the caregiver's ability to promote independence. For children who wear diapers, a full-length crotch opening with a zipper or Velcro

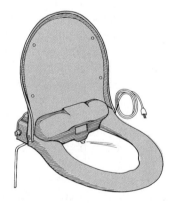

figure**16-3** Electrically powered bidet makes it possible to clean the perineal area independently without hands or paper.

closure makes changes easier. As children mature, they may be responsible for changing their own diapers or caring for their appliances and equipment. Girls may wear wrap-around or full skirts because these are easy to put on and adjust for diaper changes or toileting. The child can reach and drain leg bags with greater ease when his or her pants have zippers or Velcro closures along the seams. Flies with long zippers or Velcro closures make it easier for boys to urinate or catheterize themselves when in wheelchairs.

Adaptations for unstable posture

When children sit on the toilet, they need to feel posturally secure. When toilet seats are low enough that the feet rest firmly on the floor, the abdominal muscles that normally aid in defecation can effectively fulfill their function.

Small children often need reducer rings to decrease the size of the toilet seat opening and thus improve sitting support. A step in front of the toilet helps small children get onto it. Safety rails that attach to the toilet or wall may assist with balance and allow the child to freely use his or her hands. The child who has outgrown small training potties can use free-standing commodes, which may be useful when wheelchair access to the bathroom is impossible. Units that roll into place over the toilet may be an option.

Families can purchase commodes that feature such modifications as adjustable legs, safety bars, angled legs for stability, and padded, upholstered, and adjustable backrests and headrests. Commodes are also available with seat reducer rings, seat belts, and adjustable footrests.

■ DRESSING

Typical Development

Independence in dressing usually takes 4 years of practice. Characteristically, learning to undress comes before learning to dress. Caregivers introduce self-dressing in a natural way, at bedtime, by allowing the child to complete the final step in pulling off a garment. Similarly, when the child becomes more goal directed and motivated to be independent, he or she is ready to try the more difficult tasks of learning to put on clothing. Often the caregiver uses backward chaining by putting the garment on the child and allowing the child to complete the action. Gradually the child performs more of the task and the caregiver performs less. Table 16-8 gives the typical development of dressing skills.

Dressing requires children to know where their bodies are in space and how body parts relate. The visual and the kinesthetic systems guide arm and leg movements during dressing. Equilibrium is important as the child reaches

---

table 16-8 *Typical Developmental Sequence for Dressing*

Age (yr)	Self-Dressing Skills
1	• Cooperates with dressing (holds out arms and feet) • Pulls off shoes, removes socks • Pushes arms through sleeves and legs through pants
2	• Removes unfastened coat • Removes shoes if laces are untied • Helps pull down pants • Finds armholes in over-the-head shirt
2½	• Removes pull-down pants with elastic waist • Assists in pulling on socks • Puts on front-button coat or shirt • Unbuttons large buttons
3	• Puts on over-the-head shirt with minimal assistance • Puts on shoes without fasteners (may be on wrong foot) • Puts on socks (may be with heel on top) • Independently pulls down pants • Zips and unzips jacket once on track • Needs assistance to remove over-the-head shirt • Buttons large front buttons
3½	• Finds front of clothing • Snaps or hooks front fastener • Unzips zipper on jacket, separating zipper • Puts on mittens • Buttons series of three or four buttons • Unbuckles shoe or belt • Dresses with supervision (needs help with front and back)
4	• Removes pullover garment independently • Buckles shoes or belt • Zips jacket zipper • Puts on socks correctly • Puts on shoes with assistance in tying laces • Laces shoes • Consistently identifies the front and back of garment
4½	• Puts belt in loops
5	• Ties and unties knots • Dresses unsupervised
6	• Closes back zipper • Ties bow • Buttons back buttons • Snaps back snaps

Modified from Klein, M.D. (1983). *Pre-dressing skills*. Tucson: Communication Skill Builders.

and shifts his or her center of gravity. The child must reciprocally and cooperatively use the two sides of the body. The child needs balance, range of motion, strength, fine motor coordination, and control of movement. The visual and somatosensory systems enable the child to understand form and space and how clothing conforms to and fits on the body.

Typical Problems and Intervention Strategies

Perceptual problems

Children who have perceptual deficits may have difficulties in distinguishing right and left sides of the body, putting a shoe on the correct foot, or turning the heel of a sock. Identifying the front of clothing from the back or identifying the correct leg or sleeve are also difficult tasks. If the child avoids crossing the midline and performs dressing tasks on the right side of the body with the right hand and those on the left with the left hand, he or she most likely will have difficulty with tasks that require both hands to work together, such as fastening clothes and tying shoelaces. The therapist uses remedial or compensatory strategies to improve perceptual skills or to adapt the task and environment.

Cognitive limitations

Children with mental retardation may have difficulty organizing perceptual stimuli, discriminating left from right, or applying concepts such as above, behind, or in front of. The child who has intellectual limitations cannot remember instructions and has a short attention span. Behaviorally, the child may become frustrated with the complexity of certain dressing tasks. Language skills may be inefficient, which restricts the child's verbal capacity to express frustration. This may increase when the child is faced with tasks that require fine manipulations if coordination is limited (e.g., buttoning, snapping, zipping, or buckling).

Often a behavioral approach is effective to acquire independence. After making a baseline assessment, the therapist carefully analyzes each dressing task into its performance components. Once the therapist determines performance limitations and strengths, he or she uses partial participation and backward and forward chaining methods. Environmental and task adaptations include visual charts or pictures, checklists, and selection of clothing that is easy to manipulate (e.g., larger clothing, stretchy materials, pullover shirts, and loafers).

Physical limitations

Children with various conditions find dressing difficult because of the coordination and the range and strength required for pulling clothes on and off and connecting fasteners. Children with arthritis who have painful fingers frequently require assistance during a flare-up of their disease. They may be unable to move their arms freely and to reach certain areas of the body. Children with the use of only one hand find it difficult to zip trousers, tie shoelaces, and button shirts or blouses. The therapist may use a remedial approach to improve performance components, but in most cases the child learns compensatory techniques, often through his or her own experimentation or use of assistive technology. Children with cerebral palsy often have difficulty balancing and controlling arm and leg movement when donning and removing clothing. Limited dexterity may also interfere with dressing. The child can make tasks easier by using simple measures such as supportive positioning, dressing the involved extremity first, or using adaptive aids such as button hooks, rings on zippers, one-handed shoe fasteners, or Velcro closures (Figure 16-4).

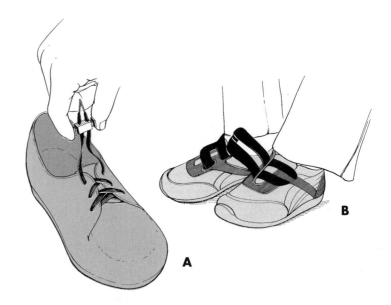

figure**16-4**   These shoelace fasteners can be managed with one hand. **A,** Spring tension blocks. **B,** Velcro fasteners.

Adaptive methods for dressing children with motor limitations

Although it is common to dress an infant while he or she is lying in the supine position, this position frequently increases extensor tone in those infants with neurologic impairment. For this reason some therapists advocate placing the infant prone across the knees with the infant's hips flexed and abducted, thus inhibiting leg extensor and adduction tone. When the infant gains head and trunk control, the caregiver can dress him or her in a sitting position with the child's back resting against and supported by the caregiver's trunk. In this position the infant has an opportunity to observe his or her own body while dressing.

When dressing an infant with stiffness, the caregiver carefully bends the infant's hips and knees before putting on shoes and socks (Figure 16-5) and brings the infant's shoulders forward before putting his or her arm through a sleeve. By flexing the child's hip and knee, postural tone is decreased and dressing becomes easier. When a child achieves sitting balance, a good way to proceed with dressing is to place the child on the floor and later on a low stool, continuing to provide support where needed from the back. Orientation to the child's body parts should remain a focus in the social interaction. The caregiver helps the child understand how his or her body relates to his or her clothes and to the various positions (e.g., "the arm goes through the sleeve" and "the head goes through the neck of a garment").

When the child is older and heavier, there may be no alternative but to dress the child while he or she is in the sidelying or supine position. Placing a hard pillow under the child's head, thus slightly raising his or her shoulders, makes it easier for the caregiver to bring the child's arms forward and to bend his or her hips and knees. If it is possible to maintain the child in a sidelying position, this posture may make it easier for the caregiver to manage the child's arms and legs and for the child to assist in the dressing task (Figure 16-6).

Adaptive methods for self-dressing

The child who has hand skills but poor balance may be able to take advantage of the function that he or she possesses when in a sidelying position with the effect of gravity lessened. For the child who can sit but is unstable, a corner of two adjoining walls or a corner seat on the floor may provide enough postural support for independent dressing. Sitting balance is more precarious as one reaches when donning overhead garments or pants and shoes; therefore the child needs additional external support. Sitting in chairs with arms or sitting on the floor against a wall may improve performance.

The occupational therapist helps improve the child's dressing skills by offering the parent and child various ways to solve problems from which the child and parents may choose. Table 16-9 offers choices in problem solving while donning and doffing different garments. Clothing selections, assistive technology, and adaptations to the task are methods for improving a child's performance in self-dressing.

Increased attention to the needs of individuals with disabilities has been shown over the last decade, with some adaptive clothing becoming available through catalog supply companies. Parents are encouraged to purchase attractive, fashionable clothing that meets functional requirements yet conforms in appearance to the child's peer group standards and fashion trends. Modifications are inconspicuous, and the appearance of the

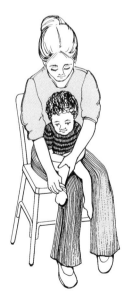

figure 16-5   When dressing the child who is hypertonic, the caregiver should carefully flex the hip and knee before putting on socks and shoes.

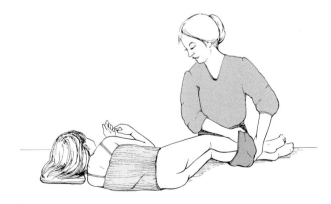

figure 16-6   The sidelying position may decrease tone and make dressing easier.

Garment	Design Features of Clothing or Assistive Technology Adaptations for Easier Dressing	Adaptations to Task Method
Pull-up garments	• Large size • Stretchy material • Loops sewn into waistband • Elastic waistbands, but not too tight • Pressure sensitive tape • Zipper pulls • Dressing sticks	• Sit on chair • Lie on floor • Lie on side and roll side to side to pull pants up • Use chair or grab bar to stabilize self while pulling up pants • Put weak or affected leg in first
Pullover garments	• Large, easy opening for head • Flexible rib knit fabric • Large armholes and sleeve openings; raglan sleeves • Elastic cuffs and waistbands	• Lay garment on lap, floor, or table, front side down; put arms in and flip over head • Pull garment over head, then put in arms • Put weak or affected leg in first
Front-opening garments	• Loose style • Fullness in back of garment • Collars on shirt or jacket; may be different color than main garment • Short-sleeve garments first, proceeding to long-sleeve garments • Raglan sleeves • Garment with no closures or one or two buttons (e.g., sweater, jacket)	• Lay garment on lap, floor, or table, with neck of garment toward the child; put in arms, duck head, extend arms, and flip garment over the head; shrug shoulders and use arms to help garment fall in place • Put weak or affected arm in first, pull up to shoulder; follow collar and then put in other arm
Buttons	• Flat, large buttons • Buttons contrast in color with garment • Buttons with shanks (easier to grasp) • Buttons sewn on loosely • Buttons sewn on one side; Velcro tape on both sides to close shirt or pants • Front buttons first, proceeding to side and back buttons	• Use pullover styles instead of buttons • Button all but the first two or three buttons and put shirt on like a pullover • Begin buttoning with bottom button (easier to see and align) • Use a button hook • Use elastic thread to sew on sleeve buttons; put on sleeve without buttoning • Use backward chaining
Zippers	• Nylon zippers (easier than metal) • Zipper tabs or rings • Zipper pulls • Velcro instead of zipper • Longer zippers (more space for donning and doffing clothes) • Front zippers first, proceeding to side and back zippers	• Sit to give stability • Stand to keep the jacket zipper flat • Hold zipper taut at the bottom of the zipper with one hand while pulling up zipper tab with other hand • For side zipper, lean against wall to hold bottom of zipper
Socks	• Soft, stretchy socks • Large size • Tube sock (no set place for heel) • Ankle socks first, proceeding to calf or over-the-calf socks • Loops sewn into socks • Sock aide or donner	• Sit on stable surface (e.g., chair, floor) • Lie on back and prop foot on opposite knee • Fold or roll sock before putting over the toes and pulling it up • Use backward chaining
Shoes	• Long-opening shoes (many eyes) with loose laces • Broad shoes (not tight) • Slip-on shoes • Velcro closures • Elastic laces already tied • Elastic curly laces that do not need tying • Tabs at heels to pull shoes on • Long-handled shoehorns	• Sit on stable surface (e.g., chair, floor) • Prop foot up on stool or chair • Lie on back and prop foot on opposite knee • Flex legs and point toes downward • Use gravity to assist pushing heel in shoe (e.g., child pushes down on a hard surface)

clothing should not single out the wearer. When possible, clothing conceals physical disabilities or at least does not attract attention to them. Clothing contributes to the wearer's sense of well being. Functionally, the design of the clothing should enable the wearer to take care of personal needs, help maintain proper body temperature, and provide freedom of movement.

Most clothing is made for individuals in a standing position. For those who spend long hours in a wheelchair, the sitting position can cause pulling and straining on some areas of the garment and a surplus of fabric in others. The caregiver can make alterations to provide more comfort in sitting (Kennedy, 1981; Kernaleguen, 1978) (e.g., pants that are cut higher in the back and lower in the front and cut larger to give additional room in the hips and thighs). A longer inseam also allows the proper hem height for pants when sitting (rests on top of shoe). Pockets in the back may cause sheering or skin breakdown with prolonged sitting. Instead, pockets can be placed on the top of the thigh or on the side of the calf for easy access. Front and side seams can be sewn with Velcro fasteners or zippers and wrist loops to assist in donning. Pullover tops with raglan and gusset sleeves allow more room when maneuvering the wheelchair. If the shirt is cut longer in the back and shorter in the front, it is easier to keep a neat appearance. Rain capes or winter capes are comfortable in a wheelchair. They are cut longer in the front to cover the child's legs and feet and shorter in the back so they do not rub against the wheel of the chair.

For children who wear orthoses for spinal support, front openings that are from the neck to the lower abdomen make self-dressing easier, whereas back openings are easier for others to dress the child (Lawrence & Niemeyer, 1994). Caregivers should use larger clothing that fits over orthoses but avoid loose sleeves for children who push wheelchairs because the sleeve may get caught in the spokes of the wheel. The child who wears an ankle-foot orthosis may need to have clothing reinforced to protect against rubbing. Ideas include sewing fabric patches inside the garment where friction and stress occur and adapting the pants with side seams and Velcro closures to help get the pants over the orthosis.

Children who are medically fragile often require clothing that has easy access for gastrostomy feedings, tracheostomy care, catheterization, or general diapering. Sweeney (1989) designed clothing for children with severe disabilities. She recommends that caregivers sew moisture-resistant fabric into the seat of pants, on collars, on attaching bibs, and on sleeve cuffs (if the child bites clothing). Jumpsuits or shirts with Velcro at the gastrostomy site, neckline or shoulder, crotch, or pant leg allow caregivers to perform medical procedures without removing the child's clothing (Lawrence & Niemeyer, 1994; Sweeney, 1989).

■ BATHING OR SHOWERING

Typical Development

A child's interest in bathing begins before 2 years of age when he or she begins to wash while in the tub. By 4 years of age, children wash and dry themselves with supervision. It is not until the child is 8 years of age when he or she can independently prepare the bath and shower water (i.e., amount and temperature) and independently wash and dry him or herself.

Good grooming habits are important for all children but take on added significance for children with disabilities. At an early age the caregiver needs to encourage and help the child with a disability to achieve cleanliness to maintain his or her health. Bathing should be a pleasurable activity, but for the parent of a child who lacks balance, it can be a tedious task that requires constant attention and alertness. The work involved multiplies as the child grows and becomes larger and heavier.

Cultural expectations and social routines for bathing vary, and the therapist should consider them when assessing a child's independence. The therapist must respect family preferences on how often a person bathes and with whom (e.g., parent and children bathing together).

Remedial Approach

Therapists often use bathing therapeutically to remediate performance components that interfere with independence. A warm bath may calm a child who is distressed and may decrease tonicity, increase range of motion, and increase independent movement (Case-Smith, 2000). When a child has hypersensitivity, washcloth rubbing, water play, and deep pressure or rubbing while drying the child may assist in reducing the child's sensitivity to touch. For children who have difficulty interacting with others or the environment, bath play may motivate the child to explore objects, engage in pretend play, and interact with a sibling or parent (Case-Smith, 2000).

For children with motor limitations, the therapist may use a remedial approach to prepare the child for self-bathing. The therapist may use activities to improve range of motion, bilateral coordination, grasp, postural control, and motor planning before teaching bathing. Activities or games (e.g., Simon Says) that require a child to reach above or behind or down to the toes may give children the body awareness and necessary movement for self-bathing.

Compensatory strategies

The caregiver's positioning and handling are prime considerations in adapting bathing of children. Children with cerebral palsy may lose their balance when startled. Keeping the child's head and arms forward when lifting and lowering him or her into the tub can prevent a reaction of full extension. The caregiver should use slow and gentle movements with the child and provide simple verbal cues about the steps of bathing. Draining the tub and wrapping the child in a towel before lifting him or her from the tub can make him or her feel more secure.

Parents often need suggestions when bathing a child who is hypersensitive to touch. This child may be avoiding bathing at all costs and is at risk of getting hurt while in the tub. Understanding the child's sensory needs and using adaptive techniques may help bathing become positive for both the parent and child. The child may prefer washing the back and extremities first, and then the stomach and face, using rhythmic, organized, deep strokes. Wrapping the child in a tight towel after bathing and holding the child with deep pressure also can help.

Special equipment that gives support can help the child feel safe and secure. Bath hammocks fully hold the body and enable the parent to wash the child thoroughly (Figure 16-7, *A*). A simple, inexpensive way for giving security is to use a plastic laundry basket lined with foam at its bottom (Figure 16-7, *B*). Commercially, a light, inconspicuous bath support (Figure 16-7, *C*) offers good design features. The front half of the padded support ring swings open for easy entry and then locks securely, holding the child at the chest to give trunk stability. Various kinds of bath seats and shower benches are available for the older child to aid bathtub seating transfers (Figure 16-7, *D*). For the child with severe motor limitations who is lying supine in the tub in shallow water, a horseshoe-shaped inflatable bath collar (Figure 16-7, *E*) serves to support the neck and keep the child's head above water level. A bath stretcher is constructed like a cot and fits inside the bathtub rim level or mid tub level to minimize the caregiver's bending while transferring and bathing the child.

Some parents and children find a hand-held shower useful in removing soap suds. A long-handled bath brush or sponge helps in reaching body parts. Children with limited grasp may be able to wash themselves using a pump soap dispenser and a bath mitt.

Parent education for safety issues

Nonslip bath mats beside the tub and in the tub are essential for safety. Grab bars and their placement require careful thought and planning in each individual case. A rubber cover for the bathtub faucet can prevent injury if the child slips and hits his or her head.

Parents are taught to use good body mechanics during bathing to prevent back injury. To lessen strain, it is best for the adult to sit on a stool beside the tub or kneel on a cushion. Lifting is done with the knees bent and back straight, using the legs for power. As children get older and heavier, a hoyer lift or easily accessed shower stall arrangement may be necessary.

Oral Hygiene

By 2 years of age, children imitate their parents when brushing their teeth. Tooth-brushing supervision continues until about 6 years of age. Tooth brushing can be especially difficult for the child with oral sensitivity. The child should use his or her preferred brushing methods until tolerance improves and he or she can accomplish more thorough cleaning. A small, soft brush is easier to move around in the mouth, especially if the child has a tongue thrust or gag reflex. When the child's gums are tender, the caregiver can substitute a soft sponge-tipped toothette for a brush. For the child who independently brushes, an electric toothbrush enables more thorough cleaning. This is a good solution for children with limited dexterity, although for children with weakness, an electric toothbrush may be too heavy to manage.

If a child has problems with a weak grasp, the caregiver can enlarge the toothbrush handle with sponge rubber or add a Velcro strap. One-handed flossing tools are available in large and small sizes and can be adapted by enlarging the size and length of the handle.

Grooming

Face washing, handwashing, and hair care are typical grooming activities taught to preschoolers and young children. The child's culture, family values, and individual interests strongly influence his or her timing for developing grooming independence. Adolescence begins at the onset of puberty and is a period of remarkable growth toward physical, sexual, emotional, and social maturity. The physiologic changes that occur at puberty are partially attributable to the increased output of hormones by the pituitary gland. For example, body hair grows and the sebaceous glands become more active, producing oily secretions. With these physical changes and different social expectations (depending on the culture), new self-maintenance tasks emerge, including skin care, hair styling, hair removal, and cosmetic application.

Intervention

Grooming is an area of self-care highly influenced by cultural values. The therapist must respect the child and family's preferences in hairstyle, cosmetics, and routines. The family and child or adolescent needs to take the lead in identifying their concerns and priorities in this self-care area. Problem solving follows the principles and approaches identified in the first sections of this chapter. The following is an example of an adolescent who desires independence in grooming:

> Josie demonstrates incoordination, poor memory, and limited judgment, but she wants to be independent in her grooming. Remedial activities are somewhat helpful, but compensatory strategies are more essential to increasing her independence in grooming. The occupational therapist recommends that Josie use a brush with

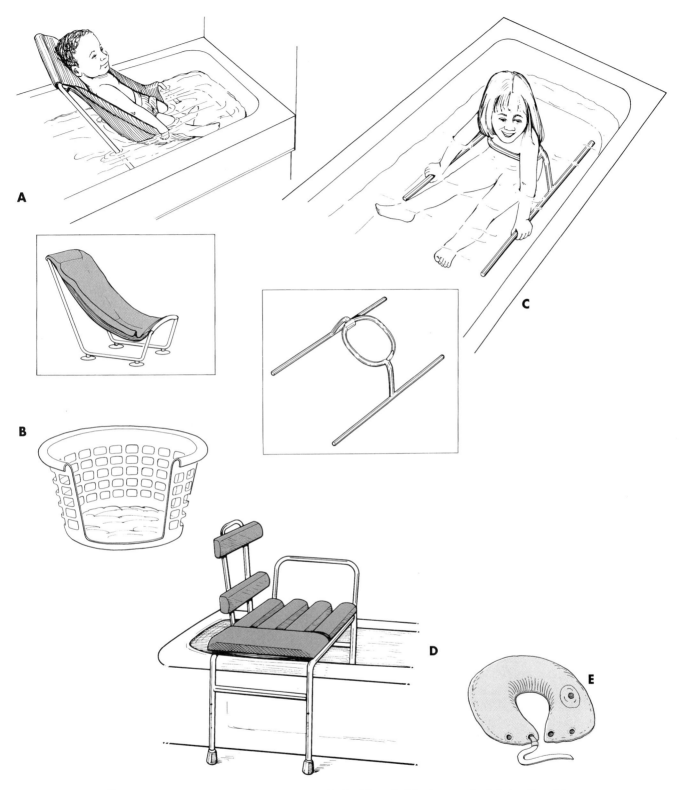

figure**16-7**   Adapted seating equipment for bathing. **A,** The hammock chair is adjustable and equipped with oversized suction feet. It fully supports the child who has no sitting balance and poor head control. **B,** The front of a plastic laundry basket is cut out to allow room for the child's legs. The basket gives security during first baths in a large tub. **C,** Trunk support is light-weight and compact and fits all bathtubs. **D,** Shower bench aids seating and transfers. **E,** Inflatable bath collar can be used when the child is in either the supine or prone position.

a built-up handle, rest her elbow on the table while brushing her hair, use a checklist and visual model, and ask a peer to help style her hair. Josie and her parents are educated about ways to incorporate grooming tasks into everyday routines by placing visual cues in the environment (e.g., deodorant left on the dresser and facial cleaning equipment left out at the sink as a visual cue to use before cosmetic application).

Health Maintenance Skills and Sexuality

Families and therapists encourage children to be responsible for all aspects of self-care. Caring for personal devices (e.g., hearing aids, wheelchairs, or splints), taking medications, and being responsible for health maintenance generally become realistic expectations for children with disabilities as they mature. Children can partially participate in any of these tasks or direct others on how to perform the task. As children make decisions about their health routines, they learn firsthand what happens if they do not follow bowel and bladder programs or develop routines for physical fitness or proper nutrition. Activities that promote the development of problem-solving skills and help children gain confidence in their abilities to be self-sufficient are critical to the child's development of self-care independence.

Children and adolescents with chronic health care needs have numerous medical tasks to learn besides general health care maintenance. Table 16-10 lists examples of health maintenance issues for children with chronic medical needs.

While working with adolescents on personal self-care tasks such as bathing or personal hygiene, sexuality questions may arise. Children and adolescents of all disabilities are sexual beings. Their parents may be receptive to discussing their child's *sexuality,* or they may feel unprepared to address these issues. When the child is less than 18 years of age, parental permission to discuss sexuality issues is necessary. Therapists need to consider the contextual aspects of the child's family and social groups. Therapists need to determine whether it is appropriate to discuss sexuality and who should discuss it (receiver and informant). If the therapist decides to enter a discourse regarding sexuality, the contextual aspects of the child's family and social groups should be considered. Occupational therapists may refer the adolescent to someone who has knowledge about and feels comfortable discussing sexuality. Responsible therapists are careful to separate personal values from the children and families' values toward sexuality.

Children and adolescents with cognitive problems related to mental retardation or a traumatic brain injury often need guidelines for expressing their sexuality appropriately within various contexts. Appropriate dress and hygiene, masturbation, touching of others, and appro-priate interactions with the opposite gender are areas that may need education. The older adolescent may question the physical and psychosocial aspects of sexuality and his or her ability to conceive. Information about contraceptive use and techniques for avoiding intercourse is essential for the adolescent to avoid unwanted pregnancies.

Functional Communication

As children mature and begin to take more responsibility for their own health maintenance and sexuality, their need to independently communicate with others increases. Children learn how to send and receive messages to and from other people through verbal, nonverbal, and graphic communication systems. Children who are nonverbal may use gestures, writing, or assistive devices to communicate their needs. This section discusses emergency systems and telephones as forms of communication (see Chapter 18 for improving handwriting skills and Chapter 19 for augmentative communication and computer access).

Emergency alert and call systems

Children with serious medical problems or with life-support systems need more frequent monitoring day and night. This need is more critical for children who have impaired mobility, dexterity, or communication skills. Intercom systems assist parents with this responsibility and give the child a way to initiate calls for help or social interaction. Call switches or buzzers that attach to the bed or wheelchair can provide an independent means of seeking assistance from individuals in other rooms. Various portable intercoms and inexpensive environmental control units are available at electronics supply stores and children's stores. Caregivers may position a wireless telephone or a cellular telephone near the child. The child can use this device as a telephone or as an intercom, depending on the model chosen.

Emergency alert systems, worn as pendants or stabilized on wheelchairs, are available for purchase with a service that places emergency calls when the system is activated. The child can use outside alarms that can be heard in the neighborhood to summon assistance. The caregivers must carefully plan arrangements and alternatives in advance. The ability to quickly exit the house is most directly influenced by the child's ability to get to the door and open it; therefore the therapist may still practice these skills in intervention sessions.

Telephones

Changes in telephone design have improved access for all persons with disabilities. Telephones may have large numbers and many features, such as redial, preprogrammed telephone numbers, and built-in intercoms or amplifiers. These features are useful for children with limited dexterity and limited abilities to sequence or remember telephone numbers. Children with auditory

table 16-10	Health Care Maintenance for Typically Developing Children and Children with Spina Bifida	

Ages (yr)	Typical Development of Health Maintenance (e.g., Medicines, Personal Devices, and Health Routines)	Additional Health Maintenance Issues for a Child with Spina Bifida
5-9	• Follows safety rules at home and school • Informs others of emergencies • Uses basic first aid techniques for minor injuries • Tells others when he or she is sick • Cares for health care items with reminders (e.g., glasses and toothbrush) • Routinely washes hands, takes a bath, and washes hair with reminders • Assists in getting medicine ready	• Does pressure reliefs and checks for skin breakdown with reminders (e.g., legs, buttocks, and feet) • Tells others when he or she is injured or feels sick (e.g., headache, pain, swelling, or change in bowel and bladder patterns) • Cares for personal adaptive devices with reminders (e.g., crutches, wheelchair, or catheters) • Catheterizes self at home and school • Carries a list of current medicines and doctors' names
10-14	• Recognizes when he or she is getting sick or needs to see a doctor • Knows emergency procedures (e.g., phone numbers, who to call, and what to do) • Cares for health care items (e.g., glasses, braces, retainers, and facial scrubs) • Uses first aid procedures • Eats nutritious meals with supervision • Exercises with supervision • Takes medicine with supervision • Avoids cigarettes, drugs, and sexual abuse	• Recognizes when he or she is injured or feels sick (e.g., headache, pain, swelling, or change in bowel and bladder patterns) • Knows dosage of medications • Knows names of doctors (e.g., primary care, urologist, neurologist, or orthopedist) • Cares for personal adaptive devices or instructs others on how to maintain the device (e.g., wheelchair, walker, or braces) • Catheterizes self in community environments • Prevents further health care problems (e.g., drinks to avoid bladder infection; exercises [push ups]; avoids latex; maintains good hygiene, eating, and exercise practices)
15-18	• Recognizes when a change in medicine or health intervention is needed • Makes appointments to see doctors • Eats nutritious meals • Exercises regularly • Cares for personal hygiene and good health habits • Uses first aid procedures for major and minor injuries • Takes medicine when needed • Uses birth control as needed	• Takes medications independently and knows side effects • Knows how to access therapy, doctors, and other health care services • Knows how to obtain and pay for medical supplies • Prevents secondary disabilities (e.g., weight management, routine medical care, skin care, and equipment maintenance)

Adapted from Ford, A., Schnorr, R., Meyer, L., Davern, L., Black, J., & Dempsey, P. (1989). *The Syracuse community-reference curriculum guide* (pp. 324-327). Baltimore: Brookes.
Peterson, P.M., Rauen, K.K., Brown, J., & Cole, J. (1994). Spina bifida: The transition into adulthood begins in infancy. *Rehabilitation Nursing, 19*(4), 229-238.

limitations can use special telephones with visual indicators (e.g., flashing light or strobe light), vibration, or hearing aid compatibility, or a telecommunication device for the deaf (TDD) (McInnes & Treffry, 1993). Telephones with remote control dialing, large illuminated letters or Braille, talk-back features (e.g., repeats last telephone number dialed or caller identification information), and voice-activated answering machines are features that assist children with limited vision.

If dexterity or endurance is problematic, the child can use a headset or a telephone that is mounted on a goose-neck or with an attached universal cuff. The child dials buttons with a T-bar or universal cuff with a pencil. Answering machines that record and save messages are helpful when writing is difficult. Some adolescents record a message asking the caller to "stay on the line until I can get to the phone!" Voice-activated answering machines and remote control dialing assist children with limited physical capabilities. Car telephones, cellular telephones, and other telephones or pagers that are portable are also beneficial to children and adolescents with disabilities. These easily accessed devices are helpful for emergencies and can be equipped with the features described previously.

Parents may not have the financial resources or an interest in changing telephone systems. Familial preferences and the environmental context often influence which telephone is selected. Sample questions for the therapist to ask are as follows:

- What is the purpose of having the telephone (e.g., safety, socialization, work)?
- In which room or rooms will the child use the telephone?
- If a child uses a headset or an environmental control unit to talk on the telephone, can other family members also access it easily?
- If the child uses a cellular telephone or a pager system, are they permitted at school?
- Can the child or will a family member be responsible for recharging the telephone or changing the batteries?

■ INSTRUMENTAL ACTIVITIES OF DAILY LIVING

Home Management Tasks

During childhood, children learn home management tasks that help them contribute to family functioning. Performing these tasks gives children a feeling of self-worth and develops skills for independent living and work environments. Home management tasks include cleaning, caring for clothing, preparing and cleaning up after meals, shopping, managing money, and maintaining a household.

Typical Developmental Sequence

As early as 18 months of age, children begin to understand what it means to "help out" in performing household chores. As children observe their parents routinely dust, sweep, set tables, or do laundry, they often initiate simple household tasks without cues from a parent (Rheingold, 1982). "Me do it" or "I want to sweep" are typical comments. As children get older, they become more capable of performing household chores, and parents often wish that enthusiasm for helping around the house will continue. Instead, adolescents become more absorbed in personal grooming or social activities and participate less in household chores (Duckett, Raffaelli, & Richards, 1989). Table 16-11 outlines the developmental sequence for learning to perform home management tasks.

Contextual considerations

Participation in home management tasks depends on the child's age and capabilities and the temporal and environmental contexts. The size of the family and accessibility of the environment can encourage or discourage

table 16-11 *Developmental Sequence for Home Management Tasks*

Age	Task
13 months	• Imitates housework
2 years	• Picks up and puts toys away with parental reminders
	• Copies parents' domestic activities
3 years	• Carries things without dropping them
	• Dusts with help
	• Dries dishes with help
	• Gardens with help
	• Puts toys away with reminders
	• Wipes spills
4 years	• Fixes dry cereal and snacks
	• Helps with sorting laundry
5 years	• Puts toys away neatly
	• Makes a sandwich
	• Takes out trash
	• Makes bed
	• Puts dirty clothes away
	• Answers telephone correctly
6 years	• Does simple errands
	• Does household chores without redoing
	• Cleans sink
	• Washes dishes with help
	• Crosses street safely
7-9 years	• Begins to cook simple meal
	• Puts clean clothes away
	• Hangs up clothes
	• Manages small amounts of money
	• Uses telephone correctly
10-12 years	• Cooks simple meal with supervision
	• Does simple repairs with appropriate tools
	• Begins doing laundry
	• Sets table
	• Washes dishes
	• Cares for pet with reminders
13-14 years	• Does laundry
	• Cooks meals

participation in household chores. Age, gender, socioeconomic status, geographic location (Light, Hertsgaard, & Martin, 1985), and customs and values about self-sufficiency (Lynch & Hanson, 1998) may influence when and how the child performs chores. Girls often participate more in chores than boys (Seymour, 1988), and they may choose more cooperative indoor chores than boys, who choose more independent outdoor chores (e.g., washing the car and lawn care) (Duckett et. al., 1989). Expectations often differ for children from low socioeconomic environments or rural versus urban areas. Families may encourage independence or they may promote interdependency among family members. Therapists need to consider these factors when working with children and their families.

The family's modeling behaviors, patience, routines, and expectations and the child's preferences influence which chores children do. This role modeling of chores by all family members is important in establishing household chores as routine and expected. If the child does household chores chaotically or rarely, he or she may not be included in "helping out" roles nor learn the typical routines or habits to complete household tasks.

When children with or without disabilities first begin to wash tables, dust, or vacuum, extra time and patience from the parent and modified expectations for performance are necessary. The parents repeat instructions and the child often must redo the tasks, taking more time than if the parents had completed the task themselves. Parents give the child time to problem solve and ideally allow him or her to learn from mistakes.

Performance Problems in Household Tasks

The medical-physical or educational needs of a child with a disability often overshadow the development of household skills. Occupational therapists collaborate with parents to set up routines and modify tasks and environments so that the child can perform all or a portion of household tasks. Often independence in household tasks is not a goal; however, some level of participation allows the child to contribute to the family's daily functions.

Children with sensorimotor problems have difficulty obtaining materials, manipulating and using typical equipment, or completing the entire task. Children with cognitive limitations have difficulty initiating and terminating the task, following and remembering the sequence, and generalizing the skills to other environments (e.g., differences in cleaning kitchen and living room floors). When a child has a low frustration level and poor impulse control, parents are often fearful to give them tasks that could potentially be unsafe.

Intervention Strategies

Environmental modifications, assistive technology, task modification, and varying levels of help from others are often the approaches that therapists use to teach home management tasks. Table 16-5 gives examples of how caregivers can adapt various environments in the home with structural changes and assistive devices to allow the child to participate in household tasks.

Natural cues within the physical or social environment assist in developing a child's IADL skills. If memory is a problem, the caregiver should keep all of the needed supplies where the child will use them. For example, the caregiver can place a sponge next to the bathroom sink to help the child find the object and remind him or her to clean the sink after tooth brushing or face washing. Artificial cues such as color-coding or labeling shelves, cabinets, and bins with pictures or words also help children locate objects within the environment. Picture charts and checklists assist the child in remembering the sequence of tasks.

Children with range of motion, strength, dexterity, or postural control problems may need modified equipment. For cleaning table surfaces, typical equipment may include dusting or wiping mitts or adapted spray bottles with cleaning solutions in them. Long-handled dustpans, dusters, or buckets on wheels with a stick attached may help the child who cannot bend forward. Broom, mop, and vacuum handles can be enlarged or adapted with additional pieces to allow the child to hold them.

Children with intellectual limitations may encounter problems with sequencing, judging, and performing the tasks on a regular basis (Browder & Snell, 1993). These children need pictorial cues in the form of a chart on the wall or a flip-card book. The charts list the steps of a task or a sequence of tasks (e.g., task analysis), and the child checks off each step or task when he or she completes it. The picture helps the child remember the sequence and helps him or her judge whether he or she has done the task correctly. For example, a pictorial recipe allows the child to see how many cups of cheese to use and whether he or she has put the cheese correctly on top of the pizza. If these materials have an acetate or plastic covering, the child can use them routinely with a washable marker. The caregiver should fade the use of pictorial cues as the child learns the task.

The caregiver should use verbal, gestural, or physical cues when child is first learning a task. For example, the caregiver can use verbal cues to tell the child how many times to "squirt" a solution when cleaning tables or mirrors. An example of a gestural cue is pointing to bed corners so the child can check if a bed is made properly.

Most families are interdependent in performing home management tasks. Although independent performance is highly valued, complete self-reliance in a task may not be achievable or even desirable if the task requires too much time and energy or if it exacerbates abnormal behaviors or movement patterns. Dependence in some tasks is appropriate at times and may permit completion of other more readily achieved independent living skills.

Children with disabilities participate in home management tasks at different levels. Some may never be independent in cooking, but the caregiver can include them in an activity through partial participation. For example, a child with athetoid cerebral palsy may not have the coordination to control stirring strokes, but he or she can participate in the task of making a cake or cutting vegetables by using an automated learning device (ALD) with an electric mixer (Levin & Scherfenberg, 1987). An ALD is a control unit with a switch that activates an appliance. The ALD reduces the voltage of the appliance to a lower voltage at the switch. It may have a timer that allows the appliance to remain on for a set amount of time without the child activating the switch during this time.

Safety in household tasks

Many parents fear allowing their children with disabilities to perform household tasks. Safety while using appliances, utensils, and other equipment is of utmost importance. For example, children with myelomeningocele may not have sensation in their lower extremities. They need to be aware of potential burns from hot plates or pots carried on their lap or touching a stove, dryer, or other hot items. Fire alarms, carbon monoxide detectors, gas detectors, and propane detectors can have amplified sound, flashing lights, and/or vibration to alert children and adolescents with sensory impairments. Children also need to be ready to respond if an emergency occurs. Access to the telephone and the correct telephone numbers and the ability to get in and out of the house are key skills. An accessible telephone station, combined with knowledge of how to contact emergency services or a designated helper, is also important.

Therapists consider cultural characteristics in relation to safety issues. In some cultures, parents are expected to protect their children until they are married and leave the house; they may not want children (with or without disabilities) exposed to uncertain or potentially risky situations. In addition, safety knowledge may be lacking for some families. For example, recently immigrated families may not have experience with electricity or plumbing and may not be aware of safety issues with water and electricity (Lynch & Hanson, 1998).

Caring for pets and others

As children grow, they are given responsibilities for caring for others. This responsibility typically begins with an animal and later may include caring for younger siblings. Table 16-12 lists typical development of caregiving skills for children and adolescents. Children and adolescents with disabilities are often cared for by others and have few opportunities to reciprocate this caring to others. Others model caregiving in social and cultural environments. With grading, prompting, and guidance, some children with disabilities learn how to do errands or favors, clean up, share materials, baby-sit, and perform volunteer work (Ford et. al., 1989). For example, children with significant delays in development can learn how to complete an errand or help their mother or a sibling feel better by rubbing her shoulders or bringing her a blanket. Visual, verbal, gestural, and physical cues may assist the child in learning caregiving occupations.

table 16-12	**Typical Development of Caring for Others**
Ages	**Caring for Others**
5-9 yrs	• Shares toys, personal belongings, or materials • Helps clean up or get materials for parent or teacher • Helps sibling or classmate learn new game or new skill • Does errands for teacher or parent • Cares for pets with reminders (e.g., feeding, exercise, play)
10-14 yrs	• Babysits siblings (e.g., first in backyard, then for longer periods) and begins babysitting neighbor children • Cares for sick sibling, parent, or friend • Does favors for peers or family • Helps neighbor with chore or errand • Cares for pets
15-18 yrs	• Babysits siblings and other children • Cares for others' pets or houses • Volunteers within community • Helps take others on errands • Nurtures others without prompting

Adapted from: Ford, A., Schnorr, R., Meyer, L., Davern, L., Black, J., & Dempsey, P. (1989). The Syracuse community-reference curriculum guide. (pp. 327-328). Baltimore: Brookes.

Community activities and skills

Shopping, eating in restaurants, banking, and attending sports and recreational events involve many similar skills, including achieving mobility, communicating with strangers, handling money and packages, reading and writing, and performing self-care skills within various settings. The therapist performs an ecological assessment to target the tasks and skills that are necessary, to identify where adaptations or skill development is needed, and to develop and analyze what instructional strategies will "fit" the environmental demands. The therapist teaches children these tasks in the community setting (Falvey, 1986; York-Barr et. al., 1996). The use of assistive devices in public depends on the degree of portability, ease of use, and attitudes of the child and family.

Managing money during shopping tasks is often difficult for the child with physical or cognitive disabilities. These children can use small zipper purses (i.e., fanny packs) that go around the waist or are hooked to the wheelchair instead of wallets. These are adapted with a large zipper pull and can be attached with Velcro to a lapboard for stability. The child can hand the fanny pack to the store clerk and ask them to get the money out or put their change in the fanny pack. When purchasing an item, children can also instruct clerks to put their change in the paper bag that is given to them. The child can use a calculator to help with arithmetic and carry cue cards to remind himself or herself of the value of money. For children with visual limitations, a money brailler, coin sorter, or specific folding technique or placement of money can help the child identify denominations of money.

Community Mobility

Functional mobility in the community is critical to the child's development and to the family's ability to be active outside the home. Community participation ranges from the early stages when the child accompanies his or her parents on errands to the time when the child goes out on his or her own. The therapist addresses transportation of the child with disabilities from functional and safety standpoints. Furthermore, when the therapist selects new equipment for a child, he or she considers the methods used for home, school, and community mobility to ensure that the child can use and transport the device as necessary. The following is an example of a child who uses a mobility device:

A power wheelchair is ordered for a child to maneuver around school and to participate in community outings. This chair gives the child tremendous capabilities when she is at school. However, at home the power wheelchair stays on the porch because it does not fit inside the front door. The family vehicle is inadequate in transporting the chair. If the therapist had considered these variables at the time of assessment, these problems would not have occurred.

Environmental factors affecting mobility

Environmental factors that affect mobility include other people and crowds, street crossings, use of personal or public transportation and elevators, and architectural barriers. Occupational therapists often are involved with a team to select the most appropriate mobility device for a child. (Chapter 20 elaborates on the devices that are available for children.) Once the therapist identifies problems in mobility, he or she may consult with or teach the child, parent, and other caregivers remedial and compensatory techniques for improving mobility in various community settings. The therapist can use his or her expertise to educate the child and caregivers on how to get in and out of doorways and elevators, get up and down curbs, and maneuver within tight spots. The therapist also uses his or her knowledge about sensory modifications, energy conservation, time management, and positive behavior supports to help children move within routine environments such as school or home. The following is an example of a child who is taught to overcome environmental barriers:

Geoff is a 16-year-old sophomore in high school with spastic cerebral palsy. He wants to hang out with his friends at a fast food restaurant but has mostly depended on his family to take him places and to get his food. Geoff uses an augmentative communication device and a power wheelchair with a laptray. As a consultant, the therapist visits the community site to perform an ecological evaluation. After assessing Geoff in the fast food restaurant, the therapist uses task analysis to determine six steps for Geoff to accomplish.

As a consultant, the therapist collaborates with Geoff, the Certified Occupational Therapy Assistant (COTA) and the teacher to determine compensatory strategies for Geoff to succeed in this community activity. Table 16-13 summarizes the approaches and adaptations that Geoff can use to improve his performance. Using systematic record keeping, the team determines the steps that Geoff does consistently and the strategies that need modification. Graphing Geoff's progress also cues the COTA, teacher, and family to reduce prompting, eliminate unnecessary adaptive equipment, and increase the level of performance expected from Geoff.

Geoff completes several IADLs during the community outing. Besides preplanning an activity and eating out, Geoff experiences getting on and off public transportation, crossing a street, asking for help, making transactions, manipulating money, choosing the most nutritious meal with the least amount of fat, and interacting with others without disabilities.

If Geoff was given a standardized upper-extremity assessment, he would have scored below the first percentile in coordination, strength, and function. This assessment is inappropriate because it does not predict or capture how Geoff's performance is influenced by a contextually based occupation that has meaning to him. In spite of Geoff's spastic cerebral palsy with quadriplegia, he independently manipulates money, puts his food on a laptray, selects a napkin and straw, and carries his food to the table. The most difficult task for Geoff is initiating the task and ordering the food. Would this outcome have been predictable if the therapist only knew Geoff's diagnoses?

Independent driving

Adolescents with or without disabilities are often excited about being able to drive. This ability gives the child more independence from his or her parents. The therapist usually consults with adapted driving program specialists unless he or she has had specialized training in driving adaptations and instruction. The therapist considers strength, range of motion, sensation, coordination, reach, reaction time, balance, and perceptual abilities in functional terms related to driving.

Automobile adaptations for the teenage driver with a disability range from simple add-on components to those that convert a car or van permanently. Add-on

table 16-13 *An Example of Instructional Procedures and Adaptations to Build Successful Occupational Performance in the Community*

Objective: Geoff will be able to purchase and eat a meal at a fast food restaurant by completing each subskill and criteria as established.

Instructional Goals and Procedures	Materials/ Assistive Technology	Task Method and Environmental Adaptations	Time	Motivational Strategies
6 Throws away trash and exits fast food restaurant, asking for help, if needed in 5-min period 1:1; prompt; wait outside for him	Power wheelchair, lapboard, augmentative communication device, watch; push open doors and trash can	Wads up trash before moving to trash can; chooses trash container not in the "main flow" of the restaurant traffic; exits door closest to table area where people may be seated; has Epson programmed to say, "Please open the door for me." "Thank you." Try automatic and manual doors	5 minutes	Being able to socialize with others with preprogrammed message; working toward independence; "beat the clock"
5 Opens or requests help to open packages and eats food independently 1:1; begin with drink, add one item each time	Drink; French fries; finger foods	Eats at the table on his lap tray; chooses items he can open (i.e., in paper, not box) and hold on to; preprogrammed Epson: "Please help me open this."	2-3 items per visit	Eating; time to socialize 1:1
4 Gets food, napkin, straw, and utensils and carries to table area on his lapboard without spilling items 1:1; verbal and gestural cues to maneuver wheelchair	Power wheelchair, lapboard, possibly dycem	Goes to restaurant at nonpeak hrs; therapist or friend may put tray on lapboard; goes to table with removable chairs	Independent	Wants to do independently
3 Independently manipulates money and pays for food 1:1; stand behind Geoff; verbal or gestural cues	Puts money in side pocket of wheelchair; uses lapboard on which to place money	Practices money skills in classroom; uses preprogrammed Epson message to ask clerk to put his return change on tray	Practices money skills for 2 wks before outing	Wants to be able to do this at other businesses
2 Uses augmentative communication device independently to order food 1:1; decides on what to eat before coming; preprogram device; timer on watch to clue him; added peer to eat with him	Epson augmentative communication device; lapboard	Hands clerk card that says, "I use this machine to talk to you." Does not go to counter until ready; does on "off times" so it is not extremely busy	2 minutes	Wants to eat food different from cafeteria at school; wants to do with friends; can choose own food!
1 Determines his order and if he has enough money 1:1; verbal prompting; counts money before going out & writes it down; timer on watch to clue him	Lapboard, side pocket for wheelchair; watch; calculator	Practices rounding numbers and counting money in math class; talks about what he thinks items will cost before going to restaurant; uses calculator to add money	3 minutes	Given certain amount of money to spend; he can keep the change

adaptations that do not affect others' use of the car are preferred when feasible. Steering knobs facilitate grasping and turning the wheel. Built-up brakes and accelerator pedals or left-footed accelerators are useful for adolescents with range of motion, weakness, or coordination difficulties. Right- or left-hand controls or relocation of the horn and dimmer switches are examples of other adaptations for the family automobile. For children with quadriplegia or significant upper-extremity weakness, zero-effort steering may be useful.

Teenagers may learn to drive with adapted controls, but independence is limited if they cannot transfer themselves and equipment, such as wheelchairs, into and out of the car. Therapists teach various transfer techniques depending on the child's capabilities, especially strength and postural control. Car door openers, enlarged controls (e.g., door locks), transfer boards, webbing loops, modified dressing sticks (to close the door), or wooden jigs to guide wheelchairs into a specific space (i.e., trunk or back seat) are examples of assistive devices that the adolescent may use. Teenagers who ambulate for short distances may be able to put a chair into the trunk or side door of a car. Other teenagers who are nonambulatory may also place the chair in the back seat of the car or may get in the front seat on the passenger side of the car and pull the wheelchair in with them. Wheelchair carriers and lifts that go on the rear or top of the car may be another option.

■ SUMMARY

This chapter presented the reader with a wide range of options for enhancing self-care and IADL skills in children and adolescents with disabilities. Typical developmental sequences and special methods for evaluating self-care and IADL skills were presented. The temporal and environmental context in which self-care tasks and IADL occur and parent and child preferences are used to plan evaluation and intervention. Personal preferences and motivational levels of the child and caregivers are important factors for the therapist to consider.

Performance in self-care tasks and IADLs is enhanced through developmental, remedial, compensatory, and educational approaches. Examples of assistive technology and environmental modifications were given. The importance of positioning and orienting the child to the work surface was stressed. As technology changes and outcome data become available, a responsibility of the occupational therapist is to remain knowledgeable about the range of current methods and equipment that promote independent function in children with disabilities.

STUDY QUESTIONS

1. Linda is 2 years old and has high tone with numerous spasms. Her mother has asked for suggestions for dressing and diapering. Linda's mother tells you that she feels like she has a morning struggle pulling her legs apart. What do you suggest?

2. Mark is 7 months old and has Down syndrome. His mother has just returned to work, and his grandmother is taking care of him. She is having difficulty with dressing Mark. She complains that her back is hurting her and that Mark is like a rag doll. What do you suggest?

3. Hank is 16 years old and has diabetes. He is cognitively intact but has peripheral neuropathies, low endurance, and poor coordination. He is in a wheelchair and lives in a wheelchair-accessible home. Hank wants to be able to stay by himself when he comes home from school, but his mother is leery. He needs to be able to take his medicine and fix himself a snack. As Hank's therapist, what things do you need to think about? What adaptations may he need?

4. Andy is 2½ years old and has begun toilet training. He has below-average equilibrium reactions for his age and has difficulty with fasteners. What suggestions do you have for his day care providers as they begin to address toilet training?

5. Colin is 5 years old and has been identified with severe perceptual problems and low tone and endurance. What do you hypothesize will be his problems with dressing? What can you do to make the task easier?

6. Nine-year-old Jeffrey has poor postural control and tactile defensiveness. Bath time is difficult for his mother because Jeffrey particularly hates to have his hair washed. What suggestions do you have for her?

7. Twelve-year-old Melinda has difficulty with balance, but she is motivated to dress herself. What positions could help facilitate her independent performance in putting on pants, shoes, or a shirt?

8. Mario is an 8-year-old child who has a strong startle reaction and is low tone. His mother is having difficulty getting him into the tub. What positions and equipment do you suggest to Mario's mother once Mario is in the tub?

9. Jay is 3 years old and has myelomeningocele. Mobility is difficult for him. Currently, he scoots himself around the floor. What suggestions do you have to improve functional mobility? What precautions do you need to think about?

Continued

STUDY QUESTIONS—cont'd

10. The principal at your school has announced that a new elementary school will be built and it is expected to have approximately 20 students who are in wheelchairs. He asks you, "What should I consider for environmental adaptations?" Thinking of this age range, what do you suggest?

11. Gary is 10 years old and was placed in traction for 4 months because of a severe break in his femur. He is modest and wants to be able to wash and dress himself. What suggestions do you give to Gary and his caregivers?

References

Bayzak, S. (1989). Changes in attitude beliefs regarding parent participation in home programs. *The American Journal of Occupational Therapy, 43,* 723-728.

Bergen, A.F., & Colangelo, C. (1985). *Positioning the client with CNS deficits: The wheelchair and other adapted equipment* (2nd ed.). Valhalla, NY: Valhalla Rehabilitation Publications.

Bergen, A.F., Presperin, J., & Tallman, T. (1990). *Positioning for function: Wheelchairs and other assistive devices.* Valhalla, NY: Valhalla Rehabilitation Publications.

Boehme, R. (1988). *Improving upper body control: An approach to assessment and treatment of tonal dysfunction.* Tucson: Therapy Skill Builders.

Brollier, C., Shepherd, J., & Markley, K. (1994). Transition from school to community living. *The American Journal of Occupational Therapy, 48* (4), 346-353.

Browder, M., & Snell, M. (1993). Daily living and community skills. In M.E. Snell (Ed.), *Instruction of students with severe disabilities* (4th ed.). (pp. 480-525). New York: Macmillan.

Brown, L., Schwarz, P., Udvari-Solner, A., Kampschroer, E., Johnson, F., Jorgensen, J., & Gruenewald, L. (1991). How much time should students with severe intellectual disabilities spend in regular education classrooms and elsewhere? *Journal of the Association for Persons with Severe Handicaps, 16,* 39-47.

Brown, M., & Gordon, W.A. (1987). Impact of impairment on activity patterns of children. *Archives of Physical Medicine and Rehabilitation, 68,* 828-832.

Bryze, K., & Curtin, C. (1993). A top-down approach: Relationships to research and occupational performance. *Developmental Disabilities Special Interest Section Newsletter, 2,* 2-4.

Case-Smith, J. (2000). Self-care strategies for children with developmental deficits. In C. Christiansen (Ed.), *Ways of living: Self-care strategies for special needs* (pp. 83-122). Bethesda, MD: American Occupational Therapy Association.

Chan, S. (1998). Families with Asian roots. In E.W. Lynch & M.J. Hanson (Eds.). *Developing cross-cultural competence: A guide for working with children and their families* (2nd ed.). (pp. 251-354). Baltimore: Brookes.

Coley, I. (1978). *Pediatric assessment of self care assessment* (pp. 145, 149). St. Louis: Mosby.

Coster, W.J. (1998). Occupation-centered assessment of children. *The American Journal of Occupational Therapy, 52* (5), 337-344.

Duckett, E., Raffaelli, M., & Richards, M. (1989). Taking care: Maintaining the self and the home in early adolescence. *Journal of Youth and Adolescence, 18* (6), 549-565.

Dunn, W., Brown, C., & McGuigan, A. (1994). Ecology of human performance: A framework for considering the effect of context. *The American Journal of Occupational Therapy, 48* (7), 595-607.

Erickson, M.L. (1976). *Assessment and management of developmental changes in children.* St. Louis: Mosby.

Eriksson, B., Gawell, A., Munthe, K., Riddar, A., Rygaard, K., Windling, U., & Zachrisson, G. (1987). *Activities using headsticks and optical pointers: A description of methods.* Stockholm, Sweden: Swedish Institute for the Handicapped.

Falvey, M. (1986). *Community based curriculum: Instructional strategies for students with severe handicaps.* Baltimore: Brookes.

Ferguson, D.L., & Baumgart, D. (1991). Partial participation revisited. *Journal of the Association for Persons with Severe Handicaps, 16,* 218-227.

Fisher, A. (1994). *Assessment of motor and process skills* (version 8.0). Unpublished test manual. Fort Collins, CO: Colorado State University.

Ford, A., Schnorr, R., Meyer, L., Davern, L, Black, J., & Dempsey, P. (1989). *The Syracuse community-reference curriculum guide.* Baltimore: Brookes.

Furuno, S., O'Reilly, K., Hosaka, C.M., Zeisloft, B., & Allman, T. (1984). *Hawaii Early Learning Profile.* Palo Alto, CA: Vort.

Geyer, L.A., Kurtz, L.A., & Byram, L.E. (1998). Promoting function in daily living skills. In J.P. Dormans & L. Peliegrino (Eds.), *Caring for children with cerebral palsy: A team approach* (pp. 323-346). Baltimore: Brookes.

Giangreco, M., Cloninger, C., & Iverson, V. (1997). *Choosing options and accommodations for children (COACH)* (2nd ed.). Baltimore: Brookes.

Haley, S.M., Coster, W.J., Ludlow, L.H., Haltiwanger, J., & Andrellos, P. (1992). *Administration manual for the Pediatric Evaluation of Disability Inventory.* San Antonio: Psychological Corporation.

Hamilton, B.B., & Granger, C.U. (1991). *Functional Independence Measure for Children (WeeFIM).* Buffalo, NY: Research Foundation of the State University of New York.

Hanson, M. (1998). Families with Anglo-European roots. In E.W. Lynch & M.J. Hanson (Eds.). *Developing cross-cultural competence* (2nd ed.). (pp. 93-126). Baltimore: Brookes.

Holm, M.B., Rogers, J.C., & James, A.B. (1998). Treatment of occupational performance areas: Section 1, treatment of activities of daily living. In M.E. Neistadt & E.B. Crepeau (Eds.), *Willard and Spackman's occupational therapy* (9th ed.). (pp. 323-364). Philadelphia: J.B. Lippincott.

Johnson-Martin, N., Jens, K.G., Attermeier, S.M., & Hacker, B. (1991). *The Carolina curriculum for handicapped infants and infants at risk.* Baltimore: Brookes.

Kangas, K. (1998). *Using your head: Access and integration of independent mobility and communication "Head First".* Presentation at TechKnowledgy '98 Conference, Richmond, VA: Children's Hospital.

Kellegrew, D. (1998). Creating opportunities for occupation: An intervention to promote the self-care independence of young children with special needs. *The American Journal of Occupational Therapy, 52* (6), 457-465.

Kennedy, E. (1981). *Dressing with pride* (vol. 1.). Groton, CT: PRIDE Foundation.

Kernaleguen, A. (1978). *Clothing designs for the handicapped.* Edmonton, Canada: The University of Alberta Press.

King, G., Law, M., King, S., & Rosenbaum, P. (1998). Parents' and service providers' perceptions of the family-centeredness of children's rehabilitation services. *Physical and Occupational Therapy, 18* (1), 21-40.

Koegel, L.K., Koegel, R.L., Kellegrew, D., & Mullen, K. (1996). Parent education for prevention and reduction of severe problem behaviors. In L.K. Koegel, R.L. Koegel, & G. Dunlap (Eds.), *Positive behavioral support: Including people with difficult behavior in the community* (pp. 3-30). Baltimore: Brookes.

Kramer, P., & Hinojosa, J. (1999). *Frames of reference for pediatric occupational therapy* (2nd ed.). Baltimore: Lippincott Williams & Wilkins.

Lambert, N.M., & Windmiller, M. (1981). *AAMD Adaptive Behavior Scale, school edition.* East Aurora, NY: Slosson Educational Publications.

Law, M., Baptiste, S., Carswell, A., McColl, M.A., Polotajiko, H., & Pollock, N. (1994). *Canadian Occupational Performance Measure* (2nd ed.). Toronto: Canadian Association of Occupational Therapists.

Law, M., & Usher, P. (1988). Validation of the Klein-Bell Activities of Daily Living Scale with children. *Canadian Journal of Occupational Therapy, 55,* 63-68.

Lawrence, K.E., & Niemeyer, S. (Eds.). (1994). *Home care issues/activities of daily living: Caregiver education guide for children with developmental disabilities* (pp. 4:31-4:46). Gaithersburg, MD: Aspen.

Levin, J., & Scherfenberg, L. (1987). *Selection and use of simple technology in home, school, work, and community settings.* Minneapolis: Ablenet.

Light, H., Hertsgaard, D., & Martin, R. (1985). Farm children's work in the family. *Adolescence, 20* (7), 425-432.

Lynch, E., & Hanson, M. (1998). *Developing cross-cultural competence* (2nd ed.). Baltimore: Brookes.

McGavin, H. (1998). Planning rehabilitation: A comparison of issues for parents and adolescents. *Physical and Occupational Therapy, 18* (1), 69-82.

McInnes, J.M., & Treffry, J.A. (1993). *Deaf-blind infants and children: A developmental guide.* Toronto: University of Toronto Press.

Newborg, J., Stock, J.R., Wnek, L., Guidubaldi, J., & Szinicki, J. (1984). *Battelle developmental inventory.* Chicago: Riverside Publishers.

Orelove, F., & Sobsey, D. (1996). Self-care skills. In F. Orelove & D. Sobsey (Eds.), *Educating children with multiple disabilities* (3rd ed.). (pp. 333-375). Baltimore: Brookes.

Reese, G.M., & Snell, M.E. (1991). Putting on and removing coats and jackets: The acquisition and maintenance of skills by children with severe multiple disabilities. *Education and Training in Mental Retardation, 26,* 398-410.

Rheingold, H. (1982). Little children's participation in the work of adults: A nascent prosocial behavior. *Child Development, 53,* 114-125.

Sailor, W., Halvorsen, A., Anderson, J., Goetz, L., Gee, K., Doering, K., & Hunt, P. (1986). Community intensive instruction. In R. Horner, L. Meyer, & B. Fredericks (Eds.), *Education of learners with severe handicaps* (pp. 251-288). Baltimore: Brookes.

Seymour, S. (1988). Expressions of responsibility among Indian children: Some precursors of adult status and sex roles. *Ethos, 17* (4), 355-370.

Smith, R., Benge, M., & Hall, M. (1994). Technology for self-care. In C. Christiansen (Ed.), *Ways of living: Self-care strategies for special needs* (pp. 379-422). Rockville, MD: American Occupational Therapy Association.

Snell, M.E., & Vogtle, L.K. (2000). Methods for teaching self-care skills. In C. Christiansen (Ed.), *Ways of living: Self-care strategies for special needs* (pp. 57-82). Bethesda, MD: American Occupational Therapy Association.

Snell, M.E., & Brown, F. (1993). Instructional planning and implementation. In M.E. Snell (Ed.), *Instruction of students with severe disabilities* (4th ed.). (pp. 99-151). New York: Macmillan.

Sparrow, S., Balla, D., & Cicchetti, D. (1984). *Vineland Adaptive Behavior Scales.* Circle Pines, MN: American Guidance Services.

Spencer, K., Murphy, M., Bean, G., & Schelly, C. (1991). Vocational needs assessment: A functional, community referenced approach. In K. Spencer (Ed.), *From school to adult life: The role of occupational therapy in the transition process* (pp. 185-213). Fort Collins: Department of Occupational Therapy, Colorado State University.

Sweeney, J. (1989). *Clothing for children with severe disabilities: A guide to adaptive garments for use in the institutional setting.* Alexandria: Special Clothes.

Trombly, C.A. (1995). Occupation: Purposefulness and meaningfulness as therapeutic mechanisms, 1995 Eleanor Clarke Slagle lecture. *The American Journal of Occupational Therapy, 47,* 253-257.

Trombly, C.A., & Quintana, L.A. (1989). Activities of daily living. In C.A. Trombly (Ed.), *Occupational therapy for physical dysfunction* (3rd ed.). (pp. 386-410). Baltimore: Williams & Wilkins.

Turnbull, A.P., & Turnbull, H.R. (1997). *Families, professionals, and exceptionality: A special partnership* (3rd ed.). Columbus, OH: Merrill/Prentice Hall.

Ward, D. (1983). *Positioning the handicapped child for function.* St. Louis: Diane E. Ward.

Willis, W. (1998). Families with African-American roots. In E.W. Lynch & M.J. Hanson (Eds.), *Developing cross-cultural competence* (2nd ed.) (pp. 165-208). Baltimore: Brookes.

York-Barr, J., Rainforth, B., & Locke, P. (1996). Developing instructional adaptations. In F.P. Orelove & D. Sobsey (Eds.), *Educating children with multiple disabilities* (3rd ed. pp. 119-159). Baltimore: Brookes.

Zuniga, M.E. (1998). Families with Latino roots. In E.W. Lynch & M.J. Hanson (Eds.), *Developing cross-cultural competence* (2nd ed.) (pp. 209-250). Baltimore: Brookes.

chapter **17**

Play

Christine Doyle Morrison
Peggy Metzger

key terms

Play skills
Playfulness
Intrinsic motivation
Internal reality
Locus of control

■ CHAPTER OBJECTIVES

1. Explain definitions of play.
2. Recognize the importance of play to children's development.
3. Define the criteria of play.
4. Understand playfulness and apply the concept of playfulness to intervention.
5. Identify different methods for using play in occupational therapy intervention.
6. Apply play skill and playfulness concepts to intervention with children with specific play deficits.

■ SCOPE OF PLAY IN OCCUPATIONAL THERAPY

Because play is the primary occupation of children, occupational therapists must recognize the importance of play when working with young clients. This chapter describes the role of play in both the assessment and intervention of children. It begins with a review of the historical role of play, examining the way early practitioners influenced current theory and practice of play. A definition of play is then provided to assist therapists in incorporating play into assessment and treatment of children. Next, assessments that measure (1) play skills, (2) traits of playfulness, and (3) developmental skills in a play environment are described. Finally, the role of play and playfulness during therapy sessions is explained, distinguishing between the use of play as a therapeutic modality to improve skills and a form of therapy focused on improving play skills and interactions.

Historical Perspective

During the early part of the twentieth century, the perspective of play as diversion was prevalent in the occupational therapy literature. Play was viewed as a means of recruiting the mind-body connection in the effort toward wellness. For example, Susan Tracy (1912), in a book designed to train nurses in the "treatment of occupation," provided lengthy descriptions for making toys from common objects when working with children who were sick. The goal of this treatment was to alter the environment of the sick room and to "divert" children from thoughts of illness by engaging them in the occupation of creating toys. Play as diversion was an integral part of occupational therapy intervention with children during this time.

Kielhofner and Burke (1983) suggested that the field of occupational therapy entered a period of crisis during the 1940s and 1950s. Because the medical community at the time was focused on identifying the internal mechanisms that underlie bodily functions, "medicine did not recognize as scientific the holistic concepts which characterized the paradigm of occupation" (p. 27).

In addition, secondary to advances in medical technology, occupational therapists were working with people with a variety of new and unfamiliar diagnoses (Slagle & Robeson, 1941). Therefore the paradigm of occupation could no longer provide practitioners with answers to all of their questions. In a search for answers to these questions, competing points of view were presented in the prevalent literature of the time.

During the beginning of this crisis period, Slagle and Robeson (1941) described play as synonymous with recreation and as equal in importance to crafts and habit training. The diversional focus of play and the dominance of the mind over the body were also seen in their writings. However, over the next 20 years, play began to take on the role of a therapeutic modality. Play was described as "activities not only to maintain status quo, but also to serve as a stimulus for normal growth and development" (Richmond & Lis, 1949, p. 186). It was also seen as the mechanism through which children develop their muscles and learn to use their bodies (Alessandrini, 1949). Thus play moved from a diversional role in the mind-body connection to healing, and it began to be viewed as a treatment modality for facilitating development.

Kielhofner and Burke (1983) proposed that occupational therapy entered into a second paradigm by the end of the 1950s; they called this the *inner mechanisms paradigm*. During this second paradigm, occupational therapists were no longer focused on the ideas of occupation, mind-body unity, and diversion. Instead, they were focused on scientific principles of practice to explain why interventions worked.

During this paradigm shift the practice theory of neurodevelopmental treatment (NDT) became widely used and the theory of sensory integration (SI) originated. Fiorentino (1966) captured this change when stating that the aim of occupational therapy was "purposeful function; the development and/or restoration of such function to the maximum ability of the child" (p. 251).

Occupation was no longer mentioned and, while "function" was the stated endpoint of occupational therapy treatment, the main goal was to "suppress or inhibit the primitive, abnormal tonic reflexes and facilitate higher, integrated righting and equilibrium reactions" (Fiorentino, 1966, p. 99). Through therapy, the child was expected to learn to move using more normal patterns and function was expected to improve automatically. The therapist did not necessarily attend to function during treatment sessions. Instead, he or she applied a developmental frame of reference. Thus play was no longer viewed as a relevant focus of pediatric occupational therapy.

Kielhofner and Burke (1983) suggested that a second crisis period emerged in the 1970s that was "precipitated by recognition of the limitations of reductionism for science and of technology for the needs of the chronically disabled and by the internal confusion and incoherence of occupational therapy" (p. 46). During this period, play resurfaced as a topic in the occupational therapy literature.

Reilly (1974) explored the complexities of play and its application to assessment and treatment of children. Play was viewed as the primary occupation of children and thus a primary focus of pediatric therapists. A variety of assessment tools were developed that applied the theory of play to pediatric practice. Several are described later in this chapter. Below the basic tenets of Reilly and her students are briefly reviewed (Table 17-1).

This work "became a stimulus for a new generation of clinicians and scholars who are intrigued by the mystery of play's power and who, benefiting from the foundation laid by Reilly and her students, are no longer embar-

table 17-1	*Occupational Therapists' Play Definitions*
Theorists	**Definition**
Reilly (1974)	*Exploratory play:* Generalized interest is in the environment and basic urge to explore. *Competency play:* Child learns not just skills but the ability to generate skilled action. *Achievement behavior:* Play bridges gap between childhood and adult occupational behavior.
Takata (1974)	Play is a complex set of behaviors characterized by a dynamic process that involves a particular attitude and action. It involves exploration, experimentation, repetition of experience, and imitation of child's surroundings.
Florey (1971)	Play is action on human and nonhuman objects.
Missiuna & Pollack (1991)	Free play is spontaneous, intrinsically motivated, self-regulated, and requires personal involvement of child. It includes exploration, mastery, decision making, achievement, increased motivation, and competency.

rassed to claim play both as a therapeutic agent and a critical outcome of intervention (Parham & Fazio, 1997, p. xi). Thus the foundation for play as primary focus of pediatric occupational therapists was created.

A. Jean Ayres (1979), who described how a child's sensory systems integrate during play activities, further reinforced the importance of play. Play became a therapeutic modality in the treatment of children with sensory integrative dysfunction (SID), because (when used in SI therapy) it provides the "just right challenge" for the child.

Characteristics of and Contexts for Play

Psychologists have also contributed to our understanding of play. Rubin, Fein, and Vandenberg (1983) combined the work of their predecessors (Piaget, Smilansky, and Parten) to define characteristics and contexts of play. First, play is defined by the traits that distinguish it from other types of behaviors. There are six commonly cited characteristics that distinguish play from nonplay:

1. Play is an intrinsically motivated behavior.
2. In play, the player pays more attention to the means than to the ends, to the process than to the product.
3. The child or organism, not the stimulus, guides the play (i.e., "What can I do with this object?" rather than "What does this object do?").
4. Play is comprised of nonserious renditions of activities.
5. In play, the player is free from externally imposed rules.
6. When playing, the player is actively engaged in the play activity, rather than a passive participant.

A second way that psychologists define play is as observable categories of behavior (Rubin et. al., 1983). For example, Piaget, Smilansky, and Parten developed categories of play-defining social and cognitive play (Table 17-2).

Another approach to defining play is by the context in which the play occurs. Rubin and others (1983, p. 701) listed five contextual elements that promote play:

1. An array of familiar peers, toys, or other materials interesting to the child.
2. An agreement between the child and adult that the child is free to choose whatever he or she may want to do.
3. Adult behavior that is minimally intrusive or directive.
4. An atmosphere that makes children feel comfortable and safe.
5. Scheduling that reduces the likelihood of the children being tired.

Neumann (1971) identified common themes in the literature that defined play. The common criteria of children's play were (1) intrinsic motivation, (2) internal reality, and (3) internal locus of control. According to Neumann, when all three of these criteria were present, a child was engaged in a play interaction.

table 17-2	Theorists and Play Categories
Theorist	**Play Categories**
Piaget (1962)	*Practice play:* Playing of infants, when child repeats actions that have been acquired
	Symbolic play: Involves manipulation of tools
	Games with rules: Involves practice with rules
Smilansky (cited in Rubin, Maioni, & Homung, 1976)	*Functional play:* Sensorimotor or practice play that consists of simple repetitive movements
	Constructive play: Manipulation of objects to construct or create something
	Dramatic play: Recognition, acceptance, and conformity to rules imposed on an activity
Parten (cited in Rubin et. al., 1976)	*Unoccupied play:* Playing with child's own body; random activity
	Solitary play: Playing with toys differently from children within speaking distance; interest centered on own play and independent activity
	Onlooker play: Watching others but not entering into situation
	Parallel play: Playing independently beside, not with, others
	Associative play: Group play with group agreement on common activities and interests
	Cooperative play: Group is organized to achieve some goal; highly organized group activity

Bundy: Playfulness

Based on the work of Rubin and Neumann, Bundy (1987) proposed a definition of play to help occupational therapists effectively evaluate and promote play. She developed a working definition of play that helps therapists understand the prerequisites of play and recognize when a child is engaged in genuine play. She defined play as a continuum:

Play is a transaction between the child and the environment which is intrinsically motivated, internally controlled, and not bound by objective reality . . . Acknowledging that it is not always possible for children to be in complete control of their environments or to fully determine their own reality, play is considered to be a continuum of behaviors which are more or less playful depending on the degree to which the criteria are present (Bundy, 1987, p.16).

To fully understand Bundy's definition of play, it is important to understand the individual criteria present in the definition. According to Bundy, there are three criteria (1) intrinsic motivation, (2) suspension of reality, and (3) internal locus of control.

Intrinsic motivation

Play theorists agree that intrinsic motivation is an important criterion of play. Neumann (1971) defined intrinsic motivation as the player being self-motivated and concerned with the purpose and process inherent in the activity. Similarly, Levy (1978) defined intrinsic motivation as "the drive to become involved in an activity originating from within the person or the activity: the reward is generated by the transaction itself" (p. 6).

Rubin and others (1983) defined intrinsic motivation by contrasting it with what it is not. A behavior that is intrinsically motivating is not governed by appetite drives, compliance with social demands, or inducements external to the behavior itself. Occupational therapy theorists have also defined intrinsic motivation through contrast. Florey (1971) defined an intrinsic motive as one that does not depend on rewards outside the activity. Takata (1971) indicated that play is not associated with a particular end or an eventual gain or profit; the player is more concerned with the process of the activity than with the product. In other words, an intrinsically motivating activity is, in itself, motivating to the child.

A child who is intrinsically motivated is the child who is so absorbed in an activity that he or she may be unaware of other activities going on around him or her. The child is also more involved in the process of the activity than in the outcome. For example, the child who is finger painting and changes the picture continually as he or she adds different colors and strokes is intrinsically motivated.

Suspension of reality

Freedom to suspend reality, the second of Bundy's criteria, is defined slightly differently by different theorists. Neumann (1971) defined internal reality as the player's being free to suspend reality to establish the rules, procedures, and content of play. That is, play behaviors are not serious renditions of the activities they resemble (Bateson, 1972). Internal reality also pertains to the individual's being able to do whatever he or she wants with objects (Rubin et. al., 1983). Focusing on the imaginative aspect of suspending reality, Levy (1978) defined internal reality as "the loss of the 'real self' and the temporary acceptance of an 'illusory self' or 'imaginative self'" (p. 12).

Bundy (1991) stated that the individual's ability to pretend (i.e., create an internal reality) was only one aspect of a larger construct of play, the suspension of reality. Included in suspension of reality is the elimination of consequences that might normally be associated with the activity if performed in "real life" (Vandenberg & Kielhofner, 1982). For example, the child may be suspending reality when he or she answers, "Whatever I want" to the question "What can I do with this object?" Because this question (1) guides play, (2) is the basis of internal locus of control, and (3) may reflect suspension of reality, the theoretical link between the ability to suspend reality and locus of control during a play transaction becomes more evident.

A child who is free to suspend reality is the child who creates play situations without needing the structure provided by specific toys or objects. Further, the child who is free to suspend reality plays in a fluid and flexible way. For example, a child might sometimes use a car as a car, but later imagine that a box is a car or boat. After a time, he or she might turn the same box over and imagine it to be a house or tunnel.

Internal locus of control

An individual's degree of internal versus external locus of control relates to his or her initiative, interaction patterns, motivation, and determination. Neumann (1971) defined locus of control as the player's determining exactly what occurs during the transaction. Similarly, Levy (1978) defined internal locus of control as "the degree to which individuals perceive they are in control of their actions and outcomes" (p. 15).

Rubin and others (1983) contrasted internal control with exploratory behavior. When a child is exploring, his or her behavior seems to answer, "I don't know" to the question, "What can I do with this object?" This behavior suggests that the child lacks control over the transaction. Hutt (1976, 1979), Rubin (1980), and Rubin and others (1983) stated that children need to explore objects and environments before they gain control and truly play. As the child becomes comfortable with the environment, he or she will use objects in a variety of ways for the purposes of play. Conversely, the child who is exploring is limited to obtaining information regarding the object.

A child who is in control of the transaction is one who is able to decide with what and whom he or she plays. This child is also able to decide what he or she is going to do with either the object or the person. In addition, this child can determine and negotiate the steps necessary to accomplish his or her desired outcome for the play scenario.

Play Transaction as a Continuum

Intrinsic motivation, freedom to suspend reality, and internal locus of control are not mutually exclusive and, as stated previously, are each part of a continuum. No transaction can be totally intrinsically motivating, internally controlled, and free to suspend reality. However, every transaction has a combination of the criteria present to greater or lesser degrees. Depending on the extent to which each of the criteria is present, the transaction becomes more playful or less playful.

Bundy (1991) presented a pictorial scale for examining the relationship between perception of control, source of motivation, and suspension of reality in any given play scenario. The information presented below can be used to conceptualize where a transaction falls on the continuum of play to nonplay (Figure 17-1).

Two other important aspects need to be addressed in expanding the definition of play. The first aspect is the transaction and framing of the play scenario, which includes giving and reading cues (Bateson, 1972). Recognizing the relationship that play creates between the child and the environment, Neumann (1971) defined transaction as a "relationship entered into by the child and his environment . . . during which specific aspects of the environment and of the child are manipulated by the child" (p. 137). This notion of a transaction is also supported by Rubin and others (1983), who stated that a player must be active for a behavior to be considered play. This active engagement or manipulation of the environment infers a constant awareness of, and response to, the immediate surroundings by the child.

The child determines the play frame by communicating a message that states: "This is play" and "This is how I am going to act" (Bateson, 1972). The child gives verbal and nonverbal cues indicating "I'm playing now" and "This is how you should act toward me." As a successful player, the child also responds appropriately to the cues of playmates.

Prerequisites to Play

It is proposed that cue giving and reading are a necessary foundation for play. Therefore it is also proposed that teaching an infant to give and read cues early may be an important first step in the development of a playful child. This can be done in infancy by responding to the infant's cues. For example, when an infant extends his arms and legs and turns his eyes away from the adult talking to him, it generally means that the infant needs to break the transaction. The adult can respond to those cues by not talking or allowing the infant to look away, that is, breaking the transaction. In a similar way, when the infant cues his mother that he is hungry by fussing and sucking on his fist, she responds by feeding the infant. In both of these instances, the adult is giving the infant the message that his cues are valued and that the infant is important and in control.

Infant's cues also provide the adult with information regarding the infant's likes and dislikes in relation to the environment. For example, when being held, the infant that molds his or her body to the mother's communicates that physical contact is enjoyable. Conversely, the infant who fusses, squirms, and pulls away each time he or she is touched may be expressing that touch is not pleasant. Responding to an infant's cues (by adapting the environment to minimize unpleasant experiences) gives the infant the message that the environment is safe and pleasant.

When they developed the Test of Playfulness (ToP), Bundy (1997) and colleagues found that if children did not feel safe, they did not play. A feeling of safety also encourages the child to explore the environment and gather sensory information, which precedes and evolves into play. This is the time during which the child learns everything he or she can about an object or the environment

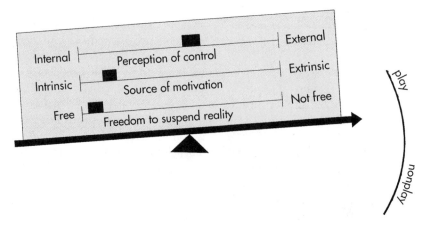

figure**17-1** Elements of play and nonplay. *(Modified from Bundy, A.C. [1991]. In A.G. Fisher, E.A. Murray, & A.C. Bundy [Eds.],* Sensory integration: Theory and practice *[p. 60]. Philadelphia: F.A. Davis.)*

before using that knowledge in play. These environmental components have been supported by various authors (Cohen, 1987; Hutt, 1976; Rubin, 1977; Schwartzman, 1984), all of whom have suggested that when a child feels comfortable and safe in the environment, he or she will be able to play.

Play Assessments

Several play assessments have been developed by occupational therapists (e.g., The Play History, The Play Scale, and the ToP). With the exception of the ToP, developmental hierarchies make up the organizational framework of these assessments. Information is presented regarding the developmental hierarchy of play behaviors, along with activities and toys that may facilitate the various stages (Table 17-3).

In The Play History, Takata (1974) used an extensive method of history taking and observation to evaluate the play development of children. The interview also gathers information about the play environment, including what toys the child uses, as well as when, where, and with whom the child plays. The Play History shows assets and limitations in the child's ability to play and in the available play opportunities (Takata, 1974). Information is gathered regarding: (1) general information about the child, (2) previous play experiences, (3) actual play examination, (4) play description, and (5) play prescription. After gathering this information, the therapist is able to put together a picture of the child's play development, analyze it for any problems, and make a prescription to minimize problems.

Bryze (1997) suggested using The Play History, not as a strict interview, but as a framework for gathering narrative information about a child's play from his or her family. A narrative approach is contrasted with an interview, which may be less flexible and "limit the meaningfulness and breadth of information obtained" (p. 26). Burke and Schaaf (1997) also suggested the use of a narrative or a storytelling approach to gathering data about the play of a child and his or her family throughout the assessment process.

The assessment that has been used and cited most often in occupational therapy literature is The Play Scale (Knox, 1974). Knox intended The Play Scale to be used to determine the child's play age as well as his or her play profile. To do this, she used descriptions of normal play behavior of preschool children in yearly increments.

Knox divided play development and play characteristics into four dimensions comprised of specific categories relating to each particular dimension: (1) *space management,* focused on gross-motor skills; (2) *material management,* defined as the manner in which a child manipulates objects and materials and the purpose for which the child uses them; (3) *imitation,* described as the manner in which the child demonstrates an understanding of the social environment and feelings; and (4) *participation,* explained as the degree and manner in which the child interacts with people in the environment.

Knox found the scale useful for measuring the everyday play behavior of children and suggested that it be evaluated for validity and reliability. In 1982, Bledsoe and Shepherd revised and renamed Knox's Play Scale, the Preschool Play Scale (PPS) and examined its reliability and validity. The results of their study suggested that the PPS yields objective, stable, and valid measurement of play behavior. However, they recommended that the PPS be used in "conjunction with an assessment of playfulness or degree of involvement in play. This aspect of play is vital to a total assessment of play behavior" (p. 788).

Knox (1997) has recently revised the PPS and renamed it the Revised Knox Preschool Play Scale. The revised scale maintains the organizational framework of the original tool, with expansion of the age ranges from birth to 3 (now 6-month increments). The dimension definitions and factor descriptions were revised based on current research in developmental play, and the name of the *imitation* dimension was changed to the *pretense-symbolic* dimension. Standardization, reliability, and validity studies are in process for the revised tool.

The previous assessments of play measure a child's skills within a play situation. Studies have found that the PPS does not adequately capture differences in play among age groups and diagnoses (Bundy, 1987; Bledsoe & Shepherd, 1982; Morrison, Bundy, & Fisher, 1991). Assessment of playfulness in conjunction with assessment of developmental skills within the context of play may better objectify the play differences observed among children.

Bundy (1997) uses the three criteria (intrinsic motivation, suspension of reality, and internal locus of control), in her definition of play as the basis of the Test of Playfulness (ToP). The ToP also incorporates the aspects of framing and giving and reading cues previously described. Development of the ToP began in 1992. The following year, an analysis of the original 60-item observational assessment resulted in a revision by Bundy and colleagues (Bundy, 1997). The second version was in use for over 4 years, during which time data were collected on almost 400 children. In 1997, Bundy and colleagues made modest revisions, resulting in the present version of the ToP.

The ToP is administered while the player is engaged in free play, as this seems to best promote playfulness. Playmates may vary in age from peers to adults. It is important for the play area and the people in it to be familiar to the child (to ensure that the child feels safe and encouraged to play).

table 17-3	*Types and Examples of Play Activities*		
Category/ Characteristic Age	**Description**	**Properties of Activities**	**Representative Toys and Activities**
Exploratory play 0 to 2 years	*Play:* Recreational experiences through which child develops body scheme, sensory integrative and motor skills, and concepts of sensory characteristics and actions of human and nonhuman objects	*Material and objects:* ▪ Child's own body ▪ Significant others ▪ Environmental textures ▪ Infant toys with distinct sensory characteristics and actions ▪ Everyday household objects *Human relationships:* ▪ Strongest relationships occur through play between child and parents	Auditory toys (rattles, play piano); balls (all sizes and textures); bells, blocks, busy boxes; containers and nesting toys; dolls and stuffed animals; hammer and pegs; imitative hand-body games; inflatables; language play with parents; mirrors; mobiles; pop-up toys; pots and pans; rolling, crawling, and cruising activities; sand and water toys and activities; brightly colored scarves; scooter boards; scribbling with crayons; "See 'N' Say," sensory play with parents; shape boxes; empty spice bottles; squeeze toys; teething toys; textured surfaces; 1- to 3-piece puzzles
Symbolic play 2 to 4 years	Play and recreational experiences through which child formulates, tests, classifies, and refines ideas, feelings, and combined actions Associated with development of language Objects are given importance according to child's ability to symbolize, control, change, and master	*Materials and objects:* ▪ Gross motor play equipment ▪ Simple construction toys ▪ Simple art materials ▪ Toys for fantasy-imaginative play *Human relationships:* ▪ Play with peers begins with parallel imitation and develops into cooperative interaction	Balance-rocker boards, blocks, beads, blowing bubbles, cars, trucks, trains, chalk and blackboard activities, clay, modeling dough, colorforms, construction kits, crayons, paints, paper, dolls and stuffed animals, dollhouses, dramatic songs, "dress up" materials, fingerpaints, hand puppets, household play items, inflatables, magnets, miniature figures, musical instruments, nesting toys, play tunnel, put-together toys, puzzles, records, rocking horse, rolling in the grass, sand and water toys, sewing cards, simple story books, slides, space stations, stacking toys, swings, toy telephones, tricycle riding

Modified from Pratt, P.N. (1989). Play and recreational activities. In P.N. Pratt & A.S. Allen (Eds.). *Occupational therapy for children*, (pp. 295-310). St. Louis: Mosby.

A supplemental tool can be used to assess the impact of the environment on the level of playfulness. The Test of Environmental Supportiveness (TOES) was developed to examine whether the human environment (e.g., caregivers and playmates) and the nonhuman environment (e.g., space and objects) facilitate or detract from the child's ability to play and to be playful. It has been recommended that the TOES and the ToP be administered simultaneously to best determine the child's level of playfulness.

■ INTERVENTION

The earlier discussion regarding children's attempts at communication suggested that when the therapist responds to the child's cues about what he or she likes and dislikes, the message to the child is that he or she is important and in control. This reciprocal communication forms the basis of a trust relationship between the child and therapist. This trust relationship is imperative if therapy is to challenge the child.

table 17-3	*Types and Examples of Play Activities—cont'd*		

Category/ Characteristic Age	Description	Properties of Activities	Representative Toys and Activities
Creative play 4 to 7 years	Play and recreational experiences through which child refines sensory, motor, cognitive, and social skills; explores combinations of actions on multiple objects; and develops interests and competencies that promote performance of school-related and work-related activities	*Materials and objects:* • Arts and crafts • Complex construction toys • Dramatic play materials • Household activities such as cooking, simple woodworking, pet care, and gardening *Human relationships:* • Play begins in cooperative peer groups with gradual emergence of competitive atmosphere; peer validation of play products becomes increasingly important • Parents assist and validate in absence of peers	Baking cookies, stringing beads, bicycle riding, craft kits, cutting and pasting, finger painting, gardening, origami, painting, paperdolls, playing house, simple weaving (placemats and pot holders), simple woodworking, stencils
Games 7 to 12 years	Play and recreational experiences that have distinct rules and involve skill development and social interaction in competitive atmosphere. Actions and results of actions are compared against those of peers	*Materials and objects:* • Arts and crafts • Complex construction toys • Dramatic play materials • Household activities such as cooking, simple woodwork, pet care, and gardening *Human relationships:* • Play begins in cooperative peer groups with gradual emergence of competitive atmosphere; peer validation of play products becomes increasingly important • Parents assist and validate in the absence of peers	Board games, card games, checkers, clubs, collections, computer games, field days (races and tug-of-war), hangman, jacks, marbles, jump rope, organized outdoor games, ping pong, roller skating and ice skating, school plays, performances, scooter board races, team sports, trading cards

Occupational therapy intervention specific to play has three perspectives:
1. Intervention uses play as a therapeutic modality when the treatment goals are to improve specific component skills (e.g., fine-motor, gross-motor, cognitive skills).
2. Intervention focuses on improving play skills.
3. Intervention focuses on facilitating playfulness.

■ USE OF PLAY AS A THERAPEUTIC MODALITY

Bundy stated that "If play is the vehicle by which individuals become masters of their environments, then play should be among the most powerful of therapeutic tools" (Bundy, 1991, p. 61). To effectively use play as a therapeutic tool, it is important to remember that play is (1) a transaction between the child and the environment which is intrinsically motivated, internally controlled, and free

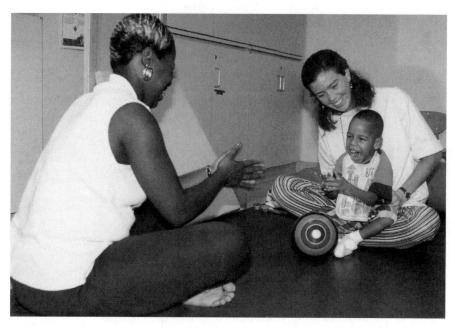

figure**17-2** Therapist uses play as a therapeutic modality to increase child's involvement in a task focused on improving bilateral use of hands.

from objective reality; and (2) a continuum of behaviors from play to nonplay. The therapist can then turn a nonplayful interaction into a playful one by altering the perception of control, the source of motivation, or the suspension of reality of the situation (Figure 17-2).

Case Study: Intervention with a Child with Cerebral Palsy

Jake is a 4 year old who loves to play and is ingenious in persisting with his play despite significant motoric challenges. Jake has spastic cerebral palsy (CP), which affects his ability to move both of his legs. Although he has functional use of both of his arms, movement of his arms increased his overall muscle tone, making it difficult for him to reach for and manipulate toys and objects This difficulty is manifested in his attempts to play with his action figures (Jake calls them his "guys"), and in his difficulty with lower extremity dressing.

Jake's occupational therapy goals are to (1) improve accuracy and aim of reach, (2) improve manipulation skills, and (3) improve his dressing skills (i.e., don pants, shoes and socks). Treatment activities involving hand-over-hand repeated practice of reach to target were frustrating and demotivating for Jake. His perception of these therapist-designed activities is shown in Figure 17-3.

Without changing the occupational therapy goals, the occupational therapist decided that the first objective was to engage Jake in play. She set up the environment with a variety of toys and activities before encouraging Jake to actively explore the entire area and choose what he would like

to do. (In designing the environment, the therapist applied information gathered from Jake's mother regarding his favorite toys at home.) Jake chose to play with his "guys."

The therapist and Jake began to engage in a play scenario in which the "guys" visit different planets, each with a variety of objects to explore. This play scenario successfully altered both the motivation (i.e., Jake chose one of his favorite toys and activities) and the reality (i.e., different surfaces requiring arm placement to a variety of planes became the planets of the play scenario).

Inherent in this play transaction are many opportunities for practicing arm placement in different planes (planets) and for manipulating different sized and shaped objects (present on the different planets). This therapy activity was no longer frustrating for Jake. In fact, he found it to be enjoyable (Figure 17-4).

The therapist has successfully used play in the orchestration of a treatment session that is both fun for Jake and allows him to practice difficult arm placement and manipulation tasks. By considering the child's perception of control, source of motivation for participating in a task, and the reality of the situation, it is possible to use play as a powerful therapeutic tool in planning and implementing intervention sessions.

Motor impairment may often prevent the child's full participation in play. Through careful selection of activities that are in line with the child's interests and capacities, the occupational therapist can design a treatment program that improves motor function. At the same time, the therapist can promote continuity in the child's development of play and related skills. The techniques

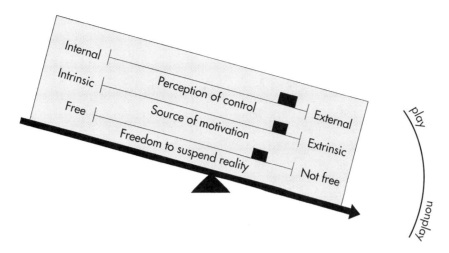

figure**17-3**   Nonplay transaction. *(Modified from Bundy, A.C. [1991]. In A.G. Fisher, E.A. Murray, & A.C. Bundy [Eds.],* Sensory integration: Theory and practice *[p. 60]. Philadelphia: F.A. Davis.)*

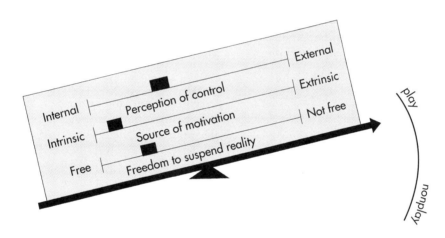

figure**17-4**   Play transaction. *(Modified from Bundy, A.C. [1991]. In A.G. Fisher, E.A. Murray, & A.C. Bundy [Eds.],* Sensory integration: Theory and practice *[p. 60]. Philadelphia: F.A. Davis.)*

that are used most with children who have motor problems include adaptation of position (of the body and work surface) and adaptation of the tools, materials, and equipment used for an activity. Information regarding toys appropriate for various developmental levels is presented (see Table 17-3).

■ INTERVENTION FOCUSED ON IMPROVING PLAY SKILLS

· The second way in which play is important to pediatric occupational therapy intervention is when a child demonstrates a play deficit. A few occupational therapy research studies have found the play of children with special needs to be different from the play of their peers without special needs (Gralewicz, 1973; Gray, 1972; Kielhofner & Burke, 1983), highlighting the importance of assessing play skills. If a play deficit is revealed, a goal of intervention is improvement of play skills.

Assessment of a child may reveal play deficits in one or more of the following ways:

1. The child demonstrates play skills that are developmentally immature for his or her chronologic age.
2. The child has a preference for types of play for which he or she does not have the necessary skills. In this situation there is a mismatch between the child's skills and his or her play preferences.

Child with Immature Play Skills

Administering assessments (e.g., The Play History or the PPS) based on developmental hierarchies provides an occupational therapist with important information concerning a child's developmental play level. A play level below the child's chronologic age is considered to indicate immature play skills and therefore a play skills deficit. The goal of any intervention program for a child with this problem should include activities designed to facilitate play skills that are more age appropriate. This type of intervention would also be aimed at expanding the child's play repertoire or ability to interact with his or her environment through play.

One approach to intervention might be to use a developmental frame of reference to treat the performance components (e.g., social, fine motor, gross motor) that impede the child's play performance. The assumption of this approach to intervention is that play skills automatically improve once improvement in performance components is achieved.

However, research suggests that the correlation between performance components and performance areas (i.e., play, for the purposes of this discussion) is not always direct. In addition, research has also shown that improvement in functional tasks or play may not occur when the underlying performance components are the focus of intervention (Bundy, 1989; Case-Smith, 1995, 1996; Morrison, Bundy, & Fisher, 1991). Therefore an alternative approach that combines interventions focused on deficits in performance components with interventions for specific developmental play deficits may be more effective.

Case Study: Intervention with a Child with Sensory Integrative Dysfunction

John is a 5-year-old-boy with SID. His difficulty in planning and sequencing unfamiliar motor tasks interferes with his ability to enjoy playground equipment and to play soccer with the other children in his class. Part of John's occupational therapy is aimed at improving his underlying dyspraxia. However, the other part of his treatment focuses on providing him with the opportunity to practice playing soccer and practice playing on the playground equipment.

The therapy sessions in which John practices his play skills allow him to do so in a safe and positive environment in which he is allowed to fail without consequences. By working on motor-planning skills and simultaneously allowing him to practice difficult play tasks, the sessions build toward improved developmental performance during play.

Part of the overall plan for John includes his family taking him to practice climbing on neighborhood playground equipment that is known to be safe and to have unusual, motivating climbing structures. Recommendations for safe playground play involve the entire family and help them understand principles for promoting John's skills and confidence.

Mismatch Between Preference and Skill

Both a child's preference and his or her play skills need to be assessed (Clifford & Bundy, 1989). Children whose play skills do not match their play preferences have been described in the literature. For example, Clifford and Bundy (1989) examined the play preferences of two groups of 4- to 6-year-old boys. They compared boys who were typically developing to boys diagnosed with SID. Both the typically developing boys and the boys with SID expressed a preference for sensorimotor play. When the relationship between play skill and play preference was examined for individual boys, however, many of the boys with SID had adapted their preference in play to reflect their skills.

Play preferences may be assessed by asking the child about his or her interests, by interviewing the child's parents, or by observing the child's choice in natural environments (e.g., home and school). It is suggested that children who (1) have the skills to play in the way that they prefer or (2) have altered their preferences for play to reflect their play skills do not require intervention focused on improving either play skills or altering preference. (This is not to say that these same children may not have other functional goals to which the occupational therapist would contribute).

However, children who prefer more complex play for which they do not have the necessary skills may have a play deficit. For example, if Jake, discussed in the earlier case study, preferred to play with his "guys" by moving their tiny arms and placing the various tools in their hands, he would have a mismatch between his play preference and his play skills (creating a play deficit). Although he had the skill for imaginary play with his "guys," he did not have the fine-motor skills for precise manipulation needed to do so. Therefore he often became frustrated when attempting to play.

In this instance, therapy with Jake could take one or more of three approaches. The occupational therapist could (1) focus treatment on improving fine-motor skills and hope to improve Jake's ability to play with his "guys" in his preferred manner, (2) expose Jake to a variety of other types of play for which he has the play skills and hope to alter his preference, or (3) alter the environment in some way to facilitate Jake's play with the toys he prefers.

Focus on Altering Preference

When working with any child whose play skills are insufficient for his or her preferred type of play (e.g., pretend play or gross-motor play), it is important to explore why the child prefers that type of play. The therapist must determine what is it about that type of play that motivates the child. It may then be possible to find other play scenarios that can meet the same need or are just as motivating for the child.

For example, Jake may prefer to play with his "guys" by moving their arms and legs and manipulating the small tools because he likes to play with his older brother and best friend when they play with their toys in this way. The motivating factor for Jake may be the social interaction with his brother and his friend. In this case it may be possible to include Jake's older brother in the treatment sessions and to explore (with both Jake and his brother) ways to play with the action figures that both of the boys are able to master.

Another scenario may be to explore with Jake and his brother types of play (e.g., computer games, playing with cars and trucks in the sand box, or playing with play dough), which require less fine-motor dexterity than manipulating the tools and extremities of the action figures. The goal of this type of intervention would be to provide Jake with an activity that satisfies his intrinsic motivation, but for which he has the skills to be in control. By exploring Jake's motivation for and preferred method of play, and by providing play scenarios in which both Jake and his brother play together, it would be possible to help Jake to develop play preferences that reflect his play skills, instead of preferences beyond his skill level.

Altering the Environment to Facilitate a Match Between Preference and Skills

The final approach to treatment when the child's play skills do not match his or her preferences and interests is to examine the environment in which the child is playing and to determine which aspects of the environment afford the child to play in the preferred manner (Vandenberg, 1981). Environmental affordance refers to the possibilities or potentials for achieving various forms of occupational behavior, along with the concept that the environment provides us with a range of opportunities for occupational behaviors (Kielhofner, 1995). An assessment described earlier, TOES, may be used to evaluate both the physical and the human characteristics of the environment.

After identifying which aspects of the physical and the human environment support or afford the child to play in his or her preferred manner, the occupational therapist (1) constructs play environments that contain these characteristics (i.e., certain playmates or positioning devices), (2) facilitates the practice of play skills in these supportive environments, and (3) generalizes the specific physical

and human characteristics affording the preferred play to other environments in the child's world, allowing the child to play in his or her preferred manner in a variety of settings.

Case Study: Intervention with a Child with Athetoid Cerebral Palsy

Darrius is a 2 year old with a diagnosis of athetoid CP. He is playful but has difficulty playing with all of the toys that interest him. Darrius' human environment is supportive of his play, however, his physical environment requires adaptations for him to play with the toys he prefers. For example, Darrius is unable to sit independently and has difficulty reaching for toys. By having him sit on a bolster and providing him with proximal stability at his trunk (with facilitation at his shoulder while reaching), he is able to reach for and play with the toys he prefers (Figure 17-5).

Equipment and materials are provided to generalize his play with preferred toys within the preschool environment. Darrius is placed in a Rifton® chair with full back support, armrests, tray, and foot support. Toys are made available that have physical characteristics that facilitate his control of movement. Heavier toys provide greater proprioceptive input and are used in activities for building and constructing. Toys with magnetic pieces are used so that he can create designs and play scenarios by simply pushing pieces along the surface.

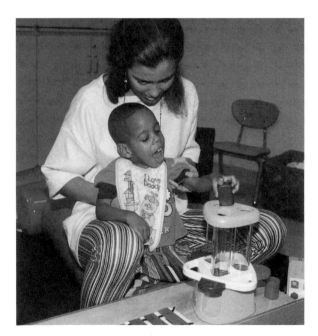

figure 17-5 Therapist's support at child's shoulders and upper trunk enables the child to reach for and play with his preferred toys.

■ INTERVENTION TO FACILITATE PLAYFULNESS

Child Who Is Not Playful

A final way in which a play deficit may be manifested is when a child is not playful. Approaching intervention from this perspective is less familiar to pediatric occupational therapists. Unlike performance areas such as work and self-care, the play activities in which individuals engage seem less important than how they approach those activities. "It may be playfulness rather than play activities that, when evaluated, provides therapists with the information they seek regarding their young clients' development" (Bundy, 1997, p. 53). Therefore in addition to promoting performance of play skills, intervention should address playfulness (Bundy, 1997).

The more playful child may generalize this flexible approach to environmental interaction beyond play and into other aspects of his or her life. For the child with a condition that impedes his or her ability to interact with the social or physical environment, a flexible (playful) approach may enable the child to succeed more frequently in difficult situations.

The ToP (Bundy, 1997) provides a way of examining playfulness in a particular child, because it gives therapists information regarding the quality of a child's play. Bundy suggested that after assessing a child with the ToP, a playfulness profile should be constructed for that child. The playfulness profile consists of information regarding the child's intrinsic motivation, internal control, suspension of reality, and framing observed during the play situations. Intervention is then based on this information.

Case Study: Intervention with a Child with Failure to Thrive

Alexis, an 18-month-old-girl, had a diagnosis of failure to thrive and developmental delay. She received weekly occupational therapy and had followed a fairly typical developmental course, with delays in all developmental areas.

The occupational therapy room where Alexis received her therapy had a variety of toys arranged in no particular fashion. Each week, Alexis sat in the middle of a therapy mat and did not initiate movement toward any of the toys. Her mother continually brought a variety of toys into her immediate environment and put them in her hands. Once the toys were in her hands, Alexis put them in her mouth. Occasionally, she waved the toys in the air or banged them against another toy within her reach.

Throughout most play sessions, Alexis did not make eye contact with her mother, her therapist, or other people in the room. She did not verbalize through babbling, and she did not gesture to indicate her wants or make her needs known. Typically, Alexis' mother directed all of the interaction between herself and Alexis. Periodically Alexis scooted away from her mother and the therapist by pulling herself along on her buttocks, with her legs straight out in front of her. During these times, Alexis either moved into the middle of the therapy room and turned around in circles or she left the room and went into the hallway. Once Alexis left the play environment, she did not typically return to play with the toys.

Alexis' play profile can be developed by placing markers along the continuum representing motivation, control, and suspension of reality (see Figure 17-1). Specific information for Alexis is provided (Figure 17-6).

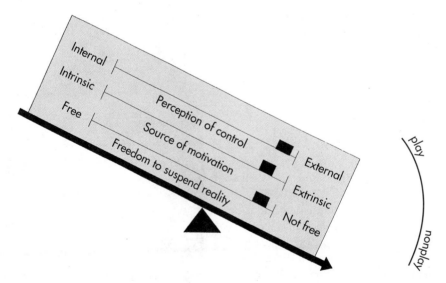

figure**17-6**   Alexis' playfulness profile. *(Modified from Bundy, A.C. [1991]. In A.G. Fisher, E.A. Murray, & A.C. Bundy [Eds.], Sensory integration: Theory and practice [p. 60]. Philadelphia: F.A. Davis.)*

Intrinsic motivation

The marker representing Alexis's source of motivation was placed closer to the "extrinsic" side of the continuum (from intrinsic to extrinsic motivation). At times Alexis appeared to be mildly engaged in the process of mouthing and banging toys.

Throughout the play sessions, Alexis' affect was flat. The only occasions during which she demonstrated any manifest joy was when she left the treatment room and went into the hall. However, it was unclear from observing Alexis exactly what her motivation was during any of these interactions.

Locus of control

The marker for locus of control was placed closer to the "external" than to the "internal" end of the continuum. Alexis initiated little play with the toys in her environment. Alexis' mother appeared to be in control of which toys Alexis played with and when she played with them. The one behavior that Alexis consistently initiated was leaving the treatment environment. However, when Alexis did interact with the toys she appeared to be exploring them more than playing with them.

As discussed earlier, several theorists have suggested that when the child is exploring objects instead of playing with them, it is because he or she is not in control of the transaction (Rubin, 1980; Rubin et. al., 1983) and is attempting to gain control (Hutt, 1976, 1979). This suggests that Alexis was not operating from an internal locus of control. Finally, Alexis demonstrated minimal modification of her interaction with the toys, again suggesting that she did not feel sufficiently self-empowered to alter the situation.

Suspension of reality

The marker for freedom to suspend reality was placed almost completely toward the "not free" end, because all of the interactions observed appeared to be bound by objective reality. Pretending was not observed. The way in which Alexis played with the toys (mouthing and banging) is more typical of a younger child. Therefore the lack of pretending could be related to her overall play age (see Table 17-3).

Framing, giving, and reading cues

When observed during therapy, Alexis did not appear to enter into a play frame. She provided few cues that indicated she was playing. In fact, she provided very few verbal or nonverbal indications of how others should act toward her at all. The few cues that Alexis did give are not typical of an 18-month-old child (e.g., moving toward the therapist backwards, instead of approaching her with face forward). In addition, Alexis' cues were difficult to interpret as play cues; her clearest cue was when she completely withdrew from the play environment.

Play profile

When assessing playfulness, it is important to differentiate between play skill performance and playfulness. It is possible for children whose play skills are developmentally delayed to execute those skills in a playful manner. This is not the case with Alexis. Her performance during play was delayed and was more typical of a 6- to 8-month-old child. In addition, Alexis showed some deficits in performance components, such as difficulty picking up and manipulating toys, and poor ideation regarding what to do with the toys once she grasped them. Alexis' level of play (using her current skills) was not playful. For this reason, her most significant play deficit appeared to be related to her low level of playfulness. Although therapy goals did include improvement in play skills and improvement in the component skills that were impacting play, the primary therapy goal was to facilitate more playful execution of her current level of play.

Intervention

Setting the environment and facilitating internal locus of control. The first step in intervention for a child like Alexis, whose playfulness profile indicates that he or she is not playful, is to establish an intervention environment to facilitate play. When a child feels safe, it is most likely that he or she will explore the environment and the toys in the environment before initiating play. Therefore increasing the child's sense of control over the situation can facilitate a transition from exploration to play.

It may be possible to do this by giving the child verbal and nonverbal cues indicating that he or she is free to select any of the play objects available and to determine how the play will unfold. The assumption is that the child will choose toys and play scenarios that are intrinsically motivating, thus incorporating a second criterion of the definition of playfulness into intervention.

As the child guides the play interaction, he or she also guides the therapist's role in his or her play. The therapist enters the play frame only when he or she is invited to enter by the child. The child invites the therapist into the play frame by providing either verbal or nonverbal cues that signal the therapist's involvement (e.g., making eye contact with the therapist or reaching toward the therapist with toys, arms, or movement of any kind).

When the therapist reads and responds to the child's cues, the message is given that the child is important and in control. To substantiate this message, the therapist should follow the child's lead when entering the play frame in an attempt to emphasize the child's strengths. By consistently doing this, a relationship based on trust develops between the child and the therapist.

In the case of Alexis, the therapy room was set up with a variety of toys placed randomly around a therapy mat. The therapist and Alexis' mother sat on the far edges of the mat, and Alexis was placed in the middle of the toys.

Several of the toys were within easy reach. After approximately 5 minutes, Alexis reached for and picked up a rattle and began shaking it. However, she initiated no interaction with either her mother or the therapist. Both the therapist and the mother stayed on the edges of the therapy mat and did not interact with Alexis. After 10 to 15 minutes of shaking and mouthing the rattle, Alexis reached for and picked up a bucket of plastic blocks. However, she still did not initiate interaction with the therapist or her mother. Her play with the blocks was also mouthing and banging. This continued for approximately 15 minutes before Alexis scooted to toys that were between herself and her mother. She then proceeded to scoot to her mother, to touch her knee briefly, and then to move quickly away.

When Alexis briefly touched her mother, her mother acknowledged the contact by saying, "Hi," but she did not suggest other play. Alexis then moved toward toys closer to the therapist, backed up toward the therapist, and touched a rattle to the therapist's leg. The therapist picked up a rattle and began shaking it in imitation of Alexis's play. Sessions continued in this manner for several weeks, with Alexis guiding the interaction with both the toys (physical) and the people (social) in her environment.

Building trust and challenging the child. Once the therapist is able to respond to the child's cues, it is possible to build on the child's strengths and to begin the process of expanding the child's repertoire of playful behaviors. To do this (while maintaining the child's trust), the therapist provides the child with the just right challenge (Ayres, 1979), in which he or she builds the play frame precisely where the child's skills are sufficient to meet the challenge of the activity. Throughout this process, it is important that the environment remain safe and that there are no negative consequences for the child's performance. That is, the child is free to practice activities without fear of failure.

Csikszentmihalyi (1975) suggested that optimal performance occurs at the point where the challenge of the activity is such that the individual must use a significant portion of his or her skill to perform the activity. When the challenge of the activity is higher than the skill of the individual, the situation can cause anxiety. When the challenge is significantly less than the individual's skill, the situation can result in boredom (Csikszentmihalyi, 1975). Therapy that both responds to the child's cues

and adapts situations to continually challenge the child's newly acquired skills may facilitate increasingly playful behaviors.

Incorporating the playful attitude into other aspects of intervention. Once the child demonstrates playful behaviors during play transactions, therapy sessions may begin to focus on the treatment of other component or developmental play skills and on generalizing this playful approach to other situations. This is done by incorporating the approach of play as a therapeutic modality and by providing the child with the just right challenge (Ayres, 1979). In addition, the concepts regarding determination and generalization of aspects of the environment that facilitate the child's optimal performance are considered.

It is clear that Alexis' play skills and ability to both give and respond to cues were quite limited. Therefore therapy sessions progressed slowly (both in terms of the cues given to Alexis by the therapist and in terms of challenging her underlying play, fine-motor, and praxis problems). When Alexis indicated an activity was too challenging by leaving the play environment, she was allowed to leave. When she returned, the level of challenge was slightly decreased. When Alexis was close to them and made eye contact, the therapist and Alexis' mother modeled how to play with a variety of simple cause-and-effect toys. In addition, they encouraged all of her attempts to play.

■ SUMMARY

Through play, a child learns about his or her world and integrates sensorimotor, cognitive, perceptual, and social skills. Occupational therapists evaluate both play skills and playfulness in children to determine what interventions will promote social and physical play, enhancing overall function and mastery of the environment. With an understanding of the child's play skills and play preferences, the therapist designs interventions that promote mastery and appeal to the child's play interests. They construct environments that afford and challenge the child's play skills. They also support the child's sense of control, intrinsic motivation, and ability to suspend reality by their own playful approaches. Skillful use of play is a powerful therapeutic modality that engages the child, motivates him or her to accept a challenge, and promotes a positive sense of self.

STUDY QUESTIONS

1. Describe how you would use the pictorial scale of playfulness to orchestrate a treatment session for Susan in which play is used as a therapeutic modality. Susan is an 18-month-old child with spastic quadraparesis who loves *Barney*. Occupational therapy long-term goals are for independent feeding from a cup. Component skills impeding this task performance are (a) decreased head and trunk control in sitting and (b) difficulty reaching with both arms simultaneously.

2. Identify which of the following scenarios describes a child(ren) who is(are) more intrinsically motivated and which describes a child(ren) who is(are) more extrinsically motivated:

   a. A group of children running around an open field chasing each other.

   b. A group of children engaged in relay races in the same field.

   c. The child playing with playdough who creates one object after the other with minimal interest in the outcome. The child may even squash the object as soon as he or she completes it and immediately begins making something else.

   d. The child who is making a teapot out of playdough and alters it until she gets it just right before presenting it to the teacher.

3. Identify which of the following scenarios describes a child who is more internally controlled and which describes a child who is more externally controlled:

   a. The child who decides to play Candy Land, convinces his parents to play with him, then proceeds to decide that instead of using the gingerbread markers that come with the game, they will use dinosaurs as game pieces.

   b. The child who decides to play Barbie dolls and to have the dolls go out to dinner, then go home and feed the baby.

   c. The child who is playing T-ball because mom and dad say he has to do so.

   d. The group of children on the playground who are playing dodge ball because the gym teacher says it is time to play dodge ball, even though they would rather play kickball.

4. Identify which of the following scenarios describes a child who is suspending reality and which describes a child who is not:

   a. The child who decides that the small child's table is a ship, the chairs that are placed on the table are the captain's chairs, he is the captain, the teddy bear in the chair is the assistant, and the pillows around the table are the water.

   b. The child who insists on keeping the same chairs on the floor next to the table and uses the table only for coloring.

References

Alessandrini, N.A. (1949). Play—A child's world. *American Journal of Occupational Therapy, 3,* 9-12.

Anderson, J., Hinojosa, J., & Strauch, C. (1987). Integrating play in neurodevelopmental treatment. *American Journal of Occupational Therapy, 41,* 421-426.

Ayres, A.J. (1979). *Sensory integration and the child.* Los Angeles: Western Psychological Corp.

Barnett, L.A., & Kleiber, D.A. (1982). Concomitants of playfulness in early childhood: Cognitive abilities and gender. *The Journal of Genetic Psychology, 141,* 115-127.

Barnett, L.A. (1991). The playful child: Measurement of a disposition to play. *Play & Culture, 4,* 51-74.

Barnett, L.A. (1990). Playfulness: Definition, design, and measurement. *Play & Culture, 3,* 319-336.

Bateson, G. (1972). Toward a theory of play and fantasy. In G. Bateson, *Steps to an ecology of the mind* (pp. 14-20). New York: Bantam.

Bledsoe, N.P., & Shepherd, J.T. (1982). A study of reliability and validity of a preschool play scale. *American Journal of Occupational Therapy, 36,* 783-788.

Bryze, K. (1997). Narrative contributions to the play history. In L.D. Parham & L.S. Fazio (Eds.), *Play in occupational therapy for children* (pp. 23-34). St. Louis: Mosby.

Bundy, A.C. (1997). Play and playfulness: What to look for. In L.D. Parham & L.S. Fazio (Eds.), *Play in occupational therapy for children* (pp. 52-66). St. Louis: Mosby.

Bundy, A.C. (1993). Assessment of play and leisure: Delineation of the problem. *American Journal of Occupational Therapy, 47,* 217-222.

Bundy, A.C. (1991). Play theory and sensory integration. In A.G. Fisher, E.A. Murray, & A.C. Bundy (Eds.), *Sensory integration: Theory and practice* (pp. 46-68). Philadelphia: F.A. Davis.

Bundy, A.C. (1989). A comparison of play skills of normal boys and boys with sensory integrative dysfunction. *Occupational Therapy Journal of Research, 9,* 84-100.

Bundy, A. (1987). *The play of preschoolers: Its relationship to balance, motor proficiency, and the effect of sensory integrative dysfunction.* Unpublished doctoral dissertation, Boston University.

Burke, J., & Shaaf, R. (1997). Family narratives and play assessment. In L.D. Parham & L. Fazio (Eds.). *Play in occupational therapy for children* (pp. 67-87). St. Louis: Mosby.

Case-Smith, J. (1995). The relationships among sensorimotor components, fine motor skills, and functional performance in preschool children. *American Journal of Occupational Therapy, 49,* 642-652.

Case-Smith, J. (1996). Fine motor outcomes in preschool children who receive occupational therapy services. *American Journal of Occupational Therpy, 50,* 52-61.

Clifford, J.M., & Bundy, A. (1989). Play preference and performance in normal preschool boys and preschool boys with sensory integrative dysfunction. *Occupational Therapy Journal of Research, 9,* 202-217.

Csikszentmihalyi, M. (1975). *Beyond boredom and anxiety: The experience of play in work and games.* San Francisco: Jossey-Bass.

Cohen, D. (1987). *The development of play.* New York: New York University Press.

Fiorentino, M. (1966). The changing dimension of occupational therapy. *American Journal of Occupational Therapy, 20,* 251-252.

Florey, L. (1981). Studies of play: Implications for growth, development, and for clinical practice. *American Journal of Occupational Therapy, 35,* 519-524.

Florey, L. (1976). Development through play. In C. Schaefer (Ed.), *The therapeutic use of child's play* (pp. 61-70). New York: Jason Aronson.

Florey, L. (1971). An approach to play and play development. *American Journal of Occupational Therapy, 25,* 275-280.

Gralewicz, A. (1973). Play deprivation in multihandicapped children. *American Journal of Occupational Therapy, 27,* 70.

Gray, M. (1972). Effects of hospitalization on work-play behavior. *American Journal of Occupational Therapy, 26,* 180.

Hartley, R., & Goldenson, R. (1963). *The complete book of children's play.* New York: Thomas Y. Crowell.

Hurff, J. (1974). A play skills inventory. In M. Reilly (Ed.), *Play as exploratory learning* (pp. 267-283). Beverly Hills: Sage.

Hutt, C. (1979). Exploration and play. In B. Sutton-Smith (Ed.), *Play and learning* (pp. 175-194). New York: Gardner.

Hutt, C. (1976). Exploration and play in children. In J. Bruner, A. Jolly, & K. Sylva (Eds.), *Play and its role in development and evolution* (pp. 202-215). New York: Basic.

Kielhofner, G. (1995). *Human occupation* (2nd ed.). Baltimore: Williams & Wilkins.

Kielhofner, G., & Burke, J. (1983). The evolution of knowledge and practice in OT: Past, present and future. In G. Kielhofner (Ed.), *Health through occupation: Theory and practice in occupational therapy* (pp. 3-52). Philadelphia: F.A. Davis.

Kielhofner, G. (1982). Occupation. In H. Hopkins & H. Smith (Eds.), *Willard & Spackman's occupational therapy* (pp. 31-41). Philadelphia: J.B. Lippincott.

Knox, S. (1997). Development and Current Use of the Knox Preschool Play Scale. In L.D. Parham & L.S. Fazio (Eds.), *Play in Occupational Therapy* (pp. 35-51). St. Louis: Mosby.

Knox, S.H. (1974). A play scale. In M. Reilly (Ed.), *Play as exploratory learning* (pp. 247-266). Beverly Hills: Sage.

Kooij, R. (1989). Research on children's play. *Play & Culture, 2,* 20-34.

Levy, J. (1978). *Play behavior.* New York: John Wiley & Sons.

Lieberman, J.N. (1977). *Playfulness: Its relationship to imagination and creativity.* New York: Academic Press.

Mack, W., Lindquist, J., & Parham, L. (1982). A synthesis of occupational behavior and sensory integration, concepts in theory and practice, part 1: Theoretical foundation. *American Journal of Occupational Therapy, 36,* 365-374.

Michelman, S. (1974). Play and the deficit child. In M. Reilly (Ed.), *Play as exploratory learning* (pp. 157-208). Beverly Hills, CA: Sage.

Michelman, S. (1971). The importance of creative play. *American Journal of Occupational Therapy, 6,* 285-290.

Missiuna, C., & Pollock, N. (1991). Play deprivation in children with physical disabilities: The role of the occupational therapist in preventing secondary disability. *American Journal of Occupational Therapy, 45,* 882-888.

Morrison, C.D., Bundy, A.C., & Fisher, A.G. (1991). The contribution of motor skills and playfulness to play performance of preschool-aged children. *American Journal of Occupational Therapy, 45,* 687-694.

Neumann, E.A. (1971). *The elements of play.* New York: MSS Information.

Parham, L.D., & Fazio, L.S. (Eds.). (1997). *Play in occupational therapy with children.* St. Louis: Mosby.

Pratt, P.N. (1989). Play and recreational activities. In P. Pratt & A.S. Allen (Eds.), *Occupational therapy for children* (2nd ed.) (pp. 295-310). St. Louis: Mosby.

Reilly, M. (Ed.). (1974). *Play as exploratory learning.* Beverly Hills: Sage Publications.

Richmond, J.B., & Lis, E.F. (1949). Occupational therapy in pediatrics. *American Journal of Occupational Therapy, 3,* 185-189.

Rubin, K., Fein, G.G., & Vandenberg, B. (1983). Play. In P.H. Mussen (Series Ed.) & E.M. Hetherington (Vol. Ed.), *Handbook of child psychology: Vol. 4. Socialization, personality, and social development* (4th ed.) (pp. 693-774). New York: Wiley & Sons.

Rubin, K.H. (1980). Fantasy play: Its role in the development of social skills and social cognition. In K.H. Rubin (Ed.), *Children's play,* (pp. 69-83). San Francisco: Jossey-Bass.

Rubin, K.H. (1977). Play behaviors of young children. *Young Children, 32,* 16-24.

Rubin, K., Maiono, T.L., & Hornung, M. (1976). Free play behaviors in middle and lower class preschoolers: Piaget and Parten revisited. *Child development, 47,* 414-419.

Schwartzman, H.B. (1984). Imaginative play: Deficit or difference? In T. Yawkey & A. Pellegrini (Eds.), *Child's play: Developmental and applied* (pp. 49-62). New Jersey: Lawrence Erlbaum Associates.

Slagle, E.C., & Robeson, H.A. (1941). *Syllabus for training nurses in occupational therapy.* Utica: State Hospitals Press.

Sutton-Smith, B. (1968). Novel responses to toys. *Merrill-Palmer Quarterly, 14,* 151-158.

Takata, N. (1974). Play as a prescription. In M. Reilly (Ed.), *Play as exploratory learning* (pp. 209-246). Beverly Hills: Sage.

Takata, N. (1971). The play milieu—A preliminary appraisal. *American Journal of Occupational Therapy, 25,* 281-284.

Tracy, S. (1912). Typical invalids: The child of poverty and the child of wealth. In S. Tracy, *Studies of invalid occupation* (pp. 22-46). Boston: Whitcomb & Barrows.

Vandenberg. B. (1981). Environment and cognitive factors in social play. *Journal of Experimental Child Psychology, 31,* 169-175.

Vandenberg, B., & Kielhofner, G. (1982). Play in evolution, culture, and individual adaptation: Implications for therapy. *American Journal of Occupational Therapy, 36,* 20-28.

Yerxa, E.J. (1994). Dreams, dilemmas, and decisions for occupational therapy practice in a new millennium: An American perspective. *American Journal of Occupational Therapy, 7,* 586-589.

chapter 18

Prewriting and Handwriting Skills

key terms

Prewriting
Functional written
    communication
Handwriting evaluation
    tools
Domains of writing
Legibility components
Frames of reference
Remedial and
    compensatory
    strategies
Service provision

Progress monitoring

*Susan J. Amundson
(with contributions from
Marsha Weil)*

■ CHAPTER OBJECTIVES

1. Describe the role of the occupational therapist in the evaluation and intervention of children with handwriting difficulties.
2. Discuss the factors contributing to handwriting readiness for young children.
3. Examine four aspects of functional written communication that are the keys to a child's performance at school and home.
4. Discuss the performance components and the performance context that contribute to a child's handwriting.
5. Develop remedial and compensatory strategies to improve a student's performance of written communication, focusing on the occupation and the occupational context.
6. Examine the relationship of various pediatric occupational therapy frames of reference and handwriting intervention programs.

Occupational therapists view the occupational performance of children to be self-care, work, and play activities. In the area of work, school-aged children's occupations encompass academic tasks, such as reading, writing, calculation, and problem solving (Llorens, 1991), as well as nonacademic or functional tasks. Functional tasks might include navigating around classroom furniture and classmates, sharing school supplies with a peer, placing a notebook into a locker, constructing a papier-mâché globe, and writing words down on paper; all of which support a student's academic performance in the classroom (Amundson, 1998). These academic skills, functional abilities, and adaptive behaviors are expected to evolve and strengthen throughout a student's school years (Levine, 1994).

One common academic activity is writing, required when children and adolescents compose stories, complete written examinations (Benbow, Hanft, & Marsh, 1992), copy numbers for calculations (Hagin, 1983), dictate telephone messages and numbers at home, and write messages to friends and family members (Amundson, 1998). Although readily demanded of students, writing is a complex process requiring the synthesis and integration of memory retrieval, organization, problem solving, language and reading ability, ideation, and graphomotor function (Levine, 1994).

The functional skill of handwriting supports the academic task of writing and allows students to convey written information legibly and efficiently, while accomplishing written school assignments in a timely manner. Once developed, these skills continue to be used throughout adult life, as individuals write checks, schedule events on calendars, write directions to the dentist's office, scribble grocery lists, and jot down notes and messages to others.

Handwriting consumes much of a student's school day. McHale and Cermak (1992) examined the amount of time allocated to fine-motor activities and the type of fine-motor activities that school-aged children were expected to perform in the classroom. In their study of six classes, consisting of two classes from grades 2, 4, and 6 in middle-income public schools, they found that 31% to 60% of the children's school day consisted of fine-motor activities. Of those fine-motor tasks, 85% of the time consisted of paper and pencil tasks, indicating that students may possibly spend up to one quarter to one half of their classroom time engaged in paper and pencil tasks.

When children are experiencing handwriting difficulty, problems with written assignments follow. Students with neurological impairments, learning problems, attention deficits, and developmental disabilities, often expend enormous time and effort just learning to write in a legible format (Amundson, 1992; Bergman & McLaughlin, 1988; Cermak, 1991). School consequences of handwriting difficulties may include (1) teachers assigning lower marks for papers with poorer legibility but not poorer content (Chase, 1986; Sweedler-Brown, 1992); (2) students' slow handwriting speed limiting compositional fluency and quality (Graham, Berninger, Abbott, Abbott, & Whitaker, 1997); (3) students taking longer to finish assignments than their peers (Graham, 1992); (4) students having problems with taking notes in class (Graham, 1992) and problems reading them later; (5) students struggling with handwriting mechanics failing to learn other higher-order writing processes, such as planning and grammar; and (6) students laboring with handwriting that results in writing avoidance, and later, arrested writing development (Berninger, Mizokawa, & Bragg, 1991).

Occupational therapists are frequently asked to evaluate handwriting when it interferes with a student's performance of written assignments. In fact, poor handwriting is one of the most common reasons for referring school-aged children for occupational therapy (Cermak, 1991; Chandler, 1994; Oliver, 1990; Reisman, 1991). The role of the occupational therapist is to view the student's performance, in this case handwriting, by focusing on the interaction of the student, the school environment, and the school occupation.

During the evaluation and intervention processes, the practitioner stays attuned to (1) the actual task of handwriting, determining which domains of handwriting (e.g., near-point copying or dictation) and which components (e.g., spacing or letter formation) are problematic for the student; (2) the school context (e.g., the cur-

riculum or physical classroom arrangement related to the child's performance); and (3) the student's abilities, experiences, and cognitive, psychosocial, and sensorimotor skills, that are interfering with handwriting production (Amundson, 1998). Another role of the occupational therapist related to handwriting is the evaluation and intervention of children's prewriting and handwriting readiness skills (Oliver, 1990), particularly children of preschool and kindergarten age.

■ PREWRITING

Handwriting Development

Many children begin to scribble on paper shortly after they are able to grasp a writing tool. If not supervised, they will eventually write on any available surface. As children mature, their scribbling evolves into the handwriting specific to their culture. Table 18-1 provides an example of the development of prewriting and handwriting of children in the United States. Because variation in skill development is to be expected among young children, the age levels of handwriting progression shown are only approximations.

As for letter copying acquisition, very little information has been documented in the literature. One study by Tan-Lin (1981) examined the sequential stages of letter acquisition of 110 children between the ages of 3 and 5 years

table 18-1 Development of Prewriting and Handwriting in Young Children

Performance Task	Age Level
Scribbles on paper	10-12 months
Imitates horizontal, vertical, and circular marks on paper	2 years
Copies a vertical line, horizontal line, and circle	3 years
Copies a cross, right oblique line, square, left diagonal line, left oblique cross, some letters and numerals, and may be able to write own name	4-5 years
Copies a triangle, prints own name, copies most lowercase and uppercase letters	5-6 years

Modified from Bayley, N. (1993). *Bayley scales on infant development.* (Rev. ed.). San Antonio, TX: Psychological Corporation.
Beery, K.E. (1982). *The Development Test of Visual-Motor Integration.* Cleveland: Modern Curriculum Press.
Tan-Lin, A.S. (1981). An investigation into the developmental course of preschool/kindergarten aged children's handwriting behavior. *Dissertation Abstracts International*, *42*, 4287A.
Weil, M., & Amundson, S.J. (1994). Relationship between visual motor and handwriting skills of children in kindergarten. *American Journal of Occupational Therapy, 48,* 982-988.

old. Children were observed copying numbers, letters, a few words, and a sentence three times over a period of 4 months. Her findings revealed the following sequential stages of prewriting and handwriting: (1) controlled scribbles; (2) discrete lines, dots, or symbols; (3) straight-line or circular upper-case letters; (4) upper-case letters; and (5) lower-case letters, numerals, and words.

Pencil Grasp Development

The development of pencil grasp follows a predictable course for typically developing children. Children commonly begin by holding the pencil with the whole hand, pronating the forearm and using the shoulder to move the pencil. Later, children use a more mature pencil grasp, holding the pencil between the distal phalanges of the thumb, index, and middle fingers. Initially, the forearm is pronated (thumb side downward), while the fingers grasp the pencil. However, in the latter stage the forearm is usually supinated, and the fine, isolated movements of the hand move the pencil (Erhardt, 1982; Rosenbloom & Horton, 1971).

Handwriting Readiness
Evaluation of readiness for handwriting

Some controversy exists as to when children are ready for formal handwriting instruction. Differing rates of maturity, environmental experiences, and interest levels are all factors that influence children's early attempts and success copying letters. Some children may be ready for writing at 4 years of age, while others may not be ready until they are 6 years old (Lamme, 1979; Laszlo & Bairstow, 1984).

A number of authors (Alston & Taylor, 1987; Donoghue, 1975; Lamme, 1979; Wright & Allen, 1975) have stressed the importance of the mastery of writing readiness skills before handwriting instruction is initiated. These authors contend that children who are taught handwriting before they are ready may become discouraged and develop poor writing habits that may be difficult to later correct.

The readiness factors for handwriting require the integrity of a number of sensorimotor systems. Letter formation requires the integration of the visual, motor, sensory, and perceptual systems. Sufficient fine-motor coordination is also needed to form letters accurately (Alston & Taylor, 1987). Donaghue (1975) and Lamme (1979) identified the following six prerequisite skills that children must have before handwriting instruction begins: (1) small-muscle development; (2) eye-hand coordination; (3) the ability to hold utensils or writing tools; (4) the capacity to smoothly form basic strokes, such as circles and lines; (5) letter perception, including the ability to recognize forms, notice similarities and differences, infer movements necessary for the production of form, and give accurate verbal descriptions of what was seen; and (6) orientation to printed language, which involves the visual analysis of letters and words along with right-left discrimination.

Other authors define readiness for writing on the basis of a child's ability to copy geometric forms. Beery (1992) and Benbow and others (1992) suggested that instruction in handwriting be postponed until after the child is able to master the first 9 figures in the Developmental Test of Visual-Motor Integration (VMI). The 9 figures are a vertical line, a horizontal line, a circle, a cross, a right-oblique line, a square, a left-oblique line, an oblique cross, and a triangle.

A study by Weil and Amundson (1994) examined 59 kindergarten children who were typically developing (aged 54 to 64 months) and their abilities to copy letter forms as well as the geometric designs on the VMI. The findings indicated that children who were able to copy the first 9 forms of the VMI were able to copy significantly more letters than those who were not able to copy the first 9 forms, thus providing support for the opinions of Beery (1992) and Benbow and others (1992).

Weil and Amundson also found that kindergarten children were, on average, able to correctly copy 78% of the letters presented, despite not having received formal handwriting instruction. Based upon the results of the study, the authors concluded that most typically developing kindergarten children should be ready for handwriting instruction in the latter half of the kindergarten school year.

Activities to promote handwriting readiness

The occupational therapy practitioner can incorporate games and activities into the classroom or home to develop children's handwriting readiness skills. Selected activities should be aimed at improving fine-motor control and isolated finger movements, promoting prewriting skills, enhancing right-left discrimination, and improving orientation to printed language (Barchers, 1994; Benbow et. al., 1992; Lamme, 1979; Myers, 1992; Wright & Allen, 1975).

Some children with significant cognitive and/or physical impairments may not acquire many of the prerequisite components needed for writing, and they are most successful in written communication by word processing with a computer. Other children, despite lacking the prerequisite components for handwriting, may be able to learn to write their name with repeated drill and practice sessions. The occupational therapy practitioner must determine when it is appropriate for the child to work on prerequisite handwriting skills, the functional skill of handwriting, or both.

Activities are commonly used with young children to facilitate certain movements, experiences, and perception for writing development. Movements and tasks to encourage writing development should be used in the context of what is meaningful and purposeful to the child. For example, the occupational therapy practitioner is encouraging Grayson to use an open web space and thumb-to-index finger opposition when picking up raisins with a tweezers. This task alone is meaningless for Grayson, until he and the practitioner decide he must feed five raisins to an open-mouthed toy alligator before the alligator slips down a toy slide and into a miniature swimming pool. This newly derived game suddenly becomes fun and motivating for Grayson because he is engaged in a meaningful activity.

Examples of tasks *to improve children's fine-motor control and isolated finger movements* include the following: (1) rolling one-quarter to one-eighth inch balls of clay or Silly Putty between the tip of the thumb and tips of the index and middle fingers; (2) picking up small objects (e.g., Cheerios or raisins) with a tweezers; (3) pinching and sealing a Ziplock™ bag using the thumb opposing each finger, while maintaining an open web space; (4) twisting open a small tube of toothpaste with the thumb and index and middle fingers, while holding the tube with the ulnar digits; and (5) moving a key from the palm to the fingertips of one hand.

To promote prewriting skills in children, the following activities may be tried: (1) drawing lines and copying shapes using shaving cream, sand trays, or finger paints; (2) drawing lines and shapes to complete a picture story on blackboards; (3) drawing pictures of people, houses, trees, cars, or animals with visual and verbal cues from the practitioner; and (4) completing simple dot-to-dot pictures and mazes.

Activities for children of preschool and kindergarten age *to enhance right-left discrimination* include (1) playing "hokeypokey," (2) maneuvering through obstacles and focusing on the concept of turning right or left; and (3) connecting dots at the chalkboard with left-to-right strokes.

To improve children's orientation to printed language the following activities may be tried: (1) labeling children's drawings based on the child's description; (2) having children make their own books on specific topics (e.g., favorite foods, the alphabet, or special places); (3) labeling common objects in the classroom or therapy room; and (4) having adults demonstrate the utility of writing in the presence of children (e.g., writing notes for parents or teachers while the child watches).

■ HANDWRITING ASSESSMENT

When a child with poor handwriting has been referred to occupational therapy, the methods to gather assessment information must be carefully selected and sequenced. An individual assessment is needed, because each child with handwriting dysfunction varies from each

and every other child with handwriting problems. A comprehensive evaluation of a child's handwriting includes (1) examining written work samples; (2) discussing the child's performance with the teacher, parent, and other team members; (3) reviewing the child's educational and clinical records; (4) observing the child directly when he or she is writing in the natural setting; (5) evaluating the child's actual performance of handwriting; and (6) assessing any suspected performance components interfering with handwriting.

Initially, the student's performance in the context of classroom standards should be the focus (before moving toward standardized testing). Assembling data and information from various sources gives the occupational therapist an integrated picture of the child's written communication. It also allows the therapist to examine the child's ability to perform other functional school tasks, such as handling school supplies and manipulatives, managing outdoor clothing and fasteners, and organizing school materials. Although poor handwriting is a common referring concern in the classroom, poor performance of other school tasks may have gone unnoticed and should also receive attention from the occupational therapist and educational team.

Work Samples

Oftentimes the referring person (e.g., the parent or educator) approaches the occupational therapist with the child's handwritten class work or homework. Written work samples may include spelling lessons, mathematical problems, or stories. Ideally, these samples should represent a typical handwriting performance of the child. When reviewing the child's written product, a comparison of the writing samples of the child's peers is also warranted to understand the classroom standards and teacher expectations.

Interviews

Obtaining anecdotal information from the child's parents, educators, and other team members serves as a mechanism for building rapport and gathering important data (Cook, 1991). Since teachers know a great deal about their students' performance in class, they can share information about the student's abilities and achievements, the classroom standards and curricula, and interactions with the student. Therefore the educator can help provide a picture of the student's capabilities, behavior, and struggles at school. A sampling of questions to facilitate discussion between the teacher and the occupational therapist are listed in Box 18-1.

Parents are also a valuable source of information for occupational therapists; they can provide a different perspective of the child and the child's handwriting abilities. Not only can parents relate the child's developmental, medical, and familial background to the educational team, they can share invaluable information about the

18-1 *Questions to facilitate discussion among educational team members*

1. What are the student's educational strengths and concerns?
2. What is his or her handwriting performance in comparison with peers?
3. What handwriting method (D'Nealian, Zaner-Bloser, Palmer, italics) is being used? What is his or her history with this method?
4. What are the learning standards or curriculum of his or her grade?
5. What seems to be causing the poor handwriting?
6. When does he or she do his or her best written work?
7. When does the performance break down?
8. What strategies for improvement have been tried? Have they worked?
9. Is a student portfolio available on the student's writing development and progress?
10. Are there other daily tasks (e.g., using scissors, getting along with peers, keeping organized) that raise concern for the teacher?

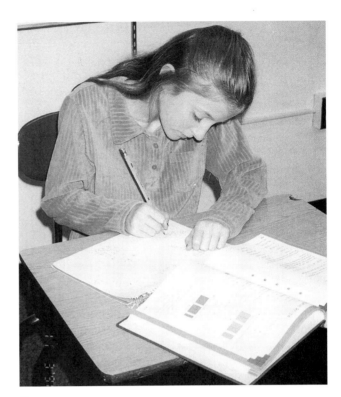

figure**18-1**   A girl completes a written assignment at her desk.

child's interests, social competence, and attitudes towards learning and school.

Parents are considered educational team members, and they provide important perspectives that give the occupational therapist a comprehensive view of the child at home and at school. Questions asked of parents related to the child and his or her writing might include the following:

1. Do parents expect the child to complete school assignments or written work at home?
2. What is the child's response to written homework?
3. How does the child perform his or her written assignments at home and school?
4. What other writing tasks are expected of the child at home (e.g., correspondence with relatives, recording of telephone messages)?

File Review

Relevant information regarding the child's past academic performance, special testing, or receipt of special services can be found in the referred child's educational cumulative file. Medical or clinical reports related to the child's education might also be located in the child's regular or special education files. For clinic- and hospital-based occupational therapists, the child's parents are a good source for academic records and reports. This documentation may trigger further discussion among the child's parents and team members.

Direct Observation

Observing the student during a writing activity is an essential step in the assessment process (Figure 18-1). The referral of the child to occupational therapy is commonly made by the teacher or parent who observes the child struggling with handwriting. Therefore occupational therapists need to examine the child in this activity. Skilled observation usually occurs in the child's classroom and focuses on task performance, attention to task, problem solving, and behavior of the child (Hanft & Place, 1996). Practitioners also note the student's organizational abilities, movement through the classroom, interactions with the teacher and peers, transitions between activities, and overall performance of other school tasks. School contextual features (e.g., the classroom arrangement, noise level, lighting, and instructional media) as well as the actual instruction from school personnel should all be considered in relationship to the student's performance.

Besides a structured protocol for direct observation, questions asked by the occupational therapist might include the following:

1. Which writing tasks (e.g., copying sentences from the chalkboard or composing a story) are most problematic for the child?
2. What avoidance behaviors (e.g., chewing on a pencil or blowing a pencil across the desktop) are manifested when the child is required to write?

3. Can the child engage in the task of writing independently, or are physical and verbal cues needed from the teacher or educational assistant?
4. Is the child easily distracted by visual and auditory stimuli (e.g., a delivery truck driving by the school) during writing?
5. Where does the child sit in the classroom?
6. What curriculum is being followed?
7. Where is the teacher located when assignment directions are given?

Measuring the Functional Performance of Handwriting

When evaluating the actual task of children's handwriting, the following areas need to be examined closely: (1) domains of handwriting, (2) legibility components, (3) writing speed, and (4) ergonomic factors (Amundson, 1992). Whether the student writes in manuscript (print), cursive (joined script), or both, examining these four aspects of the handwriting process will help the educational team to uncover problematic areas and establish a baseline of handwriting function. With accurate and comprehensive handwriting assessment data, the occupational therapist, the child's parents, and the educational or clinical team will also be able to target specific goals and objectives for the child's development of written communication.

Domains of handwriting

Evaluating the various handwriting domains allows the occupational therapist to determine which tasks the child may be having difficulty with and address those tasks in the intervention plan (Amundson, 1992). Handwriting tasks demanded of students, and helpful for intervention planning, include the following:

■ *Writing the alphabet and numerals from memory.* Writing the alphabet in both upper- and lower-case letters requires the child to remember the motor engram, form each individual letter and numeral, sequence letters and numbers, and use consistent letter cases.
■ *Copying.* Near-point copying is producing letters or words from a nearby model, commonly on the same page or on the same horizontal writing surface (e.g., copying the meaning of a word from a nearby dictionary). *Far-point copying* is producing letters or words from a distant vertical model to the writing surface (e.g., writing the words "Happy Mother's

Day" on construction paper cards from the teacher's modeled words on the class chalkboard).
■ *Manuscript-to-cursive transition.* More advanced than copying, manuscript-to-cursive transition requires a mastery of letter forms in both manuscript and cursive as the child transcribes manuscript letters and words to cursive letters and words.
■ *Dictation.* A higher-level handwriting task combines integration of auditory directions and a motoric response. Writing dictated words, names, addresses, and telephone numbers is a skill needed by children at school and at home.
■ *Composition.* The composing process (i.e., in this case, the generation of a sentence or paragraph by the child) requires the cognitive functions of planning, sentence generation, and revision (Beringer & Rutberg, 1992). Thus this writing task involves complex integration of linguistic, cognitive, organizational, and sensorimotor skills.

Legibility components

Legibility is often assessed in terms of its components (i.e., letter formation, alignment, spacing, size, and slant) (Alston, 1983; Amundson, 1995). However, the bottom line of legibility is readability. Of primary importance, is whether what was written by the child can be read by the child, parent, or teacher. Although a legibility component, such as poor text alignment, interferes with appearance, a child's writing sample may still be readable. Johnson and Carlisle (1996) found that formation and size were more problematic for students with learning disabilities in grades one, two, and three, than for their typically developing peers. Decreased legibility of cursive writing with inadequate letter formation and disproportionate size of letters is shown in Figure 18-2.

Components of handwriting legibility need to be assessed. In *letter formation,* Alston (1983) identified five features impacting legibility: (1) improper letter forms, (2) poor leading in and leading out of letters, (3) inadequate rounding of letters, (4) incomplete closure of letters, and (5) incorrect letter ascenders and descenders. *Alignment,* or *baseline orientation,* refers to the placement of text on and within the writing guidelines. *Spacing* includes the dispersion of letters within words and words within sentences, along with text organization on the entire sheet of paper. Another component of legibility, *size,* refers to the letter relative to the writing guidelines and to the other letters. Finally, the uniformity or consistency of the *slant,* or the angle of the text, should be observed.

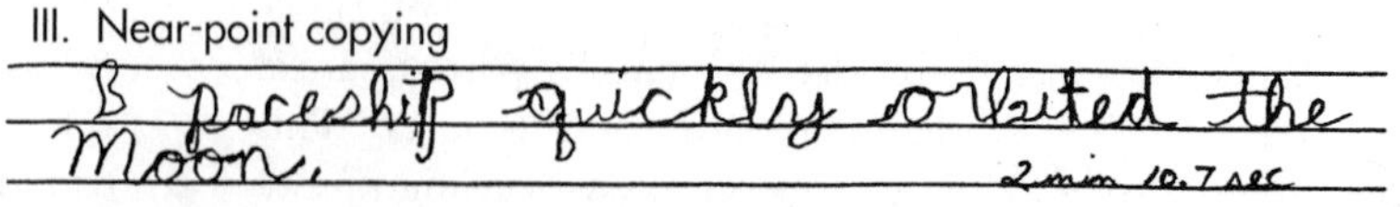

figure **18-2** Cursive handwriting sample exemplifies improper letter forms and disproportionate letter size.

III. Near-point copying

Writing speed

A child's rate of writing, or the number of letters written per minute, coupled with legibility, are the two cornerstones of functional handwriting (Amundson, 1995). Students take longer to complete written assignments, have difficulty taking notes in class (Graham, 1992), lose their train of ideas for writing (McAvoy, 1996), and become frustrated when their handwriting speed is slower than their peers. Writing speed typically decreases when the amount of written work or complexity of the writing task increases (Rubin & Henderson, 1982; Weintraub & Graham, 1998). Upper-elementary students and older children not only need an adequate writing speed, they need to be able to adjust their speed from a hurried, rough draft to a neat, well-paced, final draft (Weintraub & Graham, 1998).

Differences in methodologies, subjects, and data collection (from 1912 through 1989) have resulted in a varied baseline of writing speeds for typically developing children (Ziviani & Elkins, 1984). Table 18-2 shows different studies of children's writing speeds, along with the methodologies used in each. Handwriting speeds vary among these studies, just as they do among classrooms of children at the same grade level. Individual classroom standards and teacher expectations justify the need to compare a student's writing speed with the writing speed of his or her peers.

Ergonomic factors

Writing posture, upper-extremity stability and mobility, and pencil grasp are all ergonomic factors that must be analyzed as the child writes. Sitting posture in the classroom should be observed. Does the child rest his or her head on the forearm or desktop when writing? Is the child falling and spilling out of his or her chair? Does the child stand beside the desk or kneel in the chair? Are the desktop and chair at suitable heights?

Stability and mobility of the upper extremities refers to the stabilization of the shoulder girdle, elbow, and wrist to allow the dexterous hand to manipulate the writing instrument. Does the child write with whole-arm movements? What are the positions of the trunk and writing arm? Does the nonpreferred hand stabilize the paper? Does the child apply excessive pressure to the writing tool? Finally, a biomechanical focus for most occupational therapy practitioners is pencil grasp.

The relationship of functional writing and pencil grasp is vague throughout the educational and occupational therapy literature. Traditionally, teachers and occupational therapy practitioners have stressed the importance of a dynamic-tripod pencil grasp (Rosenbloom & Horton, 1971; Tseng & Cermak, 1993). The dynamic-tripod grasp appears with the writing utensil resting against the distal phalanx of the radial side of the middle finger, while the pads of the thumb and index finger control it (Rosenbloom & Horton, 1971).

Recent studies have found that a variety of pencil-grasp patterns exist among typical populations of adults and children, and that an atypical grasp pattern by itself does not necessarily result in handwriting difficulties (Bergmann, 1990; Schneck, 1991; Schneck & Henderson, 1990; Ziviani, 1983; Ziviani & Elkins, 1984). In their study of 320 typically developing children, Schneck and Henderson (1991) reported that by the age of 6½ to 7 years, 95% of their subjects had adopted a mature pencil grasp; either the dynamic tripod (72.5%) or the lateral tripod (22.5%).

The lateral tripod grasp may be considered an acceptable alternative to the traditionally preferred, dynamic-tripod grasp. Ziviani (1987) reported that different grasp

table 18-2 *Writing Speeds of Children (Letters Per Minute)*

Grade	Ayres (1912)*	Groff (1961)†	Phelps et. al. (1985)‡	Phelps et. al. (1987)‡	Ziviani & Elkins (1984)§	Larsen & Hammill (1989)‖
1				32		<20
2				35		20-25
3			25		32	26-33
4	55	35	37		34	34-40
5	64	41	47		38	41-46
6	71	50	57		46	47-55
7			62		52	56-65
8			72			>65

*Children were to copy passage until familiar with it; then write for speed.
†Children were to read a passage aloud until familiar with it; then write for speed.
‡Near-point passage presented: children were then to copy passage for speed.
§Near-point symbols, letters, and words presented; children were to copy for speed.
‖Authors do not provide source for writing speeds.

variations are expected, and that poor writers are more likely to demonstrate a variety of atypical grasp patterns than legible writers. A left-handed dynamic-tripod grasp and a right-handed lateral-tripod grasp of two elementary students is shown in Figure 18-3.

Handwriting Instruments

Formal, or standardized, tests are important for assessing the performance of children because they provide objective measures and quantitative scores. In addition, formal tests aid in monitoring a child's progress, assist professionals to communicate more clearly, and advance the field through research (Campbell, 1989). Numerous standardized handwriting instruments are commercially available.

Assessment tools commonly used by occupational therapists in the United States include:

The *Children's Handwriting Evaluation Scale* (Phelps, Stempel, & Speck, 1984)

The *Children's Handwriting Evaluation Scale-Manuscript* (Phelps & Stempel, 1987)

The *Denver Handwriting Analysis* (Anderson, 1983)

The *Diagnosis and Remediation of Handwriting Problems* (Stott, Moyes, & Henderson, 1985)

The *Evaluation Tool of Children's Handwriting* (Amundson, 1995)

The *Minnesota Handwriting Assessment* (Reisman, 2000)

The *Test of Handwriting Skills* (Gardner, 1998)

Each of these assessment tools possesses various features regarding domains of handwriting tested (e.g., farpoint or copying), age or grade of child (e.g., first or second grade), script examined (e.g., manuscript or cursive), scoring procedures of the writing performance (e.g., legibility of manuscript), and scores obtained (e.g., percentiles). Typically, tests measure handwriting legibility and speed of handwriting. Scoring procedures for legibility use rating techniques ranging from global and subjective to detailed and specific. (See Appendix A for information concerning handwriting instruments available to occupational therapists.)

For tool selection, the occupational therapist should keep in mind the characteristics of each instrument as well as the strengths and limitations of the tests regarding normative data, reliability, validity, and other psychometric properties (see Chapter 8). Critiques and lengthier descriptions of handwriting instruments by several authors (Amundson, 1992; Daniels, 1988; Reisman, 1991; Tseng & Cermak, 1991) are helpful to review when selecting a handwriting test. The instrument chosen should match the areas of concern regarding the child's handwriting and should allow for effective intervention planning among the occupational therapist, the child's parents, and other team members.

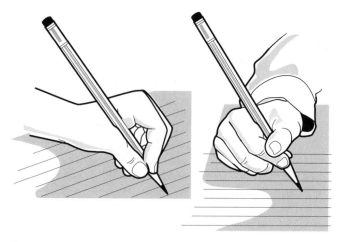

figure**18-3**   Elementary school children use a dynamic tripoid grasp and a lateral tripoid grasp for writing.

Performance Components Related to Handwriting

Concurrent with a qualitative analysis of handwriting, the occupational therapist analyzes the sensorimotor, cognitive, and psychosocial performance components that may be interfering with the child's handwriting legibility and speed. As occupational therapists build their clinical reasoning skills, they are able to observe a child struggling to write or view a child's distorted, unreadable handwriting and identify suspect performance components interfering with written communication.

For example, a 9-year-old girl with a traumatic brain injury may have an illegible script marked with overlapping letters and poor use of margins that may lead the occupational therapy practitioner to believe that she is experiencing a deficit in visual-perceptual skills. Hence, the *Developmental Test of Visual Perception - Second Edition* (Hammill, Pearson, & Voress, 1993) may be administered to the child to determine if any deficit exists (and if so, the extent of the deficit). Sensorimotor components that typically influence children's handwriting and their relationship to handwriting performance are identified in Table 18-3.

With an emphasis on sensorimotor aspects, the occupational therapy practitioner occasionally overlooks the cognitive and psychosocial performance components related to a child's handwriting dysfunction. Neglecting these factors may result in an incomplete assessment of the child and inspire an intervention program that does not recognize and address the cognitive and psychosocial needs of the child as the primary deterrents of successful performance. Cognitive skills required for handwriting include (1) attending to a writing task independently, over time, in a classroom; (2) recalling letter formations and handwriting strategies over periods of time through

table 18-3 *Sensorimotor Performance Components Influencing Handwriting*

Sensorimotor Components	Impact on Handwriting
SENSORY	
Tactile and proprioceptive	Gives information regarding grasp of writing tool, eraser, writing medium, and surface
Visual	Allows scanning the printed line, sustaining visual regard, and focusing on stationary text and formation of letters
Kinesthesia	Provides feedback related to extent, weight, and direction of movement, allowing appropriate pencil pressure and directing writing tools
Form constancy	Enables child to discriminate between numerals, letters, and words that are similar, such as *b/d* and *was/saw*
Position in space	Influences spacing between letters, words, and numerals, placing letters on and within writing lines, and using margins appropriately
Visual closure	Enables child to identify which letters have been formed completely
NEUROMUSCULAR	
Muscle tone	Allows sustaining of an upright position and upper-extremity stability and mobility
Strength	Impacts ability to firmly grasp and maintain positional consistency of the writing tool over time
Postural control	Influences ability to make postural adjustments while writing in various positions
MOTOR	
Crossing the midline	Assists child in learning to write in a horizontal plane across the midline of the body without interruption or distraction
Bilateral integration	Enables child to use symmetric and asymmetric hand movements to hold writing tool and stabilize paper
Laterality	Allows consistent and superior use of one hand for writing
Praxis	Influences capacity to plan, sequence, and execute letter forms and arrange letters to build words
Fine motor coordination, particularly in-hand manipulation	Provides moving pencil from palm to fingers (translation), adjusting pencil shaft in fingers for writing (vertical shift), and turning pencil end-over-end for erasing (complex rotation)
Visual motor integration	Impacts ability to reproduce numerals and letters accurately, to color within lines, and to trace

Modified from: Amundson, S.J. (1992). Handwriting: Evaluation and intervention in school setting. In J. Case-Smith & C. Pehoski (Eds.), *Development of hand skills in the child* (pp. 63-78). Rockville, MD: American Occupational Therapy Association.
Boehme, R. (1988). *Improving upper body control.* Tucson: Therapy Skill Builders.
Exner, C.E. (1992). In-hand manipulation skills. In J. Case-Smith & C. Pehoski (Eds.), *Development of hand skills in the child* (pp. 35-45). Rockville, MD: American Occupational Therapy Association.
Price, A. (1986). Applying sensory integration to handwriting problems. *American Occupational Therapy Association Developmental Disabilities Special Interest Section Newsletter, 9,* 4-5.

visual, verbal, orthographic, and auditory memories; and (3) generalizing handwriting from an intervention program to real-life situations, such as performing classroom assignments independently, copying a recipe, and signing checks.

Psychosocial aspects include the child's values and interests, self-regulation, self-concept, and coping skills. For the child who sees his or her handwriting as a continual visual reminder of school failure, the loss of interest and motivation to produce written text is not surprising (Pasternicki, 1987). Due to the continual criticism and judgment of their handwriting performance by educators and others, some students with poor handwriting tend to feel inadequate and their self-esteem suffers (Bailey, 1988).

■ EDUCATOR'S PERSPECTIVE

Writing Process

When educators speak of the writing or composing process, they view it as a goal-directed activity using the cognitive functions of planning, sentence generation, and revision (Hayes & Flower, 1986). Because the actual text production occurs in sentence generation, the child who needs to pay considerable attention to the mechanical requirements of writing may interrupt higher-order writing processes (e.g., planning or content generation). Hence, most educators view the mechanical requirements of handwriting as an integral subset of the writing process.

Handwriting Instruction Methods

During the past few years, an educational debate has focused on teaching handwriting systematically, through commercially prepared or teacher-developed programs, or learning it through a *"whole language"* approach. The whole language philosophy purports that both the substance (i.e., meaning) of writing is addressed as well as the form (i.e., mechanics) of writing (Graham, 1992). Thus when using the whole language method, the teacher gives advice and practice only on an individual, as-needed basis as children are learning and mastering handwriting. For example, if an educator sees a first-grader struggling to form the letter *n* while writing a story about monsters, he or she may instruct the child regarding the correct letter formation of *n* and encourage extra practice of the letter during the story composition period. Conversely, in a traditional handwriting instruction approach, students are introduced to letter formations, and they practice them outside of the context of writing. For children with learning disabilities and mild neurological impairments, regular practice in forming letters is essential in the early stages of handwriting development. However, this practice should have a meaningful context. Thus a combination of systematic handwriting instruction and whole language methods may be most beneficial to this group of children (Graham, 1992).

In the United States, traditional handwriting instruction programs vary from school district to school district. Occasionally, they vary from school to school and grade to grade. It is common for occupational therapy practitioners to receive a referral for a child with poor handwriting who has never had handwriting instruction. The most common instruction methods include Palmer, Zaner-Blöser, italics, and D'Nealian (Alston & Taylor, 1987; Duvall, 1985; Thurber, 1983) (see Appendix B for a listing of handwriting curricula used in schools). Unlike the United States, a few countries, such as the United Kingdom and New Zealand (Alston, 1991; Alston & Taylor, 1987; Jarman, 1990), have adopted national curricula for handwriting to improve the standards of handwriting assessment and instruction within their school systems.

Manuscript and Cursive Styles

A generally accepted sequence for handwriting instruction is manuscript writing for use in grades one and two, with children transitioning to cursive writing at the end of grade two or the beginning of grade three (Barchers, 1994; Bergman & McLaughlin, 1988; Hagin, 1983). The need for manuscript writing may continue throughout life, when students label maps and posters, adolescents complete job or college applications, and adults compute federal income tax forms. By junior high age, many students have blended both manuscript and cursive to form their own style of handwriting. To date, no research has decisively indicated the superiority of one script style over the other (Graham & Miller, 1980; Hagin, 1983).

Both manuscript and cursive possess complementary features, and these should be considered when the occupational therapist, child, child's parent, and educational team are collaboratively deciding which style might best serve the child. Manuscript is endorsed for the following reasons:
1. Manuscript letter forms are simpler and, hence, easier to learn.
2. It closely resembles the print of textbooks and school manuals.
3. It is needed throughout adult life for documents and applications.
4. Beginning manuscript writing is more readable than cursive.
5. Ball and stick strokes of manuscript letter formations are more developmentally appropriate than cursive letters for young children.
6. Manuscript letters are easier to discriminate visually than cursive ones (Barbe, Milone, & Wasylyk, 1983; Bergman & McLaughlin, 1988; Graham & Miller, 1980; Hagin, 1983).

Advocates of cursive writing provide the following reasons for preferring this writing style:
1. Cursive movement patterns allow for faster and more automatic writing.
2. Reversal of individual letters and transpositions of words are more difficult than in manuscript.
3. One continuous, connected line enables child to form words as units.
4. Cursive is faster than manuscript.
5. It allows the poor printer a new type of written format that may be motivating at the child's present maturity level (Armitage & Ratzlaff, 1985; Bergman & McLauglin, 1988; Graham & Miller, 1980; Hagin, 1983).

■ HANDWRITING INTERVENTION

Planning

In school settings, if the referred child's educational team decides that functional written communication is a priority for the child's academic program, the occupational therapist may be instrumental in directing and guiding this aspect of the program. Typically, the team uses either a remedial or compensatory intervention approach (or both) to better the child's written communication. Compensatory strategies improve a student's participation in school with accommodations, adaptations, and modifications for certain tasks, routines, and settings, whereas remedial strategies are used to improve a student's functional skills in a specific area.

When the team focuses on the occupation of written communication, it must generate, select, and implement strategies that help the student to be successful and functional as soon as possible. Both remedial and compensatory techniques might be employed concurrently. For example, Benjamin, a second-grader, has unreadable manuscript handwriting. About 60% of his written letters are not legible, and his writing speed is at the bottom of his class. While he participates in an intensive multisensory handwriting remediation program, he needs accommodations and strategies that assist him to be functional with his written communication in the classroom. Consequently, his teacher may need to adjust the time required to complete assignments, incorporate more oral reporting into his class assignments, or set a volume of work for Benjamin to accomplish that may be different than the volume expected from his peers. The teacher and occupational therapy practitioner might use other techniques to assist Benjamin with any legibility problems, such as spacing between words, sizing letters, and placing text on lines.

Initially, the child, the child's parents, and the educational team need to achieve consensus regarding the type of script (e.g., cursive) and the method of handwriting instruction (e.g., Zaner-Blöser) that seems most advantageous for the child. Specific intervention techniques should also be generated and selected. Subsequently, the type, frequency, and duration of service delivery, along with the need for additional service providers (e.g., a certified occupational therapy assistant) to work with the child on his or her handwriting problems may be determined during the planning meeting.

When a child's handwriting is slow and illegible, team members may decide to include computer technology, such as a portable word processor, in the intervention program (see Chapter 19). Both the student and the team, particularly the occupational therapy practitioner, must be hardworking to find a technological system that allows the student proficiency of text generation (Swinth & Anson, 1998). As with paper and pencil, computer use requires adequate attention, motor control, sensory processing, visual functioning, and self-regulation from the student. Hence, the computer is not a magical tool, but one that allows the acquisition of keyboarding and word-processing skills through planning, routine instruction, and practice (Swinth & Anson, 1998). Two studies of upper-elementary students with learning disabilities

(Lewis, Graves, Ashton, & Kieley, 1998; MacArthur & Graham, 1987) indicated that, after several months of practice, handwriting was a quicker mode of generating text than was keyboarding. Therefore while it is important for students to develop keyboarding skills as an additional academic "basic" for computer use in classrooms, work places, and homes, handwriting skills will continue to be needed throughout student and adult life.

Frames of Reference to Guide the Occupational Therapy Practitioner

Theories, strategies, and approaches of occupational therapy practitioners may seem unconventional to children, educators, parents, and other school personnel. Therefore the occupational therapist must be able to (1) clearly articulate intervention techniques, environmental arrangements, and classroom accommodations being used; (2) collaborate with the teacher and others to provide service in the least restrictive environment; (3) implement therapeutic strategies for improving written communication; (4) train others to work with children with handwriting problems; and (5) closely monitor the progress of the child and change aspects of the program to continue improvement.

The overall focus of the educational program is the improvement of student performance in a particular area (e.g., written communication). Occupational therapy frames of reference or theoretical approaches contributing to this functional outcome include (1) neurodevelopmental, (2) acquisitional, (3) sensory integration, (4) biomechanical, and (5) behavioral. When considering any intervention plan for handwriting, practitioners should consider the far-reaching parameters of each frame of reference, along with the overlap and the interplay between them. The occupational therapist must be skillful in the use of one or several frames of reference concurrently and in teaching others to implement strategies originating from these frames of reference. By remaining focused on the child's functional outcome related to handwriting and applying various frames of reference in the child's educational program, the occupational therapy practitioner can provide a conduit of opportunities for the learning and mastering of written communication skills.

Neurodevelopmental

The *neurodevelopmental theoretical approach* is based on neurological principles and normal development, focusing on an individual's ability to execute normal postural responses and movement patterns (Bobath, 1985; Bobath & Bobath, 1972). This frame of reference provides an ideal orientation for addressing problems of children who have inadequate neurodevelopmental organization exhibited by poor postural control, automatic

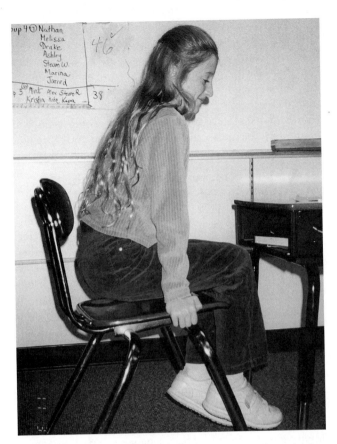

figure **18-4** A girl demonstrates an arm push-up in her school chair.

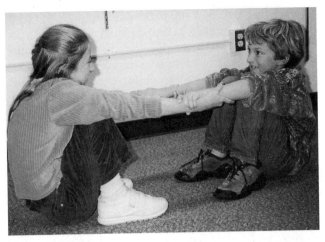

figure **18-5** Two children engage in a partner pull-up to prepare for writing.

reactions, and/or limb control (Dutton, 1993). Decreased, increased, or fluctuating muscle tone, inadequate righting and equilibrium responses, along with poor proximal stability, may interfere with successful performance in fine-motor activities (e.g., handwriting production at home and in school).

Postural and limb preparation activities are an important component of a comprehensive handwriting program for children with mild neuromuscular impairments. For these children, preparing their bodies and hands for handwriting should be the preliminary ingredient of handwriting intervention before the instructional program begins. Selecting preparatory activities to address each child's specific deficits and carefully analyzing his or her response to these activities are both critical in the preparatory phase of the handwriting intervention program. The remaining paragraphs of this section include postural and upper-extremity activities for getting children's bodies ready to write. These activities can be used in the classroom and/or pull-out therapy for (1) modulating muscle tone, (2) promoting proximal joint stability, and (3) improving hand function.

Postural preparation to modulate muscle tone may involve activities to increase, decrease, or balance muscle tone. Traditional activities to increase tone include jump-

ing while sitting on a hippity-hop ball, spinning on a "sit-and-spin," and jumping on a mini-trampoline. In the classroom, activities to build tone and strength might include students placing their hands on the sides of their chairs and bouncing in place for a "popcorn ride." They may hold that position with arms extended for a chair push-up. They may perform simple calisthenics, such as pushing down on the top of their heads and shoulders with their hands while seated in a chair (Amundson, 1998), or perform an arm push-up in a school chair (Figure 18-4).

For children whose muscle tone needs to be reduced, conventional slow rocking may be achieved by sitting astride a large bolster and moving from side to side to the rhythm of a child's poem recited aloud. Before writing, a child's postural tone may be decreased by rocking in a rocking chair to the beat of slow, rhythmical instrumental or vocal music from a headset, by snuggling into a beanbag chair, or by participating in a relaxing visual imagery exercise.

Children with poor handwriting frequently exhibit poor proximal stability. To encourage cocontraction through the neck, shoulders, elbows, and wrists, young children may enjoy animal walks, such as the crab walk, the bear walk, the inchworm creep, or the mule kick. Older children may prefer calisthenics, such as push-ups on the floor or against the wall, resistive exercises with elastic tubing or theraband, cooperatively pulling up a partner from a seated position on the floor, or yoga poses requiring weight bearing on the upper extremities. Figure 18-5 shows two children engaging in a shared exercise activity, known as a "partner pull-up." Within the school setting, proximal stability may also be improved through every day routines, such as cleaning black boards and table tops, pushing heavy external doors open, or pushing and moving classroom furniture or physical education equipment.

Alternative positions during writing activities can enhance proximal stability during writing. The prone position requires weight bearing on the forearms for writing, which increases proximal joint stability and disassociation of the hand and digits from the forearm. A student completing written schoolwork while lying in prone is shown in Figure 18-6.

When preparing to write, some children may also benefit from developing more coordinated synergies of the intrinsic and extrinsic muscles of the hand to improve overall hand function. Typically, the hand needs to be stable and strong enough to provide support for fingers to manipulate tools. In-class hand strengthening activities include carrying heavy cases with thick handles, practicing knot-tying exercises with thick rope, and participating in games, such as Felicity the Cat Scratch.

Prewriting, handwriting, and manipulative activities on vertical surfaces can assist children to develop more wrist extension stability to facilitate balanced use of the intrinsic musculature of the hand (Benbow, 1990). Activities requiring in-hand manipulation or the adjustment of an object after placement within the hand (Exner, 1989) may be appropriate for children with deficits in handwriting. (See Chapter 11 for in-hand manipulation activities). "Translation," moving the writing utensil from the palm to the fingers of the hand, "shifting" the shaft of the utensil within the hand for proper grasp, and "rotating" the pencil from the writing to the erasing position, are all in-hand manipulation skills needed for writing-tool management.

A study by Cornhill and Case-Smith (1996) of 48 first-graders indicated a moderate to high correlation between handwriting skills and in-hand manipulation, specifically translation and complex rotation. Boehme (1988) suggested that vertical excursion of the writing line is produced by the flexion and extension movements of the digits, whereas horizontal excursion originates primarily from lateral wrist movements. Hence, the balanced interaction of the intrinsic and extrinsic muscles of the hand is key to the dynamic, efficient, and fluid movements required for handwriting.

Acquisitional

Handwriting may be viewed as a complex motor skill and, like other acquisitional skills, "can be improved through practice, repetition, feedback, and reinforcement" (Holm, 1986, p. 70). Graham and Miller (1980) recommended that instructional guidance of handwriting should be (1) taught directly; (2) implemented in brief, daily lessons; (3) particularized for the individual needs of the child; (4) planned and changed, based on evaluation and performance data; and (5) overlearned and used in a meaningful manner by the child. When therapists and educators employ these conditions in a positive, interesting, and dynamic learning environment, children are more likely to become efficient, legible writ-

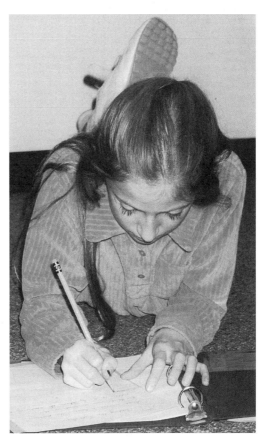

figure 18-6   A girl completes a written assignment while lying in prone.

ers (Barchers, 1994; Graham & Miller; Milone & Wasylyk, 1981).

For occupational therapy practitioners, handwriting (as a motor skill) relates to theories of motor learning that impact the instructional process. Learning a new motor skill has been described as progressing through three phases: cognitive, associative, and autonomous (Fitts & Posner, 1967). In the *cognitive phase,* the child attempts to understand the demands of the handwriting task and develop a cognitive strategy for performing the necessary motor movements. Visual control of fine-motor movements is thought to be important at this phase. A child learning handwriting in this phase may have developed some strategies for writing some of the easier manuscript letters, such as *o, l,* or *t,* but he or she may have more difficulty writing complicated letters, such as *b, q,* or *g.*

In the *associative phase,* the child has learned the fundamentals of performing handwriting and continues to adjust and refine the skill. Proprioceptive feedback becomes increasingly important during this phase, while reliance on visual cues declines. For example, in the associative phase a child may have mastered the formations of letters, but he or she is engaged in improving the handwriting product by learning to space words correctly, to write letters within guidelines, or to maintain consistent letter slant. Therefore children continue to need practice, instructional guidance, and self-monitoring strategies to improve handwriting performance during this phase.

In the final, *autonomous phase,* the child can perform handwriting automatically, with minimal conscious attention. Variability of performance is slight from day-to-day, and the child is able to detect and adjust for any small errors that may occur (Schmidt, 1982). Once the child has reached this level of handwriting, his or her attention can be expended on other higher-order elements of writing (Graham, 1992), or it can be saved to alleviate fatigue (Schmidt, 1982).

Implications and strategies for handwriting instruction and remediation evolve from reviews of handwriting studies (Bergman & McLaughlin, 1988; Graham & Miller, 1980) as well as motor-learning theory (Magill, 1985). Although many handwriting intervention programs are commercially available (see Appendix 18-C for ordering information and brief descriptions of these programs), each should contain a scope and sequence of letter and numeral formations, along with successive instructional techniques (Graham & Miller, 1980; Taylor, 1985).

The scope and sequence of the handwriting program should focus on a structured progression of introducing and teaching letter and numeral forms. Frequently, letters with common formational features are introduced as a family, such as the lower-case letters of *e, i, t,* and *l.* After a child masters these letters, they can immediately be used to write the words, *eel, tile,* and *little.* Whether the chosen handwriting intervention method is a commercially available program, or a teacher- or therapist-prepared method, each child's program should be individualized to consist of those letters that he or she has not yet mastered. Thus the focus of the child's program is to sequentially introduce new letters and use them with mastered letters; excluding letters the child is forming incorrectly or ones not known to the child, because this only reinforces unwelcomed perceptual-motor patterns (Ziviani, 1987). Combining newly acquired letters with already mastered letters provides a meaningful context, (i.e., the formation of written words and sentences). This immediate reinforcement of writing words is more powerful and purposeful for the child than writing strings of letters repeatedly.

Instructional approaches of handwriting intervention programs vary, but they tend to purport a combination of sequential techniques, including modeling, tracing, stimulus fading, copying, composing, and self-monitoring (Amundson, 1992; Bergman & McLaughlin, 1988; Milone & Wasylyk, 1987). When acquiring new letter forms, initially the child may need many visual and auditory cues. However, the service provider will want to fade the cues as soon as the child can successfully

form the letter without them. Next, the child proceeds to copying letters and words from a model to writing letters and words from memory as they are dictated. Finally, the child advances to generating words and sentences for practice. In each phase of instruction, the child should be expected to assume responsibility for correcting his or her own work, also known as self-monitoring. Older children might refer to a written checklist addressing spacing, size, alignment, letter forms, and slant during the self-assessment of their writing. However, younger children may need to verbally evaluate letter formation and overall appearance aloud to the service provider.

Acquiring handwriting skills and applying them in school life means the educational team not only focuses on teaching letter formation, it also focuses on the legibility and speed of the student's handwriting. Besides learning correct letter forms, other components of legibility include spacing, size, slant, and alignment. Spacing between letters and words, text placement on lines, and sizing letters often need direct attention.

An effective writing surface for assisting students with text placement and size is a color-coded, laminated sheet. This sheet provides immediate visual cues to the child learning letter forms, when accompanied by verbal cues from the service provider. Beneath the solid, red writing baseline, the color brown represents the "soil" or "ground;" the space above the solid baseline and dashed, black middle guideline is green, for the "grass"; and above the dashed guideline to the top solid writing line is blue, for the "sky." For example, the letter *h* would start at the top of the sky, head downward, and end in the grass. This same pictorial scheme can be applied to lined paper for classroom assignments, allowing students strong cues for learning letter placement and size (Amundson, 1998) (Figure 18-7). Various strategies for handwriting problems relating to legibility components, classroom writing assignments, and speed are listed in Table 18-4.

Sensory integration

The parameters for this frame of reference, when applied by the occupational therapist with children with handwriting problems, include controlling sensory input through selected activities to enhance the integration of sensory systems at the subcortical level (Simon, 1993). By providing various sensory opportunities, the child's nervous system may integrate information more efficiently to produce a satisfactory motor output (e.g., legible letters in a timely manner). All sensory systems, including the proprioceptive, tactile, visual, auditory, olfactory, and gustatory senses, can be tapped within a handwriting intervention program, which is thought to enhance learning. Incorporating a sensory integrative approach into handwriting intervention equates to the use of a variety of sensory experiences, mediums, and instructional materials. Additionally, providing novel and interesting materials for children to practice letter forms may keep students motivated, excited, and challenged; enhancing student success and learning. Children with handwriting difficulties, who have experienced frustration with commonly used paper and pencil drills, may be much more amenable to handwriting instruction using a unique multisensory format.

Writing tools, writing surfaces, and positions for writing are all integral parts of a sensory integrative approach. Examples of writing tools to be used include felt-tip pens (regular, overwriters, changeable-color), crayons (scented, glittered and glow-in-the-dark), paintbrushes, grease pencils or china markers, weighted pens, mechanical pencils, wooden dowels, vibratory pens, and chalk. Lamme and Ayris (1983) examined the effects of five different types of writing tools on handwriting legibility. Results indicated that the type of writing tool did not influence legibility, but the educators involved in the study reported that children's attitudes toward writing were more positive when children were able to use a felt-tip pen rather than a No. 2 pencil. This suggests that children's feelings about writing might improve when they are allowed to use a wide variety of writing tools. Writing with chalk, grease pencils, or a resistive tool also provides additional proprioceptive input to children. This is because working with these tools requires more pressure than working with the traditional medium, paper and pencil. Unconventional writing tools can be easily incorporated into classroom assignments.

Writing surfaces may be in a vertical, a horizontal, or a vertically angled plane. Common vertical surfaces for writing include the chalkboard, painting easels, or classroom assignments attached to the wall or cabinet at eye level. These surfaces, along with desktop easels set at slanted inclines, facilitate a more mature grasp of the writing tool because a child's wrist extension assists with arching of the hand and an open web space between the thumb and fingers (Benbow et. al., 1992). An upright orientation may also decrease directional confusion of early writers when learning letter formations (Hagin, 1983). On the vertical plane, "up" means "up" and "down" means "down," as opposed to working at a desktop, where the direction "up" means away from the body and "down" means toward the body. Furthermore, standing in front of a chalkboard, with the body in full extension and parallel to the writing surface, may promote more internal stability of the trunk, increase the child's arousal, provide more proprioceptive input throughout the arm and shoulder, and allow the hand to move independently or dissociate from the arm (Amundson, 1992).

Handwriting practice on a horizontal surface (e.g., at a table or on a floor) might be performed using plastic freezer bags, partially filled with colored hairstyling gel, and trays filled with sand, dry pudding mix, clay, or a light coat of hand lotion. Writing trays are baking sheets or Styrofoam™ meat-packaging trays that provide children additional tactile and proprioceptive input when forming letters, numbers, and words with isolated fingers or wooden dowels. Other writing activities might occur

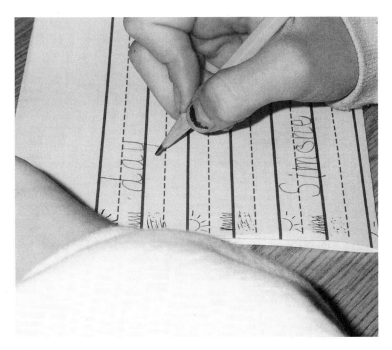

figure 18-7   Lined paper with diagrams help with letter size and placement of text.

table 18-4 *Strategies for Handwriting Problems*

Handwriting Problems	Potential Solutions
Spacing between letters	Use finger spacing with index finger.
	Use fingerprint spacing by pressing on an ink pad before finger spacing.
	Teach the "no touching rule" of letters.
Spacing between words	Use adhesive strips (e.g., Post-it Notes™) as spacers between words.
	Make spaces with a rubber stamp.
	Use a dot or dash (Morse code) between words.
Spacing on paper	Use grid paper.
	Write on every other line of the paper.
	Draw colored lines to mark (e.g., green is left, red is right).
Placing text on lines	Use pictorial schemes on writing guidelines.
	Provide raised writing lines as tactile cues for letter placement.
	Remind students that unevenly placed letters are "popcorn letters."
Sizing letters and words	Use individualized boxes for each letter.
	Call letters with ascending stems, no stems, and descending stems, "birds, skunks, and snakes," respectively.
Near-point copying	Highlight the text on the worksheet to be copied.
	Teach the student to copy two or three letters at a time.
Far-point copying	Enlarge print for better viewing.
	Start with copying from nearby vertical models.
	Position the student to face the chalkboard.
Dictation	Attach an alphabet strip to a desktop for student who cannot remember letter forms.
	Dictated spelling words would contain several but not all letters.
Composition	Be certain that students can form letters from memory.
	Provide magnetic words to write short poems or stories.
Speed	Begin assignments before peers.
	Insure student remembers letter forms.
	Allow for a separate period in the day to finish incomplete written work.

Modified from Amundson, S.J. (1998). *TRICS for written communication: Techniques for rebuilding and improving children's school skills.* Homer, AK: O.T. KIDS, Inc.

on textured wallpaper, nylon netting, finely meshed screen, or indoor-outdoor carpet squares, to again provide proprioceptive input.

Biomechanical

In the truest sense, the biomechanical frame of reference addresses occupational performance in terms of range of motion, strength, and endurance (Dutton, 1993). This discussion, however, focuses on the ergonomic factors of sitting posture, paper position, pencil grasp, writing instruments, and type of paper. Compensatory strategies, including adaptive devices, procedural adaptations, and environmental modifications to improve the interaction and fit between a child's capabilities and the demands of the handwriting task, are presented.

Sitting posture. Although standing and lying prone may be encouraged as alternative writing positions, students continue to spend much of the school day seated at a desk. Therefore the occupational therapist should im-

mediately address the student's seated position in the classroom. While writing, the student should be seated with the feet firmly planted on the floor, providing support for weight shifting and postural adjustments (Benbow, 1992). The table surface should be 2 inches above the flexed elbows when the child is seated in the chair. In this position, the student can experience both symmetry and stability while performing written work. To ensure that students are appropriately seated, the occupational therapy practitioner may recommend adjusting heights of desks and chairs, providing needed foot rests for children, adding seat cushions or inserts, or repositioning a child's desk to face the chalkboard in the classroom.

Paper position. Paper should be slanted on the desktop, so it is parallel to the forearm of the writing hand when the child's forearms are resting on the desk with hands clasped (Levine, 1991). This angle of the paper enables the student to see his or her written work and to avoid smearing his or her writing. Right-handed students may slant the top of their paper approximately 25 to 30 degrees to the left, with the paper just right of the body's midline. Conversely, a slant of 30 to 35 degrees to the right, and paper placement to the left of midline, are needed for students using a left-handed tripod grasp (Alston & Taylor, 1987). For the student with a left-handed, "hooked" pencil grasp lacking lateral wrist movements, slanting the paper to the left (as do right-handed students) is appropriate (Benbow et. al., 1992). The writing instrument should be held below the baseline, and the nonpreferred hand should hold the writing paper.

Pencil grasp. Benbow (1990) defined the ideal grasp as a dynamic tripod with an open web space. With the web space open (forming a circle), the thumb, index and middle fingers make the longest flexion, extension, and rotary excursions with a pencil (Benbow et. al., 1992) during handwriting. Variations of grasps exist with some grips, making handwriting more difficult and less functional (Tseng & Cermak, 1993). Educational team members may consider modifying a student's pencil grasp under the following conditions: (1) handwriting results in muscular tension and fatigue, also known as writer's cramp (Ziviani, 1987); (2) handwriting proficiency, such as letter formation or writing speed, is impeded (Ziviani, 1987); (3) the child's inability to use controlled and precise finger and thumb movements of the pencil stem from a tightly closed web space (Benbow, 1990); and (4) the child holds the pencil with too much pressure or exerts too much pencil-point pressure on the paper, resulting in breaking the pencil lead, making holes in the writing paper, and shaking out the writing hand repeatedly (Herrick & Otto, 1961).

When attempting to modify a grip pattern, characteristics of the child are an important consideration. The occupational therapist should encourage a mature grasp in young writers and recognize that the success in modifying a grasp pattern may be better with younger children (Ziviani, 1987). Once grip positions have been established, they are very difficult to change (Ziviani, 1987; Benbow, 1990). In fact, by the beginning of second grade, changing a child's grasp pattern may be stressful and near impossible (Benbow et. al., 1992). Therefore the educational team needs to consider a child's age, cooperation, and motivation, along with the child's acceptance of the new grip pattern or prosthetic device before attempting to reposition the child's fingers permanently.

A variety of prosthetic devices and therapeutic strategies are available to assist the child in positioning his or her digits for better manipulation of the writing instrument (Amundson, 1998). The occupational therapist should be knowledgeable of hand functions to determine the adaptive devices and techniques most appropriate for each child. Stetro™ grips, triangular pencils, moldable grips, and The Pencil Grip™ may facilitate tripod grasps.

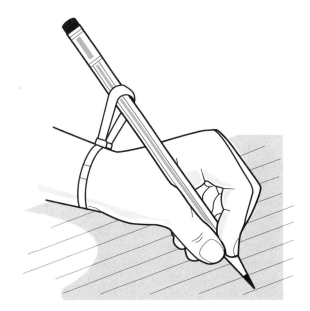

figure 18-8   A rubber band sling allows for a slanted, relaxed pencil position.

Writing muscle tension and fatigue may be reduced for some children by using pencils with wide shafts. To gain increased mobility of the radial digits, children may hold a small eraser against their palms with the ulnar digits, allowing for more dynamic movement of the pencil. For older children with hand hypotonicity, holding the pencil shaft between the web space of the index and middle fingers, with thumb opposition, may give them a viable pencil grasp (Benbow, 1990). To encourage the delicate stability-mobility balance of a functional pencil grasp, the use of external supports (e.g., rubber band pencil slings, ring splints, and neoprene splints) should be used, along with a working knowledge of hand anatomy and kinesiology. A rubber band sling that encourages the student to use a slanted and relaxed pencil position for writing is shown in Figure 18-8.

Writing tools. The type of writing instruments children use in the classroom also warrants consideration. In general, children should be allowed to choose among a variety of writing tools, and parents and teachers should help children to determine which writing utensils are most efficient and comfortable for them. Traditionally, kindergarten and primary classrooms have promoted the use of a wide, primary (or beginner's) pencil for beginning writers. Carlson and Cunningham (1990) examined tool usage among typically developing preschool children performing drawing, tracing, and writing tasks. They found that the readability of their written work was not enhanced by the use of a wider diameter pencil. This study suggests that the pervasive use of the primary pencil is probably not warranted for all kindergarten children because some children perform better with a No. 2 pencil.

Paper. Various types of writing paper are available in the educational setting. Unlined paper and lined paper with a dashed middle guideline between the lower baseline and upper line are both commonly used in the early elementary grades. For the majority of children, most of the research confirms that lined paper improves the legibility of handwriting when compared to the use of unlined paper (Pasternicki, 1987). Children typically start out using paper with wide-spaced (1-inch) guidelines. As handwriting proficiency improves, usually in grade three or four, the child begins using paper with narrow-spaced (⅜-inch) lines (Barchers, 1994). The occupational therapist and educator can allow the student the opportunity to experiment with different-lined, sized, and textured paper to determine which offers the child the best medium for handwriting.

Behavioral

The basic premise of the behavioral frame of reference is that measurable, adaptive behaviors can be learned through interaction with a reinforcing environment (Levy, 1993). In the area of handwriting, this means that a child may produce neatly written text (a measurable and adaptive behavior) when addressing an envelope to his or her residence, knowing that the occupational therapist will later use the envelope to send the child a small "surprise." Receiving a surprise, such as a bookmark, from the therapist is enjoyable and reinforcing for the child.

By sharing the importance of developing readable handwriting with children, and providing them with positive, meaningful, everyday experiences that require them to use their handwriting skills, occupational therapists encourage children's efforts to write more legibly. Simple games at school and home, such as tic-tac-toe, can be played using the newly acquired letter forms, rather than the traditional *X* and *O*. When a child presents a neatly drawn and written (relative to the child's ability) Thanksgiving Day card at home, social reinforcement can be provided by parents. In addition, teachers might reward a child with typically poor handwriting with a special certificate for improved handwriting upon receiving a readable spelling paper or class assignment. By offering children choices, success, responsibility, and encouragement within an intervention program and the natural setting, handwriting may be viewed and practiced by children as a positive functional skill.

Using the behavioral frame of reference, the occupational therapy practitioner may also enhance children's social competence within the framework of a handwriting intervention group. One such group is a handwriting club of 4 to 6 students, who work on improving handwriting, developing social skills, and monitoring their own work and behavior (Amundson, 1998). Poor social performance is common among children with learning disabilities. Behaviors that interfere with social relations include poor eye contact, physical intrusiveness, lack of greeting others, and unawareness of verbal and nonverbal social cues (Williamson, 1994). The service provider may aptly provide group experiences and teach children needed social skills, such as complimenting others, regulating the tone and volume of one's voice, accepting negative feedback, maintaining personal space, and giving and accepting apologies (Williamson, 1993), while involved with the handwriting group.

In a handwriting club, for example, when children are lying prone and practicing letter forms on a chalk mat, each of them can decide the amount of personal space they need to feel comfortable, as well as the amount of writing space required on the mat. The practitioner may introduce both of these space requirements, and he or she may give assistance to the children to aid in this problem-solving process. Another example related to building social skills in a group might occur during an in-hand manipulation preparatory activity, such as in a competitive game of "Kerplunk." While children remove plastic sticks supporting marbles from the game's cylinder, the social skills of taking turns, regulating one's behavioral state during competition, and following the rules of a game can be reinforced by the occupational therapy practitioner.

Other strategies to enhance children's social performance within an intervention group may require a proactive role of the occupational therapist. Giving an overview of the session at the beginning of the period and clearly delineating when activities are beginning and terminating may assist children who have difficulty with transitions between tasks and classes. Developing trust and a sense of cohesiveness among the children might be achieved by having the club or group members decide upon a special name, password, and/or handshake (Williamson, 1994). Finally, the interventionist should establish clear and reasonable rules and consequences, share them with the group members, and consistently and kindly manage the children's behavior. By overlaying the building of children's social skills within the framework of a handwriting intervention group, occupational therapy practitioners assist children in becoming more socially competent with their peers and adults, as well as in becoming more efficient and fluent in their handwriting.

Functional Written Communication

Some children are good candidates for improving their actual manuscript or cursive handwriting through remediation. However, other children are not. Compensatory strategies need to be considered by the occupational therapist and the child's team to allow the child with poor handwriting the greatest opportunity for functional written communication. Alternatives to handwriting include keyboarding, adapting and reducing the amount of written assignments, dictating assignments, and having study buddies to assist with written expression. In school settings, the educational team must de-will be most functional for the child and develop a short-term plan (e.g., learning essential manuscript words) and a long-term plan (e.g., learning word processing).

Service Delivery

Providing occupational therapy services to children with handwriting dysfunction should be based primarily on the needs of the individual child as determined by the educational or clinical team. More and more therapists in school-based practice are using a continuum of service delivery that allows for flexibility, fluidity, and responsiveness to an individual student's needs within the classroom (American Occupational Therapy Association, 1997).

For example, at the beginning of second grade, Tara, a girl with a learning disability, was assessed by the occupational therapist for poor handling of classroom manipulatives (e.g., glue stick, scissors, and computer mouse) and handwriting. After a comprehensive occupational therapy assessment, Tara's parents and the educational team decided to focus on assisting her to become a more proficient writer, with the occupational therapist and regular education teacher spearheading the intervention program.

The therapist and teacher met to develop classroom strategies to be implemented. These strategies included facing Tara's desk directly at the chalkboard, reducing the length of her written assignments, and providing her with an alphabet strip attached to her desktop and placed at the recommended angle of her writing paper (Figure 18-9).

therapist help her with fun exercises to get the entire class "ready to write" before their daily creative writing period. The occupational therapist scheduled a time with the teacher and spent 10 to 15 minutes per week (for 4 weeks) teaching the entire class hand-dexterity games before a classroom writing activity. She also provided the teacher a written handout of the games, so the teacher could ask questions and have a later reference.

Due to the extremely poor legibility of Tara's writing, the team chose to have her join an ongoing handwriting intervention group in the classroom. This group held 25-minute sessions, 2 times a week for 3 consecutive weeks. During this direct service time, the occupational therapist further assessed individual children. She trained the teacher's assistant to coordinate the handwriting group and address some of the individual problems. The occupational therapist returned to the handwriting intervention session once every 2 weeks to supervise the service provider, monitor the children's progress, and modify the programs when needed. A regular consultation time was established with the educator to evaluate Tara's progress in class, to strategize regarding new situations affecting her handwriting performance, and to write a progress note to her parent(s). With the case of Tara, direct service, training of an educational assistant, and consulting with the educator were implemented by the occupational therapist during the first 4 weeks after the initial team meeting. However, the provision of services was not locked into a set schedule, (e.g., two 25-minute sessions per week of direct therapy). Consequently, by

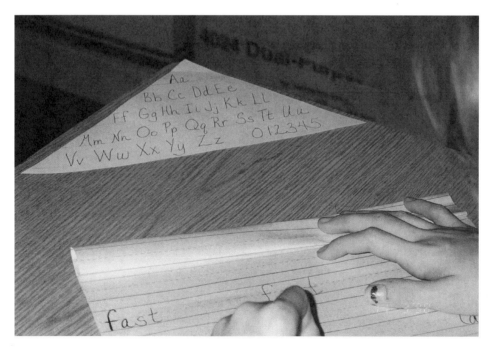

figure18-9   An angled alphabet strip is attached to a student's desktop.

cational needs by initially working with the teacher, by orchestrating an on-going intervention program that another service provider could implement after training, and by continuing regular contact with Tara and the educational team members, including Tara's parents.

Most occupational therapists are comfortable providing one-to-one or small group therapy sessions. However, they are more challenged when working directly with large groups of children, consulting, and training and supervising others to implement programs. Oftentimes, alternative service providers (i.e., educators, educational assistants, volunteers, high school students, and parents) are capable and willing to implement techniques and programs if the occupational therapist assumes responsibility for organizing and monitoring the methods and programs used. To do this, the occupational therapy practitioner must model the role of the service provider during the training, clearly articulate the rationale for the methods and approaches used in the program, and lay out the program in an organized fashion for easy use by the service provider.

By supplying (1) specific written and oral directions of the program; (2) a container, such as a basket, full of materials for the handwriting intervention (e.g., theraband, in-hand manipulation games, sequenced writing lessons, clay trays, and different writing tools); (3) data management sheets; and (4) a system to provide reinforcement and rewards; the program will be more user-friendly for the service provider. A user-friendly program may increase the likelihood that the directions provided by the occupational therapist are followed. If the occupational therapist regularly observes sessions implemented by the service provider, discusses the rationale for using specific methods, reviews the children's progress and the need for program changes, the training can be beneficial for the individual children receiving handwriting intervention. This training can also benefit other children in the classroom who may be struggling with handwriting.

■ SUMMARY

Handwriting is an important academic occupation for children. Children with mild neuromuscular impairments, learning disabilities, and developmental delays are often referred to occupational therapy, with the primary reason for referral being handwriting problems. The role of the occupational therapy practitioner includes evaluating a child's functional performance of prewriting and

also assist the educational or clinical team in determining and planning an integrated approach to promote a functional communication means for the child.

Handwriting intervention programs should be comprehensive, incorporating activities and therapeutic techniques from the neurodevelopmental, acquisitional, sensory integration, biomechanical, and behavioral frames of reference in the child's natural setting. Compensatory strategies should also be employed to provide the child a successful and efficient means for functional written communication.

STUDY QUESTIONS

1. If a 5-year-old girl cannot write her own name, is she ready for a Kindergarten class that learns letters and letter forms throughout the academic year? Give the rationale for your decision.
2. Why is it inappropriate for an occupational therapy practitioner to evaluate a child's in-hand manipulation or visual-perceptual skills as the first step of an occupational therapy assessment focusing on handwriting performance?
3. Identify the frame(s) of reference used and the rationale for its selection, when a child is involved with the following handwriting intervention activity:
   a. Miles is building small clay figurines. He is pressing modeling clay flat on the tabletop, removing tiny pieces of clay with his fingers, and rolling them into small balls within one hand.
   b. Natasha is straddling a bolster while painting letters from the day's instructional lesson with an adapted-handled paintbrush during a tic-tac-toe letter game with Jesse.
4. Jerod is having difficulty with placing cursive letters on the writing line, spacing between words, and using margins properly. Which performance component(s) seem to be interfering with his writing? What are some intervention modifications and techniques to be considered?
5. What would be the advantages of implementing a child's handwriting intervention program within the classroom in a small group setting rather than in a one-to-one "pull out" therapy session?

References

Alston, J. (1983). A legibility index: Can handwriting be measured? *Educational Review, 35*, 237-242.

Alston, J. (1991). Handwriting in the new curriculum. *British Journal of Special Education, 18*, 13-15.

Alston, J., & Taylor, J. (1987). *Handwriting: Theory, research and practice*. London: Croom Helm.

American Occupational Therapy Association. (1997). *Occupational therapy services for children and youth under the Individuals with Disabilities Education Act*. Bethesda, MD: AOTA.

Amundson, S.J. (1992). Handwriting: Evaluation and intervention in school settings. In J. Case-Smith & C. Pehoski (Eds.), *Development of hand skills in the child* (pp. 63-78). Rockville, MD: American Occupational Therapy Association.

Amundson, S.J. (1995). *Evaluation tool of children's handwriting*. Homer, AK: O.T. KIDS, Inc.

Amundson, S.J. (1998). *TRICS for written communication: Techniques for rebuilding and improving children's school skills*. Homer, AK: O.T. KIDS, Inc.

Anderson, P.L. (1983). *Denver Handwriting Analysis*. Novato, CA: Academic Therapy Publications.

Armitage, D., & Ratzlaff, H. (1985). The non-correlation of printing and writing skills. *Journal of Educational Research, 78*, 174-177.

Bailey, C.A. (1988). Handwriting: Ergonomics, assessment and instruction. *British Journal of Special Education, 15*, 65-71.

Barbe, W.B., Milone, M.J., & Wasylyk, T. (1983). Manuscript is the write start. *Academic Therapy, 18*, 397-405.

Barchers, S.I. (1994). *Teaching language arts: An integrated approach*. Minneapolis: West Publishing Company.

Bayley, N. (1993). *Bayley Scales of Infant Development—revised*. San Antonio: Psychological Corp.

Beery, K.E. (1982). *Developmental Test of Visual-Motor Integration*. Cleveland: Modern Curriculum Press.

Beery, K.E. (1992). *Developmental Test of Visual Motor Integration* (4th ed.). Austin: Pro-Ed.

Benbow, M. (1990). *Loops and other groups*. Tucson: Therapy Skill Builders.

Benbow, M., Hanft, B., & Marsh, D. (1992). Handwriting in the classroom: Improving written communication. In C.B. Royeen (Ed.), *AOTA self-study series: Classroom applications for school-based practice* (pp. 1-60). Rockville, MD: American Occupational Therapy Association.

Bergman, K.E., & McLaughlin, T.F. (1988). Remediating handwriting difficulties with learning disabled students: A review. *Journal of Special Education, 12*, 101-120.

Bergmann, K.P. (1990). Incidence of atypical pencil grasps among non-dysfunctional adults. *American Journal of Occupational Therapy, 44*, 736-740.

Berninger, V., Mizokawa, D., & Bragg, R. (1991). Theory-based diagnosis and remediation of writing disabilities. *Journal of School Psychology, 29*, 57-97.

Berninger, V.W., & Rutberg, J. (1992). Relationship of finger function to beginning writing: Application to diagnosis of writing disabilities. *Developmental Medicine and Child Neurology, 34* (3), 198-215.

Bobath, B. (1985). *Abnormal postural reflex activity caused by brain lesions* (3rd ed.). Rockville, MD: Aspen Systems.

Bobath, K., & Bobath, B. (1972). Cerebral palsy. In P.H. Pearson (Ed.), *Physical therapy services in the developmental disabilities* (pp. 31-186). Springfield, IL: Charles Thomas.

Boehme, R. (1988). *Improving upper body control*. Tucson: Therapy Skill Builders.

Campbell, S.K. (1989). Measurement in developmental therapy: Past, present, and future. *Physical and Occupational Therapy in Pediatrics, 9*, 1-14.

Carlson, K., & Cunningham, J. (1990). Effect of pencil diameter on the graphomotor skill of preschoolers. *Early Childhood Research Quarterly, 5*, 279-293.

Cermak, S. (1991). Somatosensory dyspraxia. In A. Fisher, E.A. Murray, & A.C. Bundy (Eds.), *Sensory integration: Theory and practice* (pp. 138-170). Philadelphia: F.A. Davis.

Chandler, B.E. (December, 1994). Keeping occupied at school. *OT Week, 24*.

Chase, C. (1986). Essay test scoring: Interaction of relevant variables. *Journal of Educational Measurement, 23*, 33-41.

Cook, D.G. (1991). The assessment process. In W. Dunn (Ed.), *Pediatric occupational therapy: Facilitating effective service provision* (pp. 35-72). Thorofare, NJ: Slack.

Cornhill, H., & Case-Smith, J. (1996). Factors that relate to good and poor handwriting. *American Journal of Occupational Therapy, 50*, 732-739.

Daniels, L.E. (1988). The diagnosis and remediation of handwriting problems: An analysis. *Physical and Occupational Therapy in Pediatrics, 8*, 61-67.

Donoghue, M. (1975). *The child and the English language arts* (2nd ed.). Dubuque, IA: William C. Brown Co.

Dutton, R. (1993). Biomechanical frame of reference. In H.L. Hopkins & H.D. Smith (Eds.), *Willard and Spackman's occupational therapy* (pp. 66-67). Philadelphia: Lippincott.

Dutton, R. (1993). Neurodevelopmental frame of reference. In H.L. Hopkins & H.D. Smith (Eds.), *Willard and Spackman's occupational therapy* (pp. 73-74). Philadelphia: Lippincott.

Duvall, B. (1985). *Evaluating the difficulty of cursive, manuscript, italic and D'Nealian handwriting* (No. CS 209 484). ERIC Document Reproduction Service No. ED 265 539.

Erhardt, R.P. (1982). *Developmental hand dysfunction: Theory, assessment, treatment*. Tucson: Therapy Skill Builders.

Exner, C.E. (1996). Development of hand functions. In J. Case-Smith, A.S. Allen, & P. Pratt (Eds.), *Occupational therapy for children* (3rd ed.) (pp. 268-306). St. Louis: Mosby.

Exner, C.E. (1992). In-hand manipulation skills. In J. Case-Smith & C. Pehoski (Eds.), *Development of hand skills in the child* (pp. 35-45). Rockville, MD: American Occupational Therapy Association.

Fitts, P.M., & Posner, M.I. (1967). *Human performance*. Belmont, CA: Brooks/Cole.

Gardner, M.F. (1998). *Test of Handwriting Skills*. Hydesville, CA: Psychological and Educational Publications, Inc.

Graham, S. (1992). Issues in handwriting instruction. *Focus on Exceptional Children, 25*, 1-14.

Graham, S., Berninger, V., Abbott, R., Abbott, S., & Whitaker, D. (1997). The role of mechanics in composing of elementary school students: A new methodological approach. *Journal of Educational Psychology, 89*, 170-182.

Graham, S., & Miller, L. (1980). Handwriting research and practice: A unified approach. *Focus on Exceptional Children, 13*, 1-16.

Gubbay, S.S., & deKlerk, N.H. (1995). A study and review of developmental dysgraphia in relation to acquired dysgraphia. *Brain and Development, 17*, 1-8.

Hammill, D.D., Pearson, N.A., & Voress, J.K. (1993). *Developmental Test of Visual Perception, (2nd ed)*. Austin: Pro-Ed.

Hagin, R.A. (1983). Write right or left: A practical approach to handwriting. *Journal of Learning Disabilities, 15*, 266-271.

Hanft, B.E., & Place, P.A. (1996). *The consulting therapist: A guide for OTs and PTs in Schools*. San Antonio: Psychological Corporation.

Hayes, J., & Flower, L. (1986). Writing research and the writer. *American Psychologist, 41*, 1106-1113.

Herrick, J.E., & Otto, W. (1961). Pressure on point and barrel of a writing instrument. *Journal of Experimental Education, 30*, 215-230.

Holm, M. (1986). Frames of reference: Guides for action—occupational therapist. In H.S. Powell (Ed.), *PILOT: Project for Independent Living in Occupational Therapy* (pp. 69-78). Bethesda, MD: American Occupational Therapy Association, Inc.

Jarman, C. (1990). A national curriculum for handwriting. *British Journal of Special Education, 17*, 151-153.

Johnson, D.J., & Carlisle, J.F. (1996). A study of handwriting in written stories of normal and learning disabled children. *Reading and Writing: An Interdisciplinary Journal, 8,* 45-59.

Lamme, L.L. (1979). Handwriting in an early childhood curriculum. *Young Children, 35,* 20-27.

Lamme, L.L., & Ayris, B.M. (1983). Is the handwriting or beginning writers influenced by writing tools? *Journal of Research and Development in Education, 17* (1), 33-38.

Larsen, S.C., & Hammill, D.D. (1989). *Test of legible handwriting.* Austin: Pro-Ed.

Laszlo, J.I., & Bairstow, P.J. (1984). Handwriting: Difficulties and possible solutions. *School Psychology International, 5,* 207-213.

Lee-Corbin, H., & Evans, R. (1996). Factors influencing success or underachievement of the able child. *Early Child Development and Care, 117,* 133-134.

Levine, K.J. (1991). *Fine motor dysfunction: Therapeutic strategies in the classroom.* Tucson: Therapy Skill Builders.

Levine, M. (1994). *Educational care: A system for understanding and helping children with learning problems at home and school.* Cambridge, MA: Educators Publishing Service, Inc.

Levy, L.L. (1993). Behavioral frame of reference. In H.L. Hopkins & H.D. Smith (Eds.), *Willard & Spackman's occupational therapy* (pp. 62-65). Philadelphia: Lippincott.

Lewis, R.B., Graves, A.W., Ashton, T.M., & Kieley, C.L. (1998). Word processing tools for students with learning disabilities: A comparison of strategies to increase text entry speed. *Learning Disabilities Research and Practice, 13,* 95-108.

Llorens, L.A. (1991). Performance tasks and roles throughout the life span. In C. Christiansen & C. Baum (Eds.), *Occupational therapy: Overcoming human performance deficits* (pp. 45-66). Thorofare, NJ: SLACK Incorporated.

MacArthur, A., & Graham, S. (1987). Learning disabled students' composing under three methods of text production: Handwriting, word processing, and dictation. *Journal of Special Education, 21,* 22-42.

Magill, R.A. (1985). *Motor learning concepts and applications.* Dubuque, IA: William C. Brown.

Martlew, M. (1992). Handwriting and spelling: Dyslexic children's abilities compared with children of the same chronological age and younger children of the same spelling level. *British Journal of Educational Psychology, 62,* 375-390.

McAvoy, C. (1996). Making writers. *Closing the Gap Newsletter, 15,* 1, 9.

McHale, K., & Cermak, S. (1992). Fine motor activities in elementary school: Preliminary findings and provisional implications for children with fine motor problems. *American Journal of Occupational Therapy, 46,* 898-903.

Milone, M.N., Jr., & Wasylyk, T.M. (1981). Handwriting in special education. *Teaching Exceptional Children, 14,* 58-61.

Myers, C.A. (1992). Therapeutic fine-motor activities for preschoolers. In J. Case-Smith & C. Pehoski (Eds.), *Development of hand skills in the child* (pp. 47-62). Rockville, MD: American Occupational Therapy Association.

Oliver, C.E. (1989). A sensorimotor program for improving writing readiness skills in elementary-age children. *American Journal of Occupational Therapy, 44,* 111-124.

Pasternicki, J.G. (1987). Paper for writing: Research and recommendations. In J. Alston & J. Taylor (Eds.), *Handwriting: Theory, research and practice* (pp. 68-80). London: Croom Helm.

Phelps, J., & Stempel, L. (1987). *The children's handwriting evaluation scale for manuscript writing.* Dallas: Texas Scottish Rite Hospital for Crippled Children.

Phelps, J., Stempel, L., & Speck, G. (1984). *The Children's Handwriting Evaluation Scale: A new diagnostic tool.* Dallas: Texas Scottish Rite Hospital for Crippled Children.

Reisman, J. (1991). Poor handwriting: Who is referred? *American Journal of Occupational Therapy, 45,* 849-852.

Reisman, J.E. (2000). *Minnesota Handwriting Assessment.* San Antonio: Psychological Corporation.

Rosenbloom, L., & Horton, M.E. (1971). The maturation of fine prehension in young children. *Developmental Medicine and Child Neurology, 13,* 3-8.

Rubin, N., & Henderson, S.E. (1982). Two sides of the same coin: Variations in teaching methods and failure to learn to write. *Special Education: Forward Trends, 9,* 17-24.

Schmidt, R.A. (1982). *Motor control and learning.* Champaign, IL: Human Kinetics.

Schneck, C.M. (1991). Comparison of pencil-grip patterns in first graders with good and poor writing skills. *American Journal of Occupational Therapy, 45,* 701-706.

Schneck, C.M., & Henderson, A. (1990). Descriptive analysis of the developmental progression of grip position for pencil and crayon control in nondysfunctional children. *American Journal of Occupational Therapy, 44,* 893-900.

Simon, C.J. (1993). Sensory integration frame of reference. In H.L. Hopkins & H.D. Smith (Eds.), *Willard & Spackman's occupational therapy* (pp. 74-75). Philadelphia: Lippincott.

Stott, D.H., Moyes, F.A., & Henderson, S.E. (1984). *Diagnosis and remediation of handwriting problems.* Burlington, ON: Hayes.

Sweedler-Brown, C.O. (1992). The effects of training on the appearance bias of holistic essay graders. *Journal of Research and Development in Education, 26,* 24-88.

Swinth, Y., & Anson, D. (1998). Alternatives to handwriting: Keyboarding and text-generation techniques for schools. In J. Case-Smith (Ed.), *AOTA self-study series: Making a difference in school system practice.* Bethesda, MD: American Occupational Therapy Association.

Tan-Lin, A.S. (1981). An investigation into the developmental course of preschool/kindergarten aged children's handwriting behavior. *Dissertation Abstracts International, 42,* 4287A.

Taylor, J. (1985). The sequence and structure of handwriting competence: Where are the breakdown points in the mastery of handwriting? *British Journal of Occupational Therapy, 48,* 205-207.

Thurber, D. (1983). *D'Nealian manuscript—An aide to reading development.* (No. Report No. CS 007 057). ERIC Document Reproduction Service No. ED 227 474.

Tseng, M.H., & Cermak, S.A. (1993). The influence of ergonomic factors and perceptual-motor abilities on handwriting performance. *American Journal of Occupational Therapy, 47,* 919-926.

Weil, M., & Amundson, S.J. (1994). Relationship between visual motor and handwriting skills of children in kindergarten. *American Journal of Occupational Therapy, 48,* 982-988.

Weintraub, N., & Graham, S. (1998). Writing legibly and quickly: A study of children's ability to adjust their handwriting to meet classroom demands. *Learning Disabilities Research and Practice, 13,* 146-152.

Williamson, G.G. (1993). Enhancing the social competence of children with learning disabilities. *American Occupational Therapy Association Sensory Integration Special Interest Section Newsletter, 16* (1), 1-2.

Williamson, G.G. (1994). *No one to play with: Helping kids be kids.* Handout from Maternal and Child Health Lectureship, Seattle:

Wright, J.P., & Allen, E.G. (1975). Ready to write! *Elementary School Journal, 75,* 430-435.

Ziviani, J. (1987). Pencil grasp and manipulation. In J. Alston & J. Taylor (Eds.), *Handwriting: Theory, research and practice* (pp. 24-39). London: Croom Helm.

Ziviani, J., & Elkins, J. (1986). Effect of pencil grip on handwriting speed and legibility. *Educational Review, 38,* 247-257.

Handwriting Instruments

Children's handwriting evaluation scale for manuscript writing (CHES-M)

Description:	Norm-referenced test that examines rate and quality of children's handwriting within a near-point copying task. Children's handwriting in grades one and two are examined qualitatively by letter forms, spacing, rhythm, and general appearance.
Authors:	Joanne Phelps and Lynn Stempel (1987)
Publication Information:	CHES 6031 St. Andrews Dallas, TX 75205

Children's handwriting evaluation scale (CHES-C)

Description:	Norm-referenced tool that assesses cursive writing of children in grades three through eight. Task consists of near-point copying of short paragraphs. Similar features of *CHES-M*.
Authors:	Joanne Phelps, Lynn Stempel, & Gail Speck (1984)
Publication Information:	CHES 6031 St. Andrews Dallas, TX 75205

Denver handwriting analysis

Description:	Criterion-referenced tool evaluating cursive handwriting of students in grades three through eight. Each of the following tasks has a time limit per grade: near-point copying, writing the alphabet from memory, far-point copying, manuscript-cursive transition, and dictation.
Author:	Peggy L. Anderson (1983)
Publication Information:	Academic Therapy Publications 20 Commercial Boulevard Novato, CA 94947-6191

Diagnosis and remediation of handwriting problems

Description:	Criterion-referenced test with detailed instructions and scoring criteria that requires child to generate a fable, guided by a series of 3 pictures. No age range is given, except children must have had at least 2 years of manuscript or cursive writing.
Authors:	Denis Stott, Fred Moyes, and Sheila Henderson (1985)
Publication Information:	DRAKE Educational Associates St. Fagans Road Fairwater, Cardiff CF5-3AE WALES

Evaluation tool of children's handwriting (ETCH)

Description:	Criterion-referenced test measuring a child's legibility and speed of children's handwriting in grades one through six. Domains (manuscript or cursive) include alphabet writing of lower- and upper-case letters, numeral writing, near-point copying, far-point copying, manuscript-to-cursive transition, dictation, and sentence composition.
Author:	Susan J. Amundson, MS, OTR/L (1995)
Publication Information:	O.T. KIDS, Inc. PO Box 1118 Homer, AK 99603

Minnesota handwriting assessment

Description: Norm-referenced test that looks at quality and speed of manuscript handwriting of a near-point copying task. Models are in Zaner-Bloser or D'Nealian script for children in grades one and two.

Author: Judith Reisman, PhD, OTR (1995)

Publication Information: Therapy Skill Builders
PO Box 839954
San Antonio, TX 78283
800-211-8378

Test of handwriting skills

Description: Norm-referenced test that examines both manuscript and cursive handwriting through dictation, near-point copying, and alphabet writing from memory. Normative data is provided for children 5 through 11 years old.

Author: Morrison F. Gardner (1998)

Publication Information: Psychological and Educational Publications, Inc.
PO Box 520
Hydesville, CA 95547-0520

Handwriting Curricula in Schools

D'Nealian handwriting program

Target: Manuscript, cursive
Author: Scott Foresman Co.
Vendor: Addison Wesley Longsman
Division of Scott Foresman Addison Wesley
1 Jacob Way
Reading, MA 01867
800-554-4411

Italic handwriting series

Target: Manuscript, connected script
Authors: B. Getty & I. Dubay
Vendor: Portland State University
Continuing Education Press
PO Box 1394
Portland, OR 97207-1394
800-547-8887, ext. 4891

Palmer method handwriting

Target: Manuscript, cursive
Author: McGraw-Hill
Vendor: McGraw-Hill
220 E. Danieldale Road
DeSoto, TX 75115
800-442-9685

Zaner-Blöser handwriting

Target: Manuscript, cursive
Author: Zaner-Blöser
Vendor: Zaner-Blöser
PO Box 16764
Columbus, OH 43216-6764
800-421-3018

Handwriting Intervention Programs

Callirobics

Description: A program that sets paper and pencil exercises to children's songs as preparation for manuscript and cursive handwriting. Program cassette tapes accompany the student's workbook and can be implemented either individually or in groups.

Author: Liori Laufer

Vendor: Therapro, Inc.
225 Arlington St.
Framingham, MA 01702
800-257-5376 or 508-872-9494

Big strokes for little folks

Description: A developmental training program designed for children who already recognize most letters but have difficulty forming them. Its target group is children ages 5 through 9 for spontaneous, legible manuscript writing.

Author: B. Levine Rubell

Vendor: Therapy Skill Builders
PO Box 839954
San Antonio, TX 78283
800-211-8378

Handwriting without tears

Description: A comprehensive set of manuals addressing general handwriting remediation in *Handwriting Without Tears*, manuscript writing instruction in *Printing Power* and *My Printing Book*, and cursive writing in *Cursive Handwriting*. Visual and verbal cues accompany lessons, and word and sentence writing is encouraged throughout each program.

Author: Janet Z. Olsen, OTR

Vender: Handwriting Without Tears
8802 Quiet Stream Court
Potomac, MD 90854
301-983-8409

Loops and other groups: a kinesthetic writing system

Description: This system was developed to enable second-grade children to learn the formations of all cursive lower-case letters in 6 weeks. Students learn 4 "families" of letters that share common movement patterns. Children visualize and verbalize the movement patterns while experiencing the "feel" of the letter.

Author: Mary Benbow, MS, OTR

Vendor: Therapy Skill Builders
PO Box 849954
San Antonio, TX 78283
800-211-8378

TRICS for written communication: techniques for rebuilding and improving children's school skills

Description: This resource manual provides over 400 remedial and compensatory strategies for improving students' text production in the classroom. The focus is on students who experience mechanical and organizational difficulty during writing.

Author: Susan J. Amundson, MS, OTR/L

Vendor: O.T. KIDS, Inc.
PO Box 1118
Homer, AK 99603
907-235-0688

chapter 19

Assistive Technology: Computers and Augmentative Communication

Yvonne Swinth

■ CHAPTER OBJECTIVES

1. Describe the purpose and uses of assistive technology (AT) for children with disabilities.
2. Discuss guiding theories for AT service delivery.
3. Discuss and describe the legislation related to AT service delivery.
4. Discuss how teaming, sociocultural issues, funding, and different settings influence AT service delivery.
5. Discuss an occupational therapy process in AT service delivery.
6. Describe the roles of the occupational therapist in AT service delivery.
7. Describe different input and output methods and considerations for computer use for children with disabilities.
8. Describe different considerations for augmentative communication for children with disabilities.
9. Apply knowledge about computer use and alternative and augmentative communication (AAC) to children with disabilities.

The use of assistive technology (AT) has been an important tool since the origins of the occupational therapy profession. For years, therapists have used different types of low-tech devices, such as reachers, button hooks, pencil grips, and other pieces of adaptive equipment, to promote the functional independence of their clients. However, over the past 10 to 15 years, with the technologic advances in society, occupational therapists have increasingly used a wide range of electronic devices, from simple switches to complex robotics, to promote the functional independence of their clients. Additionally, Congress has enacted legislation supporting the procurement and use of AT for individuals with disabilities. This expansion in the use of AT opens new doors, creates opportunities, and enables individuals with disabilities to realize functional goals that were previously unattainable.

The Technology-Related Assistance for Individuals with Disabilities Act of 1988 (known as the *Tech Act;* Public Law 100-407) defines *assistive technology* as "any item, piece of equipment or product system whether acquired commercially off the shelf, modified, or customized that is used to increase or improve functional capabilities of individuals with disabilities." This is the same definition used in the Individuals with Disabilities Education Act (IDEA; Public Law 101-476), the federal legislation mandating services for students with disabilities in public schools. This definition includes low-tech adaptations, such as reachers and pencil grips, and high-tech devices, such as adaptive switches, *adapted computers,* electric wheelchairs, augmentative communication devices, and environmental controls. Technology service delivery is categorized as assistive technologies, rehabilitative technologies, and learning technologies. *Assistive technologies* refers to technologies that are permanently used to compensate for a loss of skill. *Rehabilitative technologies* are used to remediate or restore function (e.g., cognitive retraining and crutches). *Learning technologies* are used to remediate or restore academic abilities (e.g., typing tutors and word banks). In this chapter, *assistive technology* is used as a broad term that includes all three concepts.

This chapter discusses general information regarding the use of AT with children, followed by specific examples on the use of computers and augmentative communication devices with children with disabilities. Other chapters in this text specifically address the other areas of AT (see Chapters 16 and 20). Many of the principles and decision-making strategies discussed in this chapter can be generalized to all areas of AT.

■ USE OF ASSISTIVE TECHNOLOGY WITH CHILDREN

Children as young as 6 months of age can learn to use simple AT devices (Swinth, Anson, & Deitz, 1993). For children with disabilities, introducing the appropriate types of technology systems as early as possible may enable the child to participate in important learning situations that otherwise, because of his or her disabilities, may not be possible. For over 10 years, researchers and clinicians have documented and discussed the unique opportunities that all types of AT offer for teaching and for advancing the life choices of children with disabilities (Behrmann, 1984; Behrmann, Jones, & Wilds, 1989; Dickey & Shealey, 1987; Douglas, Reeson, & Ryan, 1988; Foulds, 1982; Lahm, 1989; Swinth, 1998). Many types of technology are available for children with disabilities, particularly those with limited motor control. The literature suggests that integration of AT in the lives of these children allows for increased productivity and independence in the occupational performance areas of activities of daily living (ADLs), school and work, and play and leisure (Bain & Leger, 1997; Parette & VanBiervliet, 1990; Smith, 1991; Swinth, 1998; Todis & Walker, 1993). Young children with disabilities may be able to learn basic contingencies, cause-effect, discrimination, turn taking, and mobility and communication skills through the use of AT devices. All of these skills are foundational for higher-level conceptual learning. As these children grow, they can continue to use technology to develop independence in many ADLs, complete written assignments in school, develop prevocational and vocational skills, and play games or participate in leisure ac-

tivities. The use of AT can create exciting opportunities for children with special needs to explore, interact, and function in their environments.

Since technology is constantly changing, this chapter presents problem-solving strategies, principles, and frameworks for decision-making versus in-depth descriptions of specific devices or systems. Specific devices are used as examples; however, the reader is encouraged to focus on the principles versus the device itself. The frameworks and guides for decision making that are presented should not be viewed as limiting strategies. Rather, they are meant to be a starting point. Each practitioner needs to adjust the concepts given the individual needs of the client and family, teaming issues, availability of resources, and many other factors unique to each situation.

■ GUIDING THEORIES FOR DECISION MAKING

The occupational therapy practitioner must consider many factors when embarking on the AT decision-making journey. During the decision-making process, procurement, use of the AT device, and follow-up, an effective occupational therapy practitioner will consider the intrapersonal and interpersonal systems that may be acting on the client. An alarming amount of literature documents the high rate of abandonment of AT devices, even viable devices (Batavia & Hammer, 1990; Bushrow & Turner, 1994; Garber & Gregorio, 1990; Scherer & McKee, 1989; Swinth, 1997). Approximately one third of the AT devices purchased or prescribed are abandoned by the user within 2 years. This may be because the individual no longer needs the device or because something better has become available. However, too often, it appears that the high rate of abandonment is due to factors such as a mismatch between the user and the technology, complexity of the device, ineffectiveness of the device, lack of proper training on the use of the device, device failure, and amount of user input into the procurement of the device (Batavia & Hammer, 1990; Brooks & Hoyer, 1989; Bushrow & Turner, 1994; Phillips & Zhao, 1993; Scherer & McKee, 1989). By the time children with disabilities reach 21 years of age, they often have had experiences with many different types of AT devices. Given these factors, good AT decision making is crucial for the therapist to prevent device abandonment and to promote successful procurement and long-term use of AT devices by children with disabilities and their families.

The therapist must begin effective decision making by viewing the child and his or her family as a system. Throughout the process, the occupational therapist considers the child, family, environments in which the child participates, and the child's occupations (Dunn, Brown, & McGuigan, 1994; Law et. al., 1996). These person-occupation-environment models emphasize the importance of the temporal, physical, social, and cultural contexts; importance of client choice; and interactions among the child, context, tasks, performance, and therapeutic intervention (see Chapter 3).

Learned Helplessness and Self-Determination

Children with disabilities, physical or cognitive, can become passive and unmotivated because of a lack of learning opportunities and/or a lack of independent control over their environment. This can result in lack of interest or skills to interact with the environment (Douglas, Reeson, & Ryan, 1988). When children learn that they have little control over outcomes within their environments, the phenomenon of learned helplessness can result. *Learned helplessness* is a secondary disability and is the belief that one cannot exert personal control over outcomes experienced when interacting with the environment (Abramson, Seligman, & Teasdale, 1978; Gargiulo & O'Sullivan, 1986; Maier & Seligman, 1976; Weisz, 1979). Children with learned helplessness exhibit low self-esteem, directly affecting how they interact and perform functional skills. They usually demonstrate a lack of initiation and an inability to cope with the events around them. Additionally, when opportunities for integrating basic cognitive and perceptual skills are missed in early childhood, these children do not develop a foundation for learning higher-level concepts. Strategies and adaptations that allow these children the maximum amount of independence possible as early as possible decrease the chance for them to learn that they have no control over their environment.

The opposite of learned helplessness is self-determination. *Self-determination* is defined as "acting as the primary causal agent in one's life and making choices and decisions regarding one's quality of life free from undue external influence or interference" (Wehmeyer, 1996, p. 24). Self-determination is an umbrella term that encompasses several common concepts used when describing children's personal, social, and skill development. These concepts include self-efficacy (outcome and efficacy expectations), self esteem, and self-advocacy. *Efficacy expectations* are personal beliefs regarding one's capability to realize a desired behavior in a specific context (judgment of what one can do with the skills one has). *Outcome expectations* are personal beliefs about whether a particular behavior will lead to a particular consequence (being able to determine if one's goals are realistic). *Self-esteem* is the belief that one has in oneself and/or self-respect. *Self-advocacy* refers to an individual being able to speak for himself or herself, make decisions for himself or herself, and know what his or her rights are, particularly when those rights have been violated or diminished. He or she is able to take ownership of his or her needs rather than expect someone else to take responsibility for them

because he or she has a disability (Swinth, 1997; Wehmeyer, 1996). Appreciating and being able to function with a sense of interdependence also is a crucial part of self-determination.

Self-determination is a set of skills that can be taught and learned. Key characteristics and components include autonomy, self-awareness, choice making (often children with disabilities are not given the opportunities to make effective choices), decision making, problem solving, goal setting and attainment, internal locus of control, positive attributions of efficacy and outcome expectations, and self-knowledge (Wehmeyer, 1996). Often in schools and other community settings, children with disabilities have few opportunities to learn the skills needed to acquire these component elements of self-determination and limited access to experiences in which to apply the skills of self-determination.

With the increased emphasis on transition services and preparing children for life skills beyond school, occupational therapists should promote the development of self-determination for children of any age. This includes ensuring that services develop skills of interdependence and independence rather than dependence, addressing the participation and productivity of children, recognizing that self-determination can mean different things to different people, and recognizing that self-determination is a quality-of-life issue that can be addressed across settings, environments, and opportunities. AT devices, such as computers and augmentative communication devices, can help with the development, practice, and effective use of self-determining behaviors for children with disabilities.

Theories and Practice Models

The occupational therapist also uses theories and practice models to guide recommendations for procurement, implementation, and follow-up of AT intervention. Those theories and practice models most relevant to AT intervention include developmental theory and biomechanical, rehabilitation, acquisitional, and psychosocial frames of reference.

Developmental theory

The developmental perspective forms a foundational knowledge that is important to all pediatric occupational therapists. The therapist must maintain a developmental perspective when working with AT and children, especially young children, just as in any other area of pediatric practice. The child must acquire basic foundational skills before he or she can effectively use certain devices. Additionally, with some types of technology, a specific linear progression of learning and skill acquisition, both motorically and cognitively, must occur before the child can succeed with the device.

For technology to elicit an adaptive response, it must match the developmental skills of the child. For example, a child with spastic quadriparesis who requires complex adaptations to access a computer system may have the motor skills needed to access the system but may not have the cognitive skills needed to independently use the system. Introducing the complex system before the development of appropriate skills can be frustrating for both the child and family, and it may discourage future use of AT devices. Technology can also help compensate for developmental skills that a child may never obtain.

Acquisitional frame of reference

When the team decides that the child is developmentally ready to learn AT, they can apply the acquisitional frame of reference. This practice model focuses on the acquisition, or learning, of specific skills required for the optimal performance within the environment (Royeen & Duncan, 1999). The child improves his or her motor, sensory, cognitive, and psychosocial skills through practice, repetition, feedback, and reinforcement. The acquisitional frame of reference is commonly used during AT intervention. AT devices are provided when a child has significant motor or cognitive deficits that prevent him or her from performing a skill without the use of adaptations. Often the motor and/or cognitive delays prevent the child from reaching developmental milestones. Using the acquisitional frame of reference focuses on providing activities to help the child acquire specific skills both within and outside the typical developmental sequence. For example, a 14 year old with cognitive delays may be taught how to enter numbers into a computer, using a predetermined format, from a piece of paper. Once the student has developed proficiency in this task, he or she begins to work in the school's front office entering attendance data into the computer. Eventually, he or she transitions into a community job entering data for a plumbing company. However, he or she may never understand the meaning of the numbers because of cognitive delays.

Biomechanical frame of reference

The biomechanical frame of reference addresses the musculoskeletal or neuromuscular needs of a child. If a child has musculoskeletal or neuromuscular dysfunction, then he or she may have difficulty maintaining postural alignment independently. Poor postural alignment affects the child's ability to access and use most AT devices effectively and efficiently. Depending on the age of the child, the therapist may need to work on postural control before introducing a device. The therapist may need to provide external supports when the child's posture is unstable. For example, lateral supports, an H-strap, and shoulder protractors added to a wheelchair may help a child with spastic quadriparesis demonstrate improved arm control to independently access an expanded computer keyboard. When the child uses a voice recognition system, postural control is important for the child to maintain adequate voice quality. Using biomechanical principles, the therapist may also recommend or use dif-

ferent positions (e.g., standing versus sitting) to help enhance efficient AT use.

Rehabilitation frame of reference

The rehabilitation frame of reference capitalizes on a child's residual abilities as a means for compensating for a loss of skill/ability. Using this frame of reference, children adapt to their limitations by learning new methods for completing tasks. AT helps children compensate for the loss of skill. For example, a child who has had a head injury and has motor and organizational difficulties may use a computer with an adapted keyboard to complete written work at school. The computer also may be equipped with special software programs that will help the student organize his or her thoughts so that he or she can successfully write a paper.

Psychosocial frame of reference

"The theoretical base for the psychosocial frame of reference is derived from the developmental theories related to temperament, attachment, peer interactive skills, play, ability to cope, and environmental interaction" (Olson, 1999 p. 323). When working with AT, the occupational therapist must consider the psychosocial implications of the choices being made. For example, school-age children may refuse to use certain computer access systems because the system makes them look "different." The psychosocial implications of AT use become increasingly important as children mature. What children will tolerate at younger ages often becomes taboo when they reach adolescence. AT can also enable the child to successfully master his or her environment in all the performance areas. Through application of AT, the child becomes more independent and competent, which positively affects his or her motivation, initiative, self-esteem, and self-identity. For some children and their families, even though an AT device may mean increased independence and freedom, they dismiss AT device use because of how it makes them feel or because of a comment of a peer (Swinth, 1997). The therapist must consider the effect that the AT device may have on the entire family system. A complex augmentative communication system can require hours of programming by a family member as the child's communication needs and skills change. This author has worked with several families in which one parent has quit his or her job to handle the complex issues of a child's AT devices.

In most cases, therapists blend theories and practice models when designing AT intervention. For example, the therapist may use developmental and psychosocial theories when choosing an activity. The therapist uses the biomechanical frame of reference to position the child and equipment and uses the acquisitional frame of reference to develop strategies for teaching the child how to use the AT system. The therapist uses other practice models, experience, professional judgment, and the resources of other professionals to make recommendations regarding the use of AT devices.

■ BACKGROUND FOR UNDERSTANDING THE USE OF TECHNOLOGY WITH CHILDREN

Related Legislation

Since the 1970s the United States Congress has passed several legislative acts that have directly affected the availability and use of AT for individuals with disabilities. The Rehabilitation Act, which was first introduced in 1973 and then rewritten in 1986 (Public Law 99-506), supports the use of AT for individuals with disabilities to (1) have greater control over their lives; (2) participate in home, school, and work environments; (3) interact with peers who do not have disabilities; and (4) otherwise do acts taken for granted by individuals without any known disability. The enactment of the Education for All Handicapped Children Act of 1975 (Public Law 94-142) provided support for designing, adapting, and using technology in the education of students with disabilities. This act encouraged private and public sectors to market new AT and provided incentives for the dissemination of information regarding AT.

In 1990, Congress amended the Education for All Handicapped Children Act and renamed it the Individuals with Disabilities Education Act (IDEA). These amendments call for the provision of AT devices and services as required to provide an appropriate public education for children with disabilities. The law defines *assistive technology device* as any item, equipment, and system used "to increase, maintain, or improve functional capabilities of individuals with disabilities." AT services include any service that directly assists a child with a disability in the selection, procurement, and use of any AT device. Other AT services provided under the law are coordinating and using therapies, training, or technical assistance for individuals with disabilities.

The 1997 amendments to IDEA (Public Law 105-17) continue to emphasize the use of AT and AT services to enable the success of students with disabilities in their educational and school-to-career programs. These legislative acts have improved the access to and use of AT services by children with disabilities. They have also brought new options for therapeutic interventions when working with children with disabilities and their families.

Through the Tech Act (Public Law 100-407), states have established resource centers and information systems for consumers of AT. These information systems offer consumers and their families technical assistance regarding obtaining and maintaining AT. In certain states the Tech Act has supported training for consumers; other states have established central directories to facilitate access to AT. The goals of this legislation are to foster interagency cooperation, develop flexible and effective funding strategies, and promote access to AT for individuals with disabilities throughout their life spans.

Teaming

As with many other specialty areas in pediatrics, the successful implementation of AT requires a cohesive and effective team that emphasizes shared vision and ownership. *Teaming* is critical whether the team provides services in the home, clinic, or school setting. The team's input is critical in making decisions regarding AT because devices are used across the child's environments and address multiple performance goals that cross professional boundaries. Decisions based on the input of the entire team and the family are most likely to meet the multifaceted needs of the child.

The specific members of the team may be different in various situations depending on the type of device that they are introducing to the child, the expertise of the individuals involved, and the specific setting. For example, in a clinical setting, the team may include the child and family, occupational therapist, physical therapist, speech-language pathologist, doctor, nurse, rehabilitation engineer, and social worker. In a school setting, the team may include the child and family, occupational therapist, physical therapist, speech-language pathologist, educator, administrator, and psychologist. Table 19-1 illustrates the roles of some AT team members in different settings.

Often the introduction of an AT device, especially a complex device, can change the focus of a child's program. The therapist may need to spend time on training and practice within the child's educational program and at home as the family and professionals make efforts to integrate use of the device into the child's everyday activities. Thus the development of skills needed to use the device often becomes the focus of intervention. Involvement by every member of the team encourages skill generalization in various settings and situations as the child becomes increasingly proficient using the new AT device. The team's agenda may shift when the child learns a new AT system. Team input also is important to ensure that the AT device will not interfere with other priorities within the child's program. For example, if the use of an adaptive keyboard for writing limits a student's ability to complete a composition assignment, the teacher may select an alternate means for the student's completion of the assignment.

The child (if appropriate) and the family are considered members of the team in all forms of service delivery. When the team working with a child begins to consider implementing AT, they must include the family in discussion and problem-solving sessions as early as possible. The family's financial resources, time, interests, and priorities can determine the success or failure of a particular AT device (Swinth, 1997). Depending on the family's resources, the procurement of an AT system can mean de-

table 19-1 *Roles and Tasks of Some Common Assistive Technology Team Members**

Team Member	Setting	Examples of Roles in Assistive Technology (AT)
Parent or older child	Clinic or school	Communicates and advocates for needs and preferences; provides follow-through at home
Occupational therapist	Clinic or school	Assesses functional needs in daily living, physical, and environmental needs; adapts and positions adaptive control systems; trains clients in use of equipment
Physical therapist	Clinic or school	Assesses mobility, seating, and positioning as it relates to the use of AT devices
Speech or language pathologist	Clinic or school	Assesses receptive and expressive needs and abilities; determines appropriate symbol systems, techniques, and strategies; manages communication interventions
Funding specialist or social worker	Clinic	Secures funding for devices
Physician or nurse	Clinic	Manages medical needs
Rehabilitation engineer	Clinic	Designs, constructs, fits, and customizes devices and systems
Administrator	School	May become responsible to commit to district funding of systems
Special educator	School	Teaches academic and vocational skills; matches software programs with curriculum requirements
Psychologist	School	May serve as team leader; is responsible for eligibility criteria

*This is not meant to be an inclusive list of team members for any setting, nor is it meant to be set criteria for any team member's role. Often these roles overlap depending on the child's need, the service delivery systems, and the individual professionals.
Modified from Beukelman, D.R., & Mirenda, P. (1992). *Augmentative and alternative communication: Management of severe communication disorders in children and adults.* Baltimore: Brookes.
Church, G., & Glennen, S. (1992). Assistive technology programs. In G. Church & S. Glennen (Eds.), *The handbook of assistive technology* (pp. 1-26). San Diego: Singular Publishing Group.

ciding between a family vacation or the possibility of the child communicating vocally. Additionally, for some families, AT can be confusing and overwhelming. The team can eliminate this obstacle by educating the family on the uses of AT and explaining the rationale for using it with the child. The parents' acknowledgment that their child must use AT devices can increase grief because it serves as a visual reminder that their child is not like other children. Explaining that AT facilitates the development of skills and compensates for the disability allows the family to view the use of AT positively.

Setting

The structure of an AT service delivery program is influenced by the services that team members provide, type of facility, funding sources, and sometimes particular disabilities specified in the agency's mission statement. Beukelman and Mirenda (1992) identified three categories of programs for children who need AT: medical centers, regional centers, and public schools. Occupational therapists are employed in all of these settings.

Hospital or medical center

Some AT teams are based in hospitals that primarily serve children. A majority of these AT teams function in predominately an assessment role. The children may come in on an outpatient basis for a series of assessments by the AT team. The assessments may be completed in one or two visits, or they may require an inpatient stay of 2 to 3 weeks. Referrals and recommendations for specific equipment may be made to other agencies or third-party payers. After the initial assessment, team members often have limited access to the child for follow-up and training and they have limited opportunities to consult with the teachers and parents (Beukelman & Mirenda, 1992). Some AT teams in hospital settings also provide direct treatment to children with disabilities, especially for children under the age of 3 or children who have an acquired disability (e.g., a spinal cord injury).

Regional center

As a result of the Tech Act, many states have developed regional AT centers. In addition, some states have technology centers funded by the Department of Education and/or the Council for Exceptional Children. Many of these regional centers have AT lending libraries. The child, the child's school, or the professionals working with the child in the community can borrow equipment on a short-term basis. The teams working at these centers have broad-based experience with various diagnoses, resources for obtaining equipment, types of AT, and adapted methods of AT use. Many of these centers are also involved in AT advocacy, consumer awareness, focus groups, and many other activities related to efficient and effective use of AT by individuals with disabilities. Regional centers, like hospitals, often have limited follow-up care once the child has received the devices and may have minimal input into training the child, family, and educational team to use the device (Beukelman & Mirenda, 1992).

Public school

Schools are becoming the most widely used setting for providing AT services for children (Beukelman & Mirenda, 1992; RESNA, 1992). The demand for school occupational therapists to evaluate AT needs and help students learn to use AT has become a common feature of school-based practice. The large-scale growth of AT services in the school environment is part of the evolution of special education practices after the enactment of federally mandated programs and the general increase in availability of AT in schools. In school, daily problem solving related to equipment use can occur and the child can receive support in using the device in the setting in which its use is most natural and important. Children are expected to attend school every day. Thus when the entire team supports AT systems and services, practice and training in using the AT device can occur on a daily basis. Although the school-based team members have easy access to the child and the best understanding of the educational curriculum, they do not always have expertise or experience in AT. For this reason, collaboration among the school-based team and the regional and/or hospital AT teams is important.

Funding

When working in the area of AT use with children, occupational therapists are often involved in helping procure the appropriate devices, software programs, and/or adaptive peripherals. Funding can come from various sources, including Medicaid, grants, insurance, nonprofit agencies such as United Cerebral Palsy, private foundations, schools, and individual payment. In some states, funds are available through the Department of Developmental Disabilities, Department of Health, or the Department of Social Services to help purchase AT devices. As students enter high school and begin the transition to work and career sites, the state's vocational rehabilitation agency also may consider assisting with the funding of devices. Occupational therapists must consider the complexity of the funding process. No matter what the funding source, the documentation must be complete and in proper order if a system is to be funded.

Funding of AT in school districts often raises unique issues. The team often designates the occupational therapists working in schools to address specific AT or software needs of students with disabilities (e.g., a software program to teach typing or the purchase of a complex access system). The school district is the payer of last resort, but it is ultimately responsible for AT devices that the

child needs to learn in the school environment (Swinth & Anson, 1998). Public or private insurance can be applied to the provision of a student's AT devices and services when they are determined to be medically necessary (Silbert, 1997). School districts can also work with community service organizations or associations (e.g., the Muscular Dystrophy Association) to purchase AT devices or pay for services. Occupational therapists should learn about the different funding options available within their state and region to contribute to the team's effort to obtain funding for the AT device that is believed to best support the child's function.

Universal access has become an important concept that guides school and clinic purchase of new technology particularly new computer systems. Most schools and clinics have established guidelines for ensuring universal access as they update and expand their computer systems. When all children, including those with disabilities, have equal access to AT devices, costly modifications for individuals can be avoided. Often the complexity of AT is not considered when general technology is purchased, which can result in computers that do not have enough memory to support some of the software programs or adaptive peripherals needed by children with disabilities. Occupational therapists should become members of the planning team for the purchase of a computer system in a clinic or school setting by being proactive and working as consultants to the technology department.

Sociocultural Factors

Sociocultural issues also may affect the procurement, implementation, and use of an AT system. Several authors have emphasized the various cultural influences on performance (Cook & Hussey, 1995; Krefting & Krefting, 1991). Box 19-1 summarizes some examples of sociocultural factors that the therapist may need to consider when evaluating, designing, and selecting AT systems for children. Some cultures do not value the independence that AT provides individuals with disabilities, or an AT device may be abandoned if it replaces an important life function of another family member. For example, the grandmother who views communicating for a child with cerebral palsy as one of her roles may resist the use of an augmentative communication system by that child.

■ OCCUPATIONAL THERAPY PROCESS AND ASSISTIVE TECHNOLOGY

When working with AT, the occupational therapist keeps in mind the theoretic frameworks of occupational therapy and the aforementioned background information throughout the occupational therapy process. As in all areas of practice, the occupational therapy process involves evaluation, collaborative decision making, inter-

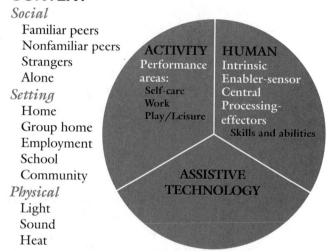

figure **19-1** The Human Assistive Technology (HAAT) model. *(From Cook, A., & Hussey, S. [1995].* Assistive technologies: Principles and practice. *St. Louis: Mosby.)*

vention planning, implementation, and discharge. In AT service delivery, two additional steps are added to this process as distinct phases: (1) procurement of devices, which occurs before and as part of intervention, and (2) follow-up. Because of the complexity of many AT systems, especially computer and augmentative communication systems, the therapist needs a systematic procedure for follow-up and adjustments to help ensure the viability of the system over time. These steps of the process are dynamic rather than linear and sequential. For example, the therapist may begin intervention by addressing prerequisite skills for AT use before completing the AT evaluation and procuring a specific device. Once a system has been chosen and purchased, components of the evaluation and decision-making processes may continue throughout intervention.

Evaluation

The AT evaluation may be completed by the team who will also provide the intervention (e.g., fitting and training of the device) or a team that has been formed specifically for the purpose of completing AT evaluations. Many hospitals, clinics, and some community agencies and schools have a designated AT team because of the complexity of many AT systems. The occupational therapist who does not work with AT on a regular basis may have difficulty maintaining expertise on all the systems and devices available because of the number of devices and the rapid development of new systems. When a team that will not be providing the intervention evaluates a

child, ideally the evaluation and intervention team collaborate to make decisions and recommendations.

Models to guide AT evaluation and service delivery have been developed (Bain & Leger, 1997; Bowser & Reed, 1998; Cook & Hussey, 1995; Scherer, 1993; Smith, 1991). Each of these models provides a framework for evaluating needs, making decisions, and implementing intervention. The model for service delivery helps ensure that the evaluation process is systematic and complete.

Human Activity Assistive Technology model

In the *Human Activity Assistive Technology (HAAT) model* (Cook & Hussey, 1995), the assessment process is dynamic and each step is interrelated. Figure 19-1 represents all the components of the model, each of which interacts with the other components and "plays a unique part in the total system" (Cook & Hussey, 1995, p. 50). In this model, the activity defines the goal of the AT system and "represents the functional result of human performance" (Cook & Hussey, 1995, p. 51). Activities are categorized within occupational performance areas. Each activity is carried out within a context, including social contexts, cultural context, physical settings, and the physical environment of a particular setting. Any of these contexts can influence how the technology is implemented. "The contexts in which the human carries out the activity are frequently forgotten when the assistive technology application is considered. However, the con-

box 19-2 *Guiding questions when evaluating a child for assistive technology*

Motor
- What body parts are capable of reliable, accurate, and controlled movement?
- Can the child be positioned adequately in and maintain an upright sitting posture?
- Does the child have sufficient range of motion, finger dexterity, strength, and endurance?
- What is the child's overall endurance and strength?
- What is the child's level of independence in daily living skills?

Sensory and perceptual
- Can the child attend to visual feedback on the monitor?
- Can the child respond to auditory feedback?
- What are the child's strengths and limitations in visual perception and visual motor skills?
- Is the child easily distracted by visual stimuli?

Cognitive and communication
- What is the child's cognitive level?
- What is the child's attention span?
- What are the child's receptive and expressive language skills? Potential?
- What are the child's face-to-face and written communication needs?
- Can the child sequence multiple-step directions?

Psychosocial
- Does the child seem motivated to use assistive technology (AT)?
- What activities does the child enjoy?
- Does the child see AT use as meaningful and rewarding?
- Will the child and family tolerate the influence of this AT device?

Context
- Where will the child use the AT device?
- How can the AT device or interface be positioned for optimal use?
- Do classroom and/or home environments allow for safe and easy access to educational materials and use of the AT devices?
- Does the child have any previous experience with AT?
- Are the individuals who work with the child (family and professionals) willing to use AT?
- What are the short- and long-term goals with the AT device?

---

text is often the determining factor in the success or failure of the assistive technology system" (Cook & Hussey, 1995, p. 55). The human component represents the user of the technology system, or the child. The therapist must be able to determine the child's skills and abilities; "an ability is a basic trait of a person, what a person brings to a new task, while a skill is a level of proficiency" (Cook & Hussey, 1995, p. 54).

The HAAT model emphasizes the need to recommend AT devices that meet the specific needs of the child and the family by considering specific skills and activities that the child can or needs to perform and the contexts in which the child will perform the activities. In summary, an AT evaluation has the following steps (Swinth, 1998):

1. A team of multidisciplinary professionals is formed.
2. The team determines family and child goals, priorities, and preferences.
3. The team identifies sociocultural considerations and concerns.
4. All team members evaluate the child. Elements of this evaluation include:
   a. Skills of the child (developmental and functional, including motor, sensory and perceptual, cognitive, communication, and psychosocial) (Box 19-2)
   b. Activities that the child needs or desires to perform
   c. Contexts in which the technology will be used (see Box 19-2)
5. The team identifies and considers types of AT devices.
6. The team provides trial opportunities for various appropriate AT devices.

Comprehensive and appropriate information gathering during the evaluation, coupled with trial periods with different types of AT, will result in a better match between the AT device or system and the child and family. The trial period may be one of the most important aspects of the AT evaluation. These trials can help prevent the costly procurement of an incorrect device. The cost of AT includes not only the purchase of the device, but also the ongoing costs for maintenance, upgrades to the system, and repairs. Figure 19-2 provides a possible format for the AT team to use to document and describe the trial processes. Other questions that the therapist should address throughout assessment and in-

ASSISTIVE TECHNOLOGY EXTENDED ASSESSMENT PLAN

Date of extended assessment planning: _____

Student Data

Student name: _____

Parent name(s): _____

Parent phone: _____

Parent e-mail: _____

Parent address: _____

_____

Date of birth: _____ CA: _____

Disability: _____

IEP date: _____

Medicaid ID # (if applicable): _____

Med. diagnosis (if applicable): _____

Social security #: _____

Grade/placement: _____

School: _____

School address: _____

_____

School phone: _____

fax: _____

Team Members

AT extended Assessment Coordinator

Name: _____

Title: _____

Phone: _____

E-Mail: _____

Other Team Members

Name: _____ Title: _____

Phone: _____

E-Mail: _____

Name: _____ Title: _____

Phone: _____

E-Mail: _____

Name: _____ Title: _____

Phone: _____

E-Mail: _____

Name: _____ Title: _____

Phone: _____

E-Mail: _____

Name: _____ Title: _____

Phone: _____

E-Mail: _____

Overall Goal for Device Use

Goal for device:

_____

_____

How will we know if the trial is successful?

_____

_____

What level of achievement is reasonable to expect during the trial period?

_____

_____

figure **19-2**   Assistive Technology Extended Assessment Plan. *(From Bowser, G., & Reed, P. [1998]. Education TECH points: A framework for assistive technology planning. Winchester, OR: Coalition for Assistive Technology in Oregon.)*

Overall Goal for Device Use—cont'd

What level of achievement is reasonable to expect during the trial period?

_____

_____

How will we know if the trial is not working? (What criteria will we use to stop?)

_____

_____

Customary Environments Where Devices Will Be Used

1. Environment: _____

   Tasks: _____

   Person responsible for implementation: _____

   Days to be used: _____

   Times to be used: _____

2. Environment: _____

   Tasks: _____

   Person responsible for implementation: _____

   Days to be used: _____

   Times to be used: _____

3. Environment: _____

   Tasks: _____

   Person responsible for implementation: _____

   Days to be used: _____

   Times to be used: _____

Specific Devices for Trial

Device #1 _____

Date of trial initiation: _____   Minimum length of trial period: _____

Device trial review date: _____

Source of device for trial: _____

Contact person for technical assistance for trial: _____

Manufacturer: _____   Manufacturer technical assistance number: _____

Comments: _____

Device #2 _____

Date of trial initiation: _____   Minimum length of trial period: _____

Device trial review date: _____

Source of device for trial: _____

Contact person for technical assistance for trial: _____

Manufacturer: _____   Manufacturer technical assistance number: _____

Comments: _____

figure **19-2, cont'd**

Specific Devices for Trial—cont'd

Device #3 _____

Date of trial initiation: _____ Minimum length of trial period: _____

Device trial review date: _____

Source of device for trial: _____

Contact person for technical assistance for trial: _____

Manufacturer: _____ Manufacturer technical assistance number: _____

Comments: _____

Extended Assessment Summary *(to be completed at the end of the assessment)*

How did the child's performance change when using the devices?

How did the student like using each device? Did the student prefer one of the devices?

What are the advantages of using the devices?

What are the disadvantages of using the devices?

How long can the child be expected to use the devices?

Extended Assessment Team Recommendations

figure **19-2, cont'd**   Assistive Technology Extended Assessment Plan. *(From Bowser, G., & Reed, P. [1998]*. Education TECH points: A framework for assistive technology planning. *Winchester, OR: Coalition for Assistive Technology in Oregon.)*

tervention in relationship to cost include the following (Swinth, 1998):

1. What financial resources are available to the family?
2. When the AT device is in need of repair, does the family have access to services?
3. Does the AT device significantly increase the child's level of independence and function?
4. Can the AT device be adapted to enable higher levels of function as the child grows and matures?
5. Can a less complex device meet the same needs just as well?

The team discusses these issues and others unique to each family in deciding whether the system is a reasonable and appropriate investment for the family that will result in increasing the child's functional independence. The team should present the child and family with objective and realistic information regarding investment in and use of AT. Given a complete description of the options and alternatives, the family makes the final decision as to what AT is implemented and how it is implemented into the child's program. Box 19-3 presents 11 criteria, developed by over 700 consumers of AT, that the team should use to evaluate different AT devices.

Decision Making

Occupational therapists use problem-solving and clinical reasoning skills throughout the process of procurement, implementation, and follow-up with AT. Effective problem solving is the basis for all clinical reasoning. Problem solving should involve defining the situation or problem, determining the short- and long-term goals, and brainstorming potential processes to reach the determined goals. The therapist is often tempted to define the situation or problem and immediately jump to possible strategies for fixing the problem. However, if the therapist does not consider the short- and long-term goals before discussing potential solutions, the strategies implemented may not have a long-term benefit for the child.

When working with children of any age, the occupational therapist should consider short- and long-term goals in terms of what the child's needs are at that time, 1 year later, 3 to 5 years later, and 7 to 10 years later. This can be difficult when working with young children, but the information can help facilitate decision-making, especially when addressing AT needs. When working with an adolescent, this long-term planning is even more critical. It leads to the development of a successful transition plan, which may in turn result in increased independence in many life roles. The therapist should not view these short- and long-term goals as permanent, but as a dynamic process that will change over time. The team should revisit and rewrite goals systematically as the child grows and matures, as contexts change, as child and family needs and desires change, and if the child's medical condition changes.

Device Procurement

Device procurement can take months to accomplish. When funding issues stall the process, members of the team may be involved in writing letters of justification to insurance companies and other third party payers. Careful documentation during the trial periods with different devices can help with this process. Documentation can include videos or pictures of the child using the system that demonstrates how the system helps improve function.

box 19-3 *Criteria for evaluating assistive technology devices*

1. *Effectiveness.* How much the device improves the user's living situation and enhances functional capability and independence
2. *Affordability.* The extent to which a person can purchase, maintain, and repair a device without financial hardship
3. *Reliability.* The degree to which a device is dependable, consistent, and predictable in its performance and levels of accuracy for reasonable amount of time
4. *Portability.* The influence of the device's size and weight on the user's ability to move, carry, relocate, and operate it in varied locations
5. *Durability.* The extent to which a device delivers continued operation for an extended period of time
6. *Securability.* How well a consumer believes that a device affords physical control and is secure from theft or vandalism
7. *Safety.* How well a device protects the user, care provider, or family member from potential harm, bodily injury, or infection
8. *Learnability.* The perspective of the device's ease of assembly, initial learning requirements, and time and effort to master use
9. *Comfort and acceptance.* The extent to which a user feels physically comfortable with the device and does not experience pain or discomfort with use; how aesthetically appealing the user finds the device and the user's psychologic comfort when using it in private or public
10. *Maintenance and repairability.* The degree to which the device is easy to maintain and repair (either by the consumer, a local repair shop, or a supplier)
11. *Operability.* The extent to which the device is easy to use, is adaptable and flexible, and affords easy access to controls and displays

From Scherer, M.J., & Lane, J.P. (1997). Assessing consumer profiles of "ideal" assistive technologies in ten categories: An integration of quantitative and qualitative methods. *Disability and Rehabilitation, 19* (12), 528-535.

Once the system has arrived, the therapist and team work to put the system together, test the system, and begin training. Some companies provide vendors that can help with the process, and others have videos that come with the system. However, it is not uncommon for a system to be delivered with minimal instructions. This can be daunting to the family if the system is delivered directly to their home and they are unsure how to use it. Comprehensive intervention and education are needed to help the child and family incorporate the device into their daily lives.

Intervention

Occupational therapy intervention has many facets when working with AT. The long-term goal of AT use should be social participation and productivity in the child's life roles and occupations of choice. However, to reach this goal the therapist needs to address performance, activity, and complex task components (Coster, 1998). Occupational therapists provide intervention to address difficulties in each of these areas of performance. As a result, the therapist may initially be using a computer system to motivate a child to work on reaching. However, the therapist knows that the long-term goal is for the child to use the same computer system to complete classroom assignments in a general education classroom. Reaching is one of the component processes that the child must learn before learning efficient use of the system.

Several authors have attempted to define specific prerequisite skills when introducing children to AT. However, empirical studies that define the skills that are needed to effectively use AT remain limited (Bowser, 1989; Symington, 1990). Behrmann and others (1989) categorized the skills that children need to successfully use AT into four areas: motor skills, cognitive-language skills, visual perceptual skills, and social-emotional skills (Box 19-4). These skills are not prerequisites to using an AT device; the child can develop these skills while using the device.

AT services are provided through direct services, consultation, education, and advocacy.

---

box 19-4 *Categories of skills needed to use technology*

Motor skills
- Range of motion
- Strength and endurance
- Press and release
- Reliable and consistent motor movement

Cognitive-language skills
- Cause-effect relationships
- Attention span (sustained or selective)
- Object permanence
- Means-ends causality
- Imitation
- One-to-one correspondence
- Intentional behavior (desire to communicate)
- Symbolic representation (recognize pictures)
- Reliable yes and no response
- Receptive understanding of commands
- Decision making

Visual perceptual skills
- Visual tracking and scanning
- Figure-ground
- Form discrimination

Social emotional skills
- Initiating and terminating interactions
- Turn taking and waiting for turn
- Attending to an object or person
- Following one-step directions

Reprinted from Behrmann, M.M., Jones, J.K., & Wilds, M.L. (1989). Technology intervention for very young children with disabilities. *Infants and Young Children, 1* (4), 66-77.

Direct service delivery

Direct service delivery may or may not involve specialized training on the part of the occupational therapist. Therapists who are specialized in AT may provide services to children for specified amounts of time that focus on helping the child develop proficiency with a system. Therapists who are not highly trained in AT should collaborate with specialists as needed. Frequently settings designate one therapist or a team of professionals to be the "AT experts." This designated expert can take a leadership role in learning how to operate the complex systems and in acquiring and reviewing updated information on AT for potential use by the team.

Direct intervention may also include training the child and family how to use the device, customizing a system, and working on prerequisite skill acquisition so the child can successfully use the system. Whenever possible, training should occur in the environments in which the system will be used. This may require the therapist to travel or at times to function in a consultative role when travel is not possible. Depending on the age, disability, program, and other child or family needs, the therapist provides direct intervention on regular or intermittent schedules for weeks, months, or in some settings, years.

Consultation

Often after the occupational therapist has completed the assessment process and set up the system, his or her services are primarily those of a consultant. For any child to be able to successfully use a system, the system must be implemented into his or her daily routine. For example, if a child is going to use a Tracker and an on-screen keyboard to complete written assignments, the child must begin using the system in the classroom once the initial training is complete. The therapist may work with the teachers to design a program so that the child can use the system in school. In addition, the therapist may design a home program so that the child can practice and develop increased proficiency with the system. The therapist then collaborates with the child, teacher, and family if any problems arise. Additionally, the therapist may systematically monitor the child's program at home and school and make changes, when needed, based on teacher, parent, or student input. If the therapist works in a preschool, he or she may help the teacher obtain a Touch Window and software program for the child to use to work on developing an understanding of cause-effect relationships and beginning computer skills. Once the therapist sets up the equipment and software programs, he or she consults with the preschool teacher as needed. As the child develops an understanding of cause-effect relationships, the therapist may help the teacher develop the next part of the technology program.

In some settings, occupational therapy assistants and aides provide some of the AT service delivery. Assistants are particularly helpful in training on a system once the therapist has set it up and established the program. Assistants and aides may also be involved in practicing use of the device with the child and helping others use the systems. Therapists working in AT service delivery must determine which activities are appropriate to delegate and which activities are specialized and require the training and skills of a therapist.

Education

Thorough training and education regarding AT systems are essential components in integrating AT into a child's daily life. Occupational therapists often function as educators for the child using the device and the family and other professionals involved in the child's program. The education that the therapist provides should be comprehensive and include use of the AT device, problem solving potential difficulties, trouble shooting when the device malfunctions, implementing the device in various settings, and when needed, obtaining maintenance or repair services. Once the child has begun to successfully use an AT system, the therapist may continue to be a resource to address any problems when they arise.

Advocacy

"Traditionally, occupational therapists have been advocates for consumers" (Trefler & Hobson, 1997, p. 501). Advocacy is part of the direct service, consultation, and educator roles of the occupational therapist. Occupational therapists work with other team members to increase the awareness of clients and families regarding their rights. Additionally, occupational therapists may use advocacy skills when working on funding issues and when helping other professionals understand the importance and function of AT in the lives of children with disabilities.

Discharge and Follow-up

Once the child and family have a basic understanding of the AT system and are able to begin to use it independently, the occupational therapist may discharge the child from services. However, discharge from a regular routine of intervention should include a follow-up plan. The therapist can perform follow-up in several ways, from a telephone call to an extended clinic visit. The type of follow-up and when follow-up should occur depend on the complexity of the system and the skills of the child, family, and other professionals working with the child. "Follow-up provides valuable information. First, the effectiveness of the technology intervention can be monitored and/or measured. Second, if the intervention is not working smoothly, assistance can be provided before abandonment occurs, and finally, timing for changes in technology can be anticipated" (Trefler & Hobson, 1997, p. 499). A predetermined schedule for follow-up (sometimes at intervals of 6 months or less and sometimes 1 year or more) is a component of effective service delivery.

■ APPLICATION OF ASSISTIVE TECHNOLOGY PRINCIPLES TO COMPUTERS AND AUGMENTATIVE COMMUNICATION

This section describes how the previous principles of AT intervention can be applied to computers and augmentative communication. Occupational therapists are generally core members of a multidisciplinary team when a child requires the use of a computer to play, learn, and work, or an augmentative communication device to communicate. Different types of systems are described, and examples are presented to illustrate principles in AT service delivery.

Computers

Use of personal computers by individuals of all ages is becoming more and more prevalent in schools, homes, and work settings. Most children with and without disabilities have had some exposure to a computer system by the time they enter school. With the increase in personal computer use, children with disabilities have daily opportunities to use computers at home and school. Behrmann (1984) reported that children with the cognitive and physical skills of a 3 month old have the potential of using electronic learning. In his study, 3-month-old infants activated a switch to hear their mothers' voices. A more realistic guideline is to begin cause-effect activities when the child reaches a 7-month cognitive level. The computer can be a motivating tool to help children learn and develop a large repertoire of skills. It provides simulations of experiences that cannot otherwise be experienced by children with motor disabilities. For example, some adolescents with disabilities describe social networks and friendships that they have been able to develop using the computer, Internet access, and appropriate software programs (Swinth, 1997). The computer is also infinitely patient with drill and practice and can provide the repetition needed for some children to learn.

An almost endless variety of software programs, input devices, and output devices are available to customize computers to meet the individual needs of each child (Anson, 1997). If the therapist is working with a young child, he or she can introduce a progression of systems that follows the developmental and functional needs of the child. For a child who is born with a disability, success using simple systems precedes the use of more complex systems (e.g., use of a cause-effect program before a complex writing system). The successful use of a computer system requires that the user be able to provide input into the system, receive output (or information) from the computer, and process that information to use it in a functional, meaningful manner. Table 19-2 describes different computer options, hardware, and access systems.

Various types of computers are available in the home, school, clinical, and work settings (e.g., Macintosh or IBM-compatible computers). For some children and settings, older machines are more successful than newer models because they are less complex and less visually distracting. For example, for some children with autism or certain visual-perceptual deficits, a monochrome monitor works better than some of the newer color monitors with high resolution. The newer monitors can overwhelm the child because of the high level of visual input. Macintosh computers tend to be the most commonly used systems in early intervention and grade school settings, and families, facilities, and higher grades in schools more commonly use IBM-compatible machines. Before the therapist recommends the purchase of software programs or adapted access devices, he or she must evaluate the memory and technology of the system to determine compatibility with the child.

Input

When the therapist is looking at different input systems, he or she should use a least change principle. This means that if the child can use a standard keyboard and standard workstation with some modifications, this should be done rather than purchasing an expanded keyboard or other type of input device (Table 19-3 on page 594). For some children, using an ergonomic keyboard

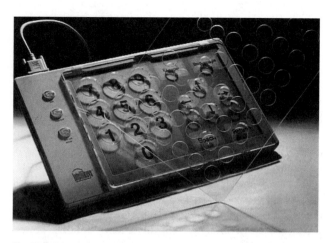

figure 19-3   An example of a keyguard on an alternative keyboard. Keyguards also are available for standard keyboards. *(Photo courtesy IntelliTools, Richmond, CA.)*

rather than a standard keyboard will increase their proficiency on the computer. For a child with slight tremors, defeating the autorepeat function or using a keyguard (plastic covers for the keyboard with a single hole) may enable independent use of the standard system (Figure 19-3). The therapist may need to consider a different type of mouse (e.g., trackball or touch pad) rather than the standard mouse. Software programs are available to redefine the keyboard versus using the standard QWERTY keyboard that comes with most computers. One commonly used keyboard is the Big Keys Plus that offers a color-coded alphabetic layout for younger children or children with cognitive delays who cannot find letters using the QWERTY layout. Additionally, the Dvorak Keyboard, on which commonly used letters are arranged so that less motion is required to access them, or a Chubon Keyboard, on which the highest frequency of use letters are placed in the center of the keyboard, can be helpful for a child with hemiplegia. Switches, adapted keyboards, and voice recognition systems offer alternative means for computer access to children with limited movement.

Some alternate input systems require interface devices, such as the Ke:nx (for the Macintosh), to access the computer (Figure 19-4 on page 593). Other alternate input systems come with their own software programs, and others are a combination of unique hardware and software adaptations. Some alternate input systems allow for *direct selection* (the use selects letters, words, or phrases by touching or pointing to the desired key), and others allow *indirect selection* (an intermediate step is used when sending a command to the computer). Direct selection offers more choices to the child, requires less cognitive skill than indirect selection, and should be the first type of system that the therapist considers.

Switches. Switches allow access with a single movement. Switches can be used for direct access (e.g., to

Text continued on p. 595

table 19-2   Computer Options, Hardware, and Access Systems*

Name of System	Requirements and Considerations	Persons Who Benefit	Ordering Information
ALTERNATE KEYBOARDS			
IntelliKeys	• Comes with some basic overlays, and customized overlays can be created using an IntelliTools program; numerous commercially produced overlays can also be used • Can be used in combination with IntelliTools to function as a talking word processer and communication tool or with IntelliPics to create accessible interactive computer programs • Can be used to run one- or two-switch programs • Works with Macintosh and IBM-compatible computers	• Individuals with limited fine motor control; access via mouth stick or head stick is possible • Individuals with decreased vision • Individuals who use a single switch to access single switch software	IntelliTools, Inc. 55 Leveroni Court, Suite 9 Novato, CA 94949 Telephone: (800) 899-6687 E-mail: info@intellitools.com Website: www.intellitools.com
Expanded keyboard: KeyLargo	• Must have Ke:nx or some other type of software that allows the keyboard to communicate with the computer • Can be customized from single choice to 128 choices	• Individuals with upper-extremity control but limited fine motor control; access via a mouth stick or head stick as well • Individuals with decreased vision	Don Johnston Developmental Equipment PO Box 639 1000 N. Rand Road, Bldg. 115 Wauconda, IL 60084 Telephone: (800) 999-4660 Website: www.donjohnston.com
Expanded keyboard: Discover:Board	• Talks so that it can be used for communication • Has basic overlays and software to create custom overlays • Can be used with educational programs • Can be used with Macintosh and IBM-compatible computers	• Individuals with limited fine motor control • Individuals with limited speech or who are auditory learners	Don Johnston Developmental Equipment PO Box 639 1000 N. Rand Road, Bldg. 115 Wauconda, IL 60084 Telephone: (800) 999-4660 Website: www.donjohnston.com
Dvorak one-handed keyboard	• Uses high-frequency keys under the fingers of the hand doing the typing (available in left-handed and a right-handed) • Can be added to mainstream computers at little or no cost	• Individuals who have one hand substantially more functional than the other; significantly diminishes finger travel as compared with the QWERTY pattern for one-handed typists; may translate into faster typing and/or increased endurance for typing	Meeting the Challenge 3630 Sinton Rd. Suite 103 Colorado Springs, CO. 80907 Telephone: (800) 864-4264 Microsoft Corporation One Microsoft Way Redmond, WA 98502 Telephone: (800) 876-4726 (ask for disk GA0650)

*This is not meant to be an inclusive list, nor is it meant to be an endorsement of any particular product.
Modified from Swinth, Y.L., & Anson, D. (1998). Alternatives to handwriting: Keyboarding and text-generation techniques for schools. In J. Case-Smith (Ed.), *AOTA self-paced clinical course: Occupational therapy: Making a difference in school system practice*. Bethesda, MD: AOTA; Contributions by J. Rogers (1999).   *Continued*

table 19-2 *Computer Options, Hardware, and Access Systems—cont'd*

Name of System	Requirements and Considerations	Persons Who Benefit	Ordering Information
ALTERNATE KEYBOARDS—cont'd			
Chord keyboard	• Uses a pattern of keys rather than a unique key for each letter • May be a replacement of the standard keyboard or an alternative driver for the standard keyboard	• Individuals with limited upper-body strength but good hand coordination; allows the individual to type with little more than pressure changes on the keys rather than moving from key to key; requires the individual to learn the keyboard completely before typing because "hunt and peck" typing does not work	AccuCorp, Inc. PO Box 66 Christiansburg, VA 24073 Telephone: (703) 961-2001 Infogrip, Inc. 1141 E. Main St. Ventura, CA 93001 Telephone: (800) 397-0921 Website: www.infogrip.com/infogrip
Mini keyboard	• Requires Ke:nx or some other type of software that allows the keyboard to communicate with the computer • Can be customized for the arrangement and size of choices	• Individuals with upper-extremity control but limited range of motion; depending on the size, requires fairly good fine motor control; access via a mouth stick or head stick	Tash International, Inc. Unit 1-91 Station Street Ajak, Ontario, CA L1S3H2 Telephone: (800) 463-5685
Big Keys Plus	• Is a simple keyboard with enlarged keys designed for young children or people who may require a large key-striking area; • Has ABC or QWERTY layout • Has color-coded keys or black or white keys	• Children with limited fine motor control, particularly limited midrange arm movement	Greystone Digital Inc. Telephone: (800) 249-5397 Website: www.bigkeys.com
Little Fingers	• Designed to fit children's smaller hands and fingers • Has trackball built into keyboard • Is only 12½ inches wide including trackball • Is compatible with Macintosh or IBM-compatible computers	• Children with small hands who need to use the keyboard as their primary method of written communication	Data Desk Website: www.datadesktech.com
MOUSE EMULATORS			
Headmaster Plus and Headmaster 2000	• Works as a mouse emulator; a unit on top of the computer senses the position of a headset that the user is wearing • Requires an on-screen keyboard for typing • Is operated when user is attached to the computer through the headset; however, infrared wireless adaptations are available	• Individuals with good-to-fair cognitive skills and no upper-extremity control; must have good head and breath control (lightly puffing into a tube connected to the headset is equivalent to mouseclick)	Prentke Romich 1022 Heyl Road Wooster, OH 44691 Telephone: (800) 262-1984

Modified from Swinth, Y.L., & Anson, D. (1998). Alternatives to handwriting: Keyboarding and text-generation techniques for schools. In J. Case-Smith (Ed.), *AOTA self-paced clinical course: Occupational therapy: Making a difference in school system practice*. Bethesda, MD: AOTA; Contribution by J. Rogers (1999).

table 19-2 *Computer Options, Hardware, and Access Systems—cont'd*

Name of System	Requirements and Considerations	Persons Who Benefit	Ordering Information
MOUSE EMULATORS—cont'd			
HeadMouse	• Works as a wireless mouse emulator; a unit on top of the computer senses the position of a small sensor "dot" that the user is wearing • Requires an on-screen keyboard for typing • User can implement key press by dwelling over a key for a set time or by using an adaptive switch	• Individuals with good-to-fair cognitive skills and no upper-extremity control; must have good head control and some motor movement to access a switch	Origin Instruments Corporation 854 Greenview Drive Grand Prarie, TX 75050 E-mail: Sales@orig.com
Tracker	• Is a wireless mouse emulator; a unit on top of the computer works as an optical head tracking sensor via a tiny sensor attached to the user • Requires an on-screen keyboard for typing	• Individuals with good-to-fair cognitive skills and no upper-extremity control	Medenta Communications, Inc. 9411A-20 Ave. Edmonton, Alberta Canada, T6N 1E5 Telephone: (800) 661-8406 E-mail: madenta@ccinet.ab.ca
Hands-free mouse	• Uses two foot pedals to control mouse direction and speed and mouse clicks	• Individuals who lack hand and arm movement but have adequate foot motion to activate pedals	Hunter Digital 11999 San Vicente Blvd, Suite 440 Los Angeles, CA 90049 Telephone: (800) 57-MOUSE
Touch Window	• Provides easy, low-cost touch access • Requires dedicated software • Is compatible with Macintosh or IBM-compatible computers • Allows user to interact directly with the computer screen; thought is not divided between the learning task and manipulating the computer	• Young children or those with limited cognitive skills	Edmark PO Box 97021 Redmond, WA 98073-9721 Telephone: (800) 362-2890 Website: www.edmark.com
OTHER INPUT SYSTEMS			
Dragon Naturally Speaking DragonDictate	• Is a voice recognition system available for MS-DOS and Windows-based computers • Can create, edit, format, and move text by voice • Can actuate a mouse by voice	• Individual with limited motor control but good voice quality; does not work well in noisy environments; takes time to train • User who can read and recognize spelling errors to recognize whether the computer is inputting the correct words	Dragon Systems, Inc. 320 Nevada St. Newton, MA 02160 Telephone: (800) TALK-TYP Website: www.dragonsy.com

Continued

table 19-2 *Computer Options, Hardware, and Access Systems—cont'd*

Name of System	Requirements and Considerations	Persons Who Benefit	Ordering Information
OTHER INPUT SYSTEMS—cont'd			
Eyegaze Computer System	• Is only available for MS-DOS computers	• User who has adequate vision to locate data on the computer screen and be able to control one eye precisely; may not work well for someone with nystagmus	LC Technologies 9455 King Court Fairfax, VA 22031 Telephone: (800) 393-4293
KEYBOARDING SYSTEMS			
AlphaSmart	• Is a small, lightweight, portable word processor for notetaking and simple compositions • Allows user to see only four lines of text at a time • Allows user to download to a Macintosh or IBM-compatible computer once he or she has entered data • Allows user to print work via downloading to a computer or directing to most printers • Can transfer data to a computer or printer using infrared	• Users with good motor control and visual perceptual skills • Users who only require the computer or word processor for simple word processing (e.g., taking notes or completing papers) • Users who need a system that they can easily transport	Intelligent Peripheral Devices, Inc. 20380 Town Center Lane, Suite 270 Cupertino, CA 95014 Telephone: (408) 252-9400 E-mail: alphasmart@eworld.com
DreamWriter	• Is a portable word processor with functions that include editing, spell checking, grammar checking, text layout and formatting, and typing tutorials • Allows user to see eight lines of text at a time • Uses an icon and Alphanumeric menu • Allows students to store, recall, rename, copy, and delete files • Comes with a calculator, calendar, electronic diary, address card system, and a world clock	• Users with good motor control and visual perceptual skills • Users who only require the computer or word processor for simple word processing (e.g., taking notes or completing papers)	NTS Computer Systems, LTD 20145 Stewart Crescent #101 Maple Ridge BC V2XOT6 Telephone: (800) 663-7163

Modified from Swinth, Y.L., & Anson, D. (1998). Alternatives to handwriting: Keyboarding and text-generation techniques for schools. In J. Case-Smith (Ed.), *AOTA self-paced clinical course: Occupational therapy: Making a difference in school system practice.* Bethesda, MD: AOTA; Contribution III J. Rogers (1999).

table 19-2   *Computer Options, Hardware, and Access Systems—cont'd*

Name of System	Requirements and Considerations	Persons Who Benefit	Ordering Information
KEYBOARDING SYSTEMS—cont'd			
Laser PC 4	• Is a portable word processor with functions that include editing, spell checking, grammar checking, text layout and formatting, and typing tutorials • Allows user to see eight lines of text at a time • Uses an alphanumeric menu • Comes with a calculator, telephone directory, a program to write programs in BASIC, a data base, and spreadsheets • Is also available with a sticky key function	• Users with good motor control and visual perceptual skills • Users of the computer or word processor for simple word processing (e.g., taking notes or completing papers), databases, spreadsheets, and/or desire to write programs in BASIC	Perfect Solutions 12657 Coral Breeze Dr. West Palm Beach, FL 33414 Telephone: (561) 790-1070
SOFTWARE			
Word Prediction (Co:Writer, KeyWiz and EZ Keys, Aurora	Co:Writer: • Is available for Macintosh or IBM-compatible computers • Allows user to type into Co:Writer window; when a sentence is finished, it is exported to a word processor • Has grammar-sensitive prediction and is customizable KeyWiz and EZ Keys: • Is available for MS-DOS and Windows • Works transparently into many word processors • Uses word frequency order of presentation Aurora: • Is available for MS-DOS and Windows • Is a word prediction package that supports large vocabularies (>100,000 words) • Offers special formatting to assist users with learning disabilities, including phonetic prediction and common misspelling prediction	• Individuals with writing or spelling impairments	Co:Writer: Don Johnston Developmental Equipment PO Box 639 1000 N. Rand Road, Bldg. 115 Wauconda, IL 60084 Telephone: (800) 999-4660 Website: www.donjohnston.com KeyWiz and EZ Keys: Words + Inc. PO Box 1229 Lancaster, CA 95354 Telephone: (805) 949-8331 Aurora: Aurora Systems 2647 Kingsway Vancouver, BC V5R 5H4 Canada Telephone: (604) 436-2694

Continued

table 19-2 *Computer Options, Hardware, and Access Systems—cont'd*

Name of System	Requirements and Considerations	Persons Who Benefit	Ordering Information
SOFTWARE—cont'd			
Biggy	• Is available for Macintosh and IBM-compatible computers	• Individuals with visual deficits and visual perceptual challenges; enlarges the cursor so individuals can find it more easily on the screen	RJ Cooper & Associates 24843 Del Prado #283 Dana Point, CA 92629 Telephone: (800) RJCooper
Write:OutLoud	• Is available for Macintosh and IBM-compatible computers • Is a word processing program with speech output • Contains a built-in Franklin spell checker and dictionary • Allows users to hear letters or words as they are typing or to have the computer read sentences to them when they are finished typing it • Highlights words as they are read • May enhance writing quality because user can hear if words are omitted or substituted • May help with comprehension	• Individuals with learning disabilities who benefit from auditory with visual input when word processing • Individuals with visual impairments.	Don Johnston Developmental Equipment PO Box 639 1000 N. Rand Road, Bldg. 115 Wauconda, IL 60084 Telephone: (800) 999-4660 Website: www.donjohnston.com
SWITCH SYSTEMS			
Discover: Switch	• Requires Ke:nx or other scanning software • Is slow and should be considered as a last resort • Allows computer to scan through various choices; user hits switch when computer reaches choice • Is available for Macintosh and IBM-compatible computers	• Individuals who can access a single switch; requires higher cognitive abilities	Don Johnston Developmental Equipment PO Box 639 1000 N. Rand Road, Bldg. 115 Wauconda, IL 60084 Telephone: (800) 999-4660 Website: www.donjohnston.com

Modified from Swinth, Y.L., & Anson, D. (1998). Alternatives to handwriting: Keyboarding and text-generation techniques for schools. In J. Case-Smith (Ed.), *AOTA self-paced clinical course: Occupational therapy: Making a difference in school system practice.* Bethesda, MD: AOTA; Contribution by J. Rogers (1999).

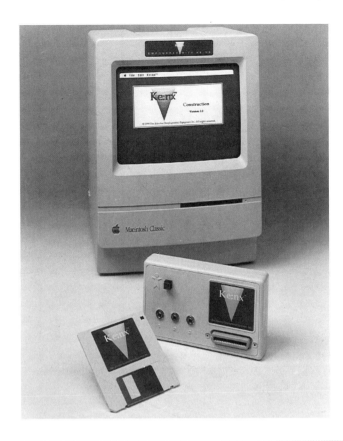

figure 19-4   Ke:nx, a keyboard emulator device. *(Photo courtesy Don Johnston, Inc., Wauconda, IL.)*

table 19-3   *Problem Solving for Computer Access (Starting with a Standard Computer Workstation)*

Problem	Potential Solutions
Difficulty pressing one or more keys	Change height of table or chair Change position of keyboard Change sensitivity of keys or activate delayed acceptance Use a keyguard Use an expanded keyboard with larger keys Use a stylus, mouthstick, or headstick Change size of letters on keyboard
Tendency to produce multiple characters rather than one	Change height of table or chair Change position of keyboard Change sensitivity of keys or activate delayed acceptance Deactivate autorepeat
Difficulty holding down more than one key simultaneously	Use Sticky Keys feature or utility Use a mechanical key latch
Ability to use only one hand	Teach student to use one-handed typing techniques for standard keyboard Use a chord keyboard Reconfigure the keyboard to use one-handed pattern Use on-screen keyboard and mouse for typing
Difficulty with the standard mouse	Use a trackball Use a Trackpad Create a mouse track template Use MouseKeys feature of operating system

From Swinth, Y.L., & Anson, D. (1998). Alternatives to handwriting: Keyboarding and text-generation techniques for schools.
In J. Case-Smith (Ed.), *AOTA self-paced clinical course: Occupational therapy: Making a difference in school system practice.* Rockville, MD: AOTA.

Continued

Problem	Potential Solutions
Slow or inefficient input	Increase keyboarding practice so that motor patterns are more automatic Set up templates for standard formats Use macros and abbreviation expansion for repeated words and phrases Use word prediction software programs
Drooling	Use a keyboard cover (Safe Skin) Use alternative keyboards that are not moisture sensitive
Difficulty seeing the screen and/or highlights	Ensure that the monitor is not facing a window or that the blinds are drawn Use an antiglare filter Reduce glare by turning down overhead lights Change size of font Change font (serif fonts are better for reading text; sans-serif fonts are better for letter recognition) Change attributes of font (bold) Change color of background and/or text for greater contrast Set screen to monochrome Use a large screen or lower screen resolution Use a screen magnifier (hardware or software)
Difficulty reading text	Ensure that the monitor is not facing a window or that the blinds are drawn Use an antiglare filter Reduce glare by turning down overhead lights Change size of font Change font (serif fonts are better for reading text; sans-serif fonts are better for letter recognition) Change attributes of font (bold) Change color of background and/or text for greater contrast Set screen to monochrome Use a large screen or lower screen resolution Use a screen magnifier (hardware or software) Use a voice output tool (screen reader)
Tendency to be distracted by sound	Turn off sound features of application Turn down volume from system control panel Use hearing protectors or noise-canceling ear protectors
Difficulty hearing feedback	Turn up volume (can use headphones) Use amplified speakers
Difficulty finding correct key on the keyboard	Use stickers or enlarged key letters to highlight correct keys Increase size or contrast of keyboard caps Use color coding for "landmark" keys Use Kids Keys Keyboard (for younger students) Mask inappropriate keys
Difficulty shifting between information on the screen, the keyboard, and/or the desktop	Use "document clip" to suspend printed page next to monitor Change position of keyboard Change position of monitor Use a Touch Window and on-screen keyboard
Difficulty remembering keyboard functions	Develop a "cheat sheet" of keyboard shortcuts to keep close by Develop keyboard mnemonics to aid memory of keyboard functions
Decreased motivation	Recheck student goals to ensure student involvement in goal-making process Try a different software program to address goal Change the purpose for which the computer is being used Change the access method Decrease the amount of time on computer Scale the activity to students's skills (up or down)

From Swinth, Y.L., & Anson, D. (1998). Alternatives to handwriting: Keyboarding and text-generation techniques for schools. In J. Case-Smith (Ed.), *AOTA self-paced clinical course: Occupational therapy: Making a difference in school system practice.* Rockville, MD: AOTA.

make a choice in a cause-effect game) or indirect access (e.g., to move the cursor to a selection on the screen). Many of the more complex switch systems use indirect selection. When considering a switch driven system, the therapist must consider the motoric and cognitive requirements of the system. For example, a child who is able to accurately and reliably hit a switch at 9 months of age does not have the cognitive skills to understand the concept of scanning. In addition, research suggests that the placement of the switch (e.g., a head switch versus a switch that is struck with the hand) may have a cognitive component that affects a child's accuracy (Glickman, Deitz, Anson, & Stewart, 1996). Many of these switch systems require additional hardware and/or software (e.g., a switch interface device or Ke:nx) to interface with the computer.

A single (or dual) switch can be used to run systems such as Morse code and scanning. Morse code is faster than scanning but requires the user to learn a new language. Scanning is the slowest of most input methods and should be considered as a last resort. Various scanning methods are available, including row-column scanning, step scanning, and automatic scanning. The method that the therapist chooses depends on the skills of the child using the system.

Alternate keyboards. *Alternate keyboards* include programmable keyboards, miniature keyboards, chord keyboards, and on-screen keyboards. Each type of alternate keyboard varies in size, layout, and complexity. The KeyLargo, Discover:Board, and Intellikeys allow the child with decreased fine motor control or cognitive delays to successfully make choices on the computer. Programmable keyboards are sometimes referred to as *expanded keyboards* and are larger than the standard keyboard.

The KeyLargo requires additional hardware and software (e.g., Ke:nx) to interface with the computer. The Discover:Board allows for customization of overlays and provides voice output. The Intellikeys (Figure 19-5) comes with interchangeable standard overlays and is compatible with Macintosh and MS-DOS computer systems. Each of these programmable keyboards allows the therapist to develop customized overlays and can be set up with "hotkeys" to allow the child to enter numbers, words, and phrases by hitting one key. Overlays are sheets of paper that have a graphic representation of a keyboard or functions of a software program (e.g., cursor keys). By changing the overlay, software program, and customization setup, the child can complete more than one activity with the same keyboard.

Miniature keyboards are smaller than the standard keyboard. An example is the Tash Mini Keyboard. These keyboards are typically lightweight and designed to be used by children with limited range of motion and/or poor endurance. However, the user must have good fine motor control since the keys are small and close together.

Chord keyboards, like miniature keyboards, are designed to minimize finger travel. Use of these keyboards, similar to playing the piano, requires multiple simultaneous keystrokes to type letters and phrases. They require good hand coordination but allow for limited range of motion. On-screen keyboards (virtual keyboards) are software programs that provide the image of a standard or modified keyboard on the computer screen. The user can access these "keys" via different input systems such as a Tracker, Touch Window, trackball, joystick, and eye gaze system.

Mouse emulators. Mouse emulators are systems that the computer reads like a standard mouse. The most common type of mouse emulators are the different head-controlled pointing devices. The Touch Window also is a mouse emulator. Using this system, the child activates the computer by touching its transparent surface. Other mouse emulators include the Headmaster, HeadMouse, and Tracker (Figure 19-6). These systems work with a virtual keyboard often located at the bottom of the monitor screen. The child looks at the letter or word that he or she wishes to select or activate. A box on top of the monitor "reads" the child's head position and sends data to the computer. The cursor rests on the specific letter or picture on the screen. The child then hits a switch to make a choice or uses a dwell typing option (leaves the cursor on the letter for a specified amount of time so that the computer will select that letter as if it had been typed).

Voice recognition. Voice (or speech) recognition systems, in which the computer recognizes and translates voice sounds into text or commands, are a good option for individuals with severe motoric limitations (e.g., high-level spinal cord injuries or spinal muscular atrophy). The user must have fair-to-good articulation to successfully operate a voice recognition system. The child speaks into a microphone to enter text, control the mouse, and execute computer commands. These systems are commonly available for IBM-compatible machines. Dragon Naturally Speaking is one example of a voice recognition system. These systems can be sensitive to environmental noise, especially in areas in which the noise level is high, such as a classroom. Voice recognition systems generally are not used with children under 12 years of age because of the complexity of the system.

Other input systems. Other types of input systems used with children include eye gaze systems, Braille, and a Tongue Touch Keypad. Eye gaze systems are costly at this time. They require the child to visually focus on a desired position on the computer monitor. An optic light on the computer "reads" where the child gazes and makes the appropriate selection. When typing, eye gaze systems use on-screen keyboards and other systems. Several programs allow a child who is blind or who has a significant visual impairment to input into the computer

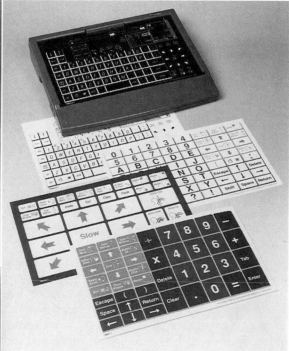

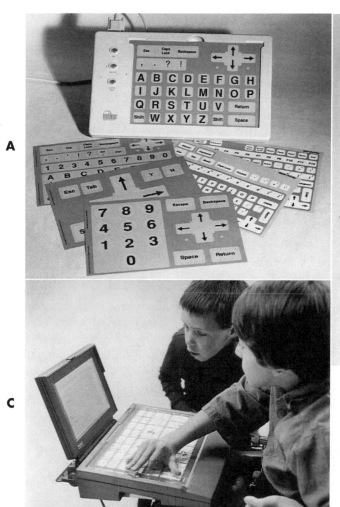

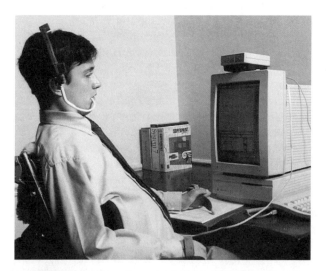

figure**19-5** Examples of alternate keyboards. **A,** IntelliKeys with alphabet overlay. *(Courtesy of IntelliTools, Richmond, CA).* **B,** KeyLargo and overlay examples. **C,** KeyLargo used with a powerbook. *(Photo courtesy Don Johnston, Inc., Wauconda, IL.)*

figure**19-6** Young man using the Headmaster with a sip and puff switch. *(Photo courtesy of Prentke Romich Co., Wooster, OH.)*

using Braille. The Tongue Touch Keypad has nine tongue-activated keys that the child activates. Once the user activates the keys, a signal is sent to an interface box connected to the computer. The keypad fits into the mouth like an orthodontic retainer.

Output systems and information processing

Computer output can also accommodate the needs of individuals with disabilities. Information (output) from the computer is visually displayed on the monitor or printed from the printer. Output can be auditory or auditory with visual. Monitors are the most common output devices, are available in various sizes, and can be mounted at various angles. For a child with a visual impairment, perceptual impairment, and/or cognitive impairment, the therapist may need to consider adaptations to the monitor. These may include the size of the monitor, whether it displays the data in color or black and white, the size of the text on the monitor, reduction of glare from the window or overhead lights, magnification of the screen, and change of contrast. The printer is the second most common way to receive information from the computer. A child with physical impairments may have difficulty managing the printer independently and thus may need assistance. A child with cognitive impairments may have difficulty learning how to independently operate the printer, and a child with visual impairments may have difficulty reading the text if the font is small. Some printers provide Braille output, and several software programs provide voice output. Some of these programs read text, whereas others provide output regarding all the functions of the computer. Voice output systems can help support learning and computer use and exploration for students with learning disabilities, cognitive delays, autism, and visual impairments.

Output and successful processing of information are often closely related. Careful attention by the occupational therapist and team can mean the difference between success or failure with a device. If children with disabilities cannot successfully process and use the information received from the computer in a meaningful and functional manner, then they will not use the system over time. Therapists often overlook the visual-perceptual demands that some software programs can place on children. With the increased screen resolution and the complexity of graphics now available in the computers, some children with visual-perceptual difficulties are finding the visual information they receive distracting or overwhelming. For example, a child who has poor figure-ground skills may have difficulty with the Living Books Programs. This software program allows the computer to read popular stories to the child, but the graphics can be cluttered and complex. The therapist can also use this software program to help improve visual-perceptual skills, but he or she needs to be careful to provide the "just right challenge" so that the child does not become overwhelmed.

Software

With the burgeoning number of software programs available, from simple to highly complex, the therapist needs to make careful decisions to find programs that match children's interests and skills. Many children with disabilities can use common software programs that are available to everyone. Often software programs require that the child make specific, discrete responses to visual, auditory, or tactile stimuli. The child must be able to attend briefly and have the interest and motivation to activate a toy or a computer purposefully. Object permanence and understanding of cause-effect relationships are typically prerequisite skills for any computer program. However, the therapist can also use computer activities and programs to teach some of these prerequisite skills, such as sustained attention and cause-effect relationships. Most computer programs also require skills in discrimination, matching, and directionality. Public domain software are available to work on cause-effect relationships and switch use.

Edmark, a software development company, has various learning programs appropriate for children of all ages. For example, the Early Learning House Series is a series of programs that work on early reading, math, science, and geography concepts through exploration and discovery. The educational version of these programs comes with a built-in single-switch scanning option. In addition to the concepts that the programs were designed to address, they also address skills such as visual perception, eye-hand coordination, visual motor skills, memory skills, sequencing skills, auditory processing, and listening skills. Another example of Edmark software is the Imagination Express Series, which works on story development and composition skills and allows children to create interactive stories using words and pictures. Sunburst, Davidson, and Laureate are other examples of software development companies that the therapist can consider when seeking different software programs appropriate for children with disabilities.

Computer software is also available that helps support the learning or computer use of children with disabilities. For example, therapists can use rate-enhancement software programs with standard or alternative input devices to increase the efficiency with which users complete written work or use alternative input devices. Examples of rate-enhancement software include abbreviation expansion and word prediction. Abbreviation expansion allows users to type in a short code that is later turned into a longer text. For example, a student with a spinal cord injury who uses a head-controlled pointing device may use abbreviation expansion to type his or her return address on college admissions applications. By typing "pra," the computer will expand this to include name, address, and phone number with correct spacing and spelling. Thus by typing three letters, the user can make an entire entry of 50 or more characters. To use abbreviated expansion, the user will need to be able to remember the codes or refer to a list of codes when needed.

Word processing programs also use word prediction to increase the speed and efficiency with which a child types by decreasing the number of keystrokes needed to complete a word. Word prediction predicts words based on 1 to 2 letters the child types. As the child types the letters, a list of words are presented on the computer screen (Figure 19-7). These words are typically a combination of commonly used words that fit the grammar of the sentence and/or the writing style of the child. For example, if the child types "s," the program lists "some," "someone," "speech," and "style." The lists of words can generally be two to eight words long and may be read to the user and presented visually. Once the program presents the list, the child either presses a number by the de-

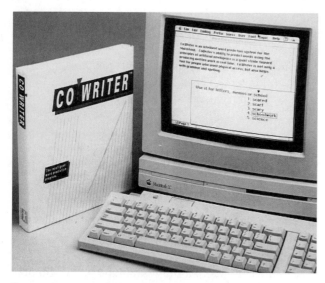

figure**19-7** Co:Writer word prediction software. *(Photo courtesy Don Johnston, Inc., Wauconda, IL.)*

sired word or continues typing until the program presents the desired word. Higher cognitive skills and a basic reading level are needed for the child to successfully use this system.

Computer Application and Intervention Techniques

With all the different input and output methods and software programs available, computers offer many ways to help children develop functional independence in life roles. The therapist should introduce children with disabilities who can benefit from the use of a computer as early as possible. They can have opportunities to use computers throughout their school careers and into their work settings. Children can also use computers as environmental control devices and for play and leisure exploration.

Early intervention

As mentioned previously, therapists are using computers with 1- and 2-year-old children. In early intervention programs, therapists typically use the computer as an educational tool to help support and develop prerequisite skills for learning. Various early learning software programs and simple input systems are available. For many young children with and without disabilities, the standard keyboard may be too complex. Input systems such as the Touch Window, a switch, and/or a mouse can simplify the cognitive and motor demands that the child faces when working on the computer. Young children can also learn simple computer functions such as putting in a disc, opening a program, and turning the computer on and off. Since many young children love to

explore, there are software programs that limit the files and programs on a computer desktop that a child can access. For example, Kids Desk by Edmark allows a second desktop to be developed specifically for the child. Thus the child cannot explore or delete any adult files or programs.

Case Study 1: Jeremy*

Jeremy is a 2 year old with Down syndrome. His family wants to provide every opportunity for him to develop cognitive skills. They plan for him to attend regular education classrooms as he gets older and have stated "with the proper stimulation and intervention, Jeremy can learn to do anything." They were recently at a conference and heard about computers as tools for supporting learning and educational performance for some children with Down syndrome. They asked the early intervention team to recommend a computer system and software to use with Jeremy. What would you recommend?

School

Computers are used to help promote learning and productivity in the classroom. This includes activities such as writing, graphic designing, and searching the World Wide Web. Many high-quality programs support children with disabilities in science and math classes. Occupational therapists working in schools support team decision making regarding computer adaptations, software recommendations, and training and implementation. Children with learning disabilities, motoric limitations, progressive illnesses, and cognitive limitations may have difficulties in written communication. It is often helpful for these children to transition from handwriting to text generation or word processing skills. Therapists combine hardware solutions (e.g., alternative keyboards) with software solutions (e.g., work prediction or write out loud) to promote students' success in written communication.

In schools it is common for various students to use one computer. This means that when changes are made to a base device, such as the addition of peripherals or software programs, the other students and teachers who use the system have to be willing to tolerate the changes. School-based occupational therapists are often involved in training other users of the systems how to work around the changes if the system is not dedicated to one student.

Case Study 2: Linnea

Linnea is a third-grade student with spinal muscular atrophy. She is fully included in her neighborhood school

*There is no one correct answer to any of the case studies in the following sections. Tables 19-6, 19-7 and Appendix A provide resources that the therapist can use when problem solving potential solutions to each case study. Appendix B provides the reader with solutions that one AT team recommended for each case study.

with support from related services as needed. Recently, she has been complaining to her parents and therapists that her hand gets tired when writing and that her handwriting looks "sloppy." Her teacher also has noticed that she seems irritable and lacks concentration during class. Linnea, her family, and her therapists have discussed using computers for written communication in the past, but Linnea and her family have always been reluctant to explore this at length because she does not want to "look different." Linnea has had experience with computers since kindergarten. Her class goes to the computer lab three times a week, and she began learning basic keyboarding skills in second grade. Her classroom has two computers that students use for drill, practice, and special projects. How would you address these concerns?

Prevocational

When students use AT in school, there is often an emphasis on inclusion and "normalcy" versus production (Dudgeon, Massagli, & Ross, 1997). This becomes an issue as students transition from the classroom to a school-to-career program. Regardless of the level of physical and/or cognitive difficulty, if a student is going to use AT within a career setting, he or she must be able to be productive and efficient with the system. Bersani, Fried-Oken, Anctil, Staehely, and Bowser (1999) stated that for an adolescent to be successful at using AT in a work setting, the occupational therapist must carefully plan the transition with AT addressed at every step of the planning process. To support AT use, the therapist may work with the educational team in determining how to adapt the environment, task, and/or computer setup. When a student with cognitive disabilities expresses interest in a job that involves computer input and simple word processing, a therapist considers hardware and software adaptations, environmental adaptations such as decreasing distractions, background color or font changes on the computer, and/or a consistent and predictable workspace. To ensure carryover with the student's caregivers and perspective employer, the therapist may develop step-by-step cheat sheets with words or pictures for directions, a drawing of a simple schematic, and/or color coding areas for attaching the peripherals. Establishing the student's success with AT is critical to his or her success in employment and community living.

Case Study 3: Margy

Margy is 17 years old and has cognitive impairments and attention-deficit hyperactivity disorder (ADHD). During her last transition individualized education program (IEP), her family expressed the desire for Margy to get a job in the family carpet cleaning business. Margy enjoys greeting people, and others enjoy her bubbly and outgoing personality, so her dad and mother felt that it would be good if she could work with the receptionist in the front office of their business. Her dad felt that she should have more responsibility than simply greeting customers. He said that Margy has always enjoyed working on the computer and recommended that she learn data entry on the computer to make productive use of her down time when she was not talking with a customer. The team agreed that this could be a reasonable expectation for Margy and worked to develop a plan to reach this goal. Describe a plan that evidences multidisciplinary input.

Environmental control

Some computer systems can double as environmental control units. Combining functions in the child's computer provides him or her with one system for several different functions and can be cost-effective since potentially fewer systems need to be purchased. Several different hardware and/or software systems support environmental control systems through the computer. These systems can be simple, such as operating a compact disc (CD) player or answering machine, or complex, such as operating several different environmental controls (e.g., unlocking and opening the front door; controlling lights and ceiling fans; and turning televisions, radios, and other small appliances on and off).

Case Study 4: Eric

Eric is 15 years old and has severe athetoid cerebral palsy. The only control that he has is dorsiflexion of his right foot. He attends general education classrooms and works independently on his computer. This year he received a new computer system. He completes all of his homework assignments via a row-column scanning system. He uses an IBM-compatible computer with Microsoft Office and word prediction software. He uses dorsiflexion of his right foot to execute the scanning. He is active on the Internet. He also writes plays for his high school football team. He would like to have some environmental control using his computer when he is in his room. What would you recommend?

Play and leisure

Many individuals who have a personal home computer use them for play and leisure activities and for work. If a student has access to a computer at home or other frequently visited settings, the therapist and educational team may want to explore whether it would be a viable tool for leisure activities. Providing opportunities for play or leisure activities may help the student become more familiar with the system and its operation. Various software programs combine learning with leisure-type activities. The occupational therapist can work with children to determine which programs and leisure activities are most interesting and recommend adaptations for access (Swinth & Anson, 1998).

Case Study 5: Ryan

Ryan is 6 years old and has autism. His family is constantly looking for appropriate play activities that he can do independently for 5 to 6 minutes at a time. Many independent play activities are not appropriate because they would lead into his self-stimulation behaviors. Ryan is intrigued when his older siblings are doing their homework on the computer. He had erased several papers from the computer when a sibling turned his or her back and Ryan happened to hit the wrong button on the keyboard. Given Ryan's interests and behaviors, what would you recommend?

■ ALTERNATIVE AND AUGMENTATIVE COMMUNICATION

Alternative and augmentative communication (AAC) is defined as communication that does not require speech and that can be individualized to the unique needs of the individual. An AAC system uses a combination of all the methods of communication available to a child. This can include "any residual speech, vocalizations, gestures, and communicative behaviors in addition to specific communication strategies and communication aids" (Doster & Politano, 1996, p. 7). The overall purpose of AAC is to enable an individual to be able to transmit a message to another individual. As stated by the National Joint Committee for the Communications of Persons with Severe Disabilities (1992), "all persons, regardless of the extent or severity of their disabilities, have a basic right to affect, through communication, the conditions of their own existence." In addition to this basic right, they have also outlined 12 specific communication rights that should be ensured during all daily communication acts with persons with disabilities (Box 19-5).

AAC devices include low-tech systems, such as communication boards and picture exchange systems, and high-tech electronic devices. Often, both speech and language pathologists and occupational therapists work together to select and train children to use AAC. Both have unique perspectives and skills to offer in this specialized area. Occupational therapists should be familiar with terminology used in the area of AAC, such as *single-switch scanning selection, encoding, directed scanning,* and *direct selection* (Angelo & Smith, 1989). Additionally, occupational therapists working in the area of AAC should be able to use strategies that facilitate communication (Box 19-6). Continuing education courses and additional training can familiarize therapists with the terminology, communication strategies, and available hardware and software.

AAC can be viewed through several continuums, including aided or unaided communication methods and low-tech or high-tech devices. Depending on their age,

contexts, and skills, children use a combination of aided and unaided communication and a combination of low- and high-tech devices. Unaided communication consists of vocalizations, gestures, facial expressions, sign language, and pantomime. All communicators use some sort of combination of unaided communication. Children with disabilities often use a higher incidence of ges-

---

box 19-5 *Basic communication rights*

1. The right to request desired objects, actions, events, and persons and to express personal preferences or feelings
2. The right to be offered choices and alternatives
3. The right to reject or refuse undesired objects, events, or actions, including the right to decline or reject all proffered choices
4. The right to request and be given attention from and interaction with another person
5. The right to request feedback or information about a state, object, person, or event of interest
6. The right to active treatment and intervention efforts to enable people with severe disabilities to communicate messages in whatever modes and as effectively and efficiently as their specific abilities will allow
7. The right to have communication acts acknowledged and responded to, even when the responder cannot fulfill the intent of these acts
8. The right to have access at all times to any needed augmentative and alternative communication devices and other assistive devices and to have those devices in good working order
9. The right to environmental contexts, interactions, and opportunities that expect and encourage persons with disabilities to participate as full communicative partners with other people, including peers
10. The right to be informed about the people, things, and events in one's immediate environment
11. The right to be communicated with in a manner that recognizes and acknowledges the inherent dignity of the person being addressed, including the right to be a part of communication exchanges about individuals that are conducted in his or her presence
12. The right to be communicated with in ways that are meaningful, understandable, and culturally and linguistically appropriate

From National Joint Committee for the Communication Needs of Persons with Severe Disabilities. (1992). Guidelines for meeting the communication needs of persons with severe disabilities. *ASHA, 34* (March, Supp. 7), 1-8.

tures, facial expressions, and/or body language as allowed by their functional skills.

Aided communication systems are also sometimes referred to as *nonelectronic* or *electronic communication aids*. Nonelectronic aids include communication boards and picture exchange systems, which use pictures, symbols, and words to communicate messages. Types of symbols include Blissymbolics, Rebus, and PicSyms (Figure 19-8). AAC users point to a picture or symbol to

communicate messages and desires. As a child becomes more proficient in the use of pictures and symbols, complex communication boards can be developed to transmit messages (Figure 19-9). These systems can be mounted to a wheelchair tray, put in a notebook that the child carries, or mounted on a series of cards that the child gives to another individual when he or she wants to communicate ideas.

High-tech electronic communication aids generally are either computer-based systems or dedicated systems. Occupational therapists often consider computer-based systems for children who are using or will be using some

---

box **19-6** *Strategies to facilitate communicative interaction*

1. Structure the environment to foster interaction.
2. Attend to the child. Solicit a shared focus.
3. Provide meaningful opportunities for communication.
4. Have realistic expectations for the child.
5. Provide appropriate language input.
6. Avoid yes/no questions and "test" questions.
7. Pace the interaction. Give the student time to communicate. WAIT.
8. Follow the child's lead. Respond to his or her attempts to communicate.
9. Provide models for the child's expressive modes of communication. Coach the child as needed.
10. Prompt if necessary. Remember to fade prompts to natural cues. Enjoy communication.

Adapted from Special Education Technology Center, Ellensburg, WA.

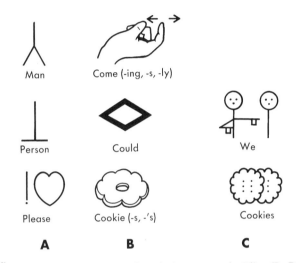

figure **19-8**   Examples of symbol systems. **A,** Bliss. **B,** Rebus. **C,** Picsyms.

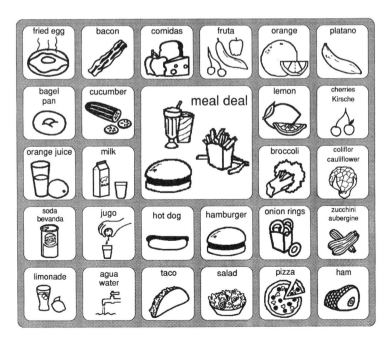

figure **19-9**   Example of a communication board that the child can use at meal time. *(Photo courtesy of Mayer-Johnson Co.)*

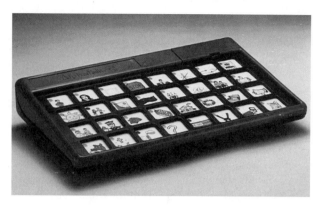

figure**19-10** This dedicated augmentative and alternative communication device uses Minspeak on its keyboard. *(Photo courtesy of Prentke Romich Co., Wooster, OH.)*

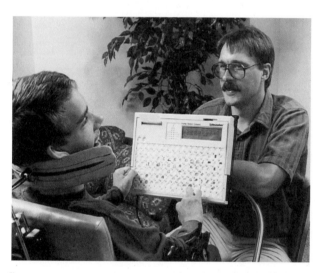

figure**19-11** Young man communicating with a Liberator. *(Photo courtesy of Prentke Romich Co., Wooster, OH.)*

sort of computer-assistive technology. Ideally, computer-based systems should be able to be mounted on wheelchairs or easily portable in some other manner. Dedicated systems operate primarily as electronic communication aids (Figure 19-10). These systems are available in various sizes and weights and provide auditory, visual, and/or printed output.

Examples of these high-tech electronic systems include devices such as the Intro Talker, the Voice Pal (Adapt Tech), the Delta Talker (formally the Touch Talker), the Vanguard and DynaVox. All electronic communication devices are programmed with individualized overlays. The board's overlays can indicate as few as 2 and as many as 128 choices to the child. The Voice Pal is easy to program, durable, portable, and inexpensive. It works via pads attached to real objects. It is a simple and effective communication system that the occupational therapist can use to reinforce the learning of cause-effect relation-

ships. The Delta Talker is activated by touch, whereas the Light Talker has numerous selection techniques, including direct selection using an optic light, row column scanning, direct scanning, and Morse code. Advanced systems include devices such as the Vanguard Liberator (Figure 19-11) or DynaVox. The Liberator is an advanced communication system with the overlay options similar to the Light Talker and Delta Talker. It is portable and flexible and can be activated either through touch or the optic light via direct selection or scanning. It is programmed similar to the Delta Talker and the Light Talker but has some additional computer-like functions, such as a notebook for taking notes. Another advanced communication system is the DynaVox (available from Sentient Systems Technology, Inc.), which has a dynamical liquid crystal display and from 1 to 60 "key" areas on a single screen. The user can input via the touch screen; single, dual, and joystick switching; and visual and auditory scanning. The dynamical display offers thousands of graphics (some that are electronically animated) and text options. Unlike other communication systems in which the user is limited to one overlay, the display on the DynaVox changes (using the same message-formation process that produces natural speech) given the choices of the user.

Computer-based and dedicated communication aids provide different types of voice outputs. Digitized speech is stored by recording the sound or message. The speech output of the system sounds like the voice of the person who dictates into the system. Synthesized speech sounds like a computerized voice but has the advantage of text-to-speech capabilities. The intelligibility of synthesized speech can vary depending on the type of system. As in computer-assistive technology, different rate enhancement options are available for high-tech, electronic communication systems. To allow a child to communicate faster than the rate of keying in text, encoding (or symbol) systems are used. A primary encoding system used in the Liberator, Vanguard, and DynaVox is Minspeak. This language uses sequenced multiple-meaning icons to retrieve words, phrases, or sentences. Like word prediction, many communication systems come with message prediction. Some of the more advanced systems can learn the communication "style" of the user and begin to predict with greater accuracy.

Case Study 6: Lisa

Lisa is a 4-year-old preschool student with spastic tetraplegia cerebral palsy. She does not have cognitive delays. Her oral motor skills are poor, making vocalizations inconsistent and unintelligible. Lisa is able to communicate basic needs through gestures and facial expressions. She also has a communication board using PicSyms mounted on her wheelchair. She is efficient with these modes of communication within her home and preschool environment, but the team is concerned about her ability to communicate more complex messages as she moves on in her educational and community settings. What might the team consider for Lisa?

Case Study 7: Jim

Jim is a 16-year-old male adolescent with a recent head injury from a motorcycle accident. He has poor expressive language, poor fine motor skills, and poor oral motor control as a result of the brain damage. He is reluctant to use any type of electronic communication device. What would you recommend for Jim?

▪ SUMMARY

Since the technology available is rapidly changing, the therapist must make an ongoing effort to stay abreast of what is available and what technology has become obsolete. By reading the current literature and research on technology for children, the occupational therapist can effectively match the needs of clients with the available technology and can prepare children and families to use it to its greatest potential. Smith (1991) presented the following as competencies and responsibilities for occupational therapists who desire to work in the area of AT:

1. To become a technology problem solver by using AT to increase an individual's functional independence
2. To see oneself as the human technology and environmental expert
3. To gain a basic comfort level with low and high technology
4. To gain a basic literacy in technology-related areas
5. To understand one's limits in the area of AT
6. To understand the ethical issues surrounding the use of AT

Various resources on the World Wide Web can help occupational therapists stay current with all the changes in AT (see Appendix A). Children who use AT at an early age have the advantage of developing with AT and using it to their benefit throughout their lives. Recent advances in AT allow many devices to grow and expand with the child during the developmental years and into adolescence and adulthood as they transition into higher education and community work experiences. With the current pace of progress and research, future AT will offer greater ease of use, wider application, assistance in additional areas of function, and more availability as a result of lower costs. Computer use, environmental control, and communication can enhance ADL skills, interaction with others, and learning capabilities of children with disabilities at all ages. Selecting and implementing an AT system for children with disabilities requires effective teaming, including the family in decision making and problem solving, and a solid match to the child's skills and limitations, the family's concerns and resources, the child's environments, and desired occupations.

STUDY QUESTIONS

1. The occupational therapist is asked to evaluate the computer lab of an elementary school for accessibility for all students. This school has a range of students with disabilities, including several with learning disabilities, mental retardation, and motor impairments. What are aspects of the environment that the therapist should evaluate? What recommendations should the therapist make regarding the computers, input devices, and output alternatives to improve accessibility for all students?

2. Give three alternative solutions so that children with ataxia and intentional tremor of their arms and hands can successfully use a computer keyboard and mouse.

3. List three types of scanning and methods of indirect selection. Describe the characteristics of a child who would benefit most from and be most successful with these methods.

4. The Touch Window is commonly available in preschool classrooms. Describe a child who would successfully use the touch window and would prefer this method of computer access over other methods.

5. List advantages of using a computer as an augmentative communication device. List disadvantages of using a computer rather than a dedicated augmentative communication device. Explore the advantages and disadvantages with a speech therapist with expertise in augmentative communication.

6. In the case study of Margy, a team of occupational, physical, and speech therapists worked with her so that she successfully entered employment. Describe potential roles of each therapist in her intervention program.

References

Abramson, L.Y., Seligman, M.E.P., & Teasdale, J.D. (1978). Learned helplessness in humans: Critique and reformation. *Journal of Abnormal Psychology, 87* (l), 49-74.

Angelo, J., & Smith, R.O. (1989). The critical role of occupational therapy in augmentative communication services. In *Technology review '89: Perspective on occupational therapy practice.* Rockville, MD: AOTA.

Anson, D.K. (1997). *Alternative computer access: A guide to selection.* Philadelphia, PA: FA Davis.

Bain, B.K., & Leger, D. (1997). *Assistive technology: An interdisciplinary approach.* New York: Churchill Livingstone.

Batavia, A.I., & Hammer, G.S. (1990). Toward the development of consumer-based criteria for the evaluation of assistive devices. *Journal of Rehabilitation Research and Development, 27* (4), 425-436.

Behrmann, M.M. (1984). A brighter future for early learning through high tech. *The Pointer, 28* (2), 23-26.

Behrmann, M.M., Jones, J.K., & Wilds, M.L. (1989). Technology intervention for very young children with disabilities. *Infants and Young Children, 1* (4), 66-77.

Bersani, H., Fried-Oken, M., Anctil, T., Staehely, J., & Bowser, G. (1999). *Transitioning from high school with assistive technology: The good, the bad and the ugly.* Paper presented at the CEC conference on assistive technology. Portland: OR.

Beukelman, D.R., & Mirenda, P. (1992). *Augmentative and alternative communication: Management of severe communication disorders in children and adults.* Baltimore: Brookes.

Bowser, G. (1989). *Computers in the early intervention curriculum.* Oregon Technology Access Project, Oregon Department of Education.

Bowser, G., & Reed, P. (1998). *Education TECH points: A framework for assistive technology planning.* Winchester, OR: Coalition for Assistive Technology in Oregon.

Brooks, N.A., & Hoyer, E.A. (1989). *Consumer evaluation of assistive devices.* (Abstract). Proceedings of the RESNA 12th Annual Conference. (pp. 358-359). New Orleans.

Bushrow, K.M., & Turner, K.D. (1994). Overcoming barriers in the use of adaptive and assistive technology in special education. In D. Montgomery (Ed.), *Rural partnerships: Working together.* Proceedings of the Annual National Conference of the American Council on Rural Special Education (ACRES). (pp. 448-454).

Church, G., & Glennen, S. (1992). Assistive technology programs. In G. Church & S. Glennen (Eds.), *The handbook of assistive technology* (pp. 1-26). San Diego: Singular Publishing Group.

Cook, A., & Hussey, S. (1995). *Assistive technologies: Principles and practice.* St. Louis: Mosby.

Coster, W. (1998). Occupation-centered assessment of children. *The American Journal of Occupational Therapy, 52* (5), 337-344.

Dickey, R., & Shealey, S.H. (1987). Using technology to control the environment. *The American Journal of Occupational Therapy, 41* (11), 717-721.

Doster, S., & Politano, P. (1996). Augmentative and alternative communication. In J. Hammel (Ed.), *AOTA self-paced clinical course: Technology and occupational therapy: A link to function.* Rockville, MD: AOTA.

Douglas, J., Reeson, B., & Ryan, M. (1988). Computer microtechnology for a severely disabled preschool child. *Child Care: Health and Development, 14,* 93-104.

Dudgeon, B.J., Massagli, T.L., & Ross, B.W. (1997). Educational participation of children with spinal cord injury. *The American Journal of Occupational Therapy, 51,* 553-561.

Dunn, W., Brown, C., & McGuigan, A. (1994). The ecology of human performance: A framework for considering the effect of context. *The American Journal of Occupational Therapy, 48,* 595-607.

Education for All Handicapped Children Act of 1975 (P.L. 94-142). 20 U.S.C. Secs. 1400-1485.

Education of the Handicapped Act Amendments of 1986 (P.L. 99-457). 20 U.S.C. Secs. 1400-1485.

Foulds, R.A. (1982). Applications of microcomputers in the education of the physically disabled child. *Exceptional Children, 49* (2),143-162.

Garber, S.L., & Gregorio, T.E. (1990). Upper extremity assistive devices: Assessment of use by spinal cord-injured patients with quadriplegia. *The American Journal of Occupational Therapy, 44* (2), 126-131.

Gargiulo, R.M., & O'Sullivan, P.S. (1986). Mildly mentally retarded and nonretarded children's learned helplessness. *American Journal of Mental Deficiency, 91,* 203-206.

Glickman, L., Deitz, J., Anson, D., & Stewart, K. (1996). Effect of switch control site on computer skills of infants and toddlers. *The American Journal of Occupational Therapy, 50* (7), 545-553.

Individuals with Disabilities Education Act. (P.L. 101-476). (1990). 20 U.S.C. Secs. 1400-1485.

Individuals With Disabilities Education Act Amendments of 1990. (P.L. 105-17). (1997). 62 Fed. Reg. 55068.

Kincaid, C. (1999). Alternative keyboards. *Exceptional Parent, Feb,* 34-35.

Krefting, L.H., & Krefting, D.V. (1991). Cultural influences on performance. In C. Christiansen & C. Baum (Eds.), *Occupational therapy: Overcoming human performance deficits* (pp. 101-124). Thorogrove, NJ: Slack Incorporated.

Lahm, E.A. (Ed.). (1989). *Technology with low incidence populations: Promoting access and learning.* Reston, VA: The Council for Exceptional Children.

Law, M., Cooper, B., Strong, S., Stewart, D., Rigby, P., & Letts, L. (1996). The person-environment-occupation model: A transactive approach to occupational performance. *Canadian Journal of Occupational Therapy, 63* (1), 9-23.

Maier, S.F., & Seligman, M.E. (1976). Learned helplessness: Theory and evidence. *Journal of Experimental Psychology: General, 105* (l), 3-46.

National Joint Committee for the Communication Needs of Persons with Severe Disabilities. (1992). Guidelines for meeting the communication needs of persons with severe disabilities. *ASHA, 34* (March, Supp. 7), 1-8.

Olson, L.J. (1999). Psychosocial frame of reference. In P. Kramer & J. Hinojosa (Eds.), *Frames of reference for pediatric occupational therapy* (2nd ed. pp. 323-376). Baltimore: Lippincott Williams & Wilkins.

Parette, H.P., & VanBiervliet, A. (1990). A prospective inquiry into technology needs and practices of school-aged children with disabilities. *Journal of Special Education Technology, 10* (4), 198-206.

Phillips, B., & Zhao, H. (1993). Predictors of assistive technology abandonment. *Assistive Technology, 5* (1), 36-45.

Rehabilitation Act Amendments of 1992. (P.L. 102-569). (October 29, 1992). Title 29, U.S.C. 701 et seq: *U.S. Statutes at Large, 100,* 4344-4488.

Rehabilitation Society of North America (RESNA). (1992). *Assistive technology and the individualized education program.* Washington, DC: RESNA Press.

Royeen, C.B., & Duncan, M. (1999). Acquisitional frame of reference. In P. Kramer & J. Hinojosa (Eds.), *Frames of reference for pediatric occupational therapy* (2nd ed. pp. 377-400). Baltimore: Lippincott Williams & Wilkins.

Scherer, M.J. (1993). *Living in the state of stuck: How technology impacts the lives of people with disabilities.* Cambridge, MA: Brookline Books.

Scherer, M.J., & Lane, J.P. (1997). Assessing consumer profiles of "ideal" assistive technologies in ten categories: An integration of quantitative and qualitative methods. *Disability and Rehabilitation, 19* (12), 528-535.

Scherer, M.J., & McKee, B.G. (1989). *But will the assistive technology device be used?* (Abstract). Proceedings of the RESNA 12th Annual Conference. (pp. 356-357). New Orleans.

Sibert, R.I. (1997). Financing assistive technology: An overview of public funding sources. *Technology Special Interest Section Newsletter, 7* (2), 1-4.

Smith, R.O. (1991). Technological applications for enhancing human performance. In C. Christiansen & C. Baum (Eds.), *Human performance deficits.* Thorofare, NJ: Slack.

Struck, M. (1996). Augmentative communication and computer access. In J. Case-Smith, A.S. Allen, & P.N. Pratt (Eds.), *Occupational therapy for children* (3rd ed.). St. Louis: Mosby.

Swinth, Y.L. (1997). *The meaning of assistive technology in the lives of high school students and their families.* Unpublished doctoral dissertation, University of Washington, Seattle.

Swinth, Y.L. (1998). Assistive technology in early intervention: Theory and practice. In J. Case-Smith (Ed), *Pediatric occupational therapy and early intervention* (2nd ed.). Woburn, MA: Butterworth-Heinemann.

Swinth, Y.L., & Anson, D. (1998). Alternatives to handwriting: Keyboarding and text-generation techniques for schools. In J. Case-Smith (Ed.), *AOTA self-paced clinical course: Occupational therapy: Making a difference in school system practice.* Rockville, MD: AOTA.

Swinth, Y.L., Anson, D., & Deitz, J., (1993). A descriptive study of young children using a single-switch system for computer access. *The American Journal of Occupational Therapy, 47* (11), 1031-1038.

Symington, L. (1990). Pre-computer skills for young children. *Exceptional Children, Jan/Feb,* 36-38.

Technology-Related Assistance for Individuals with Disabilities Act of 1988. (P.L. 100-407). 34 C.F.R. Secs. 00.16.

Trefler, E., & Hobson, D. (1997). Assistive technology. In C. Christiansen & C. Baum (Eds.), *Occupational therapy: Enabling function and well-being* (2nd ed. pp. 482-506). Thorofare, NJ: Slack.

Todis, M., & Walker, H.M. (1993). User perspectives on assistive technology in educational settings. *Focus on Exceptional Children, 46* (3), 1-16.

Wehmeyer, M.L. (1996). Self-determination as an educational outcome: Why is it important to children, youth, and adults with disabilities? In D.J. Sands & M.L. Wehmeyer (Eds.), *Self-determination across the life span: Independence and choice for people with disabilities.* (pp. 17-36). Baltimore: Paul H. Brookes.

Weisz, J.R. (1979). Perceived control and learned helplessness among mentally retarded and nonretarded children: A developmental analysis. *Developmental Psychology, 15* (3), 311-319.

Additional Resources Available on the World Wide Web

The primary goal of this chapter is to present general principles for decision making and problem solving for occupational therapy practitioners when providing assistive technology (AT) services. The author has endeavored to offer guidelines and thoughts for providing services in this area rather than a cookbook of specific strategies. Each child an occupational therapist encounters is special and unique. Thus each AT solution is as unique as the child who uses the system. New systems and software continually become available. However, because of funding issues and the appropriateness of some of the older systems, many of these systems will continue to be used by children with disabilities for years to come. Thus service delivery in this specialty area often is a blending of the old and the new.

To be an effective service provider, occupational therapy practitioners must develop and use strategies to stay current with a rapidly changing field. One way to do this is to use the vast amount of information available on the World Wide Web. The following are some websites to consider. Many of these sites have links to other sites and will support both the novice and the expert in this service area to provide quality services to the children and families with whom they work.

Apple Computer's Worldwide Disability Solutions Group
www.apple.com/disability/welcome.html

IBM's Special Needs Solutions
www.austin.ibm.com/pspinfo/snshome.html

Assistive Technology OnLine (provides extensive information on AT, including research)
www.asel.udel.edu/at-online/assistive/html

Information regarding online AT classes and other resources
snow.utoronto.ca/coursereg.html

Resource pages with links to other popular AT sites and examples of student projects
otpt.ups.edu/AT/home.html

A full resource list of websites related to disability and AT as well as links to numerous other websites
weber.u.washington.edu/~doit/Brochures/internet_resources.html

Alternate keyboards and accessories
www.cs.princeto.edu/~dwallach/tifaq/keyboards.html

Information regarding AT and links to additional resources
www.abledata.com

Center on Information Technology Accommodation
www.gsa.gov/coca

Equal Access for Software and Information
www.rit.edu/~easi

Trace Center
www.trace.wisc.edu

Canadian website with information in English and French
omeg.dawsoncollege.qc.ca/adaptech

Potential Solutions for Case Studies

Case Study 1: Jeremy

The occupational therapist began her evaluation by asking the parents if they just wanted Jeremy to use the computer at the early intervention program or if they would be using it at home. The family stated that money was not an object and that they would purchase whatever Jeremy needed. Jeremy's father said that he has an old Macintosh SE with a color monitor and CD-ROM drive at home. The therapist and team then evaluated Jeremy's skills on the computer. They found that he could touch individual keys on the standard keyboard but that he would become distracted and play with the keyboard versus watching the computer screen. They also tried several different mice but found them to be too complex for Jeremy. However, when they tried the Touch Window with Jeremy, he demonstrated sustained interaction with a cause-effect program for 4 minutes. The speech therapist commented that this was one of the longest times that she had seen Jeremy maintain on-task behavior.

The team decided to start with a Touch Window input device and use software that provided both visual and auditory output for Jeremy. His father set up his old computer, and the team had a Macintosh computer with a Touch Window that Jeremy could use when at the 0-3 center. The family and therapists decided to use various types of early learning and interactive software with Jeremy.

The parents wanted to make sure that Jeremy would have the opportunity to learn the standard keyboard and mouse as computer input systems. The occupational therapist stated that it was too early to determine if these would be viable options for Jeremy, but the team agreed to meet again in 6 months to discuss his progress and goals for computer access and use.

Case Study 2: Linnea

With the changes in Linnea's performance in the classroom, she and her family began discussing other options for written communication in addition to the traditional paper and pencil. Linnea and her family felt that her irritability and lack of concentration in the classroom may be due to fatigue, and her therapists agreed. The team decided to work with a local AT center and provide Linnea and her family with opportunities to explore different options.

Linnea's father is a computer specialist and wanted to be actively involved with the process. Because Linnea is in general education classrooms and has a full schedule when at school, the team decided to set up the trial systems to be used at home. The school occupational therapist, physical therapist, and speech therapist received permission from their administrator to provide Linnea's individualized education program (IEP) services at home to support the family's decision-making process. Linnea's teacher agreed to allow Linnea to dictate her work as needed to help prevent fatigue until a viable system is determined (some input systems require 2 to 3 weeks to achieve a level of comfort and a month to reach proficiency).

Linnea and her team explored many devices, including voice activation, a hand-held mouse system with an on-screen keyboard, scanning, and Morse code. All of the systems included word prediction and abbreviated expansion to help increase efficiency and prevent fatigue. Throughout the decision-making process, the team discussed the potential progression of her disease and future academic environments. Linnea and her family liked the voice-activated system, but they were concerned about her voice quality over time. They felt that scanning and Morse code were too time consuming, so they finally decided to use a hand-held mouse with an on-screen keyboard, word prediction, and abbreviated expansion. This system supported two of Linnea's long-term goals: word processing and Internet access.

Case Study 3: Margy

The occupational therapist, physical therapist, speech therapist, and teacher worked with Margy and her family to set up a program to help her learn simple receptionist and computer data entry skills. Margy did not have motor limitations, so she could use a standard keyboard and mouse. However, she did require external organization to complete the computer tasks. After much trial and error experimentation, the team found that a standard environmental setup that was free from extra papers and clutter and used a large font and a strong contrast on the computer monitor supported Margy's success when entering data on the computer. Margy's parents purchased a special paper holder that allowed her to keep her place on the paper when copying data so that she could quickly find her place again when she looked up to talk with customers.

Once the team found a successful system in the computer, she was registered as an office assistant as one of her classes in school. This allowed the team to be close to help problem solve any unforeseen difficulties and for Margy to practice her new skills in a familiar environment. As her skills continued to improve, she began to generalize the skills to the family business. The entire team continued to be available to problem solve any difficulties and help rearrange the reception area so that Margy could be successful. The team worked closely with Margy and her family during the transition to the family business and with the receptionist to ensure that the environmental modifications would work for Margy and the receptionist with whom Margy would work.

Case Study 4: Eric

His computer system has a CD-ROM and a phone answering machine. A family member or his assistant loads his compact discs (CDs) into his computer at his request. Once the CDs are loaded, he can turn them on and off, select the songs he wishes to hear, and control the volume. In addition, he has an answering machine hooked into his computer so that he can receive phone calls from his friends.

The occupational therapy assistant working with Eric collaborated closely with Eric, his family, and other community therapists to help come up with this system. She collaborated with the occupational therapist in drafting letters for funding and researching different options for Eric.

Case Study 5: Ryan

Because of Ryan's interest in the computer and the fact that all the other family members used the computer,

the team decided to explore computer options for play activities for Ryan. Through experimentation, the team discovered that Ryan enjoyed having the computer read different Living Books to him. He also enjoyed the exploration and cause-effect experiences when he was able to interact with pages of the book. Since Ryan seemed to enjoy being in the room when other family members worked on the computer, the family worked to use some of their respite funds from the Department of Developmental Disabilities to purchase a second computer for Ryan's use. This computer was set up in the same room as the original family computer. When siblings were working on their homework, Ryan would "work" on his computer for up to 10 minutes at a time. Ryan used earphones so that his program would not interrupt his sibling's work, but he generally resisted using them. The family referred to this as "social time" because it gave Ryan an opportunity for activity-focused interaction with the other family members.

Case Study 6: Lisa

Given Lisa's poor oral motor skills and her cognitive potential, the team has decided to begin to train her to use a Liberator. This dynamical communication system will be able to grow with her as she matures so that she can continue to communicate at increasingly more advanced levels over time. It also will support her in her academic environments and can be used as a computer interface system when she begins to work more on the computer to produce written assignments. At this time she will use direct selection with her dominant hand to access the system.

Case Study 7: Jim

Jim and his therapists work together to make a communication wallet. This wallet consists of various laminated pictures and phrases that are bound together. The occupational therapist worked with Jim and the speech pathologist to design the size and shape of the wallet and the thickness of the pages so that Jim's poor fine motor skills do not hinder his ability to communicate. In addition, the occupational therapist has worked with Jim in the clinic, community, and home settings as he has developed proficiency with the system.

chapter 20

Mobility

Christine Wright-Ott
Snaefridur Egilson

key terms

Developmental theory of mobility
Augmentative mobility
Mobility evaluation models
Alternative powered mobility devices
Manual wheelchairs
Power wheelchairs
Seating and positioning

■ CHAPTER OBJECTIVES

1. Understand the importance of mobility to development.
2. Apply a mobility assessment model to children with different levels of motor function.
3. Identify alternative methods of mobility appropriate to meet the child's developmental and functional needs.
4. Describe wheelchair features and designs that meet the needs of children with various levels of motor control.
5. Explain the biomechanical principles important to positioning and seating.
6. Identify power mobility devices currently available for children.
7. Describe power mobility assessment and intervention.
8. Describe new technology in assessing seating and positioning and new equipment available to children with unique seating and positioning needs.

The information in this chapter is intended to clarify the importance of mobility for growth and development and the implications of impaired mobility. Responsibilities of the occupational therapist for evaluating and recommending appropriate mobility devices are emphasized. Guidelines and criteria for selecting mobility equipment are defined, and descriptions of mobility devices are provided. This chapter also describes the importance of positioning and other factors that influence successful use of assistive devices.

Mobility is fundamental to an individual's overall development and functioning in the occupations of self-care, work, and leisure and is essential to quality of life. The definition of *functional mobility* includes moving from one position or place to another (e.g., bed mobility, wheelchair mobility, and transfers [wheelchair, bed, car, tub or shower, toilet, or chair]), performing functional ambulation, and transporting objects. *Community mobility* is defined as moving oneself in the community and using public or private transportation (e.g., driving or accessing buses, taxi cabs, or other public transportation systems). This chapter primarily addresses mobility as a means of locomotion, with an emphasis on evaluation and intervention principles.

■ DEVELOPMENTAL THEORY OF MOBILITY

The newborn has little independent control of any part of the body. Gradually, symmetry and midline orientation begin, followed by controlled purposeful movements and the beginning of alternating coordinated movements. The first form of mobility that the infant experiences is rolling, first from side to supine, then prone to supine, and finally in either direction. The 6-month-old infant achieves mobility by pivoting in the prone position. The infant continually becomes more active against gravity (Figure 20-1). Most 8-month-old infants creep and move from sitting to quadruped and back. By the ninth to tenth month the infant experiences a strong desire to move upward. First they pull to stand and cruise along furniture, such as a coffee table; then they hold onto someone or something as they take their first steps. The average age of independent walking is 11.2 months, and most children achieve independent upright ambulation between 9 and 15 months of age (Bly, 1994; Cech & Martin, 1995).

Developmental theorists accept that physical and psychologic development are interrelated and that early experiences influence subsequent behavior. "Through their motor interactions infants and toddlers learn about things and people in their world and also discover they can cause things to happen" (Butler, 1988b, p. 18). During the first months of life, children seek physical control of their environment and continue to do so by building and enhancing their motor skills day by day.

During the first 4 years of life, the child gains independence through mastery of important life tasks such as locomotion, ability to manipulate, bowel and bladder control, language development, and social interactions. The most fundamental of these, with the widest influence in all spheres of development, are learning to move about the environment and to use language as a communicative and information processing system.

Children gain various learning experiences as they move about. Locomotion and other motor skills, which develop rapidly during the first 3 years of life, become the primary vehicles for learning and socialization and for the healthy growth of a sense of independence and competence. Piaget (1954) viewed self-produced movement as a crucial building block of knowledge. He theorized that the intercoordination of vision and audition with movements, including locomotion, laid the basis for the child's understanding of space, objects, causality, and the self. The ability of children to influence their environment and to affect or alter it through their own actions is intrinsically motivating. Early experiences are believed to foster curiosity, exploration, mastery, and persistence and therefore are important for later intellectual functioning.

Despite theoretic agreement about the significance of locomotion, empiric research on the psychologic processes affected by the development of self-produced movement is minimal. Campos and Bertenthal (1987) believed that the psychologic domains most likely to be influenced by the development of crawling, creeping, and upright locomotion include the "development of fear of heights, changes in spatial search skills and spatial coding by the infant, and appearance of new forms of emotional communication" (p.16). These authors stressed that locomotion may be neither necessary nor sufficient for the development of other skills. Mobility appears to play at least a facilitative role as a mediator of development (Bertenthal, Campos, & Barrett, 1984).

■ IMPAIRED MOBILITY

"When development along any line is restricted, delayed, or distorted, other lines of development are adversely affected as well" (Butler, 1988a, p. 66). Children with physical disabilities who have difficulty achieving independent motor control are often deprived of self-initiated mobility experiences. Because they lack the necessary movements to engage in and act on their environment, important learning opportunities are also hindered. Restricted experiences and mobility during early childhood can have a diffuse and lasting influence.

Long-term physical restriction during infancy or early childhood can significantly alter and disrupt the entire subsequent course of emotional or psychologic development in the involved child (Becker, 1975). Such deprivation of physical and social contingencies can lead to secondary developmental problems, which are motivational. Infants born with motor impairments quickly "begin to lose interest in a world which they do not expect to control" (Brinker & Lewis, 1982, p. 113). This motivational effect is termed *learned helplessness*, a condition in which the child gives up trying to control his or her own world because of motor disability and diminished expectations of caregivers (Seligman, 1975). Butler (1988a) found that children whose mobility is limited during early childhood develop a pattern of apathetic behavior, specifically a lack of curiosity and initiative. These character traits are believed to have a critical influence on intellectual performance and social interaction.

In children with severe physical disabilities, newly gained independent mobility can have a positive effect on emotional, social, and intellectual states (Douglas & Ryan, 1987). Paulsson and Christoffersen (1984) found that children with disabilities using mobility devices became less dependent on controlling their environment through verbal commands, more interested in all mobility skills, and more active in peer activities. Increased independence through locomotion may reduce the need to use language as a control method and improve psychosocial behavior. Butler (1986) found that children who had some means of ambulation could and would make

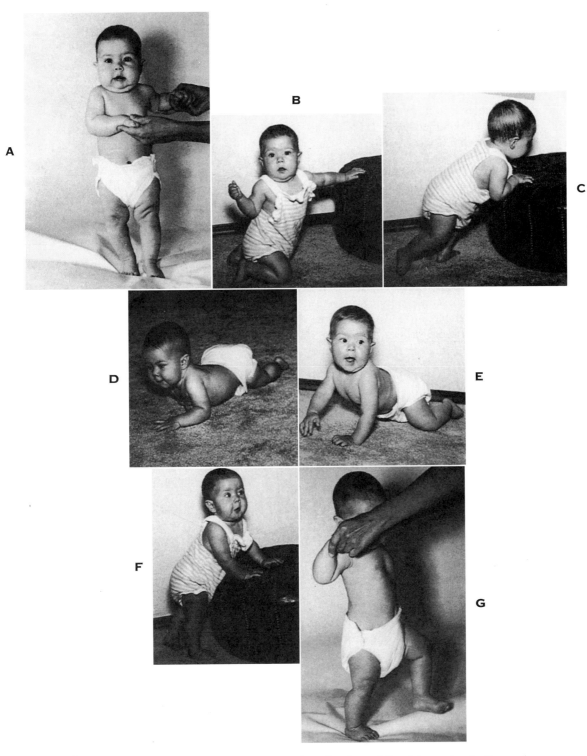

figure20-1   Development of locomotion. **A,** Infant bears full weight on feet by 7 months of age. **B,** Infant can maneuver from sitting to kneeling position. **C,** Infant can pull self to standing position. **D,** Infant crawls with abdomen on floor and pulls self forward. **E,** Infant creeps on hands and knees at 9 months of age. **F,** Infant can stand holding onto furniture at 9 months of age. **G,** While standing, infant takes deliberate steps at 10 months of age. *(From Wong, D.L. [1995]. Whaley and Wong's essentials of pediatric nursing [4th ed. p. 274]. St. Louis: Mosby.)*

choices, but those who did not ambulate were much less likely to exercise available options. The lack of ambulation appeared to severely restrict the child's opportunities to practice decision making, thus giving him or her no reason to express an opinion or desire.

Occupational and physical therapists often contribute to decision making on whether to introduce mobility devices to children with developmental delays. If the therapists determine that a mobility device is important, they then decide when it should be considered and what kind of mobility is appropriate. Whether a child should use a mobility device continues to be a topic of concern. Introduction of mobility aids to children with physical disabilities at early ages appears to facilitate psychosocial, language, and cognitive development. However, professionals lack agreement regarding use of support walkers and powered devices. A support walker provides moderate to maximum support at the pelvis, trunk, and sometimes the head. If the walker does not fit or function properly, the child may use undesirable movements to propel it. Continued use of undesirable postures and movements contradicts therapy goals and may delay or impair the quality of motor development. However, most support walkers are now designed with various adjustments and features that provide more desirable positioning than has been available in the past (Figure 20-2) (Paleg, 1997).

Research has not demonstrated that use of power mobility prevents or delays the child's acquisition of motor skills. On the contrary, researchers have found positive changes in children's development after the introduction of power mobility (Paulsson & Christoffersen, 1984). During mobility training, children with severe motor disabilities have demonstrated improved head control and trunk stability, increased motivation, and more self-confidence in movement (Butler, 1986). Nilsson and Nyberg (1997) described increased exploratory behavior and increased ability to use and integrate sensory information in various activities in two preschool children with multiple impairments after training in a powered wheelchair. In a second study, children 15 months to 5 years of age with physical disabilities who participated in a 2-week mobility exploration day camp demonstrated a variety of positive behavioral changes (Wright-Ott, 1997). The children experienced mobility by using the GoBot (formerly known as the Transitional Powered Mobility Aide [TPMA]) to explore the environment. They participated in daily 1½-hour sessions for 2 weeks. Behavioral changes that caregivers and occupational therapists observed in some children included increased eye contact, increased verbalization and communication, improved sleeping patterns, increased active arm use, and a more positive disposition.

Psychologists who have studied normal development have also observed improvements in social-emotional, cognitive, perceptual, and motor functioning in infants

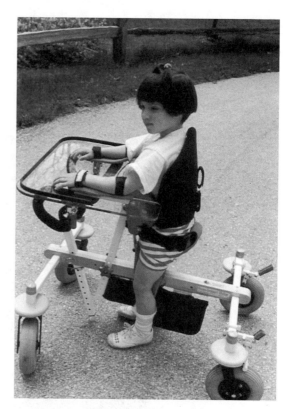

figure 20-2   Prone Support Walker with accessories. (Manufactured by Consumer Care Products, Inc.)

when they first gain mobility (Woods, 1998). Mobility appears to be a priority issue for children with disabilities and others in their environment. When researchers surveyed the occupational performance needs of school-age children with physical disabilities in the school system and community, most teachers, parents, and children identified mobility as their greatest area of concern (Pollock & Stewart, 1998).

The current trend is for mobility devices to be recommended at young ages, when typical children are first ambulating. Many professionals believe that if self-initiated mobility does not occur in the first year, the use of devices for mobility should be considered. "Clinical experience and research projects have established that powered mobility devices offer children at least as young as 17 months of age a safe and efficient method of independent locomotion" (Butler, 1988b, p. 18).

It can be a challenge for the therapist to suggest consideration of a mobility device, particularly a wheelchair, to the family of a child with a disability. Many caregivers consider the suggestion as a symbol of giving up hope for independent ambulation. The therapist must convey the concept that all children need a means of mobility and that the mobility device is intended to assist the child in achieving more independence and function until and if another method is acquired.

■ AUGMENTATIVE MOBILITY

Butler (1988b) introduced the term *augmentative mobility,* which refers to all types of mobility that supplement or augment ambulation.

> Given augmentative mobility, disabled children can experience more success in directly controlling their environment, thereby reducing or avoiding secondary social, emotional and intellectual handicaps (p. 18).

The authors of this chapter recommend that the concept of augmentative mobility be expanded to include transitional and functional mobility. Transitional mobility allows the child to use a device to experience self-initiated movement without the expectation that it must be functional. The child may not be able to move the device in a desired direction but uses it as a means for exploring the effects of movement and learning how to move. The therapist can best provide transitional mobility by allowing the child to move the device in a large room with open space where the child is free to explore. These experiences can then help the child make the transition to a more functional level of purposeful mobility. Not all children are able to achieve functional mobility; in these instances, transitional mobility remains an important means for the child to explore the environment.

The team must consider several factors before selecting the type of mobility device that is appropriate for a child. These factors include the purpose or goals for using the device, environments for intended use, and the child's physical and psychosocial abilities and limitations. When selecting a mobility device, the team considers the advantages and disadvantages of the device, the congruence to intervention goals, and the cost/benefit ratio. Ideally a mobility-impaired child should have more than one type of mobility device for use in indoor and outdoor environments. Any methods that are chosen for mobility require close cooperation among all professionals working with the child and family.

■ ASSESSMENT AND INTERVENTION

Classification of Mobility Skills

Children's mastery of functional mobility skills has been classified and categorized in several ways. Hays (1987) examined current existing diagnostic conditions of children without locomotion and divided them into four functional subgroups:

1. *Children who will never ambulate.* This includes children with cerebral palsy with severe involvement and spinal muscular atrophy types I and II. Generally, these children have no opportunity for independent mobility unless a power wheelchair is prescribed.
2. *Children with inefficient mobility who ambulate but are unable to do so at a reasonable rate of speed or with*

acceptable endurance. This includes children with cerebral palsy with less involvement and myelomeningocele with upper-extremity involvement. For these children the power wheelchair may provide an efficient means of mobility above that which they are capable of producing themselves. Warren (1990) uses the term *marginal ambulators* for this group.
3. *Children who have lost their independent mobility.* This includes victims of trauma and children with progressive neuromuscular disorders. The developmental implications may be less critical than in the first two groups, and the issue is acceptance of assisted mobility as an adaptation to the acquired disability.
4. *Children who temporarily require assisted mobility and often progress to independent mobility with age.* This includes many children with osteogenesis imperfecta and arthrogryposis. Functional considerations in this group are both developmental and practical.

There are significant differences among these groups that may have implications for mobility and its integration into the child's overall concept of disability, as well as for evaluation and intervention.

Evaluation

Evaluation of children has traditionally focused on the achievement of developmental milestones. Occupational therapists have discussed the limitation of such evaluations because underlying impairments (e.g., motor control deficits) cannot fully explain the extent and form of functional difficulties seen in children with disabilities (Coster, 1998). Furthermore, the tasks that are most relevant for daily independence in mobility function have not been well defined in traditional developmental milestone tests. Recently therapists have advocated the use of a top-down evaluation process that focuses on what the child needs or wants to do, the context in which he or she typically engages occupations, and the limitations that he or she may experience (Coster, 1998; Fisher, 1998). Therapists assess underlying performance abilities only to the extent that is needed to help clarify the possible sources of limitations in occupational performance. In mobility evaluation, occupational therapists should focus on the child's overall pattern of locomotion and transfer skills in relation to a particular performance context.

Two instruments focus on the evaluation of functional abilities, including mobility, in children. The Pediatric Evaluation of Disabilities Inventory (PEDI) (Haley, Coster, Ludlow, Haltiwanger, & Andrellos, 1992) rates two dimensions of performance—capability to perform functional skills and the level of caregiver assistance needed. The functional mobility subscale measures basic transfer skills (e.g., getting in and out of a car) and body transportation activities (e.g., walking up and down stairs). The Functional Independence Measure for Children (WeeFIM; Uniform Data System for Medical Rehabilitation, 1999) is based on the Functional Independence Measure (FIM) and is for children from 6 months to 7 years of age. It includes six subscales, three of which address mobility: transfers, locomotion, and stairs. The WeeFIM provides useful information in progress assessment, program planning, and communication with caregivers.

The Canadian Occupational Performance Measure (COPM) (Law et. al., 1994) is a semistructured interview that focuses on the identification of problems in self-care, productivity, and leisure. It provides a framework to help clients articulate the difficulties that they are encountering in their daily lives and appears to be responsive to change after occupational therapy intervention (Law et. al., 1994). In the case of mobility, the COPM can address the concerns of children and caregivers, help them identify what is important to them, and help them prioritize goals. The COPM also provides a baseline assessment for measuring outcomes on reassessment.

Occupational therapists need to evaluate several components of performance that may influence mobility control, such as motor, perceptual, and cognitive factors. This may include neuromotor status, orthopedic condition, and psychosocial considerations. The therapist must also address the performance context of chronologic and developmental age and environment. The therapist must make the mobility devices available during the evaluation process so that the child and caregivers have an opportunity to gain experience using potential mobility devices. These trials provide the caregivers and child with information and experience that will assist them in becoming informed consumers and full participants in deciding which mobility device best meets their needs.

Mobility Evaluation Models

Selection of the most appropriate positioning and mobility device requires the skills of a therapy team working in close collaboration with the school team, prescribing physician, child, parent or caregiver, and assistive technology supplier (ATS). The ATS is a specialist who is trained and experienced in providing durable medical rehabilitation equipment and is credentialed through the Rehabilitation Engineering and Assistive Technology Society of North America (RESNA). This organization also provides the assistive technology practitioner (ATP) credential for professionals. The ATS is responsible for maintaining updated knowledge of available equipment and assisting in identifying choices of mobility devices according to the features that the child requires to use it optimally.

The physical or occupational therapist, together with the child and family, identifies the needs of the child and establishes goals to identify the features and options in a mobility device or devices that will meet the desired outcomes and assist the family in setting appropriate goals

and expectations for using the mobility device. The therapist is responsible for assisting the family in becoming informed consumers who can make decisions regarding a mobility device. Once the mobility device is selected and provided to the family, the therapist is responsible for reevaluating the fit and function of the device to determine if it meets the stated goals and objectives.

Most funding agencies do not approve replacement of a mobility device, such as a wheelchair, within 3 to 5 years of the purchase date. If the equipment is not appropriate, the child and family may not have another option for several years. The limitations in reimbursement become critical when a misunderstanding during the evaluation or ordering process results in a device that does not meet the predetermined outcomes. It is imperative that the therapists, ATS, and family immediately decide on how to best resolve these issues.

Therapists can use several approaches in evaluating children for mobility devices. The most common is for the therapists to request a local supplier of durable medical equipment or ATS to bring the device under consideration to the therapy session. The ATS offers input as to what features and options are available on the device and how to properly adjust it. The difficulty encountered with this model is that one supplier typically has a limited selection of devices available for demonstration purposes, so only one device can be evaluated at each session. Therefore the therapist does not have the opportunity to compare the child's performance in various types of mobility devices. Without direct comparison of the mobility devices, decisions about which devices are optimal for the child are difficult for the therapist to make. The decision making is less risky when side-by-side comparison of each device is available during the evaluation. This method enables comparison of performance of each mobility device under consistent child and environmental conditions.

Several assistive technology (AT) centers and rehabilitation engineering centers throughout the country use a multidisciplinary team approach and side-by-side evaluation methods to assess seating and mobility needs, particularly with individuals who have severe disabilities. The teams consist of occupational therapists, physical therapists, rehabilitation engineers, speech pathologists, and ATSs working with the child's therapy team, school team, physician, and family. These centers offer the advantage of being able to consider all the needs of the child and offering a concentrated level of expertise.

■ MOBILITY DEVICES

Selection of a specific type of a mobility device depends on several factors: the purpose for using the mobility device, the indoor and outdoor environments in which it will be used, the effort required by the individual to use the device, and positioning needs. The team considers specific features and device adaptations for optimal

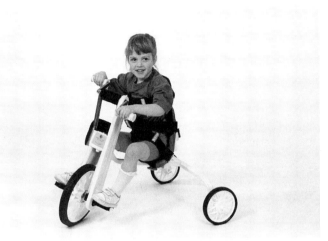

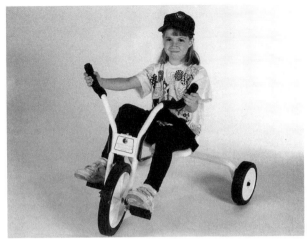

figure**20-3** **A,** The Mobility Aide Trike, hand driven. (Distributed by Consumer Care Products, Inc.) **B,** The Mobility Aide Trike, foot driven. (Distributed by Consumer Care Products, Inc.)

use in functional activities such as eating, transfers, augmentative communication, personal hygiene, and school activities. The team also considers the needs and concerns of the caregiver who will be using, transporting, and maintaining the equipment and costs versus benefits.

The occupational therapist must use the skills of an investigator during the mobility assessment process. Thoughtful planning and careful analysis of person-device-environment fit is necessary for the therapist to ensure that the child and family receive the optimal device. A wheelchair that will not fit into the family van, tips over when the augmentative communication device is mounted on it, or cannot be propelled outside because the family lives in a hilly area are examples of problems incurred when a device is ordered without comprehensive mobility evaluation. The following is an example of a child whose mobility device is not evaluated properly:

Brian is 5 years old and has severe spastic cerebral palsy. He is fully included in a kindergarten classroom. He was evaluated at the medical therapy session to determine what type of walker would provide him with mobility in the classroom. His parents expressed interest in a particular walker, and the therapist borrowed one from an ATS for Brian to use during the evaluation. The family was excited when they observed Brian slowly propelling the walker forward. The therapist recommended the walker for purchase with custom modifications, which included a higher backrest and a headrest. Brian was set up in his classroom with the new walker.

After 5 months of trying to use the walker in the classroom, he had not yet successfully used it. The therapist determined that he did not have the ability to maneuver the walker in the classroom because of the high degree of resistance from the carpeted surfaces. The therapist initially evaluated Brian in a room with linoleum, without consideration of the classroom environment. The therapist reevaluated Brian with another walker in which he was able to maneuver over carpet. At this time additional funding to purchase another walker was not available. He would have benefited from a side-by-side evaluation of several types of walkers with consideration of the characteristics of the environments in which he would use the walker.

Initial Mobility Devices for Young Children
Tricycles

Tricycles (Figure 20-3) are a means for mobility, although third-party funding is typically not available since tricycles are not considered a medical necessity. However, they can provide mobility outdoors and in hallways and corridors, such as for moving from class to class or from class to therapy. Many types of tricycles are available with adaptations, such as trunk supports, and hand propelled models are available for children who do not have the ability to pedal with their legs (e.g., children with spina bifida).

Prone scooters

Prone scooters (Figure 20-4) require use of the arms and the ability to lift the head while moving. The advantages of using a prone scooter include greater access for participating in play activities on the floor, the ability to get on and off independently, and ability to change direction more easily than with other types of manual mobility devices. Disadvantages include fatigue from maintaining neck and back extension, vulnerability of the head to hitting objects, possibility of the hands getting caught in the casters or rubbed on rough surfaces, and difficulty viewing the environment above the ground level. Children with spina bifida may find the prone scooter func-

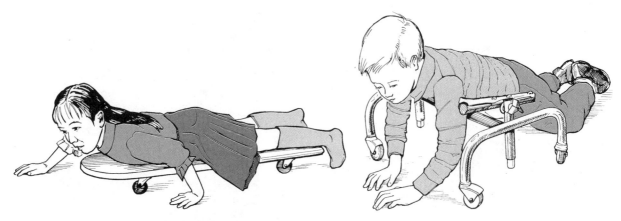

figure**20-4** Prone scooter mobility devices.

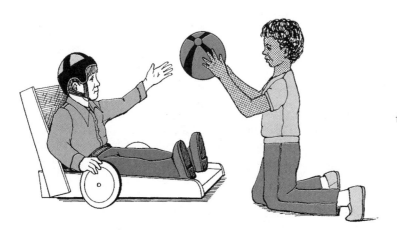

figure**20-5.** Caster cart mobility device.

tional because they have the upper-extremity function to propel it and it can support their legs.

Caster carts

Caster carts offer another means of mobility to children with upper-extremity function (e.g., those with spina bifida) (Figure 20-5). Children can use caster carts indoors or on flat outdoor surfaces, such as playgrounds. Some children may be able to transfer on and off independently because of the close proximity to the floor. The device requires a considerable amount of energy expenditure for propelling long distances because of the small diameter of the wheels. Children with lower-extremity muscle contractures or tightness, such as in the hamstring muscles, may find it difficult to sit comfortably and securely because they are often unable to tolerate long leg sitting. These children may do better with a triangular-shaped wedge placed under the knees to support their legs in knee flexion.

Aeroplane mobility device

The *aeroplane mobility device* was designed for children with cerebral palsy who can move their legs but need support of the upper body (Figure 20-6). The de-

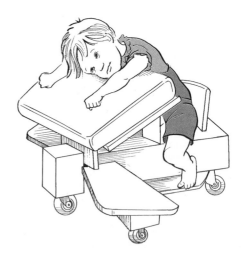

figure**20-6** Aeroplane mobility device can be handmade and is designed for children younger than 3 years of age.

vice provides developmentally appropriate positioning, particularly for children with spasticity, because the child is positioned with hip abduction and extension with knee flexion and the upper extremities are in a weight-bearing position. This position often assists in reducing muscle

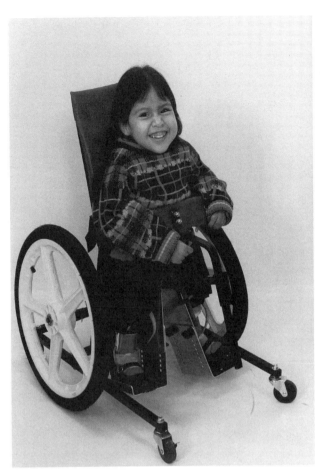

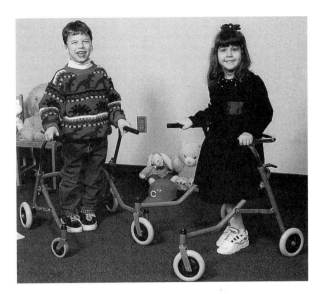

figure**20-8**   The Bugsy pediatric postural walker, by Otto Bock Rehab, incorporates a design that encourages active postural control while promoting more natural movement during ambulation.

figure**20-7**   The ABLER, a mobile stander. *(Manufactured by the Jennie Company, Bakersfield, California.)*

tone and undesirable postures in children who have spastic cerebral palsy. Other advantages include ease in viewing the environment, the handmade nature of the device, and acceptance by parents because it looks like a toy rather than an assistive device. The aeroplane mobility device is not yet commercially available but can be fabricated from wood. Disadvantages include lack of adjustability for growth, difficulty turning and moving backwards, and heaviness.

Mobile stander

If a child has upper-extremity function to push and maneuver wheels, a *mobile stander* may provide another means for mobility. These devices allow the child to experience lower-extremity weight bearing in a standing position. The child achieves mobility using large handheld wheels for self-propulsion (Figure 20-7).

Walkers

Children who have the ability to pull to a standing position and maintain a grip may be able to use a *hand-held walker.* These walkers are designed for use either in front of or behind the child *(posterior walker)* (Figure 20-8). Children with mild to moderate cerebral palsy or lower levels of spina bifida with leg bracing most commonly use hand-held walkers. Walkers can have three or four wheels and are available in various wheel sizes. The smaller the caster, the more difficult it is for use outdoors and over uneven surfaces. Posterior walkers are available with a feature in which the casters lock when the walker is pushed backwards, such as when a child leans into it. This feature enables the child to stand and lean against the walker for rest periods; however, it makes maneuvering the walker backwards more difficult.

Support walkers are designed for children who have some ability to move their legs reciprocally but need support at the pelvis, chest, and possibly the upper extremities and head (see Figure 20-2). Selection of appropriate features and adjustments that provide optimal positioning for the child are critical to functional use of these types of walkers. Support walkers that provide abduction between the legs tend to reduce muscle tone in children with spasticity, making it more efficient for the child to propel the walker. Another desirable feature in support walkers is adjustable pitch, which allows the child's upper body to be placed in a slightly forward lean position. This position places the feet behind the pelvis and trunk, which may make it easier for the child to initiate forward movement. If the feet are positioned in front of the pelvis, the child often moves backwards. Some children have a tendency to scissor or adduct their legs. A walker that is designed with a center pad between the ankles may assist in guiding the feet and reducing adduction. How-

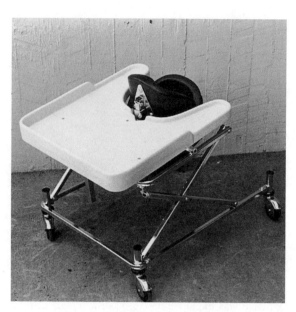

figure**20-9** Pommel Walker can be used with a tray to provide support of the upper body. *(Manufactured by the Special Services Dept., Rehabilitation Centre for Children, Winnipeg, Manitoba, Canada.)*

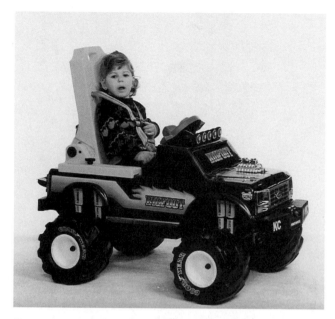

figure**20-11** Big Foot powered mobility vehicle can be maneuvered using a joystick or switches. *(Distributed by Innovative Products, Inc.)*

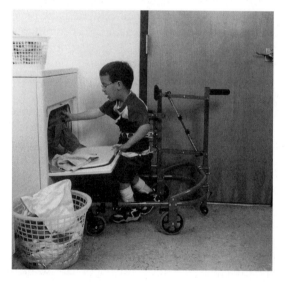

figure**20-10** Walkabout is a weight-relieving walker. *(Manufactured by Mulholland Positioning Systems, Inc.)*

ever, this feature may make it difficult for the child to turn the walker because the legs cannot cross midline to assist in maneuvering it.

Other useful features include adjustability for growth and brakes to lock the wheels for stability during transfers. Walkers with optional trays may be appropriate for children who need upper body support, such as those with muscle weakness or low muscle tone (Figure 20-9). Walkers without trays or hardware in front of the child

have the advantage of providing the child with greater access to the environment (Figure 20-10).

Support walkers can provide children with the opportunity to explore their environment in an upright, hands-free position while providing weight bearing and stretching in the hips and knees. However, support walkers have limitations in maneuverability and are difficult for some children to turn in a limited space and move backwards.

Alternative Powered Mobility Devices

Adapted motorized toy vehicles, such as the Big Foot (Figure 20-11), are available for children to provide early mobility experiences using either a joystick or up to four switches. From the caregiver's perspective, the greatest advantage for use of these toy vehicles is that they look like a toy that any other child would use rather than an assistive device. They are also an option for providing a child with the opportunity to learn how to drive a motorized device in preparation for using a power wheelchair. Disadvantages include difficulty using these vehicles indoors because of limited maneuverability; large size, which prevents the child from getting close to objects in the environment for reaching, exploring, and interacting with others; and noisy operation.

The Transitional Powered Mobility Aide (TPMA) is a new concept in mobility that was developed at the Rehabilitation Technology and Therapy Center, Lucile Packard Children's Health Services at Stanford (Figure 20-12) (Wright-Ott, 1998). The TPMA is a powered mobility device designed to enable physically challenged

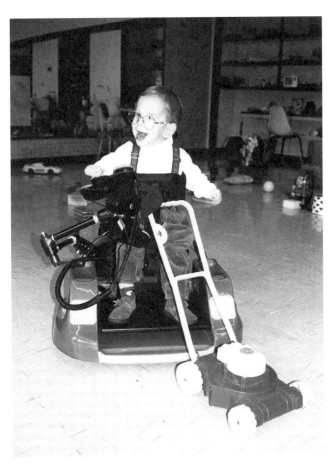

figure**20-12** A 20-month-old boy with cerebral palsy pushes a toy during exploratory play while using the Transitional Powered Mobility Aide. He operates it using switches under his right hand. (*Manufactured by Innovative Products, Inc.*)

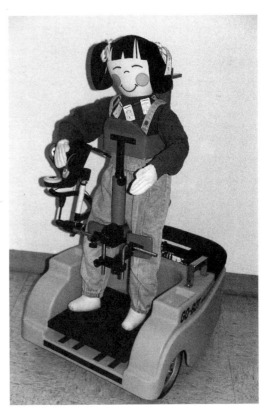

figure**20-13** The GoBot provides early, exploratory, self-initiated mobility experiences for children who are mobility impaired.

preschool children from 12 months to about 6 years of age to move in an upright position and explore the environment by getting close enough to objects and peers to reach and touch. It is intended for transitional mobility indoors or for use outdoors on flat surfaces. The child can be positioned in a standing, semistanding, or sitting position. A joystick or multiple switches can be positioned at any location at which the child can reach the controls for driving the device. The TPMA is not a power wheelchair; it is a therapeutic and educational tool intended to provide developmental opportunities equivalent to those experienced by able-bodied peers, such as pushing or pulling toys, kicking balls, moving fast, moving slowly, and problem solving. The TPMA is intended to increase the child's opportunities for hands-free exploration and provide new sensory experiences (particularly vestibular, visual motor, and spatial relations). The TPMA is now commercially available as the GoBot and is intended for children who would otherwise spend their early developmental years passively sitting in a stroller or manual wheelchair (Figure 20-13).

■ WHEELCHAIRS

Wheelchairs are either manual or powered. Manual wheelchairs depend on the user or an assistant for propulsion, whereas powered devices depend on a motorized unit that the individual accesses using a joystick or alternative control methods such as sip-and-puff or multiple switches.

Wheelchairs are available in standard or custom sizes as measured by the seat width and depth, height of the seat from the floor, and backrest height. The therapist must carefully consider features and options on wheelchairs and select the wheelchair to accommodate the child's growth and physical and functional needs as well as the needs of the caregivers. The therapist should begin selection of a wheelchair by evaluating and documenting the child's current physical and functional abilities with consideration of physical changes that may occur and the positioning and mobility goals for the child. He or she must also consider the environments in which the child will use the wheelchair, how the caregivers will transport it, and the sources of funding. The therapist is respon-

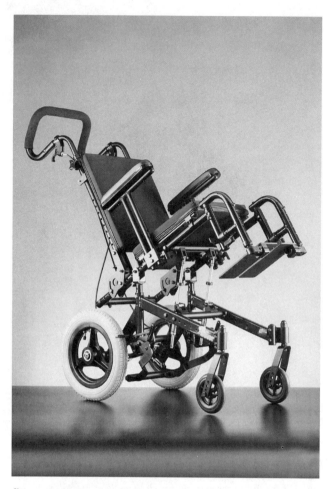

figure**20-14** The Shark is a pediatric tilt-in-space manual wheelchair that tilts 45 degrees posteriorly and 10 degrees anteriorly. Armrests drop down to seat level for barrier-free transfers, and the seat-to-back angle is adjustable. *(Distributed by Everest & Jennings.)*

sible for providing a medical justification for the seating and mobility system.

Once the therapist has identified the child's needs, he or she matches them to the specific features available in a wheelchair. For example, if a child cannot shift weight independently and is at risk for developing pressure-related problems, then a wheelchair with either a manual or powered tilt-in-space feature may be necessary to shift weight from under the buttocks to the back (Figure 20-14). The manual tilt-in-space feature allows the caregiver to press two levers, which tilts the frame of the wheelchair backwards while maintaining the same seat-to-back angle. This differs from a reclining wheelchair, which opens the seat-to-back angle so that the person is lying supine with hip extension. Powered tilt-in-space is an option available on power wheelchairs so that the user has independent control of tilting the wheelchair back. A tilt-in-space feature can also provide an anterior

tilt to position the child slightly forward, which may affect changes in muscle tone.

Specialized strollers are similar to infant strollers but are available with seating components for postural support. They are considered dependent mobility devices since the child is dependent on others for transportation. Specialized strollers are available with small casters or larger 8-inch wheels for maneuvering over rugged terrain. Parents often prefer the ease of use of a stroller and feel that its appearance is more acceptable than that of a wheelchair (Cook & Hussey, 1995).

Manual Wheelchairs

A *manual wheelchair* is appropriate for a child who has the ability to functionally and efficiently propel it. It is also used as a means of transportation by care providers or as a back-up wheelchair when the child's power wheelchair is not working. Great strides in manual wheelchair design have resulted in lightweight wheelchairs that provide higher performance during propulsion (Figure 20-15).

The therapist must consider the following wheelchair features during an evaluation:
- Style of frame (folding or rigid)
- Tilt-in-space
- Type of recline
- Type of footrest (single plate or double plate, fixed or swing away, or multiposition adjustability)
- Angle of footrest (standard, 70 degrees, 90 degrees, or less than 90 degrees)
- Style of armrest (tubular, desk arm, height adjustable, or swing away)
- Height of backrest
- Floor-to-seat height
- Height of push handles for the adult pushing the wheelchair
- Style and location of brakes
- Type and size of tires and casters
- Adjustable axle plate for placement of the wheel

Wheelchairs with large rear tires are most common, but models with large front tires and small back casters are available (Figure 20-16). Propelling a wheelchair with large front tires may be more efficient for the child because more surface area of the tire is exposed when gripping the wheel and pushing. However, the large front tires can limit access to the environment, such as when transferring and sitting at tables. The wheelchair with large front tires is also more difficult to push over curbs and uneven surfaces.

If a child will be independently propelling the wheelchair, it is critical that the equipment allows the child to use proper biomechanics for more efficient propulsion. The therapist achieves this by selecting the proper size of wheelchair frame and an appropriate seating system. Most wheelchair manufacturers include wheelchair

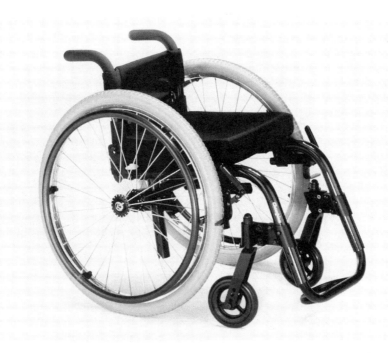

figure 20-15   The Kush/Kin 3000 lightweight rigid pediatric manual wheelchair by Everest and Jennings.

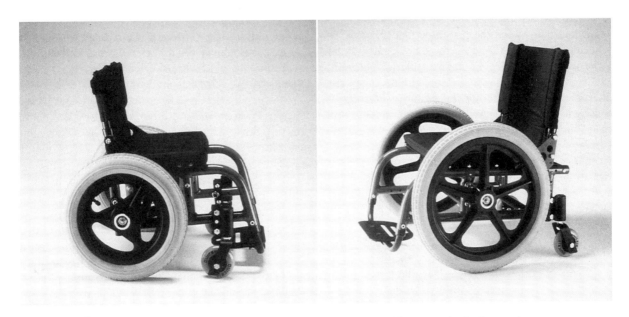

figure 20-16   Quickie Kidz manual wheelchair features wider rear wheels for maximum pushing surface and standard or reverse wheel configurations so that the chair can be propelled with either a push or pull motion. *(Manufactured by Sunrise Medical.)*

growth kits, which accommodate the need to widen or lengthen the frame without having to entirely replace the wheelchair. The therapist must select a wheelchair that fits the child's present needs rather than a wheelchair that is too large with the goal the child will grow into it. A wheelchair that is too wide is more difficult for the child to propel. If the seat is too long, the child's pelvis cannot achieve a neutral position; it will be pulled into a posterior tilt position, causing the child to sit on the sacrum with a rounded back.

The therapist simultaneously considers what type of seating or positioning system is needed and how it will

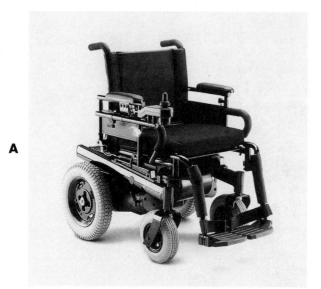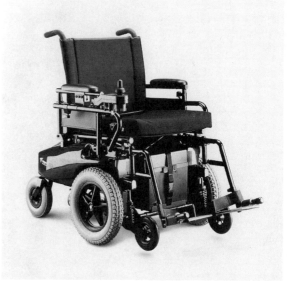

figure 20-17 **A,** Invacare Action Ranger X Storm series rear-wheel drive power wheelchair. **B,** Invacare Action Ranger II Storm series mid-wheel drive power wheelchair.

interface with the mobility base for optimal function and performance. For example, one mistake is use of a seat cushion without consideration of the frame size of the manual wheelchair. When the cushion is placed on top of the wheelchair frame, it may position the child too far from the wheels for reaching and propelling them efficiently. If the therapist had considered the height of the wheelchair seat when ordering the cushion, alternatives could have been used to prevent this situation (e.g., a narrower cushion that can be recessed into the wheelchair frame).

Another common situation that reinforces the need to assess seating and mobility simultaneously is acquiring a backrest cushion for a child after selecting the manual wheelchair. The cushion may position the child too far forward of the axle's wheel. If the child's center of gravity is forward of the rear wheels instead of directly over the rear wheel axle, propulsion is more difficult and inefficient. Many wheelchairs have a standard axle plate where the hub of the wheel is mounted to the frame and the wheels cannot be relocated within the child's reach. However, if the therapist orders an adjustable axle plate for the wheelchair in combination with the appropriate front caster size, the wheels can be relocated and mounted in the best location for the child to reach the wheels for propulsion.

Power Wheelchairs

If a child cannot propel a wheelchair long distances at the same speed and efficiency as the average person walks, then the therapist should consider ordering a *power wheelchair* to increase the child's independence and function. The advantages of a power wheelchair over a manual are increased speed capability, ease of maneuvering, and less energy expenditure required for moving. Some children who use a power wheelchair also have a manual wheelchair for use in environments that are not accessible to a power wheelchair or when the power wheelchair is being repaired.

Power wheelchairs are available in several styles with various options and are differentiated by the placement of the drive wheel, which may be front-wheel, mid-wheel, or rear-wheel drive (Figure 20-17). A few manufacturers offer the option to adjust the drive wheel by repositioning it. Attributes that are affected by the drive wheel position include maneuverability, stability, traction, and performance (speed, efficiency, obstacle climbing, and crossing a side slope). Maneuverability depends on the turning radius. The smaller the turning radius, the greater the maneuverability. Mid-wheel drive wheelchairs may have greater maneuverability because of the smaller turning radius. However, mid-wheel drive wheelchairs require a third set of stabilizing wheels that may pitch the user forward when going downhill or over curbs, affecting stability of the user.

The most common approach to selecting a power wheelchair begins by describing the environments in which the child will use it and determining which make and model offers the type of features needed to access those environments. The next consideration is to determine how the child will access or drive the power wheelchair and which models provide the access methods that the child needs now and will need in the future. Most wheelchair manufacturers provide a choice of several types of wheelchair models that are intended for joystick operation and models that include sophisticated microcomputer electronics for alternative input methods. Different models offer various features to accommodate the needs of each user. Such features include adjustments for torque, tremor dampening for children experiencing difficulty directing the joystick, a short-throw joystick option for users with muscle weakness who do not have the strength to push the joystick to its end range, speed adjustments, and acceleration settings so that the wheelchair can be set to increase speed rapidly or gradually.

A joystick is the standard and preferred method for the individual who can efficiently and accurately maneuver it. The user can operate a joystick using a hand, foot, forearm, chin, head pointer, or even the back of the head by using an adaptation that connects the joystick to a bracket that is attached to a moveable headrest. Some children may find it difficult to accurately use a joystick with a hand when the joystick is located in its traditional placement at the front end of the armrest. These children may have better motor control if the joystick is placed inside the armrest, in midline, or rotated toward their body several degrees. A remote or attendant joystick, which is smaller in size than a standard joystick, may be necessary for these types of situations and are available for most power wheelchairs. The remote joystick is easier to position in midline or under the chin. Another feature that can assist in improving control or efficiency during joystick use is a support (such as a wide armrest or trough) under the elbow, forearm, or wrist. During the evaluation for joystick operation, the therapist must consider the positioning needs of the child, placement of the joystick, type of joystick, type of joystick knob, and desired location of the on/off switch for independent access by the user.

A proportional joystick allows the driver to increase acceleration speed of the wheelchair in relationship to the distance that he or she moves the joystick. The further the user pushes the proportional joystick, the more rapidly the wheelchair moves. A nonproportional joystick (digital or microswitch) does not affect the wheelchair's speed; any amount of force used to push the joystick results in the same speed.

Joystick knobs are available in various styles, shapes, and sizes to accommodate various hand and wrist positions. The most common shapes are round, T-shaped, and I-shaped joysticks. A child with weakness of the upper extremities may find it more efficient to use a U-shaped joystick so that the hand is supported in the palm and at the sides. Selection of the most appropriate style of joystick and its placement directly affects the ability to accurately and efficiently drive a power wheelchair.

Children with severe physical disabilities may be able to operate a power wheelchair but often are not given the opportunity because they are physically unable to operate a joystick. Alternative input or access methods are avail-

able for these individuals. An input method frequently used by individuals with spinal cord injuries is sip-and-puff, which the user activates by gently inhaling or exhaling into a strawlike device held in the mouth. Another alternative is the head switch sensing array, which consists of switches embedded into a headrest that move the wheelchair by detecting head movements. A tongue touch keypad has been recently developed. This keypad is a custom-made retainer in which small switches have been imbedded. The user activates each switch by touching it with the tongue. Multiple switch access is available in which push switches are placed around the body part that is able to reach the switches. The wheelchair is driven in one of four directions, depending on which switch is activated. It is even possible for the individual to drive a power wheelchair with one switch, which operates a scanning light on a display. The following is an example of a child who uses an alternative input device.

Matthew is 14 years old and has severe spastic cerebral palsy (Figure 20-18). He uses a custom seating system composed of an antithrust seat cushion, a biangular back cushion with lateral hip and trunk pads, and an occipital neckrest with anterior chest support. This position has increased his ability to activate a push switch placed on the right side of his head. He operates his power wheel-

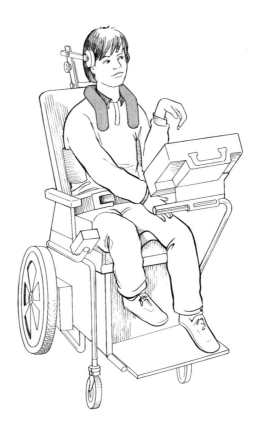

figure**21-18**   Young man with severe spastic cerebral palsy drives a power wheelchair using a switch mounted at each side of his head to operate the scanning display.

chair by using special electronic controls in the wheelchair that are connected to the switch and a small scanning light box mounted in front of him. When he presses the switch, the light begins to scan in one of four directions. Another press of the switch stops the light on the

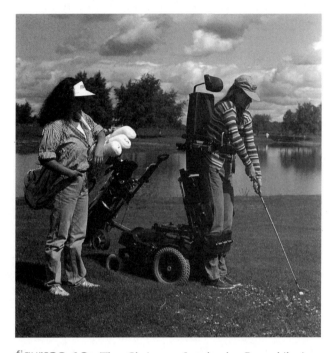

figure**20-19** The Chairman Stander by Permobile is a front-wheel drive power wheelchair that enables the user to move from a sitting to a standing position.

arrow indicating the direction of the desired movement. A third press of the switch stops the wheelchair. He uses the same switch to operate a scanning light on his augmentative communication device, mounted in front of him on his wheelchair.

Switches can be placed around any part of the body, such as the hand, head, elbows, or feet, where the child has the most reliable, accurate, and efficient movements. However, the quality of motor control and accuracy is directly dependent on the child's position and the extent to which the position influences stability, mobility, muscle tone, and energy expenditure. Therefore an evaluation of power wheelchair mobility control must include a seating evaluation to determine how the child's motor control is influenced by body position. Positioning is discussed in the final sections of this chapter.

Several features available on power wheelchairs help increase a child's function and level of independence. Technology-dependent children who require continuous oxygen support can become mobile by using portable ventilator carts attached to their wheelchair. Another recently developed feature enables the child to independently move from a sitting to a standing position and drive around while standing (Figure 20-19). A powered elevating seat, which raises the child to various heights for greater accessibility in the environment, is also available (Figure 20-20). Additional features include power tilt-in-space, which tilts the seat backwards to about 45 degrees while maintaining the same seat-to-back angle (Figure 20-21), and power recline, which places the child in the supine position by reclining the back of the chair.

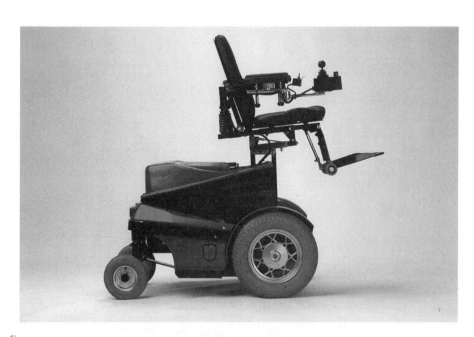

figure**20-20** Chairman Robo by Permobile is a pediatric front-wheel drive power wheelchair that can include an 8-inch seat elevator and seat-to-floor option that brings the child down to the floor level.

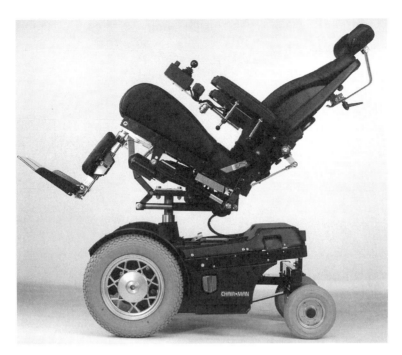

figure**20-21**   Chairman Corpus by Permobile is a front-wheel drive power wheelchair with tilt-in-space, recline with shear reduction, and an 8-inch seat elevator.

These two features are useful for individuals who need independent and frequent relief of pressure under their buttocks, such as those with spinal cord injury and muscle weakness or for those with back and neck pain.

A manual wheelchair can be converted to a power wheelchair by purchasing an add-on unit that includes two motors that are placed on the tires to rotate them, batteries, an electronic control unit, and a joystick. The electronic controls for the add-on units are not as sophisticated or adjustable as those found on standard power wheelchairs. This makes it more difficult for some children with impaired motor responses to accurately operate an add-on unit. They are also not highly recommended for individuals who use their wheelchairs outdoors and over rough terrain because they are not designed to withstand the forces that a power wheelchair must endure.

Three-wheeled scooters are another option for powered mobility. The individual who uses a scooter typically has good sitting balance, requires minimal positioning adaptation, and can understand and physically operate the tiller handle bar controls.

■ POWER MOBILITY EVALUATION AND INTERVENTION

The therapist, teacher, child, and caregivers must first define the goals for using a powered mobility device. Are the goals to provide functional and independent mobility or are the goals to provide transitional mobility experiences so that the child can have new opportunities to learn how to move, explore, and interact within the environment? Maneuverability features of the powered device are important when considering the various environments in which the device will be used (e.g., indoors, outdoors, school, home, or playground). How will the mobility device be transported? Will it need to fold to fit inside the trunk of a vehicle? If the wheelchair is to be transported in a van, is head clearance sufficient for the child when entering the vehicle? Will the environments need to be made accessible with ramps into doorways or lifts into vehicles?

The most common method for evaluating a person's ability to use a power mobility device is to have the device available for trial use during the evaluation. A facility typically cannot afford to purchase power wheelchairs for evaluation purposes. Fortunately ATSs often loan power wheelchairs to a clinical therapy unit for short-term evaluation purposes. The positioning and mobility equipment with the specific features that the child will need to use the device should be available during the evaluation. Equipment used during an evaluation should be in optimal working condition. The therapist should begin the evaluation by test driving the equipment to learn the forces and movements required to drive it, select the best speed for the client, and set any other adjustments, such as sensitivity of the controls.

The therapist begins an evaluation of the child's ability to drive a power wheelchair by evaluating the child's position to determine how to optimize motor function for efficient and accurate access of the controls. Several strategies are available to improve the ability of a child to use a joystick. If the child has difficulty moving the joystick in the desired direction, the therapist can place a template with a cross shape cut out inside the control box to limit deviation of the joystick to the desired directions. The therapist can also position the joystick with proper hardware to another location where control might be enhanced. The following is an example of a child whose position is evaluated for more accurate use of a powered mobility device.

> Erin, a 4-year-old child who is unable to communicate, was experiencing difficulty driving the power wheelchair using a joystick placed at the end of her right armrest. The teacher questioned Erin's ability to drive safely and accurately, believing that bumping into objects was purposeful. The occupational therapist observed Erin's arm and hand movements and noted that she seemed to have difficulty pushing the joystick forward and to the right side. She tended to internally rotate her arm and pull it toward her body. The joystick was mounted on an adjustable bracket that positioned it in midline, close to her chest. It also enabled the joystick box to be rotated about 30 degrees toward her body. After several more attempts at driving, her accuracy immediately improved. Once the most reliable placement was located, she became a functional driver.

If a child does not have the physical ability to control a joystick with the hand, foot, or head, the therapist can consider alternative means of switch operation, particularly for individuals with cerebral palsy. Before the therapist selects the type of switch, he or she should determine the movements that the child can use to access a switch. If the child can nod his or her head "yes" and "no", then he or she may have the ability to use switches around the back of the head.

The therapist may need to evaluate switch placement by allowing the child to first use switches to operate modified battery-operated toys (Wright & Nomura, 1991). The therapist first identifies the most reliable and efficient movements that the child can voluntarily use to access the switches. Switches are either momentary or latched. Momentary switches require the user to maintain contact on the switch to activate it. The child needs to be able to maintain contact on the switch long enough to move the wheelchair in a desired direction. A latching mode allows the individual to press the switch one time to activate it rather than holding it in the on position. A second activation turns the switch off. If the child needs to use switches to drive a power wheelchair, at least three switch sites are preferred: for driving forward, turning both directions, and moving in reverse. If the child can operate only one or two switches, the therapist may need to consider a scanning method; however, the scanning method requires a higher degree of cognitive function and concentration because of the complexity of the task.

Switch placement should begin at the hands and proceed to the head, elbows, feet, and any other location determined appropriate. An adjustable mounting bracket, such as that available through AbleNet Incorporated, is extremely helpful for positioning a switch in multiple locations. Once the therapist has determined an accurate and reliable motor response, he or she can assess the switch on a powered mobility device. Several factors can interfere with a person's ability to drive a powered mobility device. If a child has difficulty, the therapist first evaluates whether the type or placement of the controls is appropriate. The therapist then evaluates the child's position to determine if changes in the child's posture influence motor control. Other considerations include undetected visual and perceptual difficulties, impairment in response time, seizures, motivation, and behavior.

Many children may not initially be successful using a power wheelchair because of the overwhelming amount and degree of sensory input that is required. Imagine being a child with a severe disability who has difficulty with motor planning, coordination, visual perception, and communication and is experiencing movement in a powered device for the first time. It would be overwhelming to experience the excitement and vestibular sensation of moving while trying to view the surroundings, which are quickly passing by, and simultaneously listen to an adult telling you how and when to move.

The therapist should assess a young child for powered mobility, whenever feasible, by providing a method that promotes exploration and self-learning for the child. Such a method requires an open space with activities and toys strategically placed around the room to facilitate experiences in movement and exploration. The therapist should "limit physical and verbal commands as much as possible to avoid sensory overload on the part of the child" (Taylor & Monahan, 1989, p. 85). If a child is trying to move toward an object, the therapist should state the desired outcome, such as "come closer," rather than specific commands, such as "push the joystick left" or "push the red switch and come over here." Feedback should also be positive, such as "you found the wall" rather than "oops, you crashed again" (Wright-Ott, 1997). If further assistance is needed to help the child understand the operation of the control, the therapist can facilitate the proper response by physically guiding the child's movements for the desired response.

It may also be beneficial to loan or rent a power wheelchair to children and their families for an extended evaluation. This allows more time for the child to learn how to use the controls and for the family to become familiar with the features of a power wheelchair to assist them in becoming more informed consumers. It also provides an opportunity for the family to experience the responsibilities of maintaining and transporting a power wheelchair.

Computer programs are also available for powered mobility assessment and training (Taplin, 1989). R.J. Cooper and Associates have developed a joystick and mouse training program and a wheelchair simulation program. The programs display a power wheelchair on the screen that the user must navigate through a maze or room. Hasdai, Jessel, and Weiss (1998) studied whether a driving simulator would help a child master skills that are comparable with those required to drive a powered wheelchair. Their results indicated benefits from using such a program to prepare children for powered mobility.

Recently researchers have explored the use of virtual reality for assessing and training powered mobility skills (Trimble, Morris, & Crandall, 1992). The user wears a helmet that has a screen display of a three-dimensional room through which the person must navigate by using a joystick. More research is needed to determine if virtual reality is an effective means for assessing and training powered mobility and to determine if children will integrate the skills of wheelchair driving if they have not participated in the actual task.

■ POSITIONING CONSIDERATIONS

Positioning is critical to the successful use of any mobility device. How an individual is positioned in a mobility device, whether it be standing or sitting, can have an effect on several physiologic factors, including motor performance, postural control (Myhr & Wendt, 1991), ranges of movement, muscle tone (Nwaobi, 1986), endurance, comfort, respiration, and digestion. These factors can affect functional performance activities such as hand function (Nwaobi, 1987), levels of independence in mobility, self-care, activities of daily living (ADLs) such as transfers, and social interaction with others (Hulme, Poor, Schulein, & Pezzino, 1983).

Understanding the Biomechanics of Seating

To identify the positioning needs of a child, the occupational therapist must first have a thorough understanding of the biomechanical forces and physiologic factors that can influence posture and movement. Biomechanical considerations are critical to obtaining proper alignment of the pelvis, spine, and head. The position and stability of the pelvis is critical to movements that occur above and below the pelvis. Box 20-1 presents exercises that stress the importance of good alignment in sitting.

Seating Guidelines

The goal of seating is to place the pelvis and spine in a position that inhibits abnormal muscle tone, reduces undesirable biomechanical forces, and accommodates stiff postures that are no longer flexible. While accom-

---

box 20-1   *Exercises to understand the biomechanics of seating*

Sitting in posterior pelvic tilt

While in a sitting position, place your hands on the anterior crest of your pelvis (the two hip bones). Bend forward by rounding your back. You will feel your pelvis rolling backwards into a posteriorly tilted position. Hold your pelvis in this position and try to sit upright by extending your back. You may be able to move your head upright, but moving your trunk into a vertical position is dependent on placing your pelvis in a neutral or anteriorly tilted position. To view your environment with your pelvis in the posteriorly tilted position, you would either need to hyperextend your neck (an undesirable position) or slide your pelvis forward in the seat until your head achieves an upright position. Try maintaining a rounded or kyphotic back position and slide your pelvis forward in the seat. Feel the excessive pressure at the cervical and upper thoracic levels and the coccyx. Imagine being positioned like this for hours at a time and experiencing the discomfort, fatigue, and limited range of your upper extremities if you were in a wheelchair without a proper positioning system to improve or accommodate your posture.

Asymmetric pelvic position

Place your buttocks at the edge of your seat, lean only onto one side of your pelvis, and lift your feet so they are unsupported. Hold your pencil at its top edge and try to write. It is difficult to have accurate and efficient movements of your arm and hands because you do not have a stable base for the movements to occur. Imagine trying to accurately and safely operate the joystick of a power wheelchair in this position.

---

modating these postural problems, the positions should provide maximum weight distribution for stability, comfort, and skin integrity. The therapist can achieve stability at the pelvis by providing support at three contact points. The therapist first evaluates the type of support underneath the pelvis. The therapist determines whether the child can sit on a flat surface or is more stable using a contoured antithrust seat (a recessed seat that provides a recessed pocket for the pelvis and blocks forward movement of the ischial tuberosities). Some individuals require support at the sides of the pelvis to maintain a more symmetric position and reduce pelvic shift to one side. Support at the sides of the pelvis can be contoured into the seat or added as lateral hip guides. Stability can be provided above the pelvis to reduce sliding in an upward and forward direction. The therapist typically accomplishes this by placing a positioning belt at a 45-degree angle to the seat or placing it closer to the thighs. The therapist can also improve stability by ensuring that the femur is properly supported along its entire length, from the back of the pelvis to approximately 1 inch from the popliteal area under the knee. The pelvis should be supported posteriorly from the back cushion, which assists in maintaining a neutral or anteriorly tilted position. Other components, such as foot plates, lap trays, arm troughs, and neck supports, provide additional support.

The areas for the therapist to consider when evaluating the type of seating system that an individual needs in a wheelchair include (1) the angle between the seat and the back surfaces, (2) the tilt of the system in space (orientation), and (3) the type of surface on which the child will be seated (Bergen, Presperin, & Tallman, 1990, p. 17).

The three types of seating surfaces are planar, contoured, and custom molded. *Planar seating* consists of flat surfaces with no contours. This type of seating may be more appropriate for individuals with mildly affected development who require only minimal body contact with the support surfaces of the seat. *Contoured seating* systems allow the body to have more contact with the support surface because its shape conforms to the curves of the spine, buttocks, and thighs. The therapist can accomplish a contoured seat by layering various densities of foam, which respond to the height and weight of the person, thereby contouring around the bony prominences and other body curves. The therapist can purchase a contoured cushion from a manufacturer in standard sizes or it can be custom made to fit the child. It is often more advantageous to select a contoured cushion that can be opened and adjusted by adding or removing padding to fit a child's individual needs. *Custom-molded* seat cushions are designed specifically for an individual by taking an impression of the body and making a mold, which is sent to the manufacturer for fabrication of the cushions. Another method uses a computer-generated graphic picture taken from the impression, which is sent to the manufacturer, who then uses a computer-assisted milling machine to fabricate the cushions. Cushions can also be custom molded using foam-in-bag technology in which liquid foam is poured into an upholstered bag that is positioned around the person's body, providing a molded and finished cushion. This technique is more difficult to use because the individual's position must be held in place while the foam is being formed. If the child moves, the quality of the foam is negatively affected.

The use of orthotics or bracing of the extremities or body may also assist in achieving optimal positioning in the seated and standing positions. Ankle foot orthoses are most commonly recommended to align the foot and ankle and assist in either reducing muscle tone or supporting a weak limb. A thoracic lumbar sacral orthosis (TLSO), or body jacket, may be another alternative for individuals with scoliosis to use for support in the seated position.

■ METHODS FOR EVALUATING SEATING AND POSITIONING

The therapist should begin the initial assessment by observing the child using the mobility system to note posture, movements, comfort, and other factors that may affect function. The therapist should then position the child on a low mat table so that he or she can complete a postural assessment to determine whether any limitations in ranges of movement exist that may interfere with the upright seated position. The therapist obtains further information by positioning the child in a sitting position while using his or her hands to support the child to identify key points of control and positions that provide a desirable change in posture, muscle tone, and control. These key points become the necessary components of the seating system. The positions, such as the angle of hip flexion and the orientation in space of the child, become the pitches and angles of the components necessary in the seating system (Cooper, 1998).

Once the therapist gathers information from the postural assessment, other methods are also available that use evaluation equipment for assessment of a child's position to determine what components, angles, and sizes are needed in a seating system. Simulators are self-contained, adjustable fitting chairs that the therapist can adjust to fit a child or adult to determine what type of seating components and angles are appropriate (Trefler, 1999). The simulator allows the therapist to "evaluate the client in the system, alter angles of the seat to the back, try varying positions in space, and determine component sizes and accessories that are required before making recommendations for a particular system" (Trefler, Hobson, Taylor, Monshan, & Shaw, 1993, p. 73).

The therapist can use simulators to evaluate planar, contoured, and molded seating. The therapist first completes a postural evaluation of the individual to determine which seating components are necessary and then adjusts the simulator to the individual's size. The therapist selects angles, which include seat-to-back and tilt. He or she can make further adjustments to determine how position influences movement and function. The advantages of using a seating simulator include (1) use as a single evaluation tool for various ages, sizes, and diagnoses; (2) source of information about the various types of seating systems, such as planar versus molded; and (3) options to motorize simulators to evaluate powered mobility access and the effect of positioning on motor control. The problem that the assessment team often encounters when using simulators is difficulty in transferring the information from the simulator into an actual seating system and knowing how that system will integrate into a mobility base. Another disadvantage occurs when the seating system is used in a manual wheelchair; the biomechanics of propelling the wheels while positioned in the simulator cannot be assessed. Children may respond negatively to the simulator because its mechanical appearance and large size intimidate them.

Another method for evaluating seating and positioning is use of a modular "mock-up" or adjustable evaluation seat system that can be placed in a mobility base. These are typically available in planar or contoured seating devices rather than in custom-molded devices. The advantages of using this method include the ability for the child to use the mobility device while seated in the mock-up seat. This is particularly important because positioning can influence body movements and therefore functional outcomes. The disadvantages are that more equipment must be available to fit a range of individuals, and pitches and angles cannot always be accurately assessed.

Children with hypotonia, such as those with muscle diseases or cerebral palsy, have specific needs. A useful positioning system includes a back design that supports the sacrum in a neutral position but angles about 15 degrees away from the back at the posterior superior iliac spine. This provides a resting position of the trunk and accommodates the forces of gravity in the upright position. Consideration of a tilt-in-space feature in the mobility base may also provide the hypotonic or weak child with greater tolerance for sitting upright.

Children with increased muscle tone and spasticity who tend to adduct their legs and extend their hips and spine are often more difficult to position. The therapist must identify key points of control for positioning these children. For example, the therapist determines the desired degree of hip and knee flexion, hip abduction, and reduction of asymmetric positioning that positively influences muscle tone and control of extremity movement. These children may also have better postural control in the upright position rather than reclined or tilted (Nwaobi, 1986).

The therapist must frequently reevaluate a child's position, particularly in a seated mobility device, to accommodate postural, developmental, and growth changes. Once a child receives a seating mobility system, the therapist should reevaluate its fit and function every 6 months. Positioning and mobility literature and support materials are available (Cook & Hussey, 1995; Engstrom, 1993; Trefler, Hobson, Taylor, Monshan, & Shaw, 1993; Trefler, 1999), and more specific information and techniques on positioning are available through additional reading and workshops.

■ FACTORS THAT INFLUENCE SUCCESSFUL USE OF MOBILITY DEVICES

Successful use of mobility devices depends on the fit of the child, the device, and the physical and social environments. Studies have shown a significant relationship between certain standardized tests of cognition and perception and use of powered mobility. Specific functional performance tasks correlate to ability to use a power wheelchair. Preliminary findings indicate a relationship between specific cognitive scales and readiness for powered mobility (Tefft, Furumasu, & Guerette, 1992; Verburg, Field, & Jarvis, 1987).

Another factor that influences a child's ability to use a powered device is the ability of the professional or caregiver to determine the most accurate and efficient means for the child to access the device. If a child is having significant difficulty successfully maneuvering a powered mobility device, the therapist must first evaluate the access method to determine if it is the most effective means. The therapist then considers the child's positioning needs. The longer it takes a child to successfully demonstrate use of a control, the more likely it is that either the access method or position is inappropriate. The following example best describes this type of situation.

> Stephanie is a 15-month-old girl with cerebral palsy who successfully used a switch-operated toy vehicle to maneuver and explore her surroundings. It took her about 5 hours to become proficient at using a system of four hand-activated press switches and to understand the relationship to directionality. However, when she entered another therapy program, the therapist did not consider information on her ability to use switches for driving. Instead, the therapist placed her in a wheelchair training program using the only equipment available, a joystick-operated power wheelchair. After 6 months of training for 3 hours each week, Stephanie demonstrated no improvement in her ability to drive the power wheelchair. Upon reevaluation of her access method, the therapist provided her with four switches at her hand rather than a joystick, and she was immediately able to successfully drive the power wheelchair. Had the therapist provided her with the appropriate control method (four switches placed at her hand instead of a joystick, which she could not operate because of her impaired motor function), she may have demonstrated the ability to use the power wheelchair in significantly less time.

The therapist must consider changes that the child may be experiencing in the future, both unexpected and expected, when recommending equipment. For example, the therapist must determine whether the system can be readily changed as the child gains new skills, grows, or experiences other physical changes. This is particularly important for the therapist to consider when ordering a power wheelchair. For example, a child with a progressive disability may be able to operate a joystick at the time the chair is ordered. However, the therapist needs to determine whether the power wheelchair can be economically reconfigured to operate using another method, such as head switch control, as the child's strength diminishes. Several options may need to be included in the wheelchair, such as the ability to readily change the access method. It is more economical in most cases to initially order options on equipment rather than reorder the equipment at a later date.

Another issue for the therapist to consider when recommending mobility and positioning equipment is where and how augmentative communication equipment is mounted to the child's wheelchair. Selection of the appropriate mounting bracket depends on the tube size of the wheelchair frame and locations on the wheelchair where it can be attached. A problem that therapists often encounter with manual wheelchairs is positioning the child or rear wheels too far forward of the center of gravity in the wheelchair, which often causes the wheelchair to tip forward when the communication device is mounted. The most frequent problem encountered with power wheelchairs is the communication device's interference with the field of vision required for driving.

The therapy team and ATS have a responsibility to assist the family and child in selecting the most appropriate device by presenting several alternatives. The family makes the final decision on the specific type of mobility device after considering the options that the therapy team presents. The most important and significant contribution that the therapist can make is to evaluate access methods and help caregivers develop and implement strategies to meet identified goals. The therapist must reevaluate the outcome as the child progresses. This includes periodic evaluation of fit and function of the equipment.

■ SUMMARY

The literature indicates that independent mobility plays a facilitative role in cognitive and social development. Therefore when mobility is severely delayed or restricted, emotional and psychosocial development are affected. Augmentative mobility devices can provide either functional or transitional mobility. These devices can provide children with physical disabilities with greater opportunities to develop and become initiators and active participants in daily occupations and experiences. Occupational therapists emphasize methods of adapting the child's environments to maximize his or her functional mobility. The occupational therapist is responsible for ensuring that children with physical disabilities receive op-

portunities for mobility at the earliest age possible to promote participation and development more equal to their able-bodied peers.

Case Studies

These case studies include comprehensive information about the children's equipment and adapted environments. These descriptions demonstrate how mobility equipment is integrated with other assistive technology (AT) and environmental adaptations to best meet the children's functional needs.

David and Eric

David is 11 years of age, and he was diagnosed with Duchenne's muscular dystrophy at 4 years of age. Shortly afterward, his little brother, Eric, was diagnosed with the same condition at 5 months of age. The two brothers and an older sister live with their parents in a small town.

Duchenne's muscular dystrophy is an inherited X-linked disease that affects the voluntary skeletal musculature with progressive weakness and degeneration of the muscles that control movement. The muscle weakness begins in the proximal and axial musculature and slowly progresses distally. Frequently children with Duchenne's muscular dystrophy require a wheelchair by 12 years of age. Breathing becomes affected during the later stages of the disease, leading to severe respiratory problems. Respiratory infections commonly claim the patient's life during the early twenties.

When receiving David's diagnosis, the family was introduced to a team of professionals that specialize in different aspects of musculoskeletal weaknesses. The family received support to help them deal with the initial shock and necessary information about the disease. Twice a year the family continued to meet with the team for medical and orthopedic evaluations. Social and psychologic concerns were also addressed.

Last year David had an achilles tendon lengthening to release a tight heel cord. Today he walks with a long leg orthosis. It is important to lengthen the walking phase in boys with Duchenne's muscular dystrophy to delay hip and knee flexion deformities and equinovarus deformity of the foot and ankle. For 2 years David used a standard lightweight manual wheelchair for traveling long distances or when he was fatigued. Currently, the therapy team and David's family are considering a power wheelchair for David to allow him to conserve energy for social and educational activities. The team plans spinal stabilization when David's scoliosis exceeds 25 degrees and normal forced vital capacity (FVC) pulmonary function drops below 50%.

Eric is now 7 years of age. The progression of his disease is following the same course as David's, although somewhat slower. The early signs of Duchenne's muscular dystrophy are becoming prominent, such as the waddling gait, tendency to fall, and difficulty rising from a sitting or lying position.

At the time of Eric's diagnosis, the family lived in an apartment but soon decided to build a house. The occupational therapist provided recommendations for designing the house for wheelchair accessibility to maximize function and independence.

The family has been living in the house for 2 years, and they are pleased with the features that enable the boys to be independent. The outdoor surfaces (sidewalks and ramps) are firm, stable, and slip resistant. The floor plan is spacious, doorways are wide, and there are no thresholds. A few sliding doors have been installed to allow maximum door width and to eliminate floor swing space requirements. Controls, levers, and switches are placed low to be within reach from a wheelchair. The window's lower edge is only 20 inches above the floor for the same reason. The bathrooms are spacious, and there is a bathtub and a shower. The boys love taking baths because they stay warmer and move more freely in the water. The sink is free-standing so the boys can get close to the sink. An automatic faucet has been installed, which is turned on when the hands are placed under the faucet. A full-length mirror is on the wall.

The family continues to need a lot of support and assistance to adjust to new challenges. In addition to direct service to the family, the occupational therapist continues to work closely with the schools to ensure that accessibility is available.

Jason

Jason is a 7-year-old boy with cerebral palsy, which has affected his ability to speak, move his body with control, and eat. Although he demonstrates severe delays in his motor skills, he appears alert and attentive and understands what is said to him. From his early days, his family was motivated to ensure that Jason has a childhood as normal as possible. They were creative in designing simple devices and tools to accomplish these goals. His grandfather designed the first mobility device for him. It was a push cart used to hold golf clubs, but he mounted a car seat to the frame and placed foam pieces in the seat to help align Jason's body and prevent him from leaning over. His mother would use it to push him around the neighborhood during her daily jogging routine. He also used a standard stroller but required a positioning system to assist him in sitting upright by providing support at the pelvis, trunk, and head. The first seating system was made of triwall, a three-layer thickness cardboard that can be used to fabricate temporary seat inserts for children. Another seat insert was fabricated from triwall, but this one could be placed on the dining room chair so that he could eat at the family table instead of a high chair.

By the time he was 12 months of age, Jason's family built him an aeroplane mobility device (see Figure 21-6)

to use at home. When he outgrew this by 2 years of age, his therapist evaluated him for a support walker and he could effectively use the Walkabout by Mobility Plus. He continued to use this for indoor mobility and for playing in little league for special needs children when he was 5 years of age. He and his teammates used an automatic device to hit the ball, and Jason ran around the field using his walker.

When Jason was 2½ years of age, his family decided that his mobility needs were not being adequately met by the walker alone. His therapist evaluated him for a power wheelchair, and he could operate the joystick once he was positioned with maximal support at his feet, pelvis, trunk, and head. His therapist and family determined the features that he needed so that he could use a power wheelchair. They determined that he needed a molded seating system for support and alignment. To increase independence, the system needed to include the ability to elevate the seat from the floor to various heights. The therapist identified a power wheelchair with these features, and recommended a custom-molded seating system.

The family made the home environment accessible to Jason in many ways. When he was 2 years of age they decided that it was important for him to roll out of bed in the morning and try to roll on the floor. They placed a low-height mattress on the floor in the corner of his bedroom and made it his bed. They lined the sides of it with his stuffed toys to protect him from unintentionally hitting his arms against the walls. This arrangement allowed him to get out of bed on his own. They also extended the light switch in his room so that he could reach it from his walker or wheelchair.

Positioning in the bathtub when he was a toddler was a challenge, but his mother made a bath seat for him from a milk crate. She placed foam around the edges and the seat for comfort. When he outgrew this, his family acquired a bath seat designed for children with disabilities. His occupational therapist recommended an adapted toilet seat with a high backrest. It provided Jason with the ability to begin toilet training at 2 years of age. His family also installed a flip-down bar in front of the toilet so Jason could stand at the toilet "like his Dad."

During these early years, Jason's therapist introduced him to augmentative communication symbols and aids. By the time he was 12 months of age he could point to symbols in his communication book and soon progressed to using an augmentative communication device with voice output by accessing it with a light pointer on his head. The communication device was mounted on his power wheelchair. Today Jason is fully included in a second grade class. He uses AT to do his schoolwork and has an attendant with him throughout the day. Both simple and sophisticated AT devices have enabled him to function within a regular education classroom, participating in most of the activities of his peers.

STUDY QUESTIONS

1. What questions should be answered before selecting a mobility device?

2. A child with cerebral palsy (spastic diplegia) uses a push walker but needs a manual wheelchair for mobility in the community and at school. He is expected to learn how to transfer in and out of it in the future. What features will be needed on his manual wheelchair for optimal independence?

3. What type of wheelchair control would an individual with a spinal cord injury at the C3 level be most likely to use?

4. If a child has less than 90 degrees of passive range of movement in knee extension because of tight hamstring muscles, explain how this would affect his ability to sit upright in a wheelchair using standard footrest hangers (60-degree angle)?

5. Why is it important for the therapist to simultaneously consider a child's positioning needs when assessing a mobility device?

References

Becker, R.D. (1975). Recent developments in child psychiatry: The restrictive emotional and cognitive environment reconsidered: A redefinition of the concept of the therapeutic restraint. *Israel Annals of Psychiatry and Related Disciplines, 13,* 239-258.

Bergen, A., Presperin, J., & Tallman, T. (1990). *Positioning for function: Wheelchairs and other assistive technologies.* New York: Valhalla Rehabilitation Publications.

Bertenthal, B.I., Campos, J.J., & Barrett, K.C. (1984). Self-produced locomotion: An organizer of emotional, cognitive, and social development in infancy. In R.N. Emde & R.J. Harmon (Eds.), *Continuities and discontinuities in development.* New York, Plenum Press.

Bly, L. (1994). *Motor skills acquisition in the first year.* Tucson: Therapy Skill Builders.

Brinker, R.P., & Lewis, M. (1982). Making the world work with microcomputers: A learning prosthesis for handicapped infants. *Exceptional Children, 49,* 163-170.

Butler, C. (1986). Effects of powered mobility on self-initiated behaviors of very young children with locomotor disability. *Developmental Medicine and Child Neurology, 28,* 325-332.

Butler, C. (1988a). High tech tots: Technology for mobility, manipulation, communication, and learning in early childhood. *Infants and Young Children, 2,* 66-73.

Butler, C. (1988b). Powered tots: Augmentative mobility for locomotor disabled youngsters. *American Physical Therapy Association Pediatric Publication, 14,* 21.

Campos, J.J., & Bertenthal, B.I. (1987). Locomotion and psychological development in infancy. In K.M. Jaffe (Ed.), Childhood powered mobility: Developmental, technical, and clinical perspectives. In *Proceedings of the RESNA First Northwest Regional Conference* (pp. 11-42). Washington D.C: RESNA Press.

Cech, D., & Martin, A. (1995). *Functional movement development across the life span.* Philadelphia: W.B. Saunders.

Cook, A.M., & Hussey, S.M. (1995). Seating and positioning systems as extrinsic enablers for assistive technologies. In A.M. Cook & S.M. Hussey (Eds.), *Assistive technologies: Principles and practice* (pp. 235-310). St. Louis: Mosby.

Coster, W. (1998). Occupation-centered assessment of children. *The American Journal of Occupational Therapy, 52,* 337-344.

Douglas, J., & Ryan, M. (1987). A preschool severely disabled boy and his powered wheelchair: A case study. *Child Care, Health and Development, 13,* 303-309.

Engstrom, B. (1993). *Ergonomics, wheelchairs and positioning.* Hasselby, Sweden: Posturalis Books.

Fisher, A.G. (1998). Uniting practice and theory in an occupational framework. *The American Journal of Occupational Therapy, 52,* 509-521.

Haley, S.M., Coster, W.J., Ludlow, L.H., Haltiwanger, J., & Andrellos, P. (1992). *Pediatric Evaluation of Disability Inventory (PEDI).* San Antonio: Psychological Corp.

Hasdai, A., Jessel, A.S., & Weiss, P.L. (1998). Use of computer simulator for training children with disabilities in the operation of a powered wheelchair. *The American Journal of Occupational Therapy, 52,* 215-220.

Hays, R. (1987). Childhood motor impairments: Clinical overview and scope of the problem. In K.M. Jaffe (Ed.), Childhood powered mobility: Developmental, technical, and clinical perspectives. *Proceedings of the RESNA First Northwest Regional Conference.* Washington D.C: RESNA Press.

Hulme, J., Poor, R., Schulein, M., & Pezzino, J. (1983). Perceived behavioral changes observed with adaptive seating devices for multihandicapped developmentally disabled individuals. *Physical Therapy, 62* (4), 204-208.

Law, M., Baptiste, S., Carswell, A., McColl, M.A., Polatajko, H., & Pollock, N. (1994). *The Canadian Occupational Performance Measure* (2nd ed.). Toronto, ON: CAOT Publications.

Myhr, U., & Wendt, L. (1991). Improvement of functional sitting position for children with cerebral palsy. *Developmental Medicine and Child Neurology, 33,* 246-256.

Nilsson, L., & Nyberg, P. (1998). *Training two preschool children with multihandicaps to operate a powered wheelchair.* Abstract (Poster) presented at World Federation of Occupational Therapists Conference in Montreal, Quebec, Canada.

Nwaobi, O. (1986). Effects of body orientation in space on tonic muscle activity of patients with cerebral palsy. *Developmental Medicine and Child Neurology, 28,* 41-44.

Nwaobi, O. (1987). Effect of unilateral arm restraint on upper extremity function in cerebral palsy. In *Proceedings of the Annual RESNA Conference* (pp. 311-313). Washington, D.C.: RESNA Press.

Paleg, G. (July, 1997). Made for walking: A comparison of gait trainers. *Team Rehab Report,* 41-45.

Paulsson, K., & Christoffersen, M. (1984). Psychological aspects of technical aids: How does independent mobility affect the psychological and intellectual development of children with physical disabilities. In *Proceedings of the Second Annual Conference on Rehabilitation Engineering* (pp. 282-286). Washington D.C: RESNA Press.

Piaget, J. (1954). *The construction of reality in the child.* New York: Basic Books.

Pollock, N., & Stewart, D. (1998). Occupational performance needs of school-aged children with physical disability in the community. *Physical and Occupational Therapy in Pediatrics, 18* (1), 55-68.

Seligman, M. (1975). *Helplessness: On depression, development, and death.* San Francisco: W.H. Freeman.

Taplin, C.S. (1989). Powered wheelchair control, assessment, and training. In *RESNA '89: Proceedings of the 12th annual conference* (pp. 45-46.) Washington, D.C: RESNA Press.

Taylor, S., & Monahan, L. (1989). Considerations in assessing for powered mobility. In C. Brubaker (Ed.), *Wheelchair IV: Report of a conference on the state of the art of powered wheelchair mobility, December 7-9, 1988.* Washington D.C: RESNA Press.

Tefft, D., Furumasu, J., & Guerette, P. (1992). *Cognitive readiness for powered mobility in the very young child* (Unpublished manuscript). Downey, CA: Rancho Los Amigos.

Tefft, D., Furumasu, J, & Guerette, P. (1997). Pediatric powered mobility: Influential cognitive skills. In J. Furumasu (Ed.), *Pediatric powered mobility* (pp. 70-91). Washington D.C: RESNA Press.

Trefler, E. (1999). Then & now: Saving time with simulators. *Team Rehab, February,* 32-36.

Trefler, E., Hobson, D., Taylor, S., Monahan, L, & Shaw, C. (1993). *Seating and mobility.* Tucson: Therapy Skill Builders.

Trimble, J., Morris, T., & Crandall, R. (1992). Virtual reality: Designing accessible environments. *Team Rehab Report, 3,* 8-12.

Uniform Data System for Medical Rehabilitation. (1999). *Functional Independence Measure for Children (WeeFIM)* (Outpatient version 5.0.). Buffalo, NY: State University of New York at Buffalo.

Verburg, G., Field, D., & Jarvis, S. (1987). Motor, perceptual, and cognitive factors that affect mobility control. In *Proceedings of the 10th Annual Conference on Rehabilitation Technology,* Washington D.C: RESNA Press.

Warren, C.G. (1990). Powered mobility and its implications, *Journal of Rehabilitation Research and Development. Clinical Supplement* (2), 74-85.

Woods, H. (1998). Moving right along: Young disabled children can now experience the developmental benefits of moving and exploring on their own. *Stanford Medicine, Fall,* 15-19.

Wright, C., & Nomura, M. (1991). *From toys to computers, access for the physically disabled child.* San Jose, CA: Author.

Wright-Ott, C. (1997). The transitional powered mobility aid: A new concept and tool for early mobility. In J. Furumasu (Ed.), *Pediatric powered mobility.* (pp. 58-69). Washington D.C: RESNA Press.

Wright-Ott, C. (1998). Designing a transitional powered mobility aid for young children with physical disabilities. In D. Gray, L. Quatrano, & M. Lieverman (Eds). *Designing and using assistive technology: The human perspective* (pp. 285-295). Baltimore: Brooks.

section **IV**

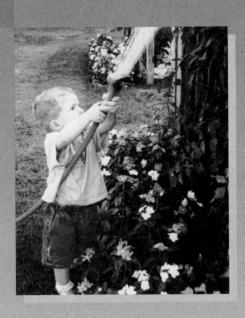

ARENAS OF PEDIATRIC OCCUPATIONAL THERAPY SERVICES

chapter **21**

Neonatal Intensive Care Unit

Jan G. Hunter

key terms

Preterm infants
Neonatal intensive care unit
Developmentally supportive care
Als' synactive theory of development
Respiratory complications
Neurologic complications and sequelae
NICU light and sound modifications

NICU caregiving patterns
Neuromotor and neurobehavioral development
Therapeutic positioning
Nonnutritive sucking patterns
Nutritive sucking patterns

■ CHAPTER OBJECTIVES

1. Understand the scope of knowledge required for competent practice in the neonatal intensive care unit (NICU).
2. Compare the traditional occupational therapy approach of rehabilitation and developmental stimulation with current concepts of individualized developmentally supportive care in the NICU.
3. Define and compute postconceptional, chronologic, and corrected age.
4. Explain why preterm infants are so susceptible to heat loss and how heat loss can occur.
5. Identify maternal medical complications and lifestyle factors that create risk to the fetus.
6. Define common medical conditions in the preterm and high-risk infant.
7. Identify potential negative effects of light, sound, and caregiving practices in the NICU.
8. Describe interventions to modify light, sound, and caregiving practices in the NICU so that preterm infants are protected from excessive stimulation.
9. Discuss the factors that complicate parenting in the NICU.

10. Describe roles and potential interventions of the NICU therapist in providing family support through family-centered neonatal care.
11. Discuss considerations when evaluating an infant in the NICU, and identify published neonatal assessments.
12. Explain the synactive theory of development proposed by Heidi Als.
13. Describe neuromotor and neurobehavioral development in preterm infants.
14. Identify and describe the six neurobehavioral states.
15. Explain the advantages and disadvantages of using different positioning techniques.
16. Describe common positional deformities of preterm infants, the potential influence on future development, and how these deformities can be prevented.
17. Explain indications for and applications of neuromotor interventions that involve range of motion and splinting.
18. Explain why nonnutritive sucking is beneficial to preterm infants.
19. Describe three nutritive sucking patterns observed during infant feeding.

20. Summarize key factors that can facilitate successful breast-feeding in the NICU.
21. Apply methods of modifying the sensory environment to a case study of an extremely preterm infant with multiple medical problems and neurobehavioral difficulties.

■ EVOLUTION OF NEONATAL INTENSIVE CARE

The *neonatal intensive care unit* (NICU) is a complex and highly specialized hospital unit designed to care for infants who are born prematurely or are critically ill (Figure 21-1). Current state-of-the-art NICUs bear little resemblance to the "Special Department for Weaklings," the first special care unit for preterm newborns established by Dr. Pierre Budin in 1893. Budin established this unit when medical care for preterm newborns consisted of providing warmth, small feedings, and protection from infection (Hodgman, 1985). Technologic advances have prompted the observation that being a newborn *preterm infant* in a modern NICU is like being abducted from a warm comfortable home by "aliens" or "terrorists" and subjected to an overwhelming barrage of continuous bright lights and jarring noises while having fruitless attempts at sleep repeatedly interrupted with frequent invasive and painful procedures by "huge creatures" (White & Newbold, 1995). Increased awareness of the influence of environmental and caregiving factors on the vulnerable newborn have enlarged the scope of NICU care to encompass developmental and family issues in addition to primary medical concerns (Als &

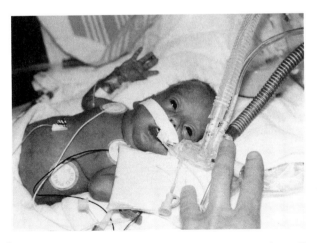

figure 21-1   Preterm infant is receiving mechanical ventilation in neonatal intensive care unit. Three cardiorespiratory leads and temperature probe are visible; a percutaneous catheter for intravenous infusions is in right arm. *(Courtesy of the Infant Special Care Unit, University of Texas Medical Branch, Galveston, TX. Photograph by Candy Cochran.)*

Gilkerson, 1997; Gottfried & Gaiter, 1985; McGrath & Conliffe-Torres, 1996). This chapter describes the knowledge and skills needed by the neonatal occupational therapist to achieve this expanded focus.

Nursery Classification and Regionalization of Care

Advances in medical technology and specialized care for preterm and high-risk infants have skyrocketed since the early 1960s. The spiraling expense and complexity of medical care created a growing discrepancy between neonatal mortality rates at major medical centers and smaller hospitals. In the early 1970s, the concept of regionalization of perinatal care emerged to provide advanced levels of health care to any mother or infant within that perinatal region while avoiding unnecessary duplication of services (American Medical Association, 1971). Patient care was generally provided at the nearest hospital, with transfer to a higher-level facility as needed for more complex problems.

Area hospitals have traditionally been designated by the level of care they provide. A level I nursery (e.g., in a small community hospital) manages uncomplicated pregnancies with expected normal deliveries and well infants. Level II nurseries are designed to care for newborn infants, including those requiring additional medical management, such as phototherapy for jaundice or intravenous (IV) antibiotics. A neonatologist is usually on staff, but these units typically lack the equipment and additional expertise, such as a pediatric surgeon or cardiologist, to care for all medical emergencies and severe neonatal problems. Level III nurseries have all of the equipment and trained personnel, in the nursery and other hospital departments, necessary to care for all potential neonatal conditions and emergencies (Korones, 1985). "Level IV" is an unofficial classification sometimes used to designate NICUs that offer "rescue" technology (e.g., nitric oxide [NO] and extracorporeal membrane oxygenation [ECMO]) for infants in respiratory failure unresponsive to conventional medical management.

Since the 1980s the economic forces of an increasingly competitive health care market have compromised the traditional concepts of regionalization of care (Pettett, Sewell, & Merenstein, 1998). The growth of managed health care and the availability of neonatal technology and specialists have encouraged many hospitals to expand their perinatal services, resulting in fragmentation of perinatal services with a wide disparity in level of care provided. Renewed analysis and modification of regionalization policies to achieve better outcomes with cost savings, such as routine provision of mechanical ventilation in Level II units, have been advocated by leading neonatologists (Meadow et. al., 1996). Achieving a balance between cost control and universal quality patient access is the current dilemma and necessity facing organizers and providers of perinatal health care.

NICU Outcome Indicators: Mortality and Morbidity

Infant survival was initially the primary indicator of NICU success. As innovations in medical science, technology, and caregiving skills increased the survival rate of younger, smaller, and sicker infants, concerns have emerged about the effects of the NICU on preterm infants and about the long-term developmental outcome of NICU survivors.

These concerns have facilitated the entry of occupational therapists and other neonatal developmental specialists into the critical care arena of the NICU. Professionals continue to explore preterm infant development, effects of acute and chronic illness, animate and inanimate NICU environmental factors, family dynamics of hospitalized infants, ultimate outcome of NICU survivors, and increase of NICU cost containment and use of resources (Peabody & Martin, 1996; Wildrick, 1997).

Sensory Deprivation Versus Stimulation

Changing theories about sensory stimulation in the NICU also promoted access for occupational therapists into the intensive care nursery. Understanding this history of stimulation in the NICU helps the therapist progress to state-of-the-art intervention:

- *Minimal stimulation*. Special care nurseries in the 1940s and 1950s were strictly minimal stimulation units with low lights, quiet environments, and restricted access by families and even doctors.
- *Sensory deprivation theory*. The scarcity of stimuli in these early nurseries precipitated the sensory deprivation theory espoused in the 1960s and 1970s.
- *Sensory stimulation programs*. Sensory deficit proponents believed that NICU infants were deprived of beneficial sensory stimuli and prescribed selected regimens of patterned stimuli in a "one size fits all" approach. These supplemental stimulation programs generally consisted of massage, stroking, passive range of motion, vestibular input, and/or auditory input. Concerns have also been raised that extra stimulation may have benefited larger stable infants but possibly stressed infants who are more fragile; behavioral responses of individual infants were not recorded.
- *Sensory overload theory*. The sensory deficit model failed to recognize that the explosion of knowledge and technology in the 1960s and 1970s actually created an abundance of noncontingent stimuli that was disorganized and disturbing to the infants. New nurseries had large, brightly lit rooms filled with noisy monitors and equipment; additional nursery staff members greatly increased the noise level and

engaged in frequent handling of infants for procedures. Sensory overload theory began to emerge in the 1970s and hypothesized that NICU infants were actually overwhelmed by various inappropriate stimuli.
- *Environmental neonatology*. Emerging concerns about the large quantity and variety of random stimuli prompted the rise in the 1980s and 1990s of "environmental neonatology," in which the influence of animate and inanimate environmental factors in NICU facilities is explored.
- *Individualized, relationship-based, family-centered developmental care*. This type of care strives to continually structure the NICU environment and caregiving practices according to ongoing neurobehavioral cues of each infant and promote the involvement of family members as primary caregivers and integrated team members for their NICU infant.

■ CHANGING FOCUS OF NEONATAL OCCUPATIONAL THERAPY

Traditional Occupational Therapy: Rehabilitation and Stimulation

Traditional neonatal occupational therapy in the 1980s (and persisting in some NICUs in the 1990s) consisted solely of rehabilitation and developmental stimulation. Infants were identified as appropriate for occupational therapy by specific risk factors (e.g., very low birth weight, prenatal drug exposure), diagnosis of pathologic condition (e.g., congenital anomalies, severe asphyxia), or performance indicators (e.g., abnormal tone, poor feeding, chronic illness with developmental delay). Therapy goals and intervention activities targeted specific problems, such as limited range of motion, high or low muscle tone, extreme irritability, poor feeding, or developmental delay (Rapport, 1992).

Rehabilitation continues to be an appropriate component of therapy for a select group of medically stable NICU infants with definitive diagnoses, such as arthrogryposis multiplex congenita (see Case Study 1) or myelomeningocele with hydrocephalus. Older chronically ill infants who need developmental stimulation may remain in some NICUs but are frequently transferred to step-down units or discharged with home health services at much earlier ages and with greater acuity than was done a decade ago.

State-of-the-Art Occupational Therapy: Developmental Support

With advances in developmental knowledge pertinent to the NICU, the parameters of neonatal occupational therapy have expanded beyond traditional rehabilitation services to encompass *developmentally supportive care.* This approach is based on the recognition that any infant young enough or sick enough to require intensive care has inherent developmental risks and vulnerabilities, parenting an infant in the NICU is stressful and difficult, and both infant and family must receive individualized support throughout the NICU hospitalization for optimal outcome (Mouradian & Als, 1994).

Developmental support includes a protective and preventive component of care that is not inherent in the traditional rehabilitation model. In contrast to the previous emphasis for direct "hands on" contact, protecting the fragile newborn from excessive or inappropriate sensory input is often a more urgent priority than direct interventions or interactions with the infant (AOTA, 2000).

Therapist Trust and Acceptance in the NICU

As the neonatal therapist expands beyond conventional stimulation and rehabilitation techniques to include the practice of individualized developmental care, closer working relationships with medical staff members result. NICU staff members are historically and rightfully protective of their tiny, vulnerable patients. Professional credentials and a patient referral may allow an unfamiliar therapist access to the unit, but the competent therapist can only earn trust and acceptance in the NICU over time. Understanding the transitional stages in developing collaborative partnerships between therapists and neonatal nurses is helpful for the therapist who is in the process of moving from "guest" to "family" in the NICU (Sweeney, 1993).

- Professional guest
  - Stage 1: Independent consultation with minimal interaction
  - Stage 2: Competitive or protective posturing while evaluating co-worker competence
- Integrated NICU team member
  - Stage 3: Building trust and mutuality in joint caregiving and problem solving
  - Stage 4: Committed partnership with peak creative experiences

Competencies for the Neonatal Therapist

Practice standards to promote relevant competencies for NICU developmental specialists have been documented (AOTA, 1993, 2000; Scull & Deitz, 1989; VandenBerg, 1993a). Occupational therapy in the NICU is considered a specialized area of practice requiring advanced knowledge and skills. Specialized knowledge requirements include familiarity with relevant neonatal medical conditions, procedures, and equipment; under-

standing of the unique developmental abilities and vulnerabilities of the infant; familiarity with theories of neonatal behavioral organization, family systems, and NICU ecology; and appreciation of the manner in which these factors interact to influence behavior. The occupational therapist develops the necessary knowledge and skills through continuing education and supervised clinical experience in assessment and intervention specific to the NICU (AOTA, 1993, 2000; Dewire, White, Kanny, & Glass, 1996; Hunter, 1996).

The remainder of this chapter is divided into four distinct but interrelated sections. The first section emphasizes development of an NICU medical foundation. The remaining three sections discuss the NICU environment, NICU family, and NICU infant; each of these sections includes foundation information, evaluation, and intervention strategies pertinent to the focus topic. Evaluation and intervention with the infant are discussed last because they are symbolic of the ethical neonatal therapist who conscientiously prepares before touching the NICU infant.

■ DEVELOPING A MEDICAL FOUNDATION

Abbreviations and Terminology

Learning the language of the NICU is essential for the neonatal occupational therapist. Documentation typically contains many abbreviations, as illustrated by this medical summary:

> Cody is a 39 wk pca wm born at 25 WBD, 27 WBE by SVD to a 18 y/o now $G_2P_1Ab_1$, A+,VDRL- mom with hx of IVDA, smokes 1 PPD, PIH and PTL tx'd with $MgSO_4$, PPROM 72° PTD. Pt. had TCAN ×1 (reduced PTD), was SGA at 505 gm, Apgars $1^1,3^5,6^{10}$. Significant medical complications have included RDS, BPD, PIE, PDA (ligated), hyperbilirubinemia, anemia, MRSE sepsis, NEC (∅ surgery), AOP, BIH, R gr. 3 and L gr.4 IVH with PVL, ROP stage III OD (regressing) and stage III+ OS (s/p laser OS). Pt. was on SIMV for 41 days, NCPAP for 32 days, and remains on FiO_2 1.0 at .5L by NC.

Understanding abbreviations and the terms they represent is a prerequisite to beginning a neonatal practice. Appendix 21-A lists some common NICU abbreviations.

Classifications for Age

Gestational age (GA) refers to the total number of weeks that the infant was in utero before birth. Determination of gestational age may be based on dating the last menstrual period (LMP) either by ultrasound (USG) or physical examination of the infant (Clopton, 1993). The range used for a full-term pregnancy is 38 to 42 weeks at some hospitals and 37 to 42 weeks at others. An infant born before 37 to 38 weeks is considered preterm; an infant born after 42 weeks is postterm. Once the infant is born, the GA remains the same.

Postconceptional age (PCA) refers to the infant's age in relation to when conception occurred and thus continually changes over time. PCA is obtained by adding the weeks since birth to the infant's gestational age. When the infant born at 27 weeks reaches his or her expected due date, the PCA is 40 weeks (27 weeks' gestation plus 13 weeks since birth to the original term due date). PCA is commonly used until 40 to 44 weeks, equivalent to term or 1 month corrected age, respectively.

Chronologic age refers to the infant's actual age since birth. Chronologically, the infant born at 27 weeks' gestation is 3 months old on the expected due date and 12 months old on the first birthday.

Chronologic age of preterm infants is usually "corrected for prematurity" to better correlate with developmental expectations and performance (i.e., the infant born at 27 weeks' gestation will not developmentally look the same at 3 months chronologic age as the infant born at term). *Corrected age* refers to how old the infant would be if born at term rather than prematurely. The number of weeks of prematurity is first determined (GA is subtracted from the term equivalent of 40 weeks) and then subtracted from the chronologic age. The infant born at 27 weeks' gestation was born 13 weeks prematurely (40 weeks−27 weeks GA=13 weeks early). The corrected age of this infant on the first birthday is 9 months because the actual birth was 3 months earlier than the expected due date. Corrected age is typically used until 2 years of age when assessing developmental status.

Classifications of Birth Weight

Infants born above 2500 grams (5.5 pounds) are considered average in size. A birth weight of 1500 to 2500 grams is termed *low birth weight* (LBW). *Very low birth weight* (VLBW) is 1000 to 1500 grams, and *extremely low birth weight* (ELBW) is less than 1000 grams.

Birth weight between the tenth and the ninetieth percentiles on a standardized growth chart is *appropriate for gestational age* (AGA). Birth weight below the tenth percentile is *small for gestational age* (SGA), and birth weight above the ninetieth percentile is *large for gestational age* (LGA). These categories apply equally to preterm, term, and postterm infants. Any infant growing normally in utero will be AGA. An infant of a mother with severe pregnancy-induced hypertension (PIH) may have experienced intrauterine growth retardation (IUGR) and may be born SGA, whereas the infant of a mother with diabetes is often LGA.

Thermoregulation

Preterm infants are predisposed to excessive heat loss and are vulnerable to cold stress from several causes. Extended posture, thin skin, and reduced insulating subcutaneous fat in very premature infants allow heat to transfer from the body to the air. A specialized *brown fat* used by newborns to metabolize heat is not produced until the last trimester of gestation. Pulmonary dysfunction, central nervous system (CNS) immaturity, and frequent caregiving interventions may also contribute to heat loss. The infant may lose heat by convection (heat loss to surrounding air), conduction (body contact with cooler solid surface), radiation (heat loss to cooler solid object not in direct contact with the infant, such as incubator walls), and evaporation (heat lost as liquid from the respiratory tract and permeable skin, which is converted into a vapor).

Radiant warmers, incubators, and swaddling in open cribs help conserve heat in NICU infants (Seguin & Vieth, 1996). The neonatal therapist must diligently protect NICU infants from heat loss during all evaluations and interventions. Cold stress can burn calories needed for growth and healing, cause behavioral and physiologic complications, and result in death in severe cases.

Medical Conditions and Equipment

Learning NICU medical terminology is an ongoing process that progresses from familiarity with definitions to gradually understanding the pathophysiology of diseases and biomechanics of equipment. Medical complications and technology both have profound effects on preterm and high-risk infants, with subsequent implications and precautions for neonatal therapists (Hunter, Mullen, & Dallas, 1994). Developing a basic medical foundation is essential to safely addressing an infant's developmental needs. Appendix 21-B presents selected neonatal medical complications frequently encountered in the NICU. Therapists should also develop a working knowledge of maternal conditions associated with premature delivery and perinatal problems.

Table 21-1 lists common medical equipment in the NICU. In addition to life support technology listed in the table, neonatal therapists use other equipment to monitor the physiologic status of the newborn. For example, pulse oximetry is a noninvasive method of continually assessing blood oxygen saturation via a sensor wrapped around an infant's hand or foot. The cardiorespiratory monitor provides a visual tracing and numerical correlate of heart and breathing rates and an auditory and/or visual alarm if these rates are not within a preset range. Newer monitors also provide hard-copy tracings and analysis of information. Physiologic monitoring capabilities are continually increasing, with dated equipment needing replacement more often than nursery budgets allow (Figure 21-2).

table 21-1   *Common Medical Equipment in the Neonatal Intensive Care Unit*

Equipment	Description	Purpose
THERMOREGULATION EQUIPMENT		
Radiant warmer	Open bed with overhead heat source	Typically used during medical workup of new admission or for critically ill infants requiring easy access for frequent or complicated medical care
Incubator (isolette)	Clear plastic heated box enclosing mattress and infant	Used to provide warmth so available calories can be used for growth and healing; infant may or may not be dressed, depending on specific NICU's protocol; access is typical by opening portholes or a door
Open crib	Bassinet-style bed; no additional heat source provided; infant is dressed and swaddled in blankets	Used for larger and more stable infants; caregivers (including occupational therapist) must be careful to avoid cold stress during baths, assessments, and procedures
OXYGEN THERAPY WITH ASSISTED VENTILATION		
Bag and mask ventilation	Bag attached to face mask is rhythmically squeezed to deliver positive pressure and oxygen	Used for resuscitation of an infant at delivery or during acute deterioration and to increase oxygenation if necessary after an apneic spell
CPAP	Steady stream of pressurized air is given through an endotracheal tube, nasopharyngeal tube, or nasal prongs; supplemental oxygen may or may not be used	Positive pressure is used to keep the alveoli and airways from collapsing (i.e., to keep them open) in an infant who is breathing spontaneously but has a disorder such as respiratory distress syndrome, pulmonary edema, or apnea
Mechanical ventilation	Machine controls or assists breathing by mechanically inflating the lungs, increasing alveolar ventilation, and improving gas exchange	Used for infants with depressed respiratory drive, pulmonary disease with increased work of breathing and suboptimal oxygenation and ventilation (i.e., MAS, RDS), and frequent apnea despite CPAP; infant is usually orally or nasally intubated, but may on occasion have a tracheostomy
ECMO	Sophisticated life-support system that uses modified heart-lung bypass to provide nearly total lung rest and minimize barotrauma (lung damage that can occur with prolonged high ventilator settings)	Used as "rescue" technology for qualifying infants in neonatal respiratory failure who are unresponsive to conventional medical management or at times for preoperative support during cardiac surgery; these infants meet medical criteria for a ≥80% mortality risk; more than 80% survive with ECMO. Most do well developmentally; school-aged sequelae may occur
OXYGEN THERAPY WITHOUT ASSISTED VENTILATION		
Oxygen hood (oxyhood)	Plastic hood with flow of warm humidified oxygen placed over infant's head	Used for infants who are breathing independently but need a higher concentration of oxygen than the 21% room air
NC	Humidified oxygen delivered by flexible NC with small prongs that fit into the nares	Used for infants requiring low concentrations of supplemental oxygen (22% to 30%), or when oxygen will be needed for a long period; handling and portability are easier with an NC than with an oxyhood

CPAP, continuous positive airway pressure; *ECMO,* extracorporeal membrane oxygenation; *NC,* nasal cannula; *NICU,* neonatal intensive care unit; *MAS,* meconium aspiration syndrome; *RDS,* respiratory distress syndrome.

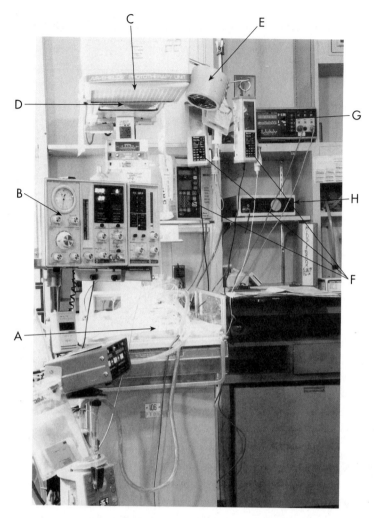

figure 21-2 Medical equipment in neonatal intensive care unit includes: **A,** radiant warmer (bed); **B,** mechanical ventilator; **C,** phototherapy lights (may also be free standing); **D,** radiant heat source; **E,** procedure light; **F,** infusion pumps for fluids and medications; **G,** cardiorespiratory monitor; **H,** pulse oximeter. *(Courtesy of the Infant Special Care Unit, University of Texas Medical Branch, Galveston, TX. Photograph by John Glow.)*

■ NICU ENVIRONMENT

"Mismatch" of Immature Infant in High-Tech Environment

Sensory components of the extrauterine environment in neonatal intensive care are different from the womb (Table 21-2). Before birth the fetus is in a warm, snug, dark environment in which basic needs are automatically met. After birth, demands are suddenly made on the newborn to breathe, regulate body temperature, move against the effects of gravity, adjust to bright light and unmuffled noise, and cope with invasive or painful procedures and frequent sleep deprivation. The preterm infant's immature CNS is generally competent for protected intrauterine life but not sufficiently developed to adjust to and organize the overwhelming stimuli and demands of the NICU. This creates a "mismatch" of the neonate with the high-tech world now necessary for survival (Als, 1986).

Continual overwhelming stimuli created by the NICU environment and caregiving practices may stress the highly sensitive preterm infant's already vulnerable and disorganized CNS. Excessive sensory stimulation can cause insults to the developing brain (e.g., from repeated hypoxic episodes related to stress) and create maladaptive behaviors that contribute to later poor developmental outcome (Als, 1986; Als et. al., 1986).

Technology has enormously increased our life support systems but has not told us how to avoid rescuing badly damaged survivors. Our facility in caring for the heart and lungs has not been matched by our ability to give intensive care and support to the brain. Intensive care nurseries have become temples of technology, with brightly gleaming hardware, bristling energetic adult caretakers,

table 21-2 *Comparison of Intrauterine and Extrauterine Sensory Environments*

System	Intrauterine	Extrauterine
Tactile	Constant proprioceptive input; smooth, wet, usually safe and comfortable	Often painful and invasive; dry, cool air; predominance of medical touching versus social touching
Vestibular	Maternal movements, diurnal cycles, amniotic fluid creates gently oscillating environment, flexed posture	Horizontal, flat postures; Influence of gravity, restraints, and equipment
Auditory	Maternal biologic sounds, muffled environmental sounds	Extremely loud, harsh, mechanical, and constant noise
Visual	Dark; may occasionally have very dim red spectrum light	Bright fluorescent lights Often no diurnal rhythm
Thermal	Constant warmth, consistent temperature	Environmental temperature variations, high risk of neonatal heat loss

ringing telephones, and flashing and beeping alarms. Sometimes lost in the transaction is the essential fragility of the tiny, immature human beings who are struggling for life and for normal integration and growth in the midst of this harsh and unnatural setting. The time has come to return to a more gentle and nurturing nursery environment without sacrificing our valuable lifesaving tools (Avery & Glass, 1989, p. 204).

Because the small, sick infant experiences significant physiologic stress (e.g., agitation, autonomic instability, excessive use of calories) when incoming stimuli exceed the immature CNS's ability to respond and adapt, it becomes a priority to help the infant avoid costly stress and remain calm. The neonatal therapist achieves this by making *NICU light and sound modifications*, reducing handling, and altering caregiver techniques so that the infant is protected from stressful stimuli and allowed to remain quiet and inactive. With environmental modifications, infants demonstrate greater physiologic and behavioral stability. These modifications also facilitate recovery in very preterm infants and improved long-term neurodevelopmental outcome (Als et. al., 1994; Buehler et. al., 1995; Fleisher et. al., 1995; VandenBerg, 1995).

Light in the NICU

The infant's visual system continues to develop during the last trimester of gestation, with significant maturation and differentiation in the retina and visual cortex (Glass, 1993; Gonzalez & Dweck, 1994). This structural and functional immaturity makes the preterm infant extremely vulnerable to light in the NICU. The eyelids remain fused until 24 to 26 weeks' gestation with minimal spontaneous eye opening until after 29 weeks, emphasizing that the eyes of the preterm infant are not yet ready to process visual input at this stage of development. Preterm infants are unable to protect themselves from room light because they are unable to close their eyelids tightly until after 30 weeks, their thin eyelids do not adequately filter light, and the iris does not significantly constrict un-

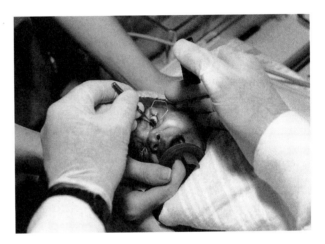

figure **21-3** Neonatal intensive care unit infant is receiving eye examination by an opthalmologist to check for development of retinopathy of prematurity. Nurse provides comfort measures for baby during examination. *(Courtesy of the Infant Special Care Unit, University of Texas Medical Branch, Galveston, TX. Photograph by John Glow.)*

til 30 to 34 weeks (Gonzalez & Dweck, 1994; Gunderson & Berns, 1995; White, 1999).

Because protection from light has not been routinely or consistently provided, concern has been expressed about the exposure of immature infants to frequent or continuous bright light from ceiling and procedure lights, phototherapy, heat lamps, and sunlight (Graven et. al., 1992) (Figure 21-3). In contrast to the dark womb and compared with standard adult office lighting of 40 to 50 footcandles (fc), the ambient lighting of modern NICUs often ranges from 30 to 150 fc, with peaks exceeding 1500 fc if sunlight is present (Glass, 1993). Continuous, intense, white fluorescent ambient light has been linked to chromosomal damage, disruption of diurnal biologic rhythms, changes in endocrine glands and gonadal function, and alteration of vitamin D synthesis in humans and other mammals (Wurtman, 1975). Small

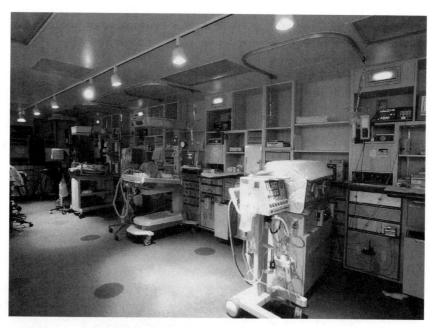

figure**21-4** An overview of neonatal intensive care unit shows an incubator and mechanical ventilator in the foreground and radiant warmers in the background. Track lighting allows option of turning off overhead ceiling lights to reduce room light levels. *(Courtesy of the Infant Special Care Unit, University of Texas Medical Branch, Galveston, TX. Photograph by John Glow.)*

preterm infants exposed to bright NICU lights may suffer retinal damage (Glass et. al., 1985). Overstimulation of the immature CNS with resultant physiologic instability and subsequent potential effects on developmental outcome has also been suggested (Gorski, Davidson, & Brazelton, 1979; VandenBerg, 1995).

Environmental Modifications of Light in the NICU

Current NICU lighting levels differ significantly among institutions and even among shifts in the same hospital, often reflecting the preferences of individual staff members and sometimes producing great potential for strife. In addition to individual work habits and lack of relevant information, the central factor in NICU lighting conflict is that the needs of adult caregivers and fragile underdeveloped infants are different. Preterm infants' obvious requirement for protection from excessive lighting has too often been sacrificed because their adult caregivers need brighter lighting for specific caregiving tasks or procedures (especially if eyesight is decreased) and to maintain arousal and avoid drowsiness.

Fortunately, creative problem solving can help meet the conflicting needs of both infants and caregivers. General lowering of ambient room light and shielding of each infant's bed space are recommended practices (National Association of Neonatal Nurses, 1995). Rheostats, track lighting, and removal of one light tube from each bank of fluorescent lights are common modifications to help con-

trol room brightness without compromising visibility in older NICUs (Figure 21-4). Individual bedside lighting, indirect and deflected lighting, and use of natural light from windows or skylights are additional options in NICUs being built or remodeled.

Additional protection from ambient room light and direct procedure lights can be achieved at each infant's bedside (e.g., shielding the infant's face, draping the isolette with a thick cover) (Figure 21-5). Use of light-filtering goggles for a minimum of 4 weeks or until the infant reaches 31 weeks' postconceptional age has also been reported (Kennedy et. al., 1997). Because infants sleep at least 80% of the time, it has been recommended that lighting at the immediate bedside be controlled to ≤ 10 footcandles (fc) at night and 25 to 30 fc during the day to promote sleep (White, 1999). Infants ≥ 32 weeks need some light for retinal stimulation, but not so bright that it wakes them up; light in the 30 to 40 fc range for intermittent periods has been suggested for these infants (White, 1999). The ability to visually attend emerges at 32 to 34 weeks' postconceptional age and is enhanced in low lighting. Providing opportunities for spontaneous eye opening in dim or dark conditions may be advantageous after this age (Glass, 1993).

The neonatal therapist should shield the infant's eyes during phototherapy (Figure 21-6) and during tasks and procedures that require increased light. Day and night cycles of light, noise, and caregiving may have implications for physiologic gains (longer sleep, less time feeding, and better weight gain) and earlier synchronization

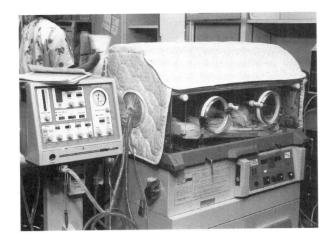

figure**21-5** Isolette cover (Children's Medical Ventures) provides infant protection from room light without eliminating visibility of the infant by neonatal intensive care unit staff. Some NICUs totally cover the isolette for maximal protection from light. *(Courtesy of the Infant Special Care Unit, University of Texas Medical Branch, Galveston, TX. Photograph by John Glow.)*

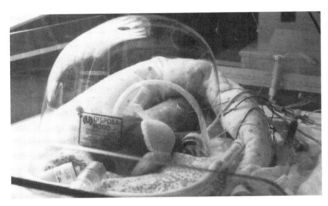

figure**21-6** Preterm infant has protective eye shields during phototherapy for the treatment of jaundice. Oxygen hood is large enough to encompass upper body and allow hand-to-face (or hand-to-mouth) movement for self-calming. In addition, Snuggle-Up provides boundaries for foot bracing, but it is left open to allow maximal skin exposure to bili lights. *(Courtesy of the Infant Special Care Unit, University of Texas Medical Branch, Galveston, TX. Photograph by Al Romeo.)*

of behavioral rhythms with the environment to establish diurnal (day-night) cycles (Gardner & Lubchenco, 1998; Mann et. al., 1986; Sisson, 1990).

NICU staff members concerned about adequate task lighting can be given the following guidelines (White, 1999):

- When writing in the patient's chart, staff members should stand away from the bedside in 25 fc lighting that is free from glare and shadows.
- Infant assessment requires light between 50 to 100 fc. Lighting of 100 to 200 fc may be necessary for tasks that require visual acuity, such as IV insertion. A proce-

dure light can focus narrowly on the task area rather than encompassing the entire infant.

- The infant's eyes should be shielded during the procedure if needed; bright lights should be turned off after the task is completed.
- Periodic "light showers" (e.g., two or three 15-minute breaks in a brightly lit room of 200 to 500 fc) can reset body clocks, restore alertness, and allow efficient functioning for staff members who become drowsy in a dim NICU (Bullough & Rea, 1996; White, 1999).

Sound in the NICU

Environmental noise can be an important cause of stress to NICU infants and a source of serious and dangerous changes in their behavioral and physiologic states. The hearing threshold has been reported as 40 decibels (dB) in the infant at 28 to 34 weeks' gestation, 30 dB at 35 to 38 weeks' gestation, and <20 dB at term; these thresholds are greatly exceeded in the NICU (American Academy of Pediatrics, 1997; Lary et. al., 1985). Typical NICU sound levels of 50 to 90 dB (comparable with street traffic and light machinery, respectively) with peaks to 120 dB (comparable with heavy machinery) have been documented (American Academy of Pediatrics, 1997). The limit that the Occupational Safety and Health Administration (OSHA) imposed in industrial standards as the highest safe level for adult workers is 90 dB for 8 hours (American Academy of Pediatrics, 1997; Lotas, 1992).

In a typical NICU, environmental noise is constant throughout the day and night—mechanical versus social—and is noncontingent to individual infants. Sound inside the isolette is characterized by continuous white noise and nonspeech sounds; harsh mechanical noises penetrate clearly, whereas speech sounds are indistinct (Newman, 1981).

Noise can be highly arousing for preterm and ill infants in the NICU, causing agitation and crying, which decrease oxygenation and increase intracranial pressure, heart rate, and respiratory rate (Long, Alistar, Phillip, & Lucey, 1980). Noise may disrupt the sleep state and sleep-wake cycle and may adversely affect the newborn's recovery and growth (DePaul & Chambers, 1995; Philbin, 1996). Loud or prolonged sounds can produce hearing loss, affecting the frequency range that corresponds to the frequency of the damaging sound. Preterm infants are at risk for hearing loss in both low-frequency (speech) and high-frequency ranges (Thomas, 1989).

Environmental Modifications of Sound in the NICU

Although definitive safety standards for sound exposure have not been established for infants (Brown & Glass, 1979; Thomas, 1989), the American Academy of Pediatrics recommends that sound levels in the NICU and within incubators be monitored and strategies be implemented to maintain a noise level of ≤45 dB (American Academy of Pediatrics, 1997). Measuring sound levels in the NICU with a sound meter can be helpful in identifying noise sources and problems, especially when done at different times throughout 24-hour days, with varying caregivers, and during different levels of activity and unit acuity.

Theoretically, sound in the NICU should be easy to reduce. However, when "people noise" is the greatest offender, change can be surprisingly difficult. Staff education, unit policies, peer pressure, and patience may be helpful; often just dimming the lights calms staff members and reduces noise.

Bacteriostatic carpet, acoustic ceiling tiles, soundproof or sound-absorbing building materials, central vacuum systems, and "pods" that divide space for use by individual or a small number of infants can be considered in remodeling and new unit design. Radios and cellular phones are often against NICU policy, although enforcement varies. Pagers should be switched to "vibrate" upon entry into the NICU. Parents and staff members can view instructional videos away from patient areas. Telephones that flash instead of ring, personal message pagers or cordless phones for nurses to enhance communication without calling across or between rooms, visual alarms, and quieter equipment (e.g., ventilators, incubators) are emerging as additional options to modify noise (White, 1996).

Implementation of a quiet hour has been suggested, during which staff members whisper at the bedside, work quietly, do not allow large equipment to enter the unit, respond quickly to alarms and crying infants, and rearrange caregiving activities to minimize infant disturbances (Strauch, Brandt, & Edwards-Beckett, 1993). A better option is to keep noise to a minimum at all times.

Nursing staff should position extremely ill or sensitive infants away from sinks, ice machines, telephones, and high-traffic areas. Staff members should reduce the volume of auditory alarms from maximal settings and silence all alarms quickly to reduce infant exposure to piercing noise; remote control devices to silence some alarms are available. Nurses and therapists can position respiratory tubing and water traps to promote drainage and empty accumulated water frequently to prevent bubbling (60 to 70 dB).

Isolette covers can significantly reduce the noise level within an incubator (Saunders, 1995). Avoidance of tapping on the isolette (80 dB), abruptly closing incubator doors and portholes (90 to 100 dB), and using the incubator top as a work surface or storage area are common recommendations (American Academy of Pediatrics, 1997; VandenBerg, 1995). Conversations, including medical rounds, should be held away from the bedside. Plastic trash cans are quietest, and trash can lids can be padded if necessary. Musical toys and tape recordings can reverberate inside the isolette; extreme caution and very low volume (if used) are recommended (Als et. al., 1986; DePaul & Chambers, 1995).

Caregiving in the NICU

NICU caregiving patterns differ significantly from the fetal intrauterine environment or the normal home setting. Touch in the NICU is usually related to medical care rather than being social in nature, with interventions constant throughout a 24-hour span (Gottfried, 1985). Examples of medical touch include physical examinations, drawing of blood, application or removal of tape, measurements (temperature, blood pressure, weight, and circumference of head or abdomen), repositioning, IV insertion, gavage feedings, transfusions, injections, bag and mask ventilation, intubation, tube adjustments, chest percussion, and suctioning.

An infant at 28 weeks' gestation can differentiate between touch and pain (Beaver, 1987); light touch increases motor movement, and painful touch causes the infant to cry and attempt to withdraw. Caregiving procedures have been related to hypoxemia (Gorski, Hole, Leonard, & Martin, 1983; Long et. al., 1980). Even social touch can be arousing and ultimately stressful to immature infants.

Caregiving based primarily on external criteria, such as fixed schedules for vital signs and feeding, often ignores or delays the caregiver's response to the infant's cues that indicate that he or she needs care. Caregiving thus becomes noncontingent to the infant's efforts to communicate. Eventually this may discourage the infant's efforts to communicate needs, lead to emotional detachment from the sensation of needs, and possibly contribute to the development of distrust (Gardner & Lubchenco, 1998).

Infants on intensive care status receive less social contact and contingent caregiving than recovering infants in step-down units. Preferred infants, described as those infants with long-term NICU status, presence of a devoted family and potential for successful outcome, tend to experience more social contact than other infants. The initiation of oral feedings also correlates with increased personal attention and social stimulation (Jones, 1982).

Sleep deprivation of NICU infants has been recognized. The fetus at 29 to 32 weeks' gestation sleeps 80% of the time in utero. Sleep cycles of prematurely born infants are less organized and of shorter duration (30 to 40 minutes) than the 50- to 60-minute sleep cycles of term infants (Anders & Keener, 1985; Dreyfus-Brisac, 1974). Some NICU infants may be disturbed 80 to 132 times per day (Gottfried, 1985; Korones, 1976). Because secretion of human growth hormone is associated with regular recurrence of sleep-wake cycles and peaks during active sleep (rapid eye movement [REM] sleep), sleep deprivation in the NICU may interfere with optimal growth and development (Gardner & Lubchenco, 1998).

Modifications of Caregiving in the NICU

Therapists should time their interventions and use appropriate techniques to minimize avoidable stress to the infant. The individual infant (rather than the nursery routines) should determine timing and sequencing of caregiving. Does the infant tolerate and benefit from caregiving procedures that are clustered together (allowing longer undisturbed periods for rest and sleep) or should caregiving procedures be interspersed because of low stress tolerance and prolonged recovery times? Often, two caregivers are needed for some procedures, with one adult attending to the task and the other adult focusing on and supporting the infant (Figure 21-7).

Caregivers must be sensitive and responsive to each infant's ongoing behavioral cues of stress, modifying caregiving pacing and techniques as necessary to facilitate infant stability and efforts at self-regulation. The caregiver should reassess necessity and frequency of all procedures and interventions based on each infant's age and medical status. For example, must weights and baths be done daily? Can some vital signs be taken from monitors? Can suctioning be on an "as needed" basis? Does the infant really need an occupational therapy evaluation requiring handling now? The caregiver should avoid unnecessary handling and movement of the infant, with sick infants handled as little as possible. The caregiver can prepare an infant for touch or movement by speaking softly first and containing extremities during movement

and lifting. Table 21-3 summarizes considerations for caregiving related to infant state of arousal.

Bath time is frequently stressful and exhausting to NICU infants (Peters, 1996, 1998). Bathing by immersion is usually more soothing than sponge bathing if the water is warm and the infant's body is well supported with extremities contained. Swaddled bathing has proven successful even with irritable and disorganized infants. The swaddled infant is immersed deeply in a tub of warm water, with only one body section unwrapped at a time for bathing and rinsing, then rewrapped before proceeding (i.e., right upper body, then left upper body, then legs and buttocks). The warmth and proprioceptive weight of a wet blanket seem calming, and infants are usually quiet and alert throughout this bath (Figure 21-8).

Even noninvasive caregiving procedures can disturb and stress vulnerable infants, requiring caregiver efforts at consoling and facilitating infant recovery. The caregiver can support the infant during routine manipulations and painful procedures by containing extremities (using Snuggle-Up, blanket swaddling, or hands of parent or second caregiver). The caregiver can allow the infant to suck on the fist or pacifier or grasp the blanket edge or a finger of a parent or caregiver. The infant's feet can be braced against nest boundaries or the caregiver's hand, and the infant's eyes can be shielded from bright procedure lights.

The caregiver should pause during a procedure to allow a stressed infant to recover when necessary and possible. After stressful interventions, caregivers should remain to help the infant calm down and stabilize. Each infant has preferred recovery methods (e.g., a facilitative tuck with the head and extremities cupped within firm but gentle caregiver hands [Figure 21-9], prone position, sucking or grasping, removal of extraneous stimuli) that the therapist can post at the bedside for consistent staff use. The therapist should always encourage and support parent involvement with caregiving.

■ FAMILIES IN THE NICU

Families in Crisis

The admission of an infant to the NICU usually puts that family in crisis. Intense and confusing emotions can result from many factors (Shellabarger & Thompson, 1993). The delivery was often unexpected, and the family unit is now separated. Some mothers have continued physical complications or illness from the pregnancy or delivery. Financial considerations can be worrisome. Parental shock, denial, and grief over loss of the ideal birth and perfect infant are compounded by concerns for the recovery of a critically ill infant. The appearance of the infant and the NICU can be frightening. Unknown staff members and unfamiliar terminology can hinder com-

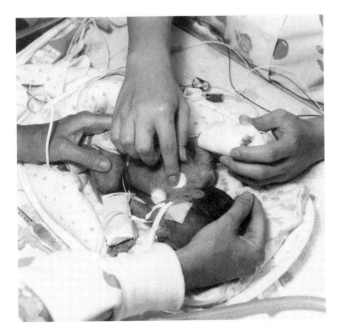

figure 21-7   Second person helps minimize stress in this preterm infant by providing containment during caregiving procedure. *(Courtesy of the Infant Special Care Unit, University of Texas Medical Branch, Galveston, TX. Photograph by John Glow.)*

table 21-3 *Newborn States and Considerations for Care Giving*

Newborn State	Comments
SLEEP STATES	

Deep sleep (non–rapid eye movement [NREM])
  Slow state changes
  Regular breathing
  Eyes closed; no eye movements
  No spontaneous activity except startles and jerky movements
  Startles with some delay and suppresses rapidly
  Lowest oxygen consumption
	Infant is very difficult if not impossible to arouse. Infant will not breastfeed or bottle-feed in this state, even after vigorous stimulation. Infant is unable to respond to environment; frustrating for caregivers.
	Term infants may exhibit a "slow" heart rate (80 to 90 beats per minute), which may trigger heart rate alarms and result in unnecessary stimulation by neonatal intensive care unit staff.
	At birth, preterm infants have altered states of consciousness: Early dominant states are light sleep, quiet, and active alert. "Protective apathy" enables the preterm to remain inactive, unresponsive, and in a sleep state to conserve energy, grow, and maintain physiologic homeostasis.

Light sleep (rapid eye movement [REM] sleep)
  Low activity level
  Random movements and startles
  Respirations irregular and abdominal
  Intermittent sucking movements
  Eyes closed; rapid eye movement
  Higher oxygen consumption
	Full-term infants begin and end sleep in active sleep; preterm infants are more responsive (than term infants) to stimuli in active sleep.
	Infants may cry or fuss briefly in this state and be awakened to feed before they are truly awake and ready to eat.
	Lower and more variable oxygenation states.

AWAKE STATES	

Drowsy or semidozing
  Eyelids fluttering
  Eyes open or closed (dazed)
  Mild startles (intermittent)
  Delayed response to sensory stimuli
  Smooth state change after stimulation
  Fussing may or may not be present
  Respirations—more rapid and shallow
	Infant may awaken further or return to sleep (if left alone).
	Quietly talking and looking at the infant, or offering a pacifier or an inanimate object to see and listen to may arouse the infant to the quiet alert state.
	Less mature infants (30 weeks) demonstrate a more drowsy than quiet alert state than older infants (36 weeks).

Quiet alert, with bright look
  Focuses attention on source of stimulation
  Impinging stimuli may break through; may have some delay in response
  Minimal motor activity
	Immediately after birth, term newborns exhibit a period of quiet alertness, their first opportunity to "take in" their parents and the extrauterine environment. Dimmed lights, quiet talking, and stroking optimize this time for parents.
	Best state for learning to occur, because infant focuses all of attention on visual, auditory, tactile, and sucking stimuli; best state for interaction with parents—baby is maximally able to attend and reciprocally respond to parents.

Active alert—eyes open
  Considerable motor activity—thrusting movements of extremities; spontaneous startles
  Reacts to external stimuli with increase in movements and startles (discrete reactions difficult to differentiate because of general higher activity level)
  Respirations irregular
  May or may not be fussy
	Infant has decreased threshold (increased sensitivity) to internal (hunger, fatigue) and external (wet, noise, handling) stimuli. Infant may quiet self, may escalate to crying, or with consolation by caretaker may become quiet, alert or go to sleep.
	Infant is unable to maximally attend to caretakers or environment because of increased motor activity and increased sensitivity to stimuli.

Crying—intense and difficult to disrupt with external stimuli Respirations rapid, shallow, and irregular	Crying is infant's response to unpleasant internal and/or external stimulation—infant's tolerance limits have been reached (and exceeded). Infant may be able to quiet self with hand-to-mouth behaviors; talking may quiet a crying infant; holding, rocking, or putting infant upright on caretaker's shoulder may quiet infant.

From Gardner, & Lubchenco. (1998). The neonate and the environment: Impact on development. In G.B. Merenstein & S.L. Garner, (Eds.), *Handbook of neonatal intensive care*, (4th ed, pp. 203-204). St. Louis: Mosby.

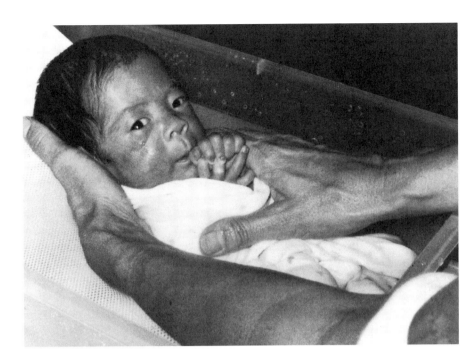

figure**21-8**　Swaddled preterm infant is immersed in a tub of warm water for a developmentally supportive bath. *(Courtesy of the NICU, Medical Center of Plano, Plano, TX. Photograph by Dana Fern.)*

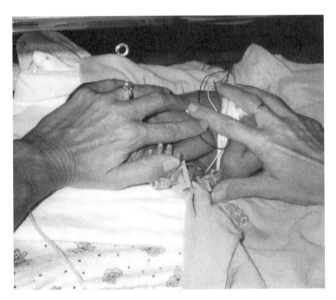

figure**21-9**　Facilitative tuck, which is gently but firmly swaddling a stressed or disorganized preterm infant in the caregiver's hands, is calming to the baby. This type of touch is well tolerated, as opposed to highly stimulating stroking. *(Courtesy of the NICU, Medical Center of Plano, Plano, TX. Photograph by Vicky Leland.)*

munication. Many areas of control are relinquished to medical staff members because the new mother and father are unprepared and uncertain how to parent an infant in the NICU.

The many facets of understanding and working with families who have an ill or special needs child are dis-

cussed in depth in Chapter 5. The primary roles of the occupational therapist with NICU families are to support them throughout the hospitalization, promote attachment between infant and family, and facilitate effective parenting within the NICU and after hospital discharge.

Identifying Needs of NICU Families

Effective and rewarding parenting of an infant in the NICU is difficult. Judgmental opinions of families in crisis are inappropriate; assessment of family concerns and priorities is solely to establish how the therapist can best offer support and facilitate a successful infant-parent relationship. General factors for the therapist to consider may include family resources and concerns (e.g., support systems, maternal health, family responsibilities, babysitting needs, finances, transportation, housing near the hospital, job issues), coping mechanisms, learning styles, personalities, and cultural background.

Occupational therapists should also assess and nurture parents' understanding and skill in recognizing and responding appropriately to their infant's cues of stress or stability, providing therapeutic positioning and developmentally supportive handling, regulating sensory input, facilitating functional oral feeding, and meeting the infant's long-term developmental needs. Nurturing parent-infant attachment and helping the family know and love their infant as a unique person is always top priority.

Collaboration with Families

Similar to community-based early intervention, the shift in the NICU has been away from "therapist as expert, child as client, parents as students" to family-centered mutual collaboration. Occupational therapy services with families in the NICU are based on relationship; the therapist talks *with* rather than *to* the parents and facilitates the family's active role on the NICU team.

Therapists support collaboration with families by creating frequent opportunities for two-way dialogue. Examples include seeking and valuing parents' opinions and insights in addition to sharing his or her own, being sensitive to possible hidden messages in parent-professional communications, addressing parent concerns, planning joint infant observations and interventions, avoiding judgments, and acknowledging that the parent has the infant's best interests at heart (Holloway, 1994). Recognizing parental skills, celebrating successes, and facilitating parent's expertise can be valuable, as illustrated by one parent's comment, "Seeing others follow through on our suggestions . . . bolstered our confidence in our parenting skills, knowledge of our baby, and ability to develop a closeness with him" (Holloway, 1994).

When parents make requests that are unusual or differ from what NICU staff members prefer, the NICU caregiver needs to remember that parents have emotional and legal rights to make decisions on behalf of their infant. Baker (1995) suggested a four-question approach to handling conflicts that allows both parents and staff members to feel respected:

1. What is the staff goal?
2. What is the parent's goal?
3. Will the parent's request harm the infant?
4. What options are available to meet both goals?

In most cases, the parent's choice will achieve the same outcome and staff members can maintain their standards for safe, effective, quality care.

Parent Perspectives

An NICU nurse whose daughter was born at 26 weeks' gestation shared her experience and offered suggestions to help staff members deal with the emotional issues of parents in the NICU (Maroney, 1994). The following are some ideas with practical applications:

■ NICU staff members should make infants as comfortable and as "normal" looking as possible. Such efforts as dressing the infant in baby clothes or a hair bow, providing a cute name tag or soft music, and using the infant's name and correct gender acknowledge that this is a real person, not just a sick premie.

■ NICU staff members should routinely ask the parents how they are feeling and validate their response. "At least" statements (e.g., "At least you have two other kids at home") are not empathetic or validating and may trigger anger.

■ Parents should have as much control as possible. They are an integral part of the team and should be involved in caregiving as much as possible (this may require

teaching). NICU staff members should ask for their opinions and insights and call them at home with an update when they cannot come in.

■ NICU staff members must recognize that the infant is part of a family unit with a distinct set of dynamics. Parents may need help to overcome intimidation of the NICU so they can participate in their child's life. NICU staff members should encourage the father, as well as the mother, to participate in discussions and caregiving.

Families as Equals

Medical care and concerns, the complexity of high-tech NICU environments, and neurobehavioral immaturity of preterm infants can undermine the role of families in the NICU (Gale & Franck, 1998; Shields-Poe & Pinelli, 1997). Conversely, providing the knowledge and fostering the skills necessary for parents to confidently nurture and care for their infant in the NICU and after discharge are the most permanent contributions that a therapist can make to any infant's developmental outcome. Implementing and integrating the concepts of family-centered neonatal care into daily caregiving philosophy and practice is a process and an adventure. This section outlines additional hints for success.

Whenever medically possible, the location of the infant's bed space should be conducive to optimal parenting (e.g., twins placed next to each other, co-bedded [both twins in same isolette or crib] rather than in separate parts of the room).

The therapist should encourage parents to ask questions and ask the parents questions about what they feel, understand, and want to know. Parents are often frustrated when information appears contradictory; much of their anxiety stems from incomplete information or a perceived lack of truth (Shellabarger & Thompson, 1993). Written information (Fern & Graves, 1996; Harrison, 1983; VandenBerg, 1993b; Zaichkin, 1996) can be available for parents in a waiting room, in a parents' library, or during individual checkout. Parent groups can also be helpful in providing information, comfort, and support.

The therapist can demonstrate to parents a behavioral and developmental assessment of the infant (Figure 21-10). The therapist can help parents learn to observe, interpret, and respond appropriately to their infant's unique behaviors. Fostering constructive parental sensitivity to the infant's behaviors is as important as any other infant care skills emphasized in discharge planning. Parents can and should learn therapeutic positioning and handling techniques (e.g., containing extremities in flexion, cupping infant's head and lower body in parent's palms, letting infant hold onto parent's finger) and sensory input to avoid (e.g., lightly stroking infant's back, giving too many kinds of stimulation at the same time).

As much as possible, feeding schedules and other types of caregiving should be arranged to accommodate par-

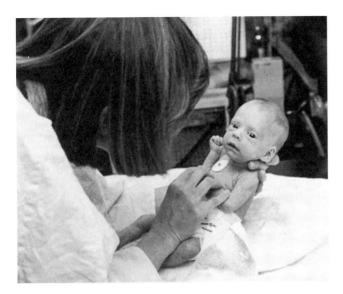

figure **21-10** Assessment of preterm infants includes evaluation of neuromotor and neurobehavioral functioning. The assessment can be a valuable teaching tool when performed jointly with the infant's parents. *(Courtesy of the Neonatal Intensive Care Unit, University of Connecticut Health Center's John N. Dempsey Hospital, Farmington, CT. Photograph by Gregory Kriss.)*

ents' schedules. The inclusion of siblings during the infant's NICU stay should be encouraged.

If parents cannot come frequently to the NICU, the therapist can make or encourage regular phone calls, send frequent photographs or notes sharing significant events or behaviors, or keep a bedside journal in which staff members can record thoughts or progress for parents to read when they arrive (Costello, Bracht, Van Camp, & Carman, 1996). Therapists can also use technology to keep these families involved and "close" to their infant. For example, the therapist can e-mail digital photographs to parents who have Internet access. One family from Africa forwarded digital photographs of their NICU infant taken by the therapist to relatives in the Congo, who then set up a web page about the infant. Future NICUs may have cameras at the bedside so that parents can log in from home and view their infant.

Skin-to-Skin Holding (Kangaroo Care)

Kangaroo care is the nickname given to the practice of parents holding their diaper-clad premature infant beneath their clothing, chest-to-chest and skin-to-skin (Anderson, 1996; Gale & VandenBerg, 1998; Luddington-Hoe et. al., 1994). During maternal holding, the mother can allow the infant self-regulatory access to breast-feeding, although this may just consist of nonnutritive suckling for the younger premie.

Kangaroo care originated in Bogota, Columbia, in response to overcrowded nurseries and insufficient medical equipment, with many infants discharged before full feedings were reached. Kangaroo care is used extensively in Western Europe and has gained acceptance in the United States during the last decade.

Initiation of kangaroo care may vary among individual institutions based on different ages, weights, and acuity of the NICU infant, but is one intervention that belongs solely to the parents. Kangaroo care supports active family involvement, satisfaction, and attachment. Benefits of skin-to-skin holding to the infant include more stable heart and breathing rates, reduced apnea, stable body temperature, decreased agitation and random motor activity, improved state control, less distress from environmental disturbances and medical interventions, and easier transition to breast-feeding. Benefits to the parents include facilitation of maternal milk production and longer duration of breast-feeding, increased awareness of their infant's cues of well-being or distress, increased parental attachment and feelings of closeness to their infant, less focus on technical care, more confidence in their own caregiving ability, and decreased maternal stress.

The therapist can actively encourage and assist with implementation of kangaroo care in the NICU. Figure 21-11 illustrates family support and participation in caregiving as a preterm infant undergoes a head ultrasound during skin-to-skin holding by his father; his mother observes while leaning on the back of the chair.

Discharge Planning

Discharge planning begins on the day of admission. Facilitating the infant's behavioral stability, sleep-wake cycle organization, and self-regulation capacities by consistent environmental modifications and sensitive caregiving will ease the transition to home for the infant and family. Including and supporting parents in active caregiving roles throughout hospitalization is beneficial. Detailed guidelines for hospital discharge of high-risk newborns (e.g., preterm infant, infant requiring technologic support, infant at risk primarily from family issues, infant whose irreversible condition will result in an early death) have been proposed (American Academy of Pediatrics, 1998).

After downsizing closed some patient care areas, one innovative hospital allowed NICU parents to stay in unoccupied rooms and thus be readily available to help care for their infant; nighttime breast-feeding was a common occurrence in their NICU. Many hospitals provide accommodations for parents to stay with their infant overnight in an NICU parent room before discharge.

Parents should be familiar with their infant's developmental strengths and needs (VandenBerg, 1999). The therapist should provide information about community resources and parent support groups and complete a referral of the infant to a local early childhood intervention program when needed. Arranging for the parents to meet community resource personnel before hospital dis-

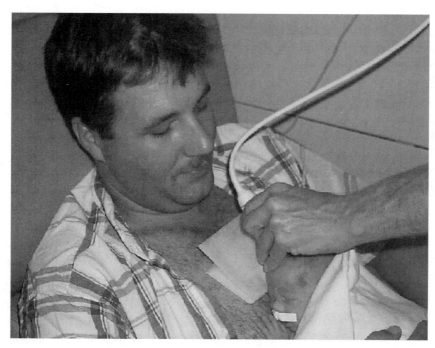

figure**21-11**   Father using skin-to-skin holding technique (Kangaroo care) while preterm infant undergoes a head ultrasound to rule-out intraventricular hemorrhage. *(Courtesy of the Infant Special Care Unit, University of Texas Medical Branch, Galveston, TX. Photograph by Jan Hunter.)*

charge and providing a follow-up telephone call from NICU staff after discharge can be helpful in reducing parental "separation anxiety" from the NICU.

It is highly recommended that neonatal therapists actively participate in NICU follow-up clinics. Besides allowing reinforcement and continuation of developmental teaching, preventing some infants from "falling through the cracks," and continuing relationships with NICU families, the therapist also gains valuable knowledge from countless opportunities to observe infant outcome from various diagnoses and clinical courses. Many infants do surprisingly well after long NICU stays, and others develop unexpected problems. This information helps the therapist appreciate the unpredictable nature of infant development and understand the variables that contribute to the developmental outcomes.

■ INFANT IN THE NICU

Evaluation

Infant assessment in the NICU

The "Golden Rule" of occupational therapy evaluation and intervention with the NICU infant is "Above all, do no harm!" Safety for the infant takes priority over convenience for the therapist in all aspects of care. The following are methods to help ensure infant protection:
1. The therapist should learn a new evaluation tool thor-

oughly (i.e., read and reread the manual, observe an experienced colleague evaluate appropriate infants of varying ages and medical status, practice on a doll and then on healthy term infants) before administering its items. Many therapists use a structured assessment that is supplemented with data gathering and clinical observations relevant to occupational therapy. Administration of several structured neonatal assessments requires that the therapist have specialized training. Others may be administered after independent study of the manual (Table 21-4 and Box 21-1).
2. The therapist should gather baseline information before performing the evaluation. This can include demographics, relevant family history (e.g., socioeconomic and cultural factors, support systems), maternal prenatal history, birth history, subsequent medical history and current status of the infant (including medical equipment in use, feeding method and schedule, current medications, and level of physiologic homeostasis).
3. The therapist should use observations extensively, including routine astute clinical observation of the infant and surrounding environment, before touching the infant. The therapist can assess very fragile infants entirely by skilled observations (Als, 1986).
4. The therapist should weigh the value of any evaluation procedures against any potential stressful effect on the infant. (What is truly necessary and impor-

table 21-4 *Neonatal Assessments Requiring Certification for Administration*

Assessment	Contact
NATURALISTIC OBSERVATIONS OF NEWBORN BEHAVIOR (NONB) Based on Als' Synactive Theory of Development For preterm and term infants too fragile for handling Structured observations of specific behaviors are repeated at 2-minute intervals before, during, and after routine caregiving. Assesses the maturation and interplay of infant neurobehavioral subsystems (autonomic, motor, state, attention and interaction, and self-regulation) as evidenced by behavioral cues to environmental and caregiving events over time. Signs of stress and stability can be catalogued as avoidance or approach behaviors, and attempts at self-organization (including failure, success, and cost of the effort) are noted. The degree of caregiver facilitation required to promote infant neurobehavioral organization may be observed if developmentally supportive care is being provided NIDCAP Level 1	Heidelise Als, PhD Enders Pediatric Research Laboratories 320 Longwood Avenue Boston, MA 02115
ASSESSMENT OF PRETERM INFANT BEHAVIOR (APIB) Based on Als' Synactive Theory of Development For stable preterm (> 30 to 32 weeks) and term infants Complex assessment that provides an integrated subsystem profile of the infant, identifying current level of functioning with varying environmental demands. The therapist handles the infant in a structured progression of test items to assess neurobehavioral organization and methods of attaining self-regulation, as well as the type and amount of caregiver support needed for the infant to achieve and maintain organized behavior Used more as a research tool than for everyday clinical purposes NIDCAP Level II	Heidelise Als, PhD Enders Pediatric Research Laboratories 320 Longwood Avenue Boston, MA 02115
NEONATAL BEHAVIORAL ASSESSMENT SCALE (NBAS) For term healthy infants (used in 36- to 44-week range) Evaluates infant neurobehavioral capabilities within the context of a dynamic relationship with the caregiver. Supplemental items can be used with high-risk infants Provided the model for the Assessment of Preterm Infant Behavior Used more as a research tool than for everyday clinical purposes	J. Kevin Nugent, PhD 300 Longwood Avenue Boston, MA 02115
INFANT BEHAVIORAL ASSESSMENT (IBA) From birth to 6 months of age; can be used for follow-up Evaluates infants within the synactive theory framework to sensitize parents or caregivers to the infant's behavioral states and organizational abilities so caregiver interactions can be modified accordingly	Rodd Hudlund, MEd Mary Tatarka, MS, PT Child Development and Mental Retardation Unit WJ-10 University of Washington Seattle, WA 98195

Note: Each certification process requires formal training and assessment of rater reliability.
NIDCAP, Neonatal Individualized Developmental Care and Assessment Program.

tant?). The therapist should not attempt specific evaluation items simply to fill in blanks on an evaluation form.

5. The bedside nurse knows recent or upcoming stressful events of which the therapist may not be aware (e.g., eye examination, placement of an IV). The therapist should appreciate the nurse's role in protecting the infant and obtain clearance for evaluation if he or she will be handling the infant.

6. The therapist should time evaluation according to the infant's sleep cycle, feeding schedule, caregiving routine, and medical status. The therapist should

---

box 21-1 *Structured neonatal assessments that do not require certification for administration*

Neurologic assessment of the preterm and full-term newborn infant (NAPFI)

Description

For preterm and term infants who can tolerate handling. Administered as per Dubowitz manual; can give partial or total assessment based on infant's specific situation.

Designed to record the functional status of an infant's nervous system by assessing habituation, posture, muscle tone, head control, spontaneous movements, abnormal movements, selected reflexes, state transition, level of arousal and alertness, auditory and visual orientation, irritability, consolability, and cry. Provides a baseline at initial assessment to which continued developmental maturation and progression can be compared during sequential assessments.

Reference

Dubowitz, L., & Dubowitz, V. (1981). The neurological assessment of the preterm and fullterm newborn infant. *Clinics in developmental medicine,* No. 79. Philadelphia: J.B. Lippincott.

Neonatal neurobehavioral evaluation (NNE)

Description

For preterm and term infants who can tolerate handling.

Closely resembles the Dubowitz, but can establish quantifiable indicators of the infant's neurobehavioral maturation over time in the areas of tone and motor patterns, reflexes, and behavioral responses. Standardization was done on term infants at 2 days of age and on preterm infants around term equivalency. Training is recommended but not mandatory; contact
Vicky L. Lee, MA, PT
University of Illinois College of Medicine at Peoria
Department of Pediatrics
320 East Armstrong Avenue
Peoria IL 61603

Reference

Morgan, A.M., Koch, V., Lee, V., & Aldag, J. (1988). Neonatal neurobehavioral examination: A new instrument for quantitative analysis of neonatal neurological status. *Physical Therapy, 68,* 1352.

Neurobehavioral assessment for preterm infants (NAPI)

Description

For medically stable preterm infants functioning in range of the 32 to 42 weeks postconceptional age. Test items were selected from existing evaluations of Amiel-Tison, Brazelton, Dubowitz, and Prechtl. Neurobehavioral areas evaluated include motor development and vigor, scarf sign, popliteal angle, alertness and orientation, irritability, vigor of crying, and percent of time sleeping.

To assess neurobehavioral maturity of infant over time and to detect neurologically suspect performance.

Reference

Korner, A.F., Constantinou, J., Dimiceli, S., & Brown, B.W., Jr. (1991). Establishing the reliability and developmental validity of a neurobehavioral assessment for preterm infants: A methodological process. *Child Development, 62,* 1200.

Neonatal neurological examination (NEONEURO)

Description

For normal and abnormal term infants during the first week of life only; cannot be used with infants born at less than 37 weeks' gestation.

Examines posture, tone, reflexes, and auditory/visual orientation to assess infant's neurologic integrity.

Reference

Sheridan Pereira, M., Ellison, P.H., & Helgeson, V. (1991). The construction of a scored neonatal neurological examination for assessment of neurologic integrity in full-term neonates. *Journal of Developmental and Behavioral Pediatrics, 12,* 25.

---

avoid unnecessary duplication of any evaluation procedures that require handling. The therapist must respect infant signs of stress during handling and therefore complete the evaluation gradually over several days. It may be delayed it to a later date if the infant does not readily return to a calm organized state even with caregiver assistance.

7. Performing an evaluation is easier than accurately analyzing the results; overinterpretation and mistak-

ing immaturity for pathology are frequent errors among new neonatal therapists. Mastery of the following sections on preterm infant development and interventions will help the neonatal therapist more accurately interpret evaluation findings. Routine ongoing reassessment in the NICU and in a follow-up clinic as infants mature and recover is essential for developing sound clinical judgment on the meaning of early clinical findings.

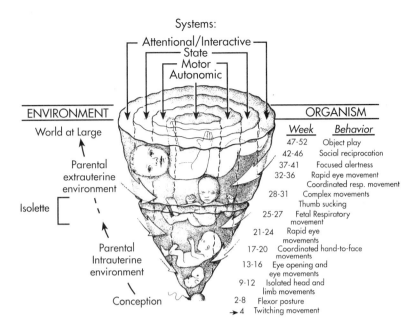

Systems:
Attentional/Interactive
State
Motor
Autonomic

ENVIRONMENT

World at Large

Parental
extrauterine
environment

Isolette

Parental
Intrauterine
environment

Conception

ORGANISM

Week	Behavior
47-52	Object play
42-46	Social reciprocation
37-41	Focused alertness
32-36	Rapid eye movement
	Coordinated resp. movement
28-31	Complex movements
	Thumb sucking
25-27	Fetal Respiratory movement
21-24	Rapid eye movements
17-20	Coordinated hand-to-face movements
13-16	Eye opening and eye movements
9-12	Isolated head and limb movements
2-8	Flexor posture
4	Twitching movement

figure 21-12 Beginning at conception, emerging and expanding capabilities of developing infant are illustrated in this model of synactive organization of behavioral development. *(From Als, H. [1982]. Toward a synactive theory of development: promise for the assessment and support of infant individuality.* Infant Mental Health Journal, 3, 229-243.)

Preterm Infant Development
Neurobehavioral organization

Synactive theory of development. Als has proposed a model for understanding the emerging capabilities of preterm infants to organize and control their behavior, since they are continually affected by and responsive to environmental influences. The synactive theory of development identifies five separate but interdependent subsystems (autonomic, motor, state, attention-interaction, and self-regulation) within the infant that are in constant interaction with one another and with the environment. Figure 21-12 illustrates the unfolding of these subsystems as the infant continues to mature before and after birth. Through recognizable approach and avoidance behaviors occurring in these subsystems, infants continually communicate their level of stress and stability in relation to what is happening to and around them (Table 21-5; Figures 21-13 and 21-14). Maturation and improved (or declining) health are reflected in sequential observation of subsystem development (Table 21-6).

Synaction refers to the process by which stable functioning or decompensation in one subsystem can affect the organization and integrity of other subsystems (Als, 1982). For example, Marissa, who is now physiologically and motorically stable and able to maintain quiet alertness for about 10 minutes, can reasonably be expected to attend to and interact with specific social stimuli. However, if the caregiver simultaneously smiles and nods

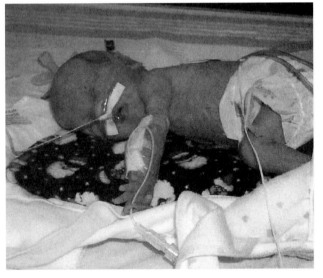

figure 21-13 Preterm infant without secure positional support showing stress cues of arm extension, finger splay, gape face, tongue protrusion, and facial grimace. *(Courtesy of the Infant Special Care Unit, University of Texas Medical Branch, Galveston, TX.)*

while talking to and stroking her, Marissa may become overwhelmed by the effort required to integrate all these incoming stimuli and respond with avoidance and stress behaviors such as gaze aversion, motor flaccidity, and possibly apnea (Figure 21-15).

Subsystem	Signs of Stress	Signs of Stability
AUTONOMIC	**Physiologic instability**	**Physiologic stability**
Respiratory	Pauses, tachypnea, gasping	Smooth, regular respiratory rate
Color	Changes to mottled, flushed, pale, dusky, cyanotic, gray or ashen	Pink, stable color
Visceral	Hiccups, gagging, spitting up, grunting, straining (as if producing bowel movement)	Stable viscera with no hiccups, gags, emesis, or grunting
Motor	Tremors, startles, twitches, coughs, sneezes, yawns, sighs, has seizures	No sign of tremors, startles, twitches, coughs, sneezes, yawns, sighs, or seizures
MOTOR	**Fluctuating tone, uncontrolled activity**	**Consistent tone, controlled activity**
Flaccidity	Gape face, low tone in trunk, limp lower extremities and upper extremities	Muscle tone consistent in trunk and extremities and appropriate for postconceptional age
Hypertonicity	Leg extensions and sitting on air; upper-extremity salutes, finger splays, and fisting; trunk arching; tongue extensions	Smooth controlled posture
Smooth movements of extremities and head
Hyperflexions	Trunk, lower extremities, upper extremities
Frantic, diffuse activity extremities	Motor control can be used for self-regulation (hand and foot clasp, leg and foot bracing, hand to mouth, grasping, tucking, sucking)
STATE	**Diffused or disorganized quality of states, including range and transition between states**	**Clear states; good, calming, focused alertness**
During sleep	Twitches, sounds, whimpers, jerky movements, irregular respiratory rate, fussy, grimaces	Clear, well-defined sleep states
Good self-quieting and consolability
Robust crying
When awake	Eye floating, glassy eyed, staring, gaze aversion, worried or dull look, hyperalert panicked expression, weak cry, irritability
Abrupt state changes	Focused clear alertness with animated expressions (e.g., frowning, cheek softening, "ooh" face, cooing, smiling)
Smooth transition between states
ATTENTION-INTERACTION	**Effort to attend and interact to specific stimulus elicits stress signals of other subsystems**	**Responsive to auditory, visual, and social stimuli**
Autonomic	Irregular respiratory rate, color changes, visceral responses, coughs, yawns, sneezes, sighs, straining tremors, twitches	Responsivity to auditory and visual stimuli is clear and prolonged
Motor	Fluctuating tone, frantic diffuse activity	Actively seeks out auditory stimulus; able to shift attention smoothly from one stimulus to another
State	Eye floating, glassy eyed, staring, worried or dull look, hyperalert panicked expression, gaze aversion, weak cry, irritability
Abrupt state changes
Becomes stressed if more than one type of stimulus is given simultaneously	Face demonstrates bright-eyed purposeful interest varying between arousal and relaxation

SELF-REGULATION: Infant's efforts to achieve, maintain, or regain balance and self-organization in each subsystem as needed. Examples include motor strategies (e.g., foot clasp, leg and foot bracing, finger folding, hand clasping, hand to mouth, grasping, tucking, sucking, postural changes); state strategies (e.g., lowers state of arousal or releases energy with rhythmic, robust crying) and attention and orientation strategies such as visual locking. The success of various strategies may vary among infants.

Modified from Als, H. (1982). Toward a synactive theory of development: Promise for the assessment and support of infant individuality. *Infant Mental Health Journal, 3*, 229-243.
Als, H. (1986). A synactive model of neonatal behavior organization: Framework for the assessment of neurobehavioral development in the premature infant and for support of infants and parents in the neonatal intensive care environment. *Physical and Occupational Therapy in Pediatrics, 6*, 3-55.

table 21-6   *Neurobehavioral Development of Preterm Infants by Gestational Age*

Neurobehavioral System	Developmental Behaviors
INFANTS AT ≤30 WEEKS' GESTATION	
Autonomic	Breathing is irregular and mainly abdominal
	Eyelids flutter; limbs twitch and tremor in jerky movements
Motor	Reflex smiling and startle response are present
	Muscle tone is flaccid. Infant has little head control or back support. Movements are jerky
	Infant is unable to coordinate sucking, swallowing, and breathing
State	Little state differentiation. Alert or drowsy states are fleeting and not robust
	Sleep states predominate, with sleep frequently in a restless undifferentiated state
	Rapid eye movement (REM) is apparent as well as continuous tonguing and mouthing
	Waking periods occur only in brief intervals
Attention/interaction	Visual acuity is poor, with little accommodation
	Infant can fixate and follow face, but this is not a common occurrence
	When visual stimuli are intense, apnea may result
	Hearing is well developed. Preference for mother's voice is possible
Self-regulation	Infant may be easily stressed by environmental stimuli
INFANTS AT ≤32 WEEKS' GESTATION	
Motor	Overall increase in motor tone with more flexion is apparent
	Smooth motor movements are evident
	Improved head control is evident
State	Regular episodes of active and quiet sleep occur
	Active sleep decreases while quiet sleep increases
	Movements are sporadic in active sleep
	Increase in alert awake time occurs with a decrease in drowsy state
INFANTS AT 34-36 WEEKS' GESTATION	
Autonomic	Color changes accompany most stimulation
Motor	Beginning coordination of sucking, swallowing, and breathing is apparent
	Head control is not complete
	Beginning of leg and trunk support can be noted when infant is held upright
State	Quiet sleep is distinguished by slow, regular respiration and little body movement
	Overall, less random activity occurs
	Active sleep and quiet sleep are clearly defined and alternate regularly
	Infant will awaken to stimulation, but awake state is brief
	Crying states are more frequent in response to discomfort, pain, or hunger
Attention/interaction	Infant can fixate up to 15 seconds on a visual stimulus
	Infant may respond briefly to auditory stimulation by turning or widening eyes
Self-regulation	Infant may become overaroused when stimulated
	Infant can be consoled by swaddling or stroking
	Infant may perform hand-to-mouth maneuvers
INFANTS 37 TO 40 WEEKS' GESTATION	
Motor	Infant may support himself or herself when placed upright
State	All states of consciousness are evident
	Quiet sleep increases with equal periods of active sleep
	Crying more closely approximates that of the term infant
Attention/interaction	Infant may maintain longer periods of alertness and shows alertness to sound
	Infant displays preferences for visual stimuli and tracks objects

Modified from Yecco, G.J. (1993). Neurobehavioral development and developmental support of premature infants. *Journal of Perinatal and Neonatal Nursing, 7,* 56-65.

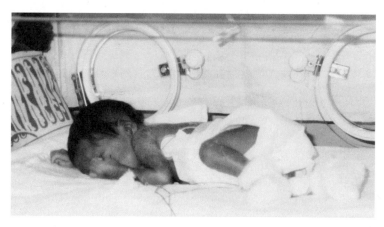

figure 21-14   Preterm infant using motor strategies of hand-to-face, extremity tucking, and foot bracing on mattress surface to maintain calm, organized state. Although competent enough to demonstrate these behaviors, this infant is expending extra energy in self-regulation because no boundaries or protection from light were provided. *(Courtesy of the Infant Special Care Unit, University of Texas Medical Branch, Galveston, TX.)*

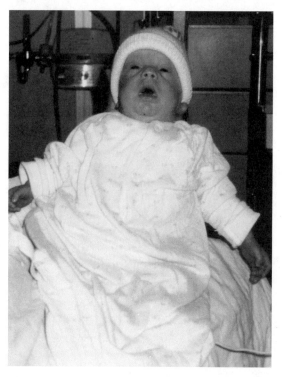

figure 21-15   Flaccid muscle tone, gape face, and low-level diffuse alertness are signs of stress in this preterm infant. *(Courtesy of the Infant Special Care Unit, University of Texas Medical Branch, Galveston, TX.)*

Synactive theory forms the basis for individualized developmentally supportive and family-centered care. Caregivers are trained to be sensitive to each infant's fragility and stress versus robustness and stability behaviors. The caregiver then uses these observations to promote modification of the immediate environment and caregiving practices to facilitate the infant's organization and well-being. The caregiver also notes and facilitates the infant's attempts to maintain or return to a calm, organized state. The infant and family are seen as an integral unit, with parents supported in assuming an active role with their infant in the NICU.

Medical, developmental, and financial gains have been attributed to provision of developmentally supportive care (Als et. al., 1986, Als et. al., 1994; Buehler et. al., 1995; Fleisher et. al., 1995; VandenBerg, 1995). These reported benefits include decreased severity of chronic lung disease, fewer days on assisted ventilation and supplemental oxygen, reduced incidence of intraventricular hemorrhage (IVH), reduced need for sedation, earlier transition to oral feedings, improved weight gain, shorter hospital stays with significant cost savings, improved cognitive and motor development as compared with control infants, and increased family involvement and confidence.

Preterm neurobehavioral organization: in-turning, coming-out, and reciprocity. Another description of preterm infant behavioral organization (Gorski, Davidson, & Brazelton, 1979) facilitates "rule of thumb" guidelines for the occupational therapist seeking to determine appropriate interventions for specific infants. Infants in the "in-turning" stage are generally immature or critically ill; these infants need minimal handling with maximal environmental and caregiving protection. Infants in the "coming-out" stage remain fragile and vulnerable but have brief periods of availability to attend to their environment; graded unimodal stimulation may be appropriate in small doses based on observed infant tolerance. The more mature and stable infant in the "reciprocity" stage is able to attend and interact when in an appropriate quiet, Alert state, but the caregiver must still respect approach and avoidance signals. Advancing postconceptional age and

Als	Gorski, Davidson, & Brazelton
Physiologic homeostasis—stabilizing and integrating temperature control, cardiorespiratory function, digestion, and elimination. Characteristics: becomes pale, dusky, cyanotic; heart and respiratory rates change—all symptoms of disorganization of autonomic nervous system.	"In turning"—physiologic stage of mere survival characterized by autonomic nervous system responses to stimuli (rapid color changes caused by swings in heart and respiratory rates); no or limited direct response; inability to arouse self spontaneously; jerky movements; asleep (and protecting the central nervous system from sensory overload) 97% of the time. Preterms (<32 weeks) are easily physiologically overwhelmed by stimuli.
Motor development may infringe on physiologic homeostasis, resulting in defensive strategies (vomiting, color change, apnea, and bradycardia). State development becomes less diffuse and encompasses full range: sleep, awake, crying. States and state changes may affect physiologic and motor stability.	"Coming out"—first active response to environment may be seen as early as 34 to 35 weeks (provided some physiologic stability has been achieved). Characteristics: remains pink with stimuli; has directed response for short periods; arouses spontaneously and maintains arousal after stimuli ceases; if interaction begins in alert state: maintains quiet alert for 5 to 10 minutes, tracks animate and inanimate stimuli; spends 10% to 15% of time in alert state with predictable interaction patterns.
Alert state is well differentiated from other states; state changes may interfere with physiologic and motor stability.	"Reciprocity"—active interaction and reciprocity with environment from 36 to 40 weeks. Characteristics: directs response; arouses and consoles self; maintains alertness and interacts with both animate and inanimate objects; copes with external stress.

Modified from Als, H. (1986). A synactive model of neonatal behavior organization: Framework for the assessment of neurobehavioral development in the premature infant and for support of infants and parents in the neonatal intensive care environment. *Physical and Occupational Therapy in Pediatrics, 6,* 3-55:
Gorski, P.A., Davidson, M.F., & Brazelton, T.B. (1979). Stages of behavioral organization in the high-risk neonate: Theoretical clinical considerations. *Seminars in Perinatology, 3,* 61-72.

medical status (acuity and chronicity) affect an individual infant's progression through these stages. Table 21-7 summarizes and compares the stages and characteristics of preterm behavioral organization of this theory and *Als' synactive theory of development.*

States of arousal. *State* refers to the infant's degree of consciousness or arousal. In a preterm infant, state significantly affects other areas such as muscle tone, feeding performance, or reaction to stimuli. State is most frequently classified into six categories (Als, 1982):

■ **State 1:** Deep sleep. Eyes are closed with no REM. Breathing is regular. Movement is absent except for isolated startles.

■ **State 2:** Light sleep. Eyes are closed; REMs may be observed under the eyelids. Breathing may be irregular. Movements are more frequent. Responsivity to external stimuli is increased.

■ **State 3:** Transitional state of dozing or drowsiness. Eyes open and close, appearing heavy-lidded. Activity level is variable. The infant in a transitional state either returns to deeper sleep or becomes increasingly alert.

■ **State 4:** Quiet and alert. Eyes are open, and movement is minimal. Quality of the quiet, alert state is im-

portant. An infant with bright-eyed "robust" alertness is in an optimal state to attend and interact with specific environmental stimuli (Figure 21-16). Conversely, an infant may be in state 4 but unavailable for interaction if the alertness is of poor quality. This is generally noted as a diffuse, low-level alertness with a dull, glassy-eyed gaze (see Figure 21-15) or hyperalertness with a wide-eyed stare that makes the infant appear somewhat panicked (Als, 1982).

■ **State 5:** Active alert. Eyes are open, and motor activity is increased. The infant may be fussy without really crying and often is unable to focus and interact with specific stimuli.

■ **State 6:** Crying. Eyes may be open or closed, motor activity is increased, and the infant is obviously distressed. The cry may be lusty with a stable or larger infant, weak in a preterm infant, or inaudible in an intubated infant. Autonomic and motor stress signals are common (see Table 21-5).

The infant's transition between states, both spontaneously and during handling, is important for the therapist to assess. The infant who cannot be aroused, who is excessively irritable, or who swings abruptly between sleep

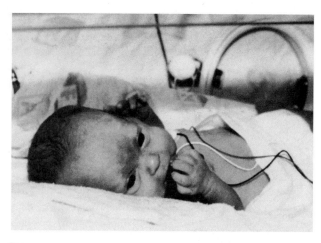

figure**21-16** This calm and alert preterm infant is in appropriate state of arousal for the therapist to assess her ability to attend and interact with specific environmental stimuli. *(Courtesy of the Infant Special Care Unit, University of Texas Medical Branch, Galveston, TX, photo by Dottie Jones.)*

and crying states with no alert periods may be demonstrating either immaturity or pathology. A gradual awakening with smooth transition from sleep to alertness and eventually back to sleep is one sign of maturation and neurologic integrity.

Individual temperament may be a variable in the infant's state of arousal; some infants are more demanding, and others are more relaxed. Therapists often initiate neurobehavioral assessments during sleep and continue them through awakening to allow observation of the infant's transition between states as the infant is handled. Noting, or charting over time, the infant's sleep-wake cycles can give important information for planning caregiving.

Neuromotor development and interventions

Reflex development. Neonatal reflex development is well documented in medical and therapy literature (Dargassies, 1977). Although reflex testing is often a popular method for therapists to assess an infant's maturation and CNS integrity, generalized reflex testing is extremely stressful for NICU infants and is unnecessary as a routine evaluation. Because sucking is the only reflex that relates directly to function, it is often sufficient to simply evaluate that reflex. Testing selected additional reflexes may be appropriate if the infant has known or suspected neuromuscular pathology (e.g., spina bifida, congenital neuropathy). The therapist can observe many reflexes (e.g., grasping, sucking, head righting) within the context of normal handling, which often provides more functional information than "formal" reflex testing.

Muscle tone. Hypotonia is present and normal for extremely preterm infants. Muscle tone in preterm infants gradually increases with age and in a caudocephalic (feet-to-head) direction; this is true for passive flexor tone seen at rest and active tone elicited by righting reactions when the infant is handled (Amiel-Tison & Grenier, 1986). However, an extremely preterm infant at term equivalency will typically demonstrate greater extension and less physiologic flexion than a full-term infant. Tremors and startles are common, but tremors should not be as prevalent as term equivalency nears.

In addition to postconceptional age, state of arousal and medical status are significant variables when assessing muscle tone. A preterm infant may be active and feisty when awake but appear hypotonic if assessed while drowsy or asleep. The therapist cannot accurately assess muscle tone in an acutely ill infant except for that point in time; the underlying muscle tone usually changes as the infant recovers. The therapist should also check medications because some have neuromotor side effects. For example, phenobarbital for seizures may initially make the infant lethargic, and some apnea medications may make the infant jittery.

The influence of muscle tone on resting posture and quantity or quality of movement has implications for positioning and caregiving needs. The therapist should note and monitor atypical findings or asymmetric responses. Often unusual movement patterns resolve with maturation and physical recovery.

Premie positional deformities. Preterm infants in the NICU are vulnerable to the effects of illness, weakness, low tone, primitive reflexes, immature motor control, and gravity. Hypotonic premies unable to counteract the effects of gravity naturally assume an extended posture, with the trunk, pelvis, and extremities flat on the bed surface (Desmond et. al., 1980; Fay, 1988) (Figure 21-17). Consequences can be observed both in the NICU and after hospital discharge. Preterm infants left in unsupported extended positions frequently exhibit increased stress and agitation with decreased physiologic stability in the NICU. Persistent and extreme extensor posturing may interfere with caregiving and with the infant's ability to attend and interact appropriately within his or her environment. Unless these susceptible infants are consistently therapeutically positioned throughout their hospitalizations (Figure 21-18), these factors may result in the gradual development of acquired positional deformities that can affect the NICU graduate's future motor development, play skills, and attractiveness.

Common positional deformities have been identified and related to inappropriate nursery positioning:

■ Shoulder external rotation and retraction with scapular adduction are common upper-extremity external rotation deformities (see Figure 21-17) (Georgieff & Bernbaum, 1986; Monfort & Case-Smith, 1997). A persistent "W" arm position can affect hand-to-mouth activity used for self-calming, interfere with forearm propping in prone and subsequent gross motor skills (e.g.,

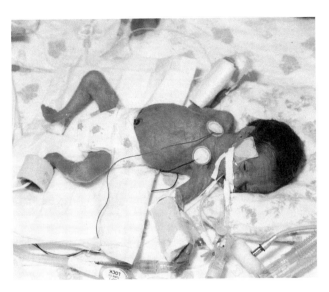

figure**21-17** Hypotonic posture of premature infant. Without therapeutic positioning, "W" configuration of arms, "frogged" posture of legs, and asymmetric head position may lead to positional deformities. Tiny premie diaper ("Wee-pee," Children's Medical Ventures) prevents forced hip abduction from diaper bulk. *(Courtesy of the Infant Special Care Unit, University of Texas Medical Branch, Galveston, TX. Photograph by John Glow.)*

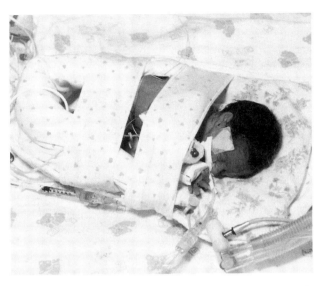

figure**21-18**   Small preterm infant (same baby as Figure 21-17) supported in sidelying position with midline orientation and flexion of extremities. Snuggle-Up bunting maintains the contained posture; Squishon I gel pillow under head facilitates comfort and minimizes head flattening. (Snuggle-Up and Squishon, Children's Medical Ventures). *(Courtesy of the Infant Special Care Unit, University of Texas Medical Branch, Galveston, TX. Photograph by John Glow.)*

sitting, hands and knees crawling, transitional movements from lying on the floor to sitting or standing), and delay the development of shoulder co-contraction.

■ Lower-extremity hip abduction, external rotation, knee flexion, and ankle eversion are common when legs rest on the surface in a "frogged" or "M" shape (see Figure 21-17); external tibial torsion (rotation of the tibia) has also been reported (Davis, Robinson, Harris, & Cartlidge, 1993; Downs et. al., 1991; Lacey et. al., 1990). These positional deformities have been implicated in various sequelae, including (1) disadvantages to the weight-bearing forefoot, leading to delays during the first year in motor skills, such as crawling and walking (Fay, 1988; Monterosso, Coenen, Percival, & Evans, 1995); (2) association with toe walking for up to 18 months of age (Fay, 1988; Bottos & Stefani, 1982); (3) persistence of out-toeing that has not resolved by 3 to 4½ years of age (Davis et. al, 1993); (4) impaired development of children with neurologic abnormalities; and (5) delayed walking in neurologically normal children because of difficulties in achieving good balance (Davis et. al., 1993). Lower-extremity positional deformities create significant concerns in parents and frequently prompt referrals to early intervention programs and/or orthopedic specialists.

■ Decreased depth of the rib cage has also been noted in NICU graduates (Semmler, 1989), which may be detrimental to infants who already experience respiratory compromise from chronic lung disease.

■ The skull of a preterm infant is thinner, softer, and more vulnerable to postural deformation than the skull of a full-term infant (Cartlidge & Rutter, 1988; Huang et. al., 1995). *Dolicephaly* refers to progressive lateral skull flattening that can result in a narrow and elongated "premie-shaped" head (Rutter, Hinchcliffe, & Cartlidge, 1993). Lateral head flattening has implications for infant attractiveness (Budreau, 1987, 1989). No effect on brain development has been reported (Elliman, Bryan, Elliman, & Starte, 1986).

■ Both preterm and full-term infants demonstrate preferential head-turning to the right spontaneously and in response to stimulation; infants with this preference keep their head to the right 70% to 80% of the time when in a supine position (Konishi, Mikawa, & Suziki, 1986). Preferential head-turning has been linked to asymmetric skull deformation (flattened occiput on preferred side, with or without a corresponding bulging of the forehead), lateral trunk curvature that does not disappear on ventral suspension, early right hand preference (because that hand is constantly in the visual field), and asymmetric gait patterns with increased external rotation of the left lower extremity (Boere-Boonekamp, vander Linden-Kuiper, & van EsP, 1997; Dias, Klein, & Backstrom, 1996). These findings are more prevalent and prolonged in preterm infants than in full-term infants and are accentuated by sudden infant death syndrome (SIDS) recommendations to place infants in a supine position for sleeping because many infants are positioned in supine when awake (Chadduck, Kast, & Donahue, 1997). Some infants with this preferential head-turning and early right hand preference have been mistakenly referred and treated in early intervention programs for a left hemiparesis, causing the parents considerable anxiety.

■ Infants may develop a grooved palate in association with prolonged oral intubation. Researchers have yet to confirm a relationship between grooved palates and prolonged oral intubation (Ash & Moss, 1987; Carillo, 1985; Erenberg & Nowak, 1984; Monteli & Bumstead, 1986; Procter, Lether, Oliver, & Cartlidge, 1998; Watterberg & Munsick-Bruno, 1986). A grooved palate may cause future problems with feeding, some speech sounds, and dental development requiring orthodontic intervention.

Therapeutic positioning. The primary purpose of *therapeutic positioning* with preterm infants is to provide secure containment with the extremities flexed and toward midline, which minimizes positional deformities and helps the infant remain calmer and more organized. Clinical experience suggests that the appropriate degree of containment is what the infant needs to remain calm and sleep peacefully. Increased freedom of movement and more upright postures become options with older, more stable infants nearing term equivalency.

Efforts at nesting infants in flexed, contained postures have historically been done with blanket and/or sheepskin rolls with variable success. Commercial positioning devices can significantly reduce variability among caregivers while improving the ease and consistency of providing therapeutic positioning. Positioning aids offer direct medical benefits and thus eventual cost savings. Therefore neonatal positioning aids are available in some NICUs by either purchasing the unit or billing the equipment to the patient. Washers and dryers are available in some units; either parents or staff may be responsible for laundering positioning items.

Because commercial devices may be unavailable in every NICU and because even the best equipment can be used inappropriately (Figure 21-19), positioning guidelines are described in the following sections. Medical and developmental advantages and disadvantages of various positioning options are summarized in Appendix 21-C.

General positioning guidelines
1. A soft surface (sheepskin, warm gel, or water mattress), secure "nesting" with deep boundaries (Snuggle-Up or high blanket rolls), and swaddling somewhat simulate the intrauterine environment and may help the infant "settle in" to rest more peacefully.
2. Motor disorganization is generally most pronounced in the supine and unsupported sidelying positions, especially if the limbs are not contained. Motor organization may be improved by the following:
   a. Prone positioning because it promotes increased physiologic stability including improved oxygen-

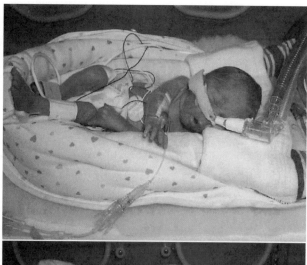
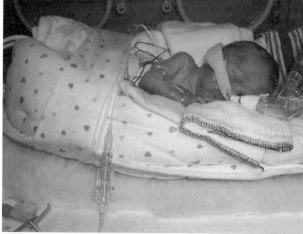

figure **21-19** Commercial positioning devices such as the Snuggle-Up (Children's Medical Ventures) make positioning easier, but the caregiver must still be aware of positioning guidelines and use positioning aides correctly to ensure secure and therapeutic positioning. Note the more relaxed posture and facial expression of this infant after suboptimal positioning was corrected. *(Courtesy of the Infant Special Care Unit, University of Texas Medical Branch, Galveston, TX. Photograph by Jan Hunter.)*

ation and ventilation, and better postural security from facilitation of trunk and extremity flexion.
   b. Sidelying is easiest to support with the infant swaddled firmly into a blanket and tucked into a Snuggle-Up or deep blanket nest; a single blanket roll behind the infant's back is inadequate. The infant's hands should be together in midline, preferably up by his or her face.
   c. Swaddling provides the easiest and most secure containment, especially when used with other positioning aids (e.g., Snuggle-Up, Bendy-Bumper), and has been successfully used with infants on warmers and in isolettes. Swaddling provides neutral warmth that helps relax the infant, reduces extraneous movement, and promotes the develop-

ment of flexor tone by containing the extremities in flexion, and it has been shown to improve the neuromuscular development of preterm infants (Short et. al., 1996). Swaddling with lightweight cotton (e.g., bandanna or handkerchief weight) can provide containment without excessive heat for infants who get too warm if blanket-swaddled in an incubator.

3. Therapists should reposition infants at least every 2 to 3 hours or when behavioral cues suggest discomfort that may be relieved by a position change.

4. Therapists must respect infant individuality and emerging capabilities, such as the occasional infant who seems to fight efforts at containment and rests better when allowed to "sprawl" or the maturing infant who can maintain a flexed posture without firm swaddling.

5. Oversized diapers on a small preterm infant passively maintain the hips in an exaggerated externally rotated and abducted "frog-leg" position. Consistent use of appropriately sized diapers combined with therapeutic positioning to maintain normal hip alignment can help reduce or prevent this typical premie positional deformity of the lower extremities.

6. The therapist should gently handle the infant with the extremities contained during and for a short period after position changes.

Supine

■ The therapist should support the infant's head in midline to relieve lateral weight-bearing pressure and secure ventilator tubing to avoid pulling the infant's head to one side or exerting traction on soft tissues (lip and palate with oral intubation; nares with nasal intubation) (Figure 21-20).

■ Unless the infant is on a waterbed (Fowler et. al., 1997), use of a gel pillow or water pillow under the head is strongly recommended. When using a gel or water pillow with a supine infant, the therapist can avoid airway occlusion from excessive neck flexion by placing the head and upper chest on the pillow to maintain neutral alignment. With very small premies, use of the gel pillow as a mattress under the head and body generally eliminates excessive neck flexion as a potential problem. The therapist should prewarm the pillow before placing it inside the Snuggle-Up or other boundary.

■ The therapist should tuck the infant's arms in by the body with elbows in flexion; this position is supported by surrounding boundaries (see Figure 21-20). Elbow flexion past 90 degrees may cause occlusion of some percutaneous lines.

■ The infant's hips should be partially flexed and adducted to near midline (not medial to neutral alignment because adduction with internal rotation

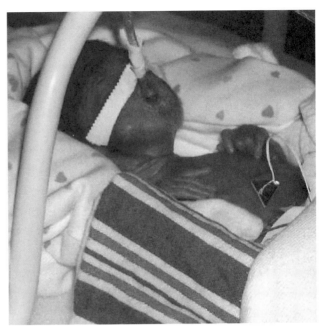

figure 21-20   The importance of attention to small details is illustrated by this extremely premature infant who is securely positioned in supine with a flexed midline orientation; tension on the endotracheal tube places deforming pressure on his gum ridge and palate. The curved bar over his body is the inner rod of a Bendy Bumper (Children's Medical Ventures) bent into a free-standing frame; a blanket is draped over this frame to shield light from infants on radiant warmers. (*Courtesy of the Infant Special Care Unit, University of Texas Medical Branch, Galveston, TX. Photograph by Jan Hunter.*)

places the newborn's hips in an unstable position that can promote dislocation).

■ The infant's knees should be partially flexed with feet *inside* surrounding boundaries (versus boundary under thighs with lower part of legs dangling over, which may compromise circulation and does not provide a support for the infant to use foot bracing as a self-regulation strategy).

Prone

■ Unless the infant is on a waterbed, the therapist should support his or her head on a gel pillow and alternately rotate the head to the right and left during position changes.

■ Extending placement of the gel or water pillow to the infant's midchest will help avoid excessive neck extension and shoulder retraction. Using the gel pillow lengthwise as a mattress under a very small premie may be a solution if the softer surface does not compromise respiratory function.

■ Use of a prone roll (e.g., gel pillow folded in half lengthwise and taped) under the infant's head and extending to the umbilicus allows the arms and legs to gently flex forward toward midline. The legs do

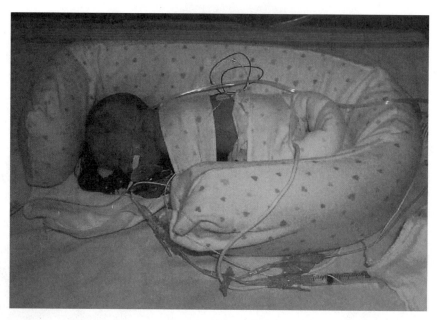

figure **21-21**   Preterm infant (same infant as in Figure 21-13) on a gel prone roll to facilitate flexed posture, with appropriately sized Snuggle-Up and Bendy Bumper (Children's Medical Ventures) making this position secure. *(Courtesy of the Infant Special Care Unit, University of Texas Medical Branch, Galveston, TX. Photograph by Jan Hunter.)*

not straddle the roll to avoid abduction. Stable external boundaries (e.g., Snuggle-Up, Bendy-Bumper) help the infant maintain a balanced and flexed position on the prone roll (Figure 21-21).

■ The therapist should provide secure lower boundaries that the infant can use for foot bracing.

Sidelying

■ Some neonatologists do not advocate prolonged sidelying for very small premies (except in treatment of specific air leaks, such as pulmonary interstitial emphysema [PIE]) because of concern that excessive time in this position may promote atelectasis of the dependent lung (lung on the underneath, weight-bearing side). The therapists should check the specific policy in each NICU and among attending neonatologists.

■ When positioned appropriately, the sidelying position decreases the extensor effects of gravity, facilitates midline orientation of the head and extremities, and encourages hand-to-hand, hand-to-mouth, or hand-to-face activity (see Figure 21-19). To maintain a sidelying position (and to avoid extremity extension and retraction, as well as increased infant stress from positional instability), the therapist should position the infant's top hip and shoulder slightly forward of the weight-bearing hip and shoulder. The therapist can achieve this with blanket rolls (firmly behind the infant, flattened between the legs, and up along the infant's front to encourage forward tucking around the roll), but the infant is more se-

cure within a Snuggle-Up. The therapist can still use small rolls as needed, such as the infant's arms tucked around a small stuffed animal to encourage forward flexion. The therapist can use a Bendy-Bumper alone or as additional support with a Snuggle-Up.

Medical considerations in positioning. Positioning may need modification to accommodate medical equipment or conditions. For example, conventional phototherapy requires a more exposed body surface, unless a fiber-optic "bili blanket" is available. The multiple lines and needs for caregiver access to a supine infant may restrict positioning options during ECMO. An infant with severe chest retractions from respiratory distress is often more stable in the prone position. Generalized edema may limit flexion of the extremities. The small jaw and recessed tongue of an infant with Pierre-Robin syndrome may result in airway obstruction if that infant is in a supine position. The prone position is not optimal for an infant with significant abdominal distention or recent abdominal surgery, and the supine position is not an option for an infant with a newly resected myelomeningocele. Extremity contractures associated with arthrogryposis multiplex congenita can make any therapeutic positioning a challenge, although use of gravity and body weight for gentle sustained stretch can make positioning a treatment option with some of these infants.

Range of motion. Passive range of motion (PROM) is primarily indicated for diagnoses that would benefit from a rehabilitation approach because of structural or neuromuscular limitation of movement (see Case Study #1) or

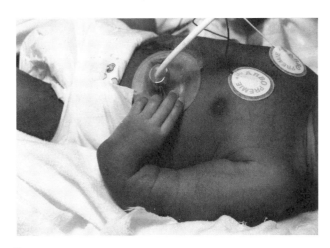

figure**21-22** Term infant with multiple congenital anomalies that require rehabilitation approach, including passive range of motion and splinting. Gastrostomy feeding tube is visible. *(Courtesy of the Infant Special Care Unit, University of Texas Medical Branch, Galveston, TX. Photograph by John Glow.)*

for infants who are demonstrating abnormal tone. PROM incorporated into therapeutic handling is preferable to conventional ranging techniques for most infants. Examples of diagnoses appropriate for PROM include congenital malformations and deformations (Figure 21-22), trauma such as a brachial plexus injury during delivery (Hunter, 1990), or hypertonicity associated with severe asphyxia. Infants usually do not need PROM after osteomyelitis because they begin to spontaneously move the affected extremity once pain and swelling subside (Hunter, 1990).

PROM may occasionally be appropriate for an infant who is sedated or chemically paralyzed for prolonged periods. However, experience suggests that prevention of positional deformities with therapeutic positioning may be sufficient intervention for infants whose movement is temporarily restricted (see Case Study #2). Therapists should *never* consider PROM a routine NICU intervention because it is unnecessary and often stressful to the general preterm population.

Splinting. Likewise, splinting is only occasionally needed with NICU infants. Significant contractures are uncommon, and infants are notably pliable over time. Therapists usually achieve significant improvement rapidly with gentle ranging, therapeutic positioning, the effects of gravity, and spontaneous movement of the infant. Conversely, spontaneous movement is inhibited while the infant is wearing a splint.

When the therapist makes the decision to splint an NICU infant, protecting skin integrity is a top priority. Thermoplastic splints may create pressure points unless well padded, including the edges. It can also be difficult to maintain correct joint alignment on a rigid splint because extremity movement of ¼ inch can significantly alter

placement of a tiny hand on a splint. A safer and still effective option is to make neonatal splints entirely from creative combinations of various foams, occasionally incorporating (enclosing) a rigid reinforcing bar if needed for some types of splints. Pliable molding compounds, such as those used in dentistry or even in children's crafts (e.g., Crayola Model Magic), may offer additional alternatives for form-fitting splints without pressure points.

The therapist should begin initial trials with the splint for short intervals to ensure tolerance, and he or she should gradually increase wearing time to correspond with other routine caregiving. Because multiple caregivers greatly increase the probability of error, the therapist should attach a photograph of proper splint application to bedside instructions. Posted written directions, wearing schedule, and precautions should be large enough to read and easy to understand. Staff and family education is essential but does not replace careful monitoring by the therapist. The therapist should provide parents of an infant going home with a splint with written and verbal instructions. The therapist must arrange follow-up appointments to monitor the splint's fit and function.

Feeding

NICU infants must be able to breathe independently, maintain a stable body temperature while still demonstrating weight gain, and successfully orally feed to allow an "uncomplicated" discharge to home. All of these variables generally improve with maturation; historically an infant simply stayed in the NICU as long as necessary. With health care changes and emphasis on cost containment during recent years, earlier discharge has become the norm and time is often no longer an ally. As more infants go home on apnea medications, monitors, and oxygen rather than outgrowing their breathing problems in the NICU, oral feeding is often the remaining obstacle to discharge. Consequently, oral feeding is routinely initiated at earlier ages. The daily challenge to caregivers is facilitation of successful oral feeding by careful balancing of the infant's maturational factors with environmental modifications and sensitive feeding techniques.

Preparation for successful oral feeding begins at birth with consistent developmentally supportive care to optimize the infant's medical, neuromotor, and neurobehavioral outcome. The infant with less severe lung disease and normal neurologic status has an advantage when mastering the complex task of feeding. Improved neurobehavioral organization, including the ability to achieve and maintain good quality alertness, contributes to feeding success. Therapeutic positioning to prevent shoulder retraction and neck hyperextension facilitates the neuromuscular control and postural alignment needed for coordinated sucking, swallowing, and breathing. Attention to minimizing aversive oral stimulation, providing pleasurable sucking experiences, and facilitating a normal sucking pattern during early weeks or months expedites transition to oral feeding.

Benefits of nonnutritive sucking

The ability to suck nonnutritively is a sign of CNS integrity (Medoff-Cooper, Verklan, & Carlson, 1993). *Nonnutritive sucking (NNS) patterns,* or "dry" sucking such as on a fist or pacifier, are present but disorganized in infants younger than 30 weeks' postconception; sucking rhythm generally improves by 30 to 32 weeks' postconception.

NNS is a self-soothing activity that improves state control, reduces stress, promotes weight gain by reducing fussing and restless activity, improves oxygenation, and increases arousal (Bernbaum, Pereira, Watkins, & Peckman, 1983; Pickler & Frankel, 1995). Caregivers frequently use NNS to support and calm an infant during stressful procedures.

NNS during gavage feedings of preterm infants is recommended to increase the maturation of the sucking reflex, decrease intestinal transit time, cause more rapid weight gain, facilitate the transition from gavage to oral feedings, and thus contribute to a shorter hospital stay (Bernbaum et. al., 1983). NNS can facilitate the initiation and duration of the first nutritive sucking burst (Pickler, Frankel, Walsh, & Thompson, 1996). Table 21-8 compares characteristics of nonnutritive and nutritive sucking.

Nutritive sucking

Nutritive sucking patterns. The most common feeding difficulties that premature and ill infants encounter are respiratory compromise and inadequate endurance. Nutritive sucking, which occurs when liquid is available to swallow, is often disorganized because of the immature infant's inability to rhythmically coordinate breathing with sustained sucking and swallowing (Glass & Wolf, 1994; Palmer, 1993; Palmer & VandenBerg, 1998). This disorganization often persists in the infant with chronic lung disease because the need to breathe supersedes the infant's efforts to suck.

Three distinct *nutritive sucking patterns* have been described (Palmer, 1993; Palmer & VandenBerg, 1998).

1. *Mature.* Typical of healthy term infants, the mature pattern demonstrates continuous sucking bursts of 10 to 30 sucks, smooth 1:1:1 suck-swallow-breathe rhythm in which respiration appears continuous and uninterrupted, and brief respiratory pauses between sucking bursts (Bu'Lock, Woolridge, & Baum, 1990; Medoff-Cooper, Verklan, & Carlson, 1993). Sucking bursts are usually longest at the beginning of a feeding (continuous sucking), followed by intermittent sucking with more opportunities for breathing as the feeding continues (Mathew, 1991).

2. *Immature.* Observed in healthy preterm infants as young as 32½ weeks' postconception, the immature nutritive sucking pattern consists of short sucking bursts (3 to 5 sucks) with respirations and swallows occurring before and after the sucking burst (Meier & Anderson, 1987). The respiratory pause is equal in length to the short sucking burst, with suck-swallow alternating with breathing in a coordinated manner (Brake & Fifer, 1988). Instead of the 1:1:1 suck-swallow-breathe coordination seen in term infants, preterm infants cluster suck and breathe together. This breath holding during sucking is believed to be related to the infant's instinct to protect the airway from penetration by the liquid bolus (Mathew, 1991; Shiao, 1997).

3. *Transitional.* Some preterm infants and older medically fragile infants (up to 45 weeks' postconception) display a disorganized pattern characterized by variable sucking bursts (generally 6 to 10 sucking bursts), with bursts and pauses of equal duration and apneic periods following longer sucking bursts (Palmer, 1993). This pattern occurs when the infant tries to use the continuous sucking burst of a mature pattern but does not yet have a smooth rhythm of suck-swallow with breathing (Palmer, 1993; Palmer & VandenBerg, 1998). Infants who demonstrate more than one sucking pattern (e.g., both long and short sucking bursts during the same feeding) are also considered transitional. Disorganized transitional sucking is the most common feeding pattern observed in NICU infants and is the pattern with the most potential for caregiver intervention.

Nutritive sucking and respiration. Oxygenation and ventilation are compromised during nutritive sucking because the airway briefly closes during every reflexive swallow (Hanlon et. al., 1997; Mathew, 1988; Shivpuri, Martin, Carlo, & Fanaroff, 1983). This compromise is more significant during continuous sucking than during intermittent sucking (Mathew, 1991; Shiao, 1997) and worse with an indwelling nasogastric tube than without the tube (Shiao, Brooker, & DiFiore, 1996; Shiao, 1997). Continuous sucking may result in blood chemistry changes that trigger the infant to change to an intermittent sucking pattern (Shivpuri et. al., 1983).

Improvement in feeding-induced apnea (deglutition apnea), often associated with multiple swallows without breathing, appears to correlate more with advancing age (maturation) than with practice (Hanlon et. al., 1997). Clinically, this means that additional time to mature is more beneficial than frequent opportunities to "practice" oral feeding for younger preterm infants. Term infants may demonstrate deglutition apnea, but its occurrence is more frequent and prolonged in preterm infants reaching term equivalency compared with term infants (Hanlon et. al., 1997).

table 21-8 *Comparison of Nonnutritive and Nutritive Sucking*

Trait	Nonnutritive Sucking (NNS)	Nutritive Sucking (NS)
Development (Progression)	**27-28 weeks:** Weak single sucks with long variable pause (random, disorganized) **30-33 weeks:** Short but stable sucking bursts (1-1.5 sucks/sec), with long irregular pauses; respiratory rate may increase; sluggish esophageal peristalsis **≥34 weeks:** Longer sucking bursts and more regular pauses; stability of sucking rate and pattern same as term infants by 37 weeks; intermittent swallowing after 6-8 sucks; smooth esophageal peristalsis	Sucking and swallowing occur in utero after the first trimester, but breathing not yet a factor Suck-swallow-breathe (s-s-b) coordination demonstrated as early as 32 weeks; smoothness and consistency of 1:1:1 s-s-b ratio improved with increasing maturity; usually mature pattern by 37 wks s-s-b coordination may be adequate for breastfeeding earlier than for bottle feeding
Rate	Two sucks per second	One suck per second
Pattern	Alternating sucking bursts (4-13 sucks) and rest periods (3-10 seconds)	Initially continuous stream of sucks (10-30); variable bursts and rest periods toward end of feed
Stimulus	Occurs in sleep as spontaneous mouthing movements or in response to "dry" stimulus (e.g., pacifier, finger)	Liquid obtainable from nipple
Arousal	Able to elicit in all states except deep sleep and crying	Occurs most efficiently in arousal episodes
Feeding	Good nonnutritive suck in a preterm infant does not imply an effective nutritive suck	Suck elicits swallow; maturation is more important than age, weight, or practice in achieving s-s-b coordination
Suck-swallow-breathe ratio	6-8 sucks before swallowing	1:1:1 ratio; may be higher (more sucks) if suck is inefficient at end of feed or with older infant Infant (preterm > term) may have multiple swallows without breathing
Respiration	Improved oxygenation in preterm infants up to 35 weeks and in noncrying term infants; breathing frequency, tidal volume, and minute ventilation remain unchanged in term infants	Breathing frequency, tidal volume, and minute ventilation become depressed in both term and preterm infants during oral feeding; apnea and cyanosis relatively common
Indicator of Neurologic Impairment	Because of its predictive and measurable qualities, NNS has been suggested as a potential early indicator of neurologic impairment in infant with perinatal distress	Because NS is sensitive to arousal and environmental distractions, it is not interchangeable with NNS as an early measurable index of neurologic function (persistent poor feeding often is ⊕ indicator)

Modified from Bosma, J.F. (1986). Development of feeding. *Clinical Nutrition, 5*, 210-218.
Bu'Lock, F., Woolridge, M.W., & Baum, J.D. (1990). Development of coordination of sucking, swallowing and breathing: Ultrasound study of term and preterm infants. *Developmental Medicine and Child Neurology, 32*, 669-678.
Comrie, J.D., & Helm, J.M. (1997). Common feeding problems in the intensive care nursery: Maturation, organization, evaluation and management strategies. *Seminars in Speech and Language, 18*, 239-261.
Daniels, H., Casaer, P., Devlieger, H., & Eggermont, E. (1986). Mechanisms of feeding efficiency in preterm infants. *Journal of Pediatric Gastroenterology and Nutrition, 5*, 593-596.
Hack, M., Eastbrook, M.M., & Robertson, S.S. (1985). Development of sucking rhythms in preterm infants. *Early Human Development, 11*, 133-140.
Hanlon, M.B., Tripp, J.H., Ellis, R.E., Flack, F.C., Selley, W.G., & Shoesmith, H.J. (1997). Deglutition apnea as indicator of maturation of suckle feeding in bottle-fed infants. *Developmental Medicine and Child Neurology, 39*, 534-542.
Harris, M.B. (1986). Oral-motor management of the high-risk neonate. *Physical and Occupational Therapy in Pediatrics, 6*, 231-253.
McCain, G. (1997). Behavioral state activity during nipple feedings for preterm infants. *Neonatal Network, 16*, 43-47.
Wolf, L.S., & Glass, R.P. (1992). *Feeding and swallowing disorders in infancy: Assessment and management.* Tucson: Therapy Skill Builders.

Feeding readiness

Traditional NICU criteria to begin oral feedings usually require the relatively stable preterm infant to reach a certain age and weight, although this target age and weight may vary considerably among physicians. Feedings are typically based on set calories and volume per kilogram of body weight and given on a set schedule around the clock.

In contrast, an individualized approach to feeding readiness considers such factors as each infant's medical status, general neurobehavioral organization (e.g., vigor, sleep and wake cycle, ability to achieve some stable alert periods), and feeding readiness cues (e.g., awakening, fussing before feedings, spontaneous rooting and sucking behaviors, gagging with gavage tube insertion) (Kinneer & Beachy, 1994; Siddell & Froman, 1994). One study reported that young preterm infants of 32 to 33 weeks' postconception showed feeding readiness cues during 92% of recorded trials, but these cues did not coincide with a scheduled feeding 70% of the time (Cagan, 1995). Cue-based feedings beginning at 32 to 33 weeks' postconception in stable preterm infants resulted in transition to full oral feedings at earlier ages and better weight gain on a lower volume of intake (Hubler et. al., 1997). The improved weight gain may be related to calorie conservation from avoidance of prolonged agitation when the infant appears ready to eat at a time when a feeding is not scheduled and to fewer interruptions of deep sleep during which growth hormone is secreted.

Clinical assessment of oral feeding

A structured format for clinical feeding evaluation of infants has been presented (Glass & Wolf, 1998; Wolf & Glass, 1992). Another feeding evaluation appropriate for the NICU population is the Neonatal Oral-Motor Assessment Scale (NOMAS), which requires training for certification to reliability (Palmer, Crawley, & Blanco, 1993). The NOMAS classifies characteristics of jaw and tongue movement into categories of normal, disorganized, and dysfunctional. Disorganization reflects a difficulty with coordinating breathing with suck-swallow coordination; it is associated with age and generally improves with maturation; dysfunction has not correlated with gestational or postconceptional age (Palmer, Crawley, & Blanco, 1993). The NOMAS can help the therapist distinguish disorganization from dysfunction during early feeding and measure intervention effectiveness with poor feeders in the NICU.

General considerations. The following are general factors for the therapist to consider during a neonatal feeding assessment:

1. Nursery environment. General level of and infant proximity to light, sound, activity, and traffic in the room
2. Seating. Comfortable for the caregiver and conducive to providing adequate support for the infant

3. Physiologic
   a. Pertinent infant medical complications (e.g., cardiopulmonary, neurologic, genetic)
   b. Baseline color, respiratory rate, heart rate, and oxygen saturation
   c. Changes from baseline during feeding
4. Anatomic
   a. Facial anomalies (e.g., micrognathia, asymmetry, cranial nerve involvement, cleft lip and/or palate)
   b. History of other anomalies or complications that can influence feeding, including gastrointestinal motility (e.g., repaired tracheoesophageal fistula, diaphragmatic hernia, duodenal or jejunal atresia or stenosis, necrotizing enterocolitis (NEC), gastrointestinal reflux)
5. Behavioral
   a. Timing, duration, and quality of arousal and alertness (spontaneous and if awakened for scheduled feeding)
   b. Sensitivity to environmental stimuli (e.g., distractibility, disorganization, shut down)
6. Response and tolerance to caregiver touch and handling. Acceptance or avoidance of pacifier or bottle nipple
7. Neuromuscular
   a. Muscle tone and posture at rest (especially head, neck, shoulders, and trunk)
   b. Differences in tone, posture, and movement with handling or change of position
   c. General activity level (Are frequency, intensity, and quality of movements normal for age?)
   d. Muscle tone and spontaneous movements of oral musculature (cheeks, lips, tongue, and jaw)

Oral-motor factors. The following questions may guide clinical observations of oral-motor function during a feeding:

- Does the infant latch on to the nipple (e.g., tongue forms central groove to cup nipple, lips close, jaw elevates)? Is the latch-on immediate or delayed? Do the infant's lips remain around the nipple (the labial seal is typically loose in young infants)? Is initiation of a sucking burst immediate or delayed? Are sucking bursts rhythmic and sustained or irregular and disorganized? Do sucking bursts alternate with rest pauses? Are rest pauses too long?
- Can the infant coordinate suck-swallow with breathing, or is external pacing by the caregiver necessary to avoid feeding-induced apnea, bradycardia, and oxygen desaturations? What changes occur in respiratory rate and saturations at the beginning and throughout the feeding? How much recovery time does the infant need to return to baseline respiratory rate and oxygen saturation? Does increasing oxygen during the feeding (if applicable) improve the infant's respiratory rate and saturation?

- Does the infant hold the tongue retracted or with the tongue tip elevated against the hard palate? Does the tongue show midline grooving and rhythmic peristalsis during sucking? Does the tongue protrude during sucking (some preterm infants who push the tongue against an endotracheal tube during prolonged oral intubation also tend to use exaggerated tongue protrusion to inadvertently push the nipple from the mouth during early oral feedings)? Are tongue movements rhythmic or disorganized?
- Are jaw movements rhythmic? Is there excessive jaw excursion (e.g., visible or smacking sound as lip seal is broken with excessive excursion)? Is the infant able to strip milk efficiently (e.g., bubbles appear in bottle and liquid is consumed at reasonable rate)? Are swallows occurring (e.g., observed, palpated, audible, heard by cervical auscultation)? Is excessive liquid lost? Is this loss by passive leakage or wet burps? Is the infant's endurance sufficient (e.g., adequate volume is consumed in a reasonable time without undue physiologic compromise)?

Facilitating feeding success in the NICU

Some preterm infants do well with oral feeding from the beginning, and many have only transient feeding difficulties that improve spontaneously with maturation. Long-term feeding problems are encountered most often, although not exclusively, in infants with persistent cardiorespiratory, gastrointestinal, and/or neurologic compromise. Box 21-2 provides multiple considerations and suggestions for the therapist to facilitate successful feeding with the preterm or high-risk infant in the NICU, but these suggestions should not be used as a "cookbook." An infant who demonstrates physiologic stability and adequate intake during oral feeding with basic environmental modifications and postural support may not need additional physical caregiver interventions, such as chin or cheek support. Caregiver manipulations during feeding should always be individualized based on demonstrated need and never done routinely with the rationale that "this is the way we feed premies."

box 21-2 *Considerations and suggestions to facilitate feeding in the NICU*

- Feeding difficulties with most preterm infants are transient, improving with maturation (most important) and practice as they learn to sustain sucking and coordinate suck-swallow with breathing.
- If excessive caregiver facilitation is required to elicit nutritive sucking, the caregiver may need to temporarily defer oral feeding; maturation is often more beneficial than "extra practice" in immature infants. Pushing an infant to do "too much, too fast" may deplete the infant's energy reserves, with a resultant setback that delays the onset of successful oral feedings.
- The caregiver should encourage pacifier sucking throughout hospitalization. The Wee Thumbie works well with small infants (Engebretson, 1997). The infant on extended nonoral feedings should transition to a pacifier shaped like a bottle nipple for NNS during later gavage feedings.
- A calm, quiet atmosphere with dimmed lighting is best. The caregiver can detect subtle physiologic color changes without bright overhead lights.
- Some preterm infants seem to feed reflexively regardless of state of arousal, but most preterm infants do better with oral feedings when awake (Figure 21-23). The caregiver should gently arouse the infant before a feeding (e.g., stroking [Gaebler & Hanzlik, 1996]), changing the diaper, talking in a soft voice, or changing the infant's position.
- Feeding the preterm infant should be nurturing but *not* overtly social. Unnecessary auditory and visual stimulation may overwhelm and disorganize the

preterm infant who is struggling to master oral feeding. The caregiver should avoid direct social interaction with a young infant and resist using feeding time with an immature or compromised infant as an opportunity to socialize with peers.
- The infant needs excellent postural support; swallowing is mechanically difficult if the neck is extended, shoulders retracted, and arms dangling. Efficient swallow is possible when the infant is swaddled with the arms and legs tucked in toward midline, the hands by the face, the neck in neutral alignment or slight flexion, and firm thoracic support (Comrie & Helm, 1997). Some infants demonstrate significantly improved sucking organization when given the opportunity to hold on to the caregiver's finger during feeding.
- The caregiver should feed the infant in a semi-upright (45 to 60 degrees) (Shaker, 1990) or upright position (Lewallen-Matthews, 1994). A semi-upright sidelying position (i.e., approximating the angle at which a breast-fed infant is held) is helpful in facilitating coordination of suck-swallow-breathing with many preterm infants (Comrie & Helm, 1997).
- The caregiver should consider a prefeeding "warm-up" of a few minutes perioral/intraoral stimulation with select infants (e.g., stroking or tapping around the mouth, stroking with pacifier or gloved finger on the tongue, pacifier sucking [Case-Smith, 1988; Gaebler & Hanzlik, 1996]).
- Firm, steady jaw support under the base of the tongue (not up-and-down pumping action of the

Continued

jaw) and firm but gentle cheek support (inward and forward) may provide helpful stability to the infant with difficulty latching, a weak lip seal, liquid loss, or excessive or poorly graded jaw excursion during the transitional stage of learning to feed (Einarsson-Backes et. al., 1994).

- Frequent twirling or twisting of the nipple in the infant's mouth creates a moving target and can prevent the infant from maintaining a firm latch-on to the nipple.
- Warm or cold temperature may increase sensory awareness of the presence of milk in the mouth. Reported effects of formula temperature are variable. One study of healthy preterm infants between 1500 and 2000 grams found gastric emptying time to be independent of cold versus warm feeding temperature (Blumenthal, Lealman, & Shoesmith, 1989). Another study of preterm infants showed significantly smaller gastric residuals after feedings with milk warmed to body temperature but no significant difference in gastric residuals when cold and room temperature milk was used (Gonzales, Duryes, Vasquez, & Geraghty, 1995). Refrigerator-chilled liquid has been suggested to improve the speed of the swallowing reflex in infants, and most young infants will take chilled formula without protest (Wolf & Glass, 1992). No significant differences in body temperature were found after using milk that was chilled, at room temperature, or warm (Gonzales et. al., 1995).
- Flow rate is often the key to failure or success. A slow-flow nipple is frequently desirable to avoid overwhelming the infant's ability to manage a liquid bolus. Some NICUs do not stock the softer, faster-flow premature nipples to reduce the occurrence of feeding-induced apnea. However, premie nipples may be helpful toward the end of a feeding if an infant fatigues or with specific low-energy infants who demonstrate poor stripping of milk from the nipple.
- The caregiver must continuously observe the infant's rhythm of sucking and breathing, noting respiratory pauses and monitoring for increased heart rate and respiratory rate with a decline in oxygen saturation.
- If sucking is vigorous and prolonged without a respiratory pause, the caregiver may need to "externally pace" the infant to provide breathing breaks and avoid feeding-induced apnea with subsequent desaturation and bradycardia. The caregiver can pace the infant by removing the nipple from the infant's mouth (VandenBerg, 1990), or if

nipple removal distresses or disorganizes the infant, tilting the bottle downward to drain milk from the nipple (Comrie & Helm, 1997) (Figure 21-24). Continuation of rhythmic external pacing that mimics an immature sucking pattern (alternating sucking bursts of three to four sucks with enforced rest pauses of 3 to 4 seconds) appears to facilitate regular breathing in infants with a transitional sucking pattern (Palmer, 1993). (There is unresolved controversy as to whether external pacing by tipping or removing the bottle is better for the infant. An air-hungry infant will respond with a gasping inhalation when the nipple is pulled out of his or her mouth, creating a risk of laryngeal penetration and/or aspiration of residual milk that has not yet been swallowed. Conversely, there are concerns that tilting the bottle will cause the infant to swallow excessive air or that air in the pharynx may be disorganizing (Shaker, 1998.)

Infants seem to have two distinct responses to bottle tilting. Some will clear milk remaining in the mouth with a swallow or two and then stop sucking for a rest pause. Other infants will keep sucking, but because fluid is the stimulus for nutritive sucking, seem to switch to a NNS pattern ("dry" sucking) (Comrie & Helm, 1997). NNS improves oxygenation (e.g., the infant can still breathe and recover), and at least 6 to 7 sucks occur before the infant elicits a swallow (see Table 21-8), suggesting that additional air intake may be minimal.

- Very short sucking bursts may be due to compromised respiratory status. The caregiver can regulate flow rate by choosing an appropriate nipple (premie and NUK nipples have faster flow than term nipples), feeding the infant in a sidelying positioning, and externally pacing to allow breathing breaks.
- Subtle, gentle outward traction on the nipple by the caregiver during the suction component of sucking may stimulate a longer, stronger suck with infants who tend to bite or suck in a rapid, inefficient pattern (Comrie & Helm, 1997).
- The caregiver can use the Haberman feeder, designed for infants with cleft lip and/or palate, with some NICU infants who do not have clefts. The benefit of the Haberman feeder is to get milk into the mouth of an infant who has an intact suck-swallow but cannot get milk adequately from the nipple (poor stripping). Infants with clefts have difficulty feeding because both negative and positive intraoral pressure (suction and compression) used in stripping milk from the nipple are compromised. Other infants who may benefit from a Haberman

box 21-2 *Considerations and suggestions to facilitate feeding in the NICU—cont'd*

feeder are those with very low energy, strength, and endurance, such as infants who are lethargic from chronic lung disease or cardiac defects. A Haberman feeder is not a good choice for a "typical" immature infant who is learning to coordinate suck-swallow with breathing or for a neurologically compromised infant with known or suspected oropharyngeal discoordination. The caregiver can use a Haberman feeder until the infant's stripping or endurance improves sufficiently to allow functional use of a regular nipple (i.e., intake of an adequate amount of milk in a reasonable time without undue fatigue).

- If possible, the caregiver should only orally feed the infant who shows readiness cues (e.g., awakening, fussing, hand to mouth, rooting, sucking) (Hubler et. al., 1997). The caregiver should avoid oral feedings after stressful procedures. The caregiver should reduce environmental distractions and avoid simultaneous physical and physiologic demands on the infant (e.g., significantly increasing feeding volume and weaning from isolette at the same time).
- The caregiver should generally complete feedings within 15 to 20 minutes for most preterm infants by discharge. Somewhat longer feeding times may be acceptable for certain infants with anomalies or chronic illness.
- For physiologically compromised infants, the caregiver should support the work of feeding by giving or increasing supplemental oxygen during oral feedings if needed, giving stable submandibular and/or cheek support, choosing an appropriate nipple (including Haberman feeder), increasing volume of gavage feedings so that oral feedings can

be smaller, using modular additives (e.g., Polycose, microlipids, corn oil), or concentrating the formula to increase caloric density and thus decrease required volume.

- Slightly thickened feedings may be a consideration for certain infants who exhibit difficulty with thin liquids. Thickened feedings as part of a gastrointestinal reflux protocol vary among hospitals and physicians. Some caregivers use commercial rice-added formula or thicken feedings slightly (1 tablespoon of standard baby rice cereal to 2 ounces of formula or breast milk, with the cereal pulverized in a blender before mixing to avoid lumps) (Wolf & Glass, 1992; Comrie & Helm, 1997). The caregiver may enlarge the nipple hole slightly to accommodate thickened milk by use of a sterilized darning needle (Comrie & Helm, 1997) or a #11 surgical blade (Wolf & Glass, 1992). Other caregivers believe that thickened feedings delay gastric emptying and thus increase the risk for reflux.
- The consistency obtained with primary nursing (or with encouraging as much parental involvement as possible) is often helpful with difficult feeders, especially if frequent disorganization or aversive behaviors are problematic. With some older chronic infants, the relationship with the caregiver becomes more important in oral feeding performance than any caregiver feeding technique.
- Documentation of oral feeding performance on the infant's nursing flow sheet should include qualitative data, not just the volume consumed and length of feeding (Ancona, Shaker, Puhek, & Garland, 1998).

Breast-feeding the preterm infant

Although breast-feeding is considered beneficial for both mothers and infants, most mothers who want to breast-feed their preterm infants give up before the infant is discharged from the NICU. Others may quit soon after going home, partly because health care trends toward shorter hospitalizations often result in the discharge of both term and preterm infants before the mother and infant establish breast-feeding success. This section presents a basic summary of breast-feeding. (See selected comprehensive texts [La Leche League International, 1997; Riordan & Auerbach, 1999] for additional information.)

Benefits of breast-feeding in the NICU. Numerous studies report significantly improved health and developmental outcomes for preterm infants fed their own mother's milk, with and without human milk fortifiers (Brown et. al, 1996). Benefits to the infant include less

physiologic stress experienced during breast-feeding (as opposed to bottle feeding) (Meier, 1988), decreased risk of NEC, decreased risk of infection, better enteral feed tolerance with quicker weaning from IV nutrition, decreased risk of later allergies, improved retinal function, and favorable effects on neurocognitive development. Maternal benefits of breast-feeding include facilitation of attachment, reduced feeling of isolation, and decreased sense of helplessness.

Challenges to breast-feeding success in the NICU. Some common obstacles to successful breast-feeding in the NICU include continued medical complications of mother and/or infant, separation of parents and infant, and maternal stress or fear. Many mothers of preterm or ill infants lack adequate breast-feeding education on access of pumps, milk expression techniques, safe collection and storage of expressed breast milk, transporting of milk

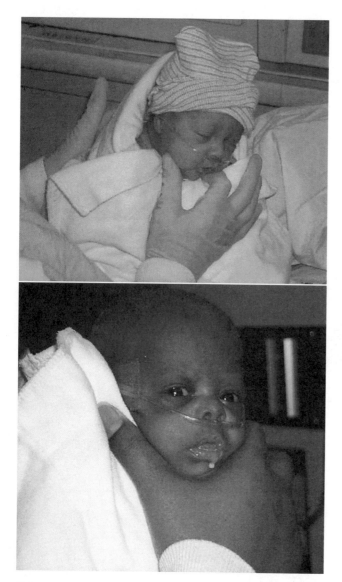

figure 21-23   Oral feeding is usually more successful once the preterm infant can achieve and maintain an awake state of arousal. *(Courtesy of the Infant Special Care Unit, University of Texas Medical Branch, Galveston, TX. Photograph by Jan Hunter.)*

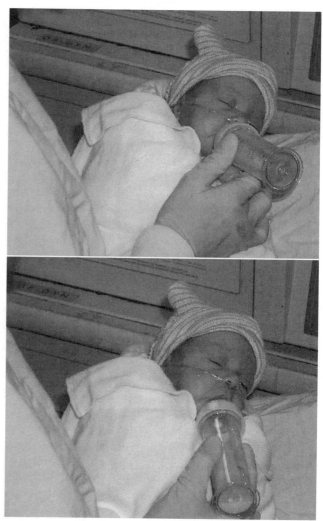

figure 21-24   Preterm infant with transitional sucking pattern being fed in modified sidelying (breast-feeding position) *(top)*, then being externally paced as the caregiver tips the bottle to force a breathing break *(bottom)*. *(Courtesy of the Infant Special Care Unit, University of Texas Medical Branch, Galveston, TX. Photograph by Jan Hunter.)*

to the hospital, and maintenance of an adequate milk supply after preterm delivery. Inadequate milk production is the most frequent reason cited for stopping breast-feeding efforts; appropriate staff interventions and support can minimize this problem.

Other difficulties include conflicting advice, lack of breast-feeding knowledge, and perceived lack of support by NICU staff members (Hill, Hanson, & Mefford, 1994). The NICU environment and policies may also not be conducive to breast-feeding. Mothers have the right to choose the type of feeding, and therapists have a responsibility to support and problem solve as needed to make breast-feeding successful if that is the mother's choice.

Facilitating breast-feeding in the NICU

Early education and pumping. Each NICU should have a consistent and efficient method to discuss options and details of breast-feeding and bottle feeding with the parents, optimally before delivery or as soon as feasible afterwards. Preterm mothers who are indecisive should begin pumping in the interim because lactation is easiest to stimulate in the early postpartum period (versus several days later) and because early milk and colostrum are highest in antiinfective properties (Meier, Brown, & Hurst, 1999). The mother can stop pumping at any time, but she will have had the opportunity and her infant will benefit. Some mothers may wish to pump and feed breastmilk by bottle to provide the benefits of breastmilk without actually putting the infant to the breast; this can be done indefinitely or on a short-term basis.

Parent education needs to include a reasonable pumping schedule and arrangements for a postdischarge pump. The goal is to obtain maximum milk volume with minimal expenditure of energy without incurring breast or nipple pain or trauma. Electric pumps and a double-pump collecting kit should be standard for NICU mothers with infants less than 1500 grams, those whose infants will not feed directly at the breast for at least 2 weeks, and those with multiple births (Auerbach & Walker, 1994).

Increasing the frequency of pumping is more effective than increasing the duration of each episode. With double pumping, the greatest milk volume is obtained within a total of about 10 to 12 minutes; double pumping facilitates more milk production than pumping each breast separately (Auerbach & Walker, 1994). Techniques that encourage rest and relaxation, reduce stress and tension, and promote pleasurable thoughts of the infant can facilitate more successful pumping (Feher, Berger, Johnson, & Wilde, 1989).

Nonnutritive nuzzling at the breast. The easiest transition to breast-feeding begins with initiation of skin-to-skin holding (kangaroo care) as soon as possible under nursery guidelines (Hurst et. al., 1997). When a stable infant reaches 30 to 32 weeks' postconception, the mother can pump her breasts just before providing kangaroo care to allow opportunities for nonnutritive suckling (nuzzling, licking, and mouthing) at the breast during skin-to-skin holding. The mother does not make an effort to get the infant to latch on and feed because this is a "get acquainted" period for the mother and infant to become familiar and comfortable with each other. Kangaroo care with nonnutritive nuzzling is also helpful in maintaining the mother's interest in breast-feeding and facilitating milk production.

Breast-feeding readiness. A good research-based clinical tool is not available for determining readiness to breast-feed. Traditional NICU criteria for beginning oral feedings (e.g., the infant has reached a predetermined age and weight) are not strictly applicable to breast-feeding. Research suggests that suck-swallow-breathe coordination may occur earlier with breast-feeding than with bottle-feeding and that early breast-feeding is physiologically less stressful (e.g., less hypoxemia, apnea, bradycardia, cyanosis) than bottle feedings for preterm infants (Meier & Anderson, 1987). The conclusion is that the mother should start breast-feedings before bottle feedings.

In some NICUs, nursing staff members follow the cues of the infant (e.g., arousal, fussing, rooting, sucking, active efforts to latch on during nonnutritive time at the breast) to determine breast-feeding readiness. Nurses in other NICUs may apply their current criteria for initiating oral (bottle) feedings to breast-feeding (e.g., start breast-feeding when bottle feedings would typically begin; refrain from any bottle use for at least 1 week while the infant learns to breast-feed).

Caregivers can alleviate concerns regarding accurate measurement of intake by weighing the infant on a sensitive scale before and after breast-feeding (Meier, Brown, & Hurst, 1999). Before and after weights are not routine for healthy term infants, but they can help the caregiver determine what a preterm infant received so that he or she can adjust other fluids and nutrients.

Methods for introducing and sustaining breast-feeding. The primary goals in early breast-feedings are for the infant to achieve proper positioning at the breast and remain physiologically stable during the session; significant volume intake is not a major objective during this phase. The mother should use a comfortable chair and pillows to raise the infant to chest height and support the mother's arm and breast. A separate breast-feeding room is ideal, but even a screen in the NICU can provide some privacy. The nurse or therapist can show the mother how to support her breast, position the infant, and help elicit latch-on to the nipple. Monitoring and documenting the infant's responses and stability during breast-feeding are important; a charting and documentation system has been developed specifically for assessment of breast-feeding (Jensen, Wallace, & Kelsay, 1994).

Optimally, some measurable nutritive intake occurs within a week after beginning early breast-feeding, as measured by test weights. Measurable intake greater than 5 ml suggests that the mother's milk has "let down" in response to the infant sucking at the breast. Once measurable intake occurs and the infant also remains physiologically stable during early breast-feeding, the goal changes to developing interventions that allow the infant to consume adequate volumes of breast milk in anticipation of hospital discharge. Interventions within this phase of breast-feeding may include test weights, transition to cue-based feeding schedules, and specific techniques for intake-related problems.

Although intake volume increases progressively from earlier to later breast-feeding, the amount of milk consumed at each breast-feeding session varies for both term and preterm infants. The nurse evaluates weights before and after feeding individually for each infant. However, a trend of inadequate volume intake at each breast-feeding over several days requires determination of the cause (e.g., low maternal milk supply, improper positioning, difficulty with milk ejection, problem with the strength, and endurance of the infant's sucking effort) and initiation of appropriate interventions (Meier et. al., 1999).

For example, if the infant has a mature sucking pattern but only sucks for a few minutes, having the mother use a breast pump at one breast while the infant feeds at the other breast will maintain the milk flow, which may encourage the infant to continue feeding. The mother can also use a supplemental feeder (bottle with breast milk hung from the mother's neck with small flexible tubing taped to extend slightly beyond the nipple) to increase milk intake during the actual sucking time. Pumping the breasts for a few minutes immediately before breast-feeding allows the infant with limited sucking time to receive calorie-rich hindmilk rather than less dense foremilk (Valentine, Hurst, & Schanler, 1994). Specific suggestions have been developed for each identified root cause of consistently inadequate milk intake (La Leche League International, 1997; Riordan & Auerbach, 1999).

Transition to cue-based feeding schedules. Term breast-fed infants are frequently fed on demand. However, the necessary self-regulation of sleep and feeding behaviors is still developing in preterm infants. If the preterm infant's need for sleep overrides the ability to feed, poor weight gain or dehydration may result. Thus the NICU staff needs to individualize and carefully monitor any transition from a 3-hour feeding schedule to cue-based feedings while the infant is still in the hospital rather than at discharge (Meier et al., 1999).

Alternative feeding methods. Nipple confusion refers to the belief held by many advocates of breast-feeding that use of artificial nipples (both bottle nipples and pacifiers) interferes with the successful initiation of breast-feeding (Neifert, Lawence, & Seacat, 1995). Nipple confusion remains a hypothesis that has not been scientifically validated but is often a passionately controversial topic (Fisher & Inch, 1996; Menaham, 1997; Neifert, Lawence, & Seacat, 1995).

Alternative feeding methods (e.g., cup, syringe with tubing, feeding tube taped to caregiver's finger, eye dropper, spoon) have been suggested to avoid bottles and prevent nipple confusion (Kuehl, 1997; Lang, Lawrence, & Orme, 1994; Neifert, 1998). Although proponents claim that these methods are safe when performed by experts, controlled clinical studies have not established safety or effect on breast-feeding outcome (Meier, et. al., 1999). A major unanswered concern is whether infants experience greater physiologic distress and risk from these devices than with bottle feedings. Wide-scale use of alternative feeding methods cannot be recommended until this type of study is completed (Shaker, 1998).

Alternative feeding methods may have evolved partially in efforts to solve a problem that may sometimes be preventable. Traditionally, bottle-feeding has been established before allowing breast-feeding in the NICU. An infant accustomed to receiving a bolus of milk with every one or two sucks from a bottle learns to expect that to happen with each feeding. When this infant is finally put to breast and that expectation is not met after four, six, or ten "unproductive" sucks at the breast, a hungry infant will often get frustrated, cry, or quit trying to feed.

However, with an emphasis on early skin-to-skin holding, nonnutritive nuzzling at the breast, and breast-feeding initiated for the first oral feedings, preterm infants have an opportunity to learn how breast-feeding works first. Once these infants are able to consistently elicit a milk ejection response and complete at least a partial feeding at the breast, clinical experience suggests that they can frequently progress to taking night feedings from a bottle (when the mother is not available) and continue breast-feeding during the day while still hospitalized. Breast-feeding is undoubtedly more complex for infants who are neurologically compromised or neurobehaviorally very disorganized.

Although mothers of term infants often want to breast-feed exclusively, most mothers of preterm infants do not object to alternating bottle and breast-feeding while their infants are hospitalized. They report that the transition from gavage to all oral feedings (breast or bottle) is a major milestone and one more step toward discharge. Many of these mothers plan for the infant to have one or more bottles daily at home, so that the father can participate, to ensure adequate intake, or to allow the mother to have an evening out. Although nurses commonly choose the NUK nipple for intermittent bottles of breast-fed infants, it is usually not the best choice; the NUK nipple does not elongate like the human nipple, has a much faster flow rate, and facilitates an up-and-down chewing motion to express milk from the nipple (Nowak, Smith, & Erenberg, 1994).

Discharge planning. Structured systematic support of breast-feeding in the hospital works, but most NICU mothers report at least one major breast-feeding problem in the first month after discharge and many stop breast-feeding during this time (Kavanaugh, Mead, Meier, & Mangurten, 1995). In-hospital support services should include preparation of the mother for breast-feeding after discharge, especially addressing common maternal concerns about her milk supply, whether the infant is getting enough milk during breast-feeding, and conflicting demands on her time (e.g., infant's medical needs, family, cooking, laundry, cleaning, job).

A frequent breast-feeding error after discharge is immediately returning the electric pump. Because the trend is toward earlier discharge of younger and smaller infants who do not yet empty the breast as efficiently as a pump, the mother's milk supply often decreases, the infant has to work harder, and the milk ejection response may be less effective. The mother should continue using the pump after each breast-feeding until the infant is emptying the breasts well and gaining weight on breast-feeding alone.

Feeding vignettes

Darian. Darian was born at 36 weeks' gestation with initial respiratory depression from maternal medications and a right cleft lip that extended through the alveolar (gum) ridge but not into the palate. He was admitted to a level II nursery and was under an oxygen hood for 48 hours and in an incubator for 8 days. Oral feedings were begun on the third day of life with good results; all feedings were taken by mouth with a regular nipple that was placed to occlude the cleft in his lip.

The occupational therapist was contacted on the tenth day of life because of an acute decline in oral feeding. He had taken less than 30 ml in the last several oral feedings, and gavage feedings had been started. Darian was lethargic and difficult to arouse, which nurses reported as a change. Darian showed no signs of illness other than lethargy and poor feeding, but a complete blood count had been done that morning with normal results and a sepsis work-up was being considered.

A trial feeding by an occupational therapist showed normal suck-swallow-breathing coordination but extremely low arousal with no active feeding effort after the first 2 minutes. His nurse related that Darian had been awake and active for about 20 minutes, 1½ hours before this scheduled feeding. Review of medical records showed two caregiving changes just before the decline in feeding performance; Darian's feeding schedule had been changed from every 3 hours to every 4 hours, and he had been weaned from his isolette to an open crib.

Collaboration with the nurse and physician produced a consensus that even though Darian was "old enough and big enough," he was possibly not ready for all the changes and "demands." The nurse and physician decided to place him back in the isolette and let him rest. Oral feedings were offered whenever Darian was awake and appeared ready to eat (cue-based feeding), with gavage feeding supplements as needed for 24 to 48 hours. Oral feedings were then advanced according to his performance. Darian was back on all oral feedings within 4 days and weaned from the incubator 2 days later. In the interim, his mother had made care arrangements for her other children and was able to stay at the nearby Ronald McDonald house. She expressed a desire to breast-feed Darian, and this transition was successfully made before his discharge on the seventeenth day of life. Darian's feeding problem was real but was related to autonomic and state factors rather than feeding mechanics; oral stimulation and specialized feeding techniques would not have been the most helpful approach.

Emile. Emile was born at 29 weeks' gestation with a birth weight of 1030 grams (2 pounds, 4 ounces). Medical complications included a patent ductus arteriosus, respiratory distress syndrome (RDS) that progressed to bronchopulmonary dysplasia (BPD), severe apnea, a bilateral grade I IVH, suspected sepsis, retinopathy of prematurity (ROP), and feeding intolerance. As she approached term equivalency, her occupational therapist was also concerned about Emile's fluctuating muscle tone, persistent tremors, irritability, and low responsiveness to auditory and visual stimuli even when held and calm.

At 39 weeks' postconceptional age, oral feedings were attempted once a day. Emile demonstrated intermittent and inefficient sucking effort; maximal caregiver support and facilitation were required to complete the feedings. A deep midline ridge in her palate was diagnosed as a submucous cleft but was not believed to be the cause of her feeding difficulty. As frequency and volume of oral feedings were slowly advanced, Emile began to desaturate during feedings.

A modified barium swallow was requested. Emile's disorganized suck expressed only small amounts of liquid from a regular nipple, so a Haberman feeder was used to complete the study. Emile demonstrated the following:
1. Oral disorganization, as observed clinically
2. Incomplete elevation of the soft palate with occasional regurgitation of barium into the nasopharynx, possibly related to the submucous cleft
3. A prompt swallow reflex with complete clearance of barium from the pharynx, even when "challenged" with large or continuous boluses squeezed from the Haberman feeder
4. One or two incidences of threatened airway penetration (a trace amount of barium entered the opening of the larynx but cleared immediately during a subsequent swallow)
5. A significant fatigue factor with increasing need for longer rest periods to allow for extra breathing and recovery of energy
6. No significant gastroesophageal reflux

Feeding recommendations included the following:
1. Continuation of oral feedings with gavage supplements as needed
2. Decreasing work of feeding by use of the Haberman feeder
3. Allowing feedings to continue 20 to 30 minutes if rest periods were needed
4. Trial of supplemental oxygen during feedings if desaturation persisted
5. Consideration of formula additives to increase calories with less volume (deferred initially because of recent feeding intolerance).

Emile's improvement was slow, but feeding became functional and weight gain occurred.

Emile's teenage married mother visited frequently and was loving toward her daughter but had difficulty with caregiving. She appeared mentally slow to the staff members, required repetitive explanations and demonstrations of all aspects of care, and needed structure and encouragement to care for Emile. At 1 month corrected age, Emile was transferred to an extended care unit where her mother could be eased into full responsibility for the infant's care under supervision.

Because concerns still existed at discharge, plans were made for the husband to drop Emile and her mother off at the grandmother's house on his way to work each morning for continued assistance and support. A check 1 week after hospital discharge showed excellent weight gain. Feeding and developmental progress were monitored at follow-up clinics, and the submucous cleft was managed by the cleft palate team, which included a speech pathologist.

Destiny. Destiny was Triplet C born SGA (420 grams) at 25 weeks' gestation. Her most significant medical complications included patent ductus arteriosus, pulmonary insufficiency, RDS, severe BPD, hypertension, bilateral IVH (right = grade 2, left = grade 3), posthemorrhagic hydrocephalus with a ventriculoperitoneal shunt, moderate ROP, and a humeral fracture secondary to bone demineralization from her body's inability to use nutrients efficiently.

Destiny remained oxygen dependent and consistently demonstrated poor growth. Her muscle tone was mildly increased but appeared related to frequent irritability. Oral feeding was delayed because of Destiny's medical status until she was nearly 5 months of age (5 weeks corrected age). Noted problems during oral feeding included difficulty latching on to the nipple, weak stripping, a humped tongue with poor intraoral bolus control, difficulty propelling a bolus posteriorly to swallow, excessive leakage that totaled 20% to 25% of the feeding, and intermittent crying. Oxygen was increased during oral feedings because of desaturations during sucking bursts and rest periods.

Several factors contributed to the therapist's growing concerns about Destiny's feeding safety. Her reduced oral control of a liquid bolus increased her risk of aspiration before a reflexive swallow. Her neurologic history (pulmonary insufficiency with resultant hypoxic episodes, IVH, and hydrocephalus) put Destiny at increased risk for neuromotor dysfunction. Mild desaturations during sucking bursts are common occurrences in the NICU, but her desaturations during rest pauses were worrisome. Destiny did not adjust easily to new caregivers, responding with increased irritability when fed by an unfamiliar person. A major concern was potential aspiration during forceful inhalation from intermittent crying during oral feedings.

A modified barium swallow was requested, during which Destiny demonstrated oral incoordination, a delayed swallow reflex, and gross silent aspiration (e.g., no changes in respirations, oxygen saturations, color; no choking or coughing). A feeding gastrostomy was subsequently placed, and Destiny went home to join her sisters as a nonoral feeder. Follow-up modified swallow studies 6 and 12 months later continued to show silent aspiration. Last seen at 2½ years of age, Destiny was orally aversive and totally gastrostomy fed. She exhibited continued failure to thrive, global developmental delays, immature play and motor patterns, and a short attention span but has not been diagnosed with cerebral palsy.

Sensory Stimulation
Sensory system development

Development of fetal sensory systems occurs in a chronologic but overlapping order. The infant's sensory systems of touch, movement, taste, smell, and hearing are all operational but functionally immature at the age of viability. The tactile system is the first to develop; even the youngest NICU infant has sophisticated perioral sensation and perceives pressure, pain, and temperature. The back and legs of a preterm infant are very sensitive to touch, especially before 32 weeks' postconception when sensory modulation improves. Because the vestibular system is structurally complete but functionally immature, movement and position changes can be overstimulating and stressful. The preterm infant withdraws from bitter taste at 26 to 28 weeks' postconception and calms to sweet taste at 35 weeks' postconception; taste can be affected by the sense of smell. NICU infants respond to odors with approach or avoidance; noxious odors can prompt physiologic instability and stress. These infants can also recognize their mother by smell.

Supplemental sensory stimulation

Much of the research on supplemental stimulation with preterm infants occurred in the 1970s and 1980s and was based on the sensory deprivation theory and the subsequent desire for intervention to prevent developmental deficits. However, this research has been criticized because of the use of small samples, exclusive use of healthy preterms, wide age span of infants treated as a homogenous group, failure to take into account individual differences of infants, and methodologic discrepancies that preclude comparisons among studies. Published reports on supplemental stimulation in the NICU have decreased in the last decade (Dieter & Emory, 1997), causing definitive guidelines to remain elusive.

When considering sensory stimulation in the NICU, protecting the fragile newborn from excessive or inappropriate sensory input is a more compelling priority than direct intervention or interaction with the infant. Stimulation is not therapeutic if it does not promote state regulation and neurobehavioral organization (Dieter & Emory, 1997). In general, an infant is not ready for "extra" stimulation until autonomic stability is present; motoric and state subsystem stability should be emerging intrinsically (e.g., under the infant's control) but may be facilitated by the caregiver during the transitional "coming-out" stage (see Table 21-7). For example, providing postural security (e.g., swaddling for limb containment and trunk support) and looking quietly at the infant without facial animation may help maintain infant alertness and minimize stress related to sensory input at this stage (Figure 21-25).

Therapists must continually modify sensory stimulation in the NICU according to the infant's postconcep-

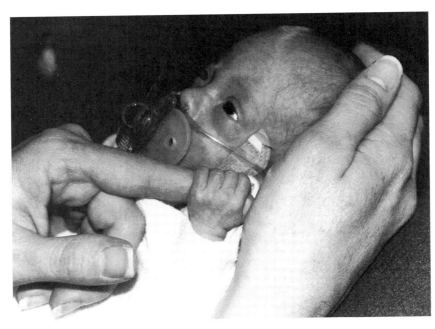

figure 21-25 The support provided by containment, sucking and grasping help this pre-term infant establish eye contact with her mother for a time of quality interaction. *(Courtesy of the NICU, Medical Center of Plano, Plano, TX. Photograph by Vicky Leland.)*

tional age, medical status, current state of readiness and responsiveness, and ongoing cues of stress or stability. In other words, the therapist provides graded sensory input when the infant is ready and seeking, not because it is "time for OT." A 32- to 35-week-old infant may respond to visual, auditory, and social stimuli, but at a physiologic cost. Early stimulation for these younger preterm infants may be safest if it replicates normal parenting activities such as being held or gently rocked, listening to the caregiver's soft voice, or looking at the caregiver's face. Thus infants tolerate stimulation best if it is unimodal (one sensory input at a time). Ideally, family members provide this contact, but the therapist can substitute if the family is absent.

Infant massage. Logically, sensory stimulation should begin with the more mature sensory systems (Dieter & Emory, 1997; Glass, 1993). Perhaps because the tactile system is the first to develop, the topic of infant massage in the NICU has generated increasing interest in recent years (Harrison, 1997; Scafidi, Field, Schanberg, 1993). Review of this literature suggests that traditional massage techniques are physiologically stressful and behaviorally disorganizing to preterm infants who are younger than 33 to 34 weeks' postconception or who are not yet medically stable (Burns et. al., 1994; White-Traut & Goldman, 1988). These younger or medically fragile infants benefit more from the firm touch and static proprioceptive input of hand swaddling ("gentle human touch" or "facilitative tuck," as demonstrated in Figure 21-26; see also Figure 21-9) than from

infant massage (Harrison et. al., 1996; Harrison & Woods, 1991).

Therapists may consider infant massage in the NICU for medically stable infants who are greater than 33 to 34 weeks' postconception or if the parent or therapist providing the massage has been appropriately trained in infant massage techniques, precautions, and warning signs. However, preterm infants with this prerequisite degree of medical stability are typically facing an eminent hospital discharge. Therapists can teach parents infant massage techniques to use with their infant at home because massage can be calming for older infants (Field, 1995). As with any type of stimulation, the therapist should closely monitor the infant's physiologic and neurobehavioral responses, with handling modified accordingly.

Auditory stimulation. Maternal heartbeat is widely assumed to be a calming familiar sound because of the infant's intrauterine exposure, but maternal heartbeat may actually not be distinct to a fetus floating in amniotic fluid. Researchers performed earlier animal studies identifying maternal heartbeat with the amniotic fluid drained to place an intrauterine sensor. This allowed the sensor to rest on the uterine wall, detecting sounds that are not as obvious when the sensor is floating in fluid (Gerhardt, 1999).

Soothing music has been recommended (Burke, Oehler, Walsh, & Gingras, 1995; Kaminski & Hall, 1996), although these samples did not include young preterm infants. When the therapist uses music with any

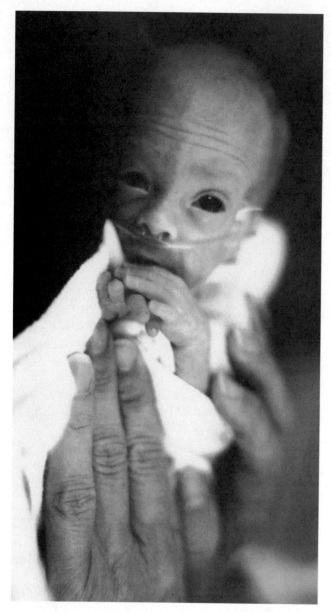

figure**21-26**   This preterm infant would be highly stressed with infant massage at this age but relaxes with the gentle pressure of hand swaddling. *(Courtesy of the NICU, Medical Center of Plano, Plano, TX. Photograph by Vicky Leland.)*

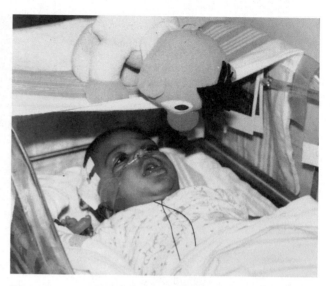

figure**21-27**   Softer, three-dimensional objects may be a more appropriate visual stimulus for preterm infants than high-contrast designs. Even though this competent infant could look at or away from "Ernie" at will, doll was removed after 2 to 3 minutes. Placement of visual stimulus that infant cannot escape is avoided. *(Courtesy of the Infant Special Care Unit, University of Texas Medical Branch, Galveston, TX. Photograph by Candy Cochran.)*

infant, he or she monitors neurobehavioral cues of stress to determine whether the effect of the music is soothing rather than distressing. Sound reverberates in an isolette and can easily be overwhelming; the volume of music for an infant in an open crib should also be soft so that neighboring infants are not disturbed. Soft human voice can be an appropriate auditory stimulus if not combined with other sensory input and if the infant is stable enough to be receptive.

Visual stimulation. Glass (1993) raises several issues regarding visual stimulation for preterm infants. An in-

fant's ability to respond to a stimulus does not necessarily mean that stimulation is beneficial. An immature infant may stare at a stimulus because of his or her inability to break away; obligatory visual attention is not a preferred behavior. Increased attention to high-contrast (black and white) stimuli does not mean that infants cannot see pastel colors. The stronger response to black and white may be obligatory rather than preferential.

The human face is the most appropriate visual stimulus in early infancy and bears no resemblance to black and white patterns. A face is three-dimensional; has some contrast at the hairline or at facial features; provides slow, contingent movement around the eyes and mouth; is situated at variable distances from the infant; changes to arouse or quiet the infant; and is not always present. It may be beneficial to incorporate some of these same features into any nonhuman visual stimuli presented to preterm infants (Figure 21-27).

Softer, simpler forms and three-dimensional objects are preferred to high-contrast designs. The therapist should avoid placement of a visual stimulus that the infant cannot escape. The infant should have opportunities for hand regard, which the therapist may provide through supportive positioning. The incubator has edges and contrasts that provide visual input. The interior of the isolette cover should be plain, and the therapist should probably place a plain blanket under a brightly colored quilt brought from home.

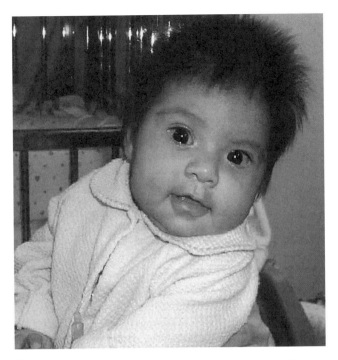

figure 21-28   This term infant remains in the NICU because of an intestinal anomaly but demands to be treated like a "real" baby! Traditional developmental stimulation is necessary and appropriate. *(Courtesy of the Infant Special Care Unit, University of Texas Medical Branch, Galveston, TX. Photograph by Jan Hunter.)*

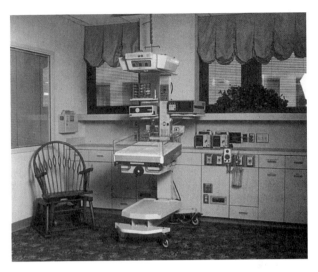

figure 21-29   Individual infant rooms provide infant protection from many environmental stressors of crowded neonatal intensive care units and facilitate development of parent-infant relationship. *(Courtesy of the Neonatal Intensive Care Unit, Baptist Medical Center of Oklahoma, Oklahoma City, OK.)*

The therapist should reserve black and white patterns for infants after term who are visually impaired, are unable to attend to a face or a toy, and have already received other forms of sensory intervention. As soon as the therapist can elicit a visual response with the high-contrast pattern, he or she should make the transition to typical infant toys.

Traditional developmental stimulation. Traditional developmental stimulation is generally not appropriate until the infant is both nearing (or past) term equivalency and sufficiently medically stable to be seeking attention and interaction (Figure 21-28). Infants vary significantly; therefore the therapist needs to be sensitive to each infant's cues.

Stable infants approaching or exceeding term postconceptional age may demand more attention with varying success; it is worrisome if prolonged crying is ignored. For auditory stimulation of these infants, the occupational therapist may provide mobiles, mirrors, or toys for visual stimulation and musical toys or tape recorders with lullabies or tapes of family members singing or reading stories. Baby swings or bouncy infant seats can provide vestibular input and a different view of the world. Even the variety of being placed in a standard infant seat may calm some infants. Portable infant carriers may be occasional options for stable infants who can be temporarily separated from their medical equipment.

Again, supporting families to be available, involved, and knowledgeable is the best way for the therapist to meet the infant's developmental and emotional needs, both in the NICU and after discharge.

■ FUTURE OF OCCUPATIONAL THERAPY IN NICU

Developmental specialists and developmentally supportive care are currently accepted standards in the NICU. Although some physicians and nurses remain reluctant or resistant to this approach, often reflecting an erroneous view of developmental intervention as "stimulation" that is not wise or proven with fragile infants (Shannon & Gorski, 1994), most NICUs are providing at least some components of developmental care. Newer NICUs are even designed and engineered to facilitate family-centered developmentally supportive care (Figure 21-29). Children's Hospital in Dayton, Ohio won a design award for their remodeled NICU; their entrance and patient bed spaces were constructed to resemble a Victorian house, helping families feel more comfortable in this "home away from home."

Ongoing changes in health care that emphasize a bottom line of cost containment and savings may be an obstacle in some NICUs. Neonatal therapists are firmly convinced that developmental care is both beneficial and cost-effective and that savings appreciated from a therapist's services are many times greater than the salary expended. Data collection and research studies that document positive outcomes are important to the long-term future of occupational therapy in the NICU.

Occupational therapists are ideal for the varied roles appropriate within the NICU because of their unique blend of psychosocial and neurophysiologic training, but occupational therapy is not the only profession that currently fulfills the role of NICU developmental specialist. As a profession of clinicians, educators, and administrators, occupational therapists must develop a more efficient system to provide training to aspiring neonatal therapists that will ensure both baseline and advanced competencies.

Case Study 1: Kevin
Medical history

Kevin was born at term to a 40-year-old married mother with two teenage children, one of whom was born with hydrocephalus 14 years earlier. Kevin was delivered by cesarean section because of an omphalocele diagnosed on prenatal ultrasound, he was SGA at 2340 grams, and his Apgar scores were $5^1/7^5$. Kevin developed respiratory distress because of severe micrognathia but was unable to be intubated because of decreased neck extension. A tracheostomy was required on his day of birth.

The following multiple congenital anomalies were noted:

1. *Omphalocele.* This was surgically repaired on his day of birth.
2. *Arthrogryposis.* Kevin has definite contractures and extreme paucity of spontaneous movement. An occupational therapist took PROM measurements at 3 days of age while Kevin remained chemically paralyzed after his tracheotomy tube placement; this allowed optimal measurements by eliminating active resistance to ranging by the infant.
   a. *Upper extremities*
      (1) Both shoulders with full extension, 90 degrees flexion, and 60 degrees external rotation
      (2) Both elbows with full extension, 90 degrees flexion, and about 20 degrees supination
      (3) Both wrists in ulnar deviation with severe flexion contractures to 90 degrees; 10 degrees (left) and 30 degrees (right) passive motion obtained
      (4) Fingers rigid in metacarpal phalangeal (MP) flexion and interphalangeal (IP) extension, which is the tenodesis position accompanying wrist flexion; fingers swollen, fusiform (muscle

atrophy make joints appear enlarged), and appeared long; both thumbs "digitalized" (high placement without true web space, appears as additional digits)
   b. *Lower extremities*
      (1) Severely deformed with legs flexed at hips (about 45 degrees) and flexed at knees (left at 90 degrees with 45 degrees passive extension, right at 110 degrees with 20 degrees passive extension, both knees fusiform) in a modified tailor position but also very adducted with the left leg overlapping the right; extremely difficult to spread the legs apart enough to insert a diaper
      (2) Greater trochanter prominent bilaterally, suggestive of teratologic hip dislocation (occurring early in fetal development and requiring surgical correction rather than treatment with a Pavlik harness) (Hunter, 1990)
      (3) Both feet rigid in talipes equinovarus, with surgical correction of his clubfeet planned at 6 to 12 months of age
3. *Cervical vertebral anomalies.* This is what limited his neck extension, requiring a tracheotomy tube for respiratory distress.
4. *Craniofacial anomalies.* These included a webbed neck, severe micrognathia, bilateral complete cleft palate, and significant ankyglossia ("tongue-tied") involving muscular connection in addition to a tight lingual frenulum. The ankyglossia was probably beneficial to Kevin after birth by preventing his tongue, already posteriorly placed because of micrognathia, from falling into his pharynx and totally obstructing his airway before the tracheotomy tube was placed.

Occupational therapy intervention

The occupational therapist was involved with Kevin from birth in multiple areas of intervention.

Tracheotomy ties. Traditional cloth ties to secure a tracheotomy tube in place frequently irritate infant skin and can be somewhat difficult to change. One solution is to make ties of Velfoam, with tapered Velcro closures, that substitute for the cotton tracheotomy ties. The therapist made Velfoam ties for Kevin in tan for the tracheotomy tube and in blue for the tracheotomy collar (small oxygen face mask held in place over the tracheotomy tube to provide humidified air, with or without supplemental oxygen). The therapist used different colors to avoid confusion and increase safety. Because the tan and blue ties were different lengths, securing the tracheotomy tube with a tie that was too long (i.e., if both sets had been the same color) may allow the tracheotomy tube to pop out. At least six Velfoam ties of each size were always at bedside; they can be hand washed, air dried, and reused.

Splinting. The therapist fabricated bilateral hand splints from 3 layers of different density foams to provide stability without pressure points. These splints encompassed the wrists and MPs, leaving the fingers free. They were well tolerated with no compromise to skin integrity. Because each took the therapist only 5 to 10 seconds to put on and just a few seconds to remove, they were worn 3 hours on and 3 hours off, around the clock. The splinting goal in NICU was to provide sustained stretch toward more normal alignment; wrist extension/radial deviation and MP extension increased to almost neutral. The therapist obtained a mild increase in IP flexion with PROM, but spontaneous finger movement was minimal. By the time of Kevin's transfer to a step-down unit, these splints maintained wrist and MP correction but no longer provided additional stretch. His therapists in the new unit would continue efforts toward further correction.

Therapeutic positioning and passive range of motion. Therapeutic positioning and PROM were major components of occupational therapy intervention with Kevin because vigorous early therapy can often achieve improvement in functional range with arthrogryposis (Hunter, 1990). The therapist wedged a thick "bolster" of rolled blankets between Kevin's legs in the supine and sidelying positions to facilitate hip abduction and hip/knee extension and to prevent skin breakdown where his legs had been folded upon each other. The therapist provided boundaries to allow proprioceptive contact for comfort with Kevin's legs as extended as possible. The therapist initiated prone positioning on a gel mattress (initially with hips dangling over the edge of the mattress because of hip flexion contractures) a few weeks after birth for variety and to use the combination of body weight and gravity to further stretch out Kevin's legs.

The therapist combined PROM with sustained stretch two to three times per day; the nurse partially did so at each diaper change. Initially the therapist coordinated these sessions with scheduled or prn (as needed) sedation and then graded them according to Kevin's tolerance. The therapist also used soft relaxation music, rest breaks, NNS, and social contact (e.g., touch, talking, eye contact) to soothe Kevin during PROM as needed. The therapist taught his family PROM techniques, but they were reluctant to assume this part of his care in the NICU. The combined effects of gravity, caregiving, some spontaneous movement, therapeutic positioning, and PROM resulted in significant increases in hip range (extension and abduction) and knee extension (Figure 21-30). The therapist noticed improvements with Kevin's hands in the splinting section. Although PROM resulted in a mild increase in finger flexion, spontaneous movement remained limited.

Development. Monitoring Kevin's neurobehavioral status with appropriate environmental and caregiving modifications and developmental stimulation as indicated were also ongoing priorities of the therapist. Although immaturity was of lesser concern because Kevin was a term infant, the NICU is still an overwhelming environment. Kevin initially required protection from avoidable stress because of environmental light, noise, and caregiving practices. He was easily stressed during caregiving but calmed to his pacifier, containment, holding, and eventually both gavage and oral feeding.

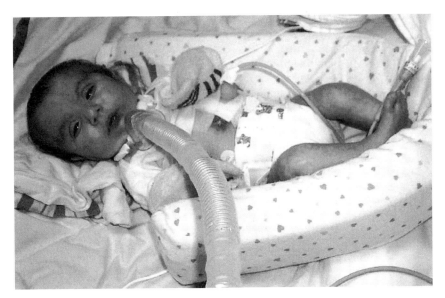

figure**21-30** Term SGA infant born with multiple anomalies, who required a combined approach of rehabilitation and developmental support, is now ready to go home. *(Courtesy of the Infant Special Care Unit, University of Texas Medical Branch, Galveston, TX.)*

Kevin's facial expression lacked variety and typically appeared "worried." He was able to visually focus, but visual tracking was limited; this was possibly due to his limited neck mobility, although the ophthalmologist also noted decreased ocular mobility during an eye examination. Kevin passed his hearing screening and calmed to gentle voices and soothing music. He enjoyed being held and recognized his family and familiar caregivers.

Feeding

The therapist began evaluation for oral feeding potential at 2 weeks of age. The nurse first thoroughly suctioned Kevin via his tracheotomy tube because excessive secretions with resultant respiratory distress and agitation were problematic. The therapist added a drop of blue food dye to his formula. Blue froth bubbling from the tracheotomy tube or blue-tinged secretions suctioned from his tracheotomy tube after nippling would be a clear indication of aspiration below the level of his vocal cords.

Kevin demonstrated normal rooting, latched on to the nipple, and had weak but rhythmic sucking bursts of 6 to 8 sucks with intermittent rest pauses. Kevin encountered the following problems:

- *Medical status.* Kevin had good days and bad days regarding physiologic stability, which invariably affected feeding.
- *Positioning.* Kevin could only orally feed when held in an upright sitting position; he became agitated and disorganized if anyone tried to feed him semi-reclined.
- *Stripping formula from the nipple.* This was due to compromised suction and compression from the cleft palate; the therapist used a Haberman feeder to compensate.
- *Ankyloglossia.* Tongue mobility (elevation, protrusion, retraction) was significantly limited, resulting in oral poor bolus control and excessive leakage during oral feeding. A plastic surgeon and the cleft palate team assessed him, but they did not consider him a candidate for surgical release during this time.
- *Endurance.* Kevin required increased oxygen during oral feeding but still consistently tired quickly.

Once he was suctioned, Kevin actually calmed to oral feeding if fed by a familiar caregiver. Kevin was fed to tolerance because of his limited and variable endurance, typically taking 30 to 35 ml in 10 minutes for the therapist and 10 ml in 10 minutes for his mother. Kevin showed good feeding potential but was unable to consume an adequate volume for nutritional needs in the NICU. A feeding gastrostomy was placed with the recommendation that it be used exclusively for night feedings (to allow the family maximal rest) and that daytime feedings include oral intake to tolerance with the remainder by gastrostomy. Once Kevin recovered from surgery for the gastrostomy placement, he was transferred from the NICU to a step-down unit to allow active family participation in preparation for discharge.

Parent support and education

Family education and support was ongoing and challenging. The family was accepting and involved but overwhelmed by Kevin's functional problems and medical needs. Because the father worked 6 days a week and Kevin's older siblings were initially still in school, the family came to the hospital most often during evenings and weekends. Once school was out for the summer, Kevin's mother and sister also came almost daily.

The family was more comfortable in observing care than participating; progress in involving the family in Kevin's routine daily care was slow and became a priority before incorporating them into his therapy needs. Kevin's mother was emotionally fragile and easily overwhelmed; she required much patient reinforcement and graded teaching over days and weeks. Kevin's sister was very attentive, willing to help care for "her baby," and perhaps the most successful in facilitating social responsiveness in Kevin.

Because Kevin's care was complex and the family was hesitant to assume full responsibility, he was transferred to a step-down unit for 5 weeks before eventual hospital discharge (see Figure 21-30). Full-time home nursing care was arranged for the first week at home to further ease the transition and to provide medical support and back-up to the family.

Referral to early intervention

Kevin's therapists completed his referral to early intervention in the step-down unit before his hospital discharge. He will also be followed by a chronic care clinic at the hospital that specializes in coordinating medical and developmental services for medically complex children who require treatment by multiple specialists. A muscle biopsy will be done at some point to assess muscle composition and assist with formulation of a realistic functional prognosis.

Case Study 2: Elizabeth
Medical history

Elizabeth was born at 27 weeks' gestation to a 27-year-old married, now G_2P_2, mother. Elizabeth demonstrated intrauterine growth retardation (IUGR), possibly caused by severe maternal pregnancy-induced hypertension (PIH) and oligohydramnios. Her birth weight was 500 grams, and her Apgar scores were $8^1/9^5$. She was orally intubated and transferred to the NICU.

Elizabeth's hospital course was complicated. Her extreme prematurity and fetal compression from maternal oligohydramnios resulted in pulmonary hypoplasia; she developed respiratory distress syndrome (RDS), which progressed to bronchopulmonary dysplasia (BPD). Hyperbilirubinemia required the initiation of phototherapy the day after birth and eventually a double-volume exchange blood transfusion. Thrombocytopenia, hypocalcemia, and electrolyte imbalances were medically managed. A right atrial mass thought to be a thrombus was discovered by an echocardiograph 6 weeks after birth but resolved spontaneously during the next several weeks. Elizabeth received several transfusions for anemia and multiple rounds of antibiotics for suspected sepsis during her hospitalization. She developed stage 3 zone I retinopathy of prematurity (ROP), undergoing successful laser surgery of both eyes to prevent retinal detachment.

Elizabeth developed abdominal distention and demonstrated feeding intolerance to enteral feedings, but her clinical picture and radiographs were not consistent with necrotizing enterocolitis (NEC). She required long-term total parenteral nutrition (TPN), which contributed to progressive cholestatic jaundice and subsequent ascites and hepatosplenomegaly. The ascites resolved, but feeding intolerance persisted. The impression from a barium enema 5 months after birth was partial obstruction caused by scarring or global dysfunction compatible with prematurity. Advancement of enteral feedings by continuous drip progressed at a conservative rate. Concerns existed about possible bone demineralization because of compromised nutritional status from severe and prolonged illness.

Elizabeth remained ventilator dependent because of severe BPD and bilateral atelectasis, which was possibly caused in part by internal compression from continued abdominal distention. Weaning from the ventilator was finally successful 6½ months after birth, with rapid subsequent medical progress and discharge to home 7 weeks later with an apnea monitor and oxygen by nasal cannula (NC). Elizabeth's chronologic age was 8 months (corrected age 5 months) at the time of discharge.

Occupational therapy intervention

First 6½ months: orally intubated and ventilator dependent. Elizabeth's medical status and neurobehavioral needs directed occupational therapy services throughout her hospitalization. Her extreme prematurity and immature CNS severely compromised her ability to cope with the extrauterine environment of the NICU. This situation was complicated by prolonged critical illness that necessitated intensive nursing care and aggressive respiratory treatments.

Neonatal Individualized Developmental Care and Assessment Program (NIDCAP) observations by the occupational therapist during Elizabeth's early life documented frequent physiologic and motoric stress signals in response to both direct caregiving and indirect environmental stimuli (e.g., monitor alarms, telephones). Her care plan emphasized protection, including efforts at modifying caregiving practices and her immediate environment. Nurses provided care with attention to Elizabeth's decreased tolerance to any stimulation and the need to protect her sleep; this balance was sometimes elusive as medical priorities emerged.

The therapist shielded Elizabeth from continuous bright light and made attempts to reduce nearby noise. The therapist transferred her to an incubator but soon returned her to a radiant warmer because of suspected sepsis. The therapist eventually moved Elizabeth to a small glass-enclosed room that allowed significantly greater flexibility in protecting her from excessive traffic and environmental stresses; she remained in "Elizabeth's room" for several months.

Therapeutic positioning was provided to reduce stress from postural insecurity, minimize positional deformities, facilitate development of extremity flexor tone, and encourage midline orientation. Elizabeth's therapist often placed her in the prone position during her first few months of life, but she developed an increasing tendency to self-extubate in this position as her energy and ability to move gradually improved. Sidelying, supine, and reclining in a bouncy infant seat were her primary positions for the next several months. Elizabeth was typically swaddled in blankets within a Snuggle-Up to conserve heat and facilitate growth, prevent self-extubation without use of arm restraints, facilitate flexion, and to provide a calming effect. Spontaneous movement was consequently restricted during this period, prompting the therapist and other caregivers to unwrap Elizabeth for supervised "exercise" periods of free movement. As her corrected age approached 3 to 4 months, the therapist added fine motor activities to Elizabeth's free play time to encourage reach, grasp, hand-to-hand, and supervised hand-to-mouth activities.

Elizabeth's state regulation, initially marked by diffuse sleep or frequent irritability when disturbed, gradually improved. As her awake periods increased, Elizabeth became responsive to auditory and visual stimuli. She appeared to recognize favorite caregivers and calmed to a human voice or soft music. The therapist changed her toys frequently to provide novelty of visual and auditory stimuli. The therapist used the bouncy infant seat more frequently to give Elizabeth a different view of her world; the therapist taped ventilator tubing to the chair for security.

Elizabeth demonstrated very low tolerance and significant stress to any tactile input, including social touch. Probable causes included months of necessary medical procedures and constant swaddling that provided proprioceptive input but minimal tactile variety. The therapist approached this problem slowly, first giving gentle pressure or patting through the swaddling and having Elizabeth hold onto an adult's finger. When Elizabeth was unswaddled for "exercise time," the therapist initially contained the extremities to prevent a startle response and then slowly removed this support. The therapist, nurses, and parents provided holding when possible.

Elizabeth became more tolerant of touch, but did not accept a pacifier readily. She exhibited tongue thrusting with no sustained or rhythmic nonnutritive sucks (NNS). Prefeeding oral stimulation and pacifier sucking were complicated by prolonged oral intubation for mechanical ventilation, an indwelling orogastric feeding tube for drip feedings, and the tape securing these tubes. The therapist anticipated that eventual transition to oral feedings would be slow.

Elizabeth's family was "attached" to her but unable to come to the hospital as often as they wanted because of transportation difficulties. Phone calls between parents and staff members were frequent, and pictures of Elizabeth were taken regularly.

From 6½ months to hospital discharge: off the ventilator. After being extubated and removed from the ventilator, Elizabeth received supplemental oxygen by an oxyhood for 4 days and then by NC. She was still on continuous drip feedings of Pregestamil with additives to increase caloric density of the formula.

Elizabeth's developmental progress and paucity of anticipated problems during this stage were impressive. She tolerated handling without difficulty. She was provided with loose boundaries but seemed to enjoy the new freedom to move. Although the therapist had been concerned about the potential effect of prolonged swaddling, the "imposed" flexion had prevented typical premie deformities and now seemed to facilitate motor skill development. Elizabeth had normal tone with good midline orientation. In the supine position she demonstrated upper-extremity antigravity flexion in midline, hand-to-hand play, mouthing of hands, and visual observation of hand movements. Leg lifting into the air developed within a month; she also had no head lag in the pull-to-sit transition at this time. Initially Elizabeth would tolerate the prone position only while sleeping, but by time of discharge 7 weeks after extubation she was propping on forearms, lifting her head consistently to 45 degrees (90 degrees with visual stimuli), and rolling purposely from the prone to supine position with appropriate quality and components of movement.

Surprisingly, Elizabeth had minimal aversive behaviors to oral stimulation. She mouthed her hands frequently, willingly mouthed toys when assisted with taking toy-in-hand to mouth, and accepted oral stimulation with a round NUK toothbrush that was used to decrease excessive tongue protrusion and increase tongue shaping (midline grooving). This strong tongue protrusion was typical

of a habitual pattern often developed by infants with prolonged oral intubation as they lick and push against the endotracheal tube. This is different from the neurologically based tongue thrust seen in cerebral palsy. Her NNS on a pacifier remained poor because of tongue protrusion.

Oral feeding, begun less than 2 weeks after extubation, was initially difficult because of her thick protruding tongue. Within a week of beginning oral feeds, the therapist was able to intermittently inhibit tongue protrusion and elicit sucking bursts of 10 to 12 sucks with good rhythm and efficient stripping. Because these sucking bursts were not consecutive, feeding time was long (40 ml in 20 minutes). Within 2 to 3 weeks, Elizabeth began her oral feeds eagerly but would abruptly stop and fight nipple insertion. The neonatologist agreed to a trial switch from Pregestamil to stock formula (initially diluted until tolerance was established); that feed was completed in 5 minutes. Elizabeth's feeding resistance vanished, suggesting taste as a factor. She continued to feed with good coordination, taking 90 ml in 20 minutes when discharged.

Although many infants with BPD tend to be irritable, Elizabeth had a delightful personality (Figure 21-31). She loved to be held or just talked to and would generally only fuss if left to entertain herself for longer than 20 to 30 minutes. The therapist frequently carried her around to visit staff members in other nursery areas and even took her outside to see a Christmas tree. The therapist initially had to elicit smiles, but they then became spontaneous and frequent, especially for her family and favorite staff members. Vocalizations remained soft and infrequent. The therapist initially anticipated transfer to a step-down unit before hospital discharge, but Elizabeth

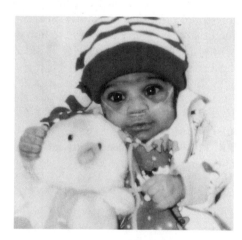

figure **21-31** Elizabeth, weighing 500 g (1 pound 1½ ounces) at birth, is finally ready to go home after 8 months in neonatal intensive care unit. Development was nearly appropriate for corrected age at time of discharge. (*Courtesy of the Infant Special Care Unit, University of Texas Medical Branch, Galveston, TX. Photograph by Jackie Lohner.*)

progressed so rapidly that the therapist decided to keep her in the NICU. After nearly 8 months, the therapist did not consider a transfer for 2 to 3 weeks to be in everyone's best interests. The entire family of mother, father, and brother came to the hospital more often as discharge approached and assumed Elizabeth's care. The staff members assembled a pictorial "biographic poster" that went home with Elizabeth. Because of Elizabeth's increased risk for developmental delay secondary to prematurity and severity of illness, the therapist referred her she to a local Early Intervention Program for developmental follow-up after discharge.

At 6 years of age, Elizabeth continues to be charming and social. She wears thick glasses for nearsightedness; demonstrates a speech delay and mild learning disabilities, and is occasionally somewhat clumsy.

STUDY QUESTIONS

1. Using the description of Cody (see description under "Developing a Medical Foundation" and Appendixes 21-A and 21-B), define the medical terms for each of the abbreviations. Explain the implications of each medical condition that represents a potential threat to Cody's development.

2. Explain how environmental light and sound levels pose a threat to the vulnerable newborn. Describe several intervention strategies that modify light and auditory input for an individual infant.

3. What issues complicate parenting in the NICU?

4. Describe published assessments and informal methods for evaluating each of the following aspects of infant function and behavior.
   a. Neurobehavioral organization
   b. Neuromotor development

5. For each general positioning goal listed below, describe how to meet the goal using a prone, supine, or sidelying position.
   a. To provide proprioceptive input to increase the infant's sense of containment
   b. To reduce premie positional deformities, increase postural flexion, and facilitate midline orientation
   c. To promote calming and behavioral organization
   d. To assist in development of hand-to-mouth movements

6. What are common feeding problems for preterm infants in the NICU? Describe appropriate interventions to help resolve these problems.

References

Als, H. (1982). Toward a synactive theory of development: Promise for the assessment and support of infant individuality. *Infant Mental Health Journal, 3,* 229-243.

Als, H. (1986). A synactive model of neonatal behavior organization: Framework for the assessment of neurobehavioral development in the premature infant and for support of infants and parents in the neonatal intensive care environment. *Physical and Occupational Therapy in Pediatrics, 6,* 3-55.

Als, H., & Gilkerson, L. (1997). The role of relationship-based developmentally supportive newborn intensive care in strengthening outcome of preterm infants. *Seminars in Perinatology, 21,* 178-189.

Als, H., Lawhon, G., Brown, E., Gibes, R., Duffy, F., McAnulty, G., & Blickman, J. (1986). Individualized behavioral and environmental care for the very low birth weight preterm infant at high risk for bronchopulmonary dysplasia: Neonatal intensive care unit and developmental outcome. *Pediatrics, 78,* 1123-1132.

Als, H., Lawhon, G., Duffy, F.H., McAnulty, G.B., Gibes-Grossman, R., & Blickman, J.G. (1994). Individualized developmental care for the very low-birth-weight preterm infant. *Journal of the American Medical Association, 272,* 853-858.

American Academy of Pediatrics, Committee on Environmental Health. (1997). Policy statement: Noise, a hazard for the fetus and newborn (RE9728). *Pediatrics, 100,* 724-727.

American Academy of Pediatrics. (1998). Policy statement: Hospital discharge of the high-risk neonate—proposed guidelines (RE9812). *Pediatrics, 102,* 411-417.

American Medical Association. (1971). *Centralized community or regionalized perinatal intensive care* (Report J). Adopted by the AMA House of Delegates, June, 1971.

American Occupational Therapy Association. (1993). Knowledge and skills for occupational therapy practice in the neonatal intensive care unit. *The American Journal of Occupational Therapy, 47,* 1100-1105.

American Occupational Therapy Association. (2000). *Knowledge and skills for occupational therapy practice in the neonatal intensive care unit* (Rev.). Bethesda, MD: AOTA, Inc.

Amiel-Tison, C., & Grenier, A. (1986). *Neurological assessment during the first year of life.* New York: Oxford University Press.

Ancona, J., Shaker, C.S., Puhek, J., & Garland, J.S. (1998). PI3: Performance improvement, ideas and innovations. Improving outcomes through a developmental approach to nipple feeding. *Journal of Nursing Care Quality, 12,* 1-4.

Anders, T.F. & Keener, M. (1985). Developmental course of nighttime sleep-wake patterns in full term and preterm infants during the first year of life. *Sleep, 8,* 173.

Anderson, G.C. (1996). Kangaroo care of the premature infant. In E. Goldson (Ed.), *Nurturing the premature infant: Developmental interventions in the neonatal intensive care nursery.* New York: Oxford University Press.

Ash, S.P., & Moss, J.P. (1987). An investigation of the features of the preterm infant palate and the effect of prolonged oral intubation with and without protective appliances. *British Journal of Ophthalmology, 14,* 253-261.

Auerbach, K.G., & Walker, M. (1994). When the mother of a premature infant use a breast pump: What every NICU nurse needs to know. *Neonatal Network, 13,* 23-29.

Avery, G.B., & Glass, P. (1989). The gentle nursery: Developmental intervention in the NICU. *Journal of Perinatology, 9,* 204-205.

Baker, J.G. (1995). Commentary: Parents as partners in the NICU. *Neonatal Network, 14,* 9-10.

Beaver, P.K. (1987). Premature infants' response to touch and pain: Can nurses make a difference? *Neonatal Network, 6,* 13-17.

Bernbaum, J.C., Pereira, G.R., Watkins, J.B., & Peckman, G.J. (1983). Non-nutritive sucking during gavage feeding enhances growth and maturation in premature infants. *Pediatrics, 71,* 41-45.

Blumenthal, I., Lealman, G., & Shoesmith, D. (1989). Effect of feeding temperature and phototherapy on gastric emptying. *Archives of Disease in Childhood, 55,* 562-574.

Boere-Boonekamp, M.M., vander Linden-Kuiper, A.T., van EsP. (1997). Preferential posture in infants: Serious demands on health care. *Nederlands Tijdschr voor Geneeskd, 141,* 769-772.

Bosma, J.F. (1986). Development of feeding. *Clinical Nutrition, 5,* 210-218.

Bottos, M., & Stefani, D. (1982). Postural motor care of the premature baby. *Developmental Medicine and Child Neurology, 5,* 706-707.

Brake, S.C., & Fifer, W.P. (1988). The first nutritive sucking responses of premature newborns. *Infant Behavior and Development, 11,* 1-19.

Brown, A.K., & Glass, L. (1979). Environmental hazards in the newborn nursery. *Pediatric Annals, 8,* 689-705.

Brown, L.P., Meier, P., Spatz, D.L., Zukowsky, K., & Spitzer, A. (1996). Use of human milk for low birthweight infants. (29 paragraphs). *Online Journal of Knowledge Synthesis for Nursing* (online serial). Available: Volume 3, Document 3, Online number 27.

Budreau, G.K. (1987). Postnatal cranial molding and infant attractiveness: Implications for nursing. *Neonatal Network, 5,* 13-19.

Budreau, G.K. (1989). The perceived attractiveness of preterm infants with cranial molding. *Journal of Obstetric, Gynecologic, and Neonatal Nursing, 18,* 38-44.

Buehler, D., Als, H., Duffy, F., McAnulty, G., & Liederman, J. (1995). Effectiveness of individualized developmental care for low-risk preterm infants: Behavioral and electrophysiologic evidence. *Pediatrics, 96,* 923-932.

Bullough, J., & Rea, M. (1996). Lighting for neonatal intensive care units: Some critical information for design. *Lighting Research Technology, 28,* 189-198.

Bu'Lock, F., Woolridge, M.W., & Baum, J.D. (1990). Development of coordination of sucking, swallowing and breathing: Ultrasound study of term and preterm infants. *Developmental Medicine and Child Neurology, 32,* 669-678.

Burke, M., Oehler, J., Walsh, J., & Gingras, J. (1995). Music therapy following suctioning: Four case studies. *Neonatal Network, 14,* 41-49.

Burns, K., Cunningham, N., White-Traut, R., Silvestri, J., & Nelson, M.N. (1994). Infant stimulation: Modification of an intervention based on physiologic and behavioral cues. *Journal of Obstetric, Gynecologic, and Neonatal Nursing, 23,* 581-589.

Cagan, J. (1995). Feeding readiness behavior in preterm infants (abstract). *Neonatal Network, 14,* 82.

Carillo, P.J. (1985). Palatal groove formation and oral endotracheal intubation. *American Journal of Diseases in Children, 139,* 859-860.

Cartlidge, P.H.T., & Rutter, N. (1988). Reduction of head flattening in preterm infants. *Archives of Disease in Childhood, 63,* 755-757.

Case-Smith, J. (1988). An efficacy study of occupational therapy with high-risk neonates. *The American Journal of Occupational Therapy, 42,* 499-506.

Chadduck, W.M., Kast, J., & Donahue, D.J. (1997). The enigma of lamboid positional molding. *Pediatric Neurosurgery, 26,* 304-311.

Clopton, N.C. (1993). Musculoskeletal and growth measures. In I.J. Wilhelm (Ed.), *Physical therapy assessment in early infancy.* (pp. 105-132). New York: Churchill Livingstone.

Comrie, J.D., & Helm, J.M. (1997). Common feeding problems in the intensive care nursery: Maturation, organization, evaluation and management strategies. *Seminars in Speech and Language, 18,* 239-261.

Costello, A., Bracht, M., Van Camp, K., & Carman, L. (1996). Parent information binder: Individualizing education for parents of preterm infants. *Neonatal Network, 15,* 43-46.

Daniels, H., Casaer, P., Devlieger, H., & Eggermont, E. (1986). Mechanisms of feeding efficiency in preterm infants. *Journal of Pediatric Gastroenterology and Nutrition, 5,* 593-596.

Dargassies, S.S. (1977). *Neurological development in the full-term and premature neonate,* New York: Excerpta Medica.

Davis, P.M., Robinson, R., Harris, L., & Cartlidge, P.H.T. (1993). Persistent mild hip deformation in preterm infants. *Archives of Disease in Childhood, 69,* 597-598.

DePaul, D., & Chambers, S.E. (1995). Environmental noise in the neonatal intensive care unit: Implications for nursing practice. *Journal of Perinatal and Neonatal Nursing, 8,* 71-76.

Desmond, M., Wilson, G., Alt, E., & Fisher, E. (1980). The very low birth weight infant after discharge from intensive care. *Current Problems in Pediatrics, 10,* 5-59.

Dewire, A., White, D., Kanny, E., & Glass, R. (1996). Education and training of occupational therapists for neonatal intensive care units. *The American Journal of Occupational Therapy, 50,* 486-494.

Dias, M.S., Klein, D.M., & Backstrom, J.W. (1996). Occipital plagiocephaly: Deformation or lamboid synostosis, Parts I and II. *Pediatric Neurosurgery, 24,* 61-68.

Dieter, J.N.I., & Emory, E.K. (1997). Supplemental stimulation of preterm infants: A treatment model. *Journal of Pediatric Psychology, 22,* 281-295.

Downs, J.A., Edwards, A.D., McCormick, D.C., Roth, S.C., & Stewart, A.L. (1991). Effect of intervention on development of hip posture in very preterm babies. *Archives of Disease in Childhood, 66,* 797-801.

Dreyfus-Brisac, C. (1974). Organization of sleep in preterms: Implications for caretaking. In M. Lewis & L.A. Rosenblu (Eds.), *The effect of the infant on its caregiver.* New York: John Wiley & Sons.

Einarsson-Backes, L.M., Deitz, J., Price, R., Glass, R., & Hays, R. (1994). The effect of oral support on sucking efficiency in preterm infants. *The American Journal of Occupational Therapy, 48,* 490-498.

Elliman, A.M., Bryan, E.M., Elliman, A.D., & Starte, D. (1986). Narrow heads of preterm infants: Do they matter? *Developmental Medicine and Child Neurology, 28,* 745-748.

Engebretson, J. (1997). Development of a pacifier for low-birth-weight infants nonnutritive sucking. *Journal of Obstetric, Gynecologic, and Neonatal Nursing, 26,* 660-664.

Erenberg, A., & Nowak, A.J. (1984). Palatal groove formation in neonates and infants with orotracheal tubes. *American Journal of Diseases in Children, 138,* 974-975.

Fay, M.J. (1988). The positive effects of positioning. *Neonatal Network, 8,* 23-29.

Feher, S.D.K., Berger, L.R., Johnson, J.D., & Wilde, J.B. (1989). Increasing breast milk production for premature infants with a relaxation/imagery audiotape. *Pediatrics, 83,* 57-61.

Fern, D., & Graves, C. (1996). *Infants in the NICU.* Weymouth, MA: Children's Medical Ventures.

Field, T. (1995). Massage therapy for infants and children. *Developmental and Behavioral Pediatrics, 16* (2), 105-111.

Fisher, C., & Inch, S. (1996). Nipple confusion: Who is confused (letter)? *Journal of Pediatrics, 129,* 174-175.

Fleisher, B., VandenBerg, K., Constantinou, J., Heller, C., Benitz, W., Johnson, A., Rosenthal, A., & Stevenson, D. (1995). Individualized developmental care for very-low-birth-weight premature infants. *Clinical Pediatrics, October,* 523-529.

Fowler, K., Kum-Nji, P., Wells, P.J., & Mangrem, C.L. (1997). Water beds may be useful in preventing scaphocephaly in preterm very low birth weight neonates. *Journal of Perinatology 17,* 397.

Gaebler, C.P., & Hanzlik, J.R. (1996). The effects of a prefeeding stimulation program on preterm infants. *The American Journal of Occupational Therapy, 50,* 184-192.

Gale, G., & Franck, L.S. (1998). Toward a standard of care for parents of infants in the neonatal intensive care unit. *Critical Care Nurse, 18,* 62-74.

Gale, G., & VandenBerg, K.A. (1998). Developmental care: Kangaroo care. *Neonatal Network, 17,* 69-71.

Gardner, S.L., & Lubchenco, L.O. (1998). The neonate and the environment: Impact on development. In S.L. Merenstein & G.B. Gardner (Eds.), *Handbook of neonatal intensive care* (4th ed.). (pp. 197-242). St. Louis: Mosby.

Georgieff, M., & Bernbaum, J. (1986). Abnormal shoulder girdle muscle tone in premature infants during their first 18 months of life. *Pediatrics, 77,* 664-669.

Glass, P. (1993). Development of visual function in preterm infants: Implications for early intervention. *Infants and Young Children, 6,* 11-20.

Glass, P., Avery, G.B., Subramanian, K.N.S., Keys, M.P., Sostek, A.M., & Friendly, D.S. (1985). Effect of bright light in the hospital nursery on the incidence of retinopathy of prematurity. *The New England Journal of Medicine, 313,* 401-404.

Glass, R.P. & Wolf, L.S. (1998). Feeding and oral-motor skills. In J. Case Smith (Ed.). *Pediatric occupational therapy and early intervention (2nd Ed.* pp. 127-166). Boston: Butterworth Heinemann.

Gonzales, I., Duryes, E.J., Vasquez, E., & Geraghty, N. (1995). Effect of enteral feeding temperature on feeding tolerance in preterm infants. *Neonatal Network, 14,* 39-43.

Gonzalez, L., & Dweck, H.S. (1994). Eye of the newborn: A neonatologist's perspective. In S.J. Isenberg (Ed.), *The eye in infancy.* (pp. 1-8). St. Louis: Mosby.

Gorski, P.A., Davidson, M.F., & Brazelton, T.B. (1979). Stages of behavioral organization in the high-risk neonate: Theoretical clinical considerations. *Seminars in Perinatology, 3,* 61-72.

Gorski, P.A., Hole, W.T., Leonard, C.H., & Martin, J.A. (1983). Direct computer recording of premature infants and nursery care: Distress following two interventions. *Pediatrics, 72,* 198-202.

Gottfried, A.W. (1985). Environment of newborn infants in special care units. In A.W. Gottfried & J.L. Gaiter (Eds.), *Infant stress under intensive care.* (pp. 23-54). Baltimore: University Park Press.

Gottfried, A.W., & Gaiter, J.L. (1985). *Infant stress under intensive care.* Baltimore: University Park Press.

Graven, S.N., Bowen, F., Brooten, D., Eaten, A., Graven, M., Hack, M., Hall, L., Hansen, N., Hurt, H., Kavavhuna, R., Little, G., Mahan, C., Morrow, G., Oehler, J., Poland, R., Ram, B., Sauve, R., Taylor, P., Ward, S., & Sommers, J. (1992). The high-risk environment. Part I. The role of the neonatal intensive care unit in the outcome of high-risk infants. *Journal of Perinatology, 12,* 164-172.

Gunderson, L.P., & Berns, S.P. (1995). Embryology and development of the infant born at 24-25 weeks of gestation. In L.P. Gunderson & C. Kenner (Eds.), *Care of the 24-25 week gestational age infant (small baby protocol).* (pp. 1-26). Petaluma CA: Neonatal Network.

Hack, M., Eastbrook, M.M., & Robertson, S.S. (1985). Development of sucking rhythms in preterm infants. *Early Human Development, 11,* 133-140.

Hanlon, M.B., Tripp, J.H., Ellis, R.E., Flack, F.C., Selley, W.G., & Shoesmith, H.J. (1997). Deglutition apnea as indicator of maturation of suckle feeding in bottle-fed infants. *Developmental Medicine and Child Neurology, 39,* 534-542.

Harris, M.B. (1986). Oral-motor management of the high-risk neonate. *Physical and Occupational Therapy in Pediatrics, 6,* 231-253.

Harrison, H. (1983). *The premature baby book: A parent's guide to caring and coping in the first years.* New York: St. Martin's Press.

Harrison, L. (1997). Research utilization: Handling preterm infants in the NICU. *Neonatal Network, 16* (3), 65-69.

Harrison, L., Olivet, L., Cunningham, K., Bodin, M.B., & Hicks, C. (1996). Effects of gentle human touch on preterm infants: Pilot study results. *Neonatal Network, 15* (2), 35-42.

Harrison, L.L., & Woods, S. (1991). Early parental touch and preterm infants. *Journal of Obstetric, Gynecologic, and Neonatal Nursing, 20* (4), 299-306.

Hill, P.D., Hanson, K.S., & Mefford, A.L. (1994). Mothers of low birthweight infants: Breastfeeding patterns and problems. *Journal of Human Lactation, 10,* 169-176.

Hodgman, J.E. (1985). Introduction. In A.W. Gottfried & J.L. Gaiter (Eds.), *Infant stress under intensive care.* (pp. 1-6). Baltimore: University Park Press.

Holloway, E. (1994). Parent and occupational therapist collaboration in the neonatal intensive care unit. *The American Journal of Occupational Therapy, 48,* 535-538.

Huang, C-S., Cheng, H-S., Lin, W-Y., Liou, J-W., & Chen, Y-R. (1995). Skull morphology affected by different sleep positions in infancy. *Cleft Palate–Craniofacial Journal, 32,* 413-419.

Hubler, E., Demare, D., Cabral, L., Stahl, G., Waber, B., & Imaizumi, S. (1997). Infant regulation of nipple feeding progression. *Pediatrics, 100,* 508S-509S.

Hunter, J.G. (1990). Orthopedic conditions. In C.J. Semmler & J.G. Hunter (Eds.), *Early occupational therapy intervention: Neonates to three years.* (pp. 72-123). Gaithersburg: Aspen.

Hunter, J.G. (1996). Clinical interpretation of "education and training of occupational therapists for neonatal intensive care units." *The American Journal of Occupational Therapy, 50,* 495-503.

Hunter, J., Mullen, J., & Dallas, D.V. (1994). Medical considerations and practice guidelines for the neonatal occupational therapist. *The American Journal of Occupational Therapy, 48,* 546-560.

Hurst, N.M., Valentine, C.J., Renfro, L., Burns, P., & Ferlic, L. (1997). Skin-to-skin holding in the neonatal intensive care unit influences maternal milk volume. *Journal of Perinatology, 17,* 213-217.

Jensen, D., Wallace, S., & Kelsay, P. (1994). LATCH: A breastfeeding charting system and documentation tool. *Journal of Obstetric, Gynecologic, and Neonatal Nursing, 23,* 27-32.

Jones, C.L. (1982). Environmental analysis of neonatal intensive care. *Journal of Nervous and Mental Diseases, 170,* 130-142.

Kaminski, J., & Hall, W. (1996). The effect of soothing music on neonatal behavioral states in the hospital newborn nursery. *Neonatal Network, 15,* 45-54.

Kavanaugh, K., Mead, L., Meier, P., & Mangurten, H.H. (1995). Getting enough: Mothers' concerns about breastfeeding a preterm infant after discharge. *Journal of Obstetric, Gynecologic, and Neonatal Nursing, 24,* 23-33.

Kennedy, K.A., Ipson, M.A., Birch, D.G., Tyson, J.E., Anderson, J.L., Nusinowitz, S., West, L. Spencer, R., & Birch, E.E. (1997). Light reduction and the electroretinogram of preterm infants. *Archives of Disease in Childhood, 76,* F168-F173.

Kinneer, M.D., & Beachy, P. (1994). Nipple feeding premature infants in the neonatal intensive-care unit: Factors and decisions. *Journal of Obstetric, Gynecologic, and Neonatal Nursing, 23,* 105-112.

Konishi, Y., Mikawa, H., & Suziki, J. (1986). Asymmetrical head-turning of preterm infants: Some effects on later postural and functional lateralities. *Developmental Medicine and Child Neurology, 28,* 450-457.

Korones, S.B. (1976). Disturbance and infants' rest. In T.D. Moore (Ed.), *69th Ross Conference on Pediatric Research: Iatrogenic Problems in Neonatal Intensive Care.* Columbus, OH: Ross Laboratories.

Korones, S.B. (1985). Physical structure and functional organization of neonatal intensive care units. In A.W. Gottfried & J.L. Gaiter (Eds.), *Infant stress under intensive care.* (pp. 7-22). Baltimore: University Park Press.

Kuehl, J. (1997). Cup feeding the newborn: What you should know. *Journal of Perinatal and Neonatal Nursing, 11,* 56-60.

Lacey, J.L., Henderson-Smart, D.J., & Edwards, D.A. (1990). A longitudinal study of early leg postures of preterm infants. *Developmental Medicine and Child Neurology, 32,* 151-163.

La Leche League International. (1997). *The breastfeeding answer book* (Rev. ed.). Schaumburg, IL: Author.

Lang, S., Lawrence, C.J., & Orme, R.L. (1994). Cup feeding: An alternative method of infant feeding, *Archives of Disease in Childhood, 71*, 365-369.

Lary, S., Briassoulis, G., de Vries, L., Dubowitz, L., & Dubowitz, V. (1985). Hearing threshold in preterm and term infants by auditory brainstem response. *Journal of Pediatrics, 107*, 593-599.

Lewallen-Matthews, C. (1994). Supporting suck-swallow-breathe coordination during nipple feeding. *The American Journal of Occupational Therapy, 48*, 561-562.

Long, J.G., Alistar, G.S., Phillip, A.G.S., & Lucey, J.F. (1980). Excessive handling as a cause of hypoxemia. *Pediatrics, 65*, 203-207.

Lotas, M.J. (1992). Effects of light and sound in the neonatal intensive care unit environment on the low-birth-weight infant. *NAACOG's Clinical Issues, 3*, 34-44.

Luddington-Hoe, S.M., Thompson, C., Swinth, J., Hadeed, A.J., & Anderson, G.C. (1994). Kangaroo care: Research results, and practice implications and guidelines. *Neonatal Network, 13*, 19-27.

Mann, N.P., Haddow, R., Stokes, L., Goodley, S., & Rutter, N. (1986). Effect of night and day on preterm infants in a newborn nursery: Randomized trial. *British Medical Journal, 293*, 1265-1267.

Maroney, D. (1994). Helping parents survive the emotional "roller coaster ride" in the newborn intensive care unit. *Journal of Perinatology, 14*, 131-133.

Mathew, O.P. (1988). Regulation of breathing pattern during feeding: Role of suck, swallow, and nutrients. In O.P. Mathew & G. Sant'Ambrogio (Eds.), *Respiratory function of the upper airway.* (pp. 535-560). New York: Marcel Dekker.

Mathew, O.P. (1991). Breathing patterns of preterm infants during bottle feeding: Role of milk flow. *Journal of Pediatrics, 119*, 960-965.

McCain, G. (1997). Behavioral state activity during nipple feedings for preterm infants. *Neonatal Network, 16*, 43-47.

McGrath, J.M., & Conliffe-Torres, S. (1996). Integrating family-centered developmental assessment and intervention into routine care in the neonatal intensive care unit. *Nursing Clinics of North America, 31*, 367-386.

Meadow, W., Mendez, D., Makela, J., Malin, A., Gray, C., & Lantos, J.D. (1996). Can and should level II nurseries care for newborns who require mechanical ventilation? *Clinics in Perinatology, 23*, 551-561.

Medoff-Cooper, B., Verklan, T., & Carlson, S. (1993). The development of sucking patterns and physiologic correlates in very-low-birth-weight infants. *Nursing Research, 42*, 100-105.

Meier, P. (1988). Bottle and breast feeding: Effects on transcutaneous oxygen pressure and temperature in preterm infants. *Nursing Research, 37*, 36-41.

Meier, P., & Anderson, G.C. (1987). Responses of small preterm infants to bottle and breast feeding. *American Journal of Maternal Child Nursing, 12*, 97-105.

Meier, P., Brown, L.P., & Hurst, N.M. (1999). Breastfeeding the preterm infant. In J. Riordan & K.G. Auerbach (Eds.), *Breastfeeding and human lactation* (2nd ed. pp. 440-481). Boston: Jones and Bartlett.

Monfort, K.P., & Case-Smith, J. (1997). The effects of a neonatal positioner on scapular rotation. *The American Journal of Occupational Therapy, 51*, 378-384.

Monteli, R.A., & Bumstead, D.H. (1986). Development and severity of palatal grooves in orally intubated newborns. *American Journal of Diseases in Children, 140*, 357-359.

Monterosso, L., Coenen, A., Percival, P., & Evans, S. (1995). Effect of a postural support nappy on 'flattened posture' of the lower extremities in very preterm infants. *Journal of Paediatric and Child Health, 31*, 350-354.

Mouradian, L.E., & Als, H. (1994). The influence of neonatal intensive care unit caregiving practices on motor functioning of preterm infants. *The American Journal of Occupational Therapy, 48*, 527-533.

National Association of Neonatal Nurses. (1995). *Infant and family-centered developmental care guidelines.* Petaluma, CA: Author.

Neifert, M.R. (1998). The optimization of breast-feeding in the perinatal period. *Clinics in Perinatology, 25*, 303-326.

Neifert, M.R., Lawrence, R., & Seacat, J. (1995). Nipple confusion: Toward a formal definition. *Journal of Pediatrics, 126*, S125-S129.

Newman, L.F. (1981). Social and sensory environment of low birth weight infants in a special care nursery: An anthropological investigation. *Journal of Nervous and Mental Disease, 169*, 448-455.

Nowak, A.J., Smith, W.L., & Erenberg, A. (1994). Imaging evaluation of artificial nipples during bottle feeding. *Archives of Pediatric and Adolescent Medicine, 148*, 40-42.

Palmer, M.M. (1993). Identification and management of the transitional suck pattern in premature infants. *Journal of Perinatal and Neonatal Nursing, 7*, 66-75.

Palmer, M.M., Crawley, K., & Blanco, I.A. (1993). Neonatal oral-motor assessment scale: A reliability study. *Journal of Perinatology, 13*, 28-35.

Palmer, M.M., & VandenBerg, K.A. (1998). A closer look at neonatal sucking. *Neonatal Network, 17*, 77-79.

Peabody, J.L., & Martin, G.I. (1996). From how small is too small to how much is too much: Ethical issues at the limits of neonatal viability. *Clinics in Perinatology, 23*, 473-489.

Peters, K.L. (1996). Dinosaurs in the bath. *Neonatal Network 15*, 71-73.

Peters, K.L. (1998). Bathing premature infants: Physiological and behavioral consequences. *American Journal of Critical Care, 7*, 90-100.

Pettett, G., Sewell, S., & Merenstein, G.B. (1998). Regionalization and transport in perinatal care. In G.B. Merenstein & S.L. Gardner (Eds.), *Handbook of neonatal intensive care* (4th ed. pp. 30-45). St. Louis: Mosby.

Philbin, M.K. (1996). Some implications of early auditory development for the environment of hospitalized preterm infants. *Neonatal Network, 15*, 71-73.

Pickler, R.H., & Frankel, H.B. (1995). The effect of non-nutritive sucking on preterm infants' behavioral organization and feeding performance (abstract). *Neonatal Network, 14*, 83.

Pickler, R.H., Frankel, H.B., Walsh, K.M., & Thompson, N.M. (1996). Effects of nonnutritive sucking on behavioral organization and feeding performance in preterm infants. *Nursing Research, 45*, 132-135.

Procter, A.M., Lether, D., Oliver, R.G., & Cartlidge, P.H.T. (1998). Deformation of the palate in preterm infants. *Archives of Disease in Childhood: Fetal and Neonatal Edition, 78*, F29-F32.

Rapport, M.J.K. (1992). A descriptive analysis of the role of physical and occupational therapists in the neonatal intensive care unit. *Pediatric Physical Therapy, 4*, 172-178.

Riordan, J., & Auerbach, K.G. (1999). Breastfeeding and human lactation (2nd ed.). Boston: Jones and Bartlett.

Rutter, N., Hinchcliffe, W., & Cartlidge, P.H.T. (1993). Do preterm infants always have flattened heads? *Archives of Disease in Children, 68*, 606-607.

Saunders, A.N. (1995). Incubator noise: A method to decrease decibels. *Pediatric Nursing, 21*, 265-268.

Scafidi, F.A., Field, T., & Schanberg, S.M. (1993). Factors that predict which preterm infants benefit most from massage therapy. *Developmental and Behavioral Pediatrics, 14* (3), 176-180.

Scull, S., & Deitz, J. (1989). Competencies for the physical therapist in the neonatal intensive care unit (NICU). *Pediatric Physical Therapy, 1*, 11-14.

Seguin, J.H., & Vieth, R. (1996). Thermal stability of premature infants during routine care under radiant warmers. *Archives of Disease in Childhood, Fetal & Neonatal Edition, 74*, F137-138.

Semmler, C. (1989). Positioning and deformities. In C. Semmler (Ed.). *A guide to care and managmenet of very low birth weight infanats: A team approach.* Tuscon: Therapy Skill Builders.

Shaker, C.S. (1990). Nipple feeding premature infants: A different perspective. *Neonatal Network, 8,* 345-350.

Shaker, C.S. (1998). Letter to the editors, re: "Cup feeding the newborn: What you should know" (JPNN 11, 56-60, September 1997). *Journal of Perinatal and Neonatal Nursing. 12,* vi.

Shannon, J.D., & Gorski, P.A. (1994). Health-care professionals attitudes toward the current level and need for developmental services in neonatal intensive care units. *Journal of Perinatology, 14,* 467-472.

Shellabarger, S.G., & Thompson, T.L. (1993). The critical times: meeting parental communication needs throughout the NICU experience. *Neonatal Network, 12,* 39-44.

Shiao, S-YPK. (1997). Comparison of continuous versus intermittent sucking in very-low-birth-weight infants. *Journal of Obstetric, Gynecologic, and Neonatal Nursing, 26,* 313-319.

Shiao, S-YPK., Brooker, J., & DiFiore, T. (1996). Desaturation events during oral feedings with and without a nasogastric tube in very low birth weight infants. *Heart and Lung, 25,* 236-245.

Shields-Poe, D., & Pinelli, J. (1997). Variables associated with parental stress in neonatal intensive care units. *Neonatal Network, 16,* 29-37.

Shivpuri, C.R., Martin, R.J., Carlo, W.A., & Fanaroff, A.A. (1983). Decreased ventilation in preterm infants during oral feeding. *Journal of Pediatrics, 103,* 285-289.

Short, M.A., Brooks-Brunn, J.A., Reeves, D.S., Yeager, J., & Thorpe, J.A. (1996). The effects of swaddling versus standard positioning on neuromuscular development of very low birth weight infants. *Neonatal Network, 15,* 25-31.

Siddell, E.P., & Froman, R.D. (1994). A national survey of neonatal intensive care units: Criteria used to determine readiness for oral feedings. *Journal of Obstetric, Gynecologic, and Neonatal Nursing, 23,* 783-789.

Sisson, R.C. (1990). Hazards to vision in the nursery. *The New England Journal of Medicine, 313,* 444-445.

Strauch, C., Brandt, S., & Edwards-Beckett, J. (1993). Implementation of a quiet hour: Effect on noise levels and infant sleep states. *Neonatal Network, 12,* 31-35.

Sweeney, J.K. (1993). Assessment of the special care nursery environment: Effects on the high-risk infant. In I.J. Wilhelm (Ed.), *Physical therapy assessment in early infancy.* (pp. 13-34). New York: Churchill Livingstone.

Thomas, K.A. (1989). How the NICU environment sounds to a preterm infant. *American Journal of Maternal Child Nursing, 14,* 249-251.

Valentine, C.J., Hurst, N.M., & Schanler, R.J. (1994). Hindmilk improves weight gain in low-birth-weight infants fed human milk. *Journal of Gastroenterology and Nutrition, 18,* 474-477.

VandenBerg, K.A. (1990). Nippling management of the sick neonate in the NICU: The disorganized feeder. *Neonatal Network, 9,* 9-16.

VandenBerg, K.A. (1993a). Basic competencies to begin developmental care in the intensive care nursery. *Infants and Young Children, 6,* 52-59.

VandenBerg, K.A. (1993b). *Homecoming for babies after the neonatal intensive care nursery: A guide for parents in supporting baby's early development.* Austin, TX: Pro-Ed.

VandenBerg, K.A. (1995). Behaviorally supportive care for the extremely premature infant. In L.P. Gunderson & C. Kenner (Eds.), *Care of the 24-25 week gestational age infant (small baby protocol).* (pp. 145-170). Petaluma, CA: Neonatal Network.

VandenBerg, K.A. (1999). Developmental care: What to tell parents about the developmental needs of their baby at discharge. *Neonatal Network, 18,* 57-59.

Watterberg, K., & Munsick-Bruno, G. (1986). Incidence and persistence of acquired palatal groove in preterm neonates following prolonged oral intubation. *Clinical Research, 34,* 113A.

White, R. (1996). Enhanced neonatal intensive care design: A physiological approach. *Journal of Perinatology, 16,* 381-384.

White, R. (1999). *Light: Use and control in the NICU.* Presented at The physical and developmental environment of the high-risk infant, Clearwater Beach, FL, January 27-30.

White-Traut, R.C., & Goldman, M.B. (1988). Premature infant massage: Is it safe?. *Pediatric Nursing, 14*(4), 285-289.

Wildrick, D. (1997). Intraventricular hemorrhage and long-term outcome in the premature infant. *Journal of Neuroscience Nursing, 29,* 281-289.

Wolf, L.S., & Glass, R.P. (1992). *Feeding and swallowing disorders in infancy: Assessment and management.* Tucson: Therapy Skill Builders.

Wurtman, R.J. (1975). The effects of light on the human body. *Scientific American, 233,* 68-77.

Zaichkin, J. (1996). *Newborn intensive care: What every parent needs to know.* Petaluma, CA: NICU, Inc.

Common Medical Abbreviations in the Neonatal Intensive Care Unit

A

A: apnea
Ab: abortions (includes spontaneous)
ABG: arterial blood gas
ABR: auditory brainstem response
AD: right ear
AEP: auditory evoked potential
AGA: appropriate for gestational age
A-line: arterial line
AOP: apnea of prematurity
AROM: assisted rupture of membranes
AS: left ear
A's & B's: apnea and bradycardia
ASD: atrial septal defect
AU: both ears

B

B: bilateral, or bradycardia
BAEP: brainstem auditory evoked potential
BAER: brainstem auditory evoked response
BIH: bilateral inguinal hernia
BPD: bronchopulmonary dysplasia
BPM: beats per minute (pulse)
BSER: brainstem evoked response (same as ABR, AEP, BAER, or BAEP)
BW: birth weight

C

CAN: cord around neck (nuchal cord)
CBC: complete blood count
CDH: congenitally dislocated hip
CHD: congenital heart disease
CHF: congestive heart failure
CLD: chronic lung disease
CMV: cytomegalovirus

CNGF: continuous nasogastric feeding
CNS: central nervous system
COGF: continuous orogastric feeding
CPAP: continuous positive airway pressure
CPT: chest physical therapy
C/S: cesarean section
CSF: cerebrospinal fluid
CTF: continuous tube feeding
CXR: chest x-ray

D

D_5W: 5% glucose solution
$D_{10}W$: 10% glucose solution
DIC: disseminated intravascular coagulation
DTGV: transposition of the great vessels

E

ECMO: extracorporeal membrane oxygenation
ELBW: extremely low birth weight (<1000 g)

F

FEN: fluids, electrolytes, nutrition
FHR: fetal heart rate
FiO_2: fraction inspired oxygen (percentage of oxygen concentration)
FT: full term

G

G: gravida (pregnancies)
GA: gestational age
GER: gastroesophageal reflux

H

HAL: hyperalimentation (same as TPN)
HC: head circumference

HFV: high-frequency ventilation
HFJV: high-frequency jet ventilation
HFOV: high-frequency oscillating ventilation
HIE: hypoxic-ischemic encephalopathy
HMD: hyaline membrane disease
HR: heart rate
HSV: herpes simplex virus
HTN: hypertension
HUSG: head ultrasound

I

ICH: intracranial hemorrhage
IDM (or IODM): infant of a diabetic mother
IDV: intermittent demand ventilation
IH: inguinal hernia
IMV: intermittent mandatory ventilation
I/O: intake/output
IPPB: intermittent positive pressure breathing
IRV: inspiratory reserve volume
IUGR: intrauterine growth retardation
IVDA: intravenous drug abuse
IVH: intraventricular hemorrhage

K

Kcal: kilocalories

L

L (or LC): living children
LA: left atrium
LBW: low–birth-weight infant (<2500 g)
LGA: large for gestational age
LMP: last menstrual period
L/S ratio: lecithin/sphingomyelin ratio
LTGV: physiologically corrected transposition of the great vessels
LV: left ventricle

M

MAS: meconium aspiration syndrome
MCA: multiple congenital anomalies
MDU: maternal drug use
MRSA: methicillin-resistant *Staphylococcus aureus*
MRSE: methicillin-resistant *Staphylococcus epidermidis*

N

NB: newborn
NC: nasal cannula
NCPAP: nasal continuous positive airway pressure
ND: nasoduodenal
NEC: necrotizing enterocolitis
NG: nasogastric
NGT: nasogastric tube
NICU: neonatal intensive care unit
NNS: nonnutritive sucking
NP: nasopharyngeal

NPCPAP: nasopharyngeal continuous positive airway pressure
NPO: nothing by mouth
NS: nutritive sucking
NTE: neutral thermal environment

O

O_2 sats: oxygen saturation
OD: oral-duodenal, **or** right eye
OG: oral gastric
OGT: oral gastric tube
OS: left eye
OU: both eyes

P

P: pulse, or para (births)
P_1: primipara (first birth)
$PaCO_2$: arterial partial pressure of CO_2 (concentration of CO_2 in peripheral arteries)
PaO_2: arterial partial pressure of O_2 (concentration of O_2 in peripheral arteries)
PCA: postconceptional age
PDA: patent ductus arteriosus
PEEP: positive end expiratory pressure
PFC: persistant fetal circulation (more correctly called persistant pulmonary hypertension of the newborn, PPHN)
PICC: percutaneously inserted central catheter (previously called PerQ cath, or percutaneous catheter)
PIE: pulmonary interstitial emphysema
PIH: pregnancy-induced hypertension (preeclampsia, eclampsia)
PIP: pulmonary insufficiency of the premature
PO: by mouth
PPD: packs per day (refers to smoking)
PPHN: persistant pulmonary hypertension of the newborn
PROM: premature rupture of membranes
PPROM: prolonged premature rupture of membranes
PS: pulmonic stenosis
PPS: peripheral pulmonic stenosis
PT: preterm
PTL: preterm labor
PVL: periventricular leukomalacia

Q

q: every
qh: every hour
qid: 4 times a day

R

RA: right atrium
RBC: red blood cell
RDS: respiratory distress syndrome
ROM: rupture of membranes

ROP: retinopathy of prematurity (formerly called retrolental fibroplasia, RLF)

RPR: rapid plasma reagin (can be used to test for syphillis)

RRR: rate, rhythm, respiration

RV: right ventricle

S

"sats": refers to oxygen saturation levels

SGA: small for gestational age

SIMV: synchronized intermittent mandatory ventilation

s/p: status post

SROM: spontaneous rupture of membranes

SVD: spontaneous vaginal delivery

T

TA: trucus arteriosus

TAPVR: total anomalous pulmonary venous return

TCAN: tight cord around neck

TCM: transcutaneous monitor

$TcPO_2$: transcutaneous oxygen pressure

TLC: total lung capacity

TOF: tetrology of Fallot

TORCH: congenital viral infections (toxoplasmosis, rubella, cytomegalovirus, or herpes)

TPN: total parenteral nutrition

TPR: temperature, pulse, respiration

TRDN: transient respiratory distress of the newborn

TTN: transient tachypnea of the newborn

U

UAC: umbilical artery catheter

UAL: umbilical artery line

URI: upper respiratory infection

USG: ultrasound

UTI: urinary tract infection

UVC: umbilical venous catheter

V

VDRL: Venereal Disease Research Laboratory

VEP (VER): vision evoked potential (response)

VLBW: very low birth weight (<1500 g)

VSD: ventricular septal defect

W

WBD: weeks by dates (for gestational age)

WBE: weeks by examination (for gestational age)

Medical Complications of Preterm and High-Risk Infants

21-B1 *Congenital cardiac defects*

Review of normal heart anatomy and physiology

The normal heart consists of two upper chambers (right and left atria) and two lower chambers (right and left ventricles) divided by septums into right and left sides, along with outflow arteries and inflow veins for both pulmonary and systemic (body) circulation. Blood flow progression is as follows:

1. From the body, returns through the inferior and superior vena cava to empty into the right atrium
2. Passes through the tricuspid valve to the right ventricle
3. Leaves the right ventricle through the pulmonary semilunar valve to the main pulmonary artery
4. Is oxygenated in the lungs and returns to the left atrium of the heart through four major pulmonary veins
5. Passes from the left atrium through the mitral valve to the left ventricle
6. Leaves the left ventricle through the aortic semilunar valve to the ascending aorta
7. Travels through the systemic vasculature network

Congenital heart disease

Congenital cardiovascular malformations occur in 8 per 1000 live births. Most of these defects are simple left-to-right shunts that are acyanotic and pose relatively low risk to the infant, such as a patent ductus arteriosus or ventricular septal defect. Approximately 25% of congenital heart disease is serious enough to require cardiac catheterization and other medical diagnostic procedures during the first year. Early surgical intervention is typically more common (and sometimes imperative) with cyanotic congenital heart disease.

Acyanotic congenital heart defects

Aortic stenosis

The aortic valve (or areas immediately above or below the actual valve) is stenosed, with resultant obstruction to outflow from the left ventricle to the aorta. Degree of stenosis is progressive (from fibrin deposits, fibrosis, and calcification) and tends to recur even after surgical correction.

Atrial septal defect (ASD)

Defect in the septum separating the right and left ventricles. Size and site of the lesion may vary. Spontaneous closure is rare unless defect is small; surgical sutures or patch is typical.

Atrioventricular (AV) canal: endocardial cushion defect

Refers to a spectrum of malformations that includes defects in the lower part of the interatrial septum, the upper part of the interventricular septum, and the portions of the AV (tricuspid and mitral) valves closest to the atrial and ventricular septa. AV valve regurgitation differentiates this anomaly from a simple ventricular septal defect or an ASD. Large defects require surgery.

Coarctation of the aorta

Narrowing or constriction of a portion of the aorta that causes elevated blood pressure proximal to the stricture and decreased blood flow or blood pressure distal to the obstruction. Surgical repair is indicated but may not be urgent.

Partial anomalous pulmonary venous return

One, but not all, of the pulmonary veins does not empty into the left atrium. The pulmonary veins on the right may connect directly to the superior vena cava, or the pulmonary veins on the left may communicate with

Daberkow-Carson, E., & Washington, R.L. (1998). Cardiovascular diseases and surgical interventions. In G.B. Gardner & S.L. Merenstein (Eds.), *Handbook of neonatal intensive care* (4th ed. pp. 437-499). St. Louis: Mosby.

Long, W.A. (1990). *Fetal and neonatal cardiology*, Philadelphia: W.B. Saunders.

Sapire, D.W. (1991). *Understanding and diagnosing pediatric heart disease*, Norwalk: Appleton & Lange.

box 21-B1 *Congenital cardiac defects—cont'd*

the inominate vein. This defect may occur in isolation or in conjunction with an ASD. Usually requires surgical correction if at least 2 veins are involved.

Patent ductus arteriosus (PDA)

A PDA is a short fetal blood vessel that connects the main pulmonary artery to the descending aorta. It is a normal component of fetal circulation, but failure of the PDA to close soon after birth allows direct shunting of blood between the main pulmonary artery and the aorta. This shunt will be right-to-left if the infant is in respiratory distress or left-to-right with potential congestive heart failure if no significant respiratory illness exists. PDA may close spontaneously or may require medication or surgical ligation.

Physiologically corrected transposition of the great vessels (LTGV)

Origins of the great vessels are reversed (aorta from the right ventricle, pulmonary artery from the left ventricle), but discordant atrioventricular and ventriculoarterial connections result in misalignment such that the right atrium drains into the left ventricle and the left ventricle drains into the right pulmonary artery. Thus systemic blood still returns to the lungs for oxygenation. Oxygenated blood proceeds to the left atrium through the right ventricle and out the aorta back into systemic circulation. LTGV frequently occurs in combination with more complex lesions. Need for surgical intervention is variable.

Pulmonic stenosis

Constriction of pulmonary artery or pulmonic semilunar valve can result in obstructed outflow from the right ventricle through the pulmonary arteries to the lungs. Stenosis is not progressive. Severe cases may need surgical intervention.

Ventricular septal defect (VSD)

Defect in the septum separating the right and left ventricles. A VSD may be an isolated defect or it may occur as part of complex heart disease; size and exact location of lesion can vary. Most VSDs close spontaneously; some require surgery.

Cyanotic congenital heart defects
Double inlet ventricle also called single ventricle

Either the right or left ventricle is incompletely formed and the remaining ventricle is dominant; the connection is described as double inlet when one, and at least 50% of the other, atrioventricular valve feeds into the dominant ventricle. Although rare, a single primitive ventricle with no dividing septum may occur.

Double outlet right ventricle

Both the aorta and the main pulmonary artery originate from the right ventricle; a VSD and varying degrees of cyanosis are always present. Surgical repair is necessary.

Ebstein's anomaly

Involves a malformation of the tricuspid valve in which leaflets of the valve are displaced downward and adhere to the inflow portion of the right ventricle. This incorporates a portion of the right ventricle into the right atrium; the remaining ventricular cavity may be small. Tricuspid insufficiency is present in varying degrees. May eventually require surgery.

Daberkow-Carson, E., & Washington, R.L. (1998). Cardiovascular diseases and surgical interventions. In G.B. Gardner & S.L. Merenstein (Eds.), *Handbook of neonatal intensive care* (4th ed. pp. 437-499). St. Louis: Mosby.
Long, W.A. (1990). *Fetal and neonatal cardiology,* Philadelphia: W.B. Saunders.
Sapire, D.W. (1991). *Understanding and diagnosing pediatric heart disease,* Norwalk: Appleton & Lange.

box 21-B1 *Congenital cardiac defects—cont'd*

Hypoplastic left heart

Left ventricle and ascending aorta are underdeveloped; mitral and aortic valves are atretic or stenotic. Multistaged surgery may be attempted (10% survival), but this defect is usually fatal without a heart transplant.

Interrupted aortic arch

The aortic arch is interrupted at some point between the inominate artery and the left subclavian artery; a VSD is typically present. Severe congestive heart failure, cyanosis, and respiratory distress appear early. Classic clinical findings are a strong pulse in the right upper extremity but weak or absent pulses from lower extremities and left upper extremity. The lower body becomes hypoxemic and acidotic; subsequent organ damage and death result if surgical repair is delayed.

Pulmonary atresia with intact ventricular septum

Forward flow through the usually hypoplastic right ventricle is not possible because of agenesis of the pulmonary valve. Blood returning from the body is shunted from the right to left atrium and mixed with whatever blood is returning from the lungs. Blood then passes into the left ventricle and back into systemic circulation. Surgical intervention is required.

Tetrology of Fallot (TOF)

Consists of a constellation of defects including a large VSD, right ventricular outflow obstruction (pulmonary stenosis), aorta overriding the VSD, and right ventricular hypertrophy. The degree of pulmonary stenosis typically dictates the severity and course of TOF. *Tet spells* refer to hypoxic episodes of suddenly increasing cyanosis and agitation that are usually associated with arising, eating, activity, or crying. Surgical intervention is usually required, although timing can vary significantly.

Total anomalous pulmonary venous return (TAPVR)

None of the four pulmonary veins empties into the left atrium; drainage occurs indirectly through various routes into the right atrium. An ASD must always be present to permit function of the left side of the heart. Early surgical correction is usually required.

Transposition of the great vessels (DTGV)

Origins of the aorta and main pulmonary artery are reversed from a normal presentation; the aorta arises from the right ventricle, and the pulmonary artery arises from the left ventricle. DTGV may occur in an isolated form or with complex heart disease. Early surgery is required.

Tricuspid atresia

The tricuspid valve between the right atrium and right ventricle is either absent or not patent, obstructing blood flow into the right ventricle. The right ventricle may be fully formed if a VSD is present, or it may be hypoplastic. Surgical repair is required.

Truncus arteriosus: Types I-IV

When normal separation of the aorta and main pulmonary artery do not occur during fetal development, both the right and left ventricles empty into a single large vessel. Types I and IV are common; Types II and III are not. The pulmonary arteries are connected to the aorta in Types I, II, and III. In Type IV the pulmonary arteries have no connection to the common trunk (single large vessel), and pulmonary perfusion occurs from collateral circulation. A VSD is always present. Surgical repair is required.

table 21-B2 *Common Respiratory Complications*

Diagnosis	Description	Implications for Occupational Therapists
Transient respiratory distress of the newborn (TRDN)	Also called transient tachypnea of the newborn (TTN), TRDN refers to delayed resorption of fetal lung fluid. It usually occurs with a term or near-term infant who has undergone a rapid delivery or cesarean section or who has neonatal depression. The baby breathes rapidly to clear excess fluid, and may require oxygen initially.	Infant typically is receiving oxygen $\leq$ 40% from an oxyhood. TRDN generally resolves within 24 to 48 hours and is not usually associated with lasting complications.
Respiratory distress syndrome (RDS)	Also called *hyaline membrane disease (HMD)*, RDS is an acute lung disease of primarily preterm infants in which the lungs cannot inflate or function correctly because of a lack of surfactant. Chronic intrauterine stress may facilitate lung maturation and decrease RDS severity; female and black infants may also be less affected. Atelectasis (incomplete expansion of lungs at birth) and collapse of lungs after expiration are primary problems. Typical symptoms of respiratory distress (tachypnea, nasal flaring, grunting, chest retractions, apnea, and cyanosis), poor air entry, and right-to-left shunting often worsen for 36 to 48 hours. RDS may plateau then improve, or it may progress to bronchopulmonary dysplasia.	Surfactant replacement therapy is common. Supplemental oxygen can be given with or without assisted ventilation. Physiologic instability is apparent; protection is indicated to facilitate recovery (Als, 1986).
Pulmonary insufficiency of the preterm (PIP)	Lung immaturity that results from extreme prematurity. The lungs are underdeveloped and need assistance to provide adequate oxygenation and ventilation for the infant.	Generally denotes an extremely premature infant, often < 1000 g. May be ventilated mechanically or under oxyhood. Protect from avoidable stress.
Meconium aspiration syndrome (MAS)	Meconium, the fecal matter passed by neonates in early bowel movements, may be released into the amniotic fluid before delivery under certain conditions of stress (e.g., postterm or IUGR infant, complicated delivery, fetal hypoxia, and acidosis). A baby may be "meconium-stained" without aspirating the tarlike substance into the tracheobronchial tree. Not all infants who aspirate meconium are symptomatic. MAS most accurately refers to those infants with meconium found below the vocal cords and typical changes on x-ray films. MAS complications may include pulmonary hypertension, need for mechanical ventilation, secondary bacterial infection, and pulmonary or cerebral hemorrhages.	Symptomatic MAS infants can be critically ill. Mechanical ventilation is required for symptomatic infants; large infants who "fight the vent" may be sedated or chemically paralyzed. Mortality increases if persistent pulmonary hypertension (PPHN) occurs; less severe cases may improve within a week. Progression to chronic lung disease is not uncommon. Acutely ill MAS infants need to be protected from avoidable stress.

Barnhart, S.L., & Czervinske, M.P. (1995). Perinatal and pediatric respiratory care. Philadelphia: W.B. Saunders.

Enzman Hagedorn, M.I., Gardner, S.L., & Abman, S.H. (1998). Respiratory diseases. In G.B. Gardner & S.L. Merenstein (Eds.), *Handbook of neonatal intensive care* (4th ed. pp. 437-499). St. Louis: Mosby.

Hazinski, T.A. Bronchopulmonary dysplasia. In V. Chernick, T.F. Boat, & E.L. Kendig, Jr. (Eds.), *Kendig's disorders of the respiratory tract in children,* (6th ed. pp. 364-385). Philadelphia: W.B. Saunders.

Kirkpatrick, B.V., & Mueller, D.G. (1998). In V. Chernick, T.F. Boat, & E.L. Kendig, Jr. (Eds.), *Kendig's disorders of the respiratory tract in children,* (6th ed. pp. 328-364). Philadelphia: W.B. Saunders.

Platzker, A.C.G. (1988). Chronic lung disease of infancy. In R.A. Ballard (Ed.), *Pediatric Care of the ICN Graduate.* (pp. 129-156). Philadelphia: W.B. Saunders.

table 21-B2 *Common Respiratory Complications —cont'd*

Diagnosis	Description	Implications for Occupational Therapists
Persistent pulmonary hypertension (PPHN)	Also called *persistent fetal circulation (PFC)*. When respiratory distress (from any cause) and the resultant hypoxia or acidosis leads to constriction of pulmonary vasculature, the increased resistance to pulmonary blood flow allows the ductus arteriosus to remain functionally open or to reopen. As blood is shunted away from the lungs, right-to-left shunting through the foramen ovale and ductus arteriosus continues and the fetal pattern of circulation persists.	Infant ventilation and oxygenation are severely compromised. This is a potentially life-threatening complication; these critically ill infants are typically on minimal stimulation protocols. Strict protection from avoidable environmental and caregiving stressors should be attempted.
Bronchopulmonary dysplasia (BPD) and chronic lung disease (CLD)	BPD occurs most commonly in infants under 1000 g and < 30 weeks gestation. BPD was originally referred to as the x-ray progression of lung changes in preterm infants with HMD. CLD includes BPD but also recognizes that chronic lung problems can occur from other causes (e.g., heart defects, diaphragmatic hernia, and MAS). The primary source of injury is barotrauma from positive pressure ventilation and prolonged high oxygen concentration.	Chronic pulmonary compromise, often with prolonged mechanical ventilation (intermittent mandatory ventilation [IMV] or synchronized intermittent mandatory ventilation [SIMV] or nasal continuous positive airway pressure. Oxygen supplements by nasal cannula may be required for months or years. Prone to recurrent respiratory infections and asthma.
	Classification of chronic lung disease: Stage I: Tachypnea Stage II: Airway obstruction: upper airway (i.e., tracheal stenosis) or lower airway Stage III: Pulmonary interstitial edema: free air from ruptured alveoli seeps into interstitial lung tissue; this may further compromise the pulmonary vascular supply and ventilation Stage IV: Hypoxia and hemoglobin desaturation (prolonged oxygen saturation less than 90%, as per oximetry) Stage V: Cor pulmonale (cardiac right ventricular hypertrophy resulting from CLD) and hypercapnia (carbon dioxide retention). May eventually be fatal. (Platzker, 1988).	Some CLD infants tend to be irritable and demonstrate increased muscle tone (aggravated by frequent agitation) while others tend to be low energy, lethargic, and difficult to arouse. Difficulty with oral feeds may occur, especially if the infant remains tachypneic, has excessive secretions, is lethargic and difficult to arouse, or has developed oral hypersensitivity. Infant usually needs extra calories for growth. Increased risk of long-term neurodevelopmental sequelae.

table 21-B2 *Common Respiratory Complications —cont'd*

Diagnosis	Description	Implications for Occupational Therapists
Apnea	Cessation of breathing occurs for more than 20 seconds. Etiology may be central (i.e., related to nervous system immaturity in preterm infant or CNS damage after asphyxia); obstructive (e.g., tracheal stenosis from repeated or prolonged intubation, micrognathia, and posterior tongue placement in Pierre-Robin sequence); associated with illness (e.g., RDS, infection, anemia, cold stress, and reflux), related to stress (e.g., after eye dilation and examination caused by hypermagnesemia or oversedation or idiopathic (cause unknown).	Infant may require prolonged mechanical ventilation or continuous positive airway pressure. Apnea medication is common. Severe apnea has increased risk of CNS damage from hypoxia and increased risk of necrotizing enterocolitis (NEC) from disturbed perfusion of intestine. Apnea in infants may result from CNS immaturity, be an early indicator of acute illness of seizures, occur during oral feeding or from gastroesophageal reflux, and is more common during periods of active sleep than when awake. May go home on apnea monitor.
Pneumonia	Infectious exposure to various organisms across the placenta or during the delivery; nosocomial infection (hospital-acquired infection, [i.e., transmission from inadequate hand washing]); or may occur in association with sepsis or meningitis. Clinical presentation may include signs of respiratory distress (grunting, flaring, retractions, tachypnea, or cyanosis), shock, and signs of sepsis (temperature instability, apnea, hypoglycemia, lethargy, poor feeding, or seizures).	Seriously or critically ill infant requires mechanical ventilation and intravenous antibiotics. Enteral feeds may be temporarily discontinued. Protect from avoidable stress.

Barnhart, S.L., & Czervinske, M.P. (1995). Perinatal and pediatric respiratory care. Philadelphia: W.B. Saunders.

Enzman Hagedorn, M.I., Gardner, S.L., & Abman, S.H. (1998). Respiratory diseases. In G.B. Gardner & S.L. Merenstein (Eds.), *Handbook of neonatal intensive care* (4th ed. pp. 437-499). St. Louis: Mosby.

Hazinski, T.A. (1998) Bronchopulmonary dysplasia. In V. Chernick, T.F. Boat, & E.L. Kendig, Jr. (Eds.), *Kendig's disorders of the respiratory tract in children,* (6th ed. pp. 364-385). Philadelphia: W.B. Saunders.

Kirkpatrick, B.V., & Mueller, D.G. (1998). In V. Chernick, T.F. Boat, & E.L. Kendig, Jr. (Eds.), *Kendig's disorders of the respiratory tract in children,* (6th ed. pp. 328-364). Philadelphia: W.B. Saunders.

Platzker, A.C.G. (1988). Chronic lung disease of infancy. In R.A. Ballard (Ed.), *Pediatric Care of the ICN Graduate.* (pp. 129-156). Philadelphia: W.B. Saunders.

table 21-B3 *Common Neurologic Complications*

Diagnosis	Description	Implications for Occupational Therapists
Brachial plexus injuries	Transient or permanent upper-extremity paralysis may result from damage to the brachial plexus during a difficult birth. Nerve roots and trunks of the plexus may be bruised, stretched, or torn.	Treatment in the acute stage is primarily aimed at preventing further damage to traumatized structures and preventing contractures of involved joints.
Erb's palsy	Damage to the upper trunk of the brachial plexus at the junction of nerve roots C-5 and C-6. Most common brachial plexus injury, best prognosis.	Caregivers are taught positioning and handling techniques that protect the extremity, as well as passive range of motion that emphasizes absent movements (Hunter, 1990a).
Erb-Duchenne-Klumpke's palsy	C-5 to T-1. Next most common injury to brachial plexus; generally good prognosis.	
Klumpke's palsy	C-8 to T-1. Least common; often less recovery.	
Intraventricular hemorrhage (IVH)	Infants <1500 g and <30 weeks' gestation are at highest risk. Most occur within the first week of life. Causes may be intravascular factors (i.e., fluctuating or increased cerebral blood flow, increased venous pressure or blood flow, platelet and coagulation disturbances); vascular factors (fragile capillaries and immature vascular network is vulnerable to rupture); extravascular factors (poor structural support of capillary bed; fibrinolytic activity extends bleed). Grades of IVH Grade I: Subepyndemal germinal matrix bleed Grade II: Bleeding extends into the ventricles Grade III: Ventricles are so full of blood they become dilated Grade IV: Bleeding extends beyond the cavity of the ventricle into the surrounding parynchema; hydrocephalus is typical	Symptoms may include apnea, temperature instability, poor sucking or feeding, vomiting, lethargy, irritability, pallor or mottling, hypotension or shock, bulging and tense fontanel, and seizures. Stress and improper handling may precipitate an IVH in a vulnerable infant (e.g., elevating hips with diaper change for a micropremie can elevate intracranial pressure). Infants with grade I or II IVH usually do well developmentally, and infants with grade III or IV IVH are more likely to have developmental problems, especially if there is associated periventricular white matter destruction (periventricular leukomalacia [PVL]) or posthemorrhagic hydrocephalus.
Periventricular leukomalacia (PVL)	PVL is a widely recognized ischemic brain lesion that occurs in 15% to 20% of preterm infants; it may happen in utero. PVL literally means the loss of white matter around the ventricles; it is characterized by necrosis and residual scarring of the white matter, and may be responsible for extension of an IVH into a grade IV bleed.	Areas of increased echodensity on head ultrasound that resolve over time are not true PVL. Repeat ultrasounds of PVL typically show cystic formation from white matter destruction. Developmental sequelae are seen in most (but not all) PVL infants.
Hydrocephalus Posthemorrhagic hydrocephalus	Inflammation from blood in the ventricles may impede the normal circulation and reabsorption of cerebrospinal fluid (CSF); fibrin or other debris may occlude the pathways for CSF drainage and thus lead to hydrocephalus.	May need ventriculoperitoneal shunt to allow drainage of CSF. If infant is too small or blood protein is too high for immediate surgery, baby may have frequent lumbar or ventricular taps to relieve accumulating pressure.

Ferriero, D., & Buescher, E.S. (1996). Central nervous system. In H.W. Taeusch, R.O. Christiansen, & E.S. Buescher, (Eds.), *Pediatric and neonatal tests and procedures*. Philadelphia: W.B. Saunders.

Medlock, M.D., & Hanigan, W.C. (1997). Neurologic birth trauma, *Perinatology, 24,* 845-857.

Moe, P., & Paige, P.L. Neurologic disorders. In G.B. Gardner & S.L. Merenstein (Eds.). *Handbook of neonatal intensive care* (4th ed. pp. 571-603), St. Louis: Mosby.

Volpe, J.J. (1995). *Neurology of the newborn* (3rd ed.). Philadelphia: W.B. Saunders.

table **21-B3** *Common Neurologic Complications —cont'd*

Diagnosis	Description	Implications for Occupational Therapists
Congenital obstructive hydrocephalus	Aqueductal stenosis: obstruction of the aqueduct of Sylvius before the fourth ventricle occludes CSF flow, causing lateral and third ventricles to dilate. Arnold-Chiari malformation: medulla is displaced inferiorly through the foramen magnum into the cervical spinal canal (type I), at times with the fourth ventricle (type II, the classic form of ACM associated with spina bifida) or the cerebellum (type III). Obstructive hydrocephalus results.	Infant may be irritable or lethargic. Brainstem dysfunction may occur with Arnold-Chiari malformation, especially after repair of the myelomeningocele and possibly several months after birth. May have silent aspiration with feeds; surgical decompression may relieve pressure on brainstem. Developmental sequelae common.
Hypoxic-ischemic encephalopathy (HIE)	Numerous maternal, placental, obstetric, and fetal and neonatal factors can decrease oxygen transfer to the baby. HIE is the neurologic syndrome resulting from perinatal asphyxia. Clinical manifestations and prognosis depend primarily on the severity and duration of asphyxia. The Sarnat classification is a common prognostic indicator, with higher staging and longer duration associated with poor outcome.	Infant may initially be on minimal stimulation protocol. Monitoring of early presentation and subsequent changes is recommended. Irritability, hyperactive tendon reflexes, and no seizures indicate mild asphyxia. Infants with moderate asphyxia show hypotonia, increased tendon reflexes, weak suck, and seizures with an abnormal EEG. Severely asphyxiated infants are unconscious with absent reflexes and unreactive pupils; prognosis is poor. Infant may show signs of more than one stage and may progress to another stage, indicating recovery or deterioration.

Ferriero, D., & Buescher, E.S. (1996). Central nervous system. In H.W. Taeusch, R.O. Christiansen, & E.S. Buescher, (Eds.), *Pediatric and neonatal tests and procedures.* Philadelphia: W.B. Saunders.

Medlock, M.D., & Hanigan, W.C. (1997). Neurologic birth trauma, *Perinatology, 24,* 845-857.

Moe, P., & Paige, P.L. Neurologic disorders. In G.B. Gardner & S.L. Merenstein (Eds.). *Handbook of neonatal intensive care* (4th ed. pp. 571-603), St. Louis: Mosby.

Volpe, J.J. (1995). *Neurology of the newborn* (3rd ed.). Philadelphia: W.B. Saunders.

table 21-B4 *Hemolytic and Infectious Complications*

Diagnosis	Description	Implications for Occupational Therapists
Anemia	Refers to low hemoglobin content of the blood. In the neonatal intensive care unit (NICU), anemia most commonly results from blood loss (i.e., frequent intermittent blood sampling or perinatal or postnatal hemorrhage) or from hemolysis (breakdown of red blood cells). Immune hemolytic disorders (e.g., ABO incompatability or Rh incompatability) or hereditary red blood cells disorders are among other causes.	Mild anemia is common; severe anemia can be life-threatening. Infant should not be disturbed during blood transfusions because of large-bore catheter in small fragile veins. Pallor is common; jaundice may occur with hemolytic anemia (i.e., bruising from delivery causes hemolysis and may subsequently result in hyperbilirubinemia). Increased lethargy is common; cardiorespiratory distress is possible.
Disseminated intravascular coagulation (DIC)	DIC is an acquired pathologic process that occurs when various underlying disorders or disease processes trigger intravascular clot formation. This clot formation consumes platelets and plasma clotting factors; additional biochemical mechanisms contribute to platelet and red blood cells destruction. DIC usually results in generalized bleeding from puncture sites, the gastrointestinal tract, the central nervous system, and skin. Anticoagulant measures to prevent major vessel thrombus or skin necrosis from thrombi can complicate medical management.	An infant with DIC is seriously or critically ill. Bruising or petechiae (tiny hemorrhages within the skin or subcutaneous layers that appear as small flat red or purple spots) are warning signs; oozing from puncture sites or hemorrhage is a definite red flag. The infant is typically on a minimal stimulation protocol to protect from avoidable stress.
Hyperbilirubinemia	Physiologic jaundice resulting from an excess of the bile pigment bilirubin in the blood. Immaturity of the liver and destruction of fetal red blood cells are common causes. Jaundice may resolve spontaneously if mild, require phototherapy if moderate, or need phototherapy and exchange blood transfusions if severe. Phototherapy converts bilirubin into a form that can be excreted; in severe cases exchange blood transfusions may be indicated to reduce blood levels of bilirubin or to correct severe anemia. In some infants, bilirubin levels may rebound after phototherapy is discontinued, and the infant is put back under the bili lights. Untreated severe neonatal hyperbilirubinemia may lead to a condition called kernicterus, which can produce mental retardation as well as sensory and motor disturbances.	Hyperbilirubinemia requiring phototherapy is common in the NICU. An infant under bili lights may appear lethargic or irritable. Unless a fiberoptic bili blanket is available to provide phototherapy when swaddled, the infant will be positioned for maximal skin exposure to the bili lights. Eyes are patched for protection (also need to protect neighboring infants from this light source). An oral feeder can generally be removed from the lights during feeds, but must remain under phototherapy the rest of the time.
Sepsis	Bacterial sepsis in neonates is characterized by systemic signs of infection associated with bacteria in the blood (bacteremia); multiple organisms can be responsible. NICU infants are susceptible to infection because of prematurity, immature immune systems, stress, medical complications, and surgical procedures. Bloodborne bacteria can localize and produce focal disease (i.e., osteomyelitis or bone infection); pneumonia, meningitis may also result from neonatal sepsis.	Inadequate hand washing is the primary cause of nosocomial infection (infection acquired during hospitalization). Symptoms vary according to severity of the disease but may include sudden deterioration, metabolic acidosis, temperature instability, apnea, and seizures. Protect from avoidable stress.

Frank, C.G., Cooper, S.C., Merenstein, & S.L. (1998). *Jaundice*. In G.B. Gardner & S.L. Merenstein (Eds.), *Handbook of neonatal intensive care* (4th ed. pp. 393-412). St. Louis: Mosby.

Johnson, M.M., Rodden, D.J., & Collins, S. (1998). Neonatal hematology. In G.B. Gardner & S.L. Merenstein (Eds.). *Handbook of neonatal intensive care* (4th ed. pp. 367-392). St. Louis: Mosby.

Merenstein, G.B., Adams, K., & Weisman, L.E. (1998). Infection in the neonate. In G.B. Gardner & S.L. Merenstein (Eds.). *Handbook of neonatal intensive care* (4th ed. pp. 413-436). St. Louis: Mosby.

table 21-B5 *Vision and Hearing Complications in Preterm/High-Risk Infants*

Diagnosis	Description	Implications for Occupational Therapists
Retinopathy of prematurity (ROP)	ROP designates a pathologic condition that occurs primarily (not exclusively) in preterm infants when injury to the still-developing blood vessels of the retina cause subsequent abnormal vascular formation. ROP is described based on location (Zone 1, innermost circle with the optic disc at its center; Zone 2, doughnut-shaped circle surrounding Zone 1; and Zone 3, crescent-shaped outer zone); on extent (retina is divided into clock hours to help describe extent of the disease); and by stage (indicates severity of vascular abnormality from least severe stage 1 to partial or total retinal detachment in stages 4 and 5). *PLUS* disease refers to increasingly dilated, tortuous peripheral retinal vessels. Prematurity with low birth weight, oxygen toxicity, vitamin E deficiency, high light intensity, blood transfusions, and infant medical complications that affect oxygen perfusion or vascular constriction and dilation have all been mentioned as potential factors in ROP.	At least 90% of infants with ROP have spontaneous regression, minimal scarring, little or no visual loss but a high incidence of subsequent refractive errors (astigmatism, myopia, or asymmetric refractive errors), amblyopia, and strabismus (i.e., esotropia and exotropia). Of the 10% that progress to fibrous scar tissue formation, about one fourth will be blind and the rest will have some degree of significant vision impairment. In general, the prognosis for vision worsens with the more posterior the location (i.e., Zone 1), the more clock hours involved (extent), and the higher the stage.
Hearing loss	The incidence of confirmed hearing loss in NICU graduates has been reported as 2% to 10%. Medical risk factors include birth weight less than 1500 g, congenital infection (cytomegalovirus, rubella, herpes, toxoplasmosis, and herpes), severe sepsis, bacterial meningitis, severe asphyxia, persistent pulmonary hypertension of the newborn, anatomic malformations of the head and neck, severe hyperbilirubinemia, and prolonged hospitalization. Certain medications can damage inner ear structures, causing permanent sensorineural hearing loss. Family history of childhood hearing impairment or parent consanguinity are additional risk factors for some infants.	Hearing screening is now routinely completed in most NICUs, often by a noninvasive technique that measures brainstem auditory pathway response to sound. Decreased infant responsiveness to auditory parental stimulation may affect optimal parent-infant relationship. Even an intermittent hearing loss (i.e., from fluid accumulation in the middle ear) or a mild hearing loss can adversely affect later speech and language development.

American Academy of Pediatrics, Committee on Environmental Health. (1997). Policy statement: Noise, a hazard for the fetus and newborn. *Pediatrics, 100,* 724-727.

Avery, G.B., & Glass, P. (1989). The gentle nursery: Developmental intervention in the NICU. *Journal of Perinatology, 11,* 216-226.

Hall, J.W. III, & Mueller, H.G. III. *The audiologists desk reference volume I.* San Diego: Singular Publishing Group. Phelps, D.L. (1994). Retinopathy of prematurity: Neonatologist's perspective. In S.J. Isenberg, (Ed.), *The eye in infancy.* (2nd ed. pp. 437-447). St. Louis: Mosby.

Rubel, E.W., Popper, A.N., & Fay, R.R. (Eds.). *Development of the auditory system.* New York: Springer-Verlag. Urrea, P.T., & Rosenbaum, A.L. (1994). Retinopathy of prematurity: Ophthalmologist's perspective. In S.J. Isenberg, (Ed.), *The eye in infancy,* (2nd ed. pp. 448-470). St. Louis: Mosby.

Volpe, J.J. (1995). *Neurology of the Newborn,* (3rd ed.) Philadelphia: W.B. Saunders.

table 21-B6 *Nutritional or Gastrointestinal Complications*

Diagnosis	Description	Implications for Occupational Therapist
Rickets of prematurity (osteopenia)	Preterm infants (especially those with very low birth weight) miss the period of most rapid intrauterine accumulation of calcium and phosphorus, which cannot be duplicated in parenteral nutrition because of insolubility. Some medications also increase urinary calcium losses. For these reasons, preterm infants are at risk for metabolic rickets of prematurity secondary to poor bone mineralization.	May be a cause of fractures in some infants, especially those with bronchopulmonary dysplasia. Caregivers must handle the infant gently and be alert for signs of possible fractures (e.g., bruising, swelling, and tenderness).
Necrotizing entercolitis (NEC)	NEC occurs primarily (90%) in preterm infants, and is a major cause of mortality in the NICU. The exact cause and pathogenesis of NEC is still unknown; infection, enteral feedings, and local vascular compromise (ischemia, e.g., secondary to cold stress or persistent apnea) of the gastrointestinal tract have all been implicated in the resultant mucosal injury. Bacterial invasion and formation of gas bubbles in the intestinal linings are common. Some cases respond to medical management, although sequelae may still occur. Surgery is indicated if the intestine ruptures or if portions of the intestine become gangrenous.	"NEC watch": Enteral feeds will be stopped; antibiotics and total parenteral nutrition (TPN) are started. The infant is positioned for comfort if abdominal distention is present. Comfort measures with gentle handling are appropriate. An infant with actual NEC will stop enteral feeds, have continuous gastric suction, be on TPN and antibiotics, and may be on a vent. Functional or structural obstruction may occur with or without surgery. Short bowel syndrome with failure to thrive may result, depending on amount and location of bowel surgically removed.
Gastroschisis	Results from a defect in the abdominal wall of the embryo, usually on the right side near, but not involving, the umbilicus. The intestines and possibly other abdominal organs (stomach, liver, and spleen) develop outside the body and are exposed at birth with no membranous covering. Gastroschisis often has an associated intestinal malrotation and occasionally there are atretic portions of the externalized bowel but not typically malformations of other organ systems.	Surgery is usually done on day of birth but may be "staged" if not all the organs can fit inside the abdominal cavity immediately (i.e., remainder is sterilely wrapped and suspended above supine infant in a "silo"; gravity and manual manipulation gradually reduce contents, with final surgical repair around 1 week of age). Increased risk of infection. Residual problems with gastrointestinal motility or absorption may affect feeding.

From Cox, J.M., Oliva, M.M., & Perman, J.A. (1993). Nutrition and gastrointestinal problems. In F.W. Witter & L.G. Keith (Eds.), *Textbook of prematurity*. Boston: Little, Brown.
Holland, R.M., Price, F.N., & Bensard, D.D. (1998). Neonatal surgery. In G.B. Gardner & S.L. Merenstein (Eds.), *Handbook of neonatal intensive care* (4th ed. pp. 625-646). St. Louis: Mosby.
Korones, S.B., & Bada-Elizey, H.S. (1993). *Neonatal decision making*. St. Louis: Mosby.

table **21-C** *Medical and Developmental Considerations of Positioning Options in the NICU*

Prone

MEDICAL ADVANTAGES

Improved oxygenation & ventilation (despite increased "work" of breathing) in infants with and without ventilatory support[1,6,20,28,37,39,48]

Better gastric emptying than in supine or on left side (unless feeds pool irregardless)[50]

Reduced reflux, especially if head of bed is elevated 30 degrees[7,40,43]

Decreased episodes of bradycardia and hypoxemia with head of bed elevated 15 degrees vs. prone horizontal[16,30]

Decreased risk of aspiration[25]

Term and preterm infants sleep more and cry less when prone rather than supine[9,11]

Less energy expenditure in prone vs. supine[38]

Less sleep apnea in prone vs. supine in term infants[28] and preterm infants[24,33]

Can expose diaper rash to air or heat lamp

MEDICAL DISADVANTAGES

Access for some acute medical procedures is more difficult

Agitated or active infant may self-extubate

Increased risk of SIDS (see SIDS section)

DEVELOPMENTAL ADVANTAGES

Facilitates development of flexor tone[2]

Facilitates hand-to-mouth activity for self-calming

Facilitates active neck extension and head raising

Improved coping with extrauterine environment (i.e., if sleep more, cry less)[9]

May decrease persistent head turning to right, with subsequent skull asymmetry

Can be used to reduce gently occasional hip flexion contractures (without extra handling for passive range of motion) by combined effect of body weight and gravity when legs are extended in neutral alignment

DEVELOPMENTAL DISADVANTAGES

Flattened "frogged" posture if not adequately supported[17,42]

Visual exploration more difficult for baby

Face-to-face social contact more difficult between infant and caregiver

Supine

MEDICAL ADVANTAGES

Easier access to infant for medical care

Supine (in hammock) increases sleep time for preterm infants (vs. "flat" spine)[8]

Recommended position to reduce risk of SIDS

DEVELOPMENTAL ADVANTAGES

Easier visual exploration by infant

Facilitates face-to-face social contact between infant and caregiver

Supine (in hammock) may facilitate midline position

Easier to position head in midline (than in prone)

table 21-C *Medical and Developmental Considerations of Positioning Options in the NICU—cont'd*

Supine

MEDICAL DISADVANTAGES

Decreased arterial oxygen tension, lung compliance, and tidal volume than in prone[1,37,48]

More reflux than in prone at any time, or than in upright sitting if infant is awake[40,43]

Greater risk of aspiration than in prone or right sidelying[25]

Term and preterm infants sleep less and cry more in supine than prone[9,11]

Supine in hammock may decrease respiration if infant has decreased lung compliance (i.e., respiratory distress syndrome)[8]

Greater energy expenditure in supine vs prone[38]

DEVELOPMENTAL DISADVANTAGES

Encourages extension rather than flexion (i.e., increased muscle tone with hyperextension of head, neck and shoulders)[2]

Encourages external rotation positional deformities of arms and legs (with subsequent delay in hands-to-midline and reaching activities, plus out-toeing gait)

Supine sleep position (as per SIDS recommendations) has been correlated to later developmental delays in motor skills[29,41] and potentially a flattened occiput[27,31]

Sidelying

MEDICAL ADVANTAGES

Right side: Better gastric emptying than supine or left sidelying (about same as prone)[50]

Infant with unilateral lung disease has better oxygenation with good lung positioned uppermost[10,23]

Can be used to treat pulmonary interstitial emphysema by placing affected lung in dependent (bottom) position[15,44]

MEDICAL DISADVANTAGES

Left side: Decreased gastric emptying compared to prone or right side[50]

May contribute to atelectasis of dependent (bottom) lung in micropremie

Side sleeping linked to increased risk of SIDS (see SIDS reference list in following section)

DEVELOPMENTAL ADVANTAGES

Encourages midline orientation of head and extremities

Counteracts external rotation of limbs; promotes extremity flexion and adduction

Facilitates hand-to-mouth pattern for self-calming

Facilitates hand-to-hand activity

DEVELOPMENTAL DISADVANTAGES

May be difficult to maintain flexed sidelying position with active, irritable, and/or hypertonic extended infant

Semi-Reclined/Sitting

MEDICAL ADVANTAGES

Alternative position (i.e., for variety, skin integrity)

Increased lung compliance and decreased pulmonary resistance (possibly due to increased pulmonary functional residual capacity) in semi-sitting vs. supine[12]

MEDICAL DISADVANTAGES

Infant seat or car seat elevated 60° increased frequency and duration of reflux[43]

More upright (95°) increases heart rate and mean arterial pressure in preterm infants, as compared to more reclined car seat positions of 110° and 140°[46]

Decreased oxygen saturation, apnea and bradycardia may occur in smaller premature infants and some healthy term infants in semi-reclined/car seat positioning[3,4]

DEVELOPMENTAL ADVANTAGES

Upright is an alerting posture

Encourages infant visual exploration

Encourages social interaction

May allow use of swing for older NICU infants

May help temporarily inhibit (relax) high tone (i.e., with hips flexed ≥90°)

DEVELOPMENTAL DISADVANTAGES

May be difficult to maintain proper head, neck, and trunk alignment as baby is more upright

Neck flexion (if it occurs) increases airway resistance and predisposes infant to obstructive apnea[12,47]

table 21-C *Medical and Developmental Considerations of Positioning Options in the NICU—cont'd*

Head Position/Head in Midline

MEDICAL ADVANTAGES

Head in midline seems to decrease intracranial pressure and intraventricular hemorrhage[22]

Elevation of head of bed 30° may reduce intracranial pressure[22]

DEVELOPMENTAL ADVANTAGES

Head in midline may improve head shape

Midline positioning reduces postural asymmetry and encourages development of antigravity flexion

Waterbeds (and water pillows) may reduce head flattening (dolichocephaly, scaphocephaly)[18,19,32,36,45]

MEDICAL DISADVANTAGES

May create pressure sore on occiput if head remains in midline too long on firm surface without pressure relief

DEVELOPMENTAL DISADVANTAGES

Head midline positioning is not practical in prone

1. Alastair, A.H., Ross, K.R., & Russell, G. (1979). The effect of posture on ventilation and lung mechanics in preterm and light-for date infants. *Pediatrics, 64,* 429-432.
2. Anderson, J., & Auster-Liebhaber, J. (1984). Developmental therapy in the neonatal intensive care unit. *Physical and Occupational Therapy in Pediatrics, 4,* 89-106.
3. Bass, J.L., Mehta, K.A., & Camara, J. (1993). Monitoring premature infants in car seats: Implementing the American Academy of Pediatrics policy in a community hospital. *Pediatrics, 91,* 1137-1141.
4. Bass, J.L., & Mehta, K.A. (1995). Oxygen saturation of selected term infants in car seats. *Pediatrics, 96,* 288-290.
5. Beckmann, C.A. (1997). Use of neonatal boundaries to improve outcomes. *Journal of Holistic Nursing, 15* (1), 54-67.
6. Bjornson, K., Deitz, J., Blackburn, S., Billingsly, F., Garcia, J., & Hays, R. (1992). The effect of body position on the oxygen saturation of ventilated preterm infants. *Pediatric Physical Therapy,* 109-115.
7. Blumenthal, I., & Lealman, G.T. (1982). Effect of posture on gastroesophageal reflux in the newborn, *Archives of Disease in Childhood, 57* (7), 555-556.
8. Bottos, M., Pettenazzo, A., Giancola, G., Stefani, D., Pettena, G., Viscolani, B., & Rubaltelli, F.F. (1985). The effect of a containing position in a hammock versus the supine position on the cutaneous oxygen level in premature and term babies. *Early Human Development, 11,* 265-273.
9. Bottos, M., & Stafani, D. (1982). Letter. Postural and motor care of the premature baby. *Developmental Medicine and Child Neurology, 24,* 706-707.
10. Bozynski, M., Naglie, R., Nicks, J., Burpee, B., & Johnson, R.V. (1988). Lateral positioning of the stable ventilated very low birthweight infant. *American Journal of Diseases in Children, 142,* 200-202.
11. Brackbill, Y., Douthitt, T., & West, H. (1973). Psychophysiologic effects in the neonate of prone versus supine placement. *Journal of Pediatrics, 82,* 82-83.
12. Carlo, W.A., Beoglos, A., Siner, B.S., & Martin, R.J. (1989). Neck and body position effects on pulmonary mechanics in infants. *Pediatrics, 84* (4), 670-674.
13. Cartilidge, P.H.T., & Rulter, N. (1988). Reduction of head flattening in preterm infants. *Archives of Disease in Childhood, 63,* 755-757.
14. Chan, J.S.L., Kelley, M.L., & Khan, J. (1995). Predictors of postnatal head molding in very low birth weight infants. *Neonatal Network, 14* (4), 47-52.
15. Cohen, R., Smith, D., Stevenson, D., Moskowitz, P.S., & Graham, B.C. (1984). Lateral decubitus position as therapy for persistent focal pulmonary interstitial emphysema in premature infants. *Pediatrics, 74,* 354-357.
16. Dellagrammatics, H., Kapetanakes, J., Papadimitriou, M., & Kourakis, G. (1991). Effect of body tilting on physiological functions in stable very low birthweight neonates. *Archives of Disease in Childhood, 66,* 429-432.
17. Downs, J.A., Edwards, A.D., McCormick, D.C., Roth, S.C., & Stewart, A.L. (1991). Effect of intervention on the development of hip posture in very preterm babies. *Archives of Disease in Childhood, 66,* 197-201.
18. Fay, M.J. (1988). The positive effects of positioning. *Neonatal Network, 8,* 23-28.
19. Fowler, K., Kum-Nji, P., Wells, P.J., & Mangrem, C.L. (1997). Water beds may be useful in preventing scaphocephaly in preterm very low birth weight neonates. *Journal of Perinatology, 17* (5), 397.
20. Fox, M. & Molesky, M. (1990). The effects of prone and supine positioning on arterial oxygen pressure. *Neonatal Network, 8* (4), 25-29.
21. Fox, R., Viscardi, R., Tackiak, V., Niknafs., H. & Cinoman, M.I. (1993). Effect of position on pulmonary mechanics in healthy preterm newborn infants. *Journal of Perinatology, 13,* 205-211.
22. Goldberg, R.N., Joshi, A., Moscoso, P., & Castillo, T. (1983). The effect of head position on intracranial pressure in the neonate. *Critical Care Medicine, 11* (6), 428-430.
23. Heaf, D.P., Helms, P., Gordon, I., & Turner, H.M. (1983). Postural effects of gas exchange in infants. *New England Journal of Medicine, 308,* 1505-1508.
24. Heimler, R., Langlois, J., Hodel, D., Nelin, L., & Sasidharan, P. (1992). Effect of positioning on the breathing pattern in premature infants. *Archives of Disease in Childhood, 67,* 312-314.
25. Hewitt, V. (1976). Effect of posture on the presence of fat in tracheal aspirate in neonates. *Australian Pediatric Journal, 12,* 267.
26. Hoshimoto, T. et. al. (1983). Postural effects on behavioral states of newborn infants: A sleep polygraphic study. *Brain Development, 5,* 286-291.
27. Hunt, C.E., & Puczynski, M.S. (1996). Does supine sleeping cause asymmetric heads? *Pediatrics, 98,* 127-129.
28. Hutchinson, A., Ross, K., & Russell, G. (1979). The effects of posture on ventilation and lung mechanics in preterm and light-for-date infants. *Pediatrics, 64,* 429-432.
29. Jantz, J.W., Blosser, C.D., & Fruechting, L.A. (1997). A motor milestone change noted with a change in sleep position. *Archives of Pediatric and Adolescent Medicine, 151,* 565-568.
30. Jenni, O.G., von Siebenthal, K., Wolf, M., Keel, M., Duc, G., & Bucher, H.U. (1997). Effect of nursing in the head elevated tilt position (15°) on the incidence of bradycardic and hypoxemic episodes in preterm infants. *Pediatrics, 100,* 622-625.

31. Kane, A.A., Mitchell, L.E., Craven, K.P., & Marsh, J.L. (1996). Observations on a recent increase in plagiocephaly without synostosis. *Pediatrics, 97,* 877-885.

32. Kramer, L.I., & Pierpont, M.E. (1976). Rocking waterbeds and auditory stimuli to enhance growth of preterm infants. *Journal of Pediatrics, 88,* 297-299.

33. Kurlak, L.O., Ruggins, N.R., & Stephenson, T.J. (1994). Effect of nursing position on incidence, type, and duration of clinically significant apnea in preterm infants. *Archives of Disease in Childhood, 71,* F16-F19.

34. Long, T., & Soderstrom, E. (1995). A critical appraisal of positioning infants in the neonatal intensive care unit. *Physical and Occupational Therapy in Pediatrics, 15* (3), 17-31.

35. Mansell, A., Bryan, C., & Levison, H. (1972). Airway closure in children. *Journal of Applied Physiology, 33,* 711-714.

36. Marsden, D.J. (1980). Reduction of head flattening in preterm infants. *Developmental Medicine and Child Neurology, 22,* 507-509.

37. Martin, R.J., Herrell, N., Rubin, D., & Fanaroff, A. (1979). Effect of supine and prone positions on arterial oxygen tension in the preterm infant. *Pediatrics, 63,* 528-531.

38. Masterson, J., Zucker, C., & Schulze, K. (1987). Prone and supine effects on energy expenditure and behavior of low birth weight neonates. *Pediatrics, 80,* 689-692.

39. Mendoza, J., Roberts, J., & Cook, L. (1991). Postural effects on pulmonary function and heart rate of preterm infants with lung disease. *Journal of Pediatrics, 118,* 445-448.

40. Meyers, W.F., & Herbst, J.J. (1982). Effectiveness of position therapy for gastroesophageal reflux. *Pediatrics, 69,* 768-772.

41. Mildred, J. et. al. (1995). Play position is influenced by knowledge of SIDS sleep position recommendations. *Journal of Pediatric Child Health, 31,* 499-502.

42. Monfort, K.P., & Case-Smith, J. (1997). The effects of a neonatal positioner on scapular rotation. *American Journal of Occupational Therapy, 51,* 378-384.

43. Orenstein, S., Whitington, P., & Orenstein, D. (1983). The infant seat as treatment for gastroesophageal reflux. *New England Journal of Medicine, 309,* 760-763.

44. Schwartz, A., & Graham, B. (1986). Neonatal tension pulmonary interstitial emphysema in bronchopulmonary dysplasia: Treatment with lateral decubitus positioning. *Radiology, 161,* 351-354.

45. Schwirian, P., Eesley, T., & Cuellar, L. (1986). Use of water pillows in reducing head shape distortion in preterm infants. *Research in Nursing and Health, 9,* 203-207.

46. Smith, P., & Turner, B. (1990). The physiologic effects of positioning premature infants in car seats. *Neonatal Network, 9,* 11-15.

47. Tcach, B.T., & Stark, A.R. (1979). Spontaneous neck flexion and airway obstruction during apneic spells in preterm infants. *Journal of Pediatrics, 94,* 275-281.

48. Wagaman, M.J., Shutack, J.G., Moomjian, A.S., Schwartz, J.G., Shaffer, T.H., & Foz, W.W. (1979). Improved oxygenation and lung compliance with prone positioning of neonates. *Journal of Pediatrics, 94,* 787-791.

49. Willett, L., Leuschen, M.P., Nelson, L.S., & Nelson, R.M. (1986). Risk of hypoventilation in premature infants in car seats. *Journal of Pediatrics, 109,* 245-248.

50. Yu, V.Y.H. (1975). Effect of body position on gastric emptying in the neonate. *Archives of Disease in Childhood, 50,* 500-504.

chapter **22**

Early Intervention

Linda C. Stephens
Susan K. Tauber

key terms

Early intervention
Part C of the Individuals with Disabilities
  Education Act
Family-centered intervention
Team models of interaction
Developmentally appropriate
Service coordination

■ CHAPTER OBJECTIVES

1. Describe the early intervention legislation and program regulations.
2. Explain family-centered early intervention philosophy and principles.
3. Define the components of an individualized family service plan (IFSP).
4. Explain models of evaluation, and describe specific assessments.
5. Describe developmentally appropriate and family-centered intervention approaches.
6. Define areas of emphasis in occupational therapy.
7. Explain strategies and activities used by occupational therapists in working with infants and children.

■ WHAT IS EARLY INTERVENTION?

The term *early intervention* connotes different meanings to different professionals. In this chapter, *early* refers to the most critical period of a child's development between birth and 3 years of age. *Intervention* refers to program implementation designed to maintain or enhance the child's development in natural environments and as a member of a family. The authors also use early intervention to describe services for children from birth to 3 years

of age who have an established risk, have a developmental delay, or are considered to be environmentally or biologically at risk.

■ LEGISLATION RELATED TO EARLY INTERVENTION

The 1980s brought widespread acceptance and support for family-centered care for children with special needs (Shonkoff & Meisels, 1990). Family-centered care is based on the principle that an infant is dependent on his or her mother and other family members for daily care and meeting his or her physical and emotional needs. At the same time, the birth of an infant with special health care needs affects the entire family emotionally, socially, and economically. In 1986, amendments to the Education of the Handicapped Act (EHA) established incentives for states to develop systems of coordinated care for infants with disabilities and their families. In 1990, the EHA was further amended and retitled the Individuals with Disabilities Education Act (IDEA; P.L. 101-476). IDEA has strengthened the incentives for establishing early intervention services and clarified how these services are to be implemented. In addition to its strong emphasis on family-centered intervention, IDEA strengthens the importance of prevention rather than remediation (Johnson, 1994) and promotes well-planned and well-coordinated transitions of children from preschool or school programs.

Part C of IDEA: Infants and Toddlers with Disabilities

Part C of the Individuals with Disabilities Education Act delineates the policies and regulations that participating states must follow in establishing early intervention services and systems. Table 22-1 summarizes the differences between Part C, which defines early intervention services for children between birth and 3 years of age, and Part B, which defines school programs for eligible students between 3 and 21 years of age (see Chapter 23 and 24). Part C is an entitlement program, and Part B defines mandated services. An entitlement simply acknowledges one's rights to something; a mandate establishes programs and services that are obligatory by law.

The purpose of Part C of IDEA is to give each state support in maintaining and implementing comprehensive, coordinated, multidisciplinary, interagency systems of early intervention services for infants and toddlers with disabilities and their families. Each state is required to establish a system that meets the following requirements:

1. Officially defines *developmental delay*
2. Establishes a state policy that ensures that appropriate early intervention services are available to all infants and children with disabilities and their families
3. Provides timely, comprehensive, multidisciplinary evaluations of the functioning of each infant and toddler with a disability
4. Allows the families of children who are recipients of early intervention services to identify their family priorities
5. Establishes a process for implementing individualized family service plans (IFSPs) that include service coordination
6. Develops a comprehensive child find system
7. Implements a public awareness program
8. Creates a central directory with information on early intervention services, resources, and experts and makes it available to families and others
9. Designs and implements a comprehensive system of personnel development; establishes policies and procedures for personnel standards
10. Puts procedure safeguards into place
11. Designates and establishes a single line of authority in a lead agency; establishes a policy for contracting or coordinating with local service providers
12. Establishes procedures for timely reimbursement of funds
13. Designs and implements a system for compiling data regarding early intervention programs
14. Defines policies and procedures to ensure that a) to the maximum extent appropriate, early intervention services are provided in a natural environment and b) provision of early intervention services occurs in a setting other than the infant's natural environment only when early intervention cannot be achieved

table 22-1 Comparison of Educational Programs by Age Group

	0 to 2 Years	3 to 5 Years	6 to 21 Years
Legislation	IDEA, Part C	IDEA, Part B	IDEA, Part B
Program	Early Intervention	Special education	Special education
Type	Entitlement	Mandate	Mandate
Eligibility	Noncategorical	Categorical	Categorical
Services Provided	16 primary services, including occupational therapy, physical therapy, speech therapy, and special instruction	Related services only as support to special education	Related services only as support to special education
	Interdisciplinary and transdisciplinary assessment	Discipline-specific assessment	Discipline-specific assessment as related to education
	Individualized Family Service Plan	Individualized Education Program	Individualized Education Program
	Family centered	Family-focused in theory, child-focused in practice	Child focused with emphasis on curricular standards
	Service coordination	Service coordination recommended but not mandated	Service coordination recommended but not mandated
Location	Natural settings	Home, center, or school based	School based

IDEA, Individuals with Diabilities Education Act.

satisfactorily for the infant or child in a natural environment

15. Establishes a state interagency coordinating council composed of parents, government officials, agency representatives, and service providers (this body advises and assists the lead agency in administering and coordinating the state early intervention system)

Eligibility

Infants or toddlers are eligible for early intervention services if they fall into the following categories:

- *Established risk.* Infants and toddlers are eligible for early intervention services if they have a diagnosis associated with developmental delay, such as Down syndrome or cerebral palsy.
- *Developmental delay.* Results of an "appropriate" diagnostic instrument or procedure or informed clinical opinion indicate delay in one or more of the following developmental areas: cognitive, motor (includes vision and hearing), communication, social-emotional, and adaptive. States differ in the criteria chosen to determine "appropriate" instruments or procedures.
- *At risk.* This category is included at state discretion and refers to a child who is considered to be at risk for the occurrence of a substantial developmental delay unless early intervention services are provided. Causation may be a result of environmental or biologic risk factors (e.g., infants born to teen mothers or drug- or alcohol-addicted mothers and infants with very low birth weight [VLBW] or failure to thrive [FTT]).

Intervention strategies and programs are intended to prevent or ameliorate developmental delays and deformities, maximize each child's potential, and assist the family in adjusting to the challenges of daily living in the home and community.

Required services

Families with infants with disabilities are eligible for 16 early intervention services provided by qualified personnel under public supervision and in conformity with the IFSP. Services should be family-centered, inclusive, and culturally sensitive. The services are as follows:

1. Assistive technology devices and services
2. Audiology
3. Family training, counseling, and home visits
4. Health services
5. Medical services for diagnostics and evaluation only
6. Nursing
7. Nutrition
8. Occupational therapy
9. Physical therapy
10. Psychological services
11. Service coordination
12. Social work
13. Special instruction
14. Speech and language therapy
15. Transportation
16. Vision services

Identification

The first step in the early intervention process is public awareness and a state system of Child Find that effectively identifies children at risk for development delay who would benefit from early intervention. This system must include standard referral procedures to be used by all primary referral sources and assignment of a service coordinator for the child and family as soon as possible after receiving the referral.

Evaluation process

Evaluation is the step that determines the eligibility of a child for initial and continuing early intervention services. Occupational therapy assessment procedures should include information about the child's performance in his or her natural environments (e.g., his or her home or childcare setting). Evaluations should include recommendations for appropriate supports that will enhance the child's success in the natural environment, such as physical accommodations or caregiver assistance.

IDEA specifies that a multidisciplinary team must evaluate the child; this team includes the professionals listed previously whose services seem warranted or are desired by the family. The team must obtain parental permission before the evaluation. Assessment is the ongoing procedure to determine the child's needs and strengths and the family's concerns, priorities, and resources. The team must complete the evaluation process within 45 days of identification.

Evaluation requirements

The service coordinator is responsible for ensuring that the evaluation process (1) is conducted by trained personnel; (2) is based on the state's adopted criteria of standard deviations or informed clinical opinion; (3) includes the child's medical and health history; (4) includes levels of functioning, unique needs, and recommended services related to the five developmental areas (cognition, physical, communication, social and emotional, and adaptive); and (5) takes place in natural environments.

The therapist documents the family resources, priorities, and concerns as they relate to the child's development. Collection of this information is family directed and voluntary. The evaluation procedures must be nondiscriminatory as to race, ethnicity, and socioeconomic background and in the family's native language or mode of communication to the best extent possible.

Individualized Family Service Plan

The IFSP follows completion of the evaluation. It is a written plan that delineates the family's desired outcomes for the child and the services that will be provided to reach those outcomes. The IFSP must be written during a meeting of the parents or caregivers and the team members within 45 days after the referral. The IFSP is a map of the family's services and informs anyone who will be working with the child and family which services will be provided, where they will be provided, and who will provide them. IDEA specifies that services must be provided in the infant's natural settings. The IFSP defines the environments in which the child is to be served and provides a statement of justification if services are not provided in natural environments. The IFSP also identifies the service coordinator who will be responsible for working with the family.

The role of a service coordinator in the IFSP process is a unique Part C provision. The service coordinator assists the family in accessing information and resources and coordinates implementation of the IFSP. Box 22-1 lists the required components as they are stated in IDEA.

If the child requires preschool special education or other services, the therapist must write the services into the IFSP's transition procedures. This step requires contact with the local education agency (LEA) and requires parental consent to provide records to the LEA for continuity of services and evaluation, as well as for assessment information. The IFSP is reviewed every 6 months with an annual reevaluation.

The IFSP is not a treatment plan; it is both a planning process and a document that identifies child and family outcomes. Specific services are listed as they relate to the hoped-for outcomes. For example, occupational therapy services may be listed on the IFSP as they relate to desired developmental goals that the parents identified. The therapist often writes specific occupational therapy intervention objectives and procedures that will support the family and infant or child outcomes on a separate document. This additional document can give specific guidance to the therapist by maintaining a record of the child's performance. The therapist may also submit the document to third-party reimbursement agencies.

Procedural safeguards

The parents must be informed of their rights that underlie the early intervention process. All states that use federal funds for early intervention services have specified procedural safeguards that protect the rights of parents and infants. The procedural safeguards required in a statewide system under section 635 (1) (13) of IDEA include the following:

1. Timely administrative resolution of complaints by parents

2. Right to confidentiality of personally identifiable information, including the right of parents to written notice of and written consent to the exchange of information among agencies
3. Right of parents to determine whether they, their infant or toddler, or other family members will accept or decline any early intervention service
4. Opportunity for parents to examine records relating to assessment, screening, eligibility determinations, and the development and implementation of the IFSP
5. Written prior notice to the parents of the infant or toddler with a disability whenever a service provider pro-

box 22-1 Required components of the Individualized Family Service Plan

The IFSP shall be in writing and shall contain the following (IDEA, sec. 636).
1. A statement of the infant's or child's present level of motor, cognitive, communication, social-emotional, and adaptive development, based on objective criteria
2. A statement of the family's resources, priorities, and concerns related to enhancing the development of the their infant or child
3. A statement of the major outcomes expected to be achieved for the infant or child and the family, and the criteria, procedures, and timelines used to determine the degree to which progress toward achieving the outcomes is being made and whether modifications or revisions of the outcomes or service are necessary
4. A statement of specific early intervention services necessary to meet the unique needs of the infant or child and the family, including the frequency, intensity, and method of delivering services
5. A statement of the natural environments in which early intervention services shall appropriately be provided, including a justification of the extent, if any, to which the services will not be provided in a natural environment
6. The projected dates for initiation of service and the anticipated duration of the services
7. The identification of the service coordination from the profession most immediately relevant to the infant's or family's needs who will be responsible for the implementation of the plan and coordination with other agencies and persons
8. The steps to be taken to support the transition of the child with a disability to preschool or other appropriate services

poses to initiate or change the identification, evaluation, or placement of the infant

6. Notice of any change fully informing the parent in the parents' native language

During the pendency of proceedings or action involving a complaint by the parents, the infant or toddler continues to receive the appropriate early intervention services currently being provided.

Transition into preschool services

A transition plan should be identified and documented in the IFSP as soon as possible and as soon as relevant. A referral to the LEA should be made 6 months before the child's third birthday or at 30 months of age. This helps the school system analyze all existing evaluation and assessment information and determine if further testing or information is necessary. It also enables the LEA to determine eligibility under Part B (which in some cases may differ from Part C eligibility) and, if eligible, plan for appropriate placement. In the case of a child who may not be eligible for preschool services, with the approval of the family, the early intervention service providers should convene to discuss the appropriate services that the child may receive.

Funding

Through the Part C program, states receive federal funds based on their census of infants and toddler compared with the total number of infants and toddlers nationally. Part C funds are used as the "payer of last resort" for services for eligible children only after other available funds through another federal, state, local, or private sources have been used. The lead agency is responsible for identifying and coordinating all funding resources and must enter into formal interagency agreements with other state agencies that provide services to young children and their families. Families are entitled to the following services at no cost: Child Find, evaluation and assessment, service coordination, and administration and coordination of IFSP activities. As in Part B of IDEA, they are entitled to all procedural safeguards.

Interagency Coordinating Council

The role of the Interagency Coordinating Council (ICC) is to advise and assist the lead agency in the implementation of a statewide early intervention system. The system is to be a "comprehensive, coordinated, collaborative, multidisciplinary, program for infants and toddlers with disabilities and their families." The ICC assists the lead agency and the state education agency (SEA) in coordinating Part C and Part B of IDEA. Members of the state ICC, who are appointed by the governor, include the following:

- Parents (at least 20% of total membership)
- Public and private providers (at least 20%)
- At least one member of the legislature

- A representative from personnel preparation
- One member from each SEA involved with payment for early intervention services who has authority to participate in policy planning and implementation
- One member from the SEA who has authority to participate in policy planning and implementation
- One member from the state governance of insurance (e.g., Medicaid)
- Others selected by the governor

Meetings must be held at least quarterly, with prior public notice and invitation for public attendance. In addition to the state ICC, each district or county has a local ICC (LICC), which includes parents and public and private providers. Each LICC is responsible for identifying and coordinating services within its geographic area. The LICC or local collaborative groups often help families identify and access infant evaluation and intervention services that are available within the county or region.

■ IMPLICATIONS OF LEGISLATION FOR THE OCCUPATIONAL THERAPIST

Part C of IDEA considers occupational therapy to be a "primary service" for eligible infants and toddlers from birth through 2 years of age who qualify for early intervention services. As a primary service, occupational therapy can be provided as the only service a child receives or in addition to other early intervention services. By its legal definition, occupational therapy includes services to address the functional needs of the child related to adaptive development; adaptive behavior and play; and sensory, motor, and postural development. It includes adaptation of the environment and selection, design, and fabrication of assistive and orthotic devices to facilitate development and promote the acquisition of functional skills. The therapist designs these services to prevent or minimize the influence of initial or future impairment, delay in development, or loss of functional ability.

The practice of occupational therapy in early intervention has been influenced by public legislation in the following ways:

1. *Team coordination and interagency communication.* The occupational therapist practices as part of an interdisciplinary team and contributes occupational therapy findings and recommendations to the IFSP. With parental permission and observation of confidentiality, the therapist shares therapy reports with other agencies that are delivering services to the family.

2. *Family service plan versus child-centered treatment plan.* The occupational therapist provides services according to family priorities. The family determines the intervention goals, which may focus on the child or the family as a whole.

3. *Indirect versus direct treatment.* The occupational therapist may consider various service delivery models, including those that may be transdisciplinary or consultative in nature. The model of direct, individual, child-centered services often is not the most appropriate one in early intervention.
4. *Concern with generalization of skills.* The occupational therapist is concerned with the functional use of skills in the child's natural environment rather than the development of skills in isolation.
5. *Ability to practice role release.* Professionals in early intervention often find it advantageous to use role release in the provision of services. In role release, one professional may be trained to take over functions that traditionally have been performed by another professional.
6. *Variety of settings.* Natural environments include the home and community settings in which children without disabilities participate. Occupational therapists are more likely to provide services in community settings, such as the home or a childcare center, than in medical settings.
7. *Wide range of disabilities.* As state lead agencies and Child Find services identify children who qualify for services, the occupational therapist is expected to work with children with various special needs. These may include biologically or environmentally at-risk populations that traditionally may not have received intervention.
8. *Work in small groups.* Traditional methods of individual, or one-on-one treatment are often replaced by the delivery of services to small groups of children or small parent-infant groups.
9. *Knowledge about the educational and community service delivery models.* Occupational therapists must be competent in working outside the traditional medical model and need to understand educational and family-centered models of practice.
10. *Addressing family concerns and priorities.* The occupational therapist must be sensitive to family needs and have respect for the parents' priorities. For example, the parent who is homeless or jobless may not be concerned about occupational therapy for the child. Another parent may believe that certain skills or goals are more important than those identified by the therapist. The occupational therapist should also be cognizant of the effect of limiting factors, such as criteria imposed by third-party payers and outcome criteria.

■ FAMILY-CENTERED PROGRAMS

The early intervention system recognizes that families can be and often are knowledgeable consumers and effective change agents for the child. It also acknowledges that families have specific needs related to a child with disabilities and that families may be the recipients of services. The family's early intervention team helps each family identify its unique resources, priorities, and concerns. The team then identifies outcomes and goals that enable the family to function more effectively and help the child as a member of the family unit. Acknowledging that families are both participants and consumers of early intervention services, Simeonsson and Bailey (1990) identified four different ways in which intervention could be provided for infants with special needs and their families:

1. Therapy administered to the infant, with the parent as a passive observer
2. Parents involved as members of the intervention team, participating in the planning process and involved in the child's program
3. Parents trained to carry out therapeutic activities as co-therapists or as the primary intervention agents
4. Families viewed as important recipients of services in their own right

The nature and extent of family involvement may vary and depends on family needs, values, lifestyles, and variables within the structure of the early intervention program itself. The degree of family involvement may fluctuate and change in response to external or internal factors that affect family functioning and coping. Some examples are degree of acceptance of the child's disability, job status of one or both parents, a new infant in the family, or changes in the family's support networks, such as grandparents, friends, or church groups.

The occupational therapist who works within a family-centered model develops goals collaboratively with parents or primary caregivers. Using a family systems perspective, the therapist recognizes the influence and interrelationships of the family within various systems, such as extended family, neighborhood, and early intervention programs. By thinking broadly about families and their subsystems, the therapist can help parents communicate their concerns and identify their priorities for the child. Effective listening and interviewing skills are essential, as is the ability to communicate with sensitivity the therapist's own concerns about the child's development. Families who have children with special needs highly value services in which professionals provide clear, understandable, complete information; demonstrate respect for the child and family; provide emotional support; and provide expert, skillful intervention (Featherstone, 1980). Box 22-2 lists principles of family-centered intervention.

■ EARLY INTERVENTION TEAM

The success of an early intervention program depends largely on the integration of the child's individual program components into a comprehensive system carried out by a cooperative team of professionals. Teamwork is critical because of the interrelated nature of the problems of the developing child and the need for skills and re-

---

box 22-2 *Principles of family-centered intervention*

The following are principles that have been generally accepted in the implementation of family-centered care (McGonigel, 1991, p. 9):

1. Infants and children are uniquely dependent on their families for their survival and nurturance. This dependence necessitates a family-centered approach to early intervention.
2. States and the program should define *family* in a way that reflects the diversity of family patterns and structures.
3. Each family has its own structure, roles, values, beliefs, and coping styles. Respect for and acceptance of this diversity is a cornerstone of family-centered early intervention.
4. Early intervention systems and strategies must honor the racial, ethnic, cultural, and socioeconomic diversity of families.
5. Respect for family autonomy, independence, and decision making means that families must be able to choose the level and nature of early intervention's involvement in their lives.
6. Family and professional collaboration and partnerships are the keys to family-centered early intervention and to successful implementation of the IFSP process.
7. An enabling approach to working with families requires that professionals re-examine their traditional roles and practices and develop new practices when necessary (practices that promote mutual respect and partnerships).
8. Early intervention services should be flexible, accessible, and responsive to family-identified needs.
9. The therapist should provide early intervention services according to the normalization principle (i.e., families should have access to services provided in as normal a fashion and environment as possible and that promote the integration of the child and family within the community).
10. No one agency or discipline can meet the diverse and complex needs of infants and children with special needs and their families. Therefore a team approach to planning and implementing the IFSP is necessary.

---

sources from many professionals to meet the needs of the child and family. The emphasis of intervention should be the child within the family unit rather than the child alone and should be carried out through collaboration among all professionals involved. (Models of teamwork are described in Chapter 2.) The two models most appropriate in early intervention are interdisciplinary and transdisciplinary.

Team Models of Interaction
Interdisciplinary

In the interdisciplinary model of interaction, a team of professionals from several disciplines involved with the child collaborates with the family to develop and implement an intervention program. These professionals have continuing direct involvement with the child and collaborate with one another in carrying out the child's program. The team members perform evaluations independently or together and set goals in collaboration with professionals and parents. With this approach the child and family can receive coordinated services and are able to benefit from the expertise of professionals from several disciplines who are directly involved (Case-Smith & Wavrek, 1998).

Each member of an interdisciplinary team is accountable to the team as a whole, although the degree and amount of involvement may vary and change depending on the child and family needs. The family's service coordinator is usually the person responsible for the coordination of team members to avoid fragmentation or duplication of services. To ensure the success of this approach, the team members must respect one another's roles, develop effective formal and informal communication patterns, and be flexible in response to family preferences. This requires a willingness to share expertise and knowledge and to assume accountability for intervention procedures.

Transdisciplinary

In the transdisciplinary model of interaction, various disciplines interact as a team, but one member is usually designated to provide direct intervention with other team members who act as consultants. This approach is based on the belief that the family benefits from having intervention primarily from one professional rather than multiple interventions from several professionals. All team members contribute to assessment and program planning, and then the designated person implements the plan with consultation and training from other members of the team. Therefore the transdisciplinary model enables each professional to perform functions that are normally outside the scope of practice of his or her discipline. Implementation of this model requires role release, or the relinquishing of some or all of one professional's functions to another professional. This has been defined as a process of sharing and the exchange of certain roles and responsibilities among team members (McGonigel, Woodruff, & Roszmann-Millican, 1994).

Giangreco (1986) describes the transdisciplinary approach as "indirect, integrated, and decentralized; it limits the number of people carrying out a program but makes use of the expertise of a variety of professionals" (p. 9). However, this approach was not intended to promote a team in which each professional developed the same skills across discipline lines, but rather to promote frequent and regular sharing of knowledge and skills. For example, a transdisciplinary team evaluated a 2-year-old child with spina bifida. The team determined that the home was the preferred location for intervention and that the physical therapist would act as the direct service provider. The occupational therapist, speech pathologist, and early childhood specialist taught the physical therapist techniques to use for feeding, language stimulation, and cognitive development. As a result, the physical therapist was able to provide various intervention strategies on her weekly visits, with periodic monitoring and consultation from the other professionals on the team.

Successful functioning as a transdisciplinary team takes commitment and willingness to cross traditional discipline boundaries and effective communication and consultative skills. To implement this approach, the therapist must be highly skilled in analyzing the child's developmental function and synthesizing the family and home situation given a limited amount of information (Case-Smith & Wavrek, 1998).

Although the transdisciplinary model may seem to be the most appropriate in early intervention, several barriers or obstacles have been identified in this approach (McGonigel et. al., 1994; Orelove & Sobsey, 1991; Ottenbacher, 1983). These obstacles include philosophic and professional differences, legal liabilities and licensure limitations, variable background education of designated service providers, and inconsistent mastery of skills practiced through role release. In addition, reimbursement from third-party payers may dictate intervention based on a medical model with direct provision of services by each professional. Regardless of which approach the team uses, effective teamwork does not come easily. It requires a flexible administration based on a sound philosophic framework and honest, hard work on the part of each team member.

■ EVALUATION OF INFANTS AND TODDLERS

Teti and Gibbs (1990) traced the interest in infancy and infant assessment back to the 1800s and the Child Study Movement and the efforts of Stanley Hall, founder of normative study of child development. Normative study of development is the basis for norm-referenced assessment, which assesses a particular behavior or attribute of children of a particular age group, establishing a mean age of development and an accompanying developmental curve with which other children can be compared.

An assumption of the developmental theory is that there is continuity of function from the infancy stages of sensorimotor development through the early childhood stages of verbalization and representational functioning. However, environmental and physiologic factors influence this development. The knowledge that environmental factors influence the infant's development and the belief that neurodevelopment of the infant is plastic and malleable supports the concept of early intervention (Teti & Gibbs, 1990).

The developmental approach to infant assessment involves a multidimensional, holistic method in which each developmental domain is individually examined and then the influence that the domains have on one another and on the child as a whole is assessed. For example, infants with motor impairments are restricted in their ability to explore their environment, a critical component to sensorimotor development, which in turn can affect other developmental areas of cognition, language, and socialization.

The functional approach focuses on the child's functional abilities in interaction with environmental activities, contexts, and conditions. To implement a functional approach, the therapist gathers information about the types of activities in which the child is to participate, methods of the child's participation, and expected goals for each activity. Using this information, the therapist analyzes competencies and barriers to the child's independent participation in relevant activities.

The functional approach relies on an ecologic framework that emphasizes skills and behaviors. The developmental approach documents the child's isolated skills (e.g., motor or cognitive) by referencing developmental milestones or domains, whereas the functional approach documents the child's behaviors by referencing skill clusters that describe functions (e.g., feeding or playing).

Early intervention evaluation consists of a series of steps and is an ongoing, collaborative process of collecting, analyzing, and gathering information about the infant and the family to identify specific needs and develop goals in the IFSP (Case-Smith, 1998a; Greenspan & Meisels, 1994). The evaluation, combined with a treatment program and ongoing reassessment, is a problem-solving process that continues throughout the period that the infant or toddler is eligible for Part C services.

Therapists can use developmental evaluations for screening, diagnosing or evaluating, and program planning. These processes are defined in Section II of this book. Family involvement with the evaluation is encouraged and varies from observation to full participation.

Screening

Often, the first step in identifying a child as appropriate for early intervention is a screening evaluation. Screening instruments should demonstrate high validity and reliability; accurately identify appropriate infants; include comprehensive health, social, behavioral, and environmental components; and involve the family members as equal partners with professionals (Hanson & Lynch, 1989). Screening tools measure quantitative performance (e.g., the child does or does not do a particular behavior) and do not consider the quality of that performance (e.g., how the child approaches a task).

One of the most widely used screening tools in medical and early intervention programs is the Denver Developmental Screening Test (DDST) II (Frankenburg et. al., 1990), which looks at behaviors in four developmental areas: gross motor, fine motor, personal-social, and language. Therapists can use DDST II for children between 2 weeks and 6 years of age.

The Battelle Developmental Inventory/Screening Test (BDI/S) (a subsection of the BDI) assesses five developmental domains: personal-social, adaptive, motor (gross and fine), communication (receptive and expressive), and cognitive (Newborg, Stock, Wnek, Guidubaldi, & Svinick, 1988). Therapists can use the BDI/S for children between 6 months and 8 years of age and adapt it for children with special needs. The BDI/S takes about 30 minutes to administer.

Evaluation

The process of evaluation is the gathering and interpreting of information on the child's health status and medical background, current developmental levels of functioning, and family resources to maximize the child's development.

Eligibility determination

Part C legislation states that the evaluation must be timely and comprehensive and must include input by a multidisciplinary team. The team should be responsive to the family's needs and desires when determining the time and location of the evaluation and which individuals should be present. The family's involvement is central to the evaluation process and should validate parental choices. The focus of the evaluation should be on the process itself (i.e., engaging the child and eliciting representative performance). In addition to test scores, the evaluation should result in a list of strengths and weaknesses (Miller, 1994).

The developmental areas that the team evaluates to determine eligibility are cognition, communication, motor, social-emotional, and adaptive. Play is another area of importance for the team to assess but is not part of most assessment instruments. However, play assessments demonstrate how well the child integrates separate skill areas and how he or she playfully interacts with social and physical environments. Some of the most frequently used instruments for the team assessment approach are the Bayley Scales of Infant Development, 2nd edition (BSID-II) (Bayley, 1993) and the BDI (Newborg et. al., 1988). Several more recently developed scales are listed in Appendix 7-A. The Hawaii Early Learning Profile (HELP; Furuno et. al., 1994; Parks, 1992) is a well-used developmental curriculum-based assessment.

Standardized assessments should never be the sole source for determining eligibility for early intervention services (McLean & McCormick, 1993). Furthermore, few reliable, comprehensive standardized assessments are available for children between birth and 2 years of age. A standardized test provides merely a sampling of a child's abilities and behaviors observed at a particular time and situation, from a particular perspective, and with a particular instrument (Greenspan & Meisels, 1994). Assessment results that do not reflect the child's typical functioning or behavioral characteristics are neither meaningful nor accurate. Therefore professional judgment is a critical element of assessment.

Intervention planning

Once the therapist has declared a child eligible for early intervention services, further assessment is important for the therapist to determine what intervention strategies and services are of greatest value to the child and family. At this point, evaluation becomes a comprehensive decision-making process to identify social-emotional, cognitive, motor, and communication problems and define an early intervention program plan. Miller (1994) made the following recommendations for assessment of infants and young children:

1. The therapist must base the assessment on an integrated developmental model. Parents and professionals must observe the child's range of functions in different contexts to identify how the child can best be helped, rather than just coming up with a grade or score.
2. Assessment involves multiple sources and multiple components of information. Parents and professionals contribute to forming the total picture of the child.
3. An understanding of typical child development is essential to the interpretation of developmental differences among infants and young children.
4. The assessment should emphasize the child's functional capacities, such as attending, engaging, reciprocating, interacting intentionally, organizing patterns of behavior, understanding his or her environment representationally or symbolically, and having problem-solving abilities (Greenspan, 1992).

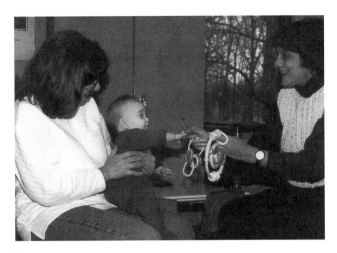

figure 22-1 Parent's presence supports the child during assessment and begins the parent-professional collaborative process.

5. The assessment process should identify the child's current abilities, strengths, and areas of need to attain desired developmental outcomes.

6. The therapist should not challenge young children during the assessment by separating them from their parents or caregivers. The parents' presence supports the child and begins the parent-professional collaborative process (Figure 22-1).

7. An unfamiliar examiner should not assess young children. The therapist should give the child a "warm-up" period. Assessment by a stranger when the parent is restricted to the role of a passive observer represents an additional challenge.

8. Assessments that are limited to easily measurable areas, such as certain motor or cognitive skills, should not be considered complete.

9. The therapist should not consider formal or standardized tests the determining factor of the assessment for the infant or young child. Most formal tests were developed and standardized on typically developing children and not on those with special needs. Furthermore, many young children have difficulty attending to or complying with the basic expectations of formal tests. Formal test procedures are not the best context in which to observe functional capacities of young children. Assessments that are intended for intervention planning should use structured tests only as part of an integrated approach.

Assessment and Team Processes

Early intervention assessment is a collaborative, cooperative, and coordinated process that involves multiple professional disciplines and the parents or primary caregivers and includes information from multiple formal and informal assessment sources. Several assessment tools are recommended for use as a "core" assessment (i.e., one to which all members of the team can contribute discipline-specific perspectives). Using developmental curricula such as the Assessment, Evaluation, and Programming System (AEPS) for Infants and Children (Bricker, 1993), the BDI, the Carolina Curriculum of Infants and Toddlers with Special Needs (Johnson-Martin, Jens, Attermeier, & Hacker, 1996) or the HELP, each team member can evaluate certain domains of performance and contribute information about that domain to the team's planning process.

The primary developmental domains evaluated are cognitive, social-emotional, motor, sensory processing, communication, and adaptive or self-help skills (Table 22-2).

One way to implement the interdisciplinary/transdisciplinary model is through the use of a play-based observational assessment. The concept of this type of assessment is to have an integrated and collaborative understanding about the child's behaviors, accomplishments, and areas of concern. The format should consist of situations that allow for both unstructured and functional play as well as structured and interactive play. One member of the team assumes the role of play facilitator with the child while another facilitates the parent's participation (Figure 22-2). The remaining team members are observers, but they can make comments or suggestions during the session. All members contribute to the interpretation of the results, including planning and recommending goals and objectives for intervention.

Videotaping the evaluation is a valuable tool for documentation, particularly when the evaluation takes place over multiple sessions and environments and perhaps with several individuals. Videotapes provide an excellent source of documenting qualitative changes over time. The transdisciplinary model allows the most pertinent information to be gathered, but it does not preclude specific evaluation by individual disciplines if further information is needed. The occupational or physical therapist often must do a more "hands-on" evaluation to assess muscle tone, movement patterns, or the infant's response to handling techniques.

Linder (1993a) has developed a play assessment process called the Transdisciplinary Play–Based Assessment (TPBA) and an accompanying intervention guide called Transdisciplinary Play–Based Intervention (TPBI) (Linder, 1993b). The TPBA includes guidelines that list the normal developmental sequence of skill acquisition in the areas of cognition, social-emotional, communication, and sensorimotor and describes procedures for conducting a transdisciplinary arena-type assessment of the child that uses a play-based format and involves the entire team

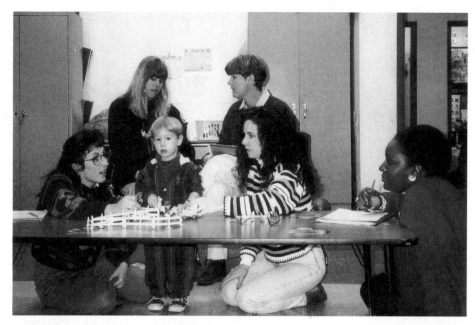

figure22-2   Transdisciplinary team uses play activities in an arena assessment.

table 22-2   *Areas of Developmental Assessment*

Performance Area	Definition	Examples of Assessment Instruments
Cognitive	The ability to acquire, store, and use information from the environment: problem solving, object permanence, cause and effect, imitation	BSID-II, BDI, HELP, TPBA
Social-emotional	The ability to regulate responses to others and the environment: temperament, ability to interact, attention, coping, activity level	BSID-II, Early Coping Inventory, TPBA, BDI, HELP
Motor	Motor patterns, muscle tone, posture, balance and equilibrium responses, hand-eye coordination, grasp and reach, manipulation	PDMS, BDI, BSID-II, Toddler and Infant Motor Evaluation, TPBA, HELP, PEDI
Communication	Receptive and expressive language skills, use of gestures	BDI, Rossetti Infant-Toddler Language Scale, Peabody Language Scale, HELP, Preschool Language Scales
Sensory	Response to tactile, vestibular, proprioceptive, auditory, and visual input	Test of Sensory Functions in Infants, sensory history
Adaptive or self-help skills	Feeding, toileting, dressing, safety	BDI, Vineland Adaptive Behavior Scales, PEDI

BDI, Battelle Developmental Inventory; *BSID-II,* Bayley Scales of Infant Development, 2nd edition; *HELP,* Hawaii Early Learning Profile; *PDMS,* Peabody Developmental Motor Scales; *PEDI,* Pediatric Evaluation of Disability Inventory; *TPBA,* Transdisciplinary Play-Based Assessment

of professionals and family members. Observation of peer interactions is recommended. The TPBA includes a preassessment and postassessment meeting, sharing of observations and identifying needs, priorities, and concerns for the child and family (Linder, 1993a).

Advantages of the TPBA are that it allows for functional play interactions with the child in a natural envi-

ronment and includes parent participation. In addition, the testing activities are flexible and can be adapted to meet the special needs of each child. Professionals can contribute their own hands-on or discipline-specific evaluations as part of the TPBA process. The TPBA is an excellent form of evaluation for children who do not comply with standardized evaluation, have difficulty managing behaviors, or demonstrate inconsistent or widely scattered skills.

An example of a child appropriate for TPBA evaluation is a 2-year-old boy with an autistic spectrum disorder who has little expressive language, has advanced gross motor skills for his age but is clumsy and fearful of movement (postural insecurity), does not like being touched by others, and is sensitive to certain textures (tactile defensiveness). He also has poor eye contact, does not socially interact with his peers or most adults, and often seems unaware of their presence in the same room. However, he is able to put together complex puzzles, knows the letters of the alphabet, and can repeat whole parts of videotapes. If the therapist were to administer a BSID-II, this child would not have related to the materials or to the examiners and therefore would have passed few, if any, items. The score obtained would be an unreliable reflection of his ability and, if presented to parents, would serve no purpose and may be discouraging. Using the TPBA, his performance as whole, including skills and limitations, becomes the basis for understanding his functional ability.

Role of the Occupational Therapist in the Assessment Process

Occupational therapists are actively involved in all levels of the evaluation process, from diagnosis to program planning and intervention. When working in the area of early intervention, the occupational therapist must use a holistic perspective as opposed to a single-discipline or domain-specific perspective. The occupational therapist may administer a core developmental assessment for diagnostic purposes or assume the leadership role in an arena assessment. Occupational therapists bring to the assessment process a unique understanding of the interdependence and relationship between the child's functional and developmental skills and of sensory perception, behavior, and neurodevelopmental processes (Case-Smith, 1998a).

During a diagnostic evaluation, the occupational therapist may use informal measures and observations to assess muscle tone, strength, coordination, motor planning, and sensory processing. The therapist can accomplish this by directly handling the child, if appropriate, or observing the child's reactions to being handled by his or her parent or a familiar adult. Evaluation to develop a program plan enables the occupational therapist to suggest appropriate goals and objectives and strategies for meeting them. The therapist assesses other areas, such as social-emotional, cognitive, and communication development, from the perspective of how the parents influence the child's ability to engage in functional play, move through the environment, or interact with others.

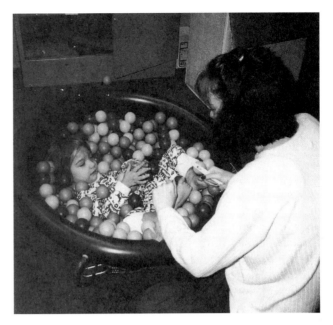

figure **22-3** Occupational therapist helps young child learn through an interactive process of sensory and motor exploration.

■ OCCUPATIONAL THERAPY INTERVENTION

Occupational therapists are important members of the early intervention team and can provide services in various settings using one of several models of intervention. The contribution of occupational therapists is described as follows:

> Occupational therapists promote a child's independence, mastery, and sense of self-worth and self-confidence in their physical, emotional, and psychosocial development. These services are designed to help families and other caregivers improve children's functioning within their environments. Therapists use a developmental framework in assessing the following domains: play, adaptive skills, sensorimotor, posture, fine motor manipulation, and oral motor feeding. Purposeful activity is then used to expand the child's functional abilities in these areas (Brown & Rule, 1993, p. 254).

Case-Smith (1998b) has identified general goals of occupational therapy intervention with infants and children:
- Facilitate change in the child's developmental function (Figure 22-3).
- Interpret and redefine behavioral responses.
- Compensate for and adapt to the effects of a disability
- Provide support to family members

Occupational therapy is provided in collaboration with other members of the team and is specified as part of the IFSP.

Settings

Early intervention legislation specifies that the therapist should provide services in the child's natural environment, including the home and community setting in which children without disabilities participate. To enable the child to remain an integral part of the family and for the family to be integral parts of the neighborhood and community, services should be community based and in locations convenient to the family (Dunst, 1991). Ideally, the therapist should offer the family a range of options so that they can choose those that best fit their priorities, lifestyle, and values. These options should include those that provide the least restrictive settings in situations that would be natural environments for a normally developing child of the same age. Some examples are a playgroup, mother's morning out program, childcare center, or Sunday School class.

The Division of Early Childhood of the Council for Exceptional Children supports the philosophy of inclusion with the following statement (DEC, 1993):

> Inclusion, as a value, supports the right of all children, regardless of their diverse abilities, to participate actively in natural settings within their communities. A natural setting is one in which the child would spend time if he or she had not had a disability (p. 4).

The philosophy of inclusion extends beyond physical inclusion to mean social and emotional inclusion of the child and family (Turnbull, Turnbull, & Blue-Banning, 1994). The implications for occupational therapists are that they provide services within the natural setting (e.g., the home or childcare center) rather than in an outpatient center, hospital, or rehabilitation center.

The inclusion model has many advantages. When the child attends the community childcare program, he or she gains opportunities for interaction with typically developing peers (Figure 22-4). Participation in community programs gives the family common experiences for relating to friends and neighbors and helps them view their child as one with differing abilities rather than one with disabilities. To be successful, the inclusion program should ensure that (1) the child's individual needs are met with appropriate aids and support services, (2) the child with special needs benefits from the typical program, and (3) the needs of the typical children are not compromised.

Several obstacles can negatively influence the benefits of inclusive programs. The child who needs intense, specialized intervention may be unable to develop his or her potential to the greatest extent because the needed individualization is not possible in a community program. For example, a child with significant acting-out behaviors may require far more attention from the teacher than the teacher is able to provide because of his or her responsibilities to the other typical children in the group. In

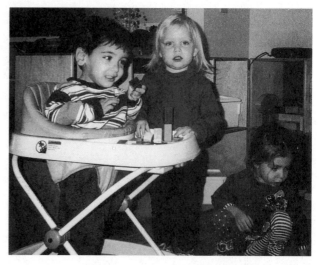

figure**22-4**   A child who attends a community childcare program benefits from interaction with typically developing peers.

addition, personnel may not have adequate training to provide the intervention needed. For some children, inclusion programs must provide a great deal of on-site support to facilitate interaction or provide adaptations for function. This may not be cost-effective when only one or two children are in one location. In areas that have shortages of occupational therapists to provide intervention, it may be impractical for the therapists to spend a great deal of travel time to provide services in the home or in childcare centers.

Occupational therapy services are provided in various settings that represent a continuum from the most restrictive (e.g., residential care facility) to the least restrictive (e.g., inclusion programs). The setting should reflect family preferences and should be consistent with the needs of the child and the goals identified on the IFSP. For example, one child with significant and acute medical problems may be best served in the hospital-based program, whereas another with similar problems may be best served in the home. One child with Down syndrome may function best in a mother's morning out program with normally developing peers, whereas another with the same diagnosis may make more developmental gains and exhibit more independence in a center-based early intervention program. Early intervention legislation provides for interagency cooperation, thus families can choose the most appropriate settings and services from either private or public providers.

Cultural Diversity

To provide appropriate intervention within the family-focused model, the occupational therapist must be aware of and respect differences in beliefs and values based on culture. "Perhaps no set of programs or services interacts with cultural views and values more than early intervention because of the focus on the very young child with a disability and the family" (Hanson, 1990, p. 116). The therapist who provides intervention in the home has an intimate view of such things as customs, eating habits, and childrearing practices that may vary among cultures. The family's beliefs and views of disability and its cause, their view of the health care system, and their sources of medical information affect their attitude toward early intervention. Based on individual cultural backgrounds, the family may view the therapist as either a helper or one who interferes.

Many of the areas in which occupational therapists provide intervention and suggestions involve caregiving and are closely tied to values and beliefs about parenting and cultural views of children. Practices regarding feeding, toileting, and bathing may vary among cultures. The therapist is urged to evaluate various health beliefs to determine whether the effects are beneficial, harmless, harmful, or uncertain before making recommendations for change (Hanson, 1998).

Early intervention legislation requires that the therapist administer assessments in the family's native language if feasible and conduct evaluation procedures in a manner that is not racially or culturally discriminatory (IDEA, 1990). Intervention methods and procedures should recognize and be sensitive to cultural differences. The following are some suggestions for the therapist (Vohs, 1989, p. 3):

- Learn about other cultures.
- Learn how persons of other cultures view children with disabilities.
- Invite members of minority cultures to become involved with your organization.
- Learn at least a few words of different languages.
- Become familiar with your community and the cultures represented.
- Examine ways to remove barriers to accessing services for minority groups.
- Recognize that everyone has prejudices and believes that his or her values are right.
- Be sensitive to problems of being a member of a minority.

Planning

Occupational therapy intervention, as with other early intervention services, is based on identified concerns and expected outcomes in the IFSP. This document specifies various services to be provided; who the provider will be; the location of the services; frequency, intensity, and duration of services; and the funding sources.

An IFSP outcome is usually stated in broad terms and reflects family priorities. An outcome is a statement of changes desired by the family that can focus on any area

of the child's development or family life as it relates to the child (Kramer, McGonigel, & Kaufman, 1991). Some examples of outcomes that relate to occupational therapy are as follows:

- Heidi will learn to eat more easily and will eat a greater variety of foods.
- Heidi will use her hands to play with toys.

The occupational therapist's intervention plan identifies the goals and objectives related to the outcomes in collaboration with the family. For example, the occupational therapy goals for Heidi include the following:

- Improve oral motor functioning for eating.
- Provide adaptations for positioning and increased function in eating and play activity.
- Increase function through developmentally appropriate sensorimotor activities.

The objectives for Heidi specifically state what is expected by the end of the time period.

- Heidi will tolerate textures provided through food or oral motor facilitation as shown by eating food of various textures with appropriate chewing and swallowing.
- The therapist will teach Heidi's mother strategies for oral motor facilitation to be implemented at home at mealtimes.
- Heidi will drink liquids independently when provided with an adapted cup.
- Heidi will be provided with seating adaptations at home and in her childcare center that will position her appropriately for feeding.

Occupational therapy's contribution to the IFSP outcomes follows *developmentally appropriate* practice and considers the child's function within her family and her environment.

Approaches
Developmentally appropriate

The occupational therapist plans and carries out therapy for the infant and child within the framework of developmental needs rather than the acquisition of isolated skills. For example, it would be inappropriate for the occupational therapist to concentrate on the development of precise fingertip prehension without consideration of how this skill contributes to the overall function of the child in the environment or how it fits into the developmental needs of the child.

Developmentally based curricula such as the HELP, the Activities-Based Intervention (AEPS for Infants and Children; Bricker, 1993) or TPBI (Linder, 1993b) provide activities matched to the developmental sequences within each domain. However, the therapist should guard against using a "cookbook" approach in intervention for specific developmental deficits.

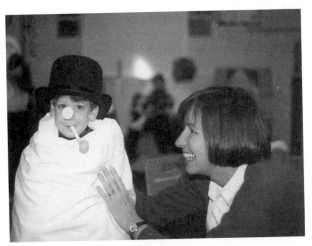

figure 22-5 Music therapist's activity of "Frosty the Snowman" helps meet occupational therapy goals of providing tactile input.

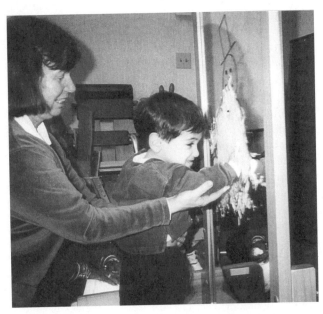

figure 22-6 Physical therapist helps a child with his standing balance while the child is involved in an activity that requires tactile input and hand function.

A team whose members have overlapping functions can effectively address developmental needs (Figures 22-5 and 22-6). When the therapist identifies a need in a specific domain (e.g., fine motor skills), he or she can implement activities that require a child to use fine motor skills. To promote generalization of the fine motor skills practiced in therapy, the therapist should employ play activities that involve the "just right" challenge to the child across domains (i.e., activities that include skill building in the cognitive and social domains). For example, stacking rings on a stick is a motor task but also involves cognitive skills such as concept of size and color. The activities also could involve social interaction, including give and take with the adult, eye contact, praise, and delight at successful attempts.

Family-centered intervention

In *family-centered intervention* the occupational therapist addresses the needs of the entire family rather than only concentrating on specific deficits in the child. The therapist should be guided by family concerns and the amount of involvement that various family members choose to have in the child's intervention program (Figure 22-7). One important way for the therapist to increase the effect of therapy is to recommend that the family implement therapy activities and exercises at home. When the child practices the activities daily at home, the child is much more likely to learn the targeted skill. However, parents vary in their desire or ability to implement structured therapy activities with their children. Time and energy, other family demands, and family support are always considerations when discussing home program with parents. One mother stated the following:

> There are times when even an acceptable amount of therapy becomes too much—when your child needs time just to be a child, or when you need time to be with the rest of the family. It is okay to say "no" at those times, for a while. Your instinct will tell you when (Simons, 1985, p. 51).

Sometimes it is more important to support the role of parent than to assume that the parent can take on the role of the therapist. Daily routines in a family with a child who has a disability can take an excessive amount of time and energy, which does not allow for carrying out a therapy home program. Suggestions that the family can incorporate into the daily routine are the most successful. For example, the caregiver can provide tactile stimulation and range of motion at bath time; an older sibling can encourage the infant to reach for toys while their mother cooks dinner.

Occupational therapists can provide support for families by listening to them, giving positive feedback regarding parenting skills, encouraging recreational activities for the family, and helping them access community resources (Case-Smith, 1998b). Often the therapist can help the family by providing intervention to make daily routines go more smoothly. Examples are suggestions for positioning and handling to make feeding more efficient or an adapted bath seat to make bathing less taxing.

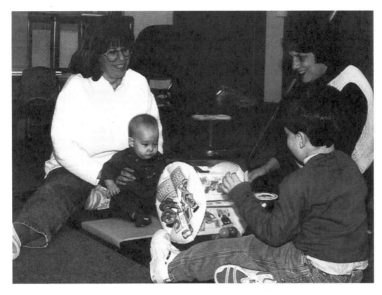

figure22-7   The older brother participates in the therapy session and learns how to play with his baby sister at home.

table 22-3 *Occupational Therapy Intervention for a 5-Month-Old Boy*

Practice Perspective	Examples of Occupational Therapy Goals and Activities
Prevention (check the negative effect of developmental problems on future abilities)	• Develop awareness of body parts through sensory input to prevent spatial orientation problems. • Increase attention and eye contact to enhance interaction with others.
Habilitation (promote developmental acquisition of future skills)	• Develop child's head control through movement, neuromuscular facilitation, and positioning. • Enhance basic oral motor functions of breathing, sucking, and swallowing in preparation for speech.
Remediation (attempt to diminish dysfunction)	• Decrease drooling through neuromuscular facilitation to mouth. • Enhance interaction through alerting techniques before play.
Compensation (substitute different skills for delayed ones)	• Encourage mother and father to carry the infant in an infant carrier ("snugli") until the infant can move on his or her own. • Position child so pacifier remains in mouth.
Maturation (use child's own developmental schedule)	• Provide appropriate toys to enhance visual attention in crib and play areas. • Offer finger foods during meals as child develops pincer grasp.

From Hanft, B. (1989). The changing environment of early intervention services: Implications for practice. In B. Hanft (Ed.), *Family-centered care: An early intervention resource manual*. Rockville, MD: American Occupational Therapy Association.

Areas of intervention

Hanft (1989) applied five practice perspectives to occupational therapy with infants and children: prevention, habilitation, remediation, compensation, and maturation (Table 22-3). The therapist can use these various perspectives at different times, depending on the child's needs and development. The therapist must determine the appropriateness of an approach at any given time. Regardless of the perspective, the therapist works in collaboration with the family and other professionals to develop functional abilities. The child is viewed in a ho-

listic manner in enhancing development; however, there are certain areas that occupational therapists have traditionally emphasized more.

Fine motor development and manipulative hand function. The occupational therapist is often concerned with delayed function or atypical function in fine motor skills. These skills include grasp and release of objects, bilateral manipulation, in-hand manipulation, hesitancy to touch and explore with the hands, lack of hand-to-mouth pattern, and other skills. Intervention begins with analyzing the quality of movement and determining un-

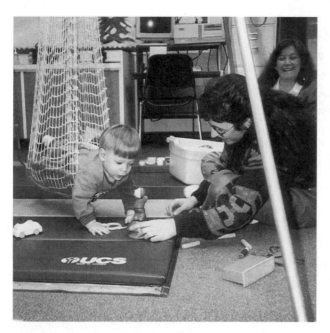

figure 22-8　Occupational therapist uses various toys and sensorimotor experiences to achieve desired results.

derlying factors, such as tactile discrimination and kinesthetic awareness.

First, the therapist observes how functional a child is in a particular skill. When a skill such as stacking blocks appears delayed or deficit, the therapist analyzes which performance components are interfering with performance. For example, the therapist notes the influence of muscle tone and proximal stability when the child attempts stacking 1-inch cubes. He or she must then determine the following:

- Is muscle tone increased?
- Are spasticity, tremor, or associated movements (mirroring) present?
- Does total body tone change with effort?
- Can the child stack the cubes while sitting unsupported on the floor?
- Does the infant slump or demonstrate lack of postural stability?
- Can the child easily disassociate the movement of the arm from the body?
- Is the child's hand-eye coordination delayed?
- Does inattention or a lack of understanding interfere with performing the task?
- Does the child have difficulty with the motor planning needed for precise release of one block on top of another?
- Does tactile defensiveness cause the child to be reluctant to handle the block or result in flinging or throwing any object in his or her hand?

A child with autistic spectrum disorder or other dysfunction that interferes with the child's ability to interact with persons and things in the environment may be unable to imitate or follow directions for a task. Therefore inability to stack blocks may not reflect a deficit in fine motor ability, but rather inexperience or disinterest in the activity. The best indication of the child's fine motor abilities may be through observation of spontaneous activity.

Stacking blocks is not an important functional skill, but it is important for developing sufficient hand skill for manipulating, placing, and releasing objects. These skills enable the child to use tools with control and with their arms unsupported. The occupational therapist uses various age-appropriate toys, games, sensorimotor experiences, and other strategies with the child to remediate underlying factors that interfere with the development of fine motor skills (Figure 22-8).

Development of play

One of the most important areas of a child's development is involvement in play. Play is open ended, self-initiated, self-directed, and unlimited in its variety. It gives the child the opportunity to develop and practice skills that will be the foundation for later occupational tasks, such as the ability to manipulate objects, problem solve, and attend to tasks (Burke, 1998). Play can be exploratory, symbolic, creative, or competitive in nature (see Chapter 18).

Sometimes therapists are so intent on remediating certain deficits that they ignore the importance of play. A toy becomes only a motivator, or a diversion, so that the therapist can elicit a certain movement pattern (Burke, 1998). Although this may sometimes be necessary, the therapist must also facilitate play skills in the child and use play as a way of enabling the child to gain function and enhance development. To use play as intervention, the occupational therapist must be playful in interactions with the child. Whether it is a game of peek-a-boo or knocking down a pretend wall when pushed on a scooter board, the activity should elicit a sense of enjoyment and fun.

Children with special needs may not have developed play skills because of long hospitalizations or medical treatments or because of the limitations imposed by a physical impairment. Other children may experience deficits in play because of cognitive limitations or difficulties in social interactions. Use of a play-based assessment can enable the occupational therapist to define the problem areas and plan intervention.

Sensory integration

Infants who have difficulty processing sensory information lack the ability to cope with environmental demands or achieve internal control. These infants may be irritable, cry frequently, be difficult to comfort, or have difficulty with changes in routine. The ability to cope "requires the ability to modulate incoming sensory information while engaged in feeding, face-to-face interactions with family, bathing, and diapering, or just being held" (Stallings-Sahler, 1998).

The therapist must recognize and address sensory integrative dysfunction in the child because of its pervasive influence on all areas of development. The therapist should use appropriate tactile, vestibular, and proprioceptive input that elicits organized behavior and simple adaptive responses on the part of the child. For example, it was determined that a 1-year-old child displayed tactile defensiveness. He refused to hold toys, refused to bear weight on his arms, was irritable when held, pulled away from touch, and avoided exploring his environment. The occupational therapist planned intervention that included proprioceptive and tactile input and midline play with textured toys. She recommended to the mother that additional tactile stimulation be provided at bath time with water play, foamy soap, and terry cloth rubs. Soon the child was clapping his hands spontaneously—a skill he had not attempted before and a nice adaptive response (see Case Study 1).

Oral motor function and feeding

Occupational therapists who work with infants and children often address problems in eating and feeding. Problem areas may include inadequate intake, excessive time for feeding, or oral motor problems associated with sucking, swallowing, and chewing (Glass & Wolf, 1998). Additional problems may center on behavioral issues such as refusals, overactivity, or messiness. Other concerns are in the area of self-feeding and drinking from a cup.

Addressing concerns in the area of feeding is also important for mother-child bonding. Glass and Wolf (1998) suggest three guiding principles of treatment for the infant:
1. Providing proper alignment of the trunk and neck
2. Providing proximal stability, especially in the head and jaw
3. Facilitating appropriate oral motor patterns through inhibitory and facilitation techniques (see Chapter 15)

Adapted equipment and positioning

The occupational therapist in early intervention can make an important contribution to the overall functioning of children through the recommendation and provision of appropriate adapted equipment (Figure 22-9). A floor sitter may enable the child with cerebral palsy to play on the floor near his or her typically developing peers. An adapted insert for a chair may make it possible for a child to begin to use his or her hands for an art project or to self-feed. As the neurologically involved child approaches preschool age and is not yet ambulating, the parents may have to face the

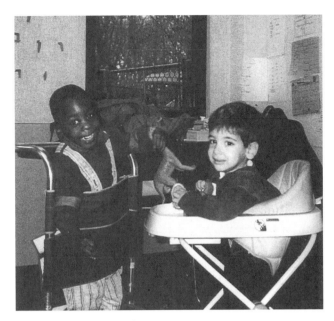

figure 22-9 Use of adapted equipment enables these children to be positioned for play.

prospect of the need for a wheelchair. The occupational therapist can assist in recommending appropriate equipment and in being sensitive to the effect that envisioning their child in a wheelchair may have on the family. The child with a neurologic impairment who can stay in an infant stroller or a high chair does not appear as "different" as the 3-year-old child who must have a wheelchair and special equipment.

■ SUMMARY

Occupational therapists use holistic approaches with children and their families that emphasize functional, developmentally appropriate approaches. By recognizing that children are part of a family system, the therapist designs programs that fit into the family's daily routine; consider sensory, motor, social, and cognitive aspects of performance; and emphasize the child's occupations of physical and social play.

Case Study 1: Alex
Background

Alex's pediatrician referred him to occupational therapy at 11 months of age because of suspected sensory integrative problems. He had a diagnosis of developmental delay and had been receiving physical therapy because of gross motor delays. Alex cried often in a distressful manner. Problem areas for Alex, as reported by his mother, included uncooperative behaviors, rages or temper tantrums, whining and fussing, feeding problems, fearfulness, poor balance, and a dislike for being on his tummy. Although he sat independently at 6 months of age, he did not reach and grasp an object until 8 months of age. He rolled from back to stomach at 9 months of age, and he was not yet crawling at 11 months of age.

Assessment

Alex was a pleasant infant who preferred not to be touched or held. He interacted with the examiner with caution after a brief period of ignoring her. His mother remained in the room and participated in the assessment. The examiner obtained a sensorimotor history by interview with Alex's mother. His mother had noticed that he had difficulty and pulled away when touched. Sometimes he stiffened and arched his back when held. Alex's mother reported that he was irritable when held and resisted having his hair or face washed. Alex seemed oversensitive to noises and was bothered by such things as a vacuum cleaner and hair dryer. Although his aversion to sound had improved, he remained apprehensive of toys with noises. Alex seemed to be fearful in situations with auditory and visual stimulation, such as a shopping mall. Alex enjoyed swinging and other movement stimuli.

The examiner administered the Test of Sensory Functions in Infants (Degangi & Greenspan, 1989) to Alex. Results showed deficiencies in reactivity to tactile deep pressure and adaptive motor functions, at-risk response to visual-tactile integration and ocular-motor control, and normal response to vestibular stimulation. Specifically, Alex exhibited a mildly defensive reaction to touch. He was not effective in his motor responses to tactile input, such as removing a mitt on his foot or a piece of tape on the back of his hand. He was more efficient using his right hand than his left. Visual-tactile response was better because he was able to locate the stimulus visually, although he could not plan the movement to remove it. However, visual tracking was delayed and inconsistent. Alex enjoyed the vestibular input as he was held and moved up and down or in circular motions. He also enjoyed upside-down positions.

The examiner observed that he avoided and resisted changing his body position (e.g., going from sitting to quadruped) and resisted the proprioceptive input of weight bearing on his upper extremities. Extensor muscle tone was increased with lower-extremity weight bearing, so much so that it was difficult to flex his hips passively for sitting. Alex went into plantar flexion and lower-extremity extension when bounced on his bare feet.

At a chronologic age of 11 months, Alex received an age equivalent of 9 months on the fine motor subtest of the Peabody Developmental Motor Scales. He used his right hand more efficiently than his left but was able to bring his hands to midline to bang cubes. However, he resisted clapping his hands. Alex removed pegs from a pegboard and briefly manipulated a piece of paper. He was able to transfer a cube from his left hand to his right when the cube was placed in his left hand. Alex had difficulty removing rings from a stand. He also displayed difficulty in deliberately releasing cubes to give to the examiner or to put them in a cup.

Summary and interpretation

Alex was a delightful infant who experienced significant difficulties in receiving and modulating sensory information. This was evident particularly in his irritability and intolerance to touch and auditory stimulation. Inadequate adaptive motor function seemed to be related to his hypersensitivity. Alex's tactile defensiveness probably contributed to his fine motor delays. Given his defensiveness, it is understandable that he was limited in his abilities to explore and manipulate objects, especially those that were new to him and in an unfamiliar environment.

Intervention

The team recommended weekly occupational therapy for Alex, which became part of his IFSP. The occupational therapist provided services in his child center once a week and at home once a month. The therapist used a sensory integrative approach with developmentally appropriate play with emphasis on increased functional hand use. Intervention included frequent brushing of the extremities and the back with a soft surgical brush followed by deep proprioceptive input. Treatment sessions included vestibular input, which Alex tolerated well, and proprioceptive and tactile input as tolerated. The therapist encouraged Alex to play with textured toys, use both hands for midline activities, and bear weight on his upper extremities. Alex's mother participated actively in each session and created additional opportunities for tactile exploration and play at home. The therapist provided his mother with reading material and a videotape to help her learn about sensory integration and understand how sensory processing affects behavior.

Alex responded well to the treatment approach and began to show indications of more efficient sensory processing and the ability to modulate sensory input. Within a few weeks, Alex began to mold to his mother when she held him and was less irritable and more relaxed in situations with auditory stimulation. After 3 months of therapy, Alex's mother reported increased cuddling and noticeable improvement in eating. He attempted a greater variety of foods and few aversions, feeding time was shorter, and it was no longer necessary to use the television as a diversion to get him to eat. Alex began to interact more with his siblings and explore his environment. Best of all, he no longer had temper tantrums when his mother left the room. His childcare provider reported that Alex tolerated the prone position and weight bearing on his hands; he had recently begun to crawl. Play skills and hand use also appeared to increase.

Case Study 2: Jeremy
Background

Jeremy's pediatric neurologist referred him for a transdisciplinary assessment at 18 months of age because of motor delays caused by his mitochondrial encephalopathy. An early intervention team, which consisted of an occupational therapist, a physical therapist, a speech-language pathologist, and an early childhood interventionist assessed him in an arena assessment. Both parents participated in the assessment. Although Jeremy had received occupational therapy and physical therapy since he was 6 months old, his parents thought he would benefit from a small group in which he could receive his therapies and special instruction in an integrated manner.

Assessment

The team chose to administer the BDI and HELP. They administered the latter through observation, direct administration of test items, and interview with the parents. The team modified portions to accommodate for Jeremy's physical limitations. Most importantly, the therapists engaged him in play activities and used their interpretation of his interactions and movements to estimate his functional abilities.

Overall, Jeremy had very low muscle tone and poor physical endurance. He needed support for sitting and could only bear some of his weight when supported in standing. He was unable to roll or crawl. Head control was poor with head stacking in a supported sitting position and lack of head righting in the prone position. He used his left hand very well to play with toys when he was positioned appropriately but did not use his right hand and protested when the therapist attempted to evaluate passive range of motion. Jeremy was alert and interested but was reluctant to leave his mother's lap. Communication skills and cognition appeared to be on age level, whereas social skills seemed immature.

Intervention

Jeremy started in the summer session of a center-based early intervention program as part of a group of six children who met twice a week. He received occupational therapy, physical therapy, speech therapy, and special instruction in a small group format with close coordination and carry over of all skills throughout the 4-hour session. The team aimed all therapies and special instruction at helping Jeremy improve social interaction with peers, improve self-help skills, and develop physical abilities to the greatest extent possible. The team obtained adapted seating and eating utensils for him and modified group activities to enable him to participate actively and as independently as possible.

Individual Family Service Plan Review

After 6 months, the service coordinator, intervention team, and family members met to review the goals on Jeremy's IFSP and to update and modify it as needed. The family and the team were pleased with Jeremy's progress and thought that he was benefiting from his intervention program. However, they also discussed Jeremy's need to be around his normally developing peers and participate in community-based activities. Jeremy was gaining confidence in a small group, developing good social and communication skills, and no longer tiring as easily. When he reached 2 years of age, the team decided to add an inclusion program to his early intervention services.

Jeremy's service coordinator arranged for him to participate in a special grant program at a local childcare center. He was enrolled in a class for 2-year-old children that met a few hours a week and had the support of an assistant who had been trained to facilitate the inclusion of children with special needs in the typical childcare setting. Although this facilitator had several other children to work with and was not in Jeremy's class all the time, she was available at any time that he needed help or that the teacher had a question or concern. After a few months, Jeremy started attending this program two times a week; meanwhile, he continued to attend the early intervention program and receive his therapies.

Annual reassessment

One year after entrance into the early intervention program, the intervention team reassessed Jeremy in preparation for the development of a new IFSP. They did not perform this assessment in a formal testing session but over a period of weeks as Jeremy participated in various activities with the group. In addition to the BDI, Jeremy's team also updated the HELP.

Results of the reassessment indicated a bright, happy, verbal 2-year-old child. Although he had gained in physical abilities, Jeremy needed a stroller-type wheelchair with special inserts for appropriate seating. The removable seat also acted as a floor sitter so that Jeremy could be close to the same level as his peers when they played on the floor. The teacher observed that Jeremy had shown considerable improvement in his play skills and that they were definitely more appropriate when he was positioned upright rather than lying on the floor. He demonstrated spontaneous interactions with his peers, he took turns with little prompting, and he began to share toys.

Jeremy continued to participate in the class at the childcare center, although the grant had ended and the facilitator was no longer there. Initially, the childcare center believed that they would be unable to take Jeremy without the support of the facilitator. The occupational therapist and the physical therapist provided on-site consultation. Through a problem-solving approach with close cooperation among the family, childcare personnel, and therapists, strategies were developed that made it possible for Jeremy to remain in the class. These strategies included providing wheelchair access to the playground (they had been carrying him), teaching principles of lifting and carrying, and making the stroller available to transport him from room to room so that the teacher had her hands free to keep up with other active 2-year-old children.

Summary

Jeremy is an example of a child who was able to benefit from a combination of programming that included center-based early intervention and inclusion in a typical childcare setting. This required close cooperation among the family, early intervention personnel, and community resources. As Jeremy grows and develops, his parents plan to place him in a total inclusion program, but they believe that, at 2½ years of age, he still needs the intense intervention that he gets in the center-based program. Meanwhile, they look forward to his graduation to the class for 3-year-old children and increasing his typical class time to 3 days a week. They have already visited the neighborhood school and hope that he will attend a regular kindergarten class when he is 5 years of age and will be supported by therapies at school. Jeremy is bright, and with the right kind of support and technology, he should be able to grow up in the mainstream of society.

STUDY QUESTIONS

1. Briefly describe the potential roles of the occupational therapist in (a) developing and writing the IFSP and (b) planning the child's transition into preschool.

2. Compare the screening process with the evaluation process. Include a comparison of the (a) purpose of each, (b) types of instruments used in each, and (c) outcomes of each process.

3. Describe developmentally appropriate and family-centered intervention approaches.

4. You are the therapist of a 2-year-old boy with severe cognitive and motor delays. The child is not yet sitting and has limited range of movement in extremities. He eats pureed food and requires thickened liquids because of delays in oral motor skills. His manipulation skills are limited to grasp and release and waving and banging. He is visually alert and seems to enjoy visual stimuli. He has no independent mobility. His family is supportive and caring. His parents have been actively involved with the occupational therapist. Describe appropriate goals and activities for (a) enhancing the child's play (see also Chapter 17), (b) improving sensory integration, (c) improving his fine motor skills, and (d) increasing the variety of food textures that he consumes (see Chapter 15).

References

Bayley, N. (1993). *Bayley Scales of Infant Development (2nd ed.).* San Antonio, TX: The Psychological Corp.

Bricker, D. (Ed.). (1993). *AEPS measurement for birth to three years.* Baltimore: Brookes.

Brown, W., & Rule, S. (1993). Personnel and disciplines in early intervention. In W. Brown, S.K. Thurman, & L.K. Pearl (Eds.), *Family-centered early intervention with infants and toddlers and innovative cross-disciplinary approaches.* Baltimore: Brookes.

Burke, J. (1998) Play: The life role of the infant and young child. In J. Case-Smith (Ed.), *Pediatric occupational therapy and early intervention.* (pp. 189-206). Boston: Butterworth-Heinemann.

Case-Smith, J. (1998a). Assessment. In J. Case-Smith (Ed.), *Pediatric occupational therapy and early intervention.* (pp. 49-82). Boston: Butterworth-Heinemann.

Case-Smith, J. (1998b). Defining the early intervention process. In J. Case-Smith (Ed.), *Pediatric occupational therapy and early intervention.* (pp. 27-48). Boston: Butterworth-Heinemann.

Case-Smith, J., & Wavrek, B. (1998). Models of service delivery and team interaction. In J. Case-Smith (Ed.), *Pediatric occupational therapy and early intervention.* (pp. 83-108). Boston: Butterworth-Heinemann.

DeGangi, G.A., & Greenspan, S.I. (1989). *Test of Sensory Functions in Infants manual.* Los Angeles: Western Psychological Services.

Division of Early Childhood. (1993). DEC position statement on inclusion. *DEC Communicator, 19,* 4.

Dunst, C.J. (1991). Implementation of the individualized family service plan. In M.J. McGonigel, R. Kaufmann, & B. Johnson (Eds.), *Guidelines and recommended practices for the individualized family service plan* (2nd ed.). (pp. 67-78). Bethesda, MD: Association for the Care of Children's Health.

Featherstone, H. (1980). *A difference in the family.* New York: Basic Books.

Folio, M.R., & Fewell, R.R. (2000). *Peabody Developmental Motor Scales and activity cards: A manual (2nd ed.).* Austin: Pro Ed.

Frankenburg, W.K., Dodds, J., Archer, P., Bresnick, B., Maschka, P., Edelman, N., & Shapiro, H. (1990). *Denver II screening manual.* Denver: Denver Developmental Materials.

Furuno, S., O'Reilly, K.A., Hosaka, C.M., Inatsuka, T.T., Allman, T.L., & Zeisloft, B. (1994). *Hawaii Early Learning Profile activity guide.* Palo Alto, CA: Vort.

Giangreco, M.F. (1986). Delivery of therapeutic services in special education programs for learners with severe handicaps. *Physical and Occupational Therapy in Pediatrics, 6,* 5.

Glass, R., & Wolf, L. (1998). Feeding and oral motor skills. In J. Case-Smith (Ed.), *Pediatric occupational therapy and early intervention.* (pp. 127-166). Boston: Butterworth-Heinemann.

Greenspan, S.I. (1992). *Infancy and early childhood.* Madison, CT: International Universities Press.

Greenspan, S.I., & Meisels, S. (1994). Toward a new vision for the developmental assessment of infants and young children. *Zero To Three, 14* (6), 2-41.

Hanft, B. (1989). The changing environment of early intervention services: Implications for practice. In B. Hanft (Ed.), *Family-centered care: An early intervention resource manual.* Rockville, MD: American Occupational Therapy Association.

Hanson, M.J. (1990). Honoring the cultural diversity of families when gathering data. *Topics in Early Childhood Special Education, 10* (1), 112-131.

Hanson, M.J. (1998). Ethnic, cultural, and language diversity in intervention settings. In E. Lynch & M. Hanson (Eds.), *Developing cross-cultural competence* (2nd ed. pp. 3-22). Baltimore: Brookes.

Hanson, M.J., & Lynch, E. (1989). *Early intervention: Implementing child and family services for infants and toddlers who are at risk or disabled.* Austin: Pro Ed.

Individuals with Disabilities Education Act of 1990 (P.L. 102-119), 20 USC Secs. 1400-1485.

Johnson, L.J. (1994). Challenges facing early intervention: An overview. In L.J. Johnson, R.J. Gallagher, M.J. La Montagne, J. Jordon, J. Gallagher, P. Hutinger, & M. Karnes (Eds.), *Meeting early intervention challenges* (pp. 1-12). Baltimore: Brookes.

Johnson-Martin, N., Jens, K., Attermeier, S., & Hacker, B. (1996). *The Carolina Curriculum for Infants and Toddlers with Special Needs (2nd ed.).* Baltimore: Brookes Publishing.

Kramer, S., McGonigel, M., & Kaufman, R. (1991). Developing the IFSP: Outcomes, strategies, activities, and services. In M. McGonigel, R. Kaufmann, & B. Johnson (Eds.), *Guidelines and recommended practices for the individualized family service plan* (2nd ed.). Bethesda, MD: Association for the Care of Children's Health.

Linder, T.W. (1993a). *Transdisciplinary play–based assessment: A functional approach to working with young children.* Baltimore: Brookes.

Linder, T.W. (1993b). *Transdisciplinary play–based intervention: Guidelines for developing a meaningful curriculum for young children.* Baltimore: Brookes.

McGonigel, M.J. (1991). Philosophy and conceptual framework. In M.J. McGonigel, R.K. Kaufmann, & B.H. Johnson (Eds.), *Guidelines and recommended practice for the Individualized Family Service Plan* (pp. 7-14). Bethesda, MD: Association for the Care of Children's Health.

McGonigel, M.J., Woodruff, G., & Roszmann-Millican, M. (1994). *The transdisciplinary team: A model for family-centered early intervention* (pp. 95-132). Baltimore: Brookes.

McLean, M., & McCormick, K. (1993). Assessment and evaluation in early intervention. In W. Brown, S.K. Thurman, & L.K. Pearl (Eds.), *Family-centered early intervention with infants and toddlers and innovative cross-disciplinary approaches.* Baltimore: Brookes.

Miller, L.J. (1994). Journey to a desirable future: A value-based model of infant and toddler assessment. *Zero To Three, 14* (6), 23-26.

Newborg, J., Stock, J.R., Wnek, L., Guidubaldi, J., & Svinicki, J. (1988). *Battelle Developmental Inventory.* Chicago: Riverside.

Orelove, F.P., & Sobsey, D. (1991). *Educating children with multiple disabilities: A transdisciplinary approach.* Baltimore: Brookes.

Ottenbacher, K. (1983). Transdisciplinary service delivery in school environment: Some limitations. *Physical and Occupational Therapy in Pediatrics, 3,* 9.

Shonkoff, J.P., & Meisels, S.J. (1990). Early childhood intervention: The evolution of a concept. In S.J. Meisels & J.P. Shonkoff (Eds.), *Handbook of early childhood intervention* (pp. 3-31). Cambridge, MA: Cambridge University Press.

Simeonsson, R.J., & Bailey, D.B. (1990). Family dimensions in early intervention. In S.J. Meisels & J.P. Shonkoff (Eds.), *Handbook of early childhood intervention.* Cambridge, MA: Cambridge University Press.

Simons, R. (1985). *After the tears.* New York: Harcourt Brace Jovanovich.

Sparrow, S., Balla, D.A., & Cicchetti, D.V. (1984). *Vineland Adaptive Behavior Scales.* Circle Pines, MN: American Guidance Service.

Stallings-Sahler, S. (1998). Sensory integration: Assessment and intervention with infants. In J. Case-Smith (Ed.), *Pediatric occupational therapy and early intervention* (pp. 309-341). Boston: Butterworth-Heinemann.

Teti, T.M., & Gibbs, E.D. (1990). Infant assessment: Historical antecedents and contemporary issues. In E.D. Gibbs & D.M. Teti (Eds.), *Interdisciplinary assessment of infants* (pp. 3-10). Baltimore: Brookes.

Turnbull, A.P., Turnbull, H.R., & Blue-Banning, M. (1994). Enhancing inclusion of infants and toddlers with disabilities and their families: A theoretical and programmatic analysis. *Infants and Young Children, 7* (2), 1-14.

Vohs, J. (1989). Recommendations for working with families and children with special needs from diverse cultures. In J. Vohs (Ed.), Organizational resources for understanding families from diverse cultures. *Coalition Quarterly: Toward Multiculturalism, 6* (2 & 3), 23.

chapter 23

Occupational Therapy in Preschool and Childcare Settings

Sharon Gartland
(with contributions from Sue Ann DuBois)

key terms

Preschool and childcare settings
Occupation-centered practice
Top-down approach
Occupational science
Collaborative teaming

■ CHAPTER OBJECTIVES

1. Describe the context of preschool and childcare settings and explain how this knowledge influences practice of occupational therapy.
2. Discuss the typical childhood occupations performed in preschool and childcare settings.
3. List the typical development of 3- to 4-year-old children in mobility, eye-hand and arm use, prewriting skills, visual-motor skills, and self-help skills.
4. Perform an activity analysis on a preschool occupation.
5. Describe the role of the occupational therapist in preschool and childcare settings.
6. Explain the various models of service delivery commonly used in preschool settings.
7. Explain a top-down approach to assessment and intervention in preschool settings.
8. Apply knowledge of therapy approaches and models of service delivery to a case study of a child with autism.

The focus of pediatric occupational therapists is helping young clients to develop the functional skills neces-

sary to perform daily occupations. Interventions to promote a child's occupations appear to be most effective when implemented in natural contexts (i.e., where the occupations are performed on a regular basis and are linked to social and physical environments that encourage child's generalization and integration of skills). This chapter examines occupational therapy services in preschools and childcare centers.

■ UNDERSTANDING THE CONTEXT OF PRESCHOOLS AND CHILDCARE CENTERS

To provide insightful and effective services, the occupational therapist must have a good grasp of the context in which those services are to be provided. Understanding the temporal, physical, cultural, and social contexts of preschools and childcare centers allows the therapist to analyze the issues and concerns surrounding specific children. This understanding is also vital to the therapist's effectiveness as a member of an educational team. In the following sections, these aspects of preschool contexts are discussed.

Temporal Context

A wide variety of scheduling options are available to the parents of children in preschool and childcare centers. Because parents often work full-time, many preschools offer childcare services before and after their more formal programs. These preschools may have a mix of children: those who attend all day and those who attend for just a few hours of formal instruction. Childcare centers may have a less-structured curriculum but continue to provide many opportunities for developing competence and independence throughout the day. In preschool settings, the caregivers may address a child's toilet training, feeding, dressing, and play skills as frequently his or her parents.

The occupational therapist works within the daily schedule of the preschool program. A typical half-day preschool might have a schedule as follows:

9:00 to 9:30 AM	Arrival time: children walk in, hang up coats, have free-choice playtime
9:30 to 10:00 AM	Group time: children sit on rug, teachers greet children, sing good morning song, read story
10:00 to 10:45 AM	Center time: children go to various tables with crafts, cooking projects, puzzles, and other activities.
10:45 to 11:00 AM	Morning clean-up time: children straighten up area and wash hands for snack
11:00 to 11:15 AM	Snack time: children pass out cups, napkins, crackers, and juice; and then sit and eat snack
11:15 to 11:45 AM	Outdoor play time: Children put on coats and go outside
11:45 AM to 12:00 PM	Clean-up time: children gather toys, sing good-bye songs
12:00 PM	Departure time: children go home

Physical Context

Childcare centers or preschools should be clean, well lit, and safe for children. There should be an array of enticing and developmentally appropriate toys available for play. Most preschools settings have the following materials and supplies available:

- Toys for fine-motor and visual-motor play: puzzles, crayons, scissors, paints, and small manipulatives such as Tinker Toys, Legos, and bristle blocks.
- Toys for gross-motor play: climbing equipment, large blocks, riding toys, balls, jump ropes, and dance music (Figure 23-1).
- Toys for imaginative and symbolic play: trucks, dolls, and dress-up clothes (Figure 23-2).
- Toys for sensory exploration: sandbox, water table, play dough, and finger paints.
- Books with pictures and simple words.

The preschool environment and space encourage the independence of young children as they perform and

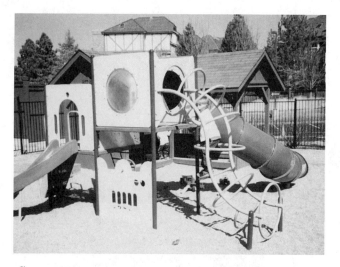

figure**23-1** Playground equipment for gross-motor play.

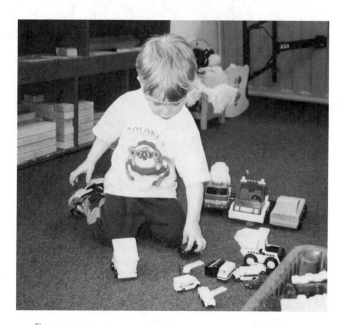

figure**23-2** Toys for imaginative and symbolic play.

master such tasks as using the toilet, washing hands, serving snacks, putting away toys, hanging up coats, and working independently at the tables. Specific features of this environment include:

- Child-sized chairs and tables
- Lowered sinks (with faucets that are easy to manipulate)
- Lowered paper towel dispensers
- Well-organized toy storage system (many schools use photos to indicate where toys belong)
- Small-sized toilets
- Low hooks and *cubbies* (individualized storage shelves)
- Small, lightweight pitchers for juice

One of the most effective ways that occupational therapists can partner with preschools and childcare centers is to make recommendations for the physical environment that will maximize the learning experience for all the children, with particular attention to accommodation for children with special needs.

Social Context

In addition to the occupational therapist, members of the preschool team often include:

- Teacher
- Aide
- Parent
- Speech–Language Pathologist
- Psychologist
- School Nurse
- Social Worker
- Physical Therapist

The qualifications and training of the teacher may vary depending on the setting. Public school settings require their teachers to have college degrees and state certification, whereas many private preschools and childcare centers employ teachers who do not have early childhood degrees. However, these private preschool teachers may be rich in experience and practical training. Childcare aides and staff may have minimal to no training in early childhood education. Typically, staff members of preschool and childcare settings receive low rates of compensation regardless of their level of education. Being sensitive to that reality, as well as understanding the background and training of all the team members, is important to the occupational therapist's ability to consult effectively in these settings.

The primary goal of most preschools is to provide a safe and motivating place for young children to gain the developmental skills they need (including social skills and motor skills) for success in later school experiences. Although some preschool programs have an academic focus, most emphasize preacademic skills such as paying attention to task when in a group, following rules, getting along with peers, participating in sensory-motor play, cutting, coloring, and writing, as well as basic self-help skills.

Cultural Context
Educational philosophy

Many preschools base their programming on a particular philosophy or theory of education. One of the most influential theorists in early childhood education is Jean Piaget. His theories supported the idea that children were active learners, who, through interactions with their environments, construct their own knowledge (Bowman, 1997). Another commonly identified preschool philosophy comes from Maria Montessori. Montessori schools place a high value on individual exploration within a highly structured environment (Richardson & Onesti, 1997).

In most preschools today, these educational philosophies are blended and the preschool staff have established their own philosophy and mission. Taking the time to discuss educational philosophy and mission with team members can enlighten occupational therapists and enhance their ability to provide quality services. Including occupational therapy's own theories on occupation and development may strengthen the teacher's ability to structure an optimal learning environment.

Religious philosophy

Many private preschools and childcare centers are located within churches and synagogues. Religious training may be part of the curriculum and should be understood and respected by the occupational therapists providing services in that setting. Examples of occupations that reflect religious philosophy include prayer before meals, kosher food during snack time, or lighting of candles during certain holy days. Many preschools with a religious foundation may use Bible stories as the basis for games, arts-and-craft activities, and other tasks.

Historical and Legal Context

It is only in the last 50 years that it has become a common experience for children in the 3- to 5-year-old age range to attend some sort of educational program outside of the home. Nursery schools developed as enrichment programs to address the needs of children in underprivileged homes (such as Head Start, which began in 1965) and as a way for middle- and upper-middle class families to increase their children's success in school (Cahan, 1985). Currently it is unusual for a child to enter kindergarten without previous learning experience outside the home environment.

Public health programs were the first to recognize the needs and civil rights of young children. The Social Security Act, enacted in 1935, authorized financial assistance to states to develop services that promoted the health of mothers and children of low socioeconomic status and crippled children. As a result, states developed Maternal and Child Health (MCH) programs and established Bureaus for Handicapped Children (Shonkoff & Meisels, 1990). These programs continue to receive federal funds and provide health services to mothers and children. In the 1940s and 1950s, occupational therapists primarily served preschoolers through nonprofit agencies such as United Cerebral Palsy and the National Easter Seal Society.

The Handicapped Children's Early Education Assistance Act of 1968 provided funds for experimental programs for children up to 8 years old who had disabilities. Several years later the Education for all Handicapped Children Act (EHA) of 1975 established programs that made available incentive funds to states that established preschool programs. This federal legislation supported the protection of the basic rights of children with disabilities to a free appropriate public education. In this law and its subsequent amendments, occupational therapy is defined as a "related service," whose purpose is to assist students with disabilities in benefiting from their special education program in public schools. Services for each preschool child are guided by a written plan called an *Individualized Education Program* (IEP). An IEP is a legal document that defines the child's goals and objectives and acts as a blueprint for each child's special education program.

In 1986, amendments to the EHA expanded the programs authorized under Part B by mandating special education services to children 3 to 5 years of age. In 1990 the EHA was reauthorized and retitled the Individuals with Disabilities Education Act (IDEA).

In the IDEA amendments of 1990 and 1997, the role of occupational therapists has remained unchanged. IDEA (1997) strengthens the role of parents in educational planning and decision making on behalf of their children. It focuses the student's educational planning process on promoting meaningful access to the general curriculum. Changes that are particularly relevant to occupational therapists include clarification of the regulations regarding discipline for children with disabilities and the inclusion of regular education teachers on the IEP team. These amendments also establish a new standard for writing team IEP goals that relate to the general curriculum.

An additional piece of legislature that affects services to preschoolers is the Americans with Disabilities Act (ADA) (1990). This is a civil rights law intended to bring individuals with disabilities into the mainstream of American life (Kalscheur, 1992). Title II of this law addresses access to public services, programs, and facilities. Segregated educational programs, recreation programs, and playgrounds administered through state and local governments for children with disabilities are prohibited (Kalscheur, 1992). Title III of the ADA requires all public accommodations and services operated by private entities to be accessible to persons with disabilities.

Federal laws and regulations, with corresponding state regulations and rules, protect rights of children with disabilities to a free and appropriate education. These laws and regulations also protect their right to all public services, programs, and facilities.

■ ROLE OF THE OCCUPATIONAL THERAPIST IN PRESCHOOL SERVICES

When working in a preschool setting, the role of the occupational therapist is to support the child's ability to successfully perform the occupations related to that environment. As a related service provider in special education, the occupational therapist's primary role is to facilitate educational outcomes, in collaboration with other professionals who are providing services for the child and family (AOTA, 1997).

Occupational therapists implement therapeutic occu-

pation to increase independence in daily activities such as play, self-care, classroom maintenance, and preacademic skills. The occupational therapist may also participate in designing environments that enhance overall development and prevent disability. In addition, the therapist may consult on and adapt curriculum and provide necessary supports (e.g., adapted equipment). With the needs of children with disabilities in mind, therapists may also serve in consultation roles regarding designing daily schedules, selecting curricula, developing behavioral plans, and adapting physical environments.

For the clinician in a preschool setting, it is important to grasp the powerful essence of occupation by valuing the ordinary stream of tasks that make-up a child's daily routines. This means that the therapist must use language, assessment tools, and intervention techniques that clearly indicate what occupation is, why it should be valued, and why it should be addressed.

Disabilities, such as cerebral palsy, developmental delay, autism, muscular dystrophy, attention deficit disorder (ADD), and pervasive developmental disorder (PDD), present unique challenges for a child's successful performance of occupations. Contextual variables, such as homelessness, poverty, abuse, and lead or drug exposure, also challenge a child's ability to successfully develop health occupations and roles. Because the goal of intervention is successful participation in the occupations of a preschool child, it is important to identify the typical occupations of children in preschool environments and to begin to analyze the many factors involved in the performance of these occupations.

Play

Play is considered to be one of the major occupations of childhood. Not only is play an activity in which children engage, it is also a primary medium for intervention and a "style we use when we approach problems and situations in a flexible manner" (Bundy, 1992, p. 217). For most preschool-age children, all action has the potential to become play, depending on the attitude and manner with which they perform the task. Research has shown that play is one of the occupations that is often significantly affected by the presence of disability (Bundy, 1989; Clifford & Bundy, 1989; Restall & Magill-Evans, 1994). Missiuna and Pollock (1991) delineated the physical, social, personal, and environmental barriers that may limit the play experiences of children with physical disabilities. These include the following:

- Limitations imposed by caregivers
- Physical and personal limitations of the child
- Environmental barriers such as steps and narrow doorways
- Difficulties in interactions with peers
- Lack of parental playfulness when interacting with the child

It is vital that play be understood and valued so that it

can be used both as therapeutic occupation and adaptive occupation (Fisher, 1998). The occupational therapist must also develop his or her own sense of playfulness to enter into the child's world. A sense of playfulness also helps the therapist plan and provide an enticing and effective treatment.

Self-Help and Classroom-Maintenance Tasks

Self-maintenance and a sense of personal responsibility develop in the preschool years. Deficits in these childhood occupations are often what prompt a referral to occupational therapy. Therefore, quality childcare centers and preschool settings should provide opportunities for a child to grow in self-help and classroom-maintenance skills (Figure 23-3). Experienced teachers may have their own adaptations and "tricks" to help children move to competency in these areas and can teach these to the therapists with whom they work. When their "bag of tricks" is exhausted, they may seek outside help from occupational therapists or other professionals. The following list of self-help and classroom-maintenance tasks are embedded in the routines of a preschool or daycare setting (Box 23-1).

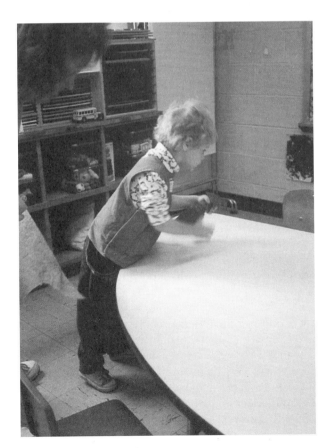

figure **23-3** Preschool settings offer opportunities to develop new skills. Table cleaning provides support for hand strength and prescissors skills.

Preacademic Skills

During the preschool years the underlying skills, which provide the foundation for good academic skills in later years, are developed. Foundational to school function is competence in motor planning, postural stability, in-hand manipulation, visual-perceptual skills, self-control, modulation of sensory input, gross-motor coordination, and many others (Ayres, 1979). Helping teachers to understand the preparatory role of a wide variety of sensorimotor tasks may help them to continue to value and incorporate them in their classroom settings. The occupational therapist can help influence and educate preschool teachers in the selection of occupations that prepare children for academic work. The following list of common preacademic skills are part of the occupations of the preschooler (Box 23-2).

---

box 23-1 Self-help and classroom-maintenance occupations

Dressing: putting on and taking off outerwear such as gloves, scarves, hat, jacket
Hanging up jacket
Toilet training
Hand washing
Nose care
Self-feeding: finger-feeding, use of utensils
Opening lunch box
Opening milk cartons
Picking up toys
Passing out crackers
Pouring liquids into cups
Passing out papers
Updating calendar
Watering plants
Washing tables
Feeding pets
Cleaning cages

---

box 23-2 Preacademic occupations

Fine-motor skills
Pencil and paper tasks: forming letters and numbers
Coloring
Cutting
Attention to tasks
Sitting in a group
Following directions
Asking for help
Completing tasks
Sensorimotor play
Constructional play

■ PROVISION OF SERVICES

Assessment Process

The following sections describe the process an occupational therapist uses to assess a child's strengths and needs in the context of the preschool environment. This process involves three main steps: (1) referral, (2) screening, and (3) evaluation.

Referral

A referral initiates the process of determining whether occupational therapy is warranted to support the child's ability to learn and function in the preschool setting. Many children are first identified as needing special education services through a screening process. The student's family, teacher, or other members of the student's educational team may generate the referral. In some cases, the referral comes through physicians, parents, or other professionals who recognize delays in a child's development and deem it best to provide services in the preschool or childcare environment.

Screening

Screening of preschool children is an initial, short-term process of data collection that is used to determine program eligibility, need for intervention, or need for further in-depth assessment of a particular area of performance. The occupational therapist may independently screen the preschooler or participate in an interdisciplinary screening. As a member of the preschool screening team, the therapist may travel to homes, agencies, and schools to complete screening procedures. In some districts, specific times of the year are dedicated to preschool screenings.

The level of interdisciplinary teaming within each school often determines how and what screening procedures are used by occupational therapists. Some schools rely on district-made developmental checklists, with assignment of specific performance areas to be administered by specific disciplines. In other school systems, the occupational therapists independently select and administer the screening instrument. The resulting information is then combined with the team's collection of data to determine if the child's performance warrants referral for further evaluation.

One screening instrument specific to preschoolers is the First STEP: Screening Test for Evaluating Preschoolers (Miller, 1993). This is an individually administered, norm-referenced screening test used to identify developmental delays in children ages 2 years, 9 months through 6 years, 2 months. It was developed to identify preschool children who are at risk in cognition, communication, physical, social and emotional, and adaptive functioning.

In many preschool settings, occupational therapists are not part of the initial screening team. Referrals may be generated once the initial IEP has been written. However, some occupational therapists in private practice provide developmental screenings in community preschools and childcare centers.

Evaluation

Occupation-centered assessment requires the use of a top-down approach. This kind of assessment begins by gathering information about what the child wants or needs to do to perform his or her occupations in a satisfactory way. Occupation-centered assessment ensures that the whole child is considered during the evaluation process (Coster, 1998). Considering the lack of standardized tools used to assess a child's occupations, therapists usually begin with informal observation and interviewing. Information about the child's preferred occupations and performance problems across environments is gathered. By asking adults who are involved with the child about his or her occupations, the therapist informs the teacher and parent about his or her interests in cultural, physical, and social contexts, which are related to the child's performance.

Interviews. It is very helpful (prior to more formal evaluation methods) to interview parents and teachers. Although the service context is the preschool setting, much can be learned about the child by seeking information about his or her ability to function in childhood occupations at home. An effective way to obtain information about the child's daily performance is to ask the parent to describe a typical day in the child's life. Seeking clarification on occupations (e.g., dressing, feeding, grooming, playing, and performing chores) as the daily routine is described, enables the therapist to easily identify areas of concern. Comparing parental perspectives with those of teachers can also help the therapist to better understand the influence of the child's environment on function. Beginning with questions about daily occupations can reveal specific component areas that need to be further explored. Taking the time to make a phone call to the parent or teacher prior to seeing a child will also assist the occupational therapist in selecting appropriate standardized tests.

File reviews. The educational file review entails a review of information and data previously collected about the child. This may include medical documents, documents of services in an early intervention program, intake procedures provided by the school, or documents of the student's performance on standardized tests. Parents of preschool children who are referred for occupational therapy may have their own file of medical reports, immunization records, and other professional evaluations (e.g., physical therapy or speech-language pathology reports). Record review is particularly useful when a child has a history of medical problems, is on medications, has received therapy services in the past, or has previously undergone evaluation for services.

Skilled observations and activity analyses. If possible, it is best to schedule time to observe the child in his or her preschool or childcare environment. Optimally, observing the child several different times a day in different settings generates the most accurate picture. It is almost always possible to take a few moments to note the objects in the room, the overall sensory stimulation of the classroom, the teacher's style, and the child's interaction with others. Observing one classroom activity, such as completing a puzzle, gives the therapist information on the child's attention span, motor skills, cognitive abilities, overall developmental level, social skills, and visual-perceptual skills (Figure 23-4). Skilled activity analysis contributes detailed, specific information that is helpful in interpreting performance. Table 23-1 presents an example of this type of activity analysis.

An activity analysis provides information about the performance components required to complete the task. Personal characteristics and environmental features must also be evaluated to complete an assessment of occupational performance. The next section provides an example of an in-depth activity analysis of a classroom occupation.

After observing occupations performed in their natural physical and temporal context, it is sometimes expedient to present the child with opportunities to play with certain toys or perform certain tasks (rather than to wait for these observations to occur naturally). The skilled therapist assesses the influence of meaning and motivation when analyzing these data. If a child is asked to wash his or her hands or hang up a coat when it is not actually necessary or natural to do so, he or she may exhibit a very different quality of skill than is seen at other times. Therefore, verifying observations with teachers and aides is always wise.

When the therapist has gained a sufficient amount of information through skilled observation, he or she may want to proceed to gathering more specific information about the child's personal characteristics. This is done through *clinical observation*. Clinical observation may include assessment of (1) muscle tone, (2) postural reaction and control, (3) range of motion, (4) movement patterns, (5) motor planning, (6) bilateral integration and sequencing, (7) manipulation, (8) ocular-motor control, (9) sensory awareness and reactivity, (10) touch and

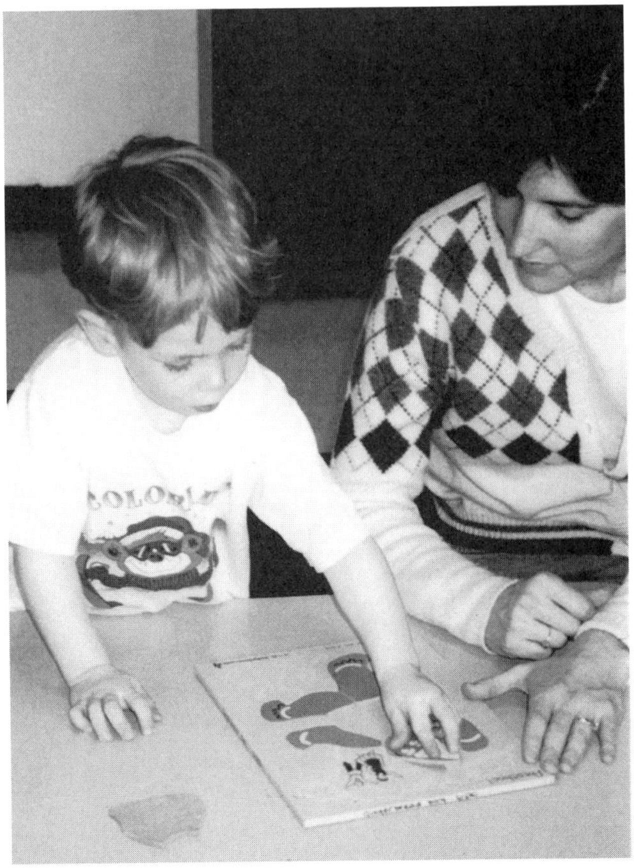

figure 23-4   Observing a child complete a puzzle gives the therapist information about attention span, motor skills, cognitive abilities, social skills, and visual-perceptual skills.

table 23-1   In-Depth Activity Analysis

Passing Out Crackers for Snack-Time: Steps Involved	Skills Needed to Complete Task Successfully
1. Teacher asks child to pass out crackers.	1. Ability to hear and follow directions
2. Child retrieves crackers from cabinet. Child passes out the crackers to the other children.	2. Values task and wants to complete it Mobility: gets to cabinet and walks around table
3. Child opens box of crackers. Child opens paper liner inside box of crackers. Child pulls out one cracker and places it on a napkin.	3. Visual-perceptual skills, such as figure-ground to locate box in cupboard
4. Child moves to next place at table and repeats until all children are served.	4. Fine-motor skills: pincer grasp, bilateral skills to hold box with one hand and pull out cracker with the other, gross grasp of box Proprioceptive awareness: such as holding cracker with appropriate pressure so as not to break it
5. Child closes box of crackers and returns box to cabinet.	5. Sequencing
	6. Self-control: does not eat crackers until snack time

proprioception reactivity, (11) vestibular function, and (12) oral-motor control.

Checklists. Checklists are often valuable tools for assessing preschoolers' performances in their educational setting. These forms should include items for evaluating functional mobility, self-help, and manipulation of classroom materials. Often checklists are generated from chronologic skills profiles. Tables 23-2, 23-3, and 23-4 provide the developmental skills of 3-, 4-, and 5-year-old children.

Using varying combinations of this information provides occupational therapists with a quick point of reference to determine whether the preschooler demonstrates isolated or generalized skill delays. If information about

table 23-2 Development Skills Profile, 3 Years

Mobility	Eye-Hand and Arm Use	Prewriting Skills	Visual-Motor Skills	Self-Help Skills
Rides tricycle Stands briefly on one foot Jumps from step with two feet Alternates feet part way walking on balance beam Alternates feet walking upstairs Runs with wide base	Isolates thumb from fist in imitation Builds nine-block tower with 1-inch cubes Catches ball with extended arms and body Demonstrates preferred hand in manipulations and tool use Supination emerges in grasp of spoon and fork Strings ½-inch beads	Holds pencil with first two fingers and thumb with good control Copies circle Imitates cross Traces square Scribbles	Imitates 3-block bridge Matches and recognizes primary colors and sizes grossly (big, little, long, and short) Identifies body parts (toes, back, stomach, chin, knee, and neck) Identifies front and behind	Unties bow Unbuttons large and small (1-inch then ⅜-inch buttons) Snaps and unsnaps Unzips separating zipper Zips and unzips non-separating zipper Dresses and undresses self fully with supervision; assistance needed in right and left shoe recognition and closures Feeds self with little or no spillage

table 23-3 Development Skills Profile, 4 Years

Mobility	Eye-Hand and Arm Use	Prewriting Skills	Visual-Motor Skills	Self-Help Skills
Stands on one foot 3 to 6 seconds Walks up and down steps reciprocally Begins to skip, using a one-foot gallop Hops on one foot 4 to 6 steps Runs more controlled with feet closer together	Uses preferred hand with better coordination More isolated finger movements to include finger spreading and opposition of thumb in sequence to all fingers Grasps spoon and fork with fingers Stacks 10 cubes Threads ¼-inch beads Cuts on lines Throws ball overhand Catches ball with arms slightly flexed	Demonstrates an open web space in tripod pencil grasp; holds distally in fingers Copies cross Imitates square and X Colors pictures but still has difficulty remaining in lines	Identifies directionality concepts of on, under, behind, and beside in relation to body Names four basic colors, shapes, and sizes Builds 6-cube pyramid Completes noninset puzzle of 3 to 5 pieces	Manages buttons completely Zips nonseparating zipper Zips separating zipper Unbuckles and buckles belt or shoes Unhooks pants Uses napkin Recognizes right shoe from left Dresses with minimal supervision Laces shoes

the child's occupational performance indicates possible sensory processing concerns, a checklist format can be sent home to be completed by parents. Team members can also complete a checklist to gather more information about the performance component and its impact on occupation (Figure 23-5).

Standardized tests. Norm- and criterion-referenced tests are widely used in preschool assessment. Used in combination with other parts of evaluation, the standardized evaluation tool can provide a comprehensive occupational therapy profile of the preschooler. Unfortunately, very few standardized tests measure the construct of occupation in pediatrics. A commonly used scale is the Pediatric Evaluation of Disability Inventory (PEDI) (Haley, Coster, Ludlow, Haltiwanger, & Andrellos, 1992). The PEDI measures three content domains: (1) self-care, (2) mobility, and (3) social function. The PEDI was developed to provide a comprehensive clinical assessment of key functional capabilities and performance of functional activities in children between the ages of 6 months and 7 years.

Standardized tests that address the occupation of play are also available. The Preschool Play Scale (Knox, 1997) is an observational assessment designed to give a developmental description of typical play behavior from birth to 6 years. The Test of Playfulness (ToP; Bundy, 1997), is a 60 item observational assessment of playfulness for children ages 2 to 10 years. (See Chapter 17 for more information about these assessments.)

Component-based standardized assessments are currently what is most often utilized in a preschool-age population. These include the following:

- *Miller Assessment for Preschoolers* (MAP) (Miller, 1988). The MAP is designed to evaluate children from ages 2 years, 9 months to 5 years, 8 months. Its purposes are to identify developmentally delayed preschoolers who need further evaluation and to provide a structured, clinical framework to identify strengths and weaknesses.

- *Peabody Developmental Motor Scales, revised* (PDMS) (Folio & Fewell, 2000). The PDMS is a standardized test for children from birth to 83 months. The test measures a child's ability to demonstrate fine- and gross-motor skills that reflect developmental milestones. The scales can be used individually or together. Because the PDMS can produce standard scores, it is often used to determine eligibility for occupational therapy.

- *Pediatric Extended Examination at Three* (PEET) (Blackman, Levine, & Markowitz, 1986) is a developmental assessment designed to aid in the early detection and clarification of problems with learning, attention, and behavior in children 3 to 4 years of age. Developmental performance areas addressed include gross-motor, language, visual-fine motor, memory and intersensory integration skills.

- *Pediatric Examination of Educational Readiness* (PEER) (Levine & Schneider, 1985) uses a set of standardized observations to gain descriptive information about the child's development and neurologic status. The PEER is designed primarily for the evaluation of children 4 to 6 years of age. Performance tasks on this evaluation include orientation, gross-motor, visual-fine motor, sequential, linguistic, and preacademic learning skills.

- *Brigance Diagnostic Inventory of Early Development* (Brigance, 1978) is designed for children from birth to 7 years of age. It contains items that measure gross and fine motor, self-help, communication, general knowledge and comprehension, reading, writing and math skills. The gross-motor, fine-motor, and self-help checklist areas best serve the preschool performance areas addressed by the occupational therapist.

table 23-4	*Developmental Skills Profile, 5 Years*			
Mobility	**Eye-Hand and Arm Use**	**Prewriting Skills**	**Visual-Motor Skills**	**Self-Help Skills**
Stands on one foot for approximately 8 seconds with arms folded Skips alternating feet Walks on balance beam without falling off Moves rhythmically to music	Preferred hand used more consistent Sews through holes in sewing card Catches large ball using two hands Uses a mature lateral grasp of spoon or fork Cuts out circle	Copies square Copies triangle Traces diamond Colors pictures neatly, staying within outlines Traces letters Begins to copy first name	Matches 10 to 12 objects Counts 10 objects Identifies body parts (shoulders and hips) Distinguishes right and left on self Builds a 6-cube step Begins to discriminate secondary colors Completes 12- to 15-piece puzzle	Zips, unzips non-separating back zipper Hooks pants Uses knife for spreading Dresses without supervision Begins to tie shoes Brushes teeth without supervision

NAME:_____

DOB:_____

PERSON COMPLETING CHECKLIST:_____

DATE:_____

Circle Y (yes) N (no) or S (sometimes) with the statement as it relates to your child

Gross and Fine Motor Skills

Difficulty riding a ride-on toy with feet propelling	Y	N	S
Difficulty pumping self on swing	Y	N	S
Dislikes playing with puzzles	Y	N	S
Dislikes playing with small manipulatives	Y	N	S
Difficulty using a spoon or cup	Y	N	S
Seems weaker or tires more easily than others of the same age	Y	N	S
Appears stiff, awkward, or clumsy in movement	Y	N	S
Seems to have much difficulty in learning new motor tasks	Y	N	S
If 4 years of age or older, has difficulty dressing self	Y	N	S
Has messy eating habits	Y	N	S

Movement and Balance Skills

Gets car sick frequently	Y	N	S
Gets nauseated or vomits from other movement experiences (e.g., playground swings, merry go rounds)	Y	N	S
Is unable to give adequate warning about feelings of nausea	Y	N	S
Seeks quantities of twirling or spinning	Y	N	S
Seeks quantities of stimulation on amusement park rides and swings	Y	N	S
Hesitates to climb or play on playground equipment	Y	N	S
Has trouble or hesitancy in learning to climb or descend stairs	Y	N	S
Dislikes being lifted up and gently tossed in the air by parent	Y	N	S
Did not or does not like being placed on his or her stomach or back as an infant	Y	N	S
Rocks himself or herself when stressed	Y	N	S
Period of crawling was absent or very brief	Y	N	S
Walks on toes now or in the past	Y	N	S

Touch

Seems unaware of being touched	Y	N	S
Seems overly sensitive to being touched, pulls away from light touch	Y	N	S
Seems excessively ticklish or strongly dislikes touch	Y	N	S
Dislikes the feeling of certain types of clothing or material or is bothered by the tags in the back of shirts	Y	N	S

figure**23-5**   Preschool sensory motor history for occupational therapy.

Standardized assessment data for the preschooler are interpreted based on their relevance to the child's occupational performance. It is possible that a child may score in the delayed range in some developmental areas, but have very little functional difficulties related to that area. Therapists need to be aware of the uneven process of development experienced in different children as well as the possibility of motivational or environmental factors that affect the testing process. The reporting of "numbers" from these tests must always be interpreted and addressed with the whole picture of the child taken into consideration.

Resists wearing short-sleeve shirts or short pants	Y	N	S
Continues to examine objects by placing them in the mouth (past age of 1½ years old)	Y	N	S
Dislikes being cuddled or hugged unless on child's terms	Y	N	S
Avoids putting hands in messy substances	Y	N	S
Strongly dislikes hair cutting or washing	Y	N	S
Strongly dislikes toe or fingernail cutting	Y	N	S
Pinches, bites, or otherwise hurts self	Y	N	S
Crawled with fisted hands	Y	N	S
Often unaware of bruises, cuts, or scrapes	Y	N	S
Seems overly sensitive to slight bumps or scrapes	Y	N	S
Tendency to touch things constantly	Y	N	S
Frequently pushes or hits other children	Y	N	S

Auditory and Language Skills

Has or has had repeated ear infections	Y	N	S
Particularly distracted by sounds, seeming to hear sounds that go unnoticed by others	Y	N	S
Often fails to listen or pay attention to what is said to him or her	Y	N	S
Is overly sensitive to mildly loud noises	Y	N	S
History of delayed speech development	Y	N	S

Bowel and Bladder Control

Late in achieving bowel and bladder control	Y	N	S
Occasionally has accidents during the day	Y	N	S
If accident occurs, does not seem to be aware ahead of time that elimination is about to occur	Y	N	S

Emotions

Does not easily accept changes in routine	Y	N	S
Becomes easily frustrated	Y	N	S
Likely to be impulsive, heedless, and accident prone	Y	N	S
Marked mood variation, tendency to outbursts or tantrums	Y	N	S
Tends to withdraw from groups; plays on outskirts	Y	N	S

Additional comments or observations that may be important to learning:

figure**23-5, cont'd**   For legend see opposite page.

■ PROGRAM PLANNING

In the public schools, the occupational therapy component of the preschooler's educational program is developed according to the IEP process outlined in the federal mandates of the IDEA. As stated earlier, the IEP is the legal document that defines the child's program of education and related services. The process of IEP development results in a collaborative program that may include specific intervention plans by the occupational therapist (see Chapter 24). These plans are made after the team identifies the child's outcomes and the team members agree that occupational therapy services would be helpful in achieving the student's outcomes.

Generating an occupational therapy plan requires the synthesis of the performance profile with home and school environments, program and curriculum outlines, and team support factors. Information gathered, related to temporal, physical, social, and cultural performance contexts, becomes vital during this process. Data on daily routines, curriculum of the classroom, and physical objects and structures in the environment guide the therapist in determining the treatment plan. The occupational therapist's scheduling needs and training also influence this planning process.

The next step in planning involves identifying the natural school or childcare center environments where occupational performance occurs in the daily routines. This may be the classroom, hallway, bathrooms, bus, or lunchroom. Intervention that addresses specific performance areas, such as hand washing, putting on jacket, or opening of food packages, should occur in the student's natural contexts. Because intervention conforms to the student's schedule, a flexible and collaborative approach to program planning is needed. Team members work together to identify what functional occupations and skill components should be prioritized. This part of program planning requires a particular sensitivity to parent concerns regarding the child.

Struck and Dubois (1993) listed the key features to program planning as follows:

- Addresses the preschooler's needs in the least restrictive environment
- Enables function within the preschool and home setting
- Allows for mutual support through collaboration in daily routine
- Allows for shared decision making with other team members
- Supports the educational program
- Reflects a team approach
- Selects activities that support occupational performance in home and preschool
- Safely implements adaptations and strategies into routines with team members
- Allows for flexibility to meet the preschooler's changing needs

■ INTERVENTION: PRINCIPLES AND STRATEGIES

Intervention entails (1) changing the task, (2) changing the environment or context, (3) changing the child's skills and abilities, or (4) some combination of the first three options.

Changing the Task

Changing the task is accomplished by decreasing the steps involved in a particular task. For example, a child who is struggling to zip her coat might receive assistance to connect the zipper and then be responsible for pulling it up. Another way of changing, or simplifying, a task is to select an easier version of a related task. A child who is unable to complete a 10-piece interlocking puzzle may be much more successful with a 6-piece inset puzzle. A third way to change the task is to provide adaptations that enhance independence. Zipper pulls that are easier for small hands and pegs added to puzzle pieces for successful motor manipulation are both simple adaptations that can be implemented in the daycare or preschool environment.

Assistive technology options also offer many ways to adapt a task and enable a child to perform it successfully. By connecting a switch to a tape recorder, a child with severe physical impairments could participate in a game of musical chairs by controlling the music. Computers can be fitted with touch screens, adapted keyboards, and special software.

Changing the Environment or Context

Changing the environment or context can be done in several ways. The therapist may recommend physical changes in the classroom or childcare setting. These changes may include selection of toys, seating and positioning devices, changes in lighting, changes in teaching methods or curriculum, as well as recommendations for organizing toys or setting up the room. For example, a boy who is having difficulty remaining seated in his own space during circle time could be encouraged to do so through the use of a carpet square. Each child could be given a square to sit on during circle time, creating a physical boundary for the child without causing him to be different from his peers (Figure 23-6).

Providing teachers and caregivers with in-service training on the relationship between sensory processing and arousal level in children, along with suggestions of how to help children modulate sensory information, is another example of changing the environment. Recommending that a child be put in a different classroom, perhaps one with fewer children or a different type of peer group, is yet another way to change the environment for the child.

Changing the Child's Skills and Abilities

Changing the child's skills and abilities is an approach that is used when it is determined that a child can gain skills, grow developmentally in a certain area, or enhance performance through changing personal characteristics such as strength, range-of-motion, visual-perceptual skills, postural stability, cognition, sensory processing skills, fine- and gross-motor skills, and oral-motor skills. This approach is also used when the therapist sees that the child can grow developmentally if he or she is provided with opportunities that enhance performance of a specific occupation, such as play skills, self-help skills, classroom-maintenance skills, and preacademic skills.

In an occupation-centered approach to treatment, the therapist typically addresses the strengthening of component skills through the use of artfully selected and adapted occupations. An example might be using the occupation of caring for a classroom pet as a time to address tactile sensitivity in a young child. One way to do would be to start by having the child feed the pet and experience the feel of dry food, then progress to exploring the texture of the animals fur (Figures 23-7 and 23-8).

This may be a highly motivating context to address tactile sensitivity because pets are fun and engaging. In this example, the desensitization should generalize to other functional tasks, but will minimally enhance the child's occupational performance of pet care. In some cases, intervention to address the growth and changing of personal skills and abilities may need to be provided outside of an occupational context.

Therapeutic interventions that decrease hypertonicity, such as weight bearing, rotation, and warmth, may need to be provided first to prepare a child with cerebral palsy or traumatic brain injury for play. Some children truly require the added repetition of fine-motor tasks and hand-strengthening exercises before they are able to integrate those skills into function. However, children are most responsive when their therapy is fun, enticing, and purposeful; it is the rare child who cooperates with repetitive exercises. A skillful therapist should be able to become a part of the child's environment and routines, enter into the spirit of play, and provide intervention, with very little awareness on the part of the child that she or he was receiving "therapy."

■ SERVICE-DELIVERY MODELS

A continuum of service models is outlined in much of the current literature on pediatric- and school-based services. Students receive direct, indirect, group monitoring, consultative, integrated, collaborative, and/or pull-out therapy services. It is generally agreed that no one model of service meets the needs of all children. An optimal service-delivery model for a specific child in a specific context is decided through the evaluation process. Sometimes parent and team members are most comfortable with one service delivery model (e.g., direct).

The occupational therapist needs to be a strong advocate for the use of flexible and appropriate service-delivery models. It is important to explain why a variety of service-delivery models are required to address childhood occupations and to ensure carryover of skills be-

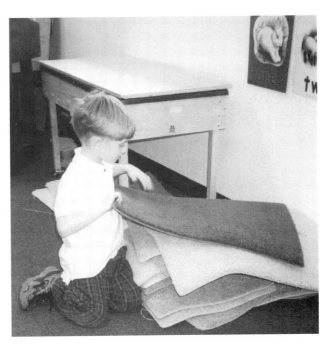

figure**23-6**   Carpet squares can provide a physical boundary for the child.

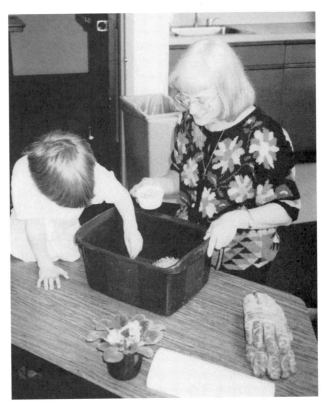

figure**23-7**   The child begins by feeding the pet and experiencing the feel of dry food.

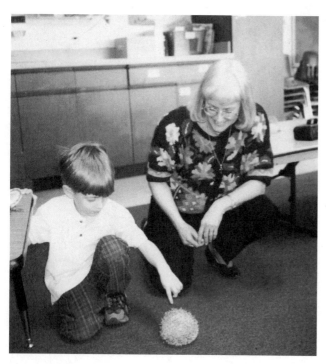

figure **23-8** He then progresses to exploring the texture of the animal's fur.

yond therapy times. Teachers may be hesitant to support a consultative approach as optimal for a certain child, because of the assumption that this will involve extra work in their already crowded days. Addressing these concerns proactively (i.e., as each opportunity presents itself) will eventually result in more flexibility in choosing service-delivery models and greater success in the implementation of them.

Recent educational trends have had significant impact on intervention for preschoolers. The current focus on inclusionary practices has supported a model for integrated services. Using this model, the occupational therapist promotes the student's performance in areas that the team has identified as priority goals (Rainforth et. al., 1992). In integrated services, occupational therapy becomes part of the child's everyday routine and environment. Therapists most often use consultation in conjunction with group and/or individual intervention sessions.

Collaborative Teaming

Collaborative teaming is essential to all service-delivery models. It combines the design of integrated therapy with the sharing of skills and information across all disciplines. It creates a child-centered program (meaning that a child's goals are at the center of decision mak-

ing and program planning), rather than a discipline-focused program.

Block scheduling is a program mechanism that promotes integrated services and collaborative teaming (Rainforth, 1992). It is a strategy for scheduling team members together in the classroom with several students who require those services. The team designs the activities, and members move in and out of activities based on the specific needs of the children. Instead of ½-hour "treatment times," the occupational therapist spends a block of time (e.g., 2 hours) in class. He or she is therefore with the children during bus-to-class transitions, circle time, and snack time. Other team members are also working with children in the classroom during this block of time. This proximity promotes collaboration on a child's behalf, and related service supports are provided within the performance routine. Providing services within the classroom is optimal for reinforcing targeted skills in the natural context of performance, and it promotes generalization of skills into multiple classroom activities (Giangreco, 1986; Giangreco, York, & Rainforth, 1989).

Consultation

Although block scheduling increases opportunities for communication between teachers and therapists, the occupational therapist can only be present for a portion of a child's day or week. However, *consultation* provides the avenue through which the child's entire day in a school setting can be influenced and changed to optimize occupational performance. However, consultation can be a complicated process: "Despite the recognized benefits of collaborating with educational staff, the art of consultation in schools remain a challenge for most therapists." (Hanft & Place, 1996).

By training the adults who are involved on a day-to-day basis with a child, the impact of occupational therapy services can have a far-reaching effect on that particular child. This training can also touch the lives of children the teachers and aids work with in the future. Hanft and Place (1996) recommend six strategies that therapists should use to providing effective consultation:

1. Work as an equal, not an authority.
2. Participate in school routines.
3. Nurture relationships with teachers and other team members.
4. Expect to learn from others and acknowledge when this happens.
5. Incorporate principles of adult learning in implementing recommendations.
6. Ask for feedback about the consultation and recommendations provided.

Possessing the skills and knowledge to successfully work with other team members is as important as providing good intervention ideas and suggestions. A teacher or aide who feels slighted or patronized during the consultation will rarely effectively carry out a therapist's recommendations, and he or she will probably not ask for consultation in the future.

A child who has poor hand strength and shoulder stability, immature fine-motor skills, and poor body awareness (all of which affect playing, drawing, coloring, cutting, and self-help skills) can exemplify the consultation model. From classroom observation, the occupational therapist noted that the classroom teacher placed a high value on individual choice during center time and free-play time, allowing each child to select his own preferred activities. This resulted in the child consistently selecting the water table, usually choosing to play with a child who was younger than he.

Explaining the importance of encouraging the child to choose gross-motor play, particularly climbing, sliding, pulling a wagon and crossing the monkey bars on a regular basis (all of which build up hand strength and shoulder girdle stability, as well as address body awareness), helped the teacher to understand the connection between gross-motor play and school-skill development. The therapist acknowledged the importance of volition in choosing tasks, and discussed ways in which the teacher could make the gross-motor play more successful and appealing to this child. Listening carefully to the teacher's concerns about this suggestion, and checking back frequently as to the success of its implementation, are important aspects of effective consultation.

Group Intervention Sessions

The group concept has been used in every aspect of educational programming. Often preschool teachers identify "motor time" as an integral part of their school day, with the emphasis on providing foundations for higher skills development through sensorimotor groups. The occupational therapist adds new perspective to these activities and helps individual children participate with greater competence. In group settings, the occupational therapist can provide activities and adaptations to promote peer interactions, motor planning, and grasp and release skills (Figures 23-9, 23-10, and 23-11).

When intervention is provided to a group of children within the classroom, collaborating with the teacher and teacher assistants in the planning and execution is essential. Part of this collaboration requires the therapist to help teachers to continue the group activities on subsequent days by providing a written record of group plans. The following is a sample plan for a preschool sensorimotor group (Figure 23-12).

It is also important for the therapist to encourage parents to attend and participate in the group. Doing this helps to develop playful and meaningful relationships with family members. Parent participation may also serve as a means to introduce toys and materials that are supportive of the preschooler's individual learning needs but have not previously been considered by the parent.

Grouping children also has the advantage of using peer modeling to elicit skills from a child. Leading a group is also a way for the occupational therapist to model differ-

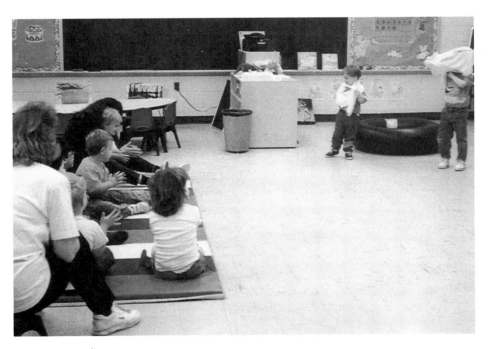

figure 23-9   Small group of peers in show-and-tell activities.

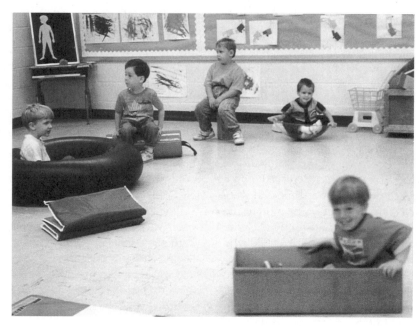

figure **23-10**   Group play.

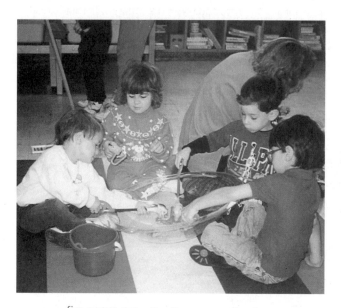

figure **23-11**   Small group exploration.

ent teaching methods and curriculum choices in a non-threatening manner. Additionally, it gives the occupational therapist a healthy respect for the challenging task of keeping 10 to 20 children engaged, productive, and learning, a task that the teacher does every day.

Grouping is a cost-effective and efficient way to provide services in preschool and childcare settings. Re-search has shown that outcomes in the school setting are the same, whether they are provided individually or in a group setting (Davies & Gavin, 1994; Dunn, 1990). Additional research is needed to support the use of alternative methods of service delivery.

Individualized Treatment

Direct, individualized treatment is a traditional service model for occupational therapists. This model includes *"pull out"* therapy, where services are provided in a separate location from the classroom as well as individualized therapeutic intervention within the classroom routines. Individual attention to a child allows the occupational therapist to get a clear sense of that child's strengths and weaknesses, and it encourages the development of a strong rapport between therapist and child. This in-depth knowledge about a child and his or her functional limitations can lead to the development of effective intervention strategies.

Individual, direct intervention times should be coupled with a consultative model. For example, after observing and working with a child directly at snack time, the occupational therapist should implement one-on-one activities to address fine-motor skills. The therapist should also provide a written plan for the teacher to carry out in the classroom routines.

The therapist must also be aware of contextual variables. For example, the therapist may first work with a child one-on-one to promote fine-motor play skills in a

Goals of the group activity
1. To enhance normal development and functional adaptive responses in the 3- to 5-year-old child
2. To provide a vehicle to assist in the development of foundational sensorimotor skills that are precursors for learning and motor skill development
3. To provide a vehicle for teacher or therapist to collaborate and to integrate sensorimotor principles into the classroom

General structure
The classroom teacher, occupational therapist, and classroom assistant direct and manage group activities cooperatively
The group meets twice a week for 25 to 30 minutes
Children participate with shoes removed
The occupational therapist and classroom teacher conduct sessions
Therapy sensorimotor equipment is used, but the focus is on the child's body and relativity to space rather than equipment
Materials and equipment used in group activity are often selected on the basis of their ability also to be used safely during free time in the class environment outside
Activities are designed to promote sensorimotor processing and neurodevelopmental foundational skills, necessary prerequisites for higher-level academic skills, and classroom performance
Specific motor skills are not emphasized, however, within select activities, dressing and manipulations for dressing are emphasized in a playful manner

Selection of activities
Activities are sequenced in a developmental continuum, as outlined in the hierarchy of neurodevelopment and the sensorimotor development process:
1. Tactile: touch
2. Vestibular: movement against gravity in linear or rotary planes
3. Proprioceptive: heavy muscle work and joint position sense
4. Postural: stabilizing the trunk and large joints
5. Bilateral: incorporating two body sides
6. Motor skill development: motor sequencing and following directions
Once sensorimotor activities are provided as a precursor to function, the remaining portion of the group stresses skills for functional outcomes, such as dressing and hand skills, for classroom tool manipulation. Functional outcome emphasis is also guided by the performance skills currently emphasized in the curriculum.

Preassessment and reassessment
1. Child's performance on selected evaluative tools or developmental class activities, selected on the basis of the child's needs
2. Teacher's observations
3. Occupational therapist's observations
4. Parents' observations

figure 23-12   Plan for preschool sensorimotor group.

separate, quiet therapy room. When the child is separated from the noisy classroom and impatient playmates, fine-motor manipulation skills may be quickly mastered. However, after an individualized session, the therapist may decide to invite another child (or small group of children) into the same room for therapeutic activities. The child can then progress to performing the activities in the class-room environment with adult support; then independently use the same play activities with peers in the regular classroom environment. The goal is to integrate the child into the regular flow of classroom experience.

The occupational therapist provides specific adaptations to classroom activities and curriculum plans, and he or she frequently seeks opportunities within the teacher-

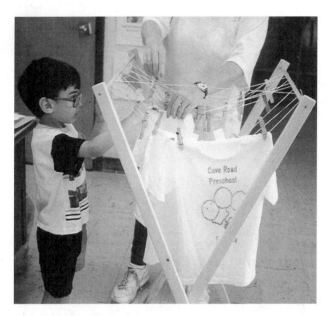

figure**23-13** Project is "hung out to dry," thus building hand strength and prehension.

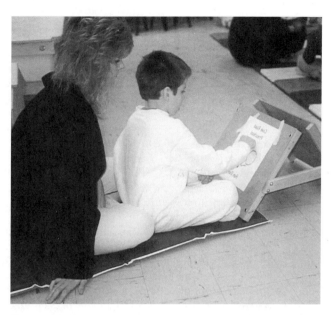

figure**23-14** Alternative positioning for a coloring project.

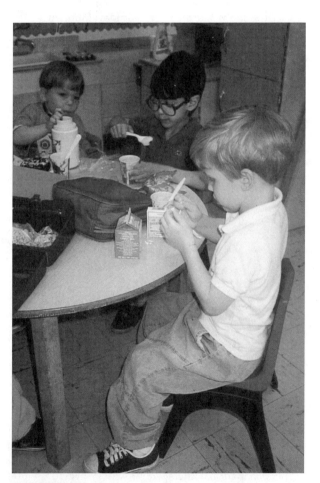

figure**23-15** Daily snacks offer opportunity to work on two-handed functions.

planned activities to help the student develop sensorimotor or perceptual motor performance components. For example, the therapist could create the opportunity for a preschooler to work on hand strength and prehension by asking the child to use a clothespin to hang a project "out to dry" on a line (Figure 23-13).

If the occupational therapist would like to support a more mature approach of forearm and wrist during a coloring project, he or she could suggest that the child use alternative positioning (Figure 23-14). Typically, this student would complete the project on a flat tabletop in a seated position. However, asking him to color on a slanted surface encourages wrist extension and efficient grasp of the crayon. Following up this session with consultation time with the teacher would facilitate consistent use of this strategy.

Accessing routines is an important way to provide occupational therapy intervention techniques, which then transition into new ways of performing tasks in the classroom. For example, the daily snack routine offers many opportunities for preschoolers to work on the two-handed functions of stabilizer and manipulator, fine-pincer grasp, and mature use of utensils (Figure 23-15). The occupational performance of snack time is also ideal for working on self-feeding and social-skill development in a natural context. The occupational therapist can give an outline to the classroom staff as a reminder for support (Figure 23-16). Letters sent home to parents containing ideas for snacks and packaging that may supplement their routines may also be helpful (Figure 23-17).

Please encourage these fine motor fundamentals

1. Opening lunch boxes independently
2. Pulling outside wrappers off straws
3. Placing straws in juice boxes or milk cartons
4. Twisting off cups and lids of a thermos independently with the preferred hand "do," nonpreferred hand "hold" method (the teacher or aide may need to slightly loosen these items)
5. Pouring liquid into the cup as needed using hand-over-hand method (older children)
6. Opening snap-and-seal containers independently (preferred hand "do," non-preferred hand "hold")
7. Collecting and properly disposing of all trash
8. Placing remaining items in a box and closing the box to be put away
9. Placing items in backpack independently
10. Each day, two children clean the tables, using a sprayer and paper towels (use preferred hand's index or middle finger or thumb to spray with the trigger and use one or two hands to wipe off tables The child should be encouraged to use pressure and good wrist extension)
11. After snack time, encourage children to wash their hands and faces, using a mirror

Ms. Smith's class-specific focus

Bobby: focus and attention, mature pinch, establish a preference, and motor plan

1. Encourage two-hand use as needed
2. Encourage use of index finger and thumb to pick up small items
3. Use firm touch pressure with hand over hand to show understanding of the action sequences to complete a task

Melissa: attention and focus, mature pinch, motor plan, and establish a preference

1. Provide hand over hand as needed to show understanding of the action sequence to complete a task
2. Encourage left "do", right "hold"
3. Allow only one food item at a time
4. Encourage use of the index finger and thumb to pinch small items
5. If the child gets off the seat during snack time, terminate snack time
6. Position items at child's midline

Jonathan: two-hand use, mature grasp, and motor plan

1. Encourage right "do", left "hold"
2. Encourage use of the index finger and thumb to pinch small items
3. Use hand-over-hand technique as needed, with firm touch pressure to show understanding of the action sequence to complete a task

figure23-16   Preschool snack-time management program.

Many preschools adopt *activity-based centers* for learning. Placed in different areas of the room, these centers have themes that define their materials and activities. The centers may include a kitchen or cooking area, an office, a zoo, a sensory area, an art area, or a construction zone. Often activity-based centers focus on manipulative tasks that support learning, and the children rotate through these centers on a daily basis.

To integrate treatment strategies within the play occupations of activity-based centers, the therapist first analyzes what skill components are naturally promoted within them. Once familiar with the materials and activities in each center, the occupational therapist can follow the child's lead and provide support of skill performance using those materials. For example, facilitation of scissors skills can be achieved in the art center, using the strategies listed in Figure 23-18.

∎ PARTNERING WITH FAMILIES

Parents are a vital component of the preschool team and should be encouraged to be involved at all levels. Their insight into their child and his or her interests and preferences is invaluable to quickly developing a therapeutic rapport and to understanding the child's roles within the family. Events and interactions within a child's home life have great impact on how the child functions at school. Simple events (e.g., not eating breakfast one

Date

Dear Parents:

As part of your child's preschool program, Ms. Smith and I are trying to encourage fine motor skill development during snack time. We encourage many of the basic hand skills necessary for school and daily routines through independent management of snack materials.

To help us with this program, we request that you send snacks in packaging containers that support skill development. Snacks wrapped in aluminum foil, plastic wrap, or zip lock bags are great! Please avoid sending snacks in sealed containers, such as the individual fruit or applesauce cups, if your child cannot currently manage these. A nice alternative to build skills is transferring these foods into small snap and seal containers. Then we can encourage the "hold-and-do" function of the hands as they open and close the container.

In the case of sealed and wrapped packages, we may be encouraging fine pinching or scissors use to open these packages.

Thank you for your cooperation and assistance as we work together for your preschooler!

Sincerely,

School Occupational Therapist

figure**23-17** Sample letter to parents.

The attached strategies and activities are provided to support the IEP fine motor goals and objectives and support the curriculum in the area of scissors skills. These include the following:
I. Prescissors experience activities
   A. Pick up relay games as demonstrated in class
   B. Squeeze play as demonstrated in class
   C. Paper punch games
II. Scissors positioning
   A. Correct finger and hand positioning as reviewed in class
   B. Use of sponge wedge or Koosh ball as outlined
   C. Cutting resistives, straws, and clay snakes
III. Directionality and control activities
   A. Cut through lines
   B. Nail head worksheets
   C. Aim for the star worksheets
Considering each child's current level of functioning, the following are recommended:
Classroom:

Student_____

Strategies suggested (list):

figure**23-18** Scissors skill development.

morning) and traumatic events in a child's life (e.g., parents going through a divorce), have a strong influence on classroom behavior. To maintain awareness of the events in a child's life, the occupational therapist should encourage communication opportunities with families through group participation, phone calls, home programs, and newsletters. These communication efforts enhance generalization and transfer of skills to other environments.

A preschool newsletter is useful for parents who do not have opportunities to visit the classroom (Figure 23-19). Providing information in this format can be helpful to parents, and it allows them to select the information that currently interests them.

The newsletter format provides a consistent program link between parents and school. It is also a vehicle for sharing the information with other team members. The written information can strengthen the team members' understanding of the occupational therapist's role with preschoolers. Common themes of the newsletters that the occupational therapist might write include (1) reinforcement of play as an important occupation of childhood, (2) home activities to promote manipulation skills, (3) sensory experiences that prepare the preschooler for learning, or (4) self-help skill development.

Tips for Growing from Occupational Therapy

May/June 2000

Focus on Motor Planning

When we first learn a new skill, we must think very carefully about how and where our movements occur. As we "learn" the movement, we find that we do not have to "think" as carefully about how the movement occurs. It becomes more "automatic." This process of motor planning is affected by the use of the sensory processes we discussed in previous newsletters. We use the systems in our body that process touch, body awareness, and sense of movement to store the memory of movements and not have to "relearn them" each time we need to call upon them. Motor planning is an important developmental consideration in young children as it forms the foundations for such things as imitation, following directions, and automatizing movements for letter formations in writing. Many of the sensory activities discussed in the previous newsletters will help develop motor planning skills. Additional activities to consider include use of constructional toys, pantomimes, follow-the-leader, catching or throwing games, and routine, simple chores at home.

Promoting Motor Planning With Playground Equipment

With the coming summer months, hours of play can be spent out-doors. The value of good playground equipment in promoting motor planning skills cannot be underestimated. I have attached some variations on standard play equipment that may provide more developmental challenges for your child. The heavy muscle work involved in negotiating playground equipment stimulates a portion of your child's brain that helps regulate balance, muscular responses, and higher challenges to the sensory systems. Encourage self-exploration. Your child will challenge his motor planning skills through the "ins and outs" and "ups and downs" of play.
Explore your nearest playground or school yard or consider creating an area in your own back yard. It is exciting to see the recent offerings in modular pieces in the home center stores.

Exciting Summer Resources

Summer can sometimes seem quite long for a young child whose attention is brief and activity level is high. You may want to consider looking at local resources to help supplement your home fun and games for the summer.

Home Activities for the Summer

Here are some simple and inexpensive ideas that incorporate many of the sensory and muscle development exercises we have focused on all year in the news letter.

Magic carpet ride
Lay a large beach blanket on the grass and have your child sit on it. Try pulling the child around on the blanket or have the child pull something on the blanket. This helps develop motor planning and stimulates body awareness and sense of movement.

Pavement painting
Let your child "paint" the pavement using a large utility paint brush and bucket of water. This helps develop hand, wrist, and finger control.

Heavy hands
Don't set large laundry containers with handles out for recycling yet. Once washed, they can be used as great containers to carry water and sand when playing at the beach. This helps to develop arm strength and control while stimulating the sensory receptors in the joints and muscles.

Bubbling Fun

Outdoor bubble games are wonderful in the summer. They are a wonderful way to promote eye-hand coordination and motor planning skills.

figure 23-19   Sample newsletter for parents.

■ DISCHARGE FROM OCCUPATIONAL THERAPY

Few guidelines are available to help in the decision to discontinue occupational therapy services in the preschool or childcare setting. Essentially, when a child is performing childhood occupations at a developmentally expected level, either independently or with the use of adaptive strategies, then it is time to discharge the child from the occupational therapy caseload. It is important to explain to parents and teachers that occupational therapy services may be initiated later (e.g., when occupational performance expectations change as a child matures).

Elementary school classrooms have additional children and involve a bigger percentage of desk time versus gross motor and/or free-play time. Children are expected to be much more independent once they enter elementary school. A child who is successfully functioning in the preschool or childcare setting may require physical and verbal assistance in the school environment. Often transitions into a kindergarten program are most successful when occupational therapy and other related services continue until the child adjusts to the new and more demanding environment.

Discharge should also be considered when goals are not met and intervention does not effect change in this child's functional skills. This can be a more difficult discharge situation to initiate with families, but occupational therapists must be ethical and realistic in monitoring the provision of services.

■ SUMMARY

This chapter has presented an overview of how occupational therapy services are provided in preschool and childcare settings. Temporal, physical, social, and cultural contexts of preschools and childcare settings were discussed in relation to current occupational therapy approaches. Common occupations, such as play, self-help, and preacademic skills, were addressed and analyzed. The assessment process, along with program planning and intervention options, was described, with an emphasis on processes consistent with an occupation-centered theory base. Finally, guidelines regarding terminating services were provided.

STUDY QUESTIONS

1. Explain the various models of service delivery used by occupational therapists in preschool settings.

2. The preschool classroom may have centers where children can explore and play in small groups. The occupational therapist may use these centers to support therapy goals for the children. Describe two activities in which children may practice bilateral hand manipulation activities in the following centers. Describe the materials used by the children and the steps they will take to complete the activities.
   - Office area
   - Kitchen or cooking area
   - Construction zone
   - Water-play area

3. List the context relevant to occupational therapy services in a preschool. Explain the importance of context in treatment planning and provide specific examples of how each context could influence intervention outcomes.

4. The preschool's occupational therapist has noticed that Ted has difficulty participating in group activities. He or she analyzed his difficulties and believes that Ted might demonstrate increased attention span if he sat on a medium-sized ball during circle time. Why did the therapist choose that intervention? What instructions and suggestions would the therapist give to the teacher and her assistant so that Ted's use of the ball is successful and will not disrupt the circle time? What other ideas could the therapist suggest to address this area of concern?

References

American Occupational Therapy Association. (1997). *Occupational therapy services for children and youth under the Individuals with Disabilities Education Act*. Bethesda: American Occupational Therapy Association.

American Occupational Therapy Association. (1994). Statement of occupational therapy referral. *American Journal of Occupational Therapy, 48*, 1034.

American Occupational Therapy Association. (1989). *Guidelines for occupational therapy services in early intervention and preschool services*. Rockville, MD: American Occupational Therapy Association.

Americans with Disabilities Act. (1990). Public Law 101-336, 42 U.S.C.

Ayres, A.J. (1979). *Sensory integration and the child*. Los Angeles: Western Psychological Services.

Blackman, J.A., Levine, M.D., & Markowitz, M. (1986). *Pediatric extended examination at three*. Cambridge, MA: Educators Publishing Service.

Bowman, B. (1994). Early childhood education, *Review of Research in Education, 2*, 25-39.

Brigance, A.H. (1978). *Brigance diagnostic inventory of early development*. Woburn, MA: Curriculum Associates.

Bruininks, G. (1978). *Bruininks-Oseretsky Test of Motor Proficiency*. Circle Pines, MN: American Guidance Service.

Bundy, A.C. (1989). A comparison of the play skills of normal boys and boys with sensory integrative dysfunction. *Occupational Therapy Journal of Research, 9*, 84-100.

Bundy, A.C. (1994). Assessment of play and leisure: Delineation of the problem. *American Journal of Occupational Therapy, 47*, 217-222.

Cahan, E.D. (1985). *Past caring: A history of U.S. preschool care and education for the poor*, (pp. 1820-1965).

Clifford, J.M., & Bundy, A.C. (1989). Play preference and play performance in normal boys and boys with sensory integrative dysfunction. *The Occupational Therapy Journal of Research, 9*, 202-217.

Coster, W. (1998). Occupation-centered assessment of children. *American Journal of Occupational Therapy ,52*, 337-344.

Davies, P., & Gavin, W. (1994). Comparison of individual and group/consultation treatment methods for preschool children with developmental delays. *American Journal of Occupational Therapy, 48*, 155-161.

Dennis, R., Edelman, S., & Giangreco, M. (1991). Common professional practices that interfere with integrated delivery of related services. *Remedial and Special Education, 12*, 16-24.

Dunn, W. (1990). A comparison of service provision models in school-based occupational therapy services: A pilot study. *Occupational Therapy Journal of Research, 10*, 300-320.

Dunn, W., Brown, C, & McGuigan, A. (1994). The ecology of human performance: A framework for considering the effect of context. *American Journal of Occupational Therapy, 48*, 595-607.

Education of the Handicapped Act Amendment. (1986). Public Law 99-457, 20 U.S.C.

Fisher, A.G. (1998). Uniting practice and theory in an occupational framework, *American Journal of Occupational Therapy, 52*, 509-521.

Folio, M.R., & Fewell, R.R. (2000). *Peabody Developmental Motor Scales* (2nd ed.). Austin, TX: Pro Ed.

Haley, S.M., Coster, W.J., Ludlow, L.H., Haltiwanger, M.A., & Andrellos., P.J. (1992). *Pediatric evaluation of disability inventory*. San Antonio: Psychological Corporation.

Hanft, B.A., & Place, P.A. (1996). *The consulting therapist*, San Antonio: Therapy Skill Builders.

Individuals with Disabilities Education Act of 1990. (1990). Public Law 101-476, 20 U.S.C. Chapter 33.

Individuals with Disabilities Education Act Amendments of 1997. (1997). Public Law 105-17, 20 U.S.C.

Kalscheur, J.A. (1992). Benefits of the Americans with Disabilities Act of 1990 for children and adolescents with disabilities. *American Journal of Occupational Therapy, 46*, 419-425.

Kielhofner, G. (Ed.). (1985). *A model of human occupation: Theory and application*. Baltimore: Williams & Wilkins.

Levine, M.D., & Schneider, E.A. (1985). *Pediatric examination of educational readiness*. Cambridge, MA: Educators Publishing Service.

McHale, K., & Cermak, S. (1992). Fine motor activities in elementary school: Preliminary findings and provisional implications for children with fine motor problems. *American Journal of Occupational Therapy, 46*, 898-903.

Missiuna, C., & Pollock, N. (1991). Play deprivation in children with physical disabilities: The role of the occupational therapist in preventing secondary disability. *American Journal of Occupational Therapy, 45*, 882-888.

Parham, L.D., & Fazio, L.S. (Eds.). (1997). *Play in occupational therapy for children*. St. Louis: Mosby.

Parham, L.D., & Primeau, L.A. (1997). Play and occupation therapy. In L.D. Parham & L.S. Fazio, (Eds.). *Play in occupational therapy for children*, St. Louis: Mosby.

Rainforth, B., York, J., & MacDonald, C. (1992). Collaborative teams for students with severe disabilities. Baltimore: Brookes.

Restall, G., & Magill-Evans, J. (1994). Play and preschool children with autism. *American Journal of Occupational Therapy, 48*, 113-120.

Richardson, A., & Onesti, S. (1997). The Montessori preschool: Preparation for writing and reading. *Annals of Dyslexia, 47*, 241-256.

Shepherd, J.T., Brollier, C.B., & Dandrow, R.L. (1994). Research report: Play skills of preschool children with speech and language delays. *Physical and Occupational Therapy in Pediatrics, 14*, 1-20.

Struck, M., & Dubois, S. (1993). *Self assessment for best practice in school based occupational therapy*. Paper presented at the American Occupational Therapy Association Annual Conference. Seattle: The Association.

Wood, W. (1996). The value of studying occupation: An example with primate play. *American Journal of Occupational Therapy, 50*, 327-337.

Case Study 1: Tomas

Tomas is a 3-year, 10-month-old child who was recently diagnosed with autism. He is the son of two physicians from Chile who are in the United States for additional training. He attends a regular private preschool, which does not have special-education services. This child has been referred to occupational therapy for support services that will enable him to succeed in his school placement. The parents would like him to remain in a classroom with nondisabled peers, because they feel he will have a better model for his language and social skills (two primary deficit areas for Tomas) when in an inclusion setting.

Case questions

What are the context areas the occupational therapist should explore when becoming familiar with Tomas? What kinds of questions does the therapist need to ask Tomas' parents and teachers to gain the appropriate context and background information? What other ways could that information be acquired?

Referral

The initial referral information reveals that Tomas has been difficult to engage in any type of purposeful, organized task during his time in school. It also reveals that he is disruptive at times: pulling hair, hugging classmates, touching everything, singing loudly at inappropriate times, and putting everything in his mouth. His most successful times during the school day have been during snack time and at the outdoor playground, where he enjoys swinging and playing in the sandbox (although rarely in an interactive manner with peers).

There are two teachers and 14 children in the class. Tomas' parents try to frequently volunteer in the classroom to support his experience there. Tomas communicates verbally, often using stereotypic phrases inserted into correct contexts. He prefers to play alone but will initiate interactions with adults when he needs something from them. The classroom teachers have expressed their concern that they are not fully equipped to educate this child and feel they often have their hands full with the other children.

Case questions

What are the typical childhood occupations a preschool child would engage in at school? At home? Given the diagnosis of autism and the little background information provided, which ones might the therapist expect Tomas to have difficulty with? What factors would contribute to his occupational performance dysfunction?

Assessment

Using an occupation-centered frame-of-reference (Fisher, 1998), the occupational therapist decided to take a top-down approach to assessment. This approach began with a review of Tomas' educational and medical files (provided by his parents). Besides a comprehensive report from the developmental neurologist (detailing the diagnosis of autism), the therapist reviewed several years of records from the speech-language pathologist who had been working with Tomas. The occupational therapist then interviewed Tomas' teachers and parents to determine their concerns and insights. These interviews also helped the therapist to compare how Tomas functioned in school and home settings.

The therapist asked the teachers and parents to describe a typical day for Tomas. This allowed the therapist to probe deeper for particular occupational performance concerns that existed and explore the influence of context on Tomas' performance. The teachers and parents were asked to fill out the sensory motor history (see Figure 23-10). Finally, the occupational therapist observed Tomas in the classroom setting during a successful time (snack) and during a more difficult occupation (completing a classroom project). The therapist then analyzed the activities and began to determine the underlying perfor-

mance components that contributed to success or failure of an occupation.

Case questions

To continue the assessment, what type of standardized evaluation tools might be appropriate to use with Tomas? Tomas has already been identified as distractible and difficult to engage unless highly motivated. What are some ways the therapist could structure the formal testing experience to elicit better cooperation and more accurate information? Where could he or she get suggestions about how to best test Tomas?

Intervention planning

After the assessment process is complete, the therapist determined that Tomas has great difficulty in many preschool occupations. The ones seen as most important to address initially are:

■ Participating in fine-motor and/or visual-motor crafts and games. (Often Tomas refuses to participate in these activities. When he does, the quality is very poor because he is not able to use scissors or write any letters. Tomas also has difficulty drawing and primarily produces only random scribbles. In addition, he is extremely messy when engaging in gluing activities and frequently destroys projects before finishing them.)

■ Socializing with peers appropriately. (Tomas has trouble initiating play, taking turns, and playing imaginatively).

■ Following classroom routines. (Tomas has trouble hanging up a coat or backpack, lining up for recess, and coming to the circle at group time. He has particular difficulty with transitions and frequent tantrums.)

Formal testing indicates that Tomas has mild gross-motor delays and moderate fine-motor delays. Self-help skills are close to age appropriate, but he appears to have difficulty consistently using his self-help skills in the correct functional context and would prefer to be dependent, particularly in dressing skills. Tomas also exhibits clinical signs of sensory defensiveness to auditory, tactile, and visual stimulation. This sensory defensiveness affects his functional abilities throughout the day because it encourages disruptive behavior (e.g., singing loudly) or a general "shutting out" of the classroom environment (e.g., closing eyes and ears and humming to himself).

Case questions

What specific occupational therapy theories and related theories might the therapist use to inform and organize treatment in this case? Write long-term (1 year) and short-term (1 month) goals for this case. How should services be provided for Tomas? Which occupations might benefit from being addressed individually, in a group, or by consulting with the teacher? List some treatment suggestions for each area of concern.

Intervention

After working with Tomas, the therapist determined that adjusting to his environment will help him focus and attend in a more organized manner. He is particularly helped by proprioceptive input, which can be provided in many ways in the classroom. Some of the adjustments that were useful for Tomas were:

- Deep pressure through shoulders provided by teacher during seated tasks
- Wearing a weighted vest for short periods throughout the day
- Encouraging Tomas to pull friends in a wagon
- Playing with modeling clay
- Hanging from the monkey bars, climbing up the slide
- Playing "squish machine" by pressing down on Tomas with beanbag chairs

Part of the therapist's consultation time was used to educate the teachers to read the cues that Tomas gave when he needed sensory input or when he began to be overloaded with too much input. The therapist trained Tomas' teachers to alternate motor activities that provide a lot of deep pressure and movement input with the fine-motor projects. The therapist also emphasized the importance of following a consistent routine each day and explained how to give Tomas visual and verbal cues that would help to anticipate transitions to new settings or activities.

Case questions

What are some group activities that the entire class can participate in which would provide proprioception and vestibular input? There is a strong need for Tomas to receive tactile input. What are some individual activities that will provide this experience for him? How can you incorporate receiving this input in a more functional task?

Transition to kindergarten

With strong support, Tomas is able to remain in his current setting and begin to make progress in all skill areas. He will continue to receive occupational therapy services for the entire time he is enrolled in this school. When he turns 5 years old, Tomas' parents may need help in determining the best kindergarten placement for Tomas.

Case questions

What might the therapist anticipate would be difficult for Tomas in a kindergarten setting? What are some suggestions the therapist could give to ease the transition to a new setting? Write a summary to include in Tomas' educational file to assist the new occupational therapist in providing services to Tomas.

chapter 24

School-Based Occupational Therapy

key terms

Individuals with Disabilities Education Act (IDEA)

Least restrictive environment

Inclusion

Multifactored evaluation

Related services

Individualized Education Program (IEP)

Collaboration

Service-delivery models

Consultation

Jane Case-Smith
Jan Rogers
Jan Haas Johnson

■ CHAPTER OBJECTIVES

1. Apply the principles and regulations of the Individuals with Disabilities Education Act to occupational therapy practice.
2. Explain the continuum of least restrictive environment.
3. Describe appropriate evaluation as defined in the Individuals with Disabilities Education Act.
4. Explain a problem-solving approach to school-based occupational therapy evaluation.
5. Define the components of and process for developing a student's Individualized Education Program.
6. Describe school-based models of service delivery, and explain when each is used.
7. Define and apply consultation models, methods, and styles.
8. Explain how occupational therapy consultation contributes to inclusive models of practice.

All children are required to spend considerable time in an educational setting in preparation for adult roles in life. *Education* has been defined as "a continuous process by which individuals learn to cope with their environments" (Pennsylvania Association for Retarded Citizens v.

Commonwealth of Pennsylvania [1971]). The occupational therapist that works in a school setting has the unique opportunity to help students become as functional as possible in their own environments. This chapter discusses schools as a context of occupational therapy practice and the roles and functions of therapists in educational settings.

■ LAWS THAT GOVERN SCHOOL-BASED PRACTICE

The role of occupational therapists in the school system has roots in the concepts of equality and civil rights that evolved from monumental changes in philosophic and political thinking during the late part of the eighteenth century. Humanitarianism and moral treatment began to be part of the public consciousness, and the new democracy of the United States enacted laws that reflected this philosophy (Hopkins, 1988). Although private institutions and organizations, such as churches and hospitals, provided ethical care and assistance to persons with disabilities, humanitarianism brought these concerns to the public. Soon Americans came to believe that ethical care of individuals with disabilities was a public responsibility and, over time, established care of, and accommodations for, individuals with disabilities as part of their civil rights.

Legislation that began in the 1930s (and continues to today) established public health programs that are available to all citizens. Federal laws have also established public education as a right of all children, regardless of privilege or power. Legal support of the right to education began with litigation related to racial desegregation, then moved on to protect the rights of students with disabilities.

In the early 1970s most states had statutes requiring educational services to be provided to certain children with disabilities. Although some states mandated services to all children with disabilities, inconsistencies were common across states and many children with disabilities were excluded from special education. At the time of enactment of the Education of the Handicapped Act (EHA) (1975), more than half of all children with disabilities in the United States did not receive appropriate educational services. In addition, more than one million children with disabilities were excluded from the public school system. Many families were forced to find services outside the public school system, often at great distance from their homes and at their own expense (EHA, 1975).

The EHA established six principles to guide the education of individuals with disabilities (Box 24-1). These principles have remained unchanged in subsequent amendments to the EHA, that is, in the Individuals with Disabilities Education Act.

Each of these concepts has significant implications for the public education system, for children with disabilities and their families, and for occupational therapists. A "free appropriate public education" refers to special education and related services that (1) have been provided at public expense, (2) are under public supervision and direction, (3) meet the standards of the state educational agency, and (4) include an appropriate education at preschool, elementary, or secondary levels. "Free" means at no cost to parents, but of course does not preclude the incidental fees that are normally charged to students without disabilities. The word "appropriate" is more difficult to define, because it does not necessarily refer to a grade level or the chronological age of a child. Appropriate is determined by the Individualized Education Program that is developed for each student by the educational team. This program is based on results of a comprehensive, multifactored assessment. As part of the educational team, occupational therapists have essential roles in these processes.

In the regulations of IDEA, occupational therapy is defined as a related service that may be required to enable a student to benefit from special education. The services

---

box 24-1 *Principles of the Individuals with Disabilities Education Act (formerly EHA [PL. 94-142])*

1. *Free Appropriate Public Education* (FAPE). Every eligible child is entitled to an appropriate education that is free to families (supported by public funds).
2. *Least Restrictive Environment.* Children with disabilities are most appropriately educated with their nondisabled peers. Special classes, separate schooling, or other removal of children with disabilities from the regular educational environment is to occur only when the nature or severity of the disability of a child is such that education in regular classes with the use of supplementary aids and services cannot be achieved satisfactorily [Section 612 (a)(5)(A)].
3. *Appropriate Evaluation.* All children with disabilities must be appropriately assessed for purposes of eligibility determination, educational programming, and individual performance monitoring.
4. *Individualized Education Program.* A document that includes an annual plan is developed, written, and (as appropriate) revised for each child with disabilities.
5. *Parent and Student Participation in Decision Making.* Parents and families must have meaningful opportunities to participate in the education of their children at school and at home.
6. *Procedural Safeguards.* Safeguards are in place to ensure that the rights of children with disabilities and their parents are protected, and that students with disabilities and their parents are provided with the information they need to make decisions. In addition, procedures and mechanisms must be in place to resolve disagreements between parents and school officials.

---

of an occupational therapist are, therefore, designed to enhance a student's abilities to participate in the educational process. The regulations of IDEA define occupational therapy as "(i) improving, developing or restoring functions impaired or lost through illness, injury or deprivation, (ii) improving ability to perform tasks for independent functioning when functions are impaired or lost, and (iii) preventing, through early intervention, initial or further impairment or loss of function." [34 C.F.R., §300.16(a)(5)]

The IDEA guarantees that each child with a disability be educated in the least restrictive environment. Children with disabilities are most appropriately educated with their nondisabled peers. Whatever the disability, the first student placement that should be considered is to assign the child to a general-education classroom, with appropriate aids and supports (Heumann & Hehir, 1994). As a result, most students with disabilities are placed in regular-education classrooms.

The amount of support provided to these students varies from a full-time aide to periodic, consultative services by an occupational therapist or special educator. When a child cannot be educated in the regular classroom, an alternative placement is considered. Accordingly, schools are required by law to ensure that a continuum of alternative placements is available to meet the needs of children with disabilities. This continuum includes a range of alternative placements such as instruction in regular classes, special classes, special schools, home instruction, and instruction in hospitals and institutions. Most children with disabilities spend at least a portion of their day in regular-education classrooms.

Inclusion is a frequently used term to describe how "least restrictive environment" is implemented. *Full inclusion* refers to a child's access to and participation in all activities of the school setting. Supports and adaptations are provided as needed to enable the child with disabilities to participate in activities with his or her peers. These services are typically provided in the child's neighborhood school. For example, Josh, a child with spina bifida and mild learning disabilities, attends his local, home elementary school in a rural community. Josh is in the regular classroom for the entire day, with a classroom aide assisting him with self-care tasks as needed. The school's special education teacher helps the classroom teacher in adapting Josh's assignments when needed.

Inclusion, also termed *integration,* can consist of a variety of learning options. A student may spend a portion of the day in a resource room and a portion in regular-education classes. For instance, Brian, who is in the 6th grade, participates in the regular-education classroom for all of his classes, except math and reading. For these subjects, he receives instruction from the resource room teacher because his performance in these classes is significantly lower than his peers, and he requires a special curriculum to progress in these areas.

Modifications are made to accommodate Brian's learning needs so that he can participate with his peers. Often the regular classroom teacher groups students for science and social studies projects so that each of the students is given a task that he or she can manage. Because Brian has difficulty with manipulation, the teacher gives manipulation tasks to the other students in the group and often selects Brian to search the Internet or oversee final-project assembly. Tests are read to Brian, and he is allowed to dictate his answers. Greg attends full-day, inclusive kindergarten with occupational therapy, physical

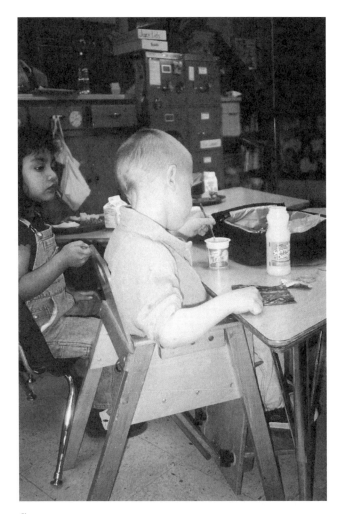

figure 24-1   Greg participates in all of the kindergarten class activities with adapted equipment (e.g., Rifton chair) and modifications to the environment (e.g., placement of activities).

therapy, and special education supporting his participation in the regular-education curriculum (Figures 24-1 and 24-2).

With more children involved in a classroom situation, inclusive experiences are primarily used for social purposes. For example, Mary, a child with cerebral palsy and significant learning disabilities, participates in the regular half-day kindergarten class in the morning. During this time, the emphasis is placed on providing socialization experiences for Mary with the students in the typical class. Mary's day is extended, and in the afternoon she is instructed in her academic subjects in the resource room.

The model for implementing "least restrictive environment" can significantly affect the delivery of occupational therapy service. Integrated, or inclusive, classrooms and resource classrooms place different demands on the student. For example, a self-contained class of eight children with special education teacher and an aide demands a different set of skills of each student than does a class of 25

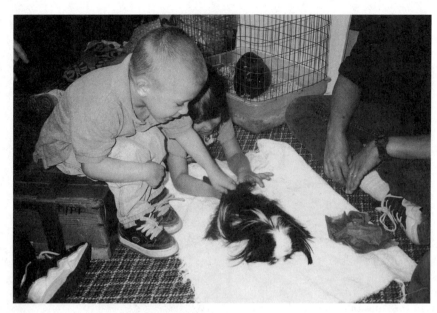

figure **24-2** Kindergarten offers a multitude of social experiences, emphasizing socially appropriate behavior, responsibility, self-maintenance, and respect and caring of others (including pets).

students taught by one teacher, who has no training in educating students with disabilities. Occupational therapists must be adept in assessing the child's performance, the context in which the child is placed, and the effects of that context on the child's performance. Therapists need to consider the difference between special education and regular-education models. Additionally, they must assess the teacher's level of expertise in working with a student and the level of support needed by the teacher. Other types of schools in which occupational therapists provide services are listed (Box 24-2). When serving students in these schools, therapists should make a specific effort to understand the mission, goals, and unique characteristics of each learning environment.

■ EVALUATION

Legal Requirement for Evaluation

The IDEA requires that a multidisciplinary team conduct a comprehensive evaluation to determine whether a child has exceptional educational needs that warrant special education services. This evaluation can be initiated by the parents or by the school team when either party notices particular problems in how the child learns or suspects that the child has a disability. This *multifactored evaluation* (MFE) is needed even when the child has an obvious disability (e.g., cerebral palsy, Down syndrome) and has received therapeutic services in the past (e.g., in an early intervention program).

Because most children with disabilities enter the school system without an educational diagnosis (or a di-

agnosis of developmental delay), a purpose of the initial MFE is to give the child a specific educational diagnosis. In most states this diagnosis (e.g., orthopedically disabled, learning disabled, multiple disabilities) is required for the child to receive specific services. Box 24-3 lists categories of disability as defined in IDEA.

The 1997 Amendments to IDEA shifted the emphasis from evaluation as the basis of a diagnostic label to evaluation focused on identifying functional problems and goals. The specific questions to be answered by the initial evaluation are:

1. What is the child's present level of educational performance?
2. What are the child's educational needs?
3. Does the child need special education and related services?
4. What additions or modifications, if any, are needed to the special education and related services to enable the child to meet annual goals in the Individualized Education Program (IEP) and to participate, as appropriate, in the general curriculum? [Section 614 (c)(2)(B)]

Students with IEPs (i.e., those who receive special education services) are considered for reevaluation every three years to determine if they continue to need special education and related services. Reevaluation determines if additions or changes need to be made to the special education and related services the child is receiving, to enable the child to meet IEP goals and to participate (as appropriate) in the general curriculum [IDEA, 20 U.S.C. 1400 et seq, Section 614 (c)(1)]. Reevaluation is not needed if sufficient information has been obtained dur-

Occupational therapists provide services to students in private and parochial schools, charter schools, and alternative schools. When indicated, and when students are eligible for special education, they are entitled to services through IDEA. This is true even when the parents elect to enroll them in private, or non-public, schools (Federal Regulations, 34 C.F.R. §300.341). When it is determined to be the most appropriate environment for a child's education, occupational therapists may also provide educationally relevant services in the home or a residential center.

Charter schools are typically small, responsive schools that allow for the development of alternative curriculum, administration of their own budgets, and autonomous decision making. They are a departure from the large public school systems and tend to put curricular and programmatic decisions in the hands of parents. Charter schools are typically unique entities and tend to reflect the interests and needs of the community they serve. They are often developed with a particular educational emphasis such as math and science, foreign languages, or the arts. Many charter schools are designed to serve children at risk for learning disabilities or school problems (Zepeda & Langenbach, 1999). Therapists working in charter schools need to learn about the focus and direction of the school as well as the types of children and families who enroll in them. By understanding the school's mission and character, the therapist can work with administrators, teachers, and families successfully.

Alternative schools are typically administered by public schools. They may be "magnet" schools that provide enriched education based upon programmatic themes such as math and science, the arts, or foreign languages. They may be schools that offer a last chance before expulsion, or they may provide remediation and rehabilitation to students with academic, social, or emotional problems (Zepeda & Langenbach, 1999). Occupational therapists may provide services in both types of alternative schools. When working in a remediation and rehabilitative school, therapists should have skills and experience in psychosocial intervention and behavioral management. Many of these schools provide a curriculum and code of conduct, with structured rules and regulations to which the therapist must adhere for the safety of staff and students.

Vocational schools may be an option for students who plan to seek immediate employment after high school graduation. They also prepare the student for the option of attending a trade school after high school graduation. Vocational schools are generally separate schools that students attend after they have obtained some of their basic high school education requirements in their home school district. The students may choose one of several career paths that may include business, health care professions, computer technology, and various trades. The emphasis of these schools tends to shift the student from an academic to a vocational perspective. Students are generally provided with specialized skills that will make them employable upon graduation. Occupational therapists assist students in developing prevocational and vocational skills. They also help students to adapt to work environments.

Occasionally medically fragile or severely impaired students receive *home-based related services*. Although a child may have extensive medical needs, the role of the school-based occupational therapist is to provide educationally relevant services. Students may also receive home-based services when suspended or expelled from school. Students with Individualized Education Programs (IEPs), who have been suspended or expelled, are entitled to the full scope of their IEP, including occupational therapy services (Federal Regulations 34 C.F.R., §300 522).

box **24-3** *Categories of disability (IDEA, 1997)*

1. Mental retardation
2. Hearing impairments (including deafness)
3. Speech or language impairments
4. Visual impairments (including blindness)
5. Emotional disturbance
6. Orthopedic impairments
7. Autism
8. Traumatic brain injury
9. Other health impairments
10. Specific learning disabilities

The term "child with a disability" may be used with a child aged 3 through 9 at the discretion of the state and the local education agency. This can be done only when a child is experiencing developmental delays (as defined by the state and as measured by appropriate diagnostic instruments and procedures), in one or more of the following areas: physical development, cognitive development, communication development, social or emotional development, or adaptive development, and who, by reason thereof, needs special education and related services [IDEA, 20 U.S.C.1400 et seq, Section 602(3) (A)(B)]

ing the course of the 3 years. The intent of this recent change in the law is to prevent unnecessary testing, such as repeated intelligence tests.

Based on current thinking and on language in IDEA, evaluation is a multidisciplinary, collaborative effort focused on function and the issues that appear to be impeding learning. Norm-referenced tests give standardized scores helpful in determining eligibility, but information from a norm-referenced test is difficult to relate to functional performance in a classroom. Although standardized tests offer an objective measure of abilities, informal observational assessment of the student in his classroom or other school environment is also important to establishing goals and objectives. These assessments are most helpful when they are criterion referenced, with the performance of peers in the same grade and the curriculum used as the criteria. For example, does the student demonstrate the same ability to attend, persist in tasks, and organize his or her materials as the other students in the classroom?

The other specific requirements for evaluation established by IDEA are listed in Box 24-4. These requirements place emphasis on using a variety of measures, including parent report, and using technically sound instruments. "Trained," "knowledgeable," and "qualified" personnel are to administer the evaluation methods; occupational therapists qualify to administer many of the evaluation methods used in schools.

Occupational Therapy Evaluation

Occupational therapy evaluation in the school focuses on the child's ability to participate in functional school activities. A problem-solving approach is used to identify the issues that are relevant to the problem and to identify strategies that may help to resolve those issues. In the first step of a problem solving approach to assessment, teacher and parent concerns are identified and primary functional problems are defined (Clark & Coster, 1998). Once the functional problems are identified, further assessment is carried out to identify the reasons for the problems and potential solutions. This process includes trial of potential solutions and intervention strategies to determine the likelihood that they will be effective. This trial helps to determine the level of change that can be expected.

A problem-solving model is circular: once decisions are made regarding intervention approaches, their effec-

---

box 24-4 *Requirements for appropriate evaluation as defined in IDEA*

Initial evaluation

The state or local education agency shall conduct a full and individual initial evaluation before initiation of services. The initial evaluation shall consist of procedures:
1. To determine whether a child has a disability.
2. To determine the educational needs of the child.

Conducting the evaluation

In conducting the evaluation:
1. A variety of assessment tools and strategies are used to gather relevant functional and developmental information. Information provided by the parent (that may assist in determining whether the child has a disability and the content of the child's individualized education program) is included. Information related to enabling the child to be involved in and progress in the general curriculum or to participate in appropriate activities is also included.
2. Any single procedure shall not constitute the sole criterion for determining whether a child has a disability or determining an appropriate educational program for the child.
3. Technically sound instruments are used to assess the relative contribution of cognitive and behavioral factors, in addition to physical or developmental factors.

Additional requirements

Each local educational agency shall ensure the following:
1. Tests and other evaluation materials used to assess a child under this section:
   a. Are selected and administered so as not to be discriminatory on a racial or cultural basis.
   b. Are provided and administered in the child's native language or other mode of communication, unless it is clearly not feasible to do so.
2. Any standardized tests that are given to the child:
   a. Have been validated for the specific purpose for which they are used.
   b. Are administered by trained and knowledgeable personnel.
   c. Are administered in accordance with any instructions provided by the producer of such tests.
3. The child is assessed in all areas of suspected disability.
4. Assessment tools and strategies that provide relevant information that directly assists persons in determining the educational needs of the child are provided.

Adapted from NICHCY (1999) www.nichcy.org.

tiveness is monitored and periodically re-evaluated to make adjustments, select alternative methods, or stay on course (See Clark & Coster, 1998; or Clark & Miller, 1996). As described in the following section, assessment begins by determining the degree to which a student *participates* in school; then it focuses on *performance* of specific school activities.

Student's level of participation

A goal of public education is that students participate in school activities to the maximum extent possible. It is expected that students demonstrate consistent progress in the curriculum or toward their individual educational goals. In addition to academic outcomes, students must demonstrate socially appropriate behaviors and functional performance that enables them to participate in nonacademic school activities (e.g., eating lunch, playground behaviors). A typical lunchroom presents multiple challenges to children with disabilities (Figure 24-3). Occupational therapists often focus on functional performance in nonacademic areas. The *School Function Assessment* (SFA) (Coster, Deeney, Haltiwanger, & Haley, 1998) provides a method for identifying a child's level of participation, assessing need for task support, and evaluating performance in school activities. This criterion-referenced tool helps to organize assessment into the primary domains of concern for occupational and physical therapists. The physical subscales identified in the SFA include travel, maintaining and changing positions, recreational movement, using materials, setup and cleanup, eating and drinking, hygiene, clothing management, written work, up and or down stairs, and computer and equipment use. The cognitive and or behavioral subscales identified in the SFA include functional communication, memory and understanding, following social conventions, task behavior and/or completion, compliance with adult directives and school rules, positive interaction, behavior regulation, personal care awareness, and safety.

To rate the SFA, the child is judged in relationship to the performance of the other students in his or her grade level or classroom. A child's participation is understood through observation of how peers perform and function relative to the curriculum and environment and what level of participation the teacher expects. To thoroughly identify the problem and to complete the SFA, the teacher is interviewed. Through her everyday observations of the student, the teacher identifies the activities in which the student struggles or fails. Informal observation by the occupational therapist validates and augments the teacher's explanation of the problem and the student's level of participation. Based on the occupational therapist's observation, the child and the context become well understood, often leading to an interpretation of the problem that sheds new light on the child's behaviors.

These three methods (i.e., use of the SFA, informal observation, and teacher-parent interview) allow for accurate identification of the problem. Using different perspectives brings the problem into focus and leads into the next steps of successful problem solving.

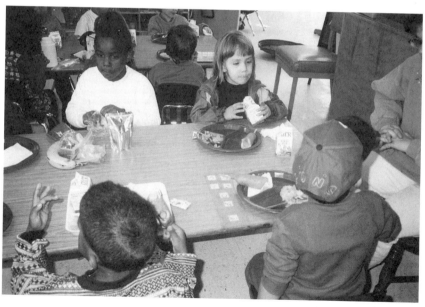

figure**24-3** Lunchtime is relatively unstructured and presents multiple challenges to children with disabilities. Participation in the lunchroom may be limited by the stimulating environment, noise levels, fine motor skills to open cartons and packages, and balance and mobility when carrying a lunch tray in a crowded environment.

Assessment of performance

Specific assessment of performance follows, using the problems observed in school functions as a basis for selecting evaluation tools. At this stage, the goal is to identify reasons for the student's difficulties. Standardized tools and structured observation are used. In addition, the environment is assessed as a possible reason for the problem and as one focus of intervention. Occupational therapists often assess the following five areas: (1) *motor performance*, (2) *sensory responsiveness*, (3) *perceptual processing*, (4) *psychosocial and cognitive abilities*, and (5) *school environment*.

Motor performance. Children in school are expected to independently travel within the school and move safely within the classroom, playground, and hallways. They must manipulate their schoolbooks, writing and cutting tools, paper, and materials; use tools such as scissors; produce legible handwriting; eat and drink independently; and use a computer. Related to their self-maintenance, they must use the toilet, wash their hands, put on and take off their jackets, and demonstrate other hygiene skills. Standardized tests to measure motor performance include the *Peabody Developmental Motor Scales (2nd ed.)* (PDMS)(Folio & Fewell, 2000) and the *Bruininks-Oseretsky Test of Motor Proficiency* (BOTMP)(Bruininks, 1978) (see Chapters 7 and 8). Although both of these tests offer a method for evaluating a child's motor performance, the items do not necessarily relate to school function and, therefore, a cautious interpretation of the scores is needed. Visual motor tests (e.g., *Developmental Test of Visual-Motor Integration* [Beery, 1997]) that require paper and or pencil skills relate to school functions, such as handwriting and tool use. These tests measure the child's skills in tracing and copying designs. The SFA has sections that measure physical performance, using a comprehensive representation of the movements and manipulation skills required to function at school.

Sensory responsiveness. A child's sensory responsiveness can be assessed using standardized interviews, inventories, or observational tests. Inventories such as the *Sensory Profile* (Dunn, 1999) rate sensory responsiveness in natural situations. Standardized observational assessments of children's sensory responsiveness and sensory integration are criterion referenced (e.g., *Sensory Integration Inventory—Revised, for Individuals with Developmental Disabilities,* [Reisman & Hanschu, 1992]) or norm referenced (e.g., the *Sensory Integration and Praxis Tests* [SIPT][Ayres, 1989]).

Perceptual processing. Assessment of a child's visual perceptual processing is particularly important to his or her school function. Standardized instruments to measure visual perception include the *Developmental Test of Visual Perception, (2nd ed.)* (DTVP-II) (Hammill, Pearson, & Voress, 1993) and the *Motor Free Visual Perception Test, Revised* (Colarusso, Hammill, & Mercier, 1995). Aspects of visual perception that relate to school function (e.g., reading, handwriting) include spatial relations, figure-ground perception, and form constancy. Other perceptual skills important to understanding performance in school activities include body scheme and body awareness, orientation to time and place, and spatial awareness (Hanft & Place, 1996).

Psychosocial and cognitive abilities. Problem solving, organizational skills, attention, and appropriate interactions with peers and adults are essential performance areas of school function. The SFA rates behavior and cognition using 10 scales. Each has high relevance to a child's success in the school environment. Behaviors are often the focus of the IEP because they determine the child's ability to function in a structured environment (e.g., classroom), to attend, demonstrate responsibility, positively interact with others, cope with new situations, and fit into the social norms of the classroom. Socially appropriate behavior is highly related to the student's academic achievement and his or her ability to succeed in environments outside school (e.g., community, work). Important elements of behavior that are often the focus of occupational therapy are attention and persistence, task completion, compliance, self-esteem and self-image, peer and adult interaction, problem solving and safety. Students frequently have difficulty transitioning from one activity to another and adapting to new situations. Adaptive behaviors are analyzed to determine the antecedents to aggressive or disruptive behaviors, or to withdrawal behaviors.

Occupational therapists are most involved in evaluation of behavior when the behaviors relate (at least in part) to the child's sensory processing. As in every other performance area, standardized tools are available. Examples include the *Behavior Evaluation Scale-2* (McCarney & Leigh, 1990), and the *Child Behavior Checklist* (Achenbach & Edelbrock, 1991). Interpretation of standardized results requires specific observations of in-classroom and out-of-classroom behaviors. It also requires the interpreter to conduct teacher and parent interviews. These interviews provide an understanding of behavioral expectations, suggest possible reasons for behaviors, define the extent of the problem, and determine desired functional outcomes.

School environment. Evaluation of functional performance includes assessment of the school environment. All of the student's school environments should be examined, including the classrooms, cafeteria, playgrounds, gymnasium, and other spaces (Figure 24-4). For children in wheelchairs or walkers, the focus of this part of the assessment may be accessibility. For children with sensory

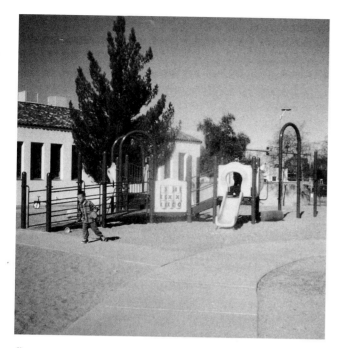

figure**24-4** The playground is one environment to be evaluated, emphasizing accessibility and safety. Although schools are constructing playgrounds with wheelchair accessibility, many remain only partially accessible. Playgrounds should include equipment that requires a range of skills and a range of sensory input.

processing problems, the focus may be the degree and types of sensory stimulation in the environment. Classrooms tend to be highly visually stimulating environments, and they can be disorganizing and overwhelming to students with sensory processing problems.

Teacher expectations and curriculum standards

To analyze the extent and the basis for a student's performance problem, the expected performance (as defined by the teacher and curriculum) must be fully understood. When teachers expect neat, precisely aligned, and well-formed handwriting, a student with poor handwriting will have a significant problem in meeting that teacher's standard. As another example, some teachers show high tolerance for disruptive behaviors and allow students to move freely about the room. A student with a high activity level and sensory seeking behaviors would have greater success in a classroom where movement was allowed, rather than one where students were expected to remain in their seats. Often a student's goals and services are based more on the discrepancy between the student's performance and classroom-teacher expectations, than on performance delays as determined by norms that reference the student's age.

Assessment as a Basis for Students' Goals

Evaluation of students is focused on the problems that seem to be affecting the child's ability to learn and function in school. Problem-based evaluation is focused and in-depth; that is, relevant performance areas are thoroughly explored in various environments and situations to determine what strategies would be most helpful in improving performance. When possible, the initial evaluation (i.e., the evaluation completed before a written plan is developed) includes a trial of possible interventions and an assessment of their effectiveness. This part of the evaluation, sometimes termed *hypothesis testing,* helps the therapist to contribute in an optimal way to the student's IEP.

Through evaluation of potential interventions, the therapist can judge:
1. The level or amount of change that can be expected in the course of the year (i.e., What goals should be established?).
2. The most appropriate intervention strategies.
3. The most effective service-delivery models (e.g., direct service, consultation, monitoring).

Because the child's plan details each of these areas of concern, trials of intervention prepare the therapist to offer valid contributions to the planning process.

■ DESIGNING INDIVIDUALIZED EDUCATION PROGRAMS

The collaborative planning process that follows comprehensive evaluation involves interpretation of the evaluation results. It also involves discussion with the parents and educational team regarding priorities and proposed interventions. This formal planning process establishes the services and program that will enable the student to participate in school and classroom activities and receive an "appropriate education." The IEP developed through this process serves as a plan and a contract; it is a legal, written statement of the child's unique educational program and a delineation of what the school will provide to help the child meet his or her educational goals.

Components of an IEP

Each IEP must include a statement of the child's present levels of performance that indicates how the child's disability affects his or her participation in the general curriculum. It also includes annual goals and objectives with accompanying criteria and evaluation procedures. Once the desired student outcomes are defined, the type and intensity of special education and related services are identified. Written statements, regarding the extent to which the student will not participate in regular

table 24-1	*Elements of the Individualized Education Program*

Component	Explanation
Present levels of educational performance	What are the student's strengths and weakness?
	What areas of skills need to be addressed?
	How does the child's disability affect his or her involvement and progress in the general curriculum?
Annual goals and short-term objectives	What educational goals are appropriate for the student, considering the areas of difficulty?
	What can the student reasonably accomplish in a year? (The goals must be annual and measurable and must relate to helping the child be "involved in and progress in the general curriculum.")
Special education and related services	What special education and related services are required to attain the annual goals?
	What supplementary aids and services are necessary to enable the student to be involved in the general curriculum, to participate in extracurricular activities, and to be educated and participate with other children?
Explanation of nonparticipation	The IEP must include an explanation of the extent, if any, to which the child or youth will *not* be participating with nondisabled children in the regular education class, in the general curriculum, and in extracurricular and nonacademic activities; this requirement emphasizes the importance of deciding the most appropriate educational setting for each student on an individual basis.
Participation in assessments	A statement must be written that outlines the specific modifications that will be made to enable the student to participate in district-wide student achievement assessments.
Dates, frequency, location, and duration of services	A statement must be written that specifies when the student's special education and related services will begin, how long they will go on, how often they will be provided, and where he or she will receive those services.
Transition services	Beginning when the student is age 14 and every year thereafter, the IEP must include a statement of that student's transition service needs in his or her courses of study.
Measuring and reporting student progress	A statement must be written that outlines how the student's progress toward the annual goals and short-term objectives will be measured.
	The parents of the child will be kept regularly informed about their child's progress toward the annual goals listed in the IEP; they must be informed at least as often as the parents of nondisabled children.

IEP, Individualized education program.

education and the need for curricular modifications and assistive technology, are also included. The elements of the IEP defined in IDEA are listed (Federal Register, 34 C.F.R. § 300.347) (Table 24-1).

IEP Team Process

The IEP team is made up of individuals who are familiar with and knowledgeable about the child. The required team members consist of at least one regular education teacher, at least one special education teacher, a local education agency representative (LEA), an individual to interpret evaluation results, parents, and any other individuals who the parents or LEA representative feel have knowledge or expertise about the child, including related service personnel such as the occupational therapist (Federal Register C.F.R. § 300.344).

Development of the IEP involves high levels of collaboration and, at times, negotiation and consensus building. The written IEP document is developed in a formal meeting, so the contents reflect the consensus of the team. Parents and other team members, including occupational therapists, contribute equally to the process. The team members discuss the student's strengths and needs and then develop goals, outcome statements, and plans through a collaborative process. Although team collaboration with parents in writing the IEP is specified in IDEA and in state policies, some districts conduct IEPs in different ways. In certain districts, team members develop goals and objectives with little input from each other. To ensure optimal participation of parents, it is helpful to send ideas to parents before the meeting, with the understanding that these suggested goals may change at the time of the meeting. By developing the student's IEP using a team process, the team assures the family that the IEP belongs to the student, and parts are not owned by the various professionals who developed them. Child outcome statements are integrated and suggest the involvement of multiple disciplines for their achievement.

Although the IEP process is ideally collaborative (from its origin to writing the goals and services to which the child is entitled), high levels of collaboration are not always possible. When several itinerant professionals are involved on the IEP team, it can be difficult, if not impossible, for school administrators to gather together or effectively communicate. This is because these professionals may only be in a school building one day a week, on different days. Additionally, IEP meetings can also be quite lengthy. For districts that have limited funds, the costs of paying contracted services or attempting to stretch the time of staff with excessively large caseloads can tempt schools to try methods to shorten the process. To avoid this, team members should encourage each other to adopt collaborative models for writing the IEP.

Educational Goals

IEP goals reflect a holistic picture of the child, an understanding of what is required to function in the school environment, and a knowledge of the curriculum. At times, the occupational therapist may feel that a particular skill is a priority for a child. However, when viewing the whole child, the team may not concur. If this is the case, some negotiation by IEP team members may be needed to select the priorities for the child. Rainforth and York-Barr (1997) suggested that for children with more severe disabilities. a comprehensive IEP should establish the following:

1. Establish overall goals to maintain a student's health and vitality.
2. Enhance a student's participation in current and future inclusive environments.
3. Increase a student's social integration, including interaction with peers and adults.
4. Refer to essential functional skills that have frequent and multiple applications across environments and activities

Educational goals are statements describing general performance, whereas objectives are usually a sequence of measurable skills that lead to the goal (Rainforth & York-Barr, 1997). Goals and objectives can be written in a variety of ways. A developmental approach assumes that skills are required in a developmental sequence. The following is an example of a developmental goal:

A *developmental approach* to writing goals and objectives assumes that skills are acquired in a developmental sequence. An example of a developmental approach is:

Goal:	1. Sally will demonstrate an appropriate grasp of a writing utensil during art activities.
Objectives:	1a. Sally will hold a marker or pencil in a digital pronated grasp during art activities.
	1b. Sally will hold a marker or pencil in a static tripod grasp during art activities.
	1c. Sally will hold a marker or pencil in a dynamic tripod grasp during art activities.

A developmental approach can create barriers to learning for students who do not master prerequisite skills in a typical developmental sequence. In the above example,

the therapist focuses on strategies to facilitate the appropriate developmental sequence of grasp. In students with neuromotor impairments, these grasping patterns may not develop. However, it may still be possible for a child with neuromotor impairments to write and draw with success, using modified grasp patterns and other compensatory strategies. When goals and objectives are written in developmental format, the targeted functional skill may be lost. In this case, facilitating effective use of tools during art activities should have priority over the type of grasping pattern demonstrated.

In the *functional curriculum approach* to writing goals and objectives, daily living skills become the focus of educational activity. Various tasks required for independence in community living or vocation are analyzed, and the performance components become the objectives for the overall goal. When the components are mastered, the student performs the functional activity. An example of a functional curriculum approach is as follows:

Goal:	1. Zach will independently don this jacket.
Objectives:	1a. Zach will independently place his arms in the sleeves and receive assistance with the zipper and snaps.
	1b. Zach will zip his coat after a classroom assistant places the zipper on track.
	1c. Zach will independently don his jacket, including all fasteners.

When specific functional performance objectives become both the methods and outcomes of the curriculum, a singular focus on specific tasks may result. Therefore, a rigid functional curriculum, where practice of established objectives is the sole focus, may limit generalization of that targeted skill to related skills areas.

In an ecological approach, teams identify the home and community environments that are important for the student, the priority activities that occur in those environments, and the skills the individual needs to participate in those activities. These become the basis for the IEP goals. All school environments are targeted (e.g., regular classroom, lunchroom, rest rooms, playground, library).

The ecological goals and objectives may reflect the educational contexts in which performance is expected. For example:

Goal:	1. Brian will improve visual-scanning and visual-memory skills to increase accuracy in copying written materials.
Objectives:	1a. Brian will accurately copy the social studies summary questions from his textbook onto notebook paper, 90% accuracy.
	1b. Brian will accurately copy homework assignments from the chalkboard during language arts class, 100% accuracy.
	1c. Brian will accurately copy math problems from his math book, 90% accuracy.

Ecological goals and objectives can also be written with goals that specify priority environments and activities. In this case, the objectives are written to specify component skills. For example:

Goals: 1. Joe will demonstrate basic word-processing skills during business education class.

Objectives: 1a. Joe will open the word-processing program, 3 of 3 sessions.

            1b. Joe will format a new document with the requested margin sets, 3 of 3 sessions.

            1c. Joe will type a simple business letter with 90% accuracy, 10 words per minute.

            1d. Joe will perform cut-and-paste functions when word processing a document, 3 of 3 sessions.

Establishing meaningful goals and objectives can be challenging and requires significant skill in evaluating both the child's needs and strengths, as well as the school environments in which the child will participate. It is important that each team member take on the perspective of the student when selecting goals. In addition, team members should always examine the relevance to school and community environments.

■ OCCUPATIONAL THERAPY IN THE SCHOOLS

The services that a child needs to achieve his or her IEP goals are determined after goals and objectives are established. The intensity and frequency of therapy (30 minutes, three times a week) and models of service delivery (direct, consultative) are specified in the written IEP. If a student participates in regular education and is not eligible for special education services, that student is not eligible for related services (under IDEA), despite the presence of a disability. Temporary impairments (e.g., a fractured bone) usually do not make a student eligible for school-based therapy, although the student may need ccupational therapy in a medical setting.

For example, a bright first-grader had mild left hemiparesis cerebral palsy. This student participated in all aspects of the educational program, including physical education, with few adaptations. The disability did not interfere with the student's educational program. Therefore, she was not eligible for occupational therapy in school, despite the fact that she did not have the full use of her left hand (Figure 24-5).

In another case, a teenager suffered traumatic amputation of the left arm in an automobile accident. He returned to his high school classes and was able to participate in everything except computer lab. The occupational therapist consulted with the computer lab instructor and recommended that a right hand keyboard be ordered and installed. The therapist gave the

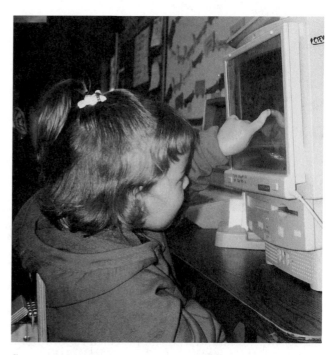

figure 24-5 A child with left hemiparesis uses a touch window on the classroom computer. Despite her left-side motor impairments, she did not qualify for related services under IDEA because she was fully functional and met all standards for kindergarten performance.

instructor resources for teaching one-hand typing. Consultation continued on an intermittent basis until the student became proficient in using the special keyboard.

Sometimes a student with a disability is not eligible for special education services, although he or she has difficulty participating in (and benefiting from) educational programs. For example, students diagnosed with attention deficit hyperactivity disorder may not be eligible for special education programs. However, these students often benefit from occupational therapy services, particularly when the student exhibits related sensory processing problems. Occupational therapy in the schools can be provided to these students under one of the civil rights acts. Section 504 of the Title V of the Rehabilitation Act of 1973 and the Title II of the Americans with Disabilities Act of 1990 (ADA) protect the rights of individuals with disabilities against discriminatory practices. Because the definition of disability is broader in these civil rights acts, a child may be eligible for occupational therapy even when he or she is not eligible for special education services. Although school personnel are not required to develop IEPs for students served under the Rehabilitation Act or the ADA, a team should develop a written plan that states goals, services, and accommodations needed to meet those goals (AOTA, 1997).

Service-Delivery Models

Acknowledging that all occupational therapy in the school must relate to the student's educational plan, three models for the delivery of occupational therapy are described in the literature: (1) *direct service,* (2) *monitoring,* and (3) *consultation.*

Direct service

According to Gilfoyle (1980), direct services are "those related services within a student's educational program for which the occupational therapy has the primary responsibility" (p. 2). Direct service can be conducted on an individual or a group basis, and is implemented personally by the practitioner. Weekly contact is usually the designated frequency of intervention. For purposes of this discussion, direct services are categorized as *"pull-out"* or *integrated therapy models.* In "pull out" services, the student is removed from the classroom and intervention occurs in a clinic or other room. In an integrated therapy model, the practitioner provides intervention within the classroom, emphasizing nonintrusive methods. The therapist's presence in the classroom benefits the instructional staff, who observe the occupational therapy intervention. Working within the classroom benefits the therapist as he or she gains a thorough understanding of the classroom environment and the behavioral and achievement expectations of its students. This integrated model of therapy also allows the student to participate in the classroom activities, with therapy support. Integrated therapy ensures that the therapist's focus has high relevance to the performance expected within the student's classroom. It also promotes the likelihood that adaptations and therapeutic techniques will be carried over into classroom activities (York, Giangreco, Vandercook, & MacDonald, 1992).

Educational proponents of inclusion support integrated models of therapy, and they suggest that pull-out services are only appropriate when students need to work on a skill that is far below the tasks presented to other students in the classroom or when the intervention activities cannot appropriately occur in a typical classroom (e.g., therapeutic use of equipment such as a swing). When intervention activities create a distraction that prevents other students from learning or the teacher from teaching, they should be performed outside the classroom (Elliot & McKenney, 1998).

Block scheduling, an alternative to traditional scheduling, is used in implementing an integrated therapy model (Rainforth & York-Barr, 1997). Therapy sessions are scheduled in longer blocks of time than usual, so the therapist has time to work within the classroom setting during the times when meaningful activities occur. The overall total therapy time in a given month may remain the same, but the students are seen every other week rather than weekly. If several students are seen in the same classroom, the therapist may continue weekly services for each by combining the students' time. The therapist remains in the classroom for the entire morning, or afternoon, and moves between students during each of the activities presented. Block scheduling gives the therapist opportunities for *co-teaching or team teaching.* In this method a therapist and classroom teacher jointly design and implement learning experiences within the classroom setting. The therapist's time is scheduled for the co-planned activities, rather than for individual sessions. Not only do the targeted students benefit from the interventions, but also the other students in the class benefit from the multidisciplinary input. For example the classroom teacher and occupational therapist may co-plan a handwriting session. The session may include both the third grade curriculum and practice of the mechanics of handwriting.

Monitoring

In service delivery that involves monitoring, the occupational therapist usually plans a program that involves specific activities for a student to be carried out with the help of other personnel (e.g., teaching assistant, aide). The person who is chosen to implement the program is trained and supervised by the therapist for specific activities. Appropriate activities to teach others to implement are those that do not require the presence of a qualified therapist to be carried out in a safe and effective manner. Regular contact is necessary to update programs and supervise the manner in which the activities are implemented. Examples of activities that can be monitored are positioning a student for written activities or implementation of assistive technology (e.g., adapted keyboard).

Consultation

Consultation supplements direct services, or it may be provided as the primary method of service delivery. In consultation, the therapist and teacher (or other professional) form a cooperative partnership and engage in a reciprocal, problem-solving process. The goal is to enhance the skills of the consultee and to improve the targeted performance area of the students. At times the focus of consultation is enhancing the teacher's knowledge and skills. At other times the focus is more directly on implementation of a specific program for the student.

To provide effective consultation, the occupational therapist needs (1) in depth knowledge and understanding of the problem, (2) knowledge of appropriate interventions, and (3) effective communication and interaction skills. The occupational therapist also must thoroughly understand the educational system so that the intervention strategies that he or she recommends are feasible within the system. Understanding the educational system also helps the therapist to ensure that appropriate classroom and student supports are identified.

An understanding of the system and school policies is particularly important when the therapist identifies curricular or environmental modifications that would benefit the student's educational program.

Various models of consultation have been defined (Hanft & Place, 1996; Idol, Paolucci-Whitcomb, & Nevin, 1987; Ross, 1995). Three models are frequently used in school settings, often in combination with direct service and monitoring models. They are (1) *the expert consultation model*, (2) *the mental-health consultation model*, and (3) *the collaborative consultation model*.

In the expert consultation model, the therapist presents the teacher or consultee with advice and recommendations to solve the problem. This directive approach is important when time does not allow for extended problem solving, when a crisis requires an immediate solution, or when a teacher is inexperienced and does not readily engage in the problem solving process. Research has shown that often teachers prefer that consultants provide specific recommendations (Werts, Wolery, Synder, Caldwell & Salisbury, 1996). The dangers in providing expert advice without entering into collaborative problem solving include:

1. The therapist is viewed as an expert, and quick advice is expected when future problems arise.
2. The teacher does not engage in a problem solving process and is less likely to be able to handle a similar problem when it occurs again.
3. Advice without deep examination of the problem is likely to be incorrect or inappropriate for the student.

The mental-health consultation model is one in which the role of the consultant is primarily that of support and encouragement. The goal of this consultation model is for the teacher to believe that he or she has the skills needed to handle the student with disabilities independently. The therapist encourages the teacher and gives positive feedback to solutions in place. The primary role of the therapist is to listen and point out the actions of the teacher that have had positive results. This type of consultation may not be helpful when practical solutions to complex issues are needed. The consultee usually desires specific information and intervention suggestions (Ross, 1995).

A third model, collaborative consultation, emphasizes that the consultant and the consultee have equally important roles. The parties agree on and work toward common goals to make decisions. Although the consultant and consultee work jointly on an equal basis, they have different roles (Zins & Erchul, 1995). The consultant structures and guides the overall process, while the consultee provides information about the problem and the expectations. The consultee generally (1) retains responsibility for the student, (2) judges treatment acceptability, and (3) implements the intervention. Because the consultee implements the intervention, it is important that he or she can accurately apply it, recognize the expected or desired response, and judge when modifications to the strategy are needed. It is the responsibility of the consultant to ensure that the consultee is well informed and sensitive to the issues. Therefore the consultant's responsibilities include (1) presenting a new or more in-depth understanding of the student's problem, (2) identifying and presenting interventions for possible implementation, (3) assisting in selecting the most appropriate and realistic solutions, and (4) developing an evaluation plan. These differing responsibilities suggest that a complementary, interdependent working relationship is needed (Zins & Erchul, 1995).

Hanft and Place (1996) described types of decision making required in the consultation role. The most appropriate intervention strategies are selected first. These decisions are based on (1) the student's and teacher's goals, (2) the student's problems, (3) the consultee's skills and interaction style, and (4) the flexibility and constraints of the environment. Examples of typical strategies recommended by occupational therapists are listed (Table 24-2).

With appropriate intervention strategies in mind, the occupational therapist selects a method for implementing the strategies. Methods range from very directive (e.g., modeling, teaching), to indirect strategies where the therapist primarily offers encouragement and support. The occupational therapist also provides specific information to help the teacher in problem solving. The method selected is based on the teacher's knowledge about and experience with children with disabilities, and his or her learning style. One teacher may be quite experienced in working with children with physical disabilities and need little support; another teacher may have minimal experience in working with students with physical disabilities and need more support.

In each model, clarity, specificity, and accuracy of the information are important. Generally a combination of methods works best. For example, the therapist can model joint compression and hand massage before writing activities or one-hand techniques in dressing. Providing written handouts and verbal cues are also helpful in guiding the teacher's facilitation of student's performance.

The third decision that the therapist must make is selection of interaction style. The occupational therapist selects an interaction style that he or she believes will be most effective with the consultee. Interaction styles are defined using different parameters. Examples of interaction styles are achiever, analyst, supporter and persuader (DeBoer, 1991).

These four styles reflect that individuals vary along a continuum of high to low people-orientation and of high to low risk-taking. Table 24-3 describes each

table 24-2 *Intervention Strategies When Consulting*

Intervention Strategies	Examples
1. Reframe the teacher's perspective	Explain the functional consequences of the perceptual problems observed in children with spina bifida.
	Identify that a child with autism is hypersensitive to tactile and auditory stimuli.
	Suggest that the reason that a child's difficulty in sitting quietly is related to his or her low arousal level and need for sensory input.
2. Improve the student's skills	Recommend that a student use carbon paper to monitor the amount of force applied with his pencil.
	Recommend that a student practice letter formation, using large-lined paper and beginning at the top of the letter.
	Recommend that a teacher provide stand-by assistance when the child practices carrying a lunch tray in the cafeteria.
3. Adapt the task	Recommend that a student begin to use a computer keyboard.
	Introduce compensatory methods for donning a jacket.
	Teach one-handed techniques during toilet training.
	Recommend that a student use earphones with music during written tests.
4. Adapt the environment	Establish a quiet area with a tent in which a student can hide and remove himself from the stimulating environment.
	Suggest that excess visual stimulation is removed from the wall in front of a student.
5. Adapt the routine	Recommend that a student have opportunities for exercise 3 times each day.
	Recommend that a student be given extra time to complete certain written assignments.
	Suggest that the student receive speech therapy after occupational therapy so that he is focused and attentive during the session.

style and the implication for consulting with an individual with each style.

As Hanft and Place (1996) have suggested, the consultant's style varies from being very directive to being primarily supportive, based on the consultee's needs and style. Also the degree of specificity and detail depends on the consultee's preference and ability to generalize concepts and principles. It is important that the occupational therapist identify his or her own style, so he or she can recognize when styles may conflict and when changes in the predominant approach are needed.

Implementing Integrated Therapy into Regular-Education Classrooms

When school-based therapists were surveyed, many believed that children were best served when they received a combination of the various service models, when therapy was integrated into the classroom, and when therapists consulted with teachers (Cable & Case-Smith, 1996). A model that appears to consider these ideas is the integrated therapy model. Integrated therapy takes place in the student's environment and focuses on priority activities for that student. Therapists evaluate students within their natural environment; then, they try the in-

tervention strategies, solve implementation problems, modify programs, and train staff members who are with the student throughout the day. They also monitor progress and support other professionals with information to ensure that intervention occurs frequently throughout the day in the student's typical environments.

When school personnel frequently collaborate and share information, discipline-specific skills become difficult to discern among professions. With experience, professionals become more knowledgeable about the methods of other disciplines. For example, eating and feeding are often areas where both the occupational therapist and speech pathologist have experience. In some instances, the occupational therapist may take the primary responsibility for a student's feeding problem. In other instances, the speech pathologist may take the leading role. For most significant functional problems, a number of professionals become involved in intervention. Goals and objectives are more likely to be successfully met when the child has an opportunity to practice the skill across many different environments and with many different people.

When working with students in a regular-education classroom, the therapist needs to have a clear understanding of the classroom expectations. This includes knowledge of classroom rules, routines, and dynamics, as well

table 24-3 *Consultation by Interaction Style*

Style	Primary Characteristics of Consultee	Implications for a Consultant
Achiever	Consultee is directive, likes to make decisions, is a risk taker, likes to be in charge, needs an end goal, and may not be sensitive to personal issues in desire to accomplish a goal.	Consultant needs to be directive and assertive; should keep recommendations short, make measurable, achievable recommendations; allow the achiever to feel in charge; should be incisive.
Analyst	Consultee is precise, detail oriented, low in people orientation, and therefore satisfied to work on own; needs lots of data to act, and needs to know that solutions are correct. Consultee implements recommendations with high precision; not a risk taker.	Consultant needs to give detailed, precise directives, and have patience with the analyst's need for information. Consultant should not push this person into decisions, respect their analytical ability. Include data collection in the plan. Consultant should encourage decision making in a timely way. The consultant should minimize risks.
Persuader	Consultee is enthusiastic, good at influencing others, relates well to almost everyone. Consultee is highly people oriented and is a high-risk taker; will sell solutions to the consultant. Consultee does not need details—likes to take action.	This consultee is fun to consult with, but follow up is necessary. Often this person will try whatever is readily available in the environment. Consultant needs to be aware that the consultee is easily influenced and may jump tracks midstream. Consultant should market ideas with enthusiasm and optimism.
Supporter	Consultee is encouraging and supportive of everyone, is high people-orientation skills; prefers that people get along rather than achieve specific goals. Consultee is good at holding together a team; may not be efficient in implementing recommendations, because this person easily becomes over committed.	Consultant's job is easy because this person is agreeable and flexible. Consultant should listen attentively and make clear recommendations that include a rationale. It is important to be positive, since this consultee is often sensitive. Follow-up is needed, because often the supporter has taken on too much. Consultee may be slow to respond to recommendations because of other commitments.

Adapted from DeBoer, A. (1991). *The art of consulting*. Chicago: Arcturus.

as knowledge of the general-education curriculum and special education adaptations. Each classroom teacher has unique teaching and classroom-management styles. Intervention techniques conducted in the classroom that may be acceptable to one teacher may not be acceptable to another teacher; they may even be considered intrusive.

Griswold (1993) recommended that therapists offer interventions that fit the existing classroom structure and culture. For example, a teacher who values child-directed learning and hands-on learning centers may respond well to a therapist's suggestions for activities to be included in the learning centers. Another teacher, who uses a strong teacher-directed classroom, may prefer to engage in team-teaching activities with the therapist.

Therapists also need to be sensitive to the regular-education schedule and not disrupt the child's and the classroom schedule, if possible. Teachers may prefer to have the therapist in the classroom at certain times or on certain days. These preferences should be negotiated with the teacher before intervention, and attempts should be made to schedule times for providing services to the child that coincide with targeted goal areas. For example, handwriting interventions can be integrated into the student's language arts time and keyboarding skills can be addressed during a student's computer or business education class.

Finally, special education teachers provide valuable resources to related service personnel. Special education teachers are usually in school buildings on a daily basis, and they know the regular-education curriculum and classroom teachers. They often function as liaisons between the regular-education teacher and the occupational therapist. Because special education teachers generally understand therapy service and the regular-education curriculum, they can be important advocates for integrated therapy services.

The support that an occupational therapist provides within the school should make both the child and the teacher's jobs easier, without placing unreasonable burdens on either the student or teacher. Although the teacher and therapist's jobs are to support the child's role as a student, at times there is a mismatch between what teachers (and parents) want and what occupational therapists want. Conflicts in point of view can be minimized or avoided if consistent communication is maintained between teachers and support personnel. The responsibility for maintaining open pathways of communication rests equally on all members of the team.

■ PROCEDURAL SAFEGUARDS

According to IDEA, parents have rights in determining what services their child receives; in accessing information about their child's evaluation results, program, and progress; and in making decisions about placement. Parents are also given a mechanism for resolving disputes with the school system about services and programs for their child. The procedural safeguards defined in IDEA do not directly involve occupational therapists. However, it is important that therapists are knowledgeable about procedures, safeguards, and parental rights so that they follow correct procedures, accurately inform parents, and guide parents to appropriate resources when a concern arises. The procedural safeguards defined in IDEA are listed in Table 24-4. Safeguards are implemented in different ways in each state, and therapists should become knowledgeable as to how his or her state interprets the federal safeguards through state laws, regulations, policies, and procedures. The procedural safeguards delineated in IDEA protect parents' rights and, at the same time, promote mediation rather than litigation. Although court cases have set important precedents for how IDEA is to be interpreted and implemented, they are costly to local and state educational agencies and disruptive to school systems. Battles over placement and services are often painful for students, professionals, and their families. IDEA appropriately emphasizes mediation as the first and most helpful method for resolving conflicts between parents and school systems. Occupational therapists must fully acknowledge and respect parents' rights. When conflicts arise between parents and school system, therapists should know the steps involved in mediation and encourage parents to seek mediation to resolve a conflict. The therapist's own skills in resolving conflict can be instrumental in helping the team and parents identify what is best for the student. These skills can also be important in negotiating what services and strategies will optimally serve the student.

table 24-4   Implications of Procedural Safeguards for Occupational Therapists

Procedural Safeguards

Parents have the right to inspect and review all of their child's educational records.

Parents have the right to obtain an IEE of their child

Parents have the right to request a due process hearing on any matter with respect to the identification, evaluation, or placement of their child or the provision of FAPE.

Parents have the right to have a due process hearing conducted by an impartial hearing officer, to appeal the initial hearing, and to bring civil action in court.

Parents must receive written notice about their rights and protections under law.

States must have a voluntary mediation process in place as a means of resolving disputes between local education agencies and parents of children with disabilities.

Parents must notify the local educational agency when they intend to remove their child from the public school and place the child in a private school at public expense.

Parents must notify the local educational agency when they intend to file a due process complaint.

Under certain circumstances, such as a child bringing a weapon to school, the child may be removed from his or her current educational placement and placed in an interim alternative education setting or suspended or expelled from school.

Attorneys' fees may, under certain circumstances, be reduced or denied.

FAPE, Free appropriate public education; *IEE,* independent educational evaluation.

■ PLANNING TO TERMINATE SERVICES

Termination of a student's occupational therapy program is often more difficult than initiation of services. It is the responsibility of the occupational therapist, in collaboration with the team, to make decisions regarding termination of services (Carver, 1998). It may be appropriate to discontinue occupational therapy when the student:

1. Has accomplished established intervention goals and objectives.
2. Performs at a standard expected of his or her typical peers.
3. Is no longer making significant progress on established objectives despite changes in intervention strategies or service-delivery models.

4. Continues to make gains but there is no evidence that the occupational therapy interventions are related to the gains.
5. The identified priority skills are no longer a concern within the student's educational context.
6. The student expresses a desire to discontinue services.

Although these examples do not imply that occupational therapy should be automatically discontinued, these are considerations that warrant examining the appropriateness and value of continuing occupational therapy services. Occasionally, when students reach adolescence and become extremely concerned about forming and maintaining peer relationships, they begin to feel self-conscious about receiving special education services. Parents, the therapists, the teachers, and the student, may need to examine the costs and benefits of intervention when the student reaches adolescence.

The occupational therapist sometimes discontinues services for a period and then resumes services when the student reaches a new developmental level or must cope with new environmental demands. For example, occupational therapy services were terminated when a student with cerebral palsy functioned adequately in an elementary school environment. However, when this student entered middle school, physical growth, psychosocial issues associated with adolescence, and the stress of learning a new environment created several functional problems, and occupational therapy services were reinitiated.

When determining the appropriateness of terminating services, the student's needs, the context for performance, and the future needs of the student should be considered (Campbell & Bain, 1991). For example, should the therapist terminate services for a second grade student who has achieved his handwriting goals at the end of the school year (with intensive therapy and teacher accommodation), knowing that in 3rd grade, the student will be expected to master cursive handwriting. When considering terminating services, the IEP team, including the parents, should be consulted. Often other team members contribute valuable insights as to why a student can benefit from continued therapy or what alternative supports should be provided when occupational therapy services are discontinued.

From the beginning of services with a student, the therapist should plan for discontinuation, that is, how could this student become more independent so that occupational therapy support is not needed. Although students may receive occupational therapy for several years, it is helpful to discuss (with parents) the scope of services, projected time lines, and expected outcomes at the time of annual review of the IEP. These discussions early in the year help a parent understand and appreciate that therapy services may not be appropriate for the child's entire school career.

Once the therapist recognizes that discontinuation of services is appropriate, he or she should begin to prepare the student and the family. Termination of occupational therapy is particularly difficult when therapists, students, and families have had long-standing relationships over several school years. Parents and students often look to the occupational therapist as the constant contact person from school year to school year, providing a sense of continuity and a watchful eye.

Families may rely on this unspoken aspect of therapy for emotional support, making its termination difficult. When possible the therapist should begin the transition months in advance to ease the sense of loss. When additional alternative supports are needed, these can also be planned for and arrangements can be made. This can help to make the actual termination a more agreeable and hopeful experience for students and families.

Case Study 1: Story of Thomas

This case study demonstrates how occupational therapy services can benefit students in educational and life goals through effective problem solving, partnerships with other educational professionals and families, and application of intervention strategies well-grounded in theory.

Thomas was a 9½-year-old child in the third grade. He had a diagnosis of autism and, at that time, attended school three partial days a week. He was placed in a classroom for children with multiple impairments without participation in a regular education classroom.

Participation: overall functional level

Thomas' strengths were his mobility skills and self-care performance. He independently ate, including cutting meat and opening cartons. He dressed independently, including buttoning and zipping. He was also independent when using the toilet. In activities that required manipulation of materials, he efficiently used two hands together and manipulated small objects within his hand. Precise prehension using fingertips was accurate and consistent. Thomas had a number of behavioral issues that are described below. However, he consistently followed routines once he had learned them. He performed structured tasks that were familiar to him on a day-to-day basis.

Thomas' limitations were in the areas of sensory modulation, language, and social interactions. He had tremendous difficulty in communication and displayed echolalic speech most of the time. He had recently begun to use 1- to 2-word statements with meaning. However, he was not able to communicate using language consistently or fluidly. His receptive language was also severely delayed, and he did not demonstrate understanding of phrases with any consistency. Thomas also had difficulty engaging in an activity for more than 10 minutes at a time (other than routine activities, such as watching "his videos," swinging, or looking at books in his quiet space). He did not interact with peers or adults consistently or meaningfully. Behavioral issues included that he had difficulty making transitions or adapting to new environments. He often had tantrums when in a highly stimulating environment, such as a gymnasium.

Evaluation of performance components

The focus of the occupational therapist's performance evaluation was on sensory processing. Thomas' behavioral and social interaction and his motor skills were also examined.

Sensory processing. As a preschooler, Thomas lacked tolerance of most activities with high sensory stimulation. He would scream and cry when students approached him quickly or unexpectedly. He was easily upset by common environmental noises. At the time of this evaluation, Thomas craved bouncing, rough play and wrestling, and swinging. He enjoyed watching videos and playing on the computer. His sensory needs seemed to fluctuate within a very short period of time. For example, one minute he withdrew and retreated to a quiet corner of the room, and the next minute he was sensory seeking (e.g., swinging, jumping, climbing).

Behavior and social interaction. Thomas did not interact with peers and adults appropriately. In preschool and kindergarten, he could not leave his mother's side. Even last year, he screamed and cried for the first hour of every day. He became upset if anyone came near him or if a peer would play along side him. By third grade, he was more tolerant of being near his peers. On occasion he initiated interaction with adults.

Motor. Gross motor skills were an asset. Thomas had good balance and demonstrated normal strength. He could climb on playground equipment and easily get in and out of a swing. Fine motor skills were also strengths, although he demonstrated some delays when compared to his peers. Although he had mastered buttoning and zipping, he continued to struggle with tying. This problem may have related to difficulty in understanding the steps involved in the process, rather than with the actual motor skill involved in tying.

Priorities

The functional priorities for Thomas were language, communication, and socialization. Another focus was improving his ability to make transitions and to change activities and environments. The team decided on the following annual goals for his Individualized Education Program: Thomas would:

1. Demonstrate understanding of and answer simple "wh" questions without prompting.
2. Demonstrate appropriate social skills in the classroom, such as greeting adults and peers.

3. When given visual cues and prompts, transition to a new environment or a new activity without outbursts.
4. Recognize and regulate his own sensory needs by requesting time out or specific sensory input.

Occupational therapy intervention

The occupational therapist recognized Thomas's need for organized sensory input and encouraged play activities that involved jumping, hopping, and climbing. Through assessing his response to these activities, she determined that proprioceptive and vestibular input helped to calm and organize Thomas and seemed to promote his ability to attend to other activities. Using these insights, she designed a sensory diet with the teacher, incorporating sensory activities into the day's routine at points when they could occur without major interruption to the other students. Together, they developed a schedule that included 2 to 3 sessions of "motor time" for Thomas, primarily implemented by the classroom aide. At these times, he and his aide visited a motor room next to the classroom, which contained swings and balls. He spent 10 to 15 minutes on the equipment, preferring rhythmical swinging and spinning. He also participated in outdoor recess, preferring to climb, jump, slide, run, and swing. He was also allowed to visit his quiet space in the classroom when needed. In the space were his rocking chair, his headset playing quiet, rhythmical music, and his videos and VCR with monitor. Initially Thomas was led to his space when he had an outburst. However, he quickly determined when and for how long he needed his space.

The occupational and speech therapists developed a picture schedule of his daily activities, so Thomas had a visual reminder of what came next (Figure 24-6). When an activity was completed, he took the picture of the activity off his activity board and placed it in a box. Then Thomas pointed to the activity that came next, and his aide or the therapist talked to him about "what comes next." This visual cueing system worked well in helping him adjust to transitions and in helping him end one activity and transition to the next.

Strategies for teamwork

These strategies were incorporated into Thomas' daily schedule, and the teacher informed the occupational therapist about the success of the various strategies once a week. Success was measured by Thomas' behavior in the classroom and his participation in classroom activities. Thomas' speech therapist discussed how these strategies appeared to be helpful to his development of communication skills and suggested modifications. The teacher felt that the sensory diet and picture board for transitioning helped Thomas do several things: tolerate school activities that were stimulating, pay attention to

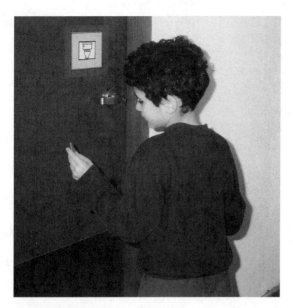

figure 24-6 Thomas is holding his picture card indicating time for a rest room break. The picture on the card matches the one on the door.

tasks, sit in his desk and perform academic skills, and work on task while near his peers. His negative behaviors decreased, and when he began to feel agitated, Thomas expressed the need to visit the motor room or his quiet space.

The speech therapist noted how Thomas' attention and spontaneous speech increased after participating in sensory modulating activities. His focus on other's verbalizations was greater, and his responses were more frequent when he had adequate sensory input that day. The strategies, therefore, appeared to positively influence the team's primary goals of communication and social interaction.

Case Study 2: Story of William

This case study emphasizes teamwork and consultation with a student preparing to enter high school. William was 13 and in middle school. He was the oldest of three children and loved nothing more than being with his younger brother and sister. At age 2, William had suffered a severe traumatic brain injury when he was injured in a car accident. He emerged from a 3-week coma with no movement on his right side and no speech. Although he regained some function in his right arm and leg, his movement remained quite impaired. William demonstrated partial range in his right shoulder and elbow but was unable to move his wrist and fingers. He used a one-hand drive wheelchair for mobility and could stand with assistance and take several steps. However, independent ambulation was not a goal.

William was essentially nonverbal in preschool. However, by age 13 he used 2- and 4-word phrases appropriately. He impulsively responded to every query with "no," when he generally meant yes, and he required a long time to think of words. The words he could produce were quite simple, his cognitive limitations were severe, and learning required many repetitions. William's primary asset was his social nature. He was friendly and cheerful; he offered everyone a smile. He tried new activities, even when they caused him discomfort. Staff in the school and his peers reported that they enjoyed being around William.

Participation in the school environment

Information about William's level of participation at school was gathered from his mother and teacher. His mother reported that he was easy going and happy. At times he demonstrated some frustration, because he had become more aware that he was different from other children. His mother's greatest concerns related to his judgment. He did not seem to understand when he was in danger and when he could hurt someone else. His mother reported that he had begun to develop some peer relations. In the past he would spend time at school by himself. However, in middle school he had established some friends and spent more time interacting with his peers.

William's teacher reported that he was a "doll, as sweet as he could be." His academic work was low level, and he required extra time to complete all work. However, he had made steady, slow progress in his reading and writing.

His teacher was concerned with his safety. She worried about his judgment, particularly outside the classroom. Currently his reading program emphasized safety words and concepts.

William had great difficulty in handling his school materials. He printed with cueing. However, his letters were poorly formed. He used a keyboard, also with verbal prompts. He independently turned on the computer and operated preschool-age storybook programs. Most of his work required assistance to keep him focused and to read difficult words. Both handwriting and keyboarding required great amounts of time and effort.

Performance in school activities

Self-maintenance. William ate independently in the cafeteria after his cartons were opened and his food was cut up. Eating was a favorite activity. He required minimal assistance to don his jacket, because he continued to neglect his right arm and only dressed his left side. William required assistance during two-hand activities and needed minimal assistance in transferring from his wheelchair to the toilet.

Manipulation of materials and writing. William required intermittent assistance to manage his school materials. He tended to neglect materials on his right side, and activities needed to be placed on his left side. He was unable to use scissors or other tools that required two hands. To help him write, William's paper was stabilized on his desk with a clipboard and dycem. In writing, his letters were large and poorly formed. He copied letters but did not compose.

Posture and mobility. William's posture had deteriorated in the last year; he leaned to the right with a rounded trunk. Poor posture had begun to interfere with eye-hand coordination and ability to move his left arm. In addition, the occupational therapist was quite concerned about the potential of developing scoliosis.

Behaviors. William was cooperative and pleasant. He followed instructions, although at times he did not attend well to classroom instructions. In addition, William continued to need one-on-one supervision for many activities, primarily due to his low cognitive level and his difficulty in problem solving the steps of a task. However, he initiated social interaction and consistently responded to others. He was motivated to try new activities and demonstrated persistence, particularly in one-on-one situations. Judgment remained a problem and seemed to relate to his impulsiveness and deficits in problem solving. Table 24-5 outlines William's annual IEP goals that required occupational therapy services.

Occupational therapy services

The occupational therapist contributed to all of these goals. She worked with William in a small group of his peers, generally on computing skills and functional mobility within the school environment. She used several typing programs that could be easily graded for beginners. William's favorite was "Slam Dunk," because he was an avid basketball fan. His family also purchased this program for practice at home.

The occupational therapist adapted William's wheelchair to improve his posture by moving his tray to a higher position and recommending a new strapping system that included a chest strap. A lateral pad on the right was tried, but it was not effective when he slumped forward in trunk flexion.

Once a month, William's therapy group planned and completed a community outing. A variety of field trips were planned, including a trip to a restaurant, a movie, a shopping trip, as well as a visit to a nearby factory and the post office. The purpose of these field trips was to increase William's ability to function in the community. Safety concepts were practiced and reinforced, including crossing the street, mobility around stairs and escalators, and care of his right arm. Appropriate social interactions with strangers and service persons were prac-

table 24-5 Goals for William

Goals	Measures
Verbalizes and demonstrates basic safety concepts regarding using his wheelchair, touching others, and appropriately positioning his right arm.	When queried on safety, he respond with 90% accuracy.
Demonstrates upright posture at his desk and in his wheelchair.	Sits with shoulders aligned directly over hips and trunk centered in chair, 80% of the time.
Demonstrates improved judgment and directionality for trial use of motorized wheelchair.	Demonstrates 80% accuracy in maneuvering his wheelchair through an obstacle course.
Independently dons his jacket by placing his right arm in its sleeve.	Puts on coat independently, 4 out of 5 times.
Demonstrates an independent standing transfer from his wheelchair to the toilet.	Demonstrates independent transfer, 5 of 5 times.
Improves his keyboarding and computing skills.	Independently operates two typing programs.

ticed. Basic concepts regarding handling money, ordering food and service, and requesting assistance were also emphasized.

These community outings were extremely helpful in identifying issues that would need to be addressed in the coming years, when William's ability to function in the community would become an important goal. Transition into community living and vocation are addressed at age 14, and these experiences helped the team establish realistic goals for the next year's IEP.

■ SUMMARY

School-based practice offers many challenges and many rewards. The Individuals with Disabilities Education Act, which defines the legal aspects of school-based therapy, frames this practice arena of occupational therapy. Although this education law establishes the scope of occupational therapy practice in the schools, the rich diversity, complexity, and significance of services provided by occupational therapists in schools extends well beyond legal definitions. Occupational therapists within schools have the potential to positively influence and enhance the lives of children by becom-

STUDY QUESTIONS

1. For a child with autism, such as Thomas (described in the case study), what intervention should be carried out in the classroom? What intervention strategies should be implemented outside the classroom?

2. Give one example of an occupational therapy evaluation tool used with children that appears to have a degree of cultural bias. What items appear to be culturally biased? What adaptations to (a) items and (b) administration procedures should be considered when using this test with a student from a minority group?

3. The primary teacher is a good resource for information concerning a child's participation in the classroom. Name other persons who may be important to interview to assess a child's overall ability to participate in school activities. Explain the benefits of using multiple informants when identifying a student's problems.

4. Using William (described in the case study), write two ecological goals for his transition to high school next year.

5. Explain a situation in which expert consultation would be the most appropriate model to implement. Describe a situation in which collaborative consultation would be the most effective model.

6. Given the scope and focus of occupational therapy and the curriculum for 3rd grade children, describe an appropriate topic for team teaching with a regular-education teacher. What therapist-teacher instructional activities could be implemented to build the students' skills related to this topic?

ing part of their everyday lives and their natural environments.

Integrating therapy services into a child's natural environment and routine requires ingenuity and adaptability. The therapist must identify the student and teacher's priorities and decide which strategies are most important to that student's ability to participate in school. Effectiveness in school-based practice relates to the therapist's ability to analyze performance, solve problems, develop effective interventions, partner with families, teachers, and other professionals. When necessary, the therapist must also advocate for children through system change.

References

Achenbach, T.M., & Edelbrock, C.S. (1991). *Child Behavior Checklist*. Burlington, VT: University of Vermont.

American Occupational Therapy Association (1997). *Occupational therapy services for children and youth under the Individuals with Disabilities Education Act*. Bethesda: American Occupational Therapy Association, Inc.

Americans with Disabilities Act of 1990, 42 U.S.C. §12134. (1990).

Ayres, A.J. (1989). *Sensory Integration and Praxis Tests*. Los Angeles: Western Psychological Services.

Beery, K.E. (1997). *Beery Development Test of Visual Motor Integration* (4th revision). Cleveland, OH: Modern Curriculum Press.

Bruininks, R.H. (1978). *Bruininks-Oseretsky Test of Motor Proficiency*. Circle Pines, MN: American Guidance Service.

Cable, J., & Case-Smith, J. (1996). Perceptions of occupational therapist regarding service delivery models in school based practice. *Occupational Therapy Journal of Research, 13*, 23-43.

Campbell, T.F., & Bain, B.A. (1991). How long to treat: A multiple outcome approach. *Language, Speech and Hearing Services in Schools, 22*, 271-276.

Carver, C. (July/August, 1998). Crossing thresholds: School based occupational therapists discuss how they move young clients into—and out of—therapy programs. *OT Practice, 3*, (7), 18-21.

Clark, G., & Coster, W. (1998). Evaluation/problem solving and program evaluation. In J. Case-Smith (Ed.), *Occupational therapy: Making a difference in school system practice*. Bethesda: AOTA, Inc.

Clark, G., & Miller, L. (1996). Providing effective occupational therapy services: Data-based decision making in school based practice. *American Journal of Occupational Therapy, 50*, 701-708.

Colarusso, R.P., Hammill, D.D., & Mercier, L. (1995). *Motor-Free Visual Perception Test-Revised (MVPT-R)*. Novato, CA: Academic Therapy Publications.

Coster, W., Deeney, T., Haltiwanger, J., & Haley, S. (1998). *School Function Assessment*. San Antonio: Psychological Corporation.

DeBoer, A.L. (1986). *The art of consulting*. Chicago: Arcturus Books.

Dunn, W.W. (1999). *Sensory Profile*. San Antonio: Psychological Corporation.

Elliot, D., & McKenny, M. (1998). Four inclusion models that work. *Teaching Exceptional Students, 30* (4), 54-58.

Federal Register. (1998). C.F.R., 34, Parts 300 to 399.

Folio, R., & Fewell, R. (2000). *Peabody Developmental Motor Scale* (2nd ed.). Austin, TX: Pro-Ed.

Gilfoyle, E. (1980). *Training occupational therapy educational management in schools* (Vol. 2-4). Rockville, MD: AOTA, Inc.

Griswold, L. (1993). Ethnographic analysis: A study of classroom environments. *American Journal of Occupational Therapy, 48*, 397-402.

Hammill, D.D., Pearson, N.A., & Voress, J.K. (1993). *Developmental Test of Visual Perception* (2nd ed.) Austin, TX: Pro Ed.

Hanft, B.E. & Place, P.A. (1996). *The consulting therapist: A guide for OTs and PTs in Schools*. San Antonio, TX: Therapy Skills Builders.

Heumann, J.E., & Hehir, T. (1994). *OSERS memorandum to Chief State School Officers: Questions and answers on the least restrictive environment requirements of the Individuals with Disabilities Education Act*. Washington, D.C: U.S. Department of Education.

Hopkins, H.L. (1988). A historical perspective on occupational therapy. In H.L. Hopkins & H. Smith (Eds.), *Willard & Spackman's occupational therapy* (7th ed.). Philadelphia: J.B. Lippincott.

Idol, L., Paolucci-Whitcomb, P., & Nevin, A. (1987). *Collaborative consultation*. Austin, TX: Pro Ed.

Individuals with Disabilities Education Act Amendments of 1990. 20 U.S.C. § 1400-1485.

McCarney, S.G., & Leigh, J.E. (1990). *The Behavior Evaluation Scale—2*. Columbia, MO: Educational Services.

NICHCY (1999). *Office of Special Education Programs' IDEA 1997 training packet*. www.nichcy.org

Pennsylvania Association for Retarded Citizens v. Commonwealth of Pennsylvania, 344 F Supp. 1257 (Pa. 1971).

Rainforth, B., & York-Barr, J. (1997). *Collaborative teams for students with severe disabilities: Integrating therapy and educational services: (2nd ed.)* Baltimore: Brookes.

Rehabilitation Act of 1973, 29 U.S.C. § 706 (8) and §794.

Reisman, J., & Hanschu, B. (1992). *Sensory Integration Inventory – Revised, for Individuals with Developmental Disabilities.* Hugo, MN: PDP Products.

Ross, (1995). Best practices in implementing intervention assistance teams. In A. Thomas & J. Grimes (Eds.), *Best practices in school psychology—III* (pp. 651-660). Washington, D.C: The National Association of School Psychologists.

Werts, M.G., Wolery, M., Snyder, E.D., Caldwell, N.K., Salisbury, C.L. (1996). Supports and resources associated with inclusive schooling: Perceptions of elementary school teachers about need and availability. *Journal of Special Education, 30,* (2), 187-203.

York, J., Giangreco, M.F., Vandercook, T., & McDonald, C. (1992). Integrating support personnel in the inclusive classroom. In S. Stainback & W. Stainback (Eds.), *Curriculum considerations in inclusive classrooms: Facilitating learning for all students.* (pp. 101-116). Baltimore: Paul H. Brookes Publishing Co.

Zepeda, S.J., & Langenback, M. (1999). *Special programs in regular schools: Historical foundations, standards, and contemporary issues.* Allyn & Bacon: Needham Heights, MD.

Zins, J.E., & Erchul, W.P. (1995). Best practice in school consultation. In A. Thomas & J. Grimes (Eds.), *Best practices in school psychology—III.* (pp. 651-660). Washington, D.C: The National Association of School Psychologists.

chapter **25**

Services for Children with Visual or Auditory Impairments

Elizabeth Snow-Russel

OCCUPATIONAL THERAPY FOR CHILDREN

key terms

Conductive hearing
  loss
Sensorineural hearing
  loss
Hearing impairments
Sign language
Total communication
American Sign
  Language
Visual Impairment
Legal blindness

Mobility training
Braille
Low-vision training

■ CHAPTER OBJECTIVES

1. Describe the role that the senses of vision and hearing play in a child's life.
2. Define terms related to visual and hearing impairment.
3. Describe the effects of visual and hearing impairments on a child's development.
4. Identify intervention goals appropriate for children with visual and hearing impairments.
5. Describe examples of occupational therapy intervention for children with visual or hearing impairments.

Hearing and vision allow us to understand what is happening in the world around us. Those with normal sensory function cannot truly understand the experience of being hearing or visually impaired. However, participating in sensory awareness activities can increase understanding of the difficulties associated with hearing or vision loss. Sensory awareness activities include eating a meal blindfolded or listening to recordings that simulate what songs sound like to an individual with a certain type of hearing loss.

However, sensory awareness activities do not give the total picture of what it is like to have a hearing- or vision-related disability. This is because people with normally functioning senses have a vast wealth of visual and auditory memories to call upon that people with some form of sensory loss do not have. It is important to note that most of the children with sensory loss seen in occupational therapy are congenitally impaired. Therefore they will have no reservoir of unimpaired information to review.

The sense organs (e.g., eyes, ears, skin, nose, tongue) are all extensions of the brain. The brain's primary function is to receive information, or sensory stimuli, from the world for processing and coding. This information is integrated and associated with past experiences. Because the nature and the intensity of stimulation to the sense organs varies greatly, one experience may take precedence over others. If a particular sense organ is not working properly, the others do not totally compensate for the loss. However, a single sensory system may take precedence over a weak or damaged system.

Ayres (1972) developed a hierarchy of sensory perceptual development that helps in the understanding of sensory impairments. The senses develop and work in an interactive manner; they do not perform in isolation but develop in a building-block manner. The *vestibular system* gives information about the body's position in space, movement or lack of movement through space, and direction of movement. It is thought that the auditory system evolved out of the more primitive vestibular system (Ayres, 1972). The receptors for the vestibular system are located in the inner ear (Figure 25-1).

The vestibular and *tactile* (touch) systems are the foundations of sensation. Visual and auditory sensations are received by the brain against a constant background of tactile stimuli and the body's position in space. It is important to think about the level of alertness required by the brain for auditory and visual perceptual processes to occur. The vestibular system and the reticular activating system have a great influence on this level of alertness. Being either overly alert or not sufficiently alert can have detrimental effects on visual and auditory perceptions.

Vision is the sense we use for understanding the relationships between people and objects. It puts the environment in perspective and precedes auditory development by building concepts and perceptual abilities. Children with visual deficits often have a diminished verbal language, because they are unable to grasp relationships and associations between people and objects. In discussing vision, it is important to differentiate between *visual acuity, visual awareness,* and *visual perception.* Impairment can occur at any or all levels, and it can occur in varying degrees within levels.

In addition to its function as the building block for speech, *audition* is the sense that conveys sound. Sound gives information on distance and direction. For example, we can hear a dog bark and, without seeing the dog, judge where and how far away it is. *Auditory perception* is the attachment of meaning to sound patterns. Sound has qualities of tone and pitch that make up auditory acuity.

As with vision, impairment can occur at the level of acuity, awareness, or perception. Although language development appears to be the most serious problem for a hearing-impaired child, the situation is much more complex. This is because language is a force in the socialization and development of the child's inner logic. In addition, the ability to use language affects personality development (Ling, 1989). Language is not innate; it is a product of the child's environment. As the child learns the language, he or she can exert greater control over this environment.

The problems of children with visual or hearing impairments can be enormous. Although these children face many shared difficulties, the differences are striking. For this reason, this chapter deals separately with the hearing impaired, the visually impaired, and the multiple-sensory impaired. Although they are usually not the primary providers of intervention for children with significant visual or hearing impairment, occupational therapists provide

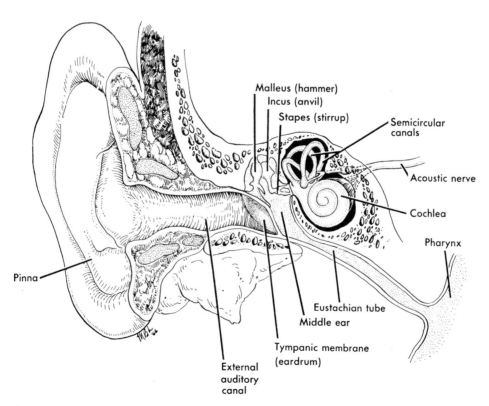

figure**25-1**   Cross section of the ear. *(From Ingalls, A.J., & Salerno, M.C. [1983].* Maternal and child health nursing *[5th ed.]. St. Louis: Mosby.)*

critical services for the associated functional problems incurred by these children. The occupational therapist is often employed in the role of consultant, providing services to individuals, entire classrooms, or institutions.

Consultation often revolves around five problems typically addressed in occupational therapy:

1. Activities of daily living (e.g., feeding, dressing, toileting)
2. Fine-motor coordination and dexterity
3. Sensory processing and perceptual skills
4. Gross-motor and body movement skills
5. Preparation for vocational training

The goal of occupational therapy services is to help the child develop typical occupations. These activities need to have meaning and purpose to the child and his or her family, and they need to occur within natural contexts of the child and family. Consultation is given to parents, teachers, and caregivers as part of the child's overall developmental and educational plan (and in conjunction with those professionals primarily involved with the child with visual and/or hearing impairment).

In providing occupational therapy for children with sensory loss, the importance of play cannot be overemphasized. Play is the means by which the child learns how to solve problems, to cope with the environment, to face the unknown, and to adapt by changing behaviors (Gunn, 1971; Michelman, 1971; Parham & Fazio, 1997). For children whose distance senses and, therefore, their abilities to perceive the environment are limited, the development of play skills, particularly active play involving use of the vestibular and proprioceptive systems, should be the highest priority.

■ HEARING IMPAIRMENT

The occupational therapist encounters children with hearing impairment in hospitals (at the time of diagnosis) or later in clinics and school settings. Prematurity increases the chances of hearing impairment (Steinberg & Knightly, 1997), and often infants leave the neonatal unit with a suspected hearing loss. Hearing loss is often identified through developmental testing in the clinic, or it is later discovered in school. With the advent of more local programs, the percentage of children with hearing impairment attending state schools for the deaf has decreased. However, a number of children with hearing impairments (particularly those with severe hearing losses or multiple sensory handicaps) still attend these schools.

In special education programs, the occupational therapist has a strategic role in the areas of self-help, socialization, fine motor, sensory integration, and perceptual motor development. The increasing number of early intervention programs allows for more therapist involvement in intervention for young children with hearing impairments and in the all-important parent-child interaction process.

Special Characteristics Relevant to Occupational Therapy

To the occupational therapist, the most important characteristic of the child with hearing-impairment is the lack of early language development and the profound problems that this delay causes in all other areas of development (Furth, 1973; Liben, 1978; Myklebust, 1964; Northern & Downs, 1992). What at first appears to be a fairly simple problem, becomes complicated when one considers the importance language plays in our society.

Language assists in environmental manipulation and gives the child labels for objects and concepts. It also plays a critical role in socialization. For example, while the typically developing infant smiles and quiets to the sounds of his or her mother, the infant with a hearing impairment does not respond to his or her mother's soft voice.

Babbling is vocal play that uses the vocal cords and muscles of the mouth, tongue, and larynx; all children do this. Children who can hear get the stimulus of hearing themselves and their parents' vocalized responses. However, children with hearing impairment get insufficient feedback, and babbling does not progress on to language development. The infant with deafness generally babbles normally up until approximately 5 months of age (Stoel-Gammon & Otomo, 1986). However, after 5 months, as the typically developing infant develops a growing repertoire of sounds, the child with hearing impairment begins to demonstrate language delay. Although early intervention is imperative in these cases, the child's hearing impairment is often not diagnosed until he or she is 2½ years of age (Goldberg, 1996).

Researchers (e.g., Meadow, 1980; Northern & Downs, 1992) believe that if intervention is delayed until 3 or 4 years of age, the most important formative period of language development is on the decline and permanent damage is done. If the child is denied cortical stimulation by organic means (because of impaired auditory stimuli), he or she may need to conceptualize by other means. Diagnostic information and description of specialized testing and intervention for children with hearing impairment can be found in Appendix A.

Occupational Therapy Assessment Procedures

The therapist can use standardized assessment tools (e.g., the Battelle Developmental Inventory, the Bayley Scales of Infant Development-revised [BSID-II], or the Hawaii Early Learning Profile [HELP]), to test a child with visual and/or hearing impairment. However, the language areas of these tests have to be modified, and standard scores should not be used. If reported, scores must acknowledge any modifications made to the test being used. If the child is using a hearing aid, cochlear implant, lip reading, or sign language, the therapist should understand the implications of these specialized devices and/or techniques. If the child uses sign language and the therapist testing the child is unable to give the commands using the type of sign the child uses, the test results should also include that information. In some instances, it is necessary to use a registered interpreter to accurately test a client with hearing-impairment. Functional developmental assessment, such as the Trandisciplinary Play Based Assessment (TPBA), is helpful in determining the child's strengths and limitations (Linder, 1993), and it avoids problems in test validity. The TPBA can be very useful with the child with hearing impairment, because the assessment setting is natural and standard responses are not expected. In this assessment, the play facilitator should be skilled in the communication system used by the child. This allows other team members, who are not skilled in the communication system used by the child, to observe the testing and request that the facilitator attempt to obtain certain information. Another advantage of TPBA is that repeated viewing of a video recording of the test allows the assessment team to pick up emerging signs and beginning language and/or communication attempts that may be too subtle to be noted initially.

Through developmental testing, the occupational therapist frequently identifies a mild problem that may have gone undiagnosed. For example, when a pediatrician recommends evaluation of a child whose language development appears delayed, a slight hearing loss may be identified. Although each child's development is unique, certain findings indicate the possibility of hearing loss and suggest referral to appropriate professionals (Box 25-1).

In most cases the parents are the keenest observers of their infants. Special attention should be given to a child whose mother or father reports that he or she does not awaken to loud noises, respond when called, or attend to noisy toys. In addition, it is important to follow-up a parental report indicating that a child gestures to communicate wants, to the exclusion of words. Therapists should attend to the parent's complaints (e.g., the child's distractibility, inattention to commands, lack of feedback to the mother or father, inappropriate responses to verbal stimuli) and recommend testing or referral to hearing specialists. Referral is also appropriate when a child with a history of recurrent ear infections or upper respiratory infections presents with a possible conductive hearing loss. Although many difficulties can be attributable to other causes, hearing impairment should be considered.

Developmental assessments of fine motor, gross motor, visual motor, sensory integration, and self-care skills can be administered to children with hearing impairments with some adaptation in instructional methods. However, written instructions should be used only if the child has the appropriate level of written comprehension, and consideration of the language demands of any

---

box 25-1 *Findings that indicate the possibility of hearing loss*

Possible hearing impairment must be considered in the following instances:

- A newborn does not awaken to sounds as expected.
- A newborn does not exhibit a startle *(Moro)* reflex in response to a sharp clap 3 to 6 feet away.
- A 3-month-old child has not developed auditory-orienting responses, as indicated by not becoming alert to noises made by certain toys.
- An 8- to 12-month-old child does not turn to a whispered voice.
- An 8- to 12-month-old child does not turn to sounds, such as a rattle, 3 feet to the rear.
- A 1-year-old child does not understand a variety of words, such as "bye-bye" and "doggie."
- A 2-year-old child is not using words.
- A 2-year-old child is unable to identify an object with a verbal cue alone, such as "Show me the ball."
- A 3-year-old child has largely unintelligible speech.
- A 3-year-old child omits beginning consonants.
- A 3-year-old child does not use two- and three-word sentences.
- A 3-year-old child mainly uses vowel sounds.
- A child of any age speaks in a voice that is too loud, too soft, of poor quality, or of a quality that does not fit his or her age and sex.
- A child always sounds as if he or she has a cold.

---

written test is important to interpreting the results. Results of testing should also note the method of communication used—oral, sign, and/or pantomime.

Objectives of Intervention and Treatment Modalities

The occupational therapist's goals must be well coordinated with the goals of those involved with the child, including the parent, early infant specialist, special educator, speech therapist, and audiologist. Generally, the occupational therapist's goals are imbedded in the team's goals for the child.

Examples of typical occupational therapy objectives include the following:

1. *To enhance sensory processing and stimulation.* The child with hearing impairment is denied adequate cortical stimulation by auditory channels and must learn to perceive and conceptualize by other means. The therapist can enhance kinesthetic, tactile, and visual processing through multisensory activities. Sensory integrative techniques are useful in developing the kinesthetic system. The tactile and proprioceptive systems

are important in the use of sign language. Tactile activities, such as having the child locate objects hidden in sand or identify objects behind a shield, are among many that can be used. Tracking exercises, perceptual motor activities, and many games or crafts can enhance the visual system.

2. *To encourage age-appropriate self-care skills.* Often the occupational therapist acts as a consultant, recommending strategies for improving the child's self-care independence. Adapted techniques or assistive devices may be needed. At times self-care skills involve concepts that require concrete cues for the child to learn. For example, the idea of left shoe and right shoe can be shown visually with color coding.

3. *To encourage fine motor and hand-coordination skills.* The movements of the hands of a fluent signer require opposition, finger and thumb flexion and extension, and finger and thumb abduction and adduction. These movements are performed by isolated digits and in total patterns, but they are all done in rapid succession and with remarkable coordination. The hand's coordination seems to be related to its sensory abilities, particularly tactile discrimination. This skill does not always come naturally to a child with hearing loss and, therefore, has to be learned. Occupational therapy's emphasis on hand skills can do much for the child with hearing loss, particularly for those children who have an identified delay in fine motor skills.

4. *To encourage socialization.* This part of occupational therapy intervention cannot be done in isolation and is of utmost importance to the child with hearing impairment. Involving the child ingroup activities with his or her peers encourages socialization. Hearing impairment is not a visible disability. A child with hearing impairment can be mistaken as being rude if he or she does not answer questions or respond to social overtures when, in fact, the child has simply not received the correct stimuli. Therefore developing the child's ability to adapt to the environment and understand social interaction and communication should also be stressed.

Special techniques

The therapist working with the child with hearing impairment becomes intimately involved with the special techniques and/or equipment used with that child (e.g., sign language, lip reading, hearing aids, and cochlear implants). In the field of hearing loss, there has been a historic battle between the *oralists* (i.e., oral language only, through the use of lip reading and speech therapy) and the *sign language users.* Many advocate *total communication,* which involves the use of all avenues of communication (e.g., oral speech, lip reading, sign language, finger spelling, gesture, and body language) simultaneously.

Sign language and total communication proponents argue that sign encourages communication and language development, and that the child with hearing impairment needs sign for early concept development (Mindel & Vernon, 1971). Proponents of total communication feel that the child will demonstrate earlier development of linguistic skills, better interpersonal relationships, and understanding of self and environment with this approach. The *bilingual-bicultural* approach entails using sign until well established, and introducing English later, as a second language (Steinberg & Knightly, 1997). Oralists maintain that if taught sign, the child may never learn to talk.

The decision of what techniques and equipment will be used with a child is the prerogative of the child's family and educational system. It is important for the occupational therapist to realize and understand the theory behind the decision and how to best facilitate the use of the techniques or equipment chosen.

At first glance, teaching the child *speech reading* (lip reading) would seem to be a good choice. However, consider that only one third of speech sounds are visible to the speech reader. In addition, many of the sounds made in English look alike. For example, *p, m,* and *b* are all made with the same lip movement (i.e., lips together). Try looking in the mirror and say *ma, pa,* and *ba* without voice; the problem is readily observed. Another example of look-alike movements would be *f* and *v,* which are both formed with the teeth to the lower lip. *Cued speech* is a system of hand signs and positions designed to help speech readers distinguish between things that look the same on the lips (Ling, 1989).

Another option, sign language, is not easily understood, and it involves many different methods. For example, in the United States, finger spelling, or *dactylology,* is done with one hand, and each configuration represents a letter in the English alphabet. Finger spelling is used by itself, or it is used in conjunction with other forms of sign language. Although it is not too difficult for the hearing person to learn to finger spell, when receiving, or listening, the tendency is to see the individual letters and not the words. With finger spelling, it is important that the hand be close enough to the face so that the person with hearing impairment can see both the lip movements and the finger spelling at the same time. For fluency and readability, the hand has to be held in a comfortable position, not stiffly.

Sign language can be divided into two categories: (1) *American Sign Language* (ASL) and (2) *Signing Exact English* (SEE) (Fant, 1971; Gustafson, Pfetzing, & Zawalkow, 1975; Klima & Bellugi, 1978). Although it is not universal, ASL is the primary language of persons with prelingual deafness in the United States. It is a language in itself and is not directly translatable to English. In addition, ASL has many abbreviations and phrases contained in a single sign, and it does not conform to the structure of English. However, SEE does conform to the structure and form of the English language.

There are many arguments for and against ASL, SEE, and other types of sign. If sign is used, it is important to become as fluent as possible in the particular system favored by the child. Many occupational therapists learn only the most simple and frequently used words and phrases; however, this is important to the child's therapy. Many good texts are available on the different types of sign. However, it is best to attend a class or practice with a friend who knows sign, because it is often difficult to correctly interpret the configuration and movement patterns of the hands.

The occupational therapist is sometimes involved with the child during the initial stages of learning sign. In this case, it is best to select the first signs to be taught from those that represent familiar objects, real-life situations, and familiar actions. The therapist should begin with what is available to the child (i.e., things to feel, handle, or do), and provide parents with a likes-dislikes checklist to determine what is appropriate for the individual child. Often a food item is used first because of its value as a reward. The adult should work at the eye level of the child, obtain eye contact, do the sign, and then physically manipulate the child's hands through the sign. Some basic suggestions for the use of total communication are listed in Box 25-2.

The occupational therapist can also be involved in the initial stages of hearing aid use. Often a history shows that the child had a hearing aid but rejected it. This can sometimes be traced to the lack of professional support for the parents and child during the difficult adjustment period, or it can be traced to the professional's lack of familiarity with the aid.

Hearing aids can be problematic because they do not allow the child to hear normally; they simply amplify the sounds in the environment. Although helpful, these devices cannot restore hearing as glasses can restore vision, and they cannot localize sounds. Instead, they amplify all sounds in the environment, thus leading to distortion. It is regrettable when an instrument that can be of help to the child is not used simply because it is not perfect. Therefore the therapist should help the parents and child by clarifying realistic expectations of the aid and explaining what it can and cannot do for the child.

Because the head is one of the most sensitive portions of the body, one of the main problems found in children with new aids is tactile defensiveness. However, the child must learn to think of the aid as a piece of clothing that is put on automatically in the morning, along with shoes and socks. Many feel that the earlier an aid is fitted to a child and put into use, the better the chances for language development (Ling, 1989).

Children using hearing aids need to adjust to the feel of the aid and recognize its importance. It is usually best for the child to begin wearing the aid during a quiet activity that involves the speech of just one person. The maximal benefit from an aid is obtained in relatively quiet settings.

Because the aid does not localize sounds, the following situations present difficulties:
- Environments with excessive background noise
- Groups with three to four people speaking at the same time
- Reamplification, such as listening to a television or tape recorder
- Distance listening

The hearing aid is a sensitive piece of equipment with several parts, and it can often be in need of repair. Everyone involved with the child should be aware of some of the common problems, because an improperly working aid is useless to the child. Four common problems are (1) dead batteries, (2) improperly placed or corroded batteries, (3) squeal (check for looseness of the cord or earmold), and (4) earmold impacted with wax that must be cleared.

The type of hearing aid prescribed for a particular child depends on the degree and configuration of the loss (Chase & Gravel, 1996; Northern & Downs, 1992). Three types of hearing aids are widely used: (1) *in-the-ear*, (2) *behind-the-ear*, and (3) *body*. The in-the-ear aid is used only for mild losses and has no external wires. The behind-the-ear aid is used for mild to profound losses and is the most-popular type of aid. It is a small unit, made up of a microphone, amplifiers, and receiver. These

---

box 25-2 *Suggestions for the use of total communication*

- Face the child squarely at eye level.
- Position yourself so that the child can easily see your face and hands at the same time.
- Make sure you have the child's attention.
- Avoid backlighting. If the child has to look into the light, he or she may be unable to see your lips.
- Use a normal tone of voice. Do not exaggerate mouth movements, because this practice tends to confuse the lip reader.
- Speak the word and give the sign at the same time, rather than in sequence.
- Use appropriate pauses between words, especially when finger spelling is used.
- Sit close to the child, rather than across the room.
- Keep instructions simple and to the point.
- Be consistent, especially with the young child.
- Talk to the child. He or she needs to receive the same amount of input as a hearing child.

components are located together, behind the ear, and connected with a short tube to a plastic earmold that has been custom formed to the shape of the child's external auditory canal. The earmold is seated directly in the ear (Figure 25-2). The microphone picks up the sound waves and converts them to electric signals. Then the am-

plifiers increase the strength of the signal, and the receiver changes the electric signals back to sound waves that are sent to the earmold.

Although it is used less frequently now than in the past, the body aid can be used for extreme hearing losses. In a body aid, the microphone, amplifier, and power sup-

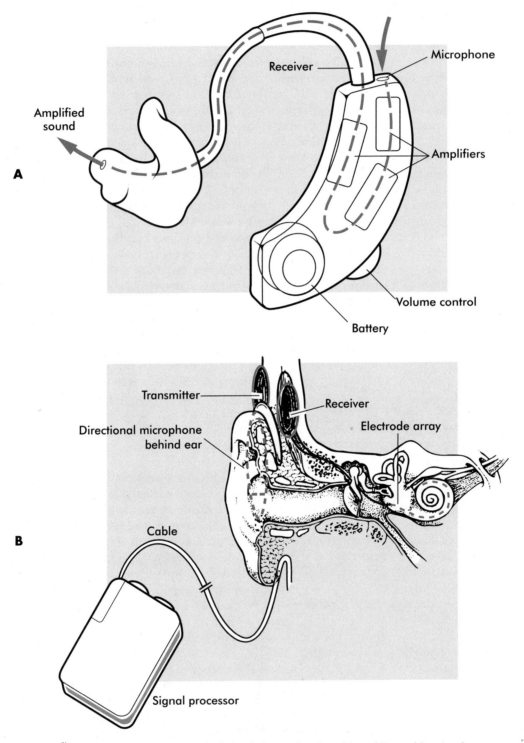

figure 25-2 **A,** Diagram of a behind-the-ear hearing aid; and **B,** cochlear implant.

ply are together in a case carried in a pocket or harness worn by the child. Small wires connect the case to the receiver, and the earmold is seated directly in the ear. A *monaural aid* refers to the use of just one aid, and *binaural aid* refers to the use of two separate aids.

Cochlear implants are recently developed and FDA-approved devices that can be surgically implanted in the cochlea of individuals with severe to profound hearing losses (Kreton & Balkany, 1991; Steinberg & Knightly, 1997). These devices provide the sensation of sound by acting as substitutes for hair cells in the organ of Corti, providing direct stimulation to the auditory nerve. Cochlear implants can now be fitted in children as young as 18 months, but only after the child has gone through a trial period with a traditional hearing aid.

The implant has four device components: (1) a receiver buried in the temporal bone, (2) an external microphone attached to a transmitter, (3) a speech processor that records and electronically codes incoming sounds, and (4) an electrode array implanted in the cochlea itself. The external transmitter is held in place on the head with a magnet that attracts to a magnet in the receiver imbedded in the temporal bone. The receiver is attached to the electrode array in the cochlea, and a cord connects the transmitter and microphone to the speech processor. The cord is usually run under the child's clothing, and the speech processor is contained in a fanny pack worn at the waist.

Sound flows from the microphone to the speech processor, where it is converted into an electrical signal. The coded signal is then sent back to the transmitter and then to the receiver, where it is decoded and delivered to the actual electrodes in the cochlea. The electrodes bypass the damaged hair cells and directly stimulate the nerve fibers in the cochlea.

Although this technique brings state-of-the-art technology to the child's functional hearing ability, the degree of hearing improvement is variable. As with the hearing aid, the implant does not restore normal hearing, but it does allow the child to hear more environmental sounds. Also, as with the hearing aid, best results are achieved if it is worn consistently. Mapping, or programming, of the speech processor is a complex process; the success of the implant depends on it.

Therapists need to be aware of the external equipment and its location during motor activities with the child. The equipment is expensive, and components worn on the child's body can be damaged by water or rough physical activity. Therefore external equipment should be removed prior to these activities. If the occupational therapist has any question about engaging the child in a specific activity, it is best to check with the parent or main service provider.

Like hearing aids, cochlear implants have external components and may cause problems with tactile defensiveness. Therefore desensitization can be an appropriate therapy goal when working with children who have been fitted with these devices. As part of the intervention team, the occupational therapist can help by providing feedback to the audiologists on the types of sounds the child appears to hear.

As with the hearing aid, the key to success with the cochlear implant is use. All adults working with the child need to check that the equipment is in good working order and the child is spoken to frequently. A normal tone of voice should be maintained, and speech volume and tones should be the same as used with any other child during therapy activities. In addition, language should be kept at age level and within the context of the situation.

In school settings, FM systems are often used with children with hearing impairments. With an FM system, the teacher wears a microphone and wireless transmitter to speak directly into the child's FM system or hearing aid. This device helps control the level of background noise in the classroom, because the teacher's voice can be amplified for the students who have hearing loss without disturbing other students in the classroom.

Preparation for adulthood

The adolescent with hearing impairment may struggle to blend into a hearing world. Universal recognition of the importance of inclusion and required accommodations in school and work settings have afforded them more opportunities, and the growing technology of communication has improved future prospects. For most adolescents, one important task is learning to drive a car. Adolescents with hearing impairment can receive special driving training. These students are taught to constantly scan the environment visually.

Another important aspect of blending into the hearing world is the use of a daily communication device often taken for granted, the telephone. Some hearing aids have a telephone setting. However, if amplification alone is not sufficient for the wearer to understand conversation, the Telephone Typewriter (TTY) is available. The TTY is a communication device that uses the telephone lines with a typewriter keyboard to "talk" and a printout device to receive the conversation. In addition, the telephone ring is replaced with a flashing light or a fan that moves back and forth to indicate an incoming call. The obvious disadvantage of the TTY is that both ends of the line need to be equipped with this system for it to work. E-mail can also be used as an alternative, and increasingly available, form of communication by the individuals with hearing impairment.

Television provides another aspect of daily life. The frequency of closed-captioned programs has increased, and all televisions manufactured after 1995 are required to have a built-in decoding device. The hearing impaired use this decoding device, known as a "black box," to view captioned versions of programs. Another technique used in broadcasts for the hearing impaired is to include a sign language interpreter in a cameo spot at the corner of the screen. However, it is often difficult to read the signs being provided when viewing programs on small television screens.

Occupational choice has always been difficult for the young adults with hearing impairment. Fortunately, today many universities offer programs designed to integrate students with hearing loss into the general student population by providing special services, such as interpreters and note takers. The Americans with Disabilities Act (ADA) (1990) requires that all public education programs provide interpreters or note takers for persons with hearing impairment when it is determined that they are required.

When an individual with hearing impairment enters a work environment, he or she is likely to miss a great deal of information transmitted in conversation as well as environmental sounds (Steinberg & Knightly, 1997). Three other factors that adversely affect occupational choice for persons with hearing loss include (Schein & Delk, 1975): (1) psychologic perception differences that affect self-perception and perception of reality, (2) restricted life space that adversely affects knowledge of areas outside of the immediate social or geographic area, and (3) limited sociocultural understanding.

Occupational therapists are aware of how important meaningful and purposeful activity is in the life and health of an individual. As part of an interdisciplinary team, therapists can help prepare the child with hearing impairment for transition to work and fuller participation in work.

Case Study 1: Ed

Ed is 2 years, 3 months old. He had bacterial meningitis during the neonatal period, with a severe degree of resultant hearing loss. Ed is the first and only child of a young couple, who are both employed. Ed attends a local early intervention program for disabled children less than 3 years of age, and he has been assessed by subjective observation and by using the Infant Developmental Assessment. Ed performed as follows:

- *Motor area:* Ed passed most of the items at the 24-month level. Although he passed items such as walking up and down stairs alone, it should be noted that he often stumbled and appeared uncoordinated. However, on subjective observation, his balance problems could be partially attributed to his "looking everywhere," that is, searching for visual output.
- *Adaptive area:* Ed passed all items at the 24-month level. Distractibility was noted.
- *Language area:* His language skills were comparable to those of a one year old. He made vowel sounds, had a receptive total communication vocabulary of five words, and had no expressive vocabulary to date. He attempted to form words verbally and with sign language.

- *Self-care:* Ed passed all items at the 24-month level, except items for toileting, communication, and social play.

As noted, Ed attends a day program with a teacher as the primary professional and with speech therapy, audiology, and occupational therapy as supportive services. Occupational and speech therapists are available on a half-time basis, and the audiologist is employed on a consulting basis.

Treatment goals

The four treatment goals were as follows:

1. Tactile desensitization of the head and face area to promote acceptance of the hearing aid: Activities included rubbing different textures; touching different parts of face on therapist, self, dolls, and felt board (this activity also promoted body identification and sign skills); and playing dress-up with different hats.
2. Improvement of fine motor coordination through use of manipulative activities, with a variety of shapes, textures, and weights: Eye-hand and tactile-discrimination were emphasized.
3. Improvement of attention to activities: Activities such as imitation games, vestibular stimulation activities (e.g., self-regulated swinging in net and using rocker board), and use of "look" sign in gross motor playground activities were used.
4. Consultation regarding toileting at both school and home, and establishment of a toileting schedule.

■ VISUAL IMPAIRMENT

Because the effects of visual impairment are evident in the development of mobility and manipulation, children with visual impairment are often referred for developmental testing and treatment by pediatricians. Therefore these children are often identified in the first year of life and soon begin to receive services from local early intervention programs. With the advent of day programs for the visually impaired, the number of children attending residential schools for the blind has been drastically reduced.

Special Characteristics Relevant to Occupational Therapy

Children with visual impairments typically incur delays in developmental skills across domains (Lampert, 1998), and they have to learn about the world with their hands. Children with normal sight develop eye-hand coordination early in life, but children with severe visual impairment must rely on ear-hand coordination, which develops at a later stage. In addition, their coordination depends on precise tactile system perception for exploration and concept development (Lampert, 1998; Lydon

& McGraw, 1973). These children manipulate objects to detect their form and shape. Therefore their concepts of objects are developed using haptic perception. Unfortunately, in association with their visual impairment, these children often exhibit tactile defensiveness.

Body movement is essential for visually impaired children to learn about spatial aspects of the environment. However, visual impairment is often associated with fear of movement. Therefore children with visual impairment have difficulty progressing through the developmental sequence of random-to-purposeful movements.

Among the limitations imposed by visual impairment, three are key to development:

1. Mobility is restricted because of the child's inability to visualize the environment, with its potential obstacles and dangers (Warren, 1994).

2. Understanding of the physical environment is limited, particularly in shape, form, distance, and object relationships (Warren, 1994).

3. Communication is often delayed because the child cannot read body language or gestures and does not see the physical cueing that accompanies speech (Dunlea, 1989; Warren, 1994).

Behaviors and mannerisms particular to visual impairment can occur; many researchers trace these to early sensory deprivation (Fraiberg, 1977; Jastrzembska, 1976). Children with visual impairment are deprived of adequate visual stimuli and, because of a lack of mobility, are often secondarily deprived of tactile, vestibular, kinesthetic, and proprioceptive stimuli. Further, because of the lack of stimuli, these children are often extremely resistant to change, setting up a cycle reinforcing resistance to new stimuli. Also, older infants with visual impairment walk late and are not as mobile as children with normal sight (Ferrell et. al., 1990).

Studies (e.g., Jastrzembska, 1976) show that sensory deprivation during formative periods can result in the failure of the deprived system to ever achieve maximal development. Multisensory deprivation has an even more pronounced effect. Diagnostic information, examples of specialized tests, and descriptions of the professionals who are involved with visually impaired children are presented in Appendix B.

Concept development is also affected by vision loss. For example, vision is normally used to identify the position of objects in space, to recognize shapes without feeling them, and to know the length of a room without pacing it. These perceptual concepts must be acquired by alternate means by the child with visual impairment.

Self-stimulatory behaviors, sometimes called blindisms, may also develop. These include eye poking and flicking hands. Such actions appeal to visually impaired children because they break up light and change what little they are able to see. These behaviors need to be evaluated closely before they are discouraged, because

they are sometimes functional behaviors, such as making repetitive sounds for echo location. At other times, they inhibit productive behaviors and need to be limited (Lampert, 1998).

Developmental Considerations

Therapists need to understand developmental differences characteristic of children with visual impairment to plan an appropriate intervention. Standardized developmental scales can be used if a notation is made as to the child's impairment. Although every area of a child's development is affected by visual impairment, generalizations may not apply.

The infant with normal sight takes hold of the world with his or her eyes in the first weeks of life (Gesell, Ilg, & Bullis, 1967). At first, all infants have monocular fixation, but by the eighth week, binocular vision is dominant in most children. The infant has sustained fixation on a nearby object (e.g., mother's face) during the first week and on more distant objects by the end of the first month. The typical infant develops eye-hand coordination by 5 months, perfecting the accuracy of visually guided reach and grasp by 12 months. This performance contrasts sharply with the infant with visual impairment, who does not develop ear-hand coordination (the ability to locate and reach for sound) until almost the end of the first year. Although ear-hand coordination in the visually impaired child begins at about the 10- to 12-month level (Fraiberg, 1977), it does not reach proficiency until the second year of life.

The typically developing child learns to associate visual experiences with symbolism (i.e., with words). The absence of the association of words with visual experiences explains why, although the child with visual impairment receives the same auditory stimuli, his or her language development is affected. Pronouns can be especially difficult for the young child with visual impairment to understand. However, he or she often learns to use language to gain attention and/or reassurance from others.

Generally, gross motor development is also affected by visual limitation. Like an infant with normally developing sight, the infant with visual impairment will cling to the parent's shoulder. However, he or she will not spontaneously turn the head like the infant with normal sight (Adelson & Fraiberg, 1974). Without sight, the prone position is not particularly interesting or comfortable; a fixed supine position is definitely preferred. If the child with visual impairment learns to creep, it is only after the development of ear-hand coordination. Often the child prefers to scoot on the back to move around.

The child with visual loss typically demonstrates a delay in crawling of approximately 6 months. Sitting usually develops within established norms because it is a static position, but the child with visual loss may have to be placed in sitting position, demonstrating difficulty with fluid movement to and from sitting. Because of the lack of the visual stimulation that motivates the child's attention, time spent in this position is also limited. Standing is also a static position and occurs roughly within the normal age range. However, walking is a dynamic movement and may be delayed by approximately 7 months (Adelson & Fraiberg, 1974).

To succeed in independent walking, the child with visual loss needs to learn the hazards and layout of the environment. Stair climbing is also delayed and often requires a great deal of guidance. The typical climbing and exploring of the 18- to 24-month-old child does not take place spontaneously in children with visual loss.

Fine motor development is strongly affected by the loss of eye-hand coordination. The child with visual loss sits and manipulates toys within reach, but once out of reach, the toy disappears. In addition, the sound of a familiar noise toy is not spontaneously connected with the feel of the toy. The child develops age-appropriate object transfer and hand play at midline, but reach for and release of objects is often delayed.

In the social-emotional area, a delay in the development of play may be anticipated in children with visual impairment. A doll or a toy truck initially has no meaning, because (as miniatures of visual objects) these objects are difficult for the child to perceive. Parallel play and mimicry are also difficult to learn without the opportunity to see and imitate others.

Development of peer relationships can be difficult because the child cannot see the smile or the frown of playmates. The child with visual impairment may find it difficult to accurately read the feelings of others without the clues of body language and facial expressions.

Feeding may be delayed by parental apprehension about the mess and by the child's initial difficulty in finding and prehending the food. Also, many children with vision loss have difficulty weaning from familiar and comforting routines, such as the use of a bottle. Feeding problems involve tactile sensitivity and the child's natural resistance to change. Difficulty in introducing new foods, storing food in cheeks, and spitting out different textures are all common feeding behaviors.

Perceptual skill development is delayed in children with vision loss. Discrimination of shape and space, which normally appears from 12 to 18 months, does not occur in the child with visual impairment until 24 to 36 months (Robbins, 1960). Concept development is problematic. The child with vision loss experiences difficulty learning that one word signifies many different tactile experiences. For example, a chair can have many different shapes, sizes, and textures, but all related forms are identified by that one word. Figure 25-3 lists some critical observations in functional assessment of children with visual impairments (Cratty, 1971; Warner, 1984). The list is not all-inclusive and would vary according to the particular situation and the child's developmental level.

Posture: Is the child's head up and held at midline? Often the head is down or the child displays unusual posturing. This needs to be noted because of its relation to the prevention of back problems and the promotion of social acceptance. Caution must be taken in interpreting unusual postures or head tilts as these may be natural ways for the child to try to see most effectively.

Balance and stability: Can the child maintain a position well? How good is his or her balance on one foot? This is important for mobility training.

Ambulation and gait: Is the gait stiff? Are the steps normal in size? How does the child manage on stairs or uneven surfaces?

Strength and tone: Is the child's tone normal, and is strength adequate for age? Such children often have low tone because of the lack of movement.

Endurance: Can the child pursue a gross or fine motor task for an appropriate length of time?

Coordination: The dexterity of children who have visual impairment can be subjectively assessed on tests, such as the Minnesota Rate of Manipulation Test (MRMT). The MRMT in particular has norms for the blind.

Identification of body planes and body parts: Does the child know front from back? Can he or she identify body parts at an age-appropriate level? The child who is visually impaired needs to know "boundaries of self."

Laterality: Can the child identify right and left on self and others and locate objects placed to either side? This is necessary in exploring the environment.

Directionality: Can the child tell which direction to go to reach an object or person, moving or stationary?

Controlled isolated body movements: Are extraneous movements present? Control is important for work and school skills, as well as social acceptance.

Tactile discrimination: Can the child use his or her hands and body to their fullest to explore?

Auditory discrimination: Can the child discriminate distances of sound and types of sound and identify different people by voice?

Spatial orientation: Is the child able to judge distances? This is important in mobility.

figure**25-3** Observation of the child with visual impairment.

The therapist may wish to administer portions of the Sensory Integration and Praxis Test (SIPT) to the child. Several parts of the test do not require sight, and others can be adapted. Although use of standard scores is not appropriate, testing results can provide important information concerning the child's spatial awareness or orientation, proprioception, and tactile awareness or orientation. Parts of the test that can be administered most readily include: Finger Identification, Graphesthesia, Localization of Tactile Stimuli, Kinesthesia, Praxis on Verbal Command, as well as parts of the Manual

Form Perception and Standing and Walking Balance sections.

Objectives and Activities of Intervention

The occupational therapist may be the primary therapist for a child with visual impairment, but most often he or she works with a team that includes the special educator, the physical therapist, and the orientation and mobility specialist. Other professionals are involved as the child's needs indicate, and the intervention plan is based on the individual assessment of the child. Lampert (1998) presents specific information on occupational therapy intervention, including illustrative case studies of children with visual impairment.

Following is a list of team goals for children with visual impairment to which the occupational therapist may contribute:

- *To develop self-care skills at age-appropriate times.* The therapist can consult with those who work with the child about the developmental sequence of self-care skills. The therapists may physically guide the child through eating and dressing activities. If abnormal eating patterns develop and are not corrected, they usually become ingrained patterns. Good supportive seating is important to the self-feeding process, and the child needs practice time with buttons and zippers. Toilet training can be facilitated in five ways: (1) a consistent schedule, (2) an established route to the bathroom, (3) the familiar sounds and smells of the room, (4) consistent use of one or two words for toileting, and (5) establishing an association between changing wet clothes and going to the bathroom.

- *To enhance sensory integration.* The child with visual impairment may benefit from vestibular stimulation using tilt boards, swings, and scooters. Sensory feedback in children who are blind is interrupted and can cause distortion of movement (deQuiros, 1976). It is important, however, that safety be maintained in the use of equipment, and that the child be allowed to control the movement. Excessive fear of falling, poor grasp of room layout, and inability to organize or cross midline are all indications of difficulty in sensory integration. Van Benschoter (1975) outlined a successful summer camp experience for children with visual impairments, aged 6 to 21 years, that stressed sensory integrative programming and had a positive effect on their movement skills.

- *To encourage movement in space.* Early in life, the infant's position must be changed frequently to counteract the resistance to movement and change. Prone positions should be encouraged. The underdevelopment of dynamic movements, such as crawling and walking, cannot be totally eliminated. However, much can be done in the therapy setting to help compensate for the underdevelopment of these movements. Crawling over different surfaces and movements on bolsters, therapy balls, and other objects are helpful activities. A push toy, riding toy, or wagon can be pushed to develop security in walking. Balance activities are helpful to decrease fear of movement. General strengthening is often indicated, because lack of mobility and passivity may cause children with visual impairment to be weak. Resisted creeping and moving heavy objects to build an obstacle course may improve strength.

- *To develop maximal tactile-perceptual abilities.* The child with visual impairment needs to maximize tactile abilities to learn about the environment and, eventually, to read Braille. Activities such as finger painting, finding and identifying objects hidden in sand or beans, and identifying gradations of textures and puzzles are among those that increase tactile awareness.

- *To decrease tactile defensiveness.* The child with visual impairment does not see the approach of people and objects and can, therefore, exhibit a defensive reaction to touch. Use of a firm touch is better than a light touch, which can be interpreted as being aversive. Techniques to decrease tactile defensiveness include activities using graded textures and exploration and play with various materials, such as sand, dried lentils, beans, and rice. Activities that include vibration or proprioceptive input are also often helpful.

- *To encourage use of hands for manipulation.* At first, the world has to come to the child. Toys should be maintained within reach (e.g., tied to the crib, walker, or table top). Practice of in-hand manipulation activities that involve rotation and translation of small objects can dynamically improve use of tools.

- *To encourage knowledge of parts of the body and body planes.* The child has to know his or her own body before understanding how it moves and fits into the environment. Body image is important to mobility and social function (Cratty, 1971). Obstacle courses can teach the child how large his or her body is in relation to other objects. Touching body parts on others is also helpful, and use of a vibrator may increase body awareness. Life-size dolls can also be used.

- *To encourage laterality and directionality.* To develop these perceptual skills, particularly for mobility, the child must learn the concepts of right-left, up-down, and in-out. The child must develop the awareness that things outside the body have sides, and he or she must be able to measure distance and direction.

- *To maximize residual vision.* The therapists should always use whatever vision the child has in the treatment program activities. The more a child uses visual pathways, the better his or her vision develops (Baker-Nobles & Rutherford, 1995). Visual awareness and discrimination activities, such as color or shape recognition and matching, are important. Activities, such as use of a flashlight in a darkened room, may also improve visual skills.

All of these goals require the occupational therapist to follow up the activities through education of (and consultation with) family members. Family members should be encouraged to handle the child with visual impairment as they would an infant without disability. Verbal and physical interaction should also be encouraged, because the child may not always demand interaction.

The family should be informed about the importance of early intervention and their options for services. Occupational therapists may consult with parents on ways to create a safe environment in which the child can play unsupervised and make recommendations for adapting the environment to optimize the independent functioning of the child.

Additional team goals to which the occupational therapist contributes include:

- *To encourage socially acceptable behaviors.* The child should be encouraged to face people when they speak, to smile appropriately, to maintain upright posture with his/her head in midline. He or she must learn how others are reacting based on voices, rather than gestures, facial expressions, or body language. By the preschool years, parents and professionals should encourage socially acceptable behaviors in children with visual impairments (Hill, 1977).
- *To encourage language and concept development.* The child must consciously be taught to develop cognitive schemes that the sighted child picks up in a relatively casual manner. This is done with verbalization and the use of the child's intact sensory systems. Those things that cannot be touched or heard, such as clouds, need to be explained.
- *To strengthen cognitive skills such as object permanence, cause and effect, object recognition, and ability to match and sort.* Games and many simple craft activities can be used to accomplish these goals. The unique abilities and limitations of the child must be considered in addressing academic goals.
- *To develop maximal auditory perceptual abilities.* The child with visual impairment has to learn to identify sounds and their meanings and react to them appropriately. Sounds come from several basic sources: toys, speech, and the environment. Active, rather than passive, listening should be emphasized. Activities, such as locating a variety of sounds in the environment, identifying sounds, and following directions from persons and recordings, are helpful.

Special techniques

Children with severe visual handicaps usually rely on Braille and talking books for their education. Braille is a system of six raised dots arranged in a cell to represent the letters of the alphabet, numbers, and words. It is produced on a special slate or on a machine, called a Braillewriter. The system was developed by a young, blind French student, Louis Braille, in 1824 and was found to be more efficient than attempting to read the raised Roman alphabet.

For the young child who will eventually use Braille in school, the importance of early tactile perceptual training cannot be overemphasized. Braille can be written in three levels, or grades, depending on the degree of contraction used. It is read left to right with one or two hands. Usually the index finger is used with a light touch. Reading speeds for Braille vary, but 104 words per minute is the average, making it useful in the educational setting.

Talking books on a wide variety of topics and for any age level are also available for the visually impaired. The development of attentive listening can be encouraged during short storytelling sessions, and adults should carefully monitor the child's attention to promote good listening skills. Scratch-and-sniff books and tactile books are also available to help in early storytelling. Those who can discriminate a large typeface can read large-print books, and enlarged letters and contrasting colors are accessible through most computer programs.

Various types of lenses are available for people with visual impairment, from the relatively common ones used to correct refractive errors to telescopic and microscopic lenses that are used as low-vision aids for certain types of blindness. There are also projection and magnifying devices, such as the opticon, which converts ink print into a readable vibrating tactile form.

Optometrists and occupational therapists have teamed up to provide vision therapy using various lenses, prisms, occlusion (patching) and other low-vision aids (Chaikin & Dowwning-Baum, 1997; Scheiman, 1997). The purpose of this vision therapy is to provide devices and activities to increase visual efficiency and visual-information-processing skills.

In mobility training, techniques such as using the "Seeing Eye dog," sighted guides, and long canes are taught (Lampert, 1998; Welsh & Blasch, 1980). The techniques of echo detection, trailing, and body protection are also important. Sighted guides usually walk a half step in front of the person with visual impairment. The visually impaired individual holds the guide's arm just above the elbow, with fingers inside (next to guide's body) and the thumb outside. A small child can hold the guide's wrist. With a sighted guide, body movement on uneven surfaces and changes of direction are easily perceived. Should the person with visual impairment need to change sides, the guide gives a verbal clue and the guided person slides over, tracing a finger along the back of the guide's waist. He or she then switches hands and grasps the guide's opposite elbow. In going through a narrow passage, the guide puts the opposite elbow behind his or her waist as a clue. The person with visual impairment then falls back a full step behind the guide, with the elbow straight and more directly in back, rather than to the side.

For stairs, the sighted guide gives a verbal indication of stairs ahead, whether they are up or down, as well as information on rail availability and placement. One technique for navigating stairs requires the guide to pause and turn at a right angle to the person with visual impairment. They take each step one at a time in a foot-to-step fashion, with the guide one step ahead of the person with visual impairment. Another technique involves using the rail, if available. In this case, the guide goes up or down the stairs without turning, one step ahead of the guided person. Cane technique is also a specialized procedure that requires the visually impaired person to obtain training from a professional.

As a rule, the orientation and mobility specialist is the one who teaches *trailing* and *body protection*. However, occupational therapists who work with individuals with visual impairment should learn the basic techniques. Trailing is the use of a wall as a guide for walking. The hand closest to the wall is extended at hip level, until the outside of the little finger touches the wall; then the back of the fingertips are used to guide the person in walking.

In the body protection technique, the upper arm is held at shoulder height and parallel to the floor, with the palm facing out to meet any obstacle before the body does. The lower arm is extended downward and forward, with the palm facing out. Another protection technique is to extend the arm palm out in front of the head, while bending down to retrieve a dropped object. The child with visual impairment can search for a lost object by touching the ground to establish a beginning point, and then he or she can search in an ever-widening concentric circle pattern.

A technique for exploring a room involves searching the parameters of the room first, then mentally dividing it into grids to be methodically searched. This is extremely helpful in introducing the child with vision loss to a new classroom or new home setup. The use of landmarks and clues, such as the grass at the edge of the sidewalk, is important for independent movement.

Some occupational therapists are involved in low-vision training (i.e., a training technique that is important to children who have poor visual acuity) (Baker-Nobles, 1997; Barraga, 1964; Fonda, 1970; Hyvarinen, 1995; Lampert & Lapolice, 1995). The basic premise of low-vision training is that the child can be taught to use his or her residual vision. Because visual acuity is, by itself, not the most important part of visual ability, planned stimulation can help a visually impaired child to increase his or her visual efficiency.

Often, light is used initially to increase focusing ability. Once fixation is achieved, the child can learn to discriminate global aspects of an image. When this happens, the child can move on to analyze discrete elements and, finally, to identify form, outline, and other aspects of an image. Although this method does not work with all children with visual impairment, it does have good results with some of them, particularly when combined with a good overall program to heighten the child's levels of perception.

With increasing use of sophisticated electronics and compact components, positive outcomes for the visually impaired are possible. For example, a light sensor can be used to train a child with low vision to detect variable light intensities. Specific training in detection of light can improve function at school or work (Schaefer & Specht, 1979).

Other advances that give individuals with visual impairment access to computers include voice-activated software and keys with Braille. Computers can increase the quantity and quality of written output and, if equipped with voice and sound capabilities, they provide opportunities for interactive learning. Given the versatility and increasing capacity of computers, this technology holds great promise for persons with visual impairments.

Gentile (1997) provides an excellent overview of the special occupational therapy techniques and treatment options used with children with visual impairment. Her text also discusses functional visual behavior and evaluation, and it includes chapters on sensory integration and visual functioning, vision therapy, visual-perceptual-motor dysfunction, visual perception, vision dysfunction from an osteopathic approach, and low-vision training.

Preparation for adulthood

As previously mentioned, the adolescent who is visually impaired faces a great challenge in selecting an appropriate occupation (Lampert, 1998). Unfortunately, visual impairment is often associated with unemployment or underemployment. However, an appropriate fit between the personality and talent areas of the adolescent can result in a successful and enduring career. Lack of exposure to many vocational options can be a problem that the occupational therapist can address (through community orientation and various activities) to give the child more prevocational experiences.

Certain mannerisms and behaviors often interfere with optimal social interaction in the work environment. Behaviors that the therapist and all the other professionals involved with the child should work to modify include:

- Standing in the personal space of others
- Rocking the body
- Blinking, rubbing, or rolling the eyes
- Stamping or shuffling the feet
- Lack of eye contact with the person who is speaking

Daily living skills, such as cooking, cleaning, and recreation, become increasingly important as the child with visual impairment reaches adolescence. The American Foundation for the Blind puts out a comprehensive list of aids and appliances that can help the visually impaired perform these skills. Devices, such as a sugar meter that dispenses one half a teaspoon of sugar at a time and an elbow-length oven mitt that is worn to protect the visually impaired cook from accidental burning, are extremely helpful. Canned goods marking kits are also available, as are self-threading needles and tools with marking gauges. Recreational activities, such as games with Braille cards and low-vision cards and table games (e.g., Scrabble and Monopoly) with Braille markings, are available.

Self-care can be facilitated by careful organization of the wardrobe and tactile clues for color of clothing. Handling money and shopping can be difficult tasks for the visually impaired and require training and assistance.

Leisure time activities are important for well-rounded adulthood. Exercise groups, weight lifting, dance classes, and bowling are all excellent physical activities that should be encouraged, because many adults with severe visual impairments lead sedentary lives. Persons with visual impairment can play ball sports with sound balls, and they can run or jog with minimal track guidance aids.

Case Study 2: Bonnie

Bonnie was 7 years, 4 months old. She had congenital cataracts removed during her first year of life. Her resultant condition was legal blindness with form perception. Bonnie is the third (and last) child of a couple who had divorced since her birth. Her mother worked while Bonnie attended a local grammar school, where she was included in a regular second grade class. The therapist had informally assessed Bonnie, and parts of the Bruininks-Oseretsky Test of Motor Proficiency had been administered to her. Bonnie performed as follows:

- Motor area: Bonnie could trail in familiar settings, such as home and school, but she needed a sighted guide for unfamiliar areas. Her gait was shuffling and hesitant, and she feared falling. Balance activities were difficult, and she could only stand on one foot momentarily. She had difficulty with motor planning but had age-appropriate grasp, pinch, and coordination skills.
- Language area: According to school testing, she was 1 to 2 years behind in vocabulary. Bonnie enjoyed music and talking books. However, her attention span was variable, and auditory discrimination was poor for sound location.
- Personal-social area: Bonnie was in an early intervention program before school placement, and she had acquired some play skills. However, she remained shy and withdrawn, especially during playground activities and physical education. She fed herself, but her mother had a great deal of difficulty getting her to dress herself. Bonnie's mother attributed this, in part, to her own inability to "let go."

As noted, Bonnie was in a regular second grade class. She received occupational therapy and special education services three times a week. She attended regular physical education with some adaptation of requirements. The occupational therapist provided consultation to the physical education instructor regarding this adaptation.

Treatment goals

The three treatment goals were as follows:
1. Increased balance, motor planning, and equilibrium skills. Swing, bolster, tilt board, and scooter activities were used. In addition, the therapist recommended that the teacher and the physical education instructor provide tactile input for planning motor activities.
2. Increased dressing skills. Consulting with Bonnie's mother regarding age-appropriate dressing skills, practicing with Bonnie on manipulation of fasteners and use of tactile strips for clothing identification, and home visits to observe and assist in arranging clothing for ease of identification were used.
3. Increased social skills. Bonnie was assisted in planning and participating in activities with small groups of classmates; cooking or craft projects were also used.

Individualized Education Program objectives

The IEP objectives for the present school year were as follows:
- Bonnie would be able to stand and balance on one foot for 10 seconds.
- Bonnie would be able to manipulate buttons, snaps, and zippers 100% of the time.
- Bonnie would plan, with the therapist, four group activities during the school year.

■ MULTIPLE SENSORY IMPAIRMENT

Clinicians appear to agree that any combination of visual and hearing impairment with cognitive and/or motor disabilities result in a multiplication of disability. A combination of sensory losses creates a difficult situation, and the interaction of problems associated with the various disabilities must be considered. A common challenge for the occupational therapist is the child whose primary problem is a physical disability or mental retardation, but who also has visual and/or hearing deficits.

Diagnostic Information

Whenever a developing brain incurs injuries, the chances of multiple resulting impairments are great. For instance, 50% of children with cerebral palsy have some visual deficit and 13% have some form of auditory problem. The percentages of visual and auditory deficits are also high for children with mental retardation. With both of these diagnoses, accurate assessment of acuity, awareness, and perception is often difficult, because these children do not always give reliable feedback to the examiner.

Embryologic studies show that the timetable of development of the eye and ear are similar (Smith, 1982).

Therefore a number of diagnoses involve both systems (e.g., cytomegalovirus infection, maternal rebella, toxoplasmosis, congenital syphilis, Hurler's syndrome, Waardenburg's syndrome, and Goldenhar's syndrome). Meningitis is a leading cause of noncongenital hearing and visual impairment in children.

Other Services

As mentioned earlier, an extraordinary number of professionals may be involved with children who have multiple sensory disabilities. Orthopedists, neurologists, and cardiologists are a few medical specialists whose expertise is often needed. As the severity of the child's disability increases, so does the chance that the occupational therapist will become involved. The occupational therapist may be a major team member, especially with the physically impaired child who has visual deficits or with the child who is both visually and hearing impaired. Often the occupational therapist's first contact with visual or hearing impairment is through a child with multiple disabilities.

■ SPECIAL CHARACTERISTICS RELEVANT TO OCCUPATIONAL THERAPY

Some behaviors are characteristic of children who have both visual and hearing impairments. Typically, they exhibit extreme tactile defensiveness. They do not like anything new or different, and changes of any type are not well accepted. Often these children exhibit oral hypersensitivity, and the change from smooth to textured foods is difficult. Neuromotor function is often affected by hypotonicity and hypermobility of the joints or by spasticity. Such children usually learn to walk, but they are delayed and cautious about giving up support. They can go from walking while holding onto a wooden stick, to walking with a smaller stick, then a piece of rope, then a piece of yarn, then a thread. However, they may still immediately fall if the thread is taken away.

Children who are visually and hearing impaired often have had difficult infancy periods, including negative reactions to parental handling that can lead to less and less parental handling. Stimuli may not make sense to children who are visually impaired and/or hearing impaired, so they ignore it or respond in a defensive manner (McInnes & Teffry, 1982). They can have many primitive withdrawal reactions similar to children with autism. Self-stimulation behaviors, such as eye poking, eye rubbing, flicking hands in front of eyes, head bumping, hair twirling, and rocking, are often present and can become self-abusive. Perseverative behaviors (e.g., teeth grinding and masturbation) are also common. Certainly, every child is different and may manifest these behaviors to a different degree.

With the child who has visual and hearing impairment, as well as physical or cognitive disabilities, characteristics such as autistic-like behaviors, tactile defensiveness, and resistance to change can be noted. Occupational therapists should remember that these children need consistent repetition to learn skills, and that progress can be made, but often it is slow. For example, a simple task, such as learning the hand-to-mouth pattern necessary for self-feeding, may require years of hand-over-hand practice with multiple clues and much consistency.

Campbell, McInerney, and Cooper (1984) found that functional patterns of movement were achieved at faster rates when children with multiple disabilities were able to practice the desired movement patterns more frequently. Therefore training of caretakers and school staff becomes extremely important. The therapist should assess the child and identify specific tasks or movements to be targeted, determine the appropriate intervention strategies, and instruct others to carry out the tasks or movements with accuracy.

The role of the occupational therapist is often that of consultant. Consultation and monitoring to promote self-care skills, such as dressing, require that the therapist develop rapport with the persons doing the training and develop the ability to encourage and reward others to help them follow the program correctly. Diagrams or pictures with clearly written directions can be helpful guides for self care programs. The therapist monitors the self-care programs by observing others implement a technique and also by directly implementing the technique with the child to receive direct feedback about the child's performance.

Occupational Therapy Assessment Procedures

Developmental scales can be used for assessment and treatment planning for children with visual and hearing impairments. Of special interest are the prehension and tactile abilities, because almost everything has to be taught in a hand-over-hand manner. The Callier-Asuza Scale (Stillman, 1978) is a checklist for use with this population. It covers developmental skills to approximately the age of 7 and is based on observations of spontaneous behaviors in structured and unstructured situations. The Callier-Asuza Scale includes five subscales: (1) motor development, (2) daily living skills, (3) language development, (4) perceptual abilities, and (5) socialization. Each subscale is further divided; for example, the daily living skills subscale consists of dressing and undressing, personal hygiene, development of feeding skills, and toileting. The directions specify that an individual familiar with the child should administer the checklist. The teacher or therapist should spend a substantial period (at least 2 weeks) working directly with the child before attempting to use the checklist. It is also suggested that aides, parents, and others be consulted about their observations to obtain the most accurate picture of the child.

A complete descriptive assessment of levels in all areas of development must be done for children who have physical or mental disabilities in addition to visual and auditory impairment. The therapist often emphasizes play and social skills, activities of daily living, arm and hand skills, and community living. The child should be observed in structured and unstructured settings, and significant others should be consulted about the child's skills. The therapist then sorts out what part each of the contributing factors plays in the total picture of the child's difficulties.

Intervention Objectives and Methods

Intervention goals depend on the individual assessment of the child and his or her identified levels of functioning. Although these goals can vary from child to child, some typical goals of the occupational therapist include:

- *To minimize tactile hypersensitivity and promote integration of the tactile system.* Because acceptance of touch is basic to any interaction, integration of the tactile system is often an initial goal. The child should be gradually introduced to a variety of tactile stimulation activities and encouraged to reach out and explore independently. Use of vibration and proprioceptive input may also be helpful.

- *To provide family members with support and education.* Family members need information about appropriate levels of stimulation and effective strategies for interaction with the child. Support groups, or parents of children with similar disabilities, can become a greatly valued resource for the parents.

- *To provide adequate positioning.* The child with multiple sensory disabilities often cannot or will not (because of fear) move by him or herself. Therefore adequate positioning of the child to interact with the environment and to prevent contractures and deformities is extremely important. Functional positioning to ensure that the child can use his or her strongest sensory systems is the aim of much treatment. For those children not moving by themselves, teaching the caretakers and special education staff different positions and encouraging them to change these positions often is important.

- *To improve movement patterns and movement opportunities.* The child may first need to be moved, and later encouraged, if able, to move by himself or herself. For the child with limited movement, efforts should be made to provide movement so that the cycle of lack of movement, contractures, and deformities is interrupted. Once a new movement pattern is introduced, practice time should be allowed and new activities introduced gradually. Activities on tilt boards, swings, and bolsters are useful, but most important is movement with another person, such as walking (holding on) or rocking together.

- *To improve self-feeding skills.* Feeding is often a problem for children who have multiple disabilities. Often they had multiple medical problems that require long periods of tube feeding. Therapy intervention with the infant should focus on obtaining good sucking skills (good rhythm and appropriate strength) and decreasing facial hypersensitivity. Later, problems such as tongue thrusting, fatigue during feeding, and poor coordination of mouth movements sometimes occur. Learning to accept textured foods and chewing usually requires intervention, and physically moving the child through self-feeding and cup placement is often necessary. Hypersensitivities and resistance to change are two major difficulties that can be intensified with the presence of increased tone and reflex patterns. Strategies need to be developed for the child who remains on a bottle or extensively drinks a high-caloric food supplement, such as Pediasure. The transition to drinking from a glass and eating table foods is a long process, and it can take several years to achieve.

- *To improve self-care skills.* Achieving as much independence as possible should be the goal for each child. Toileting is often a problem because of resistance to the task and difficulty in understanding what is required. For the child who has physical disabilities in addition to visual and auditory impairments, the use of toilet scheduling techniques may be needed. Dressing and hygiene skills are also often difficult, requiring adaptation and hand-over-hand guidance. To increase independence, adaptive equipment (e.g., a large wheelchair tray with raised edges or a scoop bowl with suction cups) is often required.

As a team member, the occupational therapist may also assist with the following goals when working with children with visual and hearing impairments:

- *To develop cause-and-effect relationships.* Many switch-activated toys (e.g., toys that include a switch that the child can press to activate a fan or a vibrator) provide sensory input that is pleasurable and motivating to the child.

- *To develop functional behaviors.* Not only must the child's perseverative, nonproductive behaviors be extinguished, but more purposeful and functional behaviors must be substituted. Otherwise, the child may develop equally undesirable behaviors. To avoid this, the child needs consistency and continuity. If tactile signs are used, they should be simple, initially, and consistent from one person to the next. The development of interpersonal and play skills is also crucial.

Special techniques

Many of the specialized techniques used with these children deal with the development of some form of communication (Hyvarinen, Gimble, & Sorri, 1990). Children with multiple sensory disabilities display a slower pace of development. Therefore task analysis and breaking a task down into its smallest component parts can be useful in setting realistic goals for therapy and in establishing objectives for the IEP.

Task analysis can be especially useful in daily living and vocational-skills activities. For example, when teaching a child with multiple sensory disabilities to butter a piece of bread, the total task can be broken down into steps; then the steps can be repeated in a backward or forward order (i.e., *chaining*). In *backward chaining*, all steps are performed for the child except the last, which is the first taught, then the next to last, and so on. In *forward chaining*, the first step is taught until it is mastered, then the second, and so on. Regardless of the instructional direction used, it is important to fade out assistance but still give as much as needed to help the child master the task in its entirety.

Another useful technique with children who have multiple sensory impairment is *behavior modification.* This is a systematic approach to alter the child's behavior through environmental programming. In behavior modification, reinforcement is often used and detailed records of the child's responses are kept. Often a positive trait (e.g., urinating when placed on the toilet) needs to be reinforced, or a negative trait (e.g., eye poking) needs to be discouraged. The therapist charts the behaviors, and the correct response is provided. Although being ignored is negative reinforcement for many children, children who have multiple sensory disabilities are often happy to be left alone. Therefore this technique may not have the desired effect.

For the child who has multiple sensory impairment and is severely physically and mentally challenged, the therapist will often focus on safety, survival, or self-care skills. These skills, even if learned in a rote manner and requiring extremely specific environmental cues to elicit, are still important to the child's ability to function. If possible, carryover should be sought. However, after weighing all factors, therapeutic judgment may support concentrating on specific skills most important to function.

Preparation for adulthood

The child with multiple sensory disabilities, as well as severe physical or mental impairment, is usually prepared for workshop employment rather than for independent living. For the most part, workshop activities are manipulative and can include folding, stamping, collating, counting, gluing, bending, sorting, assembling, wrapping, stuffing, filing, measuring, stapling, and clipping.

Eight behaviors that the adolescent has to develop for more self-sufficient living are (1) communication of basic emergency and survival words such as stop, eat, more, no, and finish; (2) social skills; (3) self-care skills; (4) telling time; (5) cooking and shopping skills; (6) home management; (7) travel and mobility; and (8) housekeeping.

If the child has remained at home with the family unit through school, adolescence is often the time when a move must be made to a residential setting. Both the family members and the child must be prepared for this. Also, the emerging sexuality of the child has to be dealt with at the level of the child's understanding.

■ SUMMARY

This chapter provided an overview of occupational therapy intervention with the child with visual and/or hearing impairment. Occupational therapy assessment emphasizes how the child's development and function are affected by loss of one or both of these senses. General intervention goals have been presented, stressing provision of activities and experiences that allow the child to develop adaptive behaviors. Brief explanations regarding specialized techniques used with these children have also been provided, including the use of hearing aids, cochlear implants, sign language, Braille, and low-vision aids. Therapists use their knowledge of adaptation, activity analysis, and developmental sequence to help children who have visual and hearing impairments develop meaningful and purposeful occupations.

STUDY QUESTIONS

1. Children with hearing impairment may use one of several basic methods to improve communication skills. List these methods and explain how each would be used in occupational therapy intervention.

2. What common problems of children with visual impairment would suggest the need for referral to occupational therapy? How can the occupational therapist help them with each of these problems?

3. How do the developmental motor skills of the 1-year-old child with severe visual impairment differ from those of a typically developing 1-year-old child?

4. How do the developmental skills of a 3-year-old child with deafness differ from those of a typically developing 3-year-old child?

5. Describe four examples of assistive technology used in occupational therapy intervention with children who have visual or hearing impairments.

References

Adelson, E., & Fraiberg, S. (1974). Gross motor development in infants blind from birth. *Child Development, 45,* 114.

Anderson, K.L., & Matkin, N.D. (1991). *Relationship of degree of long term hearing loss to psychosocial impact and educational needs.* Los Angeles: John Tracy Clinic.

Ayres, A.J. (1972). *Sensory integration and learning disorders.* Los Angeles: Western Psychological Services.

Baker-Nobles, L. (1997). Pediatric low vision. In M. Gentile (Ed.), *Functional visual behavior: A therapist's guide to evaluation and treatment options.* Bethesda, MD: American Occupational Therapy Association.

Baker-Nobles, L., & Bink M.P. (1979). Sensory integration in the rehabilitation of blind adults. *American Journal of Occupational Therapy, 33,* 559-564.

Baker-Nobles, A., & Rutherford, A. (1995). Understanding cortical visual impairment in children. *American Journal of Occupational Therapy, 49,* 899-911.

Barraga, N. (1964). *Impaired visual behavior in low vision children.* New York: The American Foundation for the Blind.

Behrman, R.E., & Vaughan, V.C. (1987). *Nelson textbook of pediatrics* (13th ed.). Philadelphia: W.B. Saunders.

Brown, D., Simmons, V., & Mathvin, J. (1984). *The Oregon project for visually impaired and blind preschool children.* Medford, OR: Jackson County Education Service District.

Bruininks, R.H. (1978). *Bruininks-Oseretsky Test of Motor Proficiency: Examiner's manual.* Circle Pines, MN: American Guidance Service.

Campbell, P.H., McInerney, W.F., & Cooper, M.A. (1984). Therapeutic programming for students with severe handicaps. *American Journal of Occupational Therapy, 38,* 594-602.

Chaikin, L.E., & Downing-Baum, S. (1997). Functional visual skills. In M. Gentile, *Functional visual behavior: A therapist's guide to evaluation and treatment options.* Bethesda, MD: American Occupational Therapy Association.

Chase, P.A., & Gravel, J.S. (1996). Hearing aids for children. In R.A. Goldberg (Ed.), *Hearing aids: A manual for clinicians.* Philadelphia: Lippincott.

Cratty, B.J. (1971). *Movement and spatial awareness in blind youth.* Springfield, IL: Charles C. Thomas.

Davidson, P.W. (1992). Visual impairment and blindness. In M.D. Levine, W.B. Carey, & A.C. Crocker (Eds.), *Developmental-behavioral pediatrics* (2nd ed.). Philadelphia: W.B. Saunders.

Davis, H., & Silverman, S. (1978). *Hearing and deafness* (4th ed.). New York: Holt, Rinehart & Winston.

deQuiros, J. (1976). *Neuropsychological fundamentals in learning disorders.* San Rafael, CA: Academic Therapy Publications.

Dickens, C.J., & Hoskins, H.D. (1989). Developmental glaucoma. In S.J. Isenberg (Ed.), *The eye in infancy.* Chicago: Year Book.

Dunlea, A. (1989). *Vision and the emergence of meaning: Blind and sighted children's early language.* New York: Cambridge University Press.

Erhardt, R.P. (1987). Sequential levels in the visual-motor development of a child with cerebral palsy. *American Journal of Occupational Therapy, 41,* 43-49.

Erhardt, R.P. (1990). *Developmental visual dysfunction: Models for assessment and management.* Tucson, AZ: Therapy Skill Builders.

Fant, L.J. (1971). *Ameslan: An introduction to American sign language.* Silver Springs, MD: The National Association for the Deaf.

Ferrell, K.A., Trief, E., Dietz, S.J., Bonner, M.A., Cruz, D., Ford, E., & Stratton, J.M. (1990). Visually Impaired Infants Research Consortium (VIIRC): First year results. *Journal of Visual Impairment and Blindness, 84,* 404-410.

Fonda, G. (1970). *Management of the patient with subnormal vision* (2nd ed.). St. Louis: Mosby.

Fraiberg, S. (1977). *Insights from the blind: Comparative studies of blind and sighted infants.* New York: Basic Books.

Furth, H.G. (1973). *Deafness and learning: A psychological approach.* Belmont, CA: Wadsworth.

Gentile, M. (1997). *Functional visual behavior: A therapist's guide to evaluation and treatment options.* Bethesda, MD: American Occupational Therapy Association.

Gesell, A., Ilg, F.L., & Bullis, G.E. (1967). *Vision: Its development in infant and child.* New York: Hafner.

Goldberg, D. (1996). Early intervention. In F. Martin & J.C. Clark (Eds.), *Hearing care for children.* Needham, MA: Allyn & Bacon.

Gunn, S.L. (1971). Play as occupation: Implications for the handicapped. *American Journal of Occupational Therapy, 25,* 285-290.

Gustafson, G., Pfetzing, D., & Zawalkow, E. (1975). *Signing exact English.* Silver Springs, MD: Modern Sign Press.

Halliday, C. (1970). *The visually impaired child: Growth, learning, development: Infancy to school age.* Louisville, KY: The American Printing House for the Blind.

Heydt, K., Clark, M.J., Cushman, C., Edwards, S., & Allon, M. (1992). *Perkins Activity and Resource Guide: A handbook for teachers and parents of students with visual and multiple disabilities.* Watertown, MA: Perkins School for the Blind.

Hiles, D.A., & Hered, R.W. (1989). Disorders of the lens. In S.J. Isenberg (Ed.), *The eye in infancy.* Chicago: Year Book.

Hill, L. (1977). Working with blind preschoolers. *American Journal of Occupational Therapy, 31,* 417-419.

Hiskey, M.S. (1983). The development, administration, scoring, and interpretation of the Hiskey-Nebraska Test of Learning Aptitude. In C.R. Reynolds & J.H. Clark (Eds.), *Assessment and programming of young children with low incidence handicaps.* New York: Plenum.

Hyvarinen, L. (1995). Considerations in evaluation and treatment of the child with low vision. *American Journal of Occupational Therapy, 49,* 891-897.

Hyvarinen, L., Gimble, L., & Sorri, M. (1990). *Assessment of vision and hearing of deaf-blind persons.* Melbourne, Australia: Royal Victorian Institute for the Blind.

Isenberg, S.J. (Ed.). (1989). *The eye in infancy.* Chicago: Yearbook.

Jastrzembska, Z.S. (1976). *The effects of blindness and other impairments on early development.* New York: The American Foundation for the Blind.

Kaarela, R., & Widerberg, L. (1970). *Basic components of orientation and movement techniques.* Kalamazoo: Western Michigan University.

Klima, E.S., & Bellugi, U. (1978). *The signs of language.* Cambridge, MA: Harvard University Press.

Kreton, J., & Balkany, T.J. (1991). Status of cochlear implantation in children. *Journal of Pediatrics, 118,* 1-7.

Lampert, J.L. (1998). Working with students with visual impairment. In J. Case-Smith (Ed.), *Occupational therapy: Making a difference in school system practice.* Bethesda, MD: American Occupational Therapy Association.

Lampert, J.L., & Lapolice, D.J. (1995). Functional considerations in evaluation and treatment of the client with low vision. *American Journal of Occupational Therapy, 49,* 885-890.

Leenenberg, E.H. (1967). *Biological foundation of language.* New York: John Wiley & Sons.

Leiter, R.G. (1969). *General instructions for the Leiter International Performance Scale.* Los Angeles: Western Psychological Services.

Liben, L.S. (1978). *Deaf children: Developmental perspectives.* New York: Academic Press.

Linder, T.W. (1993). *Transdisciplinary play based assessment.* Baltimore: Brookes.

Ling, D. (1989). *Foundations of spoken language for hearing impaired children.* Washington, D.C: A.G. Bell Association.

Lydon, W.T., & McGraw, L.M. (1973). *Concept development for the visually handicapped child.* New York: The American Foundation for the Blind.

Martin, F. (1991). *Introduction to audiology.* Englewood Cliffs, NJ: Prentice-Hall.

Martin, F., & Clark, J.G. (1996). *Hearing care for children.* Needham, MA: Allyn & Bacon.

McInnes, J.M., & Teffry, J.A. (1982). *Deaf-blind infants and children.* Toronto, Canada: University of Toronto Press.

Meadow, P.M. (1980). *Deafness and child development.* Berkely: University of California Press.

Menacker, S.J., & Batshaw, M.L. (1997). Vision: Our window to the world. In M. L. Batshaw (Ed.), *Children with disabilities.* Baltimore: Brookes.

Michelman, S. (1971). The importance of creative play. *American Journal of Occupational Therapy, 25,* 285-290.

Mindel, E.D., & Vernon, M. (1971). *They grow in silence: The deaf child and his family.* Silver Springs, MD: The National Association for the Deaf.

Myklebust, H.R. (1964). *The psychology of deafness: Sensory deprivation, learning and adjustment.* New York: Grune & Stratton.

Nelson, C. (1993). *Effective intervention for successful self-feeding.* Albuquerque: Edit Point.

Nevins, M.E., & Chase, P.M. (1996). *Children with cochlear implants in educational settings.* San Diego: Singular.

Newborg, J., Stock, J., Wneck, L., Guidubaldi, J., & Svinicki, J. (1988). *Battelle Development Inventory.* Chicago: Riverside Publishers.

Newby, H. (1972). *Audiology.* New York: Appleton-Century-Crofts.

Northern, J.L., & Downs, M.P. (1992). *Hearing in children* (4th ed.). Baltimore: Williams & Wilkins.

Palmer, E.A. (1989). Tetratogenic agents. In S.J. Isenberg (Ed.), *The eye in infancy.* Chicago: Year Book.

Parham, L.D., & Fazio, L.S. (1997). *Play in occupational therapy for children.* St. Louis: Mosby.

Perera, C.A. (1957). *May's diseases of the eye.* Baltimore: Williams & Wilkins.

Pollack, D. (1970). *Educational audiology for the limited hearing infant.* Springfield, IL: Charles C. Thomas.

Reynell, J., & Zinkin, P. (1979). *Reynell-Zinkin Developmental Scales for Young Visually Handicapped Children.* Windsor, England: NFER.

Robbins, N. (1960). *Educational beginnings with deaf-blind children.* Watertown, MA: Perkins School for the Blind.

Roid, G.H., & Miller, L.J. (1997). *General instructions for the revised Leiter International Performance Scales.* Wood Dale, IL: Stoelting.

Rugers, C.T. (1969). *Understanding Braille.* New York: The American Foundation for the Blind.

Ryan, S.J., Dawson, A.K., & Little, H.L. (1985). *Retinal diseases.* Orlando: Grune & Stratton.

Sardegna, J., & Paul, T. (1991). *The encyclopedia of blindness and vision impairment.* New York: Facts on File.

Sataloff, J., Sataloff, R.T., & Vassolo, L.A. (1980). *Hearing loss* (2nd ed.). Philadelphia: J.B. Lippincott.

Schaefer, K.J., & Specht, M.A. (1979). A light probe adapted for use in training the blind. *American Journal of Occupational Therapy, 33,* 640-643.

Scheiman, M. (1997). *Understanding and managing vision deficits: A guide for occupational therapists.* Thorofare, NJ: Slack.

Schein, J.D., & Delk, M.T. (1975). *The deaf population of the United States.* Silver Springs, MD: The National Association for the Deaf.

Silverman, W.A. (1980). *Retrolental fibroplasia: A modern parable.* New York: Grune & Stratton.

Smith, D.W. (1982). *Recognizable patterns of human malformations.* Philadelphia: W.B. Saunders.

Steinberg, A.G., & Knightly, C.A. (1997). Hearing: Sounds and silences. In M.L. Batshaw (Ed.), *Children with disabilities* (4th ed.). Baltimore: Brookes.

Stillman, R.D. (1978). *The Callier-Asuza Scale.* Dallas: Callier Center for Communication Disorders.

Stoel-Gammon, C., & Otomo, K. (1986). Babbling development of hearing-impaired and normally hearing subjects. *Journal of Speech and Hearing Disorders, 51,* 33-41.

Thurnell R.J., & Rice, D.F.G. (1970). Eye rubbing in blind children: Application of a sensory deprivation model. *Exceptional Child, 36,* 325.

Tye-Murray, N. (1992). *Hello, cochlear implant and children: A handbook for parents, teachers, and speech and hearing professionals.* Washington, D.C: A.G. Bell.

Urrea, P.T., & Rosenbaum, A.L. (1989). Retinopathy of prematurity: An ophthalmologist's perspective. In S.J. Isenberg (Ed.), *The eye in infancy.* Chicago: Year Book.

Van Benschoter, R. (1975). A sensory integration program for blind campers. *American Journal of Occupational Therapy, 29,* 615-617.

Warren, D.H. (1984). *Blindness and early childhood development.* New York: The American Foundation for the Blind.

Warren, D.H. (1994). *Blindness in children: An individual differences approach.* New York: Cambridge University.

Welsh, R.L., & Blasch, B.B. (1980). *Foundations of orientation and mobility.* New York: The American Foundation for the Blind.

Hearing Impairment

Diagnostic Information

The estimates of children with hearing impairment vary with the criteria applied. The prevalence of severe bilateral hearing loss in high-risk neonates ranges from 1.7% to greater than 5%, depending on the population surveyed. It is estimated that 8% to 10% of children from 5 to 14 years of age have a unilateral hearing loss of greater than 15 decibels (dB) (Behrman & Vaughan, 1987). However, total deafness is rare and usually only happens when there is aplasia or failure of the inner ear to develop.

A person with *deafness* is one whose hearing is so severely impaired that he or she must depend primarily on visual communication such as writing, lip reading, manual communication, or gestures. Almost all children who are deaf have some residual audition that can be used for environmental awareness (Davis & Silverman, 1978; Newby, 1972; Northern & Downs, 1992).

Ear Anatomy

To properly examine the subject of hearing loss, it is important to have a basic understanding of the nature of sound and the anatomy of the ear. Sound sets up a disturbance in the air. Air consists of more than 400 billion particles per cubic inch. As we speak or make a sound, these particles are set in motion, hitting against each other and forming a wave of sound energy.

The ear acts as a receiver, amplifier, and transmitter and is composed of three sections (see Figure 25-1). The outer ear includes the visible part *(pinna)* and the external auditory canal extending to the eardrum *(tympanic membrane)*. The function of the outer ear is to collect the sound, or acoustic energy, and channel it to the eardrum, which vibrates with the sound wave and changes the acoustic energy to mechanical energy.

The middle ear consists of the three small bones *(hammer* or *malleus, anvil* or *incus,* and *stirrup* or *stapes)* that conduct vibrations from the eardrum to the inner ear. The stapes is inserted into the oval window, beyond which is the fluid-filled vestibule of the inner ear. This fluid-filled vestibule, along with the semicircular canals found in the inner ear, make up the organs of equilibrium. The motions of the bones of the middle ear result in an increase of the mechanical energy of sound so that by the time sound travels from the eardrum to the oval window, it has been intensified many times.

The inner ear is composed of the hearing organ, cochlea, that coils off the vestibule and the *acoustic nerve* (eighth cranial nerve). The cochlea transforms the mechanical energy of the sound waves into neural energy for reception by the auditory nerve.

Hearing Loss

There are two types of hearing loss: (1) *conductive* and (2) *sensorineural.* The type of loss a child has depends on what part of his or her ear has been damaged or underdeveloped. In conductive hearing loss, the problem lies in the sound-transmitting portions, that is, the outer or middle ear. One of the most frequent conditions causing conductive hearing loss is chronic otitis media (Sataloff, Sataloff, & Vassolo, 1980). Some common causes of conductive loss are wax buildup, punctured eardrum, or inability of the middle ear bones to move properly.

We hear by bone conduction as well as by air conduction, and the relationship of these two functions gives diagnostic information about the location of the hearing loss. Diagnoses with conductive hearing loss include Treacher Collins syndrome, a hereditary underdevelopment of the external canal and middle ear, and otosclerosis, a progressive condition occurring as early as late adolescence (Steinberg & Knightly, 1997). Fortunately, when detected early many conductive losses can be corrected by medical-surgical means, such as myringotomies and the placement of *pressure equalization* (PE) tubes. Unfortunately, considerable impairment of the developmental process (e.g., poor articulation, delayed speech development, and poor school performance) can occur before the time the child's hearing loss is detected.

In sensorineural hearing loss, or nerve loss, the problem occurs in the inner ear, with damage to the cochlear hair cells or nerve fibers. A nerve loss is generally not correctable by medical-surgical means, and it requires the use of hearing aids or cochlear implants. This type of loss often produces problems with loudness and distortion of sound. Sensorineural hearing loss is often associated with infections, such as bacterial meningitis, and can be a sequela of ototoxic drugs, such as neomycin. Drugs used in early infancy to save lives can have a toxic effect on the hearing organs.

Other diagnoses include tumors of the auditory nerve. These are most usually unilateral, with the exception of von Recklinghausen's disease, in which they are bilateral. Trauma, especially repeated exposure to loud noise, can also be a factor in hearing loss later in the child's life (Steinberg & Knightly, 1997).

It is common to have a mixed hearing loss, with both conductive and sensorineural loss present. The conductive loss must be medically treated as efficiently as possible to minimize the total effect of the loss. Generally speaking, if a hearing loss is measured in the "marked loss" range, it is likely to include sensorineural components.

One medical problem of adolescents with hearing loss is of such magnitude that it should be mentioned: Usher's syndrome. This is a genetic disease that affects 3% to 6% of all individuals with congenital deafness. It is marked by the progressive blindness of retinitis pigmentosa and a degeneration of the retina that progresses from impaired night vision to the gradual constriction of the visual field (with loss of peripheral vision, to blindness, usually by 20 to 30 years of age). Because Usher's syndrome influences the education and vocational choices available to adolescents already dealing with hearing loss, emphasis is placed on early screening.

Measurement of Hearing Loss

The occupational therapist working with a child with hearing impairment must have an understanding of the measurement of hearing loss. This includes knowledge of the severity of the loss and its practical meaning to the child. The most common measuring device is the *audiogram*. This device uses a grid to record the child's response to auditory stimuli and has a vertical axis that measures decibels. The decibel level is an indication of loudness or intensity of the sound or sound pressure; it goes from 0 dB (the point at which sound is first perceived) to 140 dB (the point, or threshold, of pain).

The horizontal axis of the audiogram is the *hertz* (Hz) level. This is a measure of the frequency or number of sound vibrations per minute—the pitch or tone of sound. Pitch, or frequency, ranges from a low of 125 Hz to a high of 12,000 Hz on the audiogram. The range of 500 to 4000 Hz is the most important because it encompasses the majority of speech sounds. On the audiogram, the scores are plotted on the graph, beginning with the hearing threshold level (where the child first begins to hear sounds). In addition, the left and right ears are differentiated by use of colors or by the symbol of a circle for right and a cross for left.

Decibel level is related to the distance that a sound moves an air particle, and it is measured by a particular standard or norm, such as the 1969 American National Standards Institute (ANSI). Although it varies slightly with the norm being used, a hearing level from 0 to 25 dB is considered within normal limits. Typical loss is classified according to loudness or to decibel loss and their respective therapy-education effects, which are general in nature and, of course, vary somewhat for each child and program (Anderson & Matkin, 1991). However, they give the occupational therapist an idea of what to expect with a certain level of hearing loss (Figure 25-4).

Functional Implications and Intervention

A hearing aid can be used with mild hearing loss. However, the greatest benefit is derived when the hearing aid is used with a loss of up to 80 dB. Beyond that point, the loss is so severe that only partial help can be obtained. After hearing aids have been tried for a period of time with little or no success, individuals with a severe or profound loss may receive cochlear implants.

The child's hertz level also has implications for his or her particular hearing loss. A child may have limitation in the sound frequency that helps him or her to produce speaking tones. This, in turn, affects hearing and language development. The hair cells inside the cochlea respond best to varied levels of frequency, depending on location, with the innermost hairs responding best to the low-tone frequencies. Depending on the location and extent of damage, there may be high-tone loss, low-tone loss, or flat loss. Frequency limitations can adversely affect syllable discrimination and understanding of speech.

A high-tone loss means that the child can hear most of the vowel sounds (because they have a lower frequency) but misses the consonants. Because the consonant sounds carry most of the information needed to understand speech, receptive language is seriously impaired. This is because unlike vowels, if the consonants are deleted from words they are impossible to understand.

With a low-tone loss, the child misses vowels but hears many consonants. Voices sound weak and thin, but they are understandable if the child is close enough to the speaker. A flat loss means that all frequencies are evenly affected. Voices sound far away, and certain strong vowels, such as the *a* in ate, will be heard best.

Although the audiogram gives information on both the decibel and hertz loss of a particular child (Martin, 1991), the therapist should consult with the child's family and other professionals involved to understand how the hearing loss affects his or her functional performance.

Other Services Involved

Often many professionals provide services to a particular child with hearing impairment. Those who specialize in hearing loss include the following:

- *Otolaryngologist,* or ear, nose, and throat specialist: A physician who specializes in the anatomy, physiology,

Mild loss: 25 to 40 dB

May have difficulty hearing faint or distant speech. Needs favorable seating and lighting in therapy or school settings. May need speech therapy, special attention to vocabulary, or aid in some instances.

Moderate loss: 40 to 55 dB

Will understand face-to-face conversational speech (at a distance of 3 to 5 feet). May miss as much as 50% of group discussion if voices are low or not in the direct line of vision. May show limited vocabulary and speech anomalies. Will need hearing aid evaluation and training, speech therapy, help in vocabulary and reading, and favorable seating and lighting. May need special class placement or lipreading training.

Moderate to severe loss: 55 to 70 dB

Will have increasing difficulty in group discussions. Will show limited vocabulary and is likely to have speech anomalies and be delayed in language use and comprehension. Will need special education services, speech therapy, lipreading instruction, special help with language skills, and hearing aids. Needs to be encouraged in therapy-education settings to pay attention to visual and auditory input at all times. Use of sign language may increase understanding.

Severe loss: 70 to 90 dB

May hear loud voices about 1 foot from ear and may be able to identify environmental sounds such as a vacuum cleaner. May have speech difficulties with some ability to discriminate vowels but not all consonants. If loss is present before 1 year of age, the child will not develop spontaneous language. Will need special education services, support services, hearing aid and/or cochlear implant. Needs a comprehensive program emphasizing language and concept development, speech, lipreading, and sign language.

Profound loss: 90 dB and more

May hear some loud sounds, such as an automobile horn, very close but is aware of vibrations more than tonal patterns. Will have to rely on vision as the primary means of communication, rather than on hearing. Sign language is often the primary means of communication. Speech will be deficient and will not develop spontaneously if loss is present before 1 year of age. Will need special education on a comprehensive intensive basis.

NOTE: Shouting, talking loudly or exaggerating mouth movements, and distorted speech are not helpful techniques to increase understanding.

figure 25-4 Therapy education implications of typical hearing loss classifications.

and pathologic conditions of the head and neck, including the ears, nose, and throat, and uses medical and surgical treatment techniques.

- *Otologist:* A physician who specializes in the anatomy, physiology, and pathologic conditions of the ear, and uses medical and surgical treatment techniques.
- *Audiologist:* A specialist in the study of hearing, who performs hearing tests and provides rehabilitation and treatment, including hearing aids, for those whose impairment cannot be improved by medical-surgical means.
- *Audiometrist:* A technician trained to test and measure hearing ability.

Specialized Assessments

In the area of psychologic testing, there are several tests used with children with hearing impairment. These include the following:

- *The Hiskey Nebraska Test of Learning Abilities* (Hiskey, 1983). A test developed and standardized for the hearing impaired that covers ages 2 to 17. It consists of subtests selected to cover a broad span of intellectual abilities without language. It includes subtests, such as bead patterns, picture associations, puzzle blocks, completion of drawings, and memory for digits, and is given in an untimed fashion.
- *The Leiter International Performance Scale* (Leiter, 1969; Roid & Miller, 1997). A widely used individual IQ test administered without language with a range from 2 to 16 years. It is a performance test that was developed as a nonverbal counterpart to the Stanford-Binet test. It is used with children with hearing impairment as well as others (e.g., those who do not speak English). Directions are pantomimed, and the test is not timed. Administration begins with items below the child's estimated skill level so that the child has an opportunity to become accustomed to the testing procedure. The Leiter International Performance Scale includes numerous subtests, including items such as matching colors, number discrimination, pattern completion, similarities, classification of animals, and spatial relations.
- *The Kaufman Assessment Battery for Children* (K-ABC) (Kaufman & Kaufman, 1983). This test has a nonverbal scale with instructions that can be pantomimed. It is used for children ages 4 through 12½ and results give useful information on educational recommendations for the child with hearing impairments.
- Audiologic testing is a complicated and involved process (Martin, 1991; Martin & Clark, 1996; Newby, 1972). The occupational therapist should consult the professional administering the test on details of testing with the individual child. The most common method of testing requires the use of earphones and placement of

the child in a soundproof testing booth. The child indicates when he or she hears a sound.

- Other forms of testing are used with children who are unable to follow the specific instructions in a standardized test. Behavioral observation audiometry (BOA) is often used with young children. In BOA, the parent holds the child in his or her lap, and the audiologist notes different behavioral responses to sounds at different levels. Another test, visual reinforcement audiometry (VRA), teaches the child to orient to a sound source reinforced with light or a visual stimulus. Tangible reinforcement operant conditioning audiometry (TROCA) uses a token or candy for reinforcement when sounds are identified. In play audiometry, the child does a certain task, such as putting a cube in a bucket, when the sound is heard.

- Measurement of physiological responses is helpful in the diagnosis of hearing impairment. Auditory brain stem response (ABR) is often done with infants or unresponsive children. It uses a type of electroencephalogram machine and a computer. Earphones are placed on a sedated or quiet child, and a series of clicks or tone bursts are played into the ears. The computer records the brain wave responses and supplies information regarding the hearing mechanism response to sound.

- *Tympanometry* is a procedure to assess eardrum mobility or the presence of fluid in the middle ear. This requires the placement of a probe in the ear canal and can be difficult to perform on an uncooperative child. The acoustic reflex measurement is tested with the same instrument as the tympanogram, but it measures the response of the two middle ear muscles to the presentation of sound. Evoked otoacoustic emissions (EOAE) measures the response of the cochleae. Sound is put into the ear and will be emitted back if the child has a healthy middle ear and cochlea. Technologies continue to be developed to improve the efficiency and validity of audiological testing.

■ DIAGNOSTIC INFORMATION

Approximately 50 to 64 children per 100,000 have serious visual impairments, and at least another 100 children per 100,000 have less serious difficulties (Davidson, 1992). Total blindness is found in only a few children and is often a result of anophthalmos (i.e., absence of the eyeball). Hereditary causes account for approximately one half of all childhood blindness. Numerous low-incidence syndromes with eye and associated deformities are seen (Isenberg, 1989).

Visual deficits can be caused by neurological impairment associated with teratogenic agents, including maternal substance abuse (Palmer, 1989). Retinopathy of prematurity (ROP) occurs in 7% of infants who weigh 1200 g or less at birth (Gallo & Lennerstrand, 1991). The lower the birth weight and earlier the birth, the higher the chances of the infant developing ROP. Given the advances in medicine and the resulting increased ability of younger and smaller infants to survive, the number of infants with ROP is increasing. Once the condition has been identified, it is difficult to determine whether the process will continue and become a major problem. Various stages of severity of the condition have been identified (Urrea & Rosenbaum, 1989).

The legal definition of blindness is important to understand. In the United States it is defined as follows:

> Central visual acuity of 20/200 or less in the better eye after correction, or visual acuity of more than 20/200 if there is a field deficit in which the widest diameter of the visual field subtends to an angle distance no greater than 20 (Sardegna & Paul, 1991, p. 31).

This means that the child who is legally blind can see an object clearly at 20 feet that a child with normal vision can see at 200 feet. Acuity refers to central vision. The peripheral vision, or second part of the definition, means that the child can only see in a field of 20 degree, whereas a child with normal vision can see in a field of over 180 degree. Peripheral vision is most important in mobility and general observation of the environment. Box 25-3 lists generally accepted gradations of acuity with correction.

Acuity is not the only factor in assessing vision, and two children with equal acuity can have different visual functions. Of course, with many children it is difficult to know where and how a child sees. Spotty or irregular visual loss may occur in both the central and peripheral areas. The young child may use postural accommodation or head tilt to position to a focus point (i.e., the point from which he or she can see most clearly).

As with the ear, it is important for the occupational therapist to have a basic understanding of the anatomy and physiology of the eye to understand visual impairment. The reader should review the anatomy of the eye in Chapter 13.

Visual impairment can occur within the structures of the eyeball, at the retina, along the nerve pathway to the brain, and in the brain itself. Refractive errors occur when there is deviation in the course of the light rays as they pass through the eye, preventing sharp focus on the retina. Scheiman (1997) identified the most common refractive errors as including the following:

- *Myopia,* or nearsightedness: The child with myopia sees most clearly at close range and much less efficiently at a distance. The eyeball is too long, or refractive power is too strong, so the focus point is in front of the retina. This causes the child to have blurred vision and external strabismus is possible when looking at a distance. The child often holds printed material close to the eyes.
- *Hyperopia,* or farsightedness: The child with hyperopia has blurred vision and may have headaches when trying to focus. The eyeball is too short and underdeveloped, the refractive power is too weak, and the focus point is behind the retina. This child sees most clearly at a distance and, with constant effort to focus at close range, his or her eyes becomes fatigued.

Although these refractive errors can usually be corrected with lenses, if left undiagnosed or untreated during early school years, they can have a devastating effect on the child's development in all areas.

Cataracts are often a congenital problem that give rise to poor vision (Hiles & Hered, 1989). A cataract occurs when the lens of the eye changes from clear to

25-3 *Gradations of acuity with correction*

20/20 to 20/70 = Normal to slightly defective vision
20/70 to 20/100 = Mild visual limitation or good partial vision
20/100 to 20/200 = Moderate visual impairment or fair partial vision
20/200 to 20/1,000 = Legally blind with severe impairment
Over 20/1,000 = (1) Finger counting ability; (2) Form perception; (3) Hand movement; (4) Light perception (sees light and can tell where it is); (5) Light perception (sees light but cannot locate it)

cloudy, or opaque. After removal of the lens, the child must wear corrective lenses. Although often the result of heredity, childhood cataracts can be associated with juvenile diabetes, Down syndrome, or Hallermann-Streiff syndrome.

Glaucoma is another visual problem that can occur in childhood (Dicken & Hoskins, 1989). Glaucoma is an increase in the intraocular pressure of the eyeball, resulting in hardening of the eye and damage to the cornea. Congenital glaucoma occurs in the first year of life; it may be secondary to ocular inflammation or eye trauma. A microsurgical procedure can relieve the pressure and often preserve vision (Batshaw & Perret, 1992).

Other eye conditions and common optical terms are listed below (Isenberg, 1989; Menacker & Batshaw, 1997):

- *Amblyopia:* A condition of diminished visual acuity, sometimes called lazy eye, that usually cannot be relieved by lenses. The child may have depth perception problems and may tilt his or her head.
- *Astigmatism:* Unequal curvature of the refractive surfaces of the eye that may result in distorted images. This may result in focusing problems, because light is not sharply focused on the retina but spread over a more or less diffused area.
- *Charge:* A syndrome including coloboma, heart malformations, atresia of the nasal passage, retardation, genital abnormalities, and ear abnormalities.
- *Coloboma:* Congenital defect of the eye caused by its failure to complete growth in the affected area (usually the iris, choroid, or ciliary body).
- *Cortical Visual Impairment/Cortical Blindness:* The ocular structures are intact, but the child is functionally visually impaired or blind because of severe insult to the visual cortex of the brain. This impairment

occurs as a result of oxygen deprivation, such as in near drowning, prolonged shock, brain trauma, or infections of the central nervous system.

- *Microphthalmos:* An abnormally small eyeball.
- *Nystagmus:* Rapid involuntary movement of the eyes. May be hereditary and result in inability to fixate accurately and constantly. The movement is repetitive, and it may be lateral, vertical, rotary, or mixed.
- *Optic Atrophy:* Degeneration of the optic nerve fibers.
- *Optic Nerve Hypoplasia:* Failure of the optic nerve to fully develop.
- *Ptosis:* Drooping eyelid resulting from weak or absent muscle. This condition usually does not interfere with vision.
- *Retinoblastoma:* Malignant tumor of the retina and eye orbit that is either unilateral or, more often, bilateral.
- *Strabismus:* Squint or cross-eyes. Failure of the eyes to converge properly on an image, or both eyes not directed at the same point. This condition is often caused by muscle imbalance and frequently results in double vision. In esotropia the eye turns inward; in exotropia the eye turns outward; in vertical strabismus the eye turns up or down.
- *Toxoplasmosis:* Parasitic disease that can be congenital or acquired from household pets; causes scarring, usually on retina and choroid.

Any of these conditions may affect visual acuity. When the child is capable of understanding the directions, visual acuity is most often tested with the use of the Snellen chart. This tests central acuity with letters, numbers, or symbols in graded sizes that are drawn to Snellen measurements. Each size is labeled with the distance from which it can be seen by the normal eye. The child stands 20 feet from the chart and indicates to the examiner what he or she sees, line by line. Eye report terms include OD, which refers to the right eye, OS, to the left eye, and OU, to both eyes.

Other Services

Children with visual impairment often have a number of other professionals involved in their treatment. The most common are the following:

- *Ophthalmologist:* A physician who specializes in the diagnosis and treatment of defects and diseases of the eye, performing surgery when necessary, and prescribing other types of treatment, including corrective lenses.
- *Optometrist:* A licensed specialist in vision (OD), who is trained in the art and science of vision care. This specialist examines the eyes and preserves and restores vision through optometric means, as well as measures refractive errors and eye muscle disorders.
- *Optician:* An individual who grinds lenses, fits them into frames, and adjusts frames to the wearer.
- *Orientation and mobility specialist:* An individual specializing in orientation and mobility training of the visu-

ally impaired. Orientation is the process of using the remaining senses to establish one's position and relationship to all other significant objects in one's environment. Mobility is the ability to move safely and efficiently from one point to another in the environment.

Specialized Assessments

Standardized tests have been developed specifically for children with visual impairment. These include the following:

- *The Maxfield-Buchholz Social Maturity Scale for Blind Pre-School Children* (Maxfield & Buchholz, 1995). This test, an adapted version of the Vineland Social Maturity Scale, is of special interest to therapists and psychologists because it helps obtain an accurate developmental picture of an individual child. The Maxfield-Buchholz scale covers seven areas of the Vineland scale: (1) self-help general, (2) self-help dressing, (3) self-help eating, (4) communication, (5) socialization, (6) locomotion, and (7) occupation. The Maxfield-Buchholz scale is designed for preschoolers to children at the 5- to 6-year level. Of the 95 items on the Maxfield-Buchholz scale, 44 are from the Vineland scale. The Maxfield-Buchholz items were all standardized with children with visual impairment, and they give the examiner information about how these children compare with each other. It is administered exactly as the original Vineland scale: the parent or caregiver gives information about the performance of the child.
- *The Reynell-Zinkin Developmental Scales for Young Visually Handicapped Children* (Reynell & Zinkin, 1979). Similar to the Bayley Scales, the Reynell-Zinkin has two parts: one covering mental development and one assessing motor development. The mental scales include sections on social adaptation, sensorimotor understanding, exploration of the environment, response to sound and verbal comprehension, expressive language, and communication. The motor scales cover hand function, locomotion, and reflexes. They use a profile-type of scoring, and standard scores are not available. However, age equivalents are given for children (with and without visual impairment) who are 0 to 5 years old.
- *The Oregon Project Developmental Checklist* (Brown, Simmons, & Mathvin, 1984). This test has also been developed for assessing the child with visual impairment up to 6 years of age and for writing educational and intervention objectives. It covers the areas of cognitive, language, social, vision, compensatory, self-help, fine and gross motor development. Teaching activities are suggested for each area. This checklist

also takes into account the fact that there is a vast difference in the degree of visual impairment by indicating items that are acquired at a later age or that may not be appropriate for children with total vision loss.

- *The Perkins Activity and Resource Guide* (Heydt, Clark, Cushman, Edwards, & Allon, 1992). This test includes developmental checklists as well as developmental activities and resources for the areas of language and cognition, social development, motor development, functional academics, vocational training, daily living skills, independent-living skills, and sensory integration.
- *The Erhardt Developmental Vision Assessment* (EDVA) (Erhardt, 1987, 1990). This observational assessment measures development of ocular-motor skills from birth to 6 months. It is divided into a section on primarily involuntary visual patterns (i.e., eyelid reflexes, pupillary reactions, and doll's eye responses) and a section on voluntary patterns (i.e., fixation, localization, ocular pursuit, and gaze shift). It can be helpful to the therapist in determining the child's developmental level of functional ocular-motor abilities.

Observation of the young child's functional vision is important. In addition to a physical examination, observing the child's use of objects and toys often provides important information (Hyvarinen, 1995; Lampert & Lapolice, 1995). The subjective description of functional vision from the parent, teacher, or therapist can also add greatly to the physician's assessment.

Several intelligence tests have also been adapted for use with the visually impaired, including the Binet and the Wechsler. Other oral tests are easily adaptable. The American Foundation for the Blind publishes a comprehensive listing of psychologic, vocational, and educational tests appropriate for use with the visually impaired. As with audiologic testing, evaluation of visual acuity and visual perception has become more sophisticated with increased technology. In addition to the Snellen-type acuity examinations, other tests have been developed for young children and children with disabilities. For example, preferential looking techniques use blank versus patterned targets (Menacker & Batshaw, 1997).

Physicians use an ophthalmoscope to view the internal structure of the eye. Electroretinography (ERG) is administered with child sedated and provides a thorough examination of the retina and fundus. Visual evoked potentials (VEP) assess cortical response to light stimulation using an electroencephalogram. Results of these tests provide information about the function of the eye, the optic nerve, and the visual cortex.

chapter **26**

Hospital Services

Barbara Marin Wavrek

■ CHAPTER OBJECTIVES

1. Understand the characteristics of children's hospitals.
2. Explain the roles and functions of occupational therapists in pediatric hospitals.
3. Describe occupational therapy intervention in intensive-care units and acute-care units.
4. Explain outpatient intervention models.
5. Describe hospital-based occupational therapy services for children with burns, bone marrow transplants, and failure to thrive.

Intervention with children in hospitals presents the occupational therapist with a unique set of challenges. The demands of the evolving health care system, the varied and sometimes unusual medical conditions of the children, and the characteristics of hospitals as health care institutions all have an impact on occupational therapy practice. This chapter describes occupational therapy service provision to children in hospitals, illustrates the medical model of service delivery, and explains the roles and functions of hospital-based occupational therapy practitioners.

■ CHARACTERISTICS OF HOSPITALS AND MEDICAL SYSTEMS

Hospitals, by definition, are institutions where individuals who are ill or injured receive medical care designed to diagnose and treat the presenting problem. Over time, however, hospitals have greatly expanded their roles in the provision of health care, offering both inpatient and outpatient services for the ill and injured, as well as prevention or wellness programs designed to decrease the need for future hospitalizations and treatment.

General hospitals are institutions that serve patients of various ages and provide services for a broad range of diagnoses. General hospitals may have special facilities for children but are oriented toward meeting the broad range of community needs. Consequently, an occupational therapist employed in a general hospital is likely to be responsible for providing services to adults as well as children.

Pediatric hospitals are specialty hospitals that offer a full range of inpatient and outpatient services for infants, children, and adolescents. A wide range of pediatric diagnoses are evaluated and treated, and length of stay may be longer than in a general hospital. Children hospitalized in pediatric facilities have access to professionals in various specialties who have experience in the evaluation and treatment of complex medical problems. Because of the high volume of patient activity in hospitals, hospital personnel have the opportunity to gain experience in evaluation and treatment of medical conditions. In addition, these health care professionals learn to recognize individual differences in children's responses to similar medical problems.

Intensity of Services

Services provided to children in hospitals, whether general or specialized, tend to differ from the services provided to adults. Provision of medical intervention to children tends to be more labor intensive than provision of medical intervention to adults. "Sick children need more nursing care and therapy than sick adults, and children's care is about 30% more labor intensive. . . ." (Considine, 1994, p. 84).

Region Served

Hospitals that provide services to children may also be different in the size and location of their service regions. Children's hospitals, as specialized health care institutions, tend to serve a broader geographic region than general hospitals. This has several implications.

First, a child may be hospitalized a significant distance from home, increasing the sense of separation from family and familiar environment. Second, the distance between home and hospital may affect the family's ability to visit the child and remain in contact with the health personnel caring for the child. Third, the size of the service area, as well as the part of the country in which it is located, may mean greater cultural diversity and socioeconomic variation among those served by the hospital. This means that medical services, including occupational therapy, must be sensitive to the cultural beliefs and practices of the patient and family. Finally, the broader geographic region served by most children's hospitals usually requires hospital personnel to interact with a great number of organizations and programs in the community to plan for services after hospital discharge (Gilkerson, Gorski, & Panitz, 1990).

Health care costs

An issue of concern facing hospitals that provide service to children is the cost of health care. In recent years Heath Maintenance Organizations (HMOs) and Preferred Provider Organizations (PPOs) have proliferated; currently more than 75 million Americans are in some type of managed care plan (Dorgan, 1995). Approximately two thirds of the privately insured individuals in the United States are insured through PPOs or HMOs. These organizations have had a huge impact in how services are delivered and reimbursed, because they control costs by limiting consumers' options regarding services to in-network providers (Christiansen, 1996).

The prospective payment system, introduced through Medicare legislation in 1983, has also had a strong impact on reimbursement for services. This system uses pre-established rates of reimbursement for almost 500 diagnostic groups, and the hospital is reimbursed with the pre-established fee, regardless of the cost of treating an individual (Bailey, 1998).

Other managed-care strategies are also designed to contain costs while maintaining quality of care. Examples of cost containment strategies include requirements for patients to obtain certification or second opinions prior to obtaining desired medical intervention (Christiansen, 1996). Managed-care strategies may result in shorter hospital stays, provision of fewer services, or limited reimbursement for services provided. One result of shorter hospital stays is the increased emphasis on outpatient diagnostic and treatment services. In addition to government-sponsored institutions, hospitals may be classified as private, nonprofit institutions or private, for-profit institutions.

Critical Pathways

An external force that affects the provision of occupational therapy services for children is the development of *critical pathways* for decisions regarding the most appropriate care based on a child's diagnosis. Critical pathways are diagnosis-specific protocols that define essential medical care to be provided, or actions to be taken, within identified time-lines to achieve optimal outcomes for the client (Abreu, Seale, Podlesak, & Hartley, 1996).

These written documents often prescribe specific day-by-day caregiving, medical, and therapeutic procedures, from onset of the diagnosis (admission) to discharge. Ideally, critical pathways are designed to maintain the quality of patient care while increasing efficiency in the use of available resources. One area of concern is that adherence to critical pathways may decrease use of resources, thereby containing costs at the expense of quality of patient care.

Health Care Trends

Health care trends have the potential to affect the occupational therapy services provided to children. For example, affiliating children's hospitals may compare productivity statistics and quality improvement strategies among occupational therapy departments, or they may share program development information.

Hospitals are governed by internal policies and procedures that are usually designed to assist the institution in meeting standards of external, private accrediting agencies, government agencies, and insurance providers. Organizations such as the *Joint Commission for the Accreditation of Health Care Organizations* (JCAHO) and the

Commission for the Accreditation of Rehabilitation Facilities (CARF), as well as government agencies, such as the *Occupational Safety and Health Administration* (OSHA), have set standards regarding hospital operations. These include standards for provision of professional services, documentation of patient care activities, patient and employee safety, and quality improvement activities (Commission for the Accreditation of Rehabilitation Facilities [CARF], 1994; Joint Commission for the Accreditation of Health Care Organizations [JCAHO], 1994).

Employee education regarding safety practices (when there is risk of exposure to patient blood or body fluids) or to hazardous materials is also mandated (Occupational Exposure to Blood-Borne Pathogens, 1991). Standards such as these also influence occupational therapy department policies, procedures, and service delivery.

One trend among hospitals has been the affiliation of similar institutions, offering opportunities for consolidation of information and equipment, achievement of common goals, and program development. Pontzer (1994) noted, "Hospitals are moving in the direction of 'hospital systems' where they are serving their patients across the spectrum of placement options including acute, subacute, rehabilitation, outpatient, skilled nursing facilities, and home health care" (p. 36).

Trends in managed care that result in shorter hospital stays and limited reimbursement have the potential to restrict the occupational therapy services that may be provided or shift the emphasis to the provision of outpatient services. As part of the current trend toward decentralization of hospital-based services, many pediatric facilities have established outpatient satellite centers in the community, which may provide both medical and therapy services.

■ HOSPITAL-BASED SERVICES

Gilkerson (1990) identified the preservation of life as the most important function in a hospital and suggested that life-threatening conditions take priority in the scheme of hospital activities. Hospitals offer a range of services designed to provide medical care to children with acute or chronic illness, traumatic injury, or special needs. The method of service delivery varies according to the needs of the patient and the nature of the medical care required. For patients with burns or those who require bone marrow transplants, the hospital environment is designed to minimize the risk of infection to patients who are especially susceptible, while still enabling the completion of the medical protocol.

Acute care, intensive and critical care, special care, medical or surgical care, ambulatory or *outpatient services, and teaching and research* are just some of the hospital-based services with which occupational therapists should be familiar. Many children enter and leave the hospital system at different points along this continuum of services; others experience the full range of services.

A child with severe burns, for example, may initially be admitted to an ICU because of the life-threatening nature of the injury. Once the child's medical condition stabilizes, he or she may be transferred to a special unit for children with burns for continuation of treatment. When hospitalization is no longer necessary, the child is discharged but may be asked to return to the outpatient clinic for occupational therapy, physical therapy, or for follow-up visits with physicians, therapists, and other hospital personnel.

Most patient-care activity in hospitals is acute care. Acute care refers to short-term medical care provided during the acute phase of an illness or injury, when the symptoms are generally the most severe. Just as there are degrees of severity that categorize illnesses and injuries, there are also levels of acute care designed to meet these varied needs.

Critically ill patients who require continuous monitoring and frequent medical attention, and patients who often need special equipment to maintain or monitor vital functions, are admitted to *intensive care units* (ICUs) or *critical care units* (CCUs). Hospitals may have several intensive-care units, each of which is designated for a specific patient population or purpose. *Neonatal intensive-care units* (NICUs), *pediatric intensive-care units* (PICUs) for older children, and *surgical intensive-care units* (SICUs) are examples of intensive care units that may be found in hospitals. Personnel who provide care for patients in ICUs receive special training to enable them to respond quickly and effectively to meet the needs of medically unstable patients in this challenging environment.

A child whose illness or injury results in hospitalization, but who does not need the continuous attention, high technology, and specialized care of an ICU, may be admitted to a *medical or surgical acute-care unit*. Medical and surgical units also tend to be designated for specific types of patients. For example, patients requiring neurosurgical services may be cared for on one unit, whereas patients requiring orthopedic-related treatment may be served on another.

Although patients in a critical-care unit may share a common diagnosis, they may be at different points in their treatment and recovery. By contrast, patients with infectious conditions may have a variety of diagnoses that require treatment under isolation conditions. If this is the case, these patients are often placed in *special-care units.* Three conditions that require a child to be treated in a special care unit are (1) *acute burns,* (2) *infectious diseases,* and (3) *bone marrow transplantation.*

Medical intervention for chronically ill patients may also be provided in hospitals that emphasize acute care.

Often, chronically ill patients are admitted for an acute exacerbation of their illnesses or for treatment of complications. Diabetes, asthma, cystic fibrosis, and cancer are examples of chronic illnesses occurring in children that may require periodic hospitalization.

In some instances, chronically ill patients who are medically fragile may receive long-term care in an acute hospital setting. This long-term care may be required because the family is unable or unwilling to care for the child at home and a special placement elsewhere in the region is not readily available. DeWitt, Jansen, Ward, and Keens (1993) found that children who required ventilator assistance often remained in the hospital for nonmedical reasons after becoming medically stable. Two factors that significantly delayed hospital discharge were difficulty arranging either out-of-home placement or financial assistance to enable care in the home. However, there continues to be an increasing emphasis on arranging return to home or community placement as quickly as possible.

Ambulatory and outpatient services, or programs, are designed for patients who require medical services but whose conditions do not require hospitalization. Outpatient services may include diagnostic procedures, such as radiographs or laboratory tests. These services may also include visits to clinics (for continuity of care after discharge from the hospital) or special services, such as outpatient occupational therapy or physical therapy. In some cases, outpatient services may also include primary care.

Although most hospital services are directed toward providing medical care to the ill or injured, many hospitals also include teaching and research as part of their missions. The hospital, as a teaching institution, provides clinical education experiences for medical students, interns, residents, nursing students, and students from other health-related professions. As a research institution, a hospital often provides resources and opportunities for clinical research to advance medical knowledge and practice.

Although the primary role of the hospital-based occupational therapist is that of a clinician, occupational therapy personnel may also assume roles in education and research. For example, occupational therapists in hospitals also serve as fieldwork supervisors for occupational therapy students, and they have opportunities to educate students from other health professions about issues relevant to occupational therapy.

Hospital-based occupational therapists may also design and implement research pertinent to occupational therapy, or they may assist in multidisciplinary research efforts. However, opportunities for occupational therapists to function as educators and researchers have decreased as the emphasis on clinical productivity has increased.

■ MEDICAL MODEL AND TEAM INTERACTION

In a hospital, care of the patient focuses on the individual's medical needs and, to some extent, the family's needs. When treating children, the medical team is particularly concerned about the way certain needs affect the child's illness, recovery, and general well-being. For this reason, the composition of the medical team tends to reflect the immediate needs of the patient and family.

In general, the physician is considered the leader of the medical team for a given child, although leadership may shift to other team members during the course of the child's stay (Case-Smith & Wavrek, 1998). The child's *care manager* is often a registered nurse or other medical professional whose services have been formally requested by the physician. In some cases the parents form the remainder of the team responsible for the child's care.

Two factors that often affect the parents' participation in the child's care are (1) *the distance between the family's home and the hospital,* and (2) *the parents' other obligations, including work and child care.* These factors may limit the parents' ability to visit the hospital and therefore their ability to interact with the professionals caring for their child.

Another significant characteristic of medical teams is their dynamic nature. Because the actual health care disciplines represented in a specific case depend on the patient's needs, the medical team is continually changing. For example, a child with a feeding disorder, who is failing to grow and gain weight, may have a physician, nurses, an occupational therapist, a dietitian, and a social worker as members of his or her medical team. However, a child hospitalized with multiple injuries resulting from a motor vehicle accident may have several physicians, nurses, an occupational therapist, a physical therapist, a speech pathologist, a dietitian, a respiratory therapist, and a social worker as members of his or her medical team.

As a potential member of multiple medical teams within one hospital, the occupational therapist must communicate and collaborate with professionals from many different health-related fields. Frequently, the therapist may be required to continually redefine or explain the role of the occupational therapist to other team members, as well as to develop an understanding of the ways in which different team members' roles complement each other in the provision of services to children. With the trend toward "hospital systems," described previously, occupational therapists employed by hospitals may face the more complex challenges of defining their roles in several different settings within one integrated system of care and participating in interdisciplinary medical teams across the spectrum of care (Pontzer, 1994).

Communication of hospital team members is dependent on a number of factors. One significant factor is the limited availability of team members for scheduled meetings. Communication tends to occur *formally* through documentation in the patient's chart and *informally* during telephone calls or chance meetings throughout the day. "What appear as unplanned interactions are actually an accepted and effective way of doing business in a setting where time is at a premium, needs are immediate, and staff schedules can change daily" (Gilkerson, Gorski, & Panitz, 1990, pp. 453-454).

Communication with the patient or parent occurs at separate times for most team members. Regular team meetings, although ideal, are often not feasible in a hospital setting because of the multiple demands on hospital personnel and the likelihood of schedule changes.

■ SPECIAL NEEDS OF CHILDREN IN HOSPITALS

Hospital services, including occupational therapy, must take into consideration the child's developmental level and needs, the impact of illness or injury and hospitalization on development, and the coping strategies and needs of the family in relation to the child's medical condition. Hospitalized children are placed in a situation filled with unknowns and events over which they have little control (Gohsman, 1981). Sources of stress for the child include separation from family and the home environment, the unfamiliarity of the hospital, the increased dependency that often is associated with illness or injury and hospitalization, the unfamiliar and frequently changing hospital caregivers, and the often painful medical procedures that may be required.

Realization of potential disability or disfigurement and boredom may also add to the child's stress. The child may experience anxiety, withdrawal, regression, increased demand for parental attention, and a need for behavioral management (Knudson-Cooper, 1982; Suhr, 1986). For very young children, this is complicated by their limited ability to understand the purpose or need for the hospitalization and the anxiety produced by separation from parents or other caregivers (Wilson & Broome, 1989).

The fears provoked by hospitalization may be exacerbated by a diminished ability to cope (Gohsman, 1981). Consequently, the illness or injury and the stress of hospitalization may result in developmental regression, or it may hinder developmental progress. Petrillo and Sanger (1980) suggested that the child's successful adaptation to the overwhelming stresses of illness and hospitalization relates to his or her ability to achieve a sense of mastery over the situation.

The occupational therapist's knowledge of age-appropriate developmental tasks and understanding of the importance of purposeful activity can help the child achieve a sense of control in the foreign environment of the hospital. The occupational therapist can also help other members of the medical team understand the developmental issues of concern and suggest strategies to caregivers and family members that support normal development and help the child better cope with hospitalization.

■ CHARACTERISTICS OF HOSPITAL-BASED OCCUPATIONAL THERAPY

Many of the evaluation and treatment strategies used by occupational therapists are not unique to hospital-based practice. Instead, they tend to be the same approaches used with children in other settings. However, the diagnoses seen in hospitals challenge the occupational therapist to adapt intervention to meet specific, often acute, needs.

Examples of diagnoses and problems referred to occupational therapy include developmental delay, feeding disorders, orthopedic disorders, traumatic brain injury, or other neurologic problems, such as burns, cancer, renal disease, cardiac defects, and endocrine disorders. The occupational therapist must have a thorough understanding of the diagnosis, prognosis, contraindications, and other implications of the child's illness, injury, or medical treatment.

For most children, services are provided in a relatively brief period, requiring the occupational therapist to be highly efficient. This brief treatment requires the therapist to establish realistic treatment priorities appropriate for the patient's projected length of stay in the hospital (Freda, 1998). To do this, the evaluation process must be streamlined, and occupational therapists must prioritize treatment goals as they are identified. When possible discharge plans are articulated as part of the initial evaluation (Freda, 1998). Rausch and Melvin (1986) suggested, "A target skill for the acute-care therapist is the ability to integrate evaluation, treatment, and patient instruction into each therapy session" (p. 321).

In a children's hospital, the broad range of diagnoses requires that occupational therapists have expertise in a wide range of assessment, modalities, and interventions. However, the need for a broad range of skills does not mean a lack of specialization. "Occupational therapy services tend to be highly specialized in a pediatric facility and well-developed in specialty areas (e.g., neonatal care, upper-extremity anomalies, and burns)" (Case-Smith & Wavrek, 1998, p. 84).

Occupational therapy services for the hospitalized child vary according to the type of facility, the child's diagnosis, and the length of stay. For a child with a short or acute stay, the emphasis of occupational therapy tends to be on assessment, with program planning, recommenda-

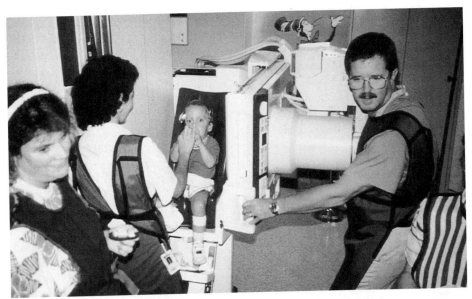

figure26-1 An interdisciplinary team uses videofluoroscopy to assess a patient's swallowing and risk for aspiration.

tions for follow-up after discharge, and equipment provision or fabrication occurring as needed.

A child hospitalized for a long time may have the benefit of receiving occupational therapy services one or two times daily, depending on the child's needs. A longer stay also provides the occupational therapist with more opportunities to interact with the family, provide parent education, and plan for discharge cooperatively with the family and other team members. Children with extended acute phases of illness or injury (e.g., those with burns, traumatic brain injury, or encephalitis), often require different and more comprehensive services than chronically ill children (e.g., those with cancer, cystic fibrosis, or diabetes) who are hospitalized frequently for exacerbations of their illness.

In some instances, services for children with acute illness or injury may be limited to provision of a piece of adaptive equipment, such as a protective helmet for a patient with neurosurgical needs or a stretcher for a patient in traction who has a fracture of the lower extremity. For patients with chronic conditions who receive occupational therapy in the community, occupational therapy services in the hospital may focus on provision of equipment or completion of evaluations that are not readily available to the occupational therapist in the community.

For example, a child with a severe developmental disability who is hospitalized with pneumonia resulting from the aspiration of food might be referred to the hospital radiology, occupational therapy, and speech pathology departments for an evaluation of feeding. This evaluation would include a videofluoroscopic swallowing

study (Figure 26-1). In situations of this type, close communication between the hospital- and community-based occupational therapists is essential and can result in better total care for the child and family.

■ SCOPE OF OCCUPATIONAL THERAPY SERVICES

Rausch and Melvin (1986) identified four types of illness or injury that require acute care from occupational therapy departments in hospitals:

1. Single injury
2. Acute illness or injury requiring extended rehabilitation
3. Chronic illness requiring periodical hospitalization for acute episodes of illness or for complications of an illness
4. Illness requiring hospitalization for diagnostic testing or adjustment of medications

In each case, occupational therapy intervention may differ according to the patient's needs and the length of stay. In some instances, level of service may be affected by staff shortages, which result in prioritizing which patients receive occupational therapy services (Rausch & Melvin, 1986).

The patient with a single injury (e.g., a hand injury) or a single episode of illness tends to have a short hospital stay with a predictable course of treatment. Patients with an acute illness or injury require extended rehabilitation. Traumatic brain injury and spinal cord injury are two examples of injuries that require both initial acute treat-

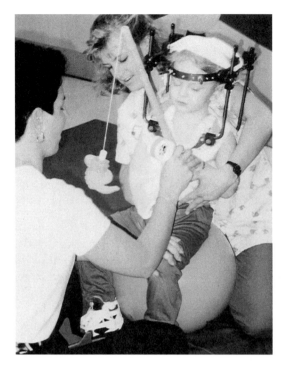

figure26-2   An occupational therapist and physical therapist collaborate on a patient evaluation.

ment and long-term rehabilitation. The length of the hospital stay for this type of patient during the acute phase of illness or injury tends to vary, because the potential for complications is greater.

The chronically ill patient is hospitalized periodically for acute episodes of an illness or complications of an illness. Children with diabetes, cancer, or cardiac conditions fall into this category. The length of hospital stay for these patients is also variable. Children hospitalized for diagnostic testing or adjustment of medications can expect a comparatively short hospital stay.

Occupational therapy evaluation in acute-care services focuses on the child's developmental or functional status within the context of the illness or injury that has resulted in hospitalization. Completion of the assessment may present a challenge for the occupational therapist, because the length of hospital stay is often short and other hospital services are competing for the patient's time.

Evaluation may begin with a chart review to obtain information about the child's medical status, the current course of medical care and goals, contraindications or precautions that may have an impact on the occupational therapy services provided, and the patient's functional level before the hospitalization. Information concerning family structure, birth history, and the child's past developmental course may also contribute to the occupational therapist's understanding of the child and family's needs.

An interview with the parents, if possible, is often the source of valuable information regarding the child's current status and the parents' goals for the child.

Before completing a functional or developmental evaluation, the occupational therapist establishes a rapport with the child and family. Increasing the comfort level of the child and family is particularly important because of the stressful and frightening nature of the hospital environment. A positive relationship between the child and therapist serves to foster cooperation, decrease the child's anxiety about the evaluation process, and enable the therapist to obtain results that reflect the child's actual functional abilities.

The choice of evaluation tools and methods depends on the child's age and needs and the protocol of the occupational therapy department. For example, a 10-year-old child with a serious hand injury might be referred for evaluation of strength, sensation, fine coordination, passive and active range of motion, independence in self-care, and the need for a splint to assist function or prevent deformity. By contrast, a 2-year-old child referred for developmental delay (secondary to chronic illness) may receive a developmental assessment that includes administration of a standardized test, such as the Bayley Scales of Infant Development, revised (BSID-II), and evaluation of sensorimotor function (e.g., muscle tone, automatic postural responses, or sensory processing), self-care, and play skills.

An evaluation of this type is often performed in collaboration or cooperation with professionals from other disciplines, such as physical therapy and speech pathology (Figure 26-2). In both instances, the occupational therapist is concerned with occupational performance areas, components, and contexts in relation to the child's age and development.

In some cases, the child's medical condition, a short length of stay, or a stressful and restrictive environment (e.g., an ICU), may prohibit the administration of a standardized evaluation. In these instances, the therapist's clinical observations of key performance areas and components may be the best alternative (Figure 26-3).

Finally, assessment in acute care also includes evaluation of the need for specialized equipment, both for use in the hospital and for use after discharge. Specialized equipment may include adapted utensils for self-feeding for a patient with a spinal cord injury, an adapted bath seat for a patient with cerebral palsy, a pressure garment to prevent hypertrophic scarring for a patient with burn injuries, a protective helmet for a patient with a skull fracture, or splints for a patient with juvenile rheumatoid arthritis. In some instances, the therapist and child may need to experiment with different pieces of equipment to determine which is best for the child's use.

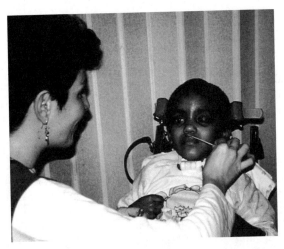

figure**26-3** An occupational therapist evaluates oral-motor skills before feeding a patient.

■ INTENSIVE CARE UNIT SERVICES

Occupational therapy services may be initiated with a patient at any point during the course of hospitalization. However, they usually occur once a patient has achieved sufficient medical stability to initiate rehabilitation. In the intensive care unit, the child is often evaluated and treated at bedside, because of the critical nature of the illness or injury and the need for constant monitoring of the child's medical status.

Occupational therapy intervention in intensive care supports the medical team's priorities and goals for the child. It is also essential that the therapist be knowledgeable about the child's diagnosis and the implications of medical procedures, the use of life-support or monitoring equipment, and contraindications for certain activities or positions. Constant monitoring of the child's status is also the responsibility of the occupational therapist during the time he or she is with the patient, making it imperative for the therapist to understand the significance of changes in the patient's vital signs, respiratory function, appearance, or symptoms.

Affleck, Lieberman, Polon, and Rohrkemper (1986) identified three problems related to the intensive care environment and child's status that affect both the child and intervention. These are (1) *immobility and the need for bed rest,* (2) *sensory deprivation and stress,* and (3) *extended mechanical ventilation.*

Prolonged bed rest and immobility often occur as a result of the critical nature of the illness, the use of high-technology equipment, or the need for restraints for the child's safety and care. The average length of stay for a child in the ICU is 4 to 6 days. However, it may be extended if the illness or injury is severe. The potential impact of extended immobility includes decreased endurance, generalized weakness, and poor tolerance for sitting. As part of an occupational therapy program, graded activities are presented and the child's participation is solicited to improve endurance and strength and to enhance functional performance.

Elements of activities that can be graded include time required to complete the task, amount and speed of active movement, level of assistance given, adaptive aids, and position and postural support. The most important parameter in grading a task is a patient's physiological response. The patient's level of activity can be upgraded only when vital signs, symptoms, and respiratory function are acceptable at the existing level of activity (Affleck et. al., 1986, p. 324).

In addition to a program of graded activity, occupational therapy intervention may include positioning recommendations or splints to preserve range of motion and prevent deformity, and specialized equipment to facilitate function.

Sensory deprivation and stress resulting from the intensive care environment may also complicate a child's illness and recovery. The lack of privacy, immobility, and the continuous sounds and lights of the intensive care unit provide the child with an atypical sensory experience. In addition, there are few indicators to orient the child to changes in time and day. Occupational therapy intervention may help counteract the effects of stress and sensory deprivation by fostering the establishment of a routine for the child and providing purposeful activities to facilitate cognitive, psychosocial, and motor functions (Affleck et. al., 1986). Positive social interaction and the use of entertainment and play activities may be especially helpful for reducing stress and promoting development of young children in the ICU.

To summarize, the occupational therapist providing services in the ICU must have a thorough understanding of the patient's condition, the purpose of intensive care, the medical priorities for the patient, and the importance of monitoring the patient's physiologic status before, during, and after occupational therapy. Two important emphases for the occupational therapist working with children in intensive care are (1) provision of graded, meaningful activities (e.g., play activities, self-care activities) to improve endurance, strength, and functional abilities (e.g., cognition, psychosocial function, and motor abilities); and (2) provision of specialized equipment, splints, and positioning recommendations as needed (Figure 26-4).

■ BURN UNIT

One of the specialty ICUs found in larger hospitals is the *burn unit.* The cause of the burn injury, the depth of the burn (e.g., partial to full thickness), the percentage of total body surface area (TBSA) affected, the location of

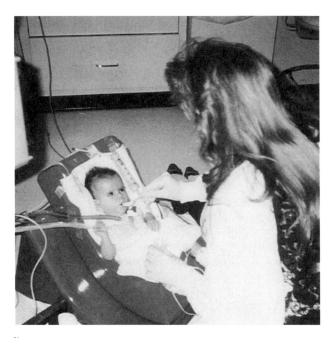

figure**26-4**   An occupational therapist assesses oral motor and feeding abilities in a patient requiring ventilator assistance for respiration.

the burn, and the age of the patient are factors considered in classifying a burn according to severity. Medical treatment for burns varies according to the severity. However, in general, burn wounds are treated with a local application of an antibacterial agent and, if needed, surgery to remove burned tissue and cover the affected area with skin grafts (Rivers & Jordan, 1998).

Parenteral hyperalimentation is often administered to maintain adequate nutrition during the early recovery periods. Major burns result in a 40% to 100% increase in energy expenditure, and good nutrition is essential for healing (Murphy, Purdue, Hunt, & Hicks, 1997). The long, often painful recovery process and the potential for lasting disfigurement and disability challenge the child and family's coping skills. For these reasons, occupational therapy with the burned child presents a special challenge.

Rivers and Jordan (1998) described three stages in the burn-injury recovery process: (1) the acute-care stage, (2) the surgical and postoperative stage, and (3) the rehabilitation stage.

The medical focus of the acute-care stage is the replacement of lost body fluids, stabilization of the patient, and care of the burn wounds. Daily wound débridement and dressing changes are needed. Occupational therapy intervention during this phase may include prevention of the loss of joint mobility, strength, and endurance; self-care activities; and education of the child and family regarding the rehabilitation process (Rivers & Jordan, 1998).

Surgical removal of burned tissue, skin grafts, and postoperative recovery characterize the surgical and post-

operative stage. Immobilization of the affected area through positioning or splints is required for approximately 3 to 7 days after surgery. In addition to the fabrication of splints and provision of positioning recommendations, serial splint placement may be used to gradually increase range of motion. The occupational therapist may provide adaptive devices to assist with self-care or other activities.

During the rehabilitation stage, wound healing continues. The patient is susceptible to scarring and contracture formation during this period. Although the rehabilitation phase begins during hospitalization, it often continues after discharge on an outpatient basis and through home programs until the patient's scars are mature. This process may take up to 2 years. Scarring, especially hypertrophic scaring, can significantly interfere with a patient's functional recovery. Hypertrophic scars tend to be thick, inflexible, and red. If they cross joints, these scars can impair joint mobility because of shortening of the skin.

Elastic wraps (e.g., Jobst™ garments), tailor-made to conform to the child's body, decrease the formation of hypertrophic scarring. Constant pressure through these Jobst™ garments, elastomer inserts, and facial masks is applied 24 hours a day for 6 to 24 months to obtain an optimal cosmetic result (Murphy et. al., 1997).

Occupational therapists contribute to the following desired outcomes:

1. Enable the child to return to his or her prior level of independence in school and the community

2. Return the child to developmentally appropriate levels of play and daily living skills

3. Assist in the prevention of deformity, contracture, and hypertrophic scar formation

4. Maintain full active range of motion, strength, functional coordination, and developmental skills

5. Support and, when needed, improve the child's emotional well-being

The following case study illustrates the complexity of intervention with a child admitted to the burn unit of a hospital:

Case Study: Intervention for Child with Burn Injuries
Presenting information

Sabrina is a 4-year-old white girl who presented with burn injuries to 60% to 70% TBSA. The burns were sustained during a house fire in which her mother and younger brother died. Sabrina's maternal grandmother and 6-year-old sister survived with no injuries. A cigarette was believed to be the cause of the fire. Sabrina received second- and third-degree burns to all areas of her body, including her face, head, hands, trunk, arms, anterior knees, and the dorsum of the feet and toes. She was referred to occupational therapy by the burn surgeon for splinting and therapeutic intervention.

Background information

Sabrina was a healthy child with no disabilities before the house fire. She resided with her mother, maternal grandmother, sister, and brother, and she attended a Head Start preschool class.

Occupational therapy and medical intervention

The burn team, consisting of the physician, occupational therapist, physical therapist, nurses, social worker, psychologist, dietitian, and child life specialist, was consulted. Initial occupational therapy involvement began when Sabrina was admitted to the ICU and focused on providing splints and guidelines for positioning.

The primary occupational therapy goal at that time was to prevent the development of contractures and deformities during burn-wound healing. The shoulders were abducted at 90 degrees using pillows or stockinette slings tied to the head of the bed. Foot drop splints were fabricated to maintain 90 degrees of ankle dorsiflexion while the patient was confined to bed and prevent hyperextension of toes. Resting hand splints were also fabricated, placing the hands in a safe position to protect damaged extensor tendons and ligaments and to provide 90 degrees of metacarpophalangeal flexion. Once Sabrina was medically stable and transferred to the Burn Unit, the occupational therapist provided daily active range-of-motion exercises to improve upper-body mobility and range of motion. Bilateral airplane splints that hold the arm in 90 degrees of shoulder abduction were fabricated for shoulder positioning, and facial expression exercises were initiated. A figure 8 clavicle strap was used for retraction of shoulders and chest. Ongoing evaluation of joint mobility and the functional limitations related to decreased joint mobility occurred throughout Sabrina's hospitalization.

The therapist used lotion to massage Sabrina's scars, particularly those on her face, one to two times per day. Stacked tongue blades were used for vertical expansion exercises to the mouth for 5 minutes before each meal. Commissure expansion was not indicated because of the location of Sabrina's burns. Pressure garments were provided for early scar management, which included elastic wrap bandages, Coban wrapping (3M Corporation, Medical-Surgical Division, St. Paul, MN) to the hands, elastinet stockings (Jobst Company, Toledo, OH), and prefabricated pressure garments. A polyform face mask with a silicone mold was fabricated to provide pressure on healed areas of her face.

Initially Sabrina required a Velcro strap on her feeding utensils. Later she became independent in self-feeding, using a large-handled spoon and fork. These adapted

utensils were not required for feeding at the time of her discharge from the hospital. She did continue to require moderate assistance in dressing and bathing. The occupational therapist provided several simple aids to improve her independence in dressing and bathing at home. The therapist also recommended types of clothing that were easy to put on and were comfortable.

In other performance areas, Sabrina quickly returned to her previous level of function. She used playground equipment with supervision, including her tricycle and scooter board. Although certain toys were difficult for her to manipulate, she played with her favorite toys without assistance. Custom pressure garments were ordered once sufficient healing had occurred, approximately 2 months post-burn. Several surgeries followed, including scar excision and skin grafting to the hands, axillae, anterior chest, and face (Figure 26-5).

Sabrina was discharged to her father's and stepmother's home, where her sister also resided. She began attending kindergarten after a school reentry program in which two members of the burn team visited the school and educated her classmates about burns, splints, and pressure garments, especially as they related to Sabrina's injuries.

After hospital discharge, Sabrina was treated by the occupational therapist on an outpatient basis three to five times per week, with additional therapy provided through a community agency near her home until she could easily achieve normal active range of movement. Sabrina continued to be measured and fitted with new pressure garments every 2 to 3 months because of

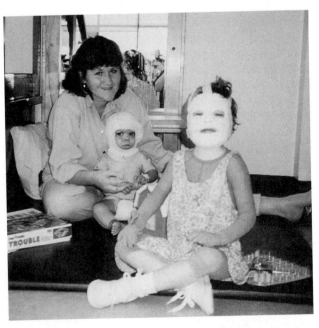

figure**26-5** Face masks and custom-fabricated pressure garments assist in scar management for children with severe burns.

growth or wear. A clear face mask was used for scar management of the face. All pressure garments were worn 23 hours a day and were expected to be worn for up to 18 months. Sabrina continued to be followed every 2 to 3 months to monitor joint mobility and to assess pressure garment needs and effectiveness.

As is evident in this case study, the preservation of joint mobility, prevention of deformity, management of scar tissue, and promotion of independence in self-care were major occupational therapy emphases in the treatment of Sabrina. The school reentry program was designed not only to educate Sabrina's classmates about burns, but also to help them become more comfortable with her disfigurement and special equipment, thus making the transition easier for Sabrina as she returned to the community.

■ BONE MARROW TRANSPLANT UNIT

Another type of highly specialized acute-care service is the *bone marrow transplant unit*. Bone marrow transplants are used as part of a medical treatment protocol for a number of life-threatening childhood illnesses, including leukemia, aplastic anemia, immunodeficiency syndromes, and tumors (Furman & Feldman, 1990; Williams, 1990; Williams & Safarimaryaki, 1990).

Transplant Procedure, Sequela, and Intervention

The procedure for bone marrow transplant involves chemotherapy, radiation, or both before the transplant. This is followed by intravenous infusion of the bone marrow taken from a compatible donor or from the patient before the pretransplant regimen of chemotherapy and radiation. The intense chemotherapy or radiation before the transplant, and the underlying disease processes, cause severe immunosuppression in patients, making them highly susceptible to life-threatening infections until the new bone marrow is established and the patient's immunohematopoietic system is once again functioning effectively (Lenarsky, 1990; Zander & Aksamit, 1990).

The *immunologic compromise* that occurs requires that the bone marrow transplant and resultant hospitalization occur in an environment designed to greatly reduce the risk of infection. The type of environment may vary among hospitals. However, common strategies to protect bone marrow transplant patients include room isolation, reverse isolation, and laminar airflow in a clean or sterile environment (Lenarsky, 1990).

Another issue of concern is the *psychosocial stress* for the patient and family. Sources of stress include the child's life-threatening illness; the risks of bone marrow

transplantation; the painful, or uncomfortable, medical procedures and extended period of isolation that the child must endure; and concern about the cost of the treatment. In addition, the transplant may occur at a hospital distant from the family's home, creating an additional burden for family members (Williams, 1990).

The many complex needs of the patient and family emphasize the importance of a collaborative team approach. The physician, nurses, occupational therapist, physical therapist, pharmacist, clinical social worker, psychologist, dietitian, chaplain, child life specialist, and a hospital-based teacher may all serve as members of a team caring for the bone marrow transplant patient and the patient's family (Spruce, 1990).

Intervention may include a pretransplant assessment of the child's development and functional abilities, as well as identification of limitations or problems caused by the underlying disease process. After the transplant, the occupational therapist's goals may be to (1) *promote normal development and age-appropriate functional skills*, (2) *enhance coping skills*, and (3) *assess for needs after discharge*.

When a child has a tumor that does not involve the bone marrow, the bone marrow transplant may be used in conjunction with large doses of chemotherapy or radiation to reduce or eradicate the tumor. The toxicity of large doses of chemotherapy and radiation has the potential to inhibit the normal functions of the patient's bone marrow, resulting in a need for a bone marrow transplant. For this purpose, some of the child's own bone marrow is removed before high-dose chemotherapy, and it is reinfused later (Williams & Safarimaryaki, 1990).

The following case study illustrates the complexity of intervention with a child who has just received a bone marrow transplant.

Case Study: Intervention for Child with Bone Marrow Transplant
Presenting information

Katie was an 8-year-old girl who had a brain tumor. After bone marrow transplantation, her oncologist referred Katie for occupational therapy. The oncologist noted that Katie exhibited decreased strength in her left arm, and that she had difficulty with fine-motor skills.

Background information

Katie resided with her mother and older sister. Although her parents are separated, her father visited regularly. Katie attended a regular public school class before her illness and transplant. Medical history included a craniotomy and excision of a right thalamic glioma, chemotherapy and radiation, placement of a broviac catheter, placement of a right ventricular-perineal shunt secondary to hydrocephalus, a history of pneumonia, and an episode of generalized tonic clonic seizures that remained under control with medication.

Medical and occupational therapy intervention

After diagnosis and initial medical and surgical intervention for the tumor, the family and oncologist determined that chemotherapy followed by a bone marrow transplant was the most desirable course of treatment. Katie's own bone marrow was excised and harvested before her admission to the hospital. After admission, she received large doses of chemotherapy, followed by reinfusion of her previously harvested bone marrow. Katie was placed in strict isolation, progressing to modified isolation as her condition improved.

Occupational therapy was provided as part of a collaborative team approach led by the physician. The team included physical therapy, dietetics, dentistry, clinical social work, child life, and other medical specialists (e.g., neurosurgeon). Daily team meetings were open to all disciplines.

Occupational therapy assessment focused on evaluation of Katie's self-care and fine-motor skills. The fine-motor evaluation included manual muscle testing, the nine-hole peg test, eye-hand coordination, in-hand manipulation skills, and clinical observations of the quality of movement and of endurance. Self-care was evaluated through an interview with her mother and observation of dressing and feeding. Her mother indicated that she was concerned about the impaired movement of Katie's left arm and hand. She was also concerned about Katie's general strength and endurance.

The fine-motor evaluation results showed full, active range of motion of the right arm, but limitations in end ranges of her left arm. Strength of her right arm was within normal limits, but was decreased in her left arm. Left-side neglect was noted. In the area of fine-motor skills, Katie demonstrated decreased coordination and in-hand manipulation in the right hand. Her left hand was significantly impaired, with decreased accuracy in gross reach-and-grasp and an inability to pick up or manipulate small objects. Katie used her left hand primarily as an assist. Her general endurance and tolerance for activity varied and ranged from an inability to sit independently to being able to get out of bed and move to sit in a chair with minimal assistance.

Based on her mother's report and clinical observation, Katie required moderate assistance with all self-care activities. Occupational therapy focused on self-care independence and age-appropriate play skills. The performance components initially emphasized improved sitting tolerance while engaged in activity, improved left arm function in bilateral tasks, and improved strength and coordination.

Because of isolation requirements, services were provided in Katie's room. Treatment equipment was limited to those items that met the criteria for prevention of infection. In addition to medical and nursing care, Katie also received services from other members of the hospital team. Physical therapy intervention was provided for strength, endurance, and gait. The dietitian was concerned with caloric needs and nutritional status. The clinical social worker assessed family dynamics and reactions to Katie's illness, provided supportive intervention, and assisted the family with financial issues.

Dentistry was concerned with the condition of Katie's teeth, mouth, and gums, because dental problems could be a source of infection. The child life specialist provided activities to assist Katie with her psychosocial adjustment to hospitalization and to help her cope with the stresses of hospitalization. Physicians from other medical specialties were involved as needed for specific problems.

After discharge, Katie returned to her mother's home, where she received home-based education services as a precaution against exposure to infections. She continued to receive occupational therapy in the bone marrow transplant day treatment program at the hospital.

In this case, the occupational therapist's role focused on arm and hand strength and on coordination, general strength, and endurance, as these variables affected functional performance. The provision of Katie's occupational therapy influenced environmental constraints designed to protect her from infection. Cooperative efforts by team members enabled services to be provided in a manner that offered Katie the greatest benefit from the individual disciplines.

■ GENERAL ACUTE-CARE UNIT

General acute-care units tend to be designated by medical specialty. For example, patients of various ages, with different types of orthopedic conditions and treatment, may be served on the same acute-care unit. Similarly, patients requiring different types of surgery may be admitted to the same general surgical unit for preoperative and postoperative care. Designating units in this manner enables physicians and other members of the medical team to use their patient-care time and equipment more efficiently. This system of designation also results in increased opportunities for formal and informal communication between team members regarding each child's care.

General acute-care units differ from ICUs in several ways. Patients tend to be more medically stable and less dependent on life-sustaining equipment as part of their medical treatment. The less serious nature of their medical conditions may enable them to receive greater benefit from occupational therapy and permit them to leave the unit for occupational therapy or other services (although services may be provided at bedside, if necessary).

Occupational therapists may be responsible for patients on one or more acute-care units, requiring them to be familiar with the procedures of each unit, the types of patients admitted to the different units, and the nurses and other hospital personnel who provide services. Patients admitted directly to an acute-care unit of this type also tend to have a shorter hospital stay than those who progress from ICU to another type of unit. Consequently, the occupational therapist often has less opportunity to develop a relationship with both the patient and family.

■ FAILURE TO THRIVE

Failure to Thrive (FTT) is a diagnosis given to children, frequently infants and young children, who fail to grow or gain weight. FTT may be designated as *organic*, arising from a diagnosable physical cause, or as *nonorganic*, which denotes impaired growth without apparent physical cause (Frank, 1985). Children with FTT often require hospitalization for acute care.

Although organic FTT can be attributed to a specific physical disorder, nonorganic FTT is primarily (but not exclusively) associated with psychosocial factors. Disturbances in parent-child interaction and development of attachment early in life, difficult infant temperament and behavior, maternal social isolation, and financial difficulties within the family are some of the variables associated with nonorganic FTT (Bithoney & Newberger, 1987; Drotar, 1985).

In some instances, FTT may be attributed to both organic and nonorganic factors. Frank (1985) suggested that children with nonorganic FTT may still have biologic risks. She identified three categories of risk: (1) *perinatal*, (2) *toxic and immunologic*, and (3) *neurodevelopmental*.

Perinatal risk refers to the potential for FTT in infants who are considered low birth weight, possibly as a result of prematurity or intrauterine growth retardation. Toxic and immunologic risks arise from significant nutritional deficiency, which has the potential to increase vulnerability to infection and increase susceptibility to lead toxicity. Neurodevelopmental risk results from effects of inadequate nutrition on the developing nervous system. Although toxic and immunologic risks are generally reversible through medical treatment, treatment may not fully reverse the neurodevelopmental consequences.

The complexity of factors implicated in FTT emphasizes the need for a coordinated team approach that offers medical, nutritional, developmental, and psychosocial intervention. As a member of the hospital-based team, the occupational therapist may contribute to both the diagnosis and treatment of the child with FTT. A comprehensive occupational therapy assessment provides the medical team with information regarding the infant's developmental status, feeding behaviors, infant-caregiver interactions during play and feeding, and infant interac-

tions with nonfamily members (e.g., the occupational therapist).

Denton (1986) differentiated between FTT in infants and children around 2 years of age, suggesting that 2-year-old children who fail to thrive present with poor feeding skills that may be the result of behavioral issues. Infant assessment emphasizes interactional issues with the caregivers, while the assessment of older children focuses more on behaviors in the feeding situation and attempts to differentiate between environmental factors and neuromotor difficulties that may be affecting feeding. A developmental and feeding history obtained from the parent is a valuable component of the occupational therapy assessment of all children with FTT.

Occupational therapy intervention goals with a child who fails to thrive may include improving oral-motor and feeding skills and facilitating development. Promoting positive parent-child interaction may also be emphasized, using strategies that help the parent understand infant behavioral cues and engage the child in positive, developmentally appropriate play experiences. This emphasis on positive parent-child interaction also encourages parents to develop behavioral expectations consistent with the child's level of functioning.

The following case study illustrates the complexity of intervention with a child with FTT:

Case Study: Intervention for Child with FTT
Presenting information

Kevin was a 3-month, 7-day-old boy transferred from a community hospital to a regional children's hospital by helicopter after suffering a seizure. He was intubated en route. Initial diagnoses included rule-out abuse, severe nonorganic FTT, anemia, rule-out sepsis and bacteremia, hyponatremia, dehydration, and seizure.

On examination, Kevin was noted to have bruising above both knees and over his right buttocks. He was also observed to have diaper rash and wasting of the left hip and extremities. Because he demonstrated poor oral feeding, the PICU attending physician referred Kevin to occupational therapy on the third day of hospitalization.

Background information

Kevin's parents brought him to the referring hospital's emergency room after a home visit by a Child Protective Services worker. He was left at the emergency room, and his parents did not visit during his 14-day hospitalization at the children's hospital. His maternal great aunt visited occasionally, and she expressed interest in adopting him.

Kevin was born at term weighing 5 pounds 12 ounces. He went home after a 48-hour hospital stay. He was hospitalized at 2 months of age for FTT, upper respiratory tract infection, and otitis media. He was discharged to his parents with home health nursing, a Child Protective Services referral, and pediatrician follow-up. Kevin's parents missed all follow-up appointments until they brought him to the emergency room.

Medical and occupational therapy intervention

A pH probe showed severe gastroesophageal reflux. An upper gastrointestinal series was performed and ruled out anatomic abnormality. Stool samples were analyzed and showed malabsorption, reducing substances, increased fatty acids, and *Giardia Lamblia,* all of which combined to reduce his level of nutrient absorption and increase fluid loss. As a result, Kevin was severely underweight and lethargic. Medical treatment for the reflux included positioning on an elevated wedge, thickened feeds, and medications.

Kevin was evaluated by occupational therapy using clinical observations for his oral-motor, feeding, and developmental skills. The Infant Neurological International Battery (INFANIB) was used to assess his reflexes, muscle tone, and posture. He demonstrated intact oral structures and sensation, with functional oral skills for safe oral feeding. He had small sucking pads with a weak suck and fair coordination of suck-swallow-breathe. His suck and coordination improved with support at his jaw and cheeks. Kevin's developmental skills were delayed, and he demonstrated poor state control with high irritability.

His score on the INFANIB indicated transient muscle tone, which is not uncommon for his age. It was the therapist's impression that Kevin's weak suck, poor feeding, and irritability were from overall weakness, malnutrition, and recent intubation, rather than from a neurologic deficit.

The occupational therapist developed a bedside plan of specific facilitation techniques to be used during feeding. These included jaw and cheek support, external tongue stimulation, flexion swaddling, decreasing external stimulation, upright and well-aligned feeding positioning, limiting oral feeding to 30 minutes, and turning off the continuous pump, feeding Kevin through a nasal gastric tube.

After implementation of occupational therapy recommendations by nursing staff, Kevin's oral intake increased dramatically over the next 3 days, with the occupational therapist feeding him once daily to monitor progress. Once the acute feeding issues were resolved, occupational therapy emphasis switched to psychosocial skills, with focus on developmental activities to improve self-calming, visual tracking, and social interactions.

Kevin was referred for outpatient occupational therapy and early intervention services before discharge. Children's Protective Services assumed custody of Kevin,

and he was discharged to a foster home with a weight increase of 2.4 lbs (follow-up weekly weight checks were scheduled with his pediatrician). The occupational therapist provided the foster parents with a home program, including positioning, feeding, and activities to promote Kevin's development.

■ OUTPATIENT SERVICES

Outpatient services are important components of the total spectrum of hospital care and may be provided at the hospital, at a hospital satellite center, or as part of an interdisciplinary hospital-based clinic (e.g., arthritis clinic, feeding clinic, or cerebral palsy clinic). Outpatient occupational therapy is generally provided for one of three purposes: (1) as part of a diagnostic assessment, (2) to provide needed intervention after hospital discharge, or (3) to provide occupational therapy intervention for individuals with disabilities or other chronic conditions (Figure 26-6).

In general, the referral base for outpatient services may extend beyond the hospital's medical staff. Patients may be referred for outpatient occupational therapy by their attending physicians in the hospital, by a community-based physician (e.g., pediatrician or family practitioner), or by a physician in a hospital-based specialty clinic. As with inpatient services, a referral from a physician determines the services to be provided.

Provision of inpatient occupational therapy services differs from provision of outpatient services in a number

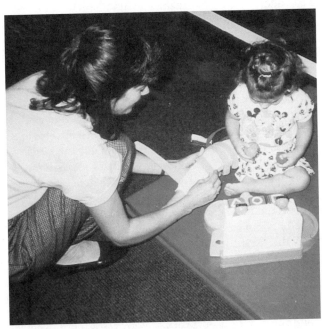

figure**26-6** An occupational therapist fabricates a splint for a young patient with juvenile rheumatoid arthritis.

of ways. Services are usually provided to outpatients less frequently (e.g., one to three times per week) and may continue for weeks or months. The longer duration provides a greater opportunity for the occupational therapist to get to know the child's family and develop a collaborative relationship. Also, children seen on an outpatient basis are essentially well, as opposed to children who are hospitalized for an acute or transient illness.

One disadvantage of outpatient therapy is the limited opportunity for collaboration and communication with other professionals who provide services to the child. In most cases the child served as an outpatient does not have a medical team with members who meet to discuss and coordinate services.

Outpatient services provided as part of an interdisciplinary medical clinic usually have a specific, well-defined purpose. In some instances the occupational therapist functions as a consultant, completing an assessment, then making recommendations to the physician. In other cases the occupational therapist is an integral part of the decision-making team and may be involved in patient assessment, treatment or equipment recommendations, or provision of splints and adaptive equipment.

One disadvantage is that children visit specialty medical clinics infrequently, one to two times a year. This limits the role of the occupational therapist in the clinic. However, children treated as patients in medical specialty clinics may also receive occupational therapy services separately, either at the hospital or in their home communities.

■ DOCUMENTATION OF OCCUPATIONAL THERAPY SERVICES

Documentation of patient care is an essential and time-consuming component of occupational therapy service provision in hospitals. Occupational therapy evaluation reports, treatment plans, patient progress notes, and discharge summaries are used to communicate occupational therapy intervention to the physician, other members of the medical team, the patient and family, and reimbursement agencies.

Format and frequency of documentation are determined by the policies and procedures of the hospital and occupational therapy department. Accreditation guidelines regarding documentation are provided to institutions by agencies such as the JCAHO and the CARF. Agencies that reimburse services, such as Medicaid or private insurance, also have requirements for documentation with which occupational therapists must comply.

Documentation of services to hospitalized patients through evaluation reports with accompanying treatment plans, progress notes, and discharge summaries occurs in the patient's medical chart. Because the medical chart remains on the unit or accompanies the patient when he or she receives services elsewhere in the hospital, information is readily available to other health professionals. Documentation of occupational therapy intervention with outpatients may take a different form, because reports are often sent to referring physicians or other agencies in the community. Copies of these outpatient reports are also retained in the patient's hospital medical record. Documentation of services in clinics may follow a different format because each clinic may have a medical chart for the patient. However, regardless of the format, documentation of services must meet the criteria established by accrediting and reimbursement agencies.

■ SUMMARY

The provision of occupational therapy services to children in hospitals is a specialized and challenging area of practice. Occupational therapists in hospitals must have a thorough understanding of the hospital's roles and characteristics in health care delivery, the numerous factors and trends that affect hospitals, and the specialized needs of hospitalized children. Occupational therapists who are employed in hospitals have the opportunity to gain expertise in assessment and treatment of children of various ages with many different diagnoses, within a dynamic, fast-paced environment. As hospitals broaden their range of services in response to a changing health care system, hospital-based occupational therapists will have opportunities to broaden their areas of expertise, apply different models of service delivery, and develop new practitioner roles.

STUDY QUESTIONS

1. Consider the child diagnosed as FTT. What occupational performance components and environmental contexts should be the focus of occupational therapy evaluation and intervention with this child?

2. List three roles of the occupational therapist with a child who has received severe burns. Give examples of occupational therapy activities at each phase of recovery (i.e., acute, surgical, and rehabilitation).

3. Describe the characteristics of occupational therapy services in a medical model. Compare these characteristics with those of occupational therapy in education settings (Chapters 23 and 24). What are advantages and disadvantages of each model of service delivery?

References

Abreu, B., Seale, G., Podlesak, J., & Hartley, L. (1996). Development of critical paths for postacute brain injury rehabilitation: Lessons learned. *American Journal of Occupational Therapy, 50,* 417-427.

Affleck, A.T., Lieberman, S., Polon, J., & Rohrkemper, K. (1986). Providing occupational therapy in an intensive care unit. *American Journal of Occupational Therapy, 40,* 323-332.

Bailey, D.M. (1998). Legislative and reimbursement influences on occupational therapy: Changing opportunities. In M.E. Neistadt & E.B. Crepeau (Eds.), *Willard & Spackman's occupational therapy* (9th ed.) (pp. 763-771). Philadelphia: Lippincott: Williams & Wilkins.

Bithoney, W.G., & Newberger, E.H. (1987). Child and family attributes of failure-to-thrive. *Developmental and Behavioral Pediatrics, 8,* 32-36.

Case-Smith, J., & Wavrek, B.B. (1998). Models of service delivery and team interaction. In J. Case-Smith (Ed.), *Pediatric occupational therapy and early intervention* (2nd ed. pp. 83-107). Boston: Butterworth-Heinemann.

Christiansen, C. (1996). Nationally speaking—managed care: Opportunities and challenges for occupational therapy in the emerging systems of the 21st century. *American Journal of Occupational Therapy, 50,* 409-416.

Commission for the Accreditation of Rehabilitation Facilities. (1994). *1994 CARF standards manual: An interpretive guideline for organizations serving people with disabilities.* Tucson: CARF.

Considine, W.H. (1994). Children's needs: A health care reform priority. *Hospital and Health Networks, 68,* 84.

Denton, R. (1986). An occupational therapy protocol for assessing infants and toddlers who fail to thrive. *American Journal of Occupational Therapy, 40,* 352-358.

DeWitt, P.K., Jansen, M.T., Ward, S.L., & Keens, T.G. (1993). Obstacles to discharge of ventilator-assisted children from the hospital to home. *Chest, 103,* 1560-1565.

Drotar, D. (1985). Failure to thrive and preventative mental health: Knowledge gaps and research needs. In D. Drotar (Ed.), *New directions in failure to thrive* (pp. 27-44). New York: Plenum Press.

Frank, D.A. (1985). Biologic risks in "nonorganic" failure to thrive: Diagnostic and therapeutic implications. In D. Drotar (Ed.), *New directions in failure to thrive* (pp. 17-26). New York: Plenum Press.

Freda, M. (1998). Facility-based practice settings. In M.E. Neistadt & E.B. Crepeau (Eds.), *Willard & Spackman's occupational therapy* (9th ed.). (pp. 803-809). Philadelphia: Lippincott: Williams & Wilkins.

Furman, W.L., & Feldman, S. (1990). Infectious complications. In F.L. Johnson & C. Pochedly (Eds.), *Bone marrow transplantation in children* (pp. 427-450). New York: Raven Press.

Gilkerson, L. (1990). Understanding institutional functional style: A resource for hospital and early intervention collaboration. *Infants and Young Children, 2,* 22-30.

Gilkerson, L., Gorski, P., & Panitz, P. (1990). Hospital-based intervention for preterm infants and their families. In S. Meisels & J. Shonkoff (Eds.), *Handbook of early childhood intervention* (pp. 445-468). Cambridge, MA: Cambridge University Press.

Gohsman, B. (1981). The hospitalized child and the need for mastery. *Issues in Comprehensive Pediatric Nursing, 5,* 67-76.

Joint Commission on the Accreditation of Health Care Organizations. (1994). *1995 comprehensive accreditation manual for hospitals.* Oakbrook Terrace, IL: JCAHO.

Knudson-Cooper, M. (1982). Emotional care of the hospitalized burned child. *Journal of Burn Care and Rehabilitation, 3,* 109-115.

Lenarsky, C. (1990). Technique of bone marrow transplantation. In F.L. Johnson & C. Pochedly (Eds.), *Bone marrow transplantation in children* (pp. 53-67). New York: Raven Press.

Levy, L.L. (1993). Occupational therapy's place in the health care system. In H.L. Hopkins & H.D. Smith (Eds.), *Willard and Spackman's occupational therapy* (pp. 357-372). Philadelphia: J.B. Lippincott.

Murphy, J.T., Purdue, G.F., Hunt, J.L., Hicks, B.A. (1997). In D.L. Levin & F.C. Morris (Eds.), *Essentials of pediatric intensive care* (2nd ed.). New York: Churchill Livingstone.

Occupational Exposure to Blood-Borne Pathogens, 56 Fed. Reg. 64175-64182 (1991).

Perinchief, J.M. (1998). Management of occupational therapy services. In M.E. Neistadt & E.B. Crepeau (Eds). *Willard & Spackman's occupational therapy* (9th ed. pp. 741-755). Philadelphia: Lippincott: Williams & Wilkins.

Petrillo, M., & Sanger, S. (1980). *Emotional care of hospitalized children.* Philadelphia: J.B. Lippincott.

Pontzer, K. (1994). Responding to managed care. *OT Week, 8,* 35-36.

Rausch, G., & Melvin, J.L. (1986). Nationally speaking: A new era in acute care. *American Journal of Occupational Therapy, 40,* 319-322.

Rivers, E.A., & Jordan, C.L. (1998). Skin system dysfunction: Burns. In M.E. Neistadt & E.B. Crepeau (Eds). *Willard & Spackman's occupational therapy* (9th ed. pp. 741-755). Philadephia: Lippincott Williams & Wilkins.

Spruce, W.E. (1990). Supportive care in bone marrow transplantation. In F.L. Johnson & C. Pochedly (Eds.), *Bone marrow transplantation in children* (pp. 69-86). New York: Raven Press.

Suhr, M.A. (1986). Trauma in pediatric populations. *Advances in Psychosomatic Medicine, 16,* 31-47.

Williams, T.E. (1990). Ethical and psychosocial issues in bone marrow transplantation in children. In F.L. Johnson & C. Pochedly (Eds.), *Bone marrow transplantation in children* (pp. 497-504). New York: Raven Press.

Williams, T.E., & Safarimaryaki, S. (1990). Bone marrow transplantation for treatment of solid tumors. In F.L. Johnson & C. Pochedly (Eds.), *Bone marrow transplantation in children* (pp. 221-242). New York: Raven Press.

Wilson, T., & Broome, M.E. (1989). Promoting the young child's development in the intensive care unit. *Heart & Lung, 18,* 274-281.

Zander, A.R., & Aksamit, I.A. (1990). Immune recovery following bone marrow transplantation. In F.L. Johnson & C. Pochedly (Eds.), *Bone marrow transplantation in children* (pp. 87-110). New York: Raven Press.

The author gratefully acknowledges the assistance of the following individuals in the completion of this chapter: Cynthia Iski, Teresa Canode, Pamela Carlson, Laura Farrel, Kimberly Lindsey, Elizabeth Loehr, and Heather Pritchard.

chapter **27**

Home-Based
Intervention

Jill Anderson
Joanne S. Schoelkopf

key terms

Home-based service
Medically fragile children
Family participation
Cultural sensitivity

■ CHAPTER OBJECTIVES

1. Describe the types of children and family circumstances that benefit from home-based services.
2. Explain the role of the occupational therapist in home-based services.
3. Identify differences between home-based and center-based intervention.
4. Define assets and limitations of occupational therapy evaluation and intervention in the home.
5. Identify examples of cultural values and differences to be respected and appreciated.
6. Describe issues in safety and universal precautions for home-based intervention.

In recent years, home-based intervention for infants and children with disabilities has expanded and proliferated (Kirk, 1997; Roberts, Akers, & Behl, 1991). Advances in medical care and a dramatic reduction of mortality rates for extremely premature and low–birth-weight infants have increased the number of children at risk for developmental disabilities (Kirk, 1997; Sandall, 1990). Prenatal detection of fetal problems and early surgical intervention has led to greater rates of survival among children with a variety of anomalies. Other advances in medi-

cal technology and life-sustaining equipment have also extended the life spans of seriously ill infants. In addition, multiple births associated with use of fertility drugs and in vitro fertilization have resulted in increased numbers of micro-premature infants, many of whom need some form of intervention service. Fortunately, the development of technology and support services over the past 20 years has made the home care of many of these children possible.

In addition to the increase in the number of infants who have or are at risk for disability, the types and nature of disabilities have changed. For example, the identified number of infants who sustained intrauterine exposure to illegal drugs (e.g., cocaine, crack) has increased. More infants in the drug-exposed population have been diagnosed as carriers of human immunodeficiency virus (HIV) (Parks, 1994; Russell & Free, 1991). Advanced neurosurgery and orthopedic interventions have enabled children with severe impairments to live, but often they can only do so with the help of life-support technology. This need for life support severely restricts the child's mobility outside the home, limiting community travel to essential, generally medically related, situations.

Occupational therapy is an integral part of home-based early intervention programs. School-aged children may continue to receive home-based occupational therapy if they have serious, chronic medical conditions (e.g., uncontrolled seizure disorders, depressed immune systems), are dependent on technology, or are acutely ill (Ahmann & Lipsi, 1991). Families may elect to supplement their children's school-based occupational therapy with private, home-based services because this form of service delivery allows greater flexibility in length and frequency of sessions and in intervention approaches.

Service delivery in the home environment appears to reduce the stress of frequent visits to a center-based program, particularly for large families and families with more than one disabled child. Home-based services also provide consistent, direct communication between parents and therapists, and may be preferred by families because they allow regular, one-on-one communication with service providers (Garbaciak, 1990).

■ NATURE OF HOME-BASED SERVICES

The Individuals with Disabilities Education Act (IDEA), Part C, provides incentives and guidance for states to develop comprehensive, multidisciplinary early intervention systems that serve developmentally delayed and at-risk infants. The original early intervention amendments (P.L. 99-457) indicated that parents were to be given choices regarding where services were to be provided. These choices included the home, which was recognized as the infant's natural environment for early development. The IDEA Amendments of 1997 (P.L. 105-17) also specify that early intervention services be provided in the infant's natural environments, which for an infant is the home. Services in the home support the social and emotional well-being of the young children and their families. The literature provides some evidence of the effectiveness of home-based services in facilitating a child's development and providing an opportunity for enhanced family decision making and parent empowerment (Raab, Davis & Trepanier, 1993; Ramey, Bryant, Sparling, & Wasik, 1984).

Initially, the costs associated with home-based services were paid directly by private clients or were reimbursed through private insurance companies. Recently the trend has shifted to public funding through Medicaid, school systems, and state-funded agencies. Home-based services may be provided by a combination of private practitioners, home health agencies, private nonprofit associations, private for-profit agencies, hospitals, schools, early intervention programs, medical personnel, and social service agencies. Competition for referrals among agencies providing home-based therapy has increased in many parts of the country.

In general, infants who are referred for home-based occupational therapy services have been identified as developmentally delayed or at risk for disability through an evaluation process. Children with specific medical diagnoses, those identified as at-risk because of birth complications, and those considered medically fragile are frequently referred for home-based services on discharge from a hospital. Many of these at-risk infants have respiratory, cardiac, and feeding problems and may be dependent on cardiac monitors and oxygen, suctioning, and feeding devices. Others have severe, uncontrolled seizure disorders that require monitoring of heart and breathing rates during the seizure and recovery period.

A family may choose home-based services when transportation to a center-based program is complicated by the need to carry medical equipment or the need for personnel to monitor the child's medical status (Del Vecchio, 1992). For example, the family of a 3-year-old child with severe seizure disorder, glaucoma, and significant developmental delay elected to continue home-based services even though the child was eligible for a center-based program. His mother was concerned that the bus ride, the lights, and the noise in the classroom might result in increased seizure activity. She also thought that it would be to the child's benefit to have therapy services at home to take advantage of his sleep and wake cycles. The home-based occupational therapist provided a program of graded sensory input that increased the child's level of alertness to his environment and decreased self-stimulatory behaviors. During the sensory activities, the child's responses were carefully monitored to prevent overstimulation or induction of seizures.

Children with acute medical conditions requiring chemotherapy, advanced surgery, or organ transplants are likely to be unable to attend school for a defined period. They often need occupational therapy to provide adaptive equipment and to develop techniques to maintain independence. A young girl who required a 3-month course of chemotherapy for leukemia received home-based occupational therapy. Because chemotherapy suppressed her immune system and significantly increased her risk of infection, the physician restricted her activity to the home during treatment. When home-based services are provided, it is important to communicate with hospital or school-based therapists to ensure continuity of care.

■ FAMILY PERSPECTIVES

For families of technology dependent children, home-based services offer many benefits and conveniences. However, the stresses on these families continue to be great. An understanding of the social, emotional, and financial impact of at-risk children on family resources is important for therapists providing home-based services.

When a child is homebound, usually at least one parent is also homebound. When children have unwieldy equipment that must be transported with them when leaving the home, travel (even within the community) requires too much effort. When this is the case, social isolation results, and the family may lose social ties held before the child's birth. Although the support of friends may be lost, the home may still bustle with the activities of professionals there to treat the child. Therefore parents may feel that they have lost their privacy while, at the same time, feeling socially isolated. When this happens, the home may lose its personal association with comfort, security, and privacy (Arras & Dubler, 1995). Therapists can show sensitivity to these issues by respecting the family's privacy and supporting the parent's need to escape the home to engage in social outings. Scheduling around the parents' opportunities to socialize with friends and blocking therapy times so that the parents also have time for privacy and family activities can be important to the family's ongoing mental health.

Therapists should also be aware of the emotional effects that around-the-clock nursing or caregiving duties have on parents. Although most children who are technology dependent have nursing care, parents express that they always have an ongoing, underlying anxiety about the child's well-being and feel that they are always "on duty." Often parents become sleep deprived, which can feed into depression. When parents provide nursing care in addition to parenting, they often feel role confusion. This is because nursing procedures can be painful or uncomfortable for children, which provokes feelings of anxiety and conflict with natural parental desires to nurture and give comfort (Kirk, 1997).

Parental emotional stress may relate to long-term responsibility, the invasion of the home by professionals, and the overall financial difficulties related to the child's ongoing medical expenses. When therapists are aware of these emotional stresses, they can respond with sensitivity, take time to listen, and provide therapy activities that prioritize the parents' needs.

■ ROLE OF THE OCCUPATIONAL THERAPIST

Occupational therapy in the home-based setting encompasses direct services, consultation services, and service coordination. The therapist must assess the impact of the child's disability on family dynamics. In the home, the therapist can be more sensitive to family issues and to the psychosocial aspects of the child's development. The home is an optimal setting for the therapist to gain an understanding of the family's interaction with the child and the effect of the environment on the child's performance (McBride & Peterson, 1997).

Direct Services

In addition to one-on-one interactions with the child, direct services include education and emotional support of caregivers. Education may include explaining the inter-

relationship of performance components (e.g., trunk control, shoulder stability, isolated finger use, flexible palmar arch) and functional skills (e.g., play, self-care). Explanation of therapy activities helps family members understand the rationale for the child's goals, and it increases the likelihood of collaboration and follow through between the child's therapist and his or her parents. Families of children with sensory integrative dysfunction (SID) also need help understanding their children's behaviors. The family may be concerned with their child's high activity level and inability to pay attention, and they may experience frustration in their daily interactions with the child. Therefore the occupational therapist explains the sensory problems that affect a child's arousal, attention, and behavior. The practitioner can also develop an individualized sensory integration program and establish a sensory diet tailored to the child and family preferences (Hanschu, 1996). Accommodations made to the sensory environment of the home can help the child modulate and organize his or her sensory responses. When infants achieve *homeostasis* (i.e., an optimal level of alertness and arousal), and when young children are comfortable in their environment, positive parent-child interactions naturally result.

When the occupational therapist is the primary health professional who has consistent contact with a family, or when a family feels most comfortable with the occupational therapist, he or she may be called on to provide emotional support and help the family deal with issues that only indirectly relate to the child's disability. Family functioning may be affected by other stressful events or situations, such as illness of another family member, substance abuse, unemployment, or financial problems. For example, the mother of an at-risk child spent part of a session speaking with the therapist about her husband's recent unemployment and alcoholism. The therapist suggested that other professionals could help in this situation and asked if she might request that the social worker contact her.

The home setting is generally more casual and informal than a center or clinic. Often the demands of caring for a special child prevent family members from taking advantage of social opportunities. Some parents express an interest in developing a social relationship with the therapist. When one infant fell asleep during the treatment session, his mother discussed other aspects of her life with the therapist. The therapist must identify the family's needs and recognize how much flexibility to allow in the relationship with the family. This must be done while continuing to provide appropriate services to the disabled child (Bryant, Lyons, & Wasik, 1990; Opacich, 1997).

The extent of a therapist's role in parent education varies according to family needs or individual parent responses to therapist recommendations. Parents who have developmental disabilities may need a concrete, problem-oriented explanation of their child's development. The therapist may also help parents select and purchase toys and introduce appropriate activities at each developmental stage in the child's life. In addition, the therapist may help parents interpret their child's behaviors. For example, the therapist may explain the causes of the child's irritability or hyperactivity. Along with explanations, the therapist can suggest methods that the parents can use to manage the child's behaviors and to promote his or her development.

Consultation

The occupational therapist collaborates with team members and parents to recommend specific positioning, adaptive equipment, and use of toys and manipulatives. For example, as part of the intervention program with a child with hemiparesis, the occupational therapist consulted with the educator to demonstrate how to position an activity to promote use of both sides of his body. She recommended that toys be placed to encourage crossing the midline and scanning the visual field on the child's affected side. This toy placement also encouraged the child to place weight on the affected side. The educator then modified how and where she presented activities to the child to encourage the use of both upper extremities.

Service Coordinator

An occupational therapist may assume the role of *service coordinator*, responsible for formal documentation and communication regarding all aspects of services being provided to the family. The service coordinator helps families access services and coordinates them so that the program goals and recommendations are cohesive and consistent with those of the family. This person takes responsibility for making phone or e-mail contacts with other service providers, and he or she arranges and schedules meetings (e.g., Individualized Family Service Plan meeting). In this expanded role, the therapist helps the family identify and contact additional services that support overall family function. For example, one mother expressed her need to learn English and indicated that she was overwhelmed with her family's problems. The therapist, who was the family's service coordinator, arranged a language class and referred her to social work and psychology services for counseling.

■ INTERVENTION PROCESS

Evaluation

During evaluation of the child in the home, the therapist must adapt to the physical environment in the home as well as the presence of family members. Many homes have space limitations or activities occurring in them that are unrelated to the intervention process. When other family members are present, the therapist may find that he or she needs to explain the evaluation process repeatedly in ways that accommodate different levels of understanding. The therapist must also be aware of the impact of these factors in the interpretation of test results. For example, a child may appear extremely distractible or hyperactive in a busy home with high activity and noise levels. Before the evaluation, the therapist may ask if the child is prepared, fed, and well rested to facilitate the child's best performance. If the child appears unusually tired or irritable, the therapist may decide to reschedule the evaluation.

Intervention

The home environment also affects the types of intervention activities that are provided. Using selected frames of reference, such as sensory integration, may be more difficult to implement in the home (Hinojosa, Anderson, & Strauch, 1988). Limitations in space, or the need for large or suspended equipment, may restrict the therapist's ability to carry out these techniques in the home. Therapists need to be creative in adapting techniques to use whatever space and equipment may be available in the home. For example, when treating a child with attention deficit hyperactivity disorder (ADHD), the therapist substituted a weighted backpack for a weighted vest. In addition, a little red wagon and a toy flying saucer were used to provide vestibular stimulation for this child. He squeezed soft rubbery toys and a Koosh ball to decrease the tactile hypersensitivity in his palms (Del Vecchio, 1992).

Many types of intervention are easily and successfully implemented in the home. For example, the family of a preschool-aged girl with a diagnosis of juvenile rheumatoid arthritis chose to continue private therapy in which myofascial release and craniosacral techniques were emphasized. The family arranged a quiet space with controlled lighting in which the therapist could implement the handling techniques without the time constraints imposed by a clinic or school setting. After the home-based intervention sessions, the therapist had time to discuss strategies for increasing the child's independence and general endurance in physical activities. The intervention techniques used with this child often are not implemented in school-based settings because of the orientation toward school-based goals and the need to schedule 30-minute, back-to-back treatment sessions.

Family-Centered Services

The presence of siblings in the home can have an impact on intervention. Therapists may set limits as to their involvement, or they may decide to include siblings in activities to motivate the child with special needs. Siblings who are close in age to the child receiving services may display disruptive behavior during intervention, because they perceive the therapy as "special attention" given to their brother or sister. Parents may need reassurance that this is a normal occurrence. For example, in a family in which the parents had marital problems and the typically developing brother had behavioral problems, the therapist was unable to limit the sibling's presence in the therapy area. To limit the brother's disruptive behavior, the therapist provided him with activities and materials during each session. This allowed the therapist to focus on the child who was receiving services. In another family, the older brother held materials at the therapist's direction to encourage his sibling's ability to reach and visually search. The older brother's participation held two advantages: (1) it freed the therapist's hands for positioning and handling, and (2) it increased the motivation of the child receiving services.

The therapist must adapt to the style the parent has chosen to use in coping with the child's disability (Figure 27-1). Some families prefer that therapists provide services without their active participation. However, others may prefer to learn and carry out therapeutic techniques used by each discipline. Some parents demonstrate their involvement by regularly communicating with each therapist, and they may be particularly eager for specific feedback regarding their child's progress. Other parents become involved in organizations or political-action groups for individuals with disabilities. In each of these circumstances, the therapist needs to adjust his or her timing, style, and mode of communication to promote an effective therapist-family relationship. Sensitivity and responsivity to the needs of family members requires ongoing listening and communication skills (Bazyk, 1989) (see Chapter 5).

One role of the therapist is to help the family include and encourage their child's participation in family activities. The therapist may concentrate on use of equipment and positioning techniques that allow the child to sit at the dinner table, watch television with siblings, or go on a family outing. For example, a child with spastic diplegia, who walked short distances in her home and in the special education setting, required assistance when traveling longer distances. The therapist helped the family select a stroller that fit in their car, was light enough to be lifted easily by all family members, and allowed them to take their child to places that required long-distance walking. Materials found in the home can also be used for positioning, particularly when financial resources are limited or when the family has difficulty accepting adaptive equipment. For example, an 8-month-old infant, born prematurely and fed with a gastric tube, required support to maintain a side-lying or sitting position. Pillows were used to reduce extensor and adductor hypertonicity in the child's legs. This allowed him to sit and work on upper-extremity skills. In addition, a commercially available ring pillow was purchased to provide support at the hips and pelvis, thus, promoting sitting independence. Other inexpensive and cosmetically appealing products are commercially available and can be recommended for positioning or sensory input. These include molded plastic floor seats with lap trays, infant carriers that hold the infant close to the mother's chest, and cloth inserts for shopping carts that abduct the legs and support the lower trunk. Figure 27-2 shows a tumble-form chair commonly used to position the child for feeding.

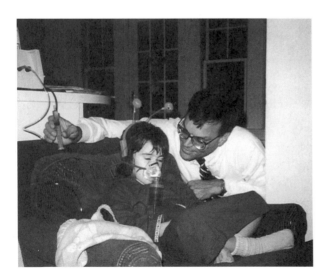

figure**27-1**   When the father is at home during a visit, the occupational therapist can solicit his concerns and perceptions. Discussions about the progress of the child, changes in goals, and family priorities should transpire on a regular basis.

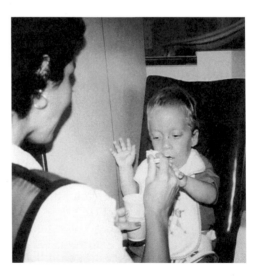

figure**27-2**   The therapist models feeding techniques. The home is an ideal environment to work on daily living skills, such as feeding, because the parent can easily replicate the positions and handling methods used by the therapist. Consistent use of handling and positioning methods by different caregivers supports the child's acquisition of new skills.

Easy access to these products and the opportunity to demonstrate their versatility in the home setting are additional benefits to the therapist providing home-based intervention.

Cultural Sensitivity

When working in the home, the therapist must be aware of and respect cultural differences. In particular, expectations for the age of achievement of self-help skills independence vary by cultural group. In some cultures, children are bottle fed for extended periods. Solid foods and drinking from a cup are introduced at different ages in different cultures, and dietary restrictions based on religion or culture must be respected. Some cultures express affection by carrying their children, even after they have learned to walk. The presence of a child with a disability may influence the way families are accepted within their community. Often these families attempt to hide the presence of intervention professionals by requesting that they not bring recognizable therapy equipment, or that they park a distance from the house. These families may also find it difficult to discuss their emotional reactions to their children's disabilities with their relatives, with community members, or with therapists providing services (Wayman, Lynch, & Hanson, 1990).

It may sometimes be difficult for female therapists to interact with fathers because of cultural or religious dictates that limit male contact with nonrelated females. There may also be styles of dress that are inappropriate to certain cultures, or styles of language that are not acceptable to them. Modern technology, such as television, electronic devices, and certain toys related to this technology, may be prohibited by a culture. If this is the case, they should not be used in therapeutic intervention activities. For example, in Hasidic or Orthodox Jewish households, only the kosher foods prepared within the home can be used for feeding. Therapists cannot bring food into the house, even if it is for their own consumption. In addition, some Jewish and Muslim families observe a conservative dress code. Therapists should respect this by avoiding shorts, short skirts, as well as sleeveless and low-cut shirts. In both of these cultures, therapies are canceled for religious holidays, which may involve extended periods.

Families who do not speak English pose a particular challenge to the therapist, and creative strategies are needed to communicate with them successfully. For example, therapists for a child of Arab parents developed a system of communicating with the child through gestures and simple English. The father, who spoke English, was not able to be present during therapy because it interfered with his work schedule. However, the therapists left notes to the father with information concerning the child, and he translated these for his wife when he came

home. The occupational therapist, in consultation with the service coordinator, helped locate an Arab-speaking pediatrician and neurologist, so the family could communicate more easily with medical personnel.

Case Study 1: Carl

This case study illustrates that a well-coordinated home-based program benefits both the child and the family, and it may be the most appropriate mode of intervention for a child who is medically fragile.

At the time of this evaluation, Carl was 12 years old. He was diagnosed with cerebral palsy and mental retardation, with onset attributed to administration of diphtheria-tetanus-pertussis injection in infancy. He was on medication for seizure disorder and was reported by his family to have many allergies and to be susceptible to illnesses when exposed to other children. He had been educated at home, with inconsistent provision of therapy services. The previous year, the school district had insisted that Carl attend school. His parents reported that during the first week of school he had suffered a seizure and had been unattended during this episode. They were called to the school, where they found him lethargic with depressed responses. After this episode, Carl never regained his previous functional level. His parents decided that they would not send him to school again for fear of further episodes. They petitioned for a full home-based program that would include all therapies, in addition to the educational services their son required.

Based on clinical assessment and interview with the family, the occupational therapist recognized the need for adaptive equipment for transportation, communication, and positioning. During the first months of intervention, after further evaluation of Carl and of the home environment, the occupational therapist recommended that the family obtain an adjustable wheelchair with environmental controls, a transportable positioner, and an augmentative communication device. She provided information regarding where and how to order the equipment and helped the family obtain funding by documenting medical necessity. The equipment met the family's needs to have Carl seated in a manner they perceived as comfortable and to allow him visual contact with family members during social activities.

Because of his previous interest in music, it was important to his family that he be able to activate a tape player and television set. Switches were provided for these purposes. A small-in-scale, lightweight wheelchair was ordered so that Carl had access to all rooms in the family's home and so that it could be put in the car easily for transport. The occupational therapist coordinated the choice of an augmentative communication device with the speech therapist so that access to the device was appropriate to Carl's visual motor and fine motor abilities.

Communication among team members and between team and family was maintained through use of a notebook. The family expressed satisfaction that home-based intervention was most appropriate for Carl's safety, and that it met their priorities for developing his ability to participate in family life.

■ OTHER CONSIDERATIONS IN HOME-BASED INTERVENTION

In addition to the cultural and psychosocial environment, physical, socioeconomic, and medical factors need to be considered when working in the home. Some homes may be unsafe. Therefore therapists need to carry disinfectants and personal cleansing items with them for infection control and general hygiene. In some states, OSHA training is required. In addition to observing universal precautions, which are primarily designed to prevent exposure to blood products, therapists must protect themselves and the children they treat from airborne diseases. Children with HIV and many other immune disorders should not be exposed to any common influenza or virus because of their increased vulnerability and the complications that may result. Therapists with allergies or asthma should carry appropriate medications with them.

Homes infested with cockroaches or mice necessitate taking precautions to seal equipment to avoid contaminating other homes. Some homes may have major structural problems that pose as hazards to the therapist. For example, stairs or flooring may be unsafe. Rusted nails and floors with splinters should be covered by transportable mats. The therapist and parents also might discuss ways to prevent injury to an infant who is learning to crawl on floor surfaces that are unsafe.

Case Study 2: Moshe

This case illustrates the way medical, cultural, and family issues affect home-based occupational therapy with a premature infant born with microcephaly and hearing impairment.

Moshe was the youngest of 5 siblings in a Hasidic family. He was born at 26 weeks gestation after a normal pregnancy. His mother's water broke at 25 weeks, and she was immediately placed on medication and bed rest to prevent contractions. He was born a week later and had respiratory distress syndrome, episodes of apnea, elevated bilirubin, and was fed through a nasogastric tube. He was on a respirator for 4 weeks and hospitalized for 8 weeks to gain weight and achieve to nipple feeding.

Moshe was referred for home-based occupational therapy when he was 3 months old (corrected age). Upon evaluation, he was noted to have elevated, tight shoulders; lack of reach and grasp patterns; poor visual focus and tracking; and weak, poorly coordinated suck-swallow-breathing pattern. He also continued to have inadequate weight gain. Initial and follow-up audiologic testing indicated severe to profound hearing loss. Occupational therapy intervention was initiated twice weekly, with the goals of improving range of motion in the shoulder girdle, improving hand function, improving responses to multisensory input, and improving efficiency of feeding.

Moshe required many follow-up visits to audiology, gastroenterology, neurology, and pediatrics. Because of the closeness of the Hasidic community, extended family was available for childcare for his other siblings.

Moshe's 20-month-old brother began to interfere with therapy as a means of demanding attention. The therapist brought novel toys in, so the brother could play alongside the therapist. She incorporated turn taking with the brother in many of the therapy activities. Toys and adapted equipment for positioning were also selected carefully to adapt to the limited space typical of city apartments and small homes in this Hasidic community. Popular toys, such as those with television or comic-book characters, were not acceptable within this community. Therefore culturally appropriate toys (e.g., puzzles with holiday symbols) were purchased at local stores. Moshe was particularly responsive to the visual stimulation provided by the toys containing pictures of familiar objects.

Because of kosher dietary restrictions and the need to have separate dishes and utensils for particular groups of food, foods and feeding utensils also had to be carefully selected. Moshe was fitted with bilateral hearing aids with an FM transmitter at 18 months old. An adapted chair was ordered to facilitate positioning for feeding and to be used during audiological training. The chair created a stable base of support for upright posture to reduce reflux, and it provided physical limits to help Moshe attend to training. The order for this adaptive equipment was coordinated among all therapists and physicians involved in Moshe's care.

■ ■ ■

Service delivery in rural areas also poses particular challenges. Families may live in isolated settings, with driving distances of 1 hour or more to different homes. Weather conditions can significantly affect frequency of therapist visits to homes located on unpaved roads. In addition, there is often limited access to supplies and equipment that are readily available in more densely populated areas. Regional values, levels of education and income, and the variety of other support services tend to differ in rural areas. Therefore therapists working in rural areas may be called on to treat a wider variety of ages and disabilities. It is important for the therapist to know where and how to access support services within each community served. Home visits in urban, high-crime areas may require therapists to work in teams and, sometimes, to make the decision to provide center-based therapy for reasons of personal safety. Parking can be a problem, and carrying equipment in elevators and to walk-up apartments requires careful planning.

Another consideration of practice in the home is the possibility for early identification of domestic violence, substance abuse, or child abuse. For example, a therapist believed that sanitary conditions were unsuitable and that nutritional needs were not being met for a medically compromised child. The therapist contacted a social worker and the service coordinator to investigate the availability of alternative housing and to provide nutrition counseling for the parents.

In most clinical and school settings, medical, transportation, and equipment emergencies are manageable, because of readily available resource personnel and procedures. In contrast, the home-based therapist must plan for emergencies or special needs and rely on what he or she can successfully transport. Investment in communication technology may be a priority for the home-based therapist. Cellular telephones, beepers, and personal computers are used to facilitate communications, for personal safety, and for record keeping. Table 27-1 lists equipment, toys, and supplies that occupational therapists frequently carry with them on home visits.

■ SUMMARY

Home-based occupational therapy is a growing area of practice. This growth has been driven by changes in IDEA and the increased survival of children with complex and severe medical problems who must receive home-based services because their health is extremely fragile or their technology support is difficult to transport. Instilled with a holistic philosophy, occupational therapists consider the family's psychosocial strengths and concerns, values, and cultural background in intervention with the child. Because respect for family values is inherent in this philosophy, occupational therapists often develop close relationships with family members.

Home-based therapy services may provide parents with a greater sense of control over their child's intervention program, because they can set limits and define parameters of behavior in their own homes. Acknowledging the family's priorities in setting therapeutic goals and objectives adds to this sense of empowerment. Home-based therapy requires a great deal of clinical expertise, flexibility, and adaptability. The case studies in this chapter illustrate methods for developing positive and productive relationships with families and providing effective intervention.

table 27-1 Examples of Equipment, Toys, and Supplies for the Home-Based Occupational Therapist

Equipment and Toys	Supplies
T-Stool	Bubbles
Scooter board	Brushes: Play Doh
Vestibular board	Textured cloths: Magna Doodle
Spinning saucer	Puzzles
Small trampoline	Different-sized balls:
Swim noodles	Dry pasta
Cardboard boxes and packing cases for tunnels	Coloring books and painting supplies
Small cuff weights	Carpet squares
Different-sized plastic buckets for a small sand or water table (family's sink)	Beanbags
Gymnastic balls	Rice, beans, and lentils
Vibrators	in containers (for
Cause-and-effect toys	tactile activities)
Laptop computer or other portable video games	
Electronic toys and switch toys	Foam balls
Corner chair or other small seating devices	

Modified from Austill-Clausen, R. (1995). Pediatric services in the home. *AOTA Home Health Guidelines.* Bethesda, MD: American Occupational Therapy Association.

STUDY QUESTIONS

1. List three types of children for whom home-based intervention would be the most appropriate form of service delivery.
2. Define two family circumstances in which some level of home-based service is appropriate.
3. Compare evaluation methods and procedures in the home versus those in the clinic (refer to Chapters 26 and 29 for comparison). What are the advantages and disadvantages of evaluation in the home?
4. What are two ways to appropriately elicit the participation of an older sibling in therapy sessions?
5. Explain two advantages of home-based care in the following instances:
   - A family in poverty
   - A family from a Middle Eastern country
   - A situation of suspected child abuse

References

Ahmann, E., & Lipsi, D.A. (1991). Early intervention for technology-dependent infants and young children. *Infants and Young Children, 3* (4), 67-77.

Arras, J., & Dubler, N. (1995). Ethical and social implications of high-tech home care. In J. Arras (Ed.), *Bringing the hospital home*. Baltimore: John Hopkins University Press.

Austill-Clausen, R. (1995). Pediatric services in the home. *In AOTA Home Health Guidelines*. Bethesda, MD: American Occupational Therapy Association.

Bailey, D.B., & Simeonsson, R.J. (1988). Home based early intervention. In S. Odem & M. Karnes (Eds.), *Early intervention for infants and children with handicaps*. Baltimore: Brookes.

Bazyk, S. (1989). Changes in attitudes and beliefs regarding parent participation and home programs: An update. *American Journal of Occupational Therapy, 43* (11), 723-728.

Bryant, D.B., Lyons, D., & Wasik, B.H. (1990). Ethical issues involved in home visiting. *Topics in Early Childhood Special Education, 10* (4), 92-107.

Del Vecchio, J.A. (1992) Home pediatric rehabilitation. *Journal of Home Healthcare Practice, 5* (1), 12-15.

Garbaciak, T. (1990). Treating kids at home. *OT Week, 4* (46), 8-9.

Hanft, B. (1988). The changing environment of early intervention services: Implications for practice. *American Journal of Occupational Therapy, 42* (11), 724-731.

Hanschu, B. (1996). *Sensory strategies for the treatment of autism and ADHD*. Paper presented at Sensory Strategies for the Treatment of Autism and ADHD: An Interactive Workshop.

Hinojosa, J., Anderson, J., & Strauch, C. (1988). Pediatric occupational therapy in the home. *American Journal of Occupational Therapy, 42* (1), 17-22.

The Individuals with Disabilities Education Act of 1990, 20 U.S.C. §1400 et seq.

The Individuals with Disabilities Act Amendments of 1997, 20 U.S.C. §1400 et seq.

Kirk, S. (1998). Families' experiences of caring at home for a technology-dependent child: A review of the literature. *Child: Care, Health and Development, 24* (2), 101-114.

McBride, S.L., & Peterson, C. (1997). Home-based early intervention with families of children with disabilities: Who is doing what? *Topics in Early Childhood Special Education, 17* (2), 209-233.

Opacich, K.J. (1997) Moral tensions and obligations of occupational therapy practitioners providing home care. *American Journal of Occupational Therapy, 51* (6), 430-435.

Parks, R.A. (1994, November). *HIV in the pediatric population: NDTA network*. Chicago: The Neurodevelopmental Treatment Association.

Raab, M., Davis, M.S., & Trepanier, A.M. (1993). Resources versus services: Changing the focus of intervention for infants and young children. *Infants and Young Children, 5*, 1-11.

Ramey, C.T., Bryant, D., Sparling, J., & Wasik, B. (1984). A biosocial systems perspective on environmental intervention for low birth-weight infants. *Clinical Obstetrics and Gynecology, 27*, 672-692.

Roberts, R.N., Akers, A.L., & Behl, D.D. (1996). Family-level service coordination within home visiting programs. *Topics in Early Childhood Special Education, 16*, 279-301.

Russell, F.F., & Free, T.A. (1991). Early intervention for infants and toddlers with prenatal drug exposure. *Infants and Young Children, 3* (4), 78-85.

Sandall, S.R. (1990). Developmental interventions for biologically at-risk infants at home. *Topics in Early Childhood Special Education, 10* (4), 1-13.

Wagner, J., Power, E.J., & Fox, H. (1988). *Technology-dependent child: Hospital versus home care*. Philadelphia: Lippincott.

Wayman, K.I., Lynch, E.W., & Hanson, M.J. (1990). Home-based early childhood services: Cultural sensitivity in a family system approach. *Topics in Early Childhood Special Education, 10* (4), 56-75.

chapter 28

The Dying Child

Margaret J. Barnstorff

■ CHAPTER OBJECTIVES

1. Understand how children of different ages view death.
2. Recognize the impact of hospitalization and the awareness of the severity of medical conditions on children.
3. Gain insight into the feelings and attitudes of families of children who are dying and the personnel working with them.

Jan was an 11-year-old girl with a distorting facial malignancy. Since the onset of her illness 2 years earlier, she had made periodic visits to various outpatient clinics, interspersed with hospital stays in her hometown and in a regional medical center. The treatment she received, as well as the disease from which she suffered, was extremely painful. As Jan was dying in the medical center, she remained in a private room that was darkened at all times. Her contacts with the outside world were few; the medical staff rarely visited her room, except during rounds or to administer medications.

Donna, a nursing student, was Jan's only meaningful contact with the outside world. Jan enjoyed Donna's visits, asked for her when she was not there, and allowed only Donna to spend extended periods with her. It was a

relationship full of meaning for both of them, and it revealed a great deal about children's perceptions of death and dying.

■ SCOPE OF THE PROBLEM

One hundred years ago, childhood deaths were common, and families had to learn to accept the loss of children as something to be expected. Today, belief in the medical system and in its ability to cure disease often leaves individuals unprepared for death. Therefore a child's death grievously affects those around the child: the family, the medical staff, and the community of friends and peers.

In the United States, tens of thousands of children die annually. However, the most prevalent cause of childhood death is not illness; it is accidents. In children, 1 to 4 years of age, accidents are followed by congenital anomalies, cancer, homicide and legal interventions, heart disease, human immunodeficiency virus (HIV), and respiratory difficulties (e.g., pneumonia, influenza). In children 5 to 14 years of age, the leading causes of death after accidents are cancer, congenital anomalies, suicide, homicide and legal interventions, heart disease, HIV, and respiratory difficulties (U.S. Bureau of the Census, 1997).

When a child is terminally ill with an acute or chronic situation, various people care for that child. The primary caregivers usually include members of the child's family and the medical staff (i.e., the primary care physician and many specialists, who work together to provide diagnosis and treatment). The nursing staff also provides care to the dying child on a daily basis, administering the medications, charting the course of the disease, and structuring opportunities for the child to use daily living skills. Allied health personnel involved in the care of dying children often include social workers, physical therapists, occupational therapists, recreational therapists, dietitians, and medical technicians. Children who are dying not only cause concern for their immediate families and health care professionals; extended family members (e.g., grandparents, aunts and uncles, siblings, cousins) and members of the community (e.g., teachers, classmates, family friends) are all affected by the child's illness and may also be involved in the care of the dying child.

Although it is typical for children who are the victims of accidents to die in the hospital, children with terminal illnesses are now more often involved in home care programs (Martinson, 1986-1987). Hospice, palliative, or respite care programs for children (e.g., the Ronald McDonald Houses affiliated with hospitals in major cities) are also becoming more common (Pizzi, 1984; Tigges, 1983; Wilson, 1988). Annually, about 5000 children (aged 1 to 14) need hospice care in the United States (Martinson, 1995). Nurses, physical therapists, occupational therapists, aides, and volunteers typically provide hospice care. Agencies that work with these children and their families include those that grant children's wishes, such as the "Make a Wish Foundation" and the "Sunshine Foundation," as well as those that provide familial bereavement counseling, such as the "Compassionate Friends" in Illinois or "the Candlelighters" in Washington, D.C. (Wessel, 1983).

Children with chronic diseases are often seen in outpatient clinics until they become too ill to remain at home. Then they are admitted to the hospital until disease remission allows them to return home. A pattern of recurrent hospitalizations is typical. In the last 10 years, an increasing number of children for whom treatment fails have been offered the option of dying at home, rather than in a hospital. This has been fostered through programs such as hospice and individually developed programs at various medical centers (Mulhern, 1983).

■ CHILDREN'S PERCEPTIONS OF DEATH

Depending on the theory chosen, there are either three or four stages in the development of a child's understanding of death. Nagy (1959), one of the first individuals to study this topic, suggested three stages: (1) from birth to 5 years, the child believes that death is a reversible process in which life activities, such as growing, hearing, and feeling, can take place; (2) from the ages of 5 to 9 years, the child personifies death as a distinct personality; and (3) from the age of 9, onward, death is understood to be a cessation of corporeal life and is a universal phenomenon.

Kane (1979) and Koocher (1973) related the development of a child's perception of death to Piaget's stages of development during the *preoperational, concrete operations,* and *formal operations states.* Their research suggested that as a child's mind matures, the cognitive stages are reflected in the child's understanding of death.

Childers and Wimmer (1971) studied children's perceptions of death, and their results indicated that differential awareness of death is a universal function of age. Among the subjects of their study, the understanding of death as being irrevocable was not demonstrated systematically until age 10.

Meliar (1973) suggested that there are four stages to the development of the concept of death: (1) Most 3- and 4-year-old children demonstrate a relative ignorance of the meaning of death; (2) Among 4- to 7-year-old children, death is seen as a temporary state; (3) Although 5- to 10-year-old children appear to function in a transitional state; these children believe that death is final but that the dead function biologically; (4) To most older children, death is a cessation of all biologic functioning.

Infants

As a child matures from infancy to adulthood, his or her concepts of self, life, and eventual death parallel Erikson's and Piaget's developmental theories. The very young infant facing death reacts only physiologically, using all of his or her strength to continue living. As the child reaches 6 months of age, he or she demonstrates an emotional reaction to the physical process of the disease symptoms and the resulting treatment procedures. At this age the infant is capable of recognizing that he or she creates stress and conflicting emotions in others, especially his or her parents. The infant may equate this with having done something wrong and may respond to treatment with anxiety and fear, which is further aggravated by separation anxiety. These reactions continue throughout the ages of 2 and 3. It is also during this period that the child learns the word *death,* but the word holds little or no meaning.

Preschool Children

Egocentricity diminishes as the child is introduced to a world larger than the one known during the toddler years. At 4 years of age, the child begins to conceptualize himself or herself as an individual. However, this concept is also accompanied by that of "not me." The preschooler must deal with feelings of being and not being. The thought of not being produces anxiety, because it means separation from family and loss of independence. Because a preschool-age child focuses on the single dimension of comparing one object with another, he or she focuses on life as "being with others on earth," and death as "separation from loved ones." To a child of this age, death also means that one becomes immobile (i.e., unable to move) (Salladay & Royal, 1981). Thus thoughts of dying suggest dependency and loss of the self-control that the child has just begun to acquire. Disease, then, threatens a child's very psychosocial existence.

Although children of ages 4 and 5 approach death with fantasy reasoning and magical thinking (Koocher 1973; Von Hug-Hellmuth, 1965), they also begin to appreciate the meaning of a diagnosis. This greatly influences their reactions to the world around them. Television, radio, magazines, books, and communications with others disclose many ideas. They hear words, view the responding emotions, and develop associations that can be applied to later experiences. Children begin this application process as they come to identify with others. Concurrently, they develop an increased curiosity about burial, dead animals and flowers, and the accidental features of death.

For 3- to 5-year-old children, death means absence or going away; it is a temporary state (Meliar, 1973). Death is seen as a continuation of life, but in a different place. Because preschool children function cognitively at the preoperational level, they are incapable of understanding the process as being irreversible. This is also true of children with developmental delays who do not have abstract thinking ability. These children are also unrealistic about the permanence or timing of death (Sternlicht, 1980). For preschool-age children, the most painful aspect of dying is the realization of separation. They often use denial to overcome feelings of helplessness and the sense of loss. Narcissism develops with the threat to life and the recognition of the reality of the situation (Cook, Renshaw, & Jackson, 1973).

School-Aged Children

Children of school age come to realize that death is irreversible, the cessation of bodily functions as we know them, and universal to the species (Speece & Brent, 1984). Children, 5 to 7 years of age, understand the prognosis and its significance. Although they may realize that death is imminent, thoughts about this are seldom vocalized; they perceive absence and death with a sense of impending tragedy. School-aged children can think of an object as a whole, as well as consider its parts. By this age, they have also mastered the concept of time. With the vivid imagination that school-aged children possess, the physical change and deterioration that occurs with death can be visualized. To them, death is specific and concrete, and it has both internal and external causes (Salladay & Royal, 1981). The prognosis becomes absolute and creates such anxiety that the child can no longer cope. As emotional and intellectual capabilities increase with age, the child's own death takes on greater meaning. A greater realization of death's meaning may lead to the child needing more assistance in coping.

Going to school full time adds to the child's continually changing social role and relationships within it. A 6- or 7-year-old child realizes that with death, previously established relationships will change. Again, death symbolizes separation from loved ones, and this potential separation breeds anxiety. The child now understands that separation cannot be avoided. Supplied with this knowledge, he or she learns to be a "good patient:" death is not mentioned and feelings of pain and emotions are repressed. The rules of life are learned. At this time there is an emotional shift from anxiety to fear of physical injury and mutilation, operations, body intrusions, and needles (Spinetta, 1974). Often these children die lonely; they pretend they will not die, while the people around them remain fully aware of the situation. In addition, they rarely ask questions related to their disease or treatment, and they tend to avoid the topic of death as if to protect their families from their approaching demise (Jeffrey & Lansdown, 1982).

From ages 5 to 9, death is personified and thought of as a contingency. Death, as a personality, is usually invisible, either having no form or going through the night so that it cannot be seen (Cook et. al., 1973). This is the time of life when children may have difficulty going to bed in the dark for fear that they may not wake the next morning. At this age children also tend to talk about the "boogeyman." Death is remote, it exists outside of one's self; through careful living, it can be kept at a distance. School-aged children also develop an interest in animate and inanimate things. This interest evolves into a transition period of superstitions and rituals about death (e.g., "Don't step on the crack, it will break your mother's back"). The child is unclear if death is funny or fearful.

It is not until children reach 8 or 9 years old that play and verbal expressions come to terms with each other. Weininger (1979) found that before this age, when children were told that a doll was sick and going to die, they tended to talk about the doll's death as being permanent. However, they continued in the play situation to have the doll recover and return to life.

Grade-school children are also aware of their own identity. This allows them to think beyond self-boundaries and to imagine. They understand about past and future concepts and fantasize about death and the idea of their own deaths. Thus they develop an alternative to death, seen in such forms as heaven, paradise, and hell. Children want their existence to continue. Through learning rules, school-age children pattern themselves after other individuals, leading to the realization that their parents are not perfect. Children therefore seek alternative heroes, groping for something to believe in and worship. These beliefs allow them to organize their worlds methodically, including a cause and purpose behind every action. This is then followed by a reward or punishment. Death, being perceived as a punishment, may cause religious guilt (Lewis & Lewis, 1973). Secondary to this perception of punishment, dying children may reject the idea of heaven, which represents only separation from family. An understanding of death increases throughout this stage, but these children tend to think that death comes suddenly and quickly. They may blot out feelings of death and, in turn, rely on parental authority (e.g., God, physicians, teachers) for final protection from death.

In the 9- and 10-year-old child, egocentricity decreases as mature concepts of time, space, quantity, and causality begin to emerge. These children appreciate life and begin to understand death as the physical finality of living. They express their anxiety about terminal illness in terms of separation and mutilation fears. Anxiety about death is characteristic in preadolescents and serves as a lead-in to adolescence (Toews, Martin, & Prosen, 1985).

Adolescents

Adolescence is the bridge from childhood to adulthood; it is a period of transition. These transitions occur not only in the physiologic, but also in the cognitive, psychodynamic, and sociocultural aspects of development. Cognitively, adolescents move into the world of abstract thought. They learn to speculate on possibilities beyond reality and what might occur, as well as what does occur (Salladay & Royal, 1981). In this exploration, adolescents delve into the limits of life and the meaning of death.

Adolescents appreciate the reality of death (O'Brien, Johnson, & Schmink, 1978). However, personal death is not accepted (McDonald & Carroll, 1981). The adolescent tends to assume the attitude of "Everyone else but me can die." Adolescence is a period of intense present, with the immediate life situation being important and past and future being pallid. More structure is given to the past than to the future, but the past represents a period of confusion. In addition, attitudes toward the future are subjective and distinctly negative. Often the future is viewed as being risky and devoid of any positive values (Cook et. al., 1973). Even if imminent, death is thought of as remote because it distorts the importance of the present.

Adolescence represents the drive for complete independence and self-sufficiency. It is a time of group identity with peers and the development of personal ideas and behavior, usually through peer-group relationships. Guilt and vague feelings of wrongdoing are felt during rejec-

tion of parental control; this rejection bothers the adolescent. Because most deaths in this age group occur secondarily to trauma or accidents (frequently resulting from the breaking of rules), death becomes a confirmation of wrongdoing and is perceived as punishment that is meted out by the unforgiving parent. This idea leads to fear of the authority figure and eventual bitterness and resentment, deepening the adolescent's guilt and accentuating his or her depression (Eason, 1970).

In dealing with death, the adolescent progresses through the five stages outlined by Dr. Elisabeth Kübler-Ross (1969): (1) denial, (2) anger, (3) bargaining, (4) depression, and (5) acceptance. Adolescents are more likely to express emotions than younger children. Death is representative of loneliness and passivity. Hospitalized adolescents fear being returned to the dependent role and may overtax their strength in an effort to seek continued independence.

Although they long for warmth and caring, they reject support. Thus they force people to withdraw from them, even while dreading loss of control. With approaching death, they become weakened and allow themselves to be loved and cared for. At this point, they rationalize that they will regain control when they regain strength. The adolescent wants to live, but at the same time may be fascinated with the concept of death (Eason, 1970).

Death in the middle teenage years defeats the newly developed self-control, self-confidence, and self-direction that led to the enjoyment of self. Older grade-school children and adolescents, who know they are dying and accept death's finality, prepare their families for the event. They gradually withdraw their expectations from the family and seemingly reject them. It is as if they are trying to comfort their families and ease them through the final phase of death with as little pain as possible. Death also means rejection by peers because it emphasizes the vulnerability of the individual, as well as the difference between individuals. The emerging independent individual cannot tolerate this rejection. Therefore death becomes a function of dependency in isolation.

Young adolescents demonstrate their anxiety through symbolization and physiologic expression. As the child gets older, death anxiety is increasingly expressed; older boys tend to act out, whereas older girls are prone to depression (Cook et. al., 1973). This expression appears to be directly related to society's role models and the difficulty on the part of men to express emotions actively. Anxiety may also appear as regression to an earlier stage of development.

It may be concluded that children at any age perceive their own death according to their developmental level and through the catalyst of some crisis event, such as a catastrophic illness. Research also indicates that the extent of understanding that children have about their own death is difficult for their parents to accept (Weber, 1985).

■ IMPACT OF HOSPITALIZATION

At some time a dying child will be hospitalized for medical intervention. Even when the child is carefully prepared, the hospital represents something fearful, simply by virtue of its difference and newness in a child's repertoire of experiences. For example, the toddler views home as the seat of security, safety, and guidance. When hospitalized, he or she experiences anxiety when separated from familiar surroundings, routine, and family. Compounding the strangeness of the hospital setting, the treatments often cause the child pain and discomfort. The child, in turn, reacts to the physical pain and his or her perceptions of his or her parents' discomfort, rather than to any understanding of the end of his or her own existence (Eason, 1970).

Erikson pointed out that with increasing age, increasing independence develops. The preschool child does not separate thinking from concrete reality. Thus hospitalization is thought of as punishment for bad thoughts (Eason, 1970). The child reacts with guilt and noncomprehension of the treatment. The child is angry with the hospitalization process, and his or her anger is usually directed toward the treatment team or other patients. In addition to anger and guilt, such a child also must deal with loneliness.

As children develop, their awareness of self increases. They begin to think in terms of "me" and "mine" versus "not me" and "not mine." The thought of not being produces anxiety; thus children react through the process of denial. Denial allows them to deal with more tolerable and productive subjects that ultimately lessen the anxiety. These children avoid speaking of death. However, their play behavior often centers around accidents and disasters as they attempt to prove to themselves that existence, like their toys, can be controlled (Eason, 1970). Frequently hospitalized children of this age show less maturity in the level of their play, as well as less playfulness when compared with nonhospitalized children (Kielhofner, Barris, Bauer, Shoestock, & Walker, 1983).

The school-aged child is busy learning rules and is expected to exert some self-control and cooperation. Intellectually, the child of this age is able to solve problems through thoughts and actions. He or she develops increased self-awareness, leading to independence from parents. Meanwhile, parental beliefs are internalized. By late grade school, the child has developed special friends, and the children play with and help each other.

Smallness, vulnerability, and inadequacy characterize the grade-school child. Such a child deals with these feelings through denial and reaction formation (Eason, 1970). For example, he or she may try to act fearless, taking unnecessary risks.

Hospitalization involves various degrees of separation from family and friends. The grade-school child may be lonely and sad, as well as fearful of the unknown. A study by Spielberger, Gorsuch, Lushene, Vagg, and Jacobs (1972) indicated strong support for the hypothesis that terminally ill children show greater awareness of their hospital experience than do children who are chronically ill. These same children also expressed more hospital- and non–hospital-related anxiety. Homesickness, anger, frustration, and anxiety are usually expressed to the treatment staff in the form of refusing to cooperate. Some children might withdraw and become obviously depressed, but the usual course of behavior is one of regression. However, these children learn quickly from others and become sensitive to the feelings of the team.

Children who are involved in activities while in the hospital may become content and cheerful. Participation in play activities with peers can improve self-image. As death approaches, they may become sad and bitter, not wanting to leave the hospital. In addition, they may feel lonely from the realization that death is one trip that must be made alone. Thus comfort and security are sought.

On the whole, then, most children recognize the severity of their own illness, whether or not they have been presented with the diagnosis (Spinetta, Rigler, & Karon, 1973). They appear aware of the serious nature of their conditions, even though no one has told them how ill they are (Spinetta, 1974). They react according to their stage of development, as well as their sociocultural expectations. For the most part, children recognize a terminal illness and the resulting thoughts of death as the removal of independence. This and the intense feelings of separation affect their response to their own deaths.

■ ASSESSING THE CHILD'S UNDERSTANDING OF DEATH

Assessing the child's understanding of death is important when working with a terminally ill child. This process helps the therapist know how to best deal with the child's understanding of what is happening to him or her. Piaget's cognitive and Erikson's psychosocial development scales are useful for this purpose, because they give an accurate assessment of the child's understanding of death (Table 28-1). Using a general assessment of cognitive level is more appropriate than interviewing the child about death, because children tend to avoid this subject with someone they have just met. Rating scales to assess cognitive understanding and anxiety toward death may be helpful in this process (Prichard & Epting, 1992; Schell, 1991).

A second consideration in assessing the child's understanding is to record the parents' understanding of death and any relevant sociocultural ideas they have (Wenestam, 1989). These sociocultural aspects color a child's perception of death and may differ from the occupational

table 28-1 *Developmental Stages: Children's Perception of Death Compared with Erikson's Psychosocial and Piaget's Cognitive Stages*

Erikson's Psychosocial Stages	Piaget's Cognitive Stages	Perception of Death
1. *Trust vs. mistrust* (birth to 1 year) Development of the sense of trust through the pairing of the infant's actions with pleasant events.	1. *Sensorimotor period* (birth to 2 years) Based on the formation of action schemas for skilled movement, language, visual perception, and object permanence.	1. *Birth to 1 year* Reacts physiologically. Without bonding there is little desire to live (failure to thrive [FTT]).
2. *Autonomy vs. doubt, shame* (1 to 3 years) The terrible twos. Beginning development of control over one's body, self, and environment.	2. *Preoperational period* (birth to 7 years) The ability to symbolize through language, thought, drawing, and play. Egocentricity. Asks questions and why? Is more able to employ past events and to consider more than one aspect of an event at a time.	2. *1 to 4 years* Responds with fear and anxiety to treatment. Death has little or no meaning.
3. *Initiative vs. guilt* (3 to 5 years) Beginning exploration of the physical environment through senses and the social, physical worlds through language.	3. *Concrete operations* (7 to 11 years) Time of real, concrete thought. Orders, counts, and thinks in terms of cause and effect. Beginning to compare own views and ideas.	3. *4 to 6 years* Has the concept of "me" and "not me." Fantasy reasoning with an increased curiosity about dead animals, flowers, burial, and so on. Death is temporary.
4. *Industry vs. inferiority* (5 to adolescence) Begins to be a worker. Wants to please. Learns the meaning of rules and uses them.	4. *Formal operations* Beginning of abstract thought and reasoning. Ability to form hypotheses and test them.	4. *6 to 8 years* Death means being separated from loved ones and causes anxiety. The child learns to be a good patient. Superstitions about death predominate.
5. *Identity vs. role diffusion* Merging of past identity with future expectations (bodily, societal, and one's own).		5. *8 to 11 years* Death is realized to be permanent.
		6. *Adolescence* Speculates about what occurs after death. Death is perceived in terms of loss of independence and identity.

therapist's. When working with terminally ill children, one should also ask what expectations the parents have, whether they are willing to have their child told that he or she is terminally ill, and what approach they are using with the child.

■ OBJECTIVES FOR OCCUPATIONAL THERAPY INTERVENTION

Determining objectives for the child with a terminal illness is often difficult for the medical team. The team members realize this is a child who will not get well and who is different from the usual pediatric patient for whom they can set goals and develop long-term expectations. Therefore their objectives are mainly psychologic in nature, placing more emphasis on quality of life and less emphasis on physical aspects of it. The focus is not only on the child, but it is also on family members and

their ability to develop adaptive responses. The objectives are as follows:

1. Understand the origin and intensity of the child's anxiety.
2. Allow thoughts or reactions to death to come into the open.
3. Encourage expressions of grief.
4. Maintain comfort and provide support.
5. Facilitate and maintain independence.
6. Facilitate and maintain participation in activities of daily living.
7. Facilitate age-appropriate play skills.
8. Facilitate adaptive child-family relationships.

■ INTERVENTION MODALITIES

When providing occupational therapy care for children with terminal illness, the underlying principle is to add quality to their remaining days. There are two performance areas that occupational therapists should address in children with terminal illness: (1) play activities and (2) activities of daily living.

Until the age of 5, children learn about their world exclusively through play. They learn and practice activities before incorporating them into practical application. The more playful and interesting the subject, the more likely they are to learn. Play encourages social and emotional expression and development of coping strategies in children with terminal illness (Gray, 1989).

Activities that are appropriate for the child's developmental level, physical level (including endurance and tolerance), intellectual level, and emotional state should be chosen. Play allows the child to work through some of the feelings that he or she cannot express (or for which he or she has no words). It also allows the child to focus his or her interest on something in the world outside of himself or herself. The occupational therapist can also suggest play activities that are appropriate for and involve family members.

The second performance area that should be addressed in therapy with children who have terminal illness is activities of daily living. Too often adults take away the independence that a sick child has acquired. Parents and staff often jump to perform an activity, such as dressing or eating, to save the child's strength. However, by doing so they take away the vestiges of independence that remain for the child. Encouraging the continuation of routine activities of daily living allows a child to look forward to consistency and to know and have some control over what is coming in the future. As the child becomes weaker, energy conservation methods can be taught to parents and introduced to children that will allow them to remain as independent as possible in self-care. These modifications can be as simple as changing from metal to plastic utensils, using Velcro fastenings on clothing, and using pushcarts so that the child does not have to carry objects as weakness progresses. Modifications allow the child to continue functioning and to feel useful, rather than force the child to spend long hours on the sofa or bed watching countless television programs. The focus of energy conservation is not only on the child but also on family members and their ability to develop adaptive responses.

■ WORKING WITH THE FAMILY OF THE DYING CHILD

Parents must deal with the loss of their child throughout the process of the illness. They must also deal with the idea that they will continue to survive after their child's death (Davies et. al., 1998). Parents often suspect the severity of the child's illness and anticipate the news (Noland, 1971). Their reaction on hearing the diagnosis may range from loss of control to outward calm. Those who display a lack of affective response do so as a defense mechanism to allow themselves to deal realistically with the problems at hand. Clinical observers, as well as parents, report that it takes several days or weeks for the realization of the diagnosis to "sink in." Typically both parents are eager to hospitalize the child once it is suggested, because hospitalization renews their hope that the diagnosis is faulty and that treatment will cure their child.

With the realization of the diagnosis and the major decisions made as to treatment, the parents are then free to react to the situation. Initially the reaction appears as shock or denial contaminated by guilt (Noland, 1971). This guilt takes the form of the parents thinking either that they are the cause of the illness or that they did not pay enough attention to the child. This reaction, combined with questioning of the medical staff, represents an attempt by the parents of the terminally ill child to search for meaning or understanding of the situation. A problem occurs, however, if feelings of guilt become prolonged in nature and lead to overindulgence or to lack of discipline.

Denial is often part of the parents' coping strategy and may be the underlying reason for seeking other opinions. This search of other opinions represents the parent's hope that the diagnosis is incorrect. Binger and others (1969) studied 23 families of terminally ill children and found that the immediate family does not usually show this reaction; rather, the grandparents and friends of the family are often the ones who search for other opinions.

Intellectualization also occurs. Parents seek information about the disease and cures, especially from other parents on the hospital ward and from support groups. Information seeking is a natural and helpful coping strategy; it gives the family an intellectual understanding of the disease and helps them deal with the situation and the decisions that surround their child's treatment (Davies et. al., 1998). However, increasing questions from parents usually indicate increasing anxiety and guilt. This anxiety and guilt are not resolved by more information and suggest that the therapist should encourage parents to share their perceptions and feelings.

Throughout the course of the child's illness, hostility and anger are expressed by parents. Initially, this reaction appears as a fight to reverse the diagnosis. Next, parents often feel resentment that they, and their child, should suffer in such a manner. This may be complicated by guilt over their feelings of resentment, which is usually channeled outward and directed toward the medical team. The parents' fear of the unknown then produces feelings of anger and hostility. Further, in the course of an illness, sick children often do not act sick, which reinforces the parents' denial (Eason, 1970).

Parents often want to stay with their child during the course of his or her hospitalization. Urging the parents to return home may add to feelings of distress and guilt. The sick child's siblings are often neglected, increasing their feelings of rivalry and resentment toward their hospitalized brother or sister. Parents feel the constant need to cheer up their sick child. However, because hospitalization promotes feelings of separation and anxiety on the part of parents and sick children, this does not acknowledge a child's true feelings. While the parents are eager to hospitalize an extremely ill child to provide medical treatment, they are fearful to let the child go because hospitalization represents a loss of control. No longer is the parent in charge; the authority is transferred to the medical personnel, and eventually the parents must come to depend on the strength and support of the hospital.

Resentment is increased if the physician is unable to provide a curative treatment. This is complicated by the child's feelings. He or she expects parents to ease the pain and make him or her well. When parents are unable to do this, the child may become angry and the parents may have feelings of failure. A remission is anticipated eagerly until the child is allowed to return home. The child's parents then realize that they are in sole care of the child, and this increases their anxieties. Overprotective behavior displayed by the parents leads to resentment by others and affects all family members (Noland, 1971).

A relapse confronts the parents with the cold reality of the situation. They may react as if they had just learned of the diagnosis. A relapse causes great stress, and effective coping behavior is needed. Emotional states fluctuate, and transient episodes of ineffective coping are common. Successful coping behavior protects the parents from being overwhelmed by environmental and psychologic stress, while they continue to function in the medical and psychologic care of their child.

Anticipatory grief is the gradual occurrence of mourning behavior, precipitated by the first acute critical phase of a terminal illness (Cook et. al., 1973). It is typically characterized by somatic symptoms: apathy, weakness, preoccupation with thoughts of the ill child, sighing, occasional crying at night, and appearing depressed. At other times, parents may demonstrate increased motor behavior and increased talk about the child. These symptoms help to reintegrate the feelings with the gradual redirection of external energies (Friedman, 1967).

Physical complaints are gradually replaced by resignation and the desire to have the situation resolved. Parents turn their energies to other matters. Visits become a duty; the parents seem detached from their own child and more interested in the remaining children on the ward (Cook et. al., 1973). This is indicative of acceptance; mourning energies are being converted to more constructive means. Exhaustion of treatment options accelerates the grieving, and parents may experience decreasing understanding and become more prone to anger.

In chronic terminal cases, the parents have had time to rehearse how they will act. They usually control their expressions of grief, taking death calmly. However, if the parents have expressed denial continually throughout the course of their child's illness, death will be a shock, an experience of immediate loss. The parents often need many months before they can speak about the child without distress.

Finally, death is experienced with relief, and guilt is tinged with remorse (Lewis & Lewis, 1973). Mourning may deepen feelings of self-value through thoughts of death. In addition, the love and warmth felt for the dead child may lead to a greater sense of self-worth. Between 3 and 6 days after the child's death, the parents' mourning becomes less pronounced. However, parents may continue to interact with the hospital staff through gift giving, initiation of research foundations, and library donations. After the child's death, the parents tend to reverbalize their guilt, which is bound up with the feelings of relief.

Binger and others (1969) found that in half of the 23 families they studied, one or more members required psychiatric help after a child's death, although none had required it before. Mulhern (1983) found that 50% of the bereaved families had at least one member who had sought psychiatric or psychologic care, that 70% reported serious marital discord after the child's death, and that 25% to 50% of the surviving siblings experienced significant emotional, behavioral, or academic difficulties. Siblings evidenced higher levels of behavior problems and social incompetencies before, and up to a year after, their sibling's death (Birenbaum, Robinson, Phillips, & Stewart, 1989-1990). Three types of unhealthy family protective maneuvers can affect the sibling's relations. The first is the *conspiracy of guilt* that occurs when parents feel the death was preventable. Communication about the lost child is shrouded to protect the living members of the family. This evasive manner tends to support the idea that if the parents had acted differently, the child would still be alive. Therefore guilt is maintained, and the issue of the child's death is not explored for fear that someone will be blamed (Krell & Rabkin, 1979). Surviving children in such a family live in a world of distrust and in constant fear of what may be in store; they are hesitant to ask for clarification of what happened to their sibling.

A second unhealthy coping maneuver is the *preciousness of the survivor*. This leads to overprotection and shielding of the surviving children, with imagined attributes and expectations placed on them. This may lead to implications of specialness and good fortune placed on the survivors. Survivors may be filled with feelings of omnipotence and the desire to test fate, which limits their ability to develop practical coping mechanisms (Krell & Rabkin, 1979).

The last type of unhealthy family protective maneuver is the *substitution for the lost child*. The chosen child is likely to be vulnerable and forced to live a dual life: one of his or her own and one of the dead sibling's. Because of this, the child is not likely to develop a secure sense of identity (Krell & Rabkin, 1979). Unhealthy coping strategies used by families require outside intervention from mental health professionals. Even in healthier families, as evidenced by their more adaptive coping patterns, one finds persisting guilt, sadness, and health fears that continue to be problematic after a child's death (Mulhern, 1983).

After their experiences, families of dying children made the following suggestions to health care professionals (Noland, 1971):

1. Listen to what the families have to say about the deaths of their children.

2. Reassure parents to calm their guilt feelings.

3. Present information to parents at their level of understanding.

4. Answer questions patiently, kindly, and realistically.

Therapists should also realize that families might be grateful *and* angry. These angry feelings are dealt with best if the treatment team does not react to them as a personal insult or attack and if the anger can be channeled productively. If information is available on support groups, the staff members should make it known to parents (Brown, 1989). According to a survey of parents of pediatric oncology patients, parents also need to (1) have their child recognized as special, while attempting to retain normalcy in their lives; (2) have a caring relationship and feel a connectedness with their health care professionals; and (3) be responsible for parenting their child (James, 1997).

After a child's death, the family also experiences difficulty relinquishing the ties with the health care personnel who have been involved with their child's treatment. Increasing numbers of agencies and facilities offer bereavement counseling to aid the family through the first year after the child's death. This is thought to be the average length of time for family grief to be resolved, but it may endure as long as 3 years (Powell, 1991; Wessel, 1983).

Case Study 1: Jan

When Jan, the 11-year-old girl described at the beginning of this chapter, first had treatment, her facial cancer was hardly noticeable. She often came to the playroom. In the playroom, occupational therapists worked with the children, allowing them to express their feelings about the medical procedures through the use of play. For example, they encouraged the children to play nurse and doctor with a doll and actual, nonharmful medical items or play with age-appropriate toys.

After several admissions and subsequent surgery, Jan began to withdraw to her room. The staff initially tried to get her to come out, but eventually they obeyed her wishes and visited her in her room. By this time, Jan preferred quieter activities, such as painting, drawing, sewing, and crafts. These activities offered recognizable end products and allowed her to feel purposeful (i.e., able to accomplish a task from the beginning to the end).

As she became weaker because of the disease and the treatment for it, activities often consisted only of talking and reading. At that time Jan was being bathed primarily by the nursing staff, although she was encouraged to perform at least part of the routine herself. She could still feed herself most of her meals, although her intake was supplemented with intravenous feedings, and she continued to refuse to leave her room.

Jan began to draw away from the majority of the staff and her parents, as if to spare them the pain of her death. She allowed only a few people within her realm, thus adding to her life an element of control respected by the staff. It was during this time that Donna, the nursing student, became important to her. Donna and Jan talked together as Jan grew weaker and lost her ability to perform activities. Treatment eventually failed to produce a response, and Jan grew weaker and died.

Case Study 2: Courtney

Courtney is an 11-year-old girl. As an infant, she was diagnosed with many allergies to everyday substances. These allergies caused her to have chronic otitis media and pulmonary difficulties. Initially, she entered the therapy setting for treatment of sensory integration difficulties. The treatment she received for her balance and praxis difficulties was considered successful. However, Courtney's endurance continued to be poor.

Further medical evaluation suggested that she suffered from an HIV-like immunologic dysfunction. She had periods of good health, usually during the summer. During winter, pulmonary problems increased and, because of her immunologic problems, she was often unable to attend school with her friends. She was susceptible to communicable diseases and, because of her allergies, she could not be treated with antibiotics; she was allergic to most of them.

Fatigue was a constant with Courtney. When at school, she put on a strong front, but her mother reported that she was often in tears at home, wishing she could be "normal." On days that she could not attend school, Courtney received homebound instruction. Her occupational therapy services emphasized energy conservation and adaptations of her home environment to accommodate her reduced energy level. Courtney's therapist consulted with her mother and the school staff to develop an intervention program that would be less taxing for Courtney while still allowing her to feel independent. They included suggestions such as using a tape recorder to record assignments and a computer to write them, rather than requiring her to write assignments by hand. Another suggestion was to purchase word-prediction software that could save Courtney time and effort by predicting her style of writing.

Suggestions were also provided to help Courtney's parents organize their multilevel home so that she did not have to go up and down the stairs needlessly. Time was spent listening to Courtney's mother and providing suggestions for community resources to help her care for her daughter. For a sick child like Courtney, the goal of occupational therapy is to allow her to participate in the remainder of her childhood to the greatest extent possible (Gray, 1989).

■ WORKING WITH PERSONNEL CLOSE TO THE DYING CHILD

Although personnel who treat a dying child and counsel his or her family may feel compassion for the individuals involved in the case, they may also feel repulsed by the inherent threat of death that the case represents. Therapists should be aware of feelings of ambivalence produced by this conflict, because the ability to resolve it determines the degree of success of the health care team.

Because the primary goal of health care professionals is to help patients get well, a dying child prevents them from reaching this goal. This results in feelings of frustration and anger on the part of the health care professional. Nursing research indicates once a nurse realizes a child's death to be inevitable, he or she begins to struggle with grief and moral distress (Davies et. al., 1996). However, one cannot get angry with a sick child, and this situation often leads to feelings of guilt and even greater anger toward the one causing the guilt. This emotional state may become cyclic.

Sack, Fritz, Krener, & Springer (1984) found that the physicians used the following coping strategies to deal with a child's death: (1) they had a tendency to try to master anxiety-provoking situations; (2) they tended to want to change the environment and not themselves; and (3) they habitually used intellect to master their anxieties. These patterns do not benefit the child, the family, or the health care team involved with the child.

Reactions of the personnel toward the terminally ill child are influenced by previous experiences with death. The health care personnel may take the approach of being overprotective toward the child. This overprotectiveness often leads to overt or covert reactions of anger by the child. On the other hand, the staff members may be overindulgent, and thereby put an added burden of guilt on the child (e.g., the child begins to wonder what he or she has done to deserve special treatment). When the staff shows both types of behaviors, the inconsistency tends to confuse the child, who may not know how to

react. When treatment fails, health care professionals may accuse each other of failure, thus redirecting the anger, frustration, and irritation they feel toward each other because they were unable to help the child.

One staff member reacted to a child's dying by hopping into his sports car and racing the highways until he had worked through his distressed feelings. Although this is one method of coping, it produced anxiety in the rest of the staff until his safe return. Methods that are more constructive can channel anger and irritation into productive actions, whether oriented to motor release or to talking. Some of the methods currently used by staff members to deal with a child's death include individual counseling, team support group meetings, and case conferences, during which a child's course of treatment and eventual death are discussed.

Although a child's death is painful to everyone involved in the case, it can also be a time of learning about life, love, and the appreciation of others. The best advice is often the hardest to take. Parents recommend trying to live each day as it comes and enjoying one's child while they are present (Binger et. al., 1969). Occupational therapists are able to provide aid and support to these special children and their families.

■ SUMMARY

In working with dying children, occupational therapists must be aware of developmental differences in the way children and their parents view death. These differences, added to the impact of hospitalization, affect children's responses to treatment and to the health care professionals who provide it. Therapists can be effective in promoting play activities and activities of daily living. When working with a dying child, it is important to understand the positive and negative emotions affecting parents, staff, and self.

STUDY QUESTIONS

1. Write down your feelings about working with children who are dying. How do you think these feelings are going to influence your ability to work professionally with dying children?

2. How would your own view of death affect your interactions with the family of a dying child?

3. Children's understanding of death varies from age to age. How would this affect occupational therapy intervention with a preschool child, a grade-school child, and an adolescent?

4. What are the major roles of the occupational therapist when working with the family of a dying child?

References

Ashby, M.A., Kosky, R.J., Laver, H.T., & Sims, E.B. (1991, February 4). An inquiry into death and dying at the Adelaide Children's Hospital: A useful model. *Medical Journal of Australia, 154 (3)*, 165-170.

Barakat, L.T., Sills, R., & LaBagnara, S. (1995). Management of fatal illness and death in children or their parents. *Pediatric Review, 16* (11), 419-423.

Bergman, A.B. (1967). Psychosocial aspects in the care of children with cancer. *Pediatrics, 40 (3)*, 492-497.

Binger, C.M., Ablin, A.R., Reuerstein, R.C., Kushner, J.H., Zoger, S., & Mikkelsen, C. (1969). Childhood leukemia: Emotional impact on patients and family. *New England Journal of Medicine, 280*, 414-418.

Birenbaum, L.K., Robinson M.A., Phillips, D.S., & Stewart, B. (1989-90). The response of children to the dying and death of a sibling. *Omega Journal of Death and Dying, 20* (3), 213-228.

Brown, P.G. (1989). Families who have a child diagnosed with cancer: What the medical caregiver can do to help them and themselves. *Issues in Comprehensive Pediatric Nursing, 12* (2-3), 247-260.

Childers, P., & Wimmer, M. (1971). The concept of death in early childhood. *Child Development, 42*, 1299-1301.

Cook, S.S., Renshaw, D.C., & Jackson, E.N. (1973). *Children and dying: An exploration and a selected bibliography.* New York: Health Sciences Publishing.

Davies, B., Cook, K., O'Loane, M., Clarke, D., MacKenzie, B., Stutzer, C., Connaughty, S., & McCormick, J. (1996). Caring for dying children: Nurses' experience. *Pediatric Nursing, 22*, 500-507.

Davies, B., Deveau, E., deVeber, B., Howell, D., Martinson, I., Papadatou, D., Pask, E., & Stevens, M. (1998). Experiences of mothers in five countries whose child died of cancer. *Cancer Nursing, 21*, 301-311.

Eason, W.M. (1970). *The dying child: The management of the child or adolescent who is dying.* Springfield, IL: Charles C. Thomas.

Friedman, S.B. (1967). Care of the family of the child with cancer. *Pediatrics, 40*, 498-507.

Gray, E. (1989). The emotional and play needs of the dying child. *Issues in Comprehensive Pediatric Nursing, 12* (2-3), 207-224.

Huffman, S.L., & Martin, L. (1994). Child nutrition, birth spacing, and child mortality. *Annuals of New York Academy of Science, 709*, 236-248.

James, L., & Johnson, B. (1997). The needs of parents of pediatric oncology patients during the palliative care phase. *Journal of Pediatric Oncology Nursing (A14), 14* (2), 83-95.

Jeffrey, P., & Lansdown, R. (1982). The role of the special school in the care of the dying child. *Developmental Medicine and Child Neurology, 24* (5), 693-697.

Kane, B. (1979). Children's concepts of death. *Journal of General Psychology, 134*, 141-153.

Kielhofner, G., Barris, R., Bauer, D., Shoestock, B., & Walker, L. (1983). A comparison of play behavior in non-hospitalized and hospitalized children. *American Journal of Occupational Therapy, 37* (5), 305-312.

Koocher, G.P. (1973). Childhood, death, and cognitive development. *Developmental Psychology, 9* (3), 369-375.

Krell, R., & Rabkin, L. (1979). The effects of sibling death on the surviving child: A family perspective. *Family Process, 18* (4), 471-477.

Kübler-Ross, E. (1969). *On death and dying.* New York: Macmillan.

Lewis, M., & Lewis, D.O. (1973). The crisis of death: A child dies. *Current Problems in Pediatrics, 3*, 1-11.

Martinson, I.M. (1995). Improving care of dying children. *Western Journal of Medicine (XN5), 163* (3), 258-262.

Martinson, I.M. (1986-1987). Home care for the dying child with cancer: Feasibility and desirability. *Loss, Grief and Care, 1* (1-2), 97-114.

McDonnald, R.T., & Carroll, J.D. (1981). Appropriate death: College students preferences vs. actuarial projections. *Journal of Clinical Psychology, 37* (1), 28-31.

Meliar, J.D. (1973). Children's conception of death. *Journal of General Psychiatry, 123*, 359-366.

Mulhern, R.K. (1983). Death of a child at home or in the hospital: Subsequent psychological adjustment of the family. *Pediatrics, 71* (5), 743-747.

Nagy, M. (1959). The child's view of death. In W.H. Feifel (Ed.), *The meaning of death.* New York: McGraw-Hill.

Noland, R.L. (1971). *Counseling parents of the ill and the handicapped.* Springfield, IL: Charles C. Thomas.

O'Brien, C.R., Johnson, J.L., & Schmink, P.D. (1978). Death education: What students want and need. *Adolescence 1* (52), 729-734.

Oleske, J., Minnefor, A., Cooper, R., Thomas, K., dela Cruz, A., Ahdieh, H., Guerrero, I., Joshi, V.V., & Desposito, F. (1983). Immune deficiency syndrome in children. *Journal of the American Medical Association, 249*, 2345-2349.

Pizzi, M. (1984). Occupational therapy in hospice care. *American Journal of Occupational Therapy, 38* (4), 252-257.

Powell, M. (1991). The psychosocial impact of sudden infant death syndrome on siblings. *Irish Journal of Psychology, 12* (2), 235-247.

Prichard, S., & Epting, F. (1992). Children and death: New horizons in theory and measurement. *Omega Journal of Death and Dying, 24* (4), 271-288.

Sack, W.H., Fritz, G., Krener, P.G., & Sprunger, L. (1984). Death and the pediatric house officer revisited. *Pediatrics, 73* (5), 676-681.

Salladay, S.A., & Royal, M.E. (1981). Children and death: Guidelines for grief work. *Child Psychiatry and Human Development, 11* (4), 203-212.

Schell, D. (1991). Development of death anxiety scale for children. *Omega Journal of Death and Dying, 23* (3), 227-234.

Speece, M.W., & Brent, S.R. (1984). Children's understanding of death. *Child Development, 55*, 1671-1686.

Spielberger, C.D., Gorsuch, R.L., Lushene, R., Vagg, P.R., & Jacobs, G.A. (1972). *Children's State-Trait Anxiety Inventory.* Palo Alto, CA: Consulting Psychologist's Press.

Spinetta, J.J. (1974). The dying child's awareness of death: A review. *Psychology Bulletin, 81*, 256-260.

Spinetta, J.J., Rigler, D., & Karon, M. (1973). Anxiety in the dying child. *Pediatrics, 52*, 841-845.

Sternlicht, M. (1980). The concept of death in preoperational retarded children. *Journal of General Psychology, 137* (2), 157-164.

Tigges, K.N., & Sherman, L.M. (1983). The treatment of the hospice patient: From occupational history to occupational role. *American Journal of Occupational Therapy, 37*, 235-238.

Toews, J., Martin, R., & Prosen, H. (1985). Death anxiety: The prelude to adolescence. *Adolescent Psychiatry, 12*, 134-144.

U.S. Bureau of the Census. (1997). *Statistical Abstract of the United States: 1997* (117th ed.). Washington D.C: U.S. Government Office of Publications.

Von Hug-Hellmuth, H. (1965). The child's concept of death. *Psychoanalysis Quarterly, 34*, 499-516.

Weber, J.A. (1985). Family support and a child's adjustment to death. *Family Relations Journal of Applied Family and Child Studies, 34* (1), 43-49.

Weininger, O. (1979). Young children's concepts of dying and death. *Psychology Report, 44*, 395-407.

Wenestam, C.G. (1989). Om barns tankade om doden [On the thoughts of children about death]. *Psykisk-Halsa, 30* (3), 229-236.

Wessel, M.A. (1983). The primary physician and the death of a child in a specialized hospital setting. *Pediatrics, 71* (3), 443-445.

Wilson, D.C. (1988). The ultimate loss: The dying child. *Loss, Grief and Care, 2* (3-4), 125-130.

Suggested Readings

Kübler-Ross, E. (1983). *On children and death.* New York: Macmillan.

Oremland, E.K., & Oremland, J.D. (1973). *The effects of hospitalization on children.* Springfield, IL: Charles C. Thomas.

Picard, H.B., & Magno, J.B. (1982). The role of occupational therapy in hospice care. *American Journal of Occupational Therapy, 36* (9), 597.

chapter 29

Pediatric Rehabilitation

Brian J. Dudgeon

key terms

Subacute rehabilitation
Acute rehabilitation
Outpatient rehabilitation
Children with acquired injury and disease
Complications of chronic disability
Adaptive techniques for activities of daily living

■ CHAPTER OBJECTIVES

1. Describe the types of children who are commonly treated within hospital-based pediatric rehabilitation units and those who typically receive specialized outpatient clinic and therapy services.
2. Discuss existing research of pediatric rehabilitation programs and of specific interventions for children with common diagnoses.
3. Identify and describe collaborative relationships with other providers in interdisciplinary and transdisciplinary practice settings.
4. Propose and apply a prioritization system for assessment and intervention planning that guides selection of therapy goals and intervention approaches.
5. Emphasize teaching strategies as an integral component of therapy designed to optimize occupational performance.
6. Describe frames of reference commonly used in pediatric rehabilitation and apply them in a complementary manner in treatment planning.
7. Recognize opportunities for family involvement and explain levels of family participation.
8. Discuss the elements of a plan for transition of care from the hospital setting to home and the community.

In the past, children who required pediatric rehabilitation often experienced long-term hospital stays or frequent hospitalizations. For some children the hospital and staff members nearly took on the roles of a home and family. These environments addressed medical care and rehabilitative intervention and often branched into programs addressing socialization, education, and vocation (Burkett, 1989; Edwards, 1992). Currently, most pediatric therapy practice is delivered through school systems. This shift in policy, along with advances in medical care and rehabilitation practice, has changed the role of hospital-based pediatric rehabilitation. In general, most hospital-based programs now focus on acute-onset problems and provision of specialized services for children and adolescents with disabilities that are of low occurrence but high complexity. Hospital-based programs are continuing to evolve, aiming to address known and newly identified health threats in a way that emphasizes a partnership with the child and family and resources in their local community.

This chapter describes the scope of occupational therapy services provided as part of hospital-based pediatric rehabilitation services. As a context for occupational therapy practice, the organization of rehabilitation services is outlined and the types of children treated in these settings are discussed. Interdisciplinary care is emphasized, with the child and family as central participants in goal setting and decision making. Case studies are used to illustrate the occupational therapist's role in family-based evaluation, goal setting, and intervention processes. This chapter stresses strategies used by occupational therapists to address activities of daily living (ADLs) and the occupations of children, which include participation in school and other community activities. Specific techniques that reduce impairment and minimize disability are prioritized to support the child's requisite and desired performance goals within the environment that he or she regard as home and community.

A primary concept in the practice of pediatric rehabilitation is the differentiation of *habilitation* and *rehabilitation*. For children, *habilitation* is the term most often used to denote attention to the child's acquisition of expected age level skill and function. *Rehabilitation* is the classic term used to reflect the process of an individual working to regain skills and functions that had been established but subsequently lost. For most practitioners in pediatrics, the term *rehabilitation* is used to encompass both concepts. This is true because disability, whether new or chronic, creates ongoing challenges to current function and future demands that evolve as part of growth and development. In this chapter the term *rehabilitation* is used to include both concepts.

Children who experience injuries, diseases or illnesses, and complications from chronic disorders often experience loss of existing functions for which rehabilitation of previous skills becomes the primary goal. Nevertheless, ongoing development of age-specific skills throughout childhood, adolescence, and young adult years necessitates frequent reappraisal and shifts in rehabilitation goals and programming to address new skill needs. Gans (1993) has cautioned that some physical medicine and rehabilitation specialists incorrectly think of children as small adults. Orientation to the developmental needs of children and an appreciation for intensive involvement with families are critical to working within hospital-based pediatric rehabilitation programs.

Described in general terms, pediatric rehabilitation might be characterized as a planned approach involving any type and number of providers who specify a mission to focus on functional and psychosocial needs of children and their families. More formally, rehabilitation services in pediatrics may be received within one or more levels of care that have evolved as part of the health care delivery system. In general, these interdisciplinary services are designed to address the management of acute disabling conditions, prevention of secondary complications, recovery or enhancement of function, and a return to home, school, and community participation. Outcomes from pediatric rehabilitation can be difficult to predict because of the complexity of factors shaping perfor-

mance. Severity of impairments and spontaneous recovery, developmental changes and maturation, use of specific rehabilitation approaches, and characteristics of families and their environments combine to influence outcomes. Rehabilitation care should always be perceived as an ongoing process that is best carried out as a partnership between family, community, school, and the hospital's specialized programs.

■ LEVELS OF SERVICES

Levels of rehabilitation services are subacute, acute, and outpatient or ongoing care. This range is best understood by reviewing typical programs of care and contrasting different purposes within and across settings.

Subacute Rehabilitation

Subacute rehabilitation services are typically organized within skilled nursing facilities (SNFs) or other long-term care settings. Such programs are designed for children and adolescents who are too medically fragile or dependent to be cared for at home but who are not yet able to tolerate or benefit from the intensive efforts of acute rehabilitation. After initial hospitalization, children and adolescents with moderate to severe head injury, multi-trauma, or other systemic illnesses may be admitted to an SNF with subacute rehabilitation services. In these settings, children may receive daily therapy to prevent secondary complications and work toward goals of greater independent function. This interdisciplinary care may culminate in admission to an acute rehabilitation program or a planned discharge to an organized home- and community-based service system of care.

Acute Rehabilitation

Acute rehabilitation is characterized by inpatient hospital units and services. Three types of programs are included in this category. The most common are dedicated rehabilitation units within children's hospitals. Another form of organization is the specification of beds and services for pediatric patients within a large rehabilitation hospital. A third setting involves the designation of pediatric beds in a large rehabilitation unit that is part of a comprehensive hospital system. Adolescents 15 years of age or older may also be admitted to rehabilitation units that commonly serve adults and older adults. Children and adolescents are admitted to acute rehabilitation from other acute or transitional care medical services within the hospital, other local hospitals, or subacute rehabilitation settings. Children and adolescents who are admitted to trauma centers may be regularly screened to identify the need for transfer to children's hospitals or other rehabilitation units. Some children are also admitted to acute rehabilitation directly from community care providers or through the hospital's outpatient clinics and services.

table 29-1 Rapid Onset

Type of Onset	Examples
Accidental injury	Traumatic brain injury (e.g., closed head injury)
	Skull fracture or penetrating head injury
	Burns and smoke inhalation
	Multitrauma
	Near drowning
	Spinal cord injury
Violence	Multitrauma
	Traumatic brain injury (e.g., gunshot wound)
	Burns, iron burns, cigarette burns, and scalding
Disease processes	Central nervous system infection (e.g., encephalitis and meningitis)
	Transverse myelitis
	Guillain Barré syndrome
	Cancer

table 29-2 Complications in Children with Chronic Disorders

Type of Onset	Examples
Neurologic	Spina bifida
	Cerebral palsy
	Mental retardation
Orthopedic	Juvenile rheumatoid arthritis
	Congenital amelia and dwarfism
	Arthrogryposis multiplex congenital
Muscular	Muscular dystrophy
Pulmonary	Bronchopulmonary dysplasia

table 29-3 Special Medical Procedures

Type of Procedure	Examples
Clinical procedure	Selective dorsal rhizotomy
	Continuous intrathecal baclofen
	Ilizarov
Medical technology	Ventilator dependence

Essential to acute rehabilitation programs is the presence of a broad range of services, including occupational therapy, and specific requirements for intensity of services to meet goals that are systematically developed. Such programs are characterized as meeting three types of needs (Tables 29-1 to 29-3):

1. Organize and implement a planned approach for the management of recovery and rehabilitation of children with rapid-onset disorders.
2. Redirect care after onset of complications in children with chronic disorders.
3. Provide an environment for specialized medical or surgical procedures that involves specific care regimens and protocols.

Children and adolescents who sustain a sudden illness or injury are the most common type of admission in acute rehabilitation. Table 29-1 indicates the common problems that affect a typically developing child who experiences injury from accidents, violence, or rapid-onset disease. Acquired injuries or diseases represent a substantial health threat to children (Moront & Eichelberger, 1994; Rodriquez & Brown, 1990). Injuries are the leading cause of death and disability among children older than 1 year of age. Traumatic brain injuries (TBIs), including closed head injury, skull fracture, and penetrating brain injuries, are an increasingly recognized problem among children and adolescents because of transportation-related crashes, falls, recreational injury, and violence. Such causes are also associated with children who sustain spinal cord injury (SCI) and multitrauma. Environmental hazards, accidents, and abuse are also implicated among children who experience burns, near drowning, smoke inhalation, carbon monoxide poisoning, or drug overdose.

Aside from known hazards, children also develop infections that involve the central nervous system (CNS); they may sustain cerebrovascular accidents or acquire other neurologic disorders such as transverse myelitis or Guillain-Barré syndrome. Cancer and its treatment may cause children and adolescents to develop problems necessitating acute rehabilitation. All of these disorders are characterized by typical development and an acute health crisis that causes a severe loss of function, a likelihood of prolonged recovery with residual disability, and chronic health complications associated with disability. For such children and their families, the purpose of rehabilitation is to prevent further deterioration or the development of complications, as well as organize and implement an approach to initial and long-term management that optimizes function in family and community life.

Children with congenital or chronic disorders may also require acute rehabilitation (see Table 29-2). Many youths with genetic disorders or other congenital abnormalities, or those who experience chronic disease, often have delayed or atypical patterns of functional skill development. These children are also at risk for complications that can create a gradual or critical loss of function. Episodes of respiratory complications, bony fractures and dislocations, skin breakdown, or other systemic complications may be associated with functional deterioration. Children with cerebral palsy, spina bifida, or other types of congenital defects are included in this at-risk group. Likewise, children with congenital limb deficiency or arthrogryposis multiplex congenital syndrome may have reconstructive surgery necessitating acute rehabilitation. Children with osteogenesis imperfecta may have episodes of curtailed functional gains after injury and require acute rehabilitation services. Juvenile rheumatoid arthritis and systemic disorders can be associated with periods of rapid decline in function. For these children, the goals of rehabilitation are to limit or prevent further losses and facilitate reacquisition of skills consistent with the pattern of functional progression that was previously shown.

The third major group of children who receive acute rehabilitation services are those who are hospitalized for treatment with special medical, surgical, or technologic procedures (see Table 29-3). For children with cerebral palsy, use of new medical interventions such as selective dorsal rhizotomy, continuous intrathecal baclofen, or other neurosurgical techniques to reduce spasticity may involve admission to acute rehabilitation (Albright, 1992). Ilizarov procedures, the surgical technique of increasing congenital limb length or repairing severe orthopedic injury, may also be associated with acute rehabilitation (Mosca, 1991). Children with severe pulmonary complications or those who are ventilator dependent may be admitted for acute rehabilitation to assist families in learning how to perform care procedures and use medical technology (Buschbacher, 1995; Richardson & Robinson, 1989). These interventions often involve the therapists in following specific evaluation and treatment protocols designed to optimize functional outcomes.

A key feature of all types of admissions to acute rehabilitation is an emphasis on the planning and facilitation of community-based care plans. Discharge planning typically begins at referral to rehabilitation. School and other community-based providers are invited to participate in discharge arrangements that ease the transition from hospital to home and school settings. Often the hospital's outpatient services or clinics are recommended to monitor care and serve as an ongoing resource to the family and local care providers who implement the greater part of rehabilitation that takes place in home and school settings.

Outpatient and Ongoing Rehabilitation

Another major component of pediatric rehabilitation exists within specialized outpatient services and clinics that provide ongoing care. Typically, as part of children's hospitals or rehabilitation hospitals, interdisciplinary outpatient clinics are organized to provide monitoring and interventions with children who experience particular types of chronic health risks and disabilities. Occupational therapists often provide follow-up and follow-along attention to children and families after hospitalization, but many of these children are never hospitalized. Therapists who work at these clinics most often focus on the child's or adolescent's health status and develop-

ment, emphasizing functional progress and participation in home, school, and community activities.

Clinic programs that most commonly involve occupational therapists are displayed in Table 29-4. Such clinic programs may be scheduled weekly, monthly, quarterly, or even annually as needed. Sometimes these programs are conducted away from the hospital facility at community sites such as schools. Often the therapists offer consultation and recommendations to the family and local therapists who know the particular child well but have limited experience with a specific disorder or type of specialized intervention. For example, school personnel may have limited experience with children who have arthrogryposis, limb deficiency, or various forms of muscular dystrophy, whereas the hospital clinic therapists would have regular (e.g., weekly) experiences with these disabilities. Rapid developments in assistive technology (AT) also limit the likelihood that all schools or local programs can remain current and effective in applying new systems and approaches. Therapists who work in specialized hospital programs are provided with unique exposure to otherwise uncommon diagnoses and clinical procedures and can pass this experience on to other families and therapists as a conduit of information and new ideas. Specific study and preparation for consultation is sug-

table 29-4	Outpatient Clinics and Programs Often Served by Occupational Therapists
Clinic Title	**Example of Clients or Services**
Congenital disorders	Spina bifida
Neuromuscular disorders	Cerebral palsy
Developmental disabilities	Down syndrome
	Fetal alcohol syndrome
Rheumatology	Juvenile rheumatoid arthritis
	Systemic lupus erythematosis
Craniofacial abnormality	Cleft lip and palate
Orthopedic	Traumatic hand injury
	Congenital limb deficiency
Rehabilitation	Traumatic brain injury
	Spinal cord injury
Muscular dystrophy	Duchenne's muscular dystrophy
	Spinal muscle atrophy
Limb deficiency	Congenital amelia
	Traumatic amputation
Cystic fibrosis	Cystic fibrosis
Assistive technology	Seating and positioning
	Wheelchair control
	Augmentative communication
	Computers and information technology

gested for entry-level therapists and can be an important skill for the therapist to develop as part of pediatric rehabilitation (Dudgeon & Greenberg, 1998).

Therapists also provide outpatient services in the form of individualized assessment and therapy trials at the hospital, home-based programs, or free-standing outpatient clinics. Outpatient services often occur concurrently with the child's return to school and school-based therapy; the former is organized around medical needs, whereas the latter addresses educational performance.

Efforts to augment function beyond the child's current development are also represented by efforts to apply uses of AT (see Chapters 19 and 20). The therapist may plan outpatient services to permit intensive evaluation and trials in use of aided and augmentative communication systems, computer access and use of information technologies, therapeutic seating, powered mobility, or other technologies that enable environmental access and control. These applications of special procedures or AT devices are characterized by preplanned and often short trials leading to prescription of devices. Efforts culminate in intensive family training and transitions to follow-up in the community often as a partnership with local providers in the environments in which AT devices are used.

Another form of outpatient pediatric rehabilitation service is characterized by residential or intensive day-treatment programs. Interdisciplinary services are most often organized for children and adolescents with brain injury. These extended care programs are geared toward direct assistance with community reentry and participation. Simulated or actual environments become the training site for skills that enable community participation and effective performance toward goals of independent living, education, and work activities.

Accrediting Agencies

Pediatric rehabilitation advocates and service providers have both influenced and been shaped by accreditation processes. For example, the Heath Care Financing Administration (HCFA), the agency responsible for administering Medicare and Medicaid programs in most states, designates requirements for services that are organized and paid to provide "medical rehabilitation." To meet HCFA guidelines for rehabilitation, rules are placed on such systems that mandate specific program emphasis, dedicated space and personnel, admission and discharge procedures, service intensity, goal setting, and monitoring of progress toward goals. Most rehabilitation programs also pursue voluntary accreditation by groups such as the Joint Commission on Accreditation of Healthcare Organizations (JCAHO) and the Commission on Accreditation of Rehabilitation Facilities (CARF). These organizations assign additional mandates that also shape program characteristics. Such guidelines may include integrated planning with community-based services and continuous quality improvement procedures. Every few

years, accreditation standards and procedures based on JCAHO and CARF shift emphasis and specification of essential requirements. Generally, after initial accreditation, reaccreditation visits are scheduled every 3 years and programs may be subject to periodic interim review and reporting about their overall performance.

Reimbursement for Services

Inpatient pediatric rehabilitation services are typically funded by a combination of private insurance carriers, Medicaid, and under some circumstances by Medicare. Preadmission review and authorization are generally required. Comprehensive rehabilitation units continue to be exempt from the prospective payment funding systems based on diagnosis-related groups (DRGs). However, new DRG equivalents called *function-related groups* specific to medical rehabilitation are being developed. Rehabilitation costs are generally regarded as difficult to predict, and additional work is underway to develop appropriate prospective payment systems for both inpatient and outpatient services. Occupational therapy has typically been recognized as a service that is reimbursed within inpatient medical rehabilitation, home health care, and less commonly in outpatient services. Medicare guidelines are generally universal across different states. However, each state's Medicaid rules and regulations, and local insurance companies, have differing provisions related to funding of occupational therapy services and supplies or assistive devices that may be used or recommended. Review of local regulations is necessary to ensure that appropriate levels of reimbursement are available and that families are informed about service options.

Lengths of stay for acute pediatric rehabilitation are varied, from as short as a few days, to weeks, or perhaps months. Like adult rehabilitation units and all inpatient hospitals, third-party payers and other regulators strive to control costs by seeking shortened lengths of stay and transfer of patients more quickly to skilled nursing facilities, home care, outpatient, or school-based services in the family's local community. Changes within and across treatment settings can be problematic, often resulting in confusion among families about entitlements and expectations for services. Clearly stated goals and time frames for outcomes in each care setting are desired. Case managers, who are familiar with funding rules and regulations, work with families and rehabilitation teams to coordinate services and prepare the family for transitions between care settings.

■ REHABILITATION TEAM

Hospital-based rehabilitation permits the child and family to benefit from a wide range of medical care specialists and services that they can access as needed. Pediatric rehabilitation teams also include various providers with differing expertise. Such teams are most often led by physicians who are trained as pediatricians and in other arenas of practice, such as neurology, orthopedics, or developmental medicine. In recent years, leadership in pediatric rehabilitation has come primarily from pediatricians jointly certified in the practice of physiatry (rehabilitation medicine).

The rehabilitation team places an emphasis on interdisciplinary teamwork, with each discipline having particular capabilities or areas of focus. Sometimes the team uses a transdisciplinary model so that only one or two professionals work directly with a particular child or family. Specific roles for each discipline within acute rehabilitation have been described for teams consisting of physicians, nurses, occupational therapists, physical therapists, speech-language pathologists, therapeutic recreational specialists, psychologists, social workers, educators, and other specialists (Blatzheim, Edberg, & Lacy, 1987; Eigsti, Aretz, & Shannon, 1990; Gardner & Workinger, 1990). In larger programs, specialty teams may develop so that the same personnel treat children grouped by diagnosis (e.g., TBI).

Team Interaction

Interdisciplinary care within pediatric rehabilitation is common and mandated by most regulatory mechanisms. The success of such collaboration often depends on a shared mission that focuses the team's energy and creativity. Team conferences that involve the family are characteristic. The team holds family conferences on admission, at key decision points during the hospitalization, and at discharge to ensure communication and clarification of care recommendations with the family and local care providers. In addition, the team conducts weekly rounds to review the progress of each child and discuss any changes in treatment plans that are designed for each problem.

The occupational therapist's holistic concerns related to health, function, and participation necessitate and are enriched by the collaborative relationships among team members of multiple disciplines. Partnerships between registered therapists and certified assistants can broaden the scope and timeliness of services. Need for frequent reevaluation and trials with new strategies necessitate dynamic and shared interventions. Team efforts are the rule rather than the exception in pediatric rehabilitation. For example, occupational and physical therapists often take a joint interest in addressing a child's gross and fine motor skills related to positioning, transfers, wheelchair seating, and functional mobility. The therapists can evaluate feeding and swallowing and augmentative communication and plan interventions in cooperation with speech-language pathologists. Nursing and occupational therapy personnel typically have collaborative roles dealing with skills such as grooming, dressing, and bathing

and training in special care routines of toileting and skin care. Occupational therapists may work together with therapeutic recreation specialists to provide adaptive play and socialization through activity and community outings.

A primary goal with children is to improve their participation and performance in educational programs. Acute rehabilitation programs and children's hospitals typically have teachers on staff. In conjunction with occupational therapists and other team members, these educators and developmental specialists can address skills and special needs that the child will have on return to school. Psychologists and those who specialize in neuropsychology also provide suggestions for school placement and may work with occupational therapists to adapt learning strategies for the child as he or she returns to the classroom. Social workers typically address issues of adjustment and coping with the child and family. Occupational therapists, like all team members, are sensitive and supportive when educating family members to assume new duties as care providers. Recommendations should seek a realistic balance within the family culture, established roles, and new responsibilities for care.

Families

The therapist must recognize that many families are dealing with tragic events or at least unexpected complications that seriously affect their life processes. The children and adolescents are also challenged to deal with changes, and this process can be further complicated by their own cognitive or behavioral impairments (Donders, 1993). An educational model may provide a helpful perspective. Recognizing that family members have a short amount of time to learn a great deal about caring for their family member who is faced with new disabilities, rehabilitation team members also need to devote their time and attention to understanding the family's priorities and learning preferences. In all cases, the normal routines of the family are severely altered by hospitalization and residual disability (Rivara, 1993). This often creates worry, grief, and financial hardships that necessitate a transformation of relationships (Guerriere & McKeever, 1997). Families function in different ways, and variations in styles appear to have a lot to do with effective coping (Rivara et. al., 1996). Healthy and resilient families may show exceptional caring, open communication, balancing of family needs, and positive problem-solving abilities. Families with limited coping skills may need increased support and help in identifying resources to meet immediate needs and in coping with problems that they will face during transitions back to managing the child at home. In either case, the needs of families often change during the rehabilitation process, requiring ongoing attention to maintain a collaborative partnership that can achieve the best outcomes for the child.

Transition from Rehabilitation to the Community

To facilitate continuity of care when the child is discharged from a pediatric rehabilitation hospitalization, the team and family should develop a comprehensive plan of transition. The child's transition from hospital to home is successful when both the sending and receiving agencies coordinate the transition (Case-Smith & Wavrek, 1998). Often a child with a TBI requires special education services after discharge from the medical center. Team and family activities and communication need to focus on the transition from rehabilitation to school and community as soon as discharge is considered. Transition activities include interagency team meetings at which school and rehabilitation team members are represented. Ideally, at least one interagency meeting occurs in the rehabilitation unit and at least one in the school. By sharing where the meeting is hosted, team members get a realistic picture of the child's environments. When the meeting is at the team's home site, most, if not all, team members who worked with the child can be involved. By meeting the child and family before discharge and learning about the child's condition and needs, the school personnel can begin to plan and prepare an educational program. Visits by the medical team to the school at which the child will receive follow-up services can promote continuity of care. Therapists from the hospital and school should share information related to concerns, priorities, and results of intervention approaches (what worked and what did not). The child's rehabilitation team can help problem solve issues in the school's accessibility, appropriate levels of sensory stimulation in the classroom, and possible modifications to the curriculum. Visits to the child's classroom can help identify accommodations that need to be in place. During these visits, the rehabilitation team can present information to the other students in the class about the child's disability, his or her rehabilitation, and the types of changes that they may expect in their peer. An inservice about the injury is most important when a child returns to his or her preinjury classroom, because the student's peers have preset expectations about his or her behavior and personality, or in the case of severe burns, about the student's appearance. In addition, before discharge, the child should visit his or her home, school, and other important environments to determine what accommodations will need to be made. Visits followed by a return to the hospital can allow both school and hospital teams to address the issues proactively.

Monitoring by the rehabilitation team during the first few months after discharge is critical. Often the child continues with outpatient services while initiating school-based services. Duplicate services can be beneficial during the period of transition as the child continues to make rapid progress while struggling to adapt to new environments. The consistent individuals in the transition are the family members, who ultimately support the child through the transition to the home. In support of the family's transition, the teams involved should provide the parents with comprehensive information about the special education system in their community, their rights as parents of a child who newly qualifies for special education services, and other community programs, supports, and resources that they can access.

■ RESEARCH ON EFFICACY OF PEDIATRIC REHABILITATION PROGRAMS

Improvements in ADLs and disposition at discharge are typically the most common measures used to document the benefits of rehabilitation with children and adults (Fuhrer, 1987; Jaffe, Okamoto, & Lemire, 1986). Most research of acute rehabilitation outcomes has been descriptive. Evidence regarding benefits of specific intervention strategies is known to be lacking because it is tremendously difficult and costly to conduct research that analyzes application of particular techniques of rehabilitation. Experimental research of rehabilitation effectiveness is particularly difficult to conduct because of the heterogeneity of participants and ethical conflicts encountered by suspending or withholding services to specific children.

In general, early referral to rehabilitation specialists is recommended, but patterns of recovery and benefits from services vary by diagnostic group. For example, after TBI, an extended period of recovery is expected. Boyer and Edwards (1991) reviewed outcomes of 220 children and adolescents with TBI who were admitted to a comprehensive pediatric rehabilitation program. They reported continued progress in mobility, ADLs, and education and cognition for up to 3 years after the injury. Physical recovery was greatest in the first year, and cognitive and language gains generally occurred later.

Researchers have studied complications from TBI by following a series of children identified in trauma registries (Coster, Haley, & Baryza, 1994; DiScala, Osberg, Gans, Chin, & Grant, 1991). Jaffe and others conducted the most thorough follow-up of children with head injury (Fay et. al., 1994; Jaffe, Fay et. al., 1993; Jaffe, Massagli et. al., 1993; Jaffe, Polissar, Fay, & Liao, 1995). In this series, researchers developed an age-matched cohort to provide a careful assessment of sequelae from mild, moderate, and severe classifications of TBI. Among these children who were 6 to 15 years of age at the time of injury, many with moderate and most with severe injury evidenced persisting and comprehensive cognitive, language, academic, behavioral, and functional deficits.

More common than appraisal of rehabilitation techniques or measurement of specific outcomes, the pediatric rehabilitation literature has addressed both inpatient and *outpatient rehabilitation* needs of specific populations. Massagli and Jaffe (1990) have described rehabilitation needs of children with SCI and report follow-up of a series of children returning to school (Dudgeon, Massagli, & Ross, 1997). Outcomes of care after SCI from achondroplasia have also been reported (Wieting & Krach, 1994). Children with a primary brain tumor who received rehabilitative care have been reported to show improved management of residual disability (Philip, Ayyangar, Vanderbilt, & Gaebler-Spira, 1994). Rehabilitative needs of other children have also been demonstrated, including burns (Herndon, Rutan, & Rutan, 1993), osteogenesis imperfecta (Binder et. al., 1993), spina bifida (Watson, 1991), asthma (Strunk, Mascia, Lipkowitz, & Wolf, 1991), pulmonary disorders (Buschbacher, 1995), and other disorders (Heery, 1992; Russman, 1990).

The service model of inpatient rehabilitation with adults shows improvements in function, with or without reductions in impairment (Roth et. al., 1998), and comparable benefits appear to be found in similar programs designed for children. However, specific analysis of different priorities within pediatric rehabilitation, mixtures of service providers, or contrasts with less intensive subacute or outpatient services have not been reported. Routine appraisal of individual benefits and overall program effectiveness are being mandated by professional organizations, the insurance industry, and government agencies involved in regulation and reimbursement of rehabilitation programs and services. Additional research of pediatric rehabilitation program outcomes experienced by children within common diagnostic groups can be expected in coming years.

▪ OCCUPATIONAL THERAPY SERVICES

Functions of Occupational Therapists

The primary focus of the occupational therapist within pediatric rehabilitation is on ADLs and other instrumental tasks associated with independent living, school performance, and community participation. Therapists use many frames of reference to develop insights about the child's function, establish priorities for treatment, and guide the organization of treatment goals with the child, family, and local care providers. In most forms of rehabilitation, the therapist follows a prioritization system that first focuses on prevention of problems associated with major trauma or disability, then resumption of the able self, and finally restoration of lost skills and functions. A key concept in rehabilitation is the recognition that therapy is learning (Schwartz, 1991). Thus the therapist employs behavioral and cognitive learning principles and the interpersonal relationship inherent in a teacher-pupil relationship. The therapist emphasizes

a blending of his or her technical competency with personal caring and mutuality of goals and efforts with children and their families.

Activity analysis is another universal strategy that therapists use to determine skill requirements of functional tasks and the therapeutic activities selected to improve skills. Such analysis leads to the breakdown of tasks into sensorimotor, cognitive, and psychologic components of performance. The therapist can reorganize or adapt functional activities so that skillful components are substituted or emphasized over those that are missing or deficit. Specific intervention techniques used to achieve priority goals combine biomechanical, sensorimotor, perceptual-cognitive, and rehabilitative treatment approaches (see Chapters 10 to 13).

Prevention

Primary prevention is a term used to denote efforts that decrease the likelihood of accidents, violence, or disease. *Secondary* and *tertiary prevention* refer to specific interventions, arrangement of care systems, and environmental modifications to prevent the onset of problems among at-risk populations. Children admitted to pediatric rehabilitation units are typically at risk for developing a number of secondary disabilities. The therapist, along with other team members, has a responsibility to be familiar with such risks. Included are concerns for safety in positioning and movement, risks of aspiration in swallowing, provision of orientation, and appropriate measures to reduce stresses experienced in an unfamiliar environment and prevent self-injurious behaviors. The therapist must be aware of risks and avoid involving the child in ADLs that would be harmful or would perpetuate impaired habits that could hamper recovery. Complications from immobilization, abnormal muscle tone, and other neuromuscular abnormalities often necessitate careful attention to maintaining range of motion, strength, and general fitness (Figure 29-1). Concern for wound healing and protection of neurogenic skin are also essential to the early planning and ongoing achievement of goals, interventions, and education of the child and his or her family.

Resumption

The second level of priority for occupational therapy is a focus on resuming the use of available skills and independence in easily accomplished tasks. Emphasizing the able self provides the individual child with an opportunity to resume doing tasks on his or her own, or at least to have a say about how he or she is assisted. Such an approach may be important in preventing the child or adolescent from developing dependent behaviors or learned helplessness. The latter has been commonly described in adults who are admitted to institutional-like settings in which supervision is abundant and behaviors are not encouraged (Raps, Peterson, Jonas, & Seligman, 1982). Efficiency demands placed on nursing may often cause the child to be-

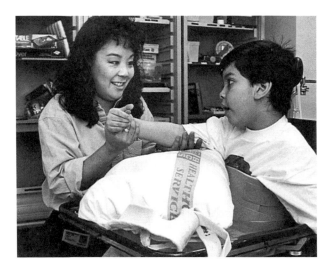

figure 29-1   Active assistive range of motion exercises are performed several times each day to prevent joint and muscle contractures with this boy who sustained a severe closed head injury. Stretch is also applied to existing contractures, along with other joint mobilization techniques.

come a passive recipient of care. The therapist should provide the child with sufficient time to perform activities on his or her own. Early emphasis on providing children with opportunities to make choices about the types of assistance they receive or activities they pursue should help them develop confidence in their returning abilities.

Restoration

Lost skills and function follow in priority, with efforts to restore abilities. The therapist uses biomechanical, sensorimotor, perceptual-cognitive, and rehabilitative approaches individually or in combination to restore function. Such approaches may necessitate extensive retraining or complex adaptation. When performance is severely impaired, reacquisition of skill is often initiated during acute rehabilitation with continuation of training as part of outpatient and ongoing rehabilitative care.

Each prioritization level may capitalize on treatment strategies drawn from frames of references that directly address performance component skills versus those that address occupational performance areas. For example, biomechanical and sensorimotor techniques are designed to improve component skills such as strength, range of motion, postural control, skilled movements, and coordination. Such approaches include use of therapeutic activities and exercise, splinting and positioning, physical handling, and use of biomedical devices like functional electric stimulation. Children with perceptual and cognitive difficulties are retrained or taught adapted methods of compensation.

Practicing activities that selectively challenge component skills are often used with the expectation that skills will transfer or generalize to ADLs and work perfor-

mance. Rehabilitative approaches contrast with biomechanic and sensorimotor techniques designed to sensorimotor, cognitive, or psychologic skill levels. In the rehabilitation approach, therapists teach clients compensatory techniques that use existing skills to maintain or restore function. In rehabilitative approaches, therapists teach clients to use adapted routines and AT devices and modify environments to promote optimal function. Initial training and use of AT devices to enable manipulation, mobility, and communication are part of restoration. Client outcomes are optimal when occupational therapists use complementary strategies to improve the child component skills, adapt functional activities, and modify environmental contexts.

Evaluation

In nearly all instances, occupational therapy services in hospital-based pediatric rehabilitation are initiated through physician's orders. Often required by law or regulatory guidelines, therapists respond to initial orders and negotiate as necessary with the physician to add specific elements to assessment and intervention activities. Most commonly, initial orders to occupational therapy involve a focus on ADLs and component skills that support function.

Multiple sources for data are available within the pediatric rehabilitation setting. Review of medical records and discussions with other providers may form the initial basis for evaluation. In general, evaluation consists of asking (e.g., clinical interview), looking (e.g., clinical observation), touching (e.g., physical examination), and testing (e.g., using standardized assessments). Most often, the therapist uses clinical interview and observation to initiate the assessment process. Observed areas of concern may necessitate a more thorough evaluation through physical examination and direct observation with the use of standardized tests. Such measures help in the diagnostic process. Impairments in performance components are likely to be implicated as causes of ADL disabilities. Once the therapist makes the hypotheses and initiates intervention plans, the repeated use of clinical examination and standardized tests serves as objective measures of skill improvement. For diagnostic purposes, the therapist judges a child's performance against normed scores, but for evaluative purposes, the therapist judges a child's scores on reassessment against his or her previous performance. Selection of a specific measure should be based on its reliability, sensitivity, and appropriateness given the child's age and diagnosis.

Evaluation of ADL skills helps prioritize which components and impairments require a more detailed evaluation. After evaluation of the child's ability to participate in functional activities, the therapist analyzes performance components to determine the skills to be targeted in intervention and the types of adaptations that may be warranted.

The therapist may organize assessment of ADLs around checklists or other reporting tools that specify activities and methods of rating the individual's level of skill. For example, the Functional Independence Measure (FIM) was developed as part of a Uniform Data System for Medical Rehabilitation for use in patient and program monitoring and outcome evaluation systems (Keith, Granger, Hamilton, & Sherwin, 1987). The FIM is generally for individuals 7 years of age and older. A pediatric version of this tool, called the *Wee-FIM,* has been developed for children of developmental age 6 months to 7 years (Msall, DiGaudio, & Duffy, 1993). Eighteen specific ADL tasks, including communication and social cognition, are rated for dependence based on the individual's need for adaptation and assistance from a helper.

Another tool that the therapist can use for rating and describing function in children is the Pediatric Evaluation of Disability Inventory (PEDI) (Haley, Coster, Ludlow, Haltiwanger, & Andrellos, 1992). Based on a combination of interview and observation, the PEDI specifies discrete levels of skills in domains of self-care, mobility, and social function. A description of needs for care provider assistance and reliance on AT devices is included with the measure. Both the FIM and PEDI are used for individualized assessment and planning; both are used in program evaluation. Although these tools focus directly on daily functional tasks, use of additional broad-based measures that assess play- and school-related performance are also encouraged in rehabilitation settings (Johnston & Granger, 1994).

Following these functional assessments, the therapists have specific directions to pursue an analysis of performance components. Tools and methods to evaluate performance components are described in Chapters 7 and 8.

Determining Intervention Goals

As stated throughout this text, goals for services must be explicitly stated, measurable, and functionally relevant. A goal to "increase ADL skills" is not adequate. For the child, family, and third-party payers, the therapist must specify clearer targets for functional outcomes. The therapist should write long-term goals to reflect the outcomes expected during the child's length of stay (e.g., acute rehabilitation admission). The therapist specifies short-term goals as interim steps toward reaching long-term goals. Goals describe specific tasks that the child will perform, conditions of performance, and the type and frequency of assistance needed. Component skills that are emphasized by the therapist may be described as goals if appropriately linked to meaningful functional outcomes (e.g., achieve hand grasp and manipulation skills sufficient for desktop activities and writing at school).

Functional goals must include specification of skills and the level of independence that is being sought. Levels of *independence* describe varying degrees of dependence on personal assistance, adaptive environments, and use of AT devices. In many cases, ADL goals describe how the child or adolescent will manage personal care assistants to achieve a self-managed dependence. On most ADL scales, level of independence is rated as the amount of physical and cognitive assistance needed as a proportion of the task (e.g., moderate assist = 50% assistance or the amount of time required for partial task, whole task, and task transition assistance by a care provider). However, when concerned with the integration of an individual back into his or her home, the concept of *interdependence* among family members may be a more important consideration. Given the negative value associated with *dependence in the Anglo-American culture,* a more positive term to express shared needs between family members is *interreliance.*

In pediatric rehabilitation, the selection of specific ADL goals is influenced by various factors. Goals based on the family's priorities are likely to garner the best motivation and support. Priorities for function are individualized and may differ from those presumed by therapists. The child's or adolescent's ability to restore skills in self-care and important everyday activities helps restore a sense of well-being. However, institutional and insurance directives also influence the selection of ADL goals. Reduction of dependence makes care possible in progressively less restrictive and less costly environments. Intervention goals most often focus on functional skill acquisition that enables the child to be discharged from inpatient hospital settings to services provided within long-term care, home health care, outpatient care, and eventually to use of nonmedical community support systems.

Intervention
Preventing secondary disability and restoring component skills

The prevention of secondary disability and reduction of existing complications is of the highest priority in a treatment plan. The therapist typically addresses neuromuscular and musculoskeletal complications by programs to maintain or regain normal passive range of motion. Through use of special handling techniques, the occupational and physical therapists carry out daily programs that can involve slow stretch and joint mobilization. The therapists can correct existing limitations by using a combination of these techniques and specialized positioning and splinting. The therapist may apply splints for various purposes, including maintaining positions (e.g., resting hand splint), correcting motions (e.g., drop-out splints, dynamic splints with spring tension forces, or serial casting), or promoting function (e.g., wrist cock-up, tenodesis splints) (Figure 29-2).

The therapist facilitates improved movement and strength by using activities and exercises that are most of-

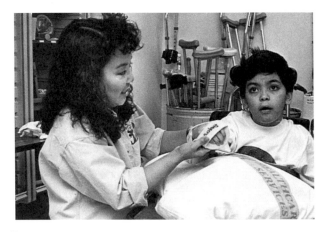

figure29-2   Splints are used to prevent or reduce contractures. Use of serial static splints requires regular monitoring and clear instructions for use to family members and other care providers.

ten incorporated into play. For children and adolescents with musculoskeletal and lower motor neuron or motor unit disorders, use of progressive exercise and activity routines may be appropriate. For those with TBI causing upper motor neuron dysfunction, muscle tone and voluntary motor control are addressed. The therapist can use various sensorimotor techniques to manage muscle tone, with the goal of promoting agonist and antagonist balance as a basis for movement (see Chapters 10 and 11).

A second major concern of pediatric rehabilitation is skin care. Pressure areas from bed positioning, static sitting, and use of orthosis and splints call for routine skin monitoring. The patient must often develop a tolerance to new positioning strategies and splint applications over several days, with skin tolerance being a critical issue in decisions to change bed positions, increase sitting time, and use splints or other orthotic devices.

Patients often experience perceptual, cognitive, and behavioral dysfunction after TBI. With a prevention emphasis, programs to ensure safety in movement and with manipulation of objects are critical. The therapist also implements methods to alleviate stresses of disorientation and memory loss, although restricted environments and restraints may be necessary initially. However, when the child is more alert and aware of his or her surroundings, the therapist may use an educational approach coupled with behavioral interventions. The therapist should inform the child of unit rules, post such rules, and emphasize strict adherence to them. The therapist may carry out reinforcement programs structured through a team and family approach to shape behaviors (Silver, Boake, & Cavazos, 1994). The therapist can use daily orientation programs and memory books to ease the burden of confusion. Teaching the family about the child's perceptual and cognitive impairments and programs in

place to ensure safety and comfort is important. Managing the environment to reduce risk and placement of family pictures and other familiar items from home create a stimulating and more comforting environment.

Resuming and Restoring Occupational Performance

Once the therapist negotiates goals for ADL performance, he or she determines what the child needs to learn, how such learning will take place, and how training can best be organized within the clinical care setting. Schwartz (1991) described the basis of natural learning versus mediated learning. By *natural learning,* the child or adolescent may discover, in one or more sessions, simple strategies to resume activity performance. If these techniques are safe and efficient, the therapist need only guide the child in determining appropriate means to achieve consistent performance. However, many times the child is unable to make natural adaptations to achieve performance. Therapists then *mediate new learning* by instructing the child or adolescent and other care providers in the principles of adaptation and engage them in joint problem solving to determine the most effective methods of performance.

Once the therapist determines what the child needs to learn, he or she organizes specific and desired routines for learning. In mediated learning, some form of instruction takes place through a combination of guided activity and use of instructional aids. For initial instruction of new or adapted tasks, the therapist may demonstrate the task to be learned and have the child copy that demonstration. The therapist may also use verbal or manual guidance cues to assist learning (Figures 29-3 and 29-4). For some tasks, predetermined scripts or learning materials are available (Pedretti 1996; Trombly, 1995).

When the therapist has determined a particular task sequence, he or she selects methods to achieve repetition, generalization, and development of new skills (Figure 29-5). For example, the therapist may help the child memorize a routine so that the child can guide his or her own performance using verbal, visual, or tactile feedback. If the child cannot memorize a routine, the therapist can use other training tools. The therapist can prepare written instructions, pictorial step cues, and audiotapes with specific directions. Whole-task instruction and the use of forward- or reverse-step sequence training are common methods. The therapist can implement training over several days that capitalizes on use of naturally occurring times when tasks are routinely performed (e.g., dressing in the morning and at night or before and after swimming). As training progresses, the therapist gradually reduces the extent of external cueing from a person or instructional aids so that only a minimal amount of such support is required for safe and efficient performance. Often the team and family plan gradual withdrawal of

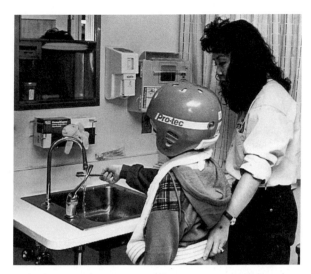

figure**29-3** The occupational therapist provides the child with cues and performance feedback while he carries out an adapted self-help sequence. A helmet is required to protect the head because of an open skull fracture.

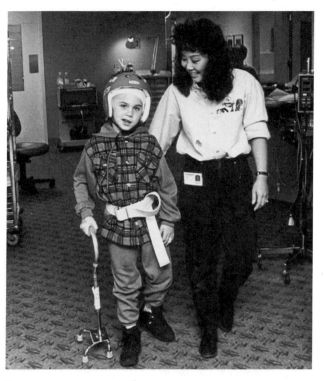

figure**29-4** Mobility is a fundamental part of self-help routines. After completing a morning care routine, this child walks to breakfast with assistance from the occupational therapist for safety and technique.

aides and assistance after discharge from the inpatient hospital setting. Strategies that will continue to promote the child's independence form the basis of family or care provider training.

The environment used for ADL training is also important. Most therapists agree that children prefer familiar environments. However, except in home health care service delivery, environments must be simulated in hospital wards or clinics. Generalization of performance from one setting to another can be difficult because familiar settings may provide unrecognized prompts that are not present in simulated settings. Home visits with the child and family to survey and collaborate in planning of organizational changes, equipment needs, and architectural modifications can facilitate the necessary transition. Day or weekend home passes for the child are desirable when possible. The therapist often develops specific goals, and feedback from the family about the time at home can be important to prioritizing goals, equipment, and family training needs.

Adaptations for ADL Skills

Basic principles apply to adapted performance of ADL skills (Box 29-1) at the end of the chapter. Safety in performance and the avoidance of abnormal or unhealthy movements are essential. New learning is generally more difficult and more energy consuming. Principles of joint protection and work simplification are commonly used, and performance is geared toward functioning in the most barrier-free environment with the use of familiar conveniences. Adaptations of a routine are aimed at reducing complexity, ensuring safety, and minimizing complications if errors occur.

Adaptive methods of ADL skills may include the use of AT devices (see Box 29-1). Reliance on AT devices may be temporary or permanent. Early use of devices can increase safety or immediate function during recovery. Permanent use of devices is also common when the child exhibits residual impairments necessitating adaptation. When selecting devices, therapists often choose to adapt existing equipment that is already familiar to the child. If such adaptation is not desirable or practical, the therapist may direct the family toward purchase of items with features more compatible with the child's or adolescent's special needs through standard shopping sources. If needs cannot be met, specialized rehabilitation devices are purchased through medical and rehabilitation equipment vendors. AT devices are generally designed to accommodate or substitute for skill limitations in gross movement, reach, prehension, manipulation, sensation, or perception. Use of devices should reduce task difficulty and complexity, although initial learning and use may be awkward.

■ SUMMARY

Hospital-based pediatric rehabilitation services play a unique role in the overall management of children with a new or chronic disability. In addressing acute and chronic problems, the emphasis of practice is nearly always on

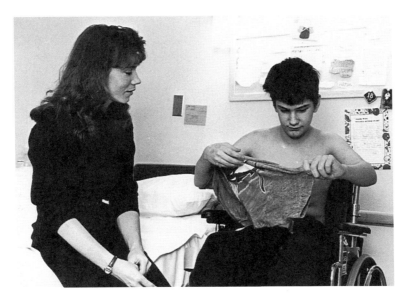

figure **29-5**   Adapted dressing routines are developed to achieve success and ease learning. For this boy, who has perceptual and cognitive deficits after brain injury, the occupational therapist cues him in a repetitive sequence of steps that accomplish the task.

function and participation in life's events at home, at school, and in the community. Both new and established impairments and disabilities pose risks for further complications, which necessitate a prevention prioritization through subacute, acute, and outpatient or ongoing rehabilitation interventions.

Services are medically oriented and delivered within constraints imposed by accreditation and regulatory agencies and third-party payers. Collaboration with school- and community-based services is critical to effective intervention and transition. The challenge of pediatric rehabilitation is to address the acute problems while considering the overall development of the child and the priorities of the family.

Using strategically placed guiding questions, the following case studies promote the student's ability to use clinical reasoning. Students should respond to the questions after each section before reading the next.

Case Study 1: Stephen

Physician prescription: 8-year-old boy with mild R HP 2° TBI, skull fracture

Precautions: Dysphagia, aphasia, falls

Treatment objectives: Evaluate and train ADL skills, PROM with RUE, facilitate use of RUE, evaluate and intervene for visual/perceptual and cognitive skill deficits

1. Given this prescription, what would you do next?
2. What information may you collect before seeing Stephen?
3. Which frames of reference may you use and why?

Referral history

Stephen is an 8-year-old boy from a two-parent, three-sibling home in a small coastal town. Stephen was described by family as being energetic and well-liked. In October he was a passenger on a three-wheel all-terrain vehicle when it rolled over. Stephen was not wearing a helmet and was reported to have struck his head. He was initially alert but soon experienced diminished wakefulness and was unresponsive when paramedics arrived. At the trauma center, Stephen was found to have a left basilar skull fracture, and a computed tomography (CT) scan showed bilateral frontal punctate lesions and an apparent left temporal-parietal focal lesion. Three days after the injury, Stephen became more responsive, demonstrating minimal movement of his right arm and leg, no vocalizations, and dysphagia. He continued to show gradual improvement in his level of consciousness and was evaluated for transfer to acute rehabilitation. His injury was classified as moderate. Twelve days after the accident, Stephen was transferred to the local children's hospital.

1. Given this information, identify your initial priorities for evaluation.
2. What specific evaluation activities do you suggest? Specify an assessment sequence and time period for evaluations.
3. Consider the relationship between referral, evaluation activities, and likely intervention priorities.

Clinical findings

On admission to rehabilitation, Stephen was following simple one-step commands and attempting to verbalize, but word finding was difficult. He was noted to be fatigued and difficult to engage for more than a few minutes at a time. He was also regarded as quiet and reserved, being fearful of separation from his mother, who stayed with him nearly full-time during the day and evenings. Diminished alertness, easy distraction, and disorientation to place and time were also noted. These impairments caused Stephen to become anxious during evaluation and treatments. Swallowing was judged safe from aspiration, although one-to-one supervision was recommended because of Stephen's tendency to overstuff food and poorly sequence his intake of fluids and solids.

During grooming and dressing tasks, Stephen was observed as being disorganized. In part because of his age, he showed poor ability to make natural adaptations to hemiplegia. Continual verbal cues were needed to initiate, set up, and proceed with grooming, dressing, and bathing tasks. Physical demonstration and cues were needed to teach adapted sequences. No perceptual deficits were found by observation or by use of standardized tests.

Further observations showed mild right hemiplegia, characterized by effortful movements of both upper and lower limbs. Little spontaneous use of his right arm was seen, and he showed characteristic synergy patterns and increased muscle tone when he attempted to grasp objects on command. Passive range of motion was normal. In sensory testing, Stephen showed impaired proprioception and localization to touch in distal portions of the arm and leg. Stephen did not ambulate but had partial weight bearing in stance with foot drop when he tried to walk. The physical therapist initiated use of a right ankle-foot orthosis (R-AFO) and a cane.

1. Based on these evaluation findings, identify specific priorities to address in interventions.
2. Suggest at least three long-term treatment goals that could be negotiated with family.
3. Specify frames of reference, intervention activities, and time planning to address each goal.
   a. Address cognitive and behavioral needs
   b. Suggest teaching and training methods for ADLs
   c. Plan strategies to promote upper-limb function and fine motor skill recovery

Intervention activities

The therapist initiated use of an orientation board in his room, regular reminders provided by staff and his mother, written schedules, and a memory book that Stephen completed after each treatment session. The therapist planned consistent routines for self-care, sequenced daily therapies, and structured play activities. The therapist uses familiar play items, pictures of family, his own clothes, his favorite music, and art supplies to enhance comfort and provide memory cues and prompts for orientation. The therapist organized visits by other family members and friends from school and used them in scheduling and memory book entries.

The therapist scheduled Stephen for one-to-one therapy sessions twice each day and planned morning self-care training and afternoon therapeutic activities. In addition to structured self-care routines and orientation-memory programs, the therapist also engaged Stephen in selected activities to facilitate use of his right arm and provide cognitive challenge in organizing steps, following sequences, and sustaining engagement in both familiar and novel tasks (Figure 29-6). The therapist taught self daily range-of-motion and whole-body stretches to maintain normal range and facilitate symmetric trunk and limb use.

Spontaneous use of his right arm improved, but poor recovery of his right hand resulted in Stephen attempting to perform activities using his nondominant left hand. Such attempts proved to be awkward and unsuccessful. The therapist trained Stephen and cued him to use both hands together (Figure 29-7), using the right hand as an assist to the left hand. This strategy improved his self-care performance so that the therapist discontinued use of

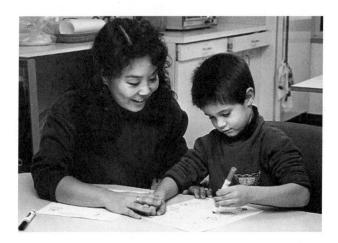

figure**29-6** The occupational therapist promotes use of the hemiparetic arm to hold the paper while the child carries out a drawing and writing activity.

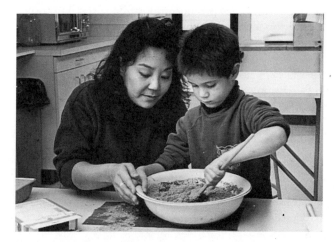

figure**29-7** The therapist provides guidance in using both arms while participating in a cookie-baking activity.

adaptive devices such as a button-aide and a rocker knife after 2 weeks. Handwriting with either the right or left hand was not satisfactory for schoolwork because of language disorders, illegibility, and slow speed. The therapist introduced a computer keyboard and initiated supplementary handwriting activities to facilitate movement and augment function. The therapist judged his physical management of other school-related tasks to be adequate, although communication and cognitive impairments posed major challenges to Stephen's return to school. Three weeks after admission, Stephen was ambulatory with use of an AFO. He continued to show evidence of topographic disorientation but otherwise was thought to be a safe ambulator, even on uneven surfaces, and stairs. He performed activities of grooming, dressing, and bathing with supervision for initiation and safety. Stephen appropriately initiated toileting, and his mother judged his hygiene after bowel movements to be adequate.

1. Determine discharge training needs with Stephen, his family, and school personnel.
2. Specify follow-up plans and extension of pediatric rehabilitation services.

Discharge follow-up plan

Discharge planning included home program suggestions for Stephen and his family. In addition to organization of ADL routines at home, the therapist wrote activities to promote fine motor skills and reviewed them with Stephen's mother. The team held meetings with school personnel to address academic program needs and potential benefits from school-based therapy services. The team determined eligibility for special education and initiated planning of assessments related to an individualized educational plan. The team scheduled interim school visits by the hospital neuropsychologist to occur after Stephen's return to a half-day school program 2 weeks after discharge. The team scheduled a Rehabilitation Medicine Outpatient Clinic follow-up visit to include occupational therapy in 6 weeks, with a plan for regular follow-along clinic visits at 2-month intervals during the next 6 months.

Case Study 2: Lydia

Physician prescription: 9-year-old girl with 2-month history of pneumonia; recent left fibular fracture; secondary diagnosis includes cerebral palsy with spastic quadriplegia, developmental delay, and seizure disorder

Precautions: Dysphagia, osteoporosis, pain, declining ADL function

Treatment objectives: Evaluate skills and retrain adaptive ADL routines with family

1. Given this prescription, what would you do next?
2. What would you do before seeing Lydia?
3. Which frames of reference may you use? (State assumptions about use of each intervention.)

Referral history

Lydia's mother brought her to the emergency room last spring because of severe pulmonary distress attributed to viral pneumonia. She was intubated with a tracheotomy and did well with medications and vigorous chest physical therapy. Extubation was performed, but she soon experienced another episode of pulmonary distress that required reintubation and use of a ventilator for about 1 week. Her respiratory problems dramatically altered her participation in school and her regular routines for over 8 weeks. Her mother's attempts to have Lydia resume walking resulted in refusals, with apparent swelling and pain in her left ankle. Orthopedic consultation determined that she had developed a stress fracture of her distal fibula. Her ankle was casted, but she was free to bear weight. Late in her second hospitalization she was evaluated for admission to acute rehabilitation. Transfer was determined to be necessary because of Lydia's deterioration in gross motor function, oral motor function, and ability to perform ADLs compared with her baseline skills when seen through the neuromuscular clinic and from school records. A short-term rehabilitation program was planned to ensure safety and adequate nutrition by oral feeding; and to reattain functional short-distance ambulation with the use of bilateral plastic AFOs and a walker, with crawling up and down stairs, and with long-distance wheelchair mobility. In addition, the program was planned to promote upper extremity endurance; to resume a routine of assisted dressing and supervision with feeding and hygiene and family use of adaptive equipment for safety in transfers; to improve speech intelligibility to preinfection status; and to facilitate transition back to school and an extended school-year program.

1. State a plan for evaluation priorities and methods.
2. Goals for the admission have been stated. Elaborate on likely ADL and performance issues that would need to be addressed in intervention.

Clinical findings

Through an interview with the family, prior therapists, and direct observation, the following information was gathered. Viewed by parents as an imaginative girl, Lydia enjoys various games and activities. She was reported to be cooperative and could normally express needs in short words and phrases, although picture boards for communication in self-care and therapy routines had been developed. Task-specific communication boards had also been used at school. She was observed to pull her hair, bite her hands, and use her wheelchair to collide with objects; these behaviors were believed to be signs of frustration and fatigue. The therapy team chose to follow Lydia's school and home behavior routine, including short-term time-out, acknowledging her emotions, and then redirect her to a new activity. Lydia's mother reported a prior level of ADL function in which Lydia ate and dressed with minimal help but received a great deal of assistance with toileting and bathing. With set-up help and supervision for quality, Lydia brushed her teeth and enjoyed other grooming tasks. While hospitalized Lydia had indicated her need to toilet but had been assisted for the most part with all functions and had not been initiating any personal care. Lydia had much more difficulty eating, and her communication attempts had diminished. Therapists observed Lydia to be withdrawn and difficult to engage in activities.

1. Consider collaborations with other rehabilitation team members to address overall admission goals.
2. Determine likely discharge goals for ADL performance and other occupational needs.
3. Outline intervention plans, including frequency and length of visits and activities to be addressed.

Intervention activities

In addition to collaborative sessions with other team members, Lydia was seen in hour long therapy sessions that included weekday morning ADL training and afternoon gross motor and fine motor activities. Occupational therapy focused on Lydia's use of sequenced routines of dressing and hygiene with the nursing staff. In conjunction with the speech pathologist, a swallowing evaluation showed microaspirations that required a change in Lydia's foods to a dysphagia mechanical diet with thick liquids. One-to-one supervision was needed to cue for bite size and complete chewing before swallow. The speech pathologist gave Lydia oral exercises to increase strength and coordination of her tongue, lips, and jaw for purposes of speech and the oral phase of feeding. Therapeutic recreation involved Lydia in play activities such as group puppet shows and construction of posters. The occupational therapist emphasized strengthening her arms through therapeutic activities emphasizing aerobic tolerance. The therapists also stressed wheelchair propulsion, wheelchair pushups for pressure relief, and crawling to help Lydia recover her baseline abilities in use of her upper extremities. The therapists noted fatigue in fine motor tasks, although skilled movements appeared similar to her prior status. The therapists stressed endurance with tabletop tasks of writing and use of manipulatives.

Lydia's mother was infrequently involved with therapy sessions because of her job responsibilities. Care provider instruction emphasizes assisted bathtub and car transfers, increasing Lydia's participation in assisted routines of bathing and toileting and organization and planning for supervision in eating, hygiene, and dressing activities. Lydia and her mother had previously developed a fast-paced care routine that allowed Lydia few opportunities to participate in or influence her care. The occupational therapist placed emphasis on having Lydia and her mother develop and follow simplified written routines, which enabled Lydia to direct more of her own care. This was thought to be important to her mother but also essential for use with other care providers like her father, with

whom she stayed every other month for a weekend. Lydia's admission to acute rehabilitation lasted 12 days. Her tolerance of bracing returned, and she was able to use a walker for up to 25 yards. She continued to need contact guarding in wheelchair-to-floor transfers and was able to crawl up and down seven carpeted steps. Manual wheelchair propulsion was limited to 100 yards on smooth and level surfaces. No complaints of arm fatigue were noted with activities of 15 minutes' duration. Lydia advanced to a regular diet, although the therapists instructed her mother to follow precautions that included use of an upright posture while eating and drinking, a slow pace of eating, and avoidance of foods with stringy texture that were difficult for her to manage as a bolus and during the pharyngeal phase of swallowing.

1. Suggest follow-up or follow-along services to recommend.

Discharge follow-up plan

The therapists made plans with the school for an extended school-year program to complete the work missed during her long absence. At discharge, follow-up clinic visits for orthopedics and pulmonary disorders were scheduled, and Lydia was scheduled to see her physiatrist as part of her routine neurodevelopmental clinic visit in 2 months.

Case Study 3: Kyle

Physician prescription: 14-year-old male adolescent with congenital limb deficiencies, undergoing second-stage orthopedic surgery to rotate and lengthen left leg
Precautions: Falls, Ilizarov protocol
Therapeutic objectives: Evaluation of ADLs and retraining with adaptive techniques and AT
1. Consider plans and actions to follow before seeing Kyle.
2. Specify frame of references likely to be used in interventions.

Referral history

Kyle has a long history of involvement with rehabilitation specialists. He was born with a unique combination of limb deficiencies. His right upper extremity amelia resulted in the equivalent of a right shoulder disarticulation, and his left upper extremity hemimelia results in a short above-elbow residual limb. His left lower extremity has femoral and tibial shortening with ankle and foot deformity. Kyle's right lower limb was comparatively normal. Multiple limb abnormalities resulted in Kyle being followed for several years through a specialized clinic for children with limb deficiency. Several attempts at prosthetic fit for his left leg proved difficult, expensive, and nonfunctional. Kyle developed good use of his right foot for prehension and used his left foot as an assist. As a teenager, Kyle had good family support, attended school with his same-aged cohort in their hometown, and was a good student.

At that time, Kyle was considered a good candidate for left leg surgery to correct a rotation deformity and lengthen the limb by the Ilizarov procedure. Kyle's balance had begun to deteriorate with growth. His leg length discrepancy became more pronounced, causing severe problems when barefoot and not using his large shoelift, which was also viewed as unsightly. Although he could walk, run, and use his lower limbs well for many ADL skills, it was believed that he would benefit from the surgical procedure, which would add approximately 6 cm of length to his left tibia. Anticipated benefits included better single-leg balance and reduced need for extensive lifts on his left shoe.

Two stages were planned for the surgical correction. The first included a left distal femoral wedge osteotomy to correct the rotation deformity of his knee and a heel cord release at the ankle. The second procedure would involve tibial lengthening with the Ilizarov technique. Kyle underwent the first part of this series with mixed results. Because of his upper limb deficiency, use of traditional crutches was not possible, and he required a lengthened period of rehabilitation to learn to walk again. He experienced several falls and had complaints of ankle pain. Because his running skills decreased after the first surgery, he became reticent about the second procedure. Anxiety and depressive reactions were seen, and referrals were made for more extensive assessment and treatment. It was determined that both Kyle and his family needed more information about the surgery and the expected course of recovery.

In planning his second surgery, which was expected to have an even longer recovery time, careful assessment of rehabilitative needs was addressed. The procedure necessitated the development of a customized crutch to be used on the right side and careful planning to address concerns he and his family had regarding his independence. A prosthetist developed a crutch device that molded to the axilla for weight bearing through the ribs and the latissimus muscle and had a detachable post modified from a Loftstrand design (Mosca, Okumura, & Jaffe, 1993). Kyle learned to use the crutch quickly. During the summer he underwent the second procedure and was admitted to acute rehabilitation. Goals after his surgery were to restore safe mobility and, before returning home, reestablish desired independence in feeding, grooming, bathing, dressing, and written communication skills. The admission also provided an opportunity to more directly evaluate and explore options for the skills that Kyle had been inconsistent in performing.

1. Consider Kyle's options for limited reach and prehension and techniques used with ADL tasks.
2. Propose options to explore in terms of AT for purposes of communication and environmental control.
3. How can Kyle's psychosocial needs be addressed during this admission.

Clinical findings

External fixation of the tibia created some difficulty in using his left foot as an assistor. An occupational therapist saw Kyle twice per day to address further adaptation of functional skills. The therapist recruited Kyle to participate in problem solving, and he willingly tried new techniques. He resumed feeding by using his regular routine of his right foot over his left thigh and handling utensils to bring food to his mouth from a specially positioned plate. He continued to have difficulty opening packaged foods because of his left foot immobility.

Intervention activities

The occupational therapist introduced adaptations to his usual AT devices that allowed him to resume independence in grooming and bathing tasks. The therapist configured a dressing board similar to the one Kyle used at home to provide him with independence in donning and doffing his clothes by use of specially placed stationary hooks. Kyle also resumed right foot writing and computer operation using a miniature keyboard and other adaptive interface features with Windows 98. The therapist introduced Internet access to Kyle and arranged it as an evening activity, along with custom access devices for video games. The therapist also explored driving with Kyle and scheduled a referral to the local adaptive drivers' training program for a time after healing and before his sixteenth birthday. The physical therapist engaged Kyle in ambulation training and specific muscle strengthening of the left lower extremity. At discharge he was able to walk with his crutch for distances up to 300 feet and bear approximately 80% of his body weight over his left leg. Transfers from seated surfaces and standing were independent, but he continued to require assistance getting up from the floor.

1. Recommend home program activities.
2. Suggest further options to address pediatric rehabilitation needs.

Discharge follow-up plan

Kyle's admission to acute rehabilitation lasted 3 weeks, with additional community-based physical therapy planned. Continued visits to the limb deficiency program at the rehabilitation clinic were scheduled along with referral to adaptive driving program and AT clinics. These systems would address with Kyle and his family his progression in needs or transitions in school, independent living, and vocational exploration.

I wish to thank the children and families involved with Children's Hospital and Regional Medical Center, Seattle, Washington, for their willingness to share their experiences. I also want to acknowledge the advice and help of colleagues from the same institution in preparation of this chapter.

box 29-1 *Basic rehabilitation strategies*

Occupational therapists use several strategies for specific types of impairments to adapt activities for children with functional limitations. In addition to these suggestions, uses of assistive technology (AT) should be reviewed (see Chapter 19 and 20).

Motor limitations

Limited range of motion

Reduced range of motion in the neck, trunk, and proximal and intermediate joints of the limbs limits ability to reach all parts of the body and objects within the immediate environment. Limitations of hand motion can reduce holding and handling of objects. To substitute for reach, the child should use extended and specially angled handles (e.g., long-handled spoon or fork, bath brush, dressing stick, or shoe horn) or devices that are more specialized, such as reachers. If a child is unable to use devices that extend reach, the therapist employs other strategies to permit function. Mounting objects on the floor, wall, or table and bringing the body part to the device (e.g., boot tree for removing shoes, friction pad on floor for socks, hook on the wall to pull pants up or down, or sponges mounted in the shower to wash) prove useful. For some tasks, devices may replace any reach requirement, such as use of a bidet for hygiene after toileting or manual or electric feeders operated by microswitches to bring food to the mouth.

When motion of the hand is limited, the therapist can assist holding and manipulating of objects by providing enlarged or differently styled handles that reduce the grasp requirement (e.g., T-handled cup). The therapist can replace holding functions by use of universal cuff or C-shaped handles. Friction surfaces may provide more secure grasp. When forearm rotation is limited, swivel spoons or angled utensils may assist bringing food to the mouth.

Limited range of motion also reduces gross motor movements, such as in bed mobility and elevation changes (moving from sitting to standing and performing transfers in bathing and toileting). The therapist typically changes surface levels (i.e., raised or lowered) to limit the extent of elevation change required. The therapist may lower the bed height to allow ease in wheelchair transfers or raise it to ease in coming up to standing from sitting. Raised chairs, toilet seats, and bath benches reduce extreme changes in elevation required in transfers.

Decreased strength and endurance

Strength and endurance limitations are common among children who are acutely ill or injured. The goals of adaptation are to reduce the effects of gravity by use of lightweight objects, movements in the horizontal plane, reduced friction, and when possible, the use of body mechanics for leverage and gravity to assist movement. Electrically powered devices may meet goals of work simplification. Efficiency of movement is essential. Similar to limited range of motion, weakness can cause inability to reach body parts or make elevation changes. Extended handles may be necessary; however, increased weight and the forces required to handle and apply leverage can increase difficulty.

A major goal with activity adaptation for decreased strength is to limit the need to sustain static postures and prolonged holding. The therapist can use surfaces to support posture and proximal limb positions in various ways (e.g., bed positioning, seating adaptations, and use of armrests and table surfaces). The therapist reduces the need for sustained holding by mounting devices or stabilizing devices with friction (e.g., Dycem or spike board) or using an enlarged lightweight object. Universal cuffs or C-cuffs are also common to limit demands for grasp. Manipulation may be impaired and necessitate use of hooks and loops on clothing and adaptation of fasteners by use of Velcro, zippers, enlarged buttons, or elastic shoelaces. Less complex movement and reduced force is required to manipulate lever handles on faucets, doors, and appliances. The therapist helps the child reduce movement against gravity in transfers by changing the heights of surfaces and using AT devices such as sliding boards, springs, or hydraulic lifts to aid movement.

For children with cardiac or pulmonary disorders, progression of ADL performance may be based on estimated metabolic equivalents levels or by direct monitoring. The therapist should schedule and pace tasks, simplify work, and use rest breaks within tasks.

Incoordination

Incoordination primarily causes difficulty with manipulation skills. The extent to which incoordination influences performance is determined by the range of movement required, weight and resistance of objects being handled, and positioning of the body in relation to objects. A primary concern is to achieve proximal stability when executing movements. Stabilizing the trunk and head while making movements of the arm and hand is thought to improve skilled movements. Likewise, the

box 29-1 *Basic rehabilitation strategies—cont'd*

therapist should stabilize the proximal segments of the limb while manipulating the hand (e.g., resting the elbow and forearm on the table while using the wrist and fingers to manipulate objects). Friction surfaces and containers that hold objects being manipulated may also be suggested for stabilization of the limb (e.g., friction pad plate or nonslip cup).

Another common strategy is to determine if increased weight dampens exaggerated movements and tremor. The therapist may select heavier objects or add weight to objects. The therapist can attach a weight to the arm or apply resistance to movement by placing devices across joints (e.g., elastic sleeves, friction feeder) to determine if more precise movements can be achieved. When such methods are inadequate, other techniques employed are similar to those for reduced range of motion and strength, including mounting devices on stable surfaces and bringing the body to these devices using gross movements.

One-handed techniques

When a child has to perform most activities with one hand, the barriers to be overcome typically involve replacing the stabilization function of the other limb, improving the skills of the hand being used, and adapting tasks that require alternating movements of two hands. Generally, the child can accomplish many tasks easily with the use of one hand. If the hand being used was not previously the preferred or dominant hand, skilled movements may take a greater amount of time to develop. For those with perceptual and cognitive impairments, learning to use one hand may be particularly difficult. For children with hemiplegia, various dressing routines have been scripted that follow the rules of dressing the affected limb first and avoiding the use of abnormal postures. The stabilization function of the impaired limb may not be entirely lost, although the child may need to learn how to assist movement in placing or positioning the limb to effectively stabilize objects. To entirely replace the stabilization function of the impaired or lost upper limb, the therapist may use mounting or friction surfaces. Some two-handed tasks require the use of specially designed devices or methods. For example, the therapist can provide the child with a rocker-knife or cutting-edged fork to help him or her cut with a knife and fork, a button hook to aid in buttoning, a special lacing technique to aid in shoe tying, and a one-handed keyboard arrangement and training program to aid in typing.

Perceptual and cognitive limitations

Sensory, perceptual, and cognitive impairments alone pose various challenges to ADL performance but are most often associated with other physical disorders previously described. If retraining of component skills is ineffective and impairment continues, the therapist should consider substitution for impaired skills by using more intact sensory, perceptual, or cognitive skills (e.g., using a bell on the hemiplegic arm to draw attention if being neglected tactually or visually). Compensation techniques may also be planned that modify the activity sequence and environment to enable the child to accomplish the challenging task.

Perceptual and cognitive deficit

Perceptual and cognitive deficits affect ADL skill routines and school performance. To compensate for perceptual or cognitive deficits, the therapist can design step-by-step routines with cueing systems and repeat them in training. The therapist employs work simplification principles and uses substitution strategies. Children with perceptual or cognitive deficits may rely on memorizing and reciting a verbal routine or follow audiotaped instruction. They may also rely on written instructions or pictorial cues. With impaired visual perception, the child may need to learn reliance on tactile feedback cues. At times, the therapist specially selects materials used in ADL to compensate for impairments. The therapist may use color-contrasted clothing, texture, or color-coding cues with objects. Sometimes the therapist can encourage the use of mirrors to give the child feedback about his or her performance.

Visual Impairment

Blindness or severe visual impairment require that the therapist employ strategies to substitute for vision by use of other sensory skills and cognitive routines. Consistent organization of the environment and storage of items is necessary. The therapist may use tactile identifiers on objects such as raised letters and locations of more transient items described by a companion or a standard technique such as analog clock location. The therapist can build sound feedback into some items to aid in orientation or search. Mobility specialists instruct individuals to use techniques such as long canes or guide dogs for ambulation or wheelchair guidance and to use a leader's arm for guidance in walking.

STUDY QUESTIONS

1. For a child with traumatic injury, suggest reasons why acute rehabilitation would be recommended. How would recommendations differ from care in subacute or outpatient rehabilitation settings? How would this differ for a child with a congenital onset disorder?

2. Considering the intensive yet comprehensive nature of acute rehabilitation, suggest types of program outcomes that would reflect the contribution of occupational therapy in this setting.

3. For a new admission to acute rehabilitation, describe how assessment and treatment planning would be prioritized. Consider how the family is involved in the process of setting goals and selecting treatment strategies.

4. For teaching adaptive methods that may involve use of assistive technology devices, suggest three alternatives for providing such instruction.

5. Short of independence, suggest long-term goals for acute rehabilitation that would be relevant to the child's function at home, at school, and in other community settings.

References

Albright, A.L. (1992). Neurosurgical treatment of spasticity: Selective posterior rhizotomy and intrathecal baclofen. *Stereotactic and Functional Neurosurgery, 58,* 3-13.

Binder, H., Conway, A., Hanson, S., Gerber, L.H., Marini, J., Berry, R., & Weintraub, J. (1993). Comprehensive rehabilitation of the child with osteogenesis imperfecta. *American Journal of Medical Genetics, 45,* 265-269.

Blatzheim, L.L., Edberg, A., & Lacy, L. (1987). Operationalizing primary nursing in the pediatric rehabilitation setting. *Journal of Pediatric Nursing, 2,* 434-437.

Boyer, M.G., & Edwards, P. (1991). Outcome 1 to 3 years after severe traumatic brain injury in children and adolescents. *Injury, 22,* 315-320.

Burkett, K.W. (1989). Trends in pediatric rehabilitation. *Nursing Clinics of North America, 24,* 239-255.

Buschbacher, R. (1995). Outcomes and problems in pediatric pulmonary rehabilitation. *American Journal of Physical Medicine and Rehabilitation, 74,* 287-293.

Case-Smith, J., & Wavrek, B. (1998). Models of service delivery and team interaction. In J. Case-Smith (Ed.), *Pediatric occupational therapy and early intervention* (pp. 83-108). Boston: Butterworth Heinemann.

Coster, W.J., Haley, S., & Baryza, M.J. (1994). Functional performance of young children after traumatic brain injury: A 6-month follow-up study. *The American Journal of Occupational Therapy, 48,* 211-218.

Di-Scala, C., Osberg, J.S., Gans, B.M., Chin, L.J., & Grant, C.C. (1991). Children with traumatic head injury: Morbidity and postacute treatment. *Archives of Physical Medicine and Rehabilitation, 72,* 662-666.

Donders, J. (1993). Bereavement and mourning in pediatric rehabilitation settings. *Death Studies, 17,* 517-527.

Dudgeon, B.J., & Greenberg, S.L. (1998). Preparing students for consultation roles and systems. *The American Journal of Occupational Therapy, 52,* 801-809.

Dudgeon, B.J., Massagli, T.L., & Ross, B.W. (1997). Educational participation of children with spinal cord injury. *The American Journal of Occupational Therapy, 51,* 553-561.

Edwards, P.A. (1992). The evolution of rehabilitation facilities for children. *Rehabilitation Nursing, 17,* 191-195.

Eigsti, H., Aretz, M., & Shannon, L. (1990). Pediatric physical therapy in a rehabilitation setting. *Pediatrician, 17,* 267-277.

Fay, G.C., Jaffe, K.M., Polissar, N.L., Liao, S., Rivara, J.B., & Martin, K.M. (1994). Outcome of pediatric traumatic brain injury at three years: A cohort study. *Archives of Physical Medicine and Rehabilitation, 75,* 733-741.

Fuhrer, M.J. (1987). *Rehabilitation outcomes, analysis and measurement.* Baltimore: Brookes.

Gans, B.M. (1993). Rehabilitation of the pediatric patient. In J.A. Delisa (Ed.), *Rehabilitation medicine, principles and practice* (2nd ed.). Philadelphia: J.B. Lippincott.

Gardner, J., & Workinger, M.S. (1990). The changing role of the speech-language pathologist in pediatric rehabilitation/habilitation. *Pediatrician, 17,* 283-286.

Guerriere, D., & McKeever, P. (1997). Mothering children who survive brain injuries: Playing the hand you're dealt. *Journal of the Society of Pediatric Nurses, 2,* 105-115.

Haley, S.M., Coster, W.J., Ludlow, L.H., Haltiwanger, J.T., & Andrellos, P.J. (1992). *Pediatric Evaluation of Disability Inventory.* Boston: New England Medical Center Hospitals.

Heery, K. (1992). Restoring childhood through rehabilitation. *Rehabilitation Nursing, 17,* 193-195.

Herndon, D.N., Rutan, R.L., & Rutan, T.C. (1993). Management of the pediatric patient with burns. *Journal of Burn Care and Rehabilitation, 14,* 3-8.

Jaffe, K.M., Fay, G.C., Polissar, N.L., Martin, K.M., Shurtleff, H.A., Rivara, J.B., & Winn, H.R. (1993). Severity of pediatric traumatic brain injury and neurobehavioral recovery at one year—a cohort study. *Archives of Physical Medicine and Rehabilitation, 74,* 587-595.

Jaffe, K.M., Massagli, T.L., Martin, K.M., Rivara, J.B., Fay, G.C., & Polissar, N.L. (1993). Pediatric traumatic brain injury: Acute and rehabilitation costs. *Archives of Physical Medicine and Rehabilitation. 74,* 681-686.

Jaffe, K.M., Okamoto, G.A., & Lemire, C. (1986). Inpatient pediatric rehabilitation: A five year review. *Rehabilitation Literature, 47,* 286-289.

Jaffe, K.M., Polissar, N.L., Fay, G.C., & Liao, S. (1995). Recovery trends over three years following pediatric traumatic brain injury. *Archives of Physical Medicine and Rehabilitation, 76,* 17-26.

Johnston, M.V., & Granger, C.V. (1994). Outcomes research in medical rehabilitation: A primer and introduction to a series. *American Journal of Physical Medicine and Rehabilitation, 73,* 296-303.

Karger, C., Guile, J.T., & Bowen, J.R. (1993). Lengthening of congenital lower limb deficiencies. *Clinical Orthopedics and Related Research, 291,* 236-245.

Keith, R.A., Granger, C.V., Hamilton, B.B., & Sherwin, F.S. (1987). The functional independence measure: A new tool for rehabilitation. *Advances in Clinical Rehabilitation, 1,* 6-18.

Massagli, T.L., & Jaffe, K.M. (1990). Pediatric spinal cord injury: Treatment and outcome. *Pediatrician, 17,* 244-254.

Moront, M., & Eichelberger, M.R. (1994). Pediatric trauma. *Pediatrics Annals, 23,* 186-191.

Mosca, V.S. (1991). The Ilizarov method: Orthopedic and rehabilitation management. *Physical Medicine and Rehabilitation Clinics of North America, 2,* 951-970.

Mosca, V.S., Okumura, R., & Jaffe, K.M. (1993). Prosthetic crutch for a patient with congenital bilateral, upper extremity deficiencies undergoing lower extremity lengthening by the Ilizarov method. *Journal of the Association of Children's Prosthetic-Orthotic Clinics, 28,* 19-20.

Msall, M.E., DiGaudio, K.M., & Duffy, L.C. (1993). Use of functional assessment in children with developmental disabilities. *Physical Medicine and Rehabilitation Clinics of North America, 4,* 517-527.

Pedretti, L.W. (Ed.). (1996). *Occupational therapy: Practice skills for physical dysfunction* (4th ed.). St. Louis: Mosby.

Philip, P.A., Ayyangar, R., Vanderbilt, J., & Gaebler-Spira, D.J. (1994). Rehabilitation outcome in children after treatment of primary brain tumor. *Archives of Physical Medicine and Rehabilitation, 75,* 36-39.

Raps, C.S., Peterson, C., Jonas, M., & Seligman, M.E. (1982). Patient behavior in hospitals: Helplessness, reactance, or both? *Journal of Personality and Social Psychology, 42,* 1036-1041.

Richardson, C.J., & Robinson, S.S. (1989). Neonatal intensive care and pediatric rehabilitation: A joint program for care of chronically ill infants. *Journal of Perinatology, 9,* 52-55.

Rivara, J.B. (1993). Family functioning following pediatric traumatic brain injury. *Pediatric Annals, 23,* 38-43.

Rivara, J.B., Jaffe, K.M., Polissar, N.L., Fay, G.C., Liao, S., & Martin, K.M. (1996). Predictors of family functioning and change 3 years after traumatic brain injury in children. *Archives of Physical Medicine and Rehabilitation, 77,* 754-764.

Rodriquez, J., & Brown, S.T. (1990). Childhood injuries in the United States, Division of Injury Control, Center for Environmental Health and Injury Control, Center for Disease Control. *American Journal of Diseases of Children, 144,* 627-646.

Roth, E.J., Heinemann, A.W., Lovell, L.L., Harvey, R.L., McGuire, J.R., & Diaz, S. (1998). Impairment and disability: Their relation during stroke rehabilitation. *Archives of Physical Medicine and Rehabilitation, 79,* 329-335.

Russman, B.S. (1990). Rehabilitation of the pediatric patient with a neuromuscular disease. *Neurology Clinics, 8,* 727-740.

Schwartz, R.K. (1991). Educational and training strategies, therapy as learning. In C. Christiansen & C. Baum (Eds.), *Occupational therapy: Overcoming human performance deficits* (pp. 664-698). Thorofare, NJ: Slack.

Silver, B.V., Boake, C., & Cavazos, D.I. (1994). Improving functional skills using behavioral procedures in a child with anoxic brain injury. *Archives of Physical Medicine and Rehabilitation, 75,* 742-745.

Strunk, R.C., Mascia, A.V., Lipkowitz, M.A., & Wolf, S.I. (1991). Rehabilitation of a patient with asthma in the outpatient setting. *Journal of Allergy and Clinical Immunology, 87* (3), 601-611.

Trombly, C.A. (Ed.). (1995). *Occupational therapy for physical dysfunction* (4th ed.). Baltimore: Williams & Wilkins.

Watson, D. (1991). Occupational therapy intervention guidelines for children and adolescents with spina bifida. *Child: Care, Health, and Development, 17,* 367-380.

Wieting, J.M., & Krach, L.E. (1994). Spinal cord injury rehabilitation in a pediatric achondroplastic patient: Case report. *Archives of Physical Medicine and Rehabilitation, 75,* 106-108.

Suggested Readings

Carney, J., & Gerring, J. (1990). Return to school following severe closed head injury: A critical phase in pediatric rehabilitation. *Pediatrician, 17,* 222-229.

Del Vecchio, J. (1992). Home pediatric rehabilitation. *Journal of Home Health Care Practice, 5,* 12-15.

DiCowden, M. (1990). Pediatric rehabilitation: Special patients, special needs. *Journal of Rehabilitation, 56,* 13-18.

Kurtz, L.A., & Scull, S.A. (1993). Rehabilitation for developmental disabilities. *Pediatric Clinics of North America, 40,* 629-643.

Matthews, D.J., Meier, R.H., & Bartholome, W. (1990). Ethical issues encountered in pediatric rehabilitation. *Pediatrician, 17,* 108-114.

Molnar, G.E. (1988). A developmental perspective for the rehabilitation of children with physical disability. *Pediatric Annals, 17,* 766, 768-776.

chapter 30

Programs and Services for Children with Psychosocial Dysfunction

Debora A. Davidson

key terms

Early childhood intervention programs
Students with behavioral disorders
Classroom-based psychosocial therapy
Outpatient mental health services
Day treatment programs
Residential treatment centers
Juvenile justice system
Inpatient psychiatric hospitals

■ CHAPTER OBJECTIVES

1. Identify the continuum of services available to children and youth with psychosocial disorders.
2. Define the roles of occupational therapists who provide services to children and youth with psychosocial disorders.
3. Explain frames of reference and intervention strategies used in psychosocial intervention.
4. Explain the variety of service delivery models used by occupational therapists in psychosocial settings.

Health care professionals who work with children and adolescents can expect to encounter clients with psychosocial problems regardless of the setting. Research on random samples of children and adolescents in the community indicates that 15% to 22% of the general population has psychosocial problems, but only about 2% receives intervention specific to mental health concerns (National Advisory Mental Health Council, 1990; Tuma, 1989). One reason for the low level of intervention is that mental health services for children and adolescents typically have been sparse and poorly funded in the United States (Knitzer, 1982; Solomon & Evans, 1992; Tuma, 1989). Another reason is the pervasive cultural bias that deters families from admitting to having and seeking help for psychosocial problems. Lastly, there is a tendency to ignore the psychosocial needs of clients who have other more visible physical and cognitive problems such as cerebral palsy or Down syndrome, despite evidence that children with chronic health problems are at increased risk for psychosocial dysfunction (Offard & Fleming, 1991).

Occupational therapists are uniquely educated and positioned to provide needed psychosocial evaluation and intervention to children and adolescents in a variety of contexts. Despite this advantage, occupational therapists have often limited their involvement in directly addressing mental health needs of referred families because of concerns about role conflicts and reimbursement regulations (Davidson & LaVessar, 1998; Schultz, 1992). Neglect of mental health needs can result in problems that range from client dissatisfaction to regression rather than progress. Contemporary leaders in occupational therapy agree that best practice includes evaluation of and intervention to help meet the psychosocial needs of all clients (Davidson & LaVessar, 1998; Florey, 1989; Peloquin, 1993; Williamson, 1993).

The purposes of this chapter are to describe ways in which occupational therapists provide psychosocial intervention in a variety of settings and to inspire therapists to use all of their skills to address the full spectrum of children's needs. These goals are approached by describing a variety of treatment settings that represent a continuum from less to more psychiatrically oriented and from less to more intensive and restrictive. The mission, clientele, services, frames of reference, and staffing patterns for each type of facility are described, as well as traditional or potential roles for occupational therapists in each setting. Case studies synthesized from the author's clinical experiences illustrate innovative ways of providing psychosocial intervention in a variety of traditional and nontraditional settings.

Therapeutic environments to be discussed in this chapter include early childhood intervention programs, public schools, outpatient mental health centers, day treatment programs, residential treatment centers, correctional facilities, and inpatient acute care hospitals. Some of these programs are designed specifically to assist children and adolescents who have identified mental health problems; other programs are oriented toward meeting more general educational or developmental needs. Occupational therapists have been well established in some of these settings and pioneers in other settings. In any case, pediatric occupational therapists have the knowledge base, the skills, and the opportunities to provide psychosocial intervention to children and adolescents in need regardless of the service setting.

■ EARLY CHILDHOOD INTERVENTION PROGRAMS

The primary mission of *early childhood intervention* (ECI) *programs* is the prevention and amelioration of developmental disabilities in children from birth to 3 years of age. Clients include infants and toddlers who are diagnosed as having developmental delay, those who are considered to be at risk for developmental problems, and their families (Individuals with Disabilities Act [IDEA], 1990). Although infants and toddlers are referred primarily to early intervention for evaluation and treatment of neurologic and physical conditions, children may be referred when their development is at risk because of parental mental health problems, such as chemical dependency, domestic violence, parental depression, or other psychiatric disorders. Occasionally the identified child may have a diagnosed mental health disorder, such as nonorganic failure to thrive, or pervasive developmental disorder (American Psychological Association, 1994; Hunter & Powell, 1990).

Professionals working in ECI programs are likely to use developmental, neurodevelopmental, rehabilitation, behavioral, interactional, and family systems as frames of reference (Table 30-1). Occupational therapists, edu-

cated to recognize and treat persons with mental illness, contribute significantly to the ECI team's effectiveness with high-risk families. For example, parents who are experiencing depression are often unable to meet their infant's needs for responsive interaction (Pickens & Field, 1993). Parents who are addicted to drugs are at increased risk of neglecting or abusing their children (Wolfner & Gelles, 1993). Occupational therapists can screen clients for problems such as depression and substance abuse and can facilitate clients' accessing evaluation and treatment by a qualified care provider. Environmental stressors such as poverty, social isolation, and community violence also need to be evaluated and addressed since they play a part in a family's ability to meet the needs of infants and children (Coulton, Korbin, Su, & Chow, 1995; Humphrey, 1995; Vondra, 1990). If the parent of a child with medical complications reports that the family is having difficulty following through with the child's care because of unemployment and marital stress, the ECI team is in a position to refer the parents for financial assistance, work placement, and counseling services. Once these concerns are resolved, parents have more energy available for childcare. If there appears to be a danger of child abuse or neglect, the occupational therapist is mandated by law to report these concerns to the State Child Protection Agency (Davidson, 1995). The following case study presents an example of family-centered early intervention.

Case Study 1: Vanessa
Part A

Vanessa, who is 16 years of age and her 4-month-old daughter Nicole, live independently in a subsidized housing development in a large city. Nicole was referred to an early childhood intervention (ECI) program by her pediatrician, who was concerned about the possibility of developmental delay related to her low birth weight and probable fetal alcohol effects. Nicole was evaluated by the center's interdisciplinary team and was found to be a passive baby who rarely interacted with people or the environment, had low muscle tone, and was slow to drink from a bottle. Because of transportation problems, Vanessa decided that she would prefer home-based intervention. The team agreed that the occupational therapist would provide therapeutic and case management services.

1. What are key personal, environmental, and occupational issues for this mother and child?
2. If you were the therapist, how could you find answers to these questions? Are there general learning issues that this case raises for you as a student? Where will you access this information?
3. As a direct service provider, what assessments would you use? What information would these tools or methods provide?

table 30-1　Settings for Psychosocial Treatment of Children and Adolescents

	Early Childhood Intervention Programs	School Systems	Outpatient and Day Treatment Programs	Residential Treatment Centers	Correctional Facilities	Inpatient Hospitals
Frames of reference	Developmental Neurodevelopmental Rehabilitation Behavioral Family systems	Educational Developmental Behavioral	Behavioral Cognitive Developmental Psychodynamic Family systems Neurobehavioral	Behavioral Developmental Milieu	Behavioral Educational	Developmental Neurobehavioral Behavioral Cognitive Psychodynamic Family systems
Clientele	Families of children aged 0 to 3 years who are diagnosed with developmental delay or are at risk for delay	Children and adolescents 2 to 18 years of age	Children and adolescents 5 to 18 years of age and their families	Children and adolescents 5 to 10 years of age, sometimes families	Children and adolescents 10 to 18 years of age	Children and adolescents 3 to 18 years of age
Staffing*	2 and 3 Special educators Speech-language pathologists Audiologists Occupational therapists Physical therapists Social workers Psychologists Nurses Nutritionists	1 and 2 Educators Special educators Speech-language pathologists Occupational therapists Physical therapists Counselors Psychologists Administrators	1, 2, and 3 Psychiatrists Psychologists Social workers Nurses Counselors Occupational therapists Art therapists Recreational therapists Music therapists	2 and 3 Houseparents Psychologists Social workers Educators	1 and 2 Guards Police officers Parole officers Lawyers Psychologists Psychiatrists Social workers Educators Counselors Occupational therapists	1 and 2 Psychiatrists Nurses Unit staff Psychologists Social workers Occupational therapists Recreational therapists Music therapists Art therapists

*Dominant team style: 1, Multidisciplinary; 2, interdisciplinary; 3, transdisciplinary.

4. What is the role of a case manager? How would you fulfill this role with Vanessa and her baby?

Part B

The therapist worked with Nicole and Vanessa individually and together. To coordinate care, she established communication with two other agencies that were also providing services to the family: the state's Department of Children and Family Services and the public school. ECI with Nicole was focused toward increasing her arousal level and responsiveness to the environment, developing motor control, and improving her efficiency in eating. Neurodevelopmental and sensory integrative therapy techniques were applied to reach these goals. The therapist provided a selection of toys each week and encouraged Vanessa to give Nicole opportunities to move and explore the environment.

Vanessa was initially shy and guarded with the therapist but became increasingly comfortable after several weeks. The therapeutic relationship was forged when the occupational therapist and Vanessa worked together to assemble a colorful mobile for the baby's crib. During that session, Vanessa confided that she was living in fear of Nicole's father, who had beaten Vanessa repeatedly during her pregnancy and was threatening her life if she did not agree to let him move into the apartment.

5. What are the therapist's legal and ethical responsibilities at this point?
6. What resources are available for this family?

The occupational therapist assisted Vanessa in contacting a battered women's service organization, which offered support groups, crisis shelter, legal services, and adult education programs. She also helped Vanessa identify family members who might be able to assist with childcare and to help with occasional transportation needs. During the course of their relationship, the occupational therapist continued to listen to Vanessa's concerns and encouraged her to pursue the resources that were available to her. She also monitored the home situation for potential violence toward Nicole, in case a referral to Child Protective Services was needed. Additionally, she maintained regular communication with the referring pediatrician, who assisted with monitoring Nicole's health and the family's progress.

Although Vanessa consistently expressed strong feelings of affection and the desire to be a good mother to Nicole, the therapist observed that the mother-infant interactions were often poorly synchronized, resulting in frustration for both.

7. What are five risk factors for child neglect or abuse that are present in this case?
8. What is the therapist's legal responsibility at this point?
9. What resources are available to the therapist/case manager?

10. What would be the long- and short-term therapy goals for this family?
11. Is there sometimes a conflict between client-centeredness and our legally mandated obligations to protect clients from abuse and neglect? How do we align client-centered values with the needs and concerns of clients who are experiencing family violence?

The occupational therapist taught Vanessa to recognize Nicole's changing states of arousal and to time her attempts to engage the baby in social play when Nicole was calm and alert. Vanessa learned to involve Nicole in developmentally appropriate interactive activities such as "peek-a-boo," gentle tickling, and "so big." She also learned the importance of providing Nicole with a variety of sensory, motor, and language experiences.

After 6 months of therapy, Vanessa was regularly attending educational and support activities sponsored by the women's shelter. She planned to enroll in her school's vocational training program. Nicole had become appropriately active and sociable, and both she and her mother interacted warmly in a manner that bespoke their mutual emotional development and attachment. Nicole's motor development was in the low-average range.

The therapist in this example helped the family address key psychosocial needs through direct intervention and community referral. The ECI team carried out its mission by providing direct assistance and coordinating the provision of services among various agencies. As with most young families, the psychosocial and physical needs of the infant could only be met fully when those of the primary caregiver were met as well.

■ PUBLIC SCHOOL SYSTEMS

The primary mission of public education is academic and social preparation for future education and work roles. Research shows that this goal has been largely unreached for students who have emotional and behavioral problems (Carson, Sitlington, & Frank, 1995; Maag & Katsiyannis, 1998; Blackorby & Wagner, 1996; Walker & Bunsen, 1995). Prevalence studies have indicated that 10.5% of secondary special education students have a primary classification of emotional disturbance, making this group the second largest after that of learning disabilities (Blackorby & Wagner, 1996). Beyond this group, many others also have behavioral problems that disrupt their performance in school. Students with moderate to severe behavioral problems are unable to take full advantage of education and experience repeated academic and social failure. As high as 40% of students with emotional or behavioral disorders drop out of high school (U.S. Department of Education, 1993). These students have a significantly increased risk for economic dependency and crime (Blackorby & Wagner, 1996; Wagner, 1995). The public schools represent an arena where occupational therapists have an unrealized opportunity to have a tremendous effect on the lives of children with psychosocial problems.

Students whose special needs are primarily of a psychosocial nature are classified by the school system as "seriously emotionally disturbed" (SED). Federal regulations of the Individuals with Disabilities Education Act (IDEA) (1990, 1997) define this special education classification as:

> . . . a condition exhibiting one or more of the following characteristics over a long period of time and to a marked degree, which adversely affects educational performance: (A) An inability to learn that cannot be explained by intellectual, sensory, or health factors; (B) An inability to build or maintain satisfactory interpersonal relationships with peers or teachers; (C) Inappropriate types of behavior or feelings under normal circumstances; (D) A general pervasive mood of unhappiness or depression; or (E) A tendency to develop physical symptoms or fears associated with personal or school problems.

Children who exhibit psychosocial disorders are included under the classification *"seriously emotionally disturbed."* This category does not include children who demonstrate socially maladjusted behavior (e.g., delinquency, school truancy, conduct disorder) in the absence of the problems previously listed. Other categories in which psychosocial problems and behavioral disorders are often present include pervasive developmental disorders, mental retardation, and traumatic brain injuries (IDEA, 1990).

A variety of school settings serves special education students with behavioral problems, depending on the school districts' and individual schools' philosophies and resources, individual students' needs, and parents' preferences. Self-contained classroom arrangements allow students whose behavior is frequently disruptive or otherwise inappropriate to receive intensive behavioral intervention while being educated in a small group setting. However, students in such classrooms are segregated from peers and role models and suffer the stigma of being identified as "different." The current trend is toward the inclusion of special education students in regular education settings as much as possible. In this model, students attend regular education classrooms with support services that may include a resource room for specific subjects, classroom aides, crisis intervention, and counseling services. Benefits of this approach include regular exposure to a normal school environment, opportunities to interact with typically developing peers, and positive experiences that reinforce learning of social skills. Problems can arise with this approach when the teachers have large numbers of students and little training in preventing or managing disruptive behaviors. Teachers and students then feel inadequate and frustrated.

Many schools incorporate social skills training programs into their regular curricula that are taught by the classroom teachers. These programs are suitable for all children, and they address areas such as communication skills (Gresham & Elliot, 1993), social problem solving (Shure & Spivack, 1982; Weissburg, 1985; Weissberg, Caplan, & Bennetto, 1988), and drug abuse prevention (Cohen, Brennan, & Sexton, 1984). Such educational programs can provide an excellent means of developing pro-social thinking and behavior in typically developing children. However, these programs do not provide the intensive guidance required by children and adolescents who have psychosocial dysfunction affecting performance in these areas.

School-based therapeutic intervention is directed toward enhancing students' academic and future vocational performance with an emphasis on both scholastic and social development. Traditionally the school psychologist, counselor, or social worker assumes responsibility for evaluating psychosocial needs and may work with students in individual or small group sessions. These professionals serve the needs of all students, not just those in special education, and may not have an extensive clinical background in psychopathology (Maag & Katsiyannis, 1996). Frames of reference usually include behavioral, cognitive, and developmental approaches (see Table 30-1).

Many leaders in education and occupational therapy believe that the services provided to behaviorally disturbed students are inadequate in quantity and quality (Florey, 1989; Maag & Katsiyannis, 1996; Martin, Lloyd, Kauffman, & Coyne, 1995). Teachers express despair as they sacrifice creative educational methods to address behavioral crises. Parents of *students with behavioral disorders* are frustrated by the paucity of services to address their children's particular needs. All parents are concerned about their children's safety and social education while they are at school.

Two similar models for providing psychosocial occupational therapy services in the school systems have been described by Agrin (1987) and Schultz (1992). Both writers described occupational therapy activity groups for elementary students who have social and behavioral difficulties. Motivating activities such as planning and preparing meals, creating craft projects, producing a newspaper, performing skits and plays, and refinishing furniture help students develop competencies in daily living skills while practicing adaptive responses to interpersonal challenges and developing self-confidence. The goals of this type of approach would facilitate improved occupational functioning in the classroom and other school settings. Agrin's (1987) experience with this type of group indicated that many times, improved behavior generalized beyond the confines of therapy, thus winning the support of educators and administrators in the school.

Agrin also speculated that the students' future success in less restrictive settings could be predicted by the development of their social skills in the activity groups.

Students who are referred for occupational therapy services to address fine motor, perceptual, or orthopedic problems may also have social and emotional needs that impair academic performance. Case Study 2 exemplifies how one student's multiple needs were addressed. With the advent of inclusion, general education teachers are working with increasing numbers of special needs children, including those who have educational diagnoses of SED. Additionally, their classrooms include children who are not enrolled in special education, but who are troubled and preoccupied with acute and/or chronic life stresses such as poverty, community violence, and family turmoil. In some schools the majority of students are trying to learn despite a climate of constant crises. Behavioral disruptions are frequent and educators feel endangered and unsupported. Occupational therapists are positioned to provide consultation to teachers who need ideas regarding environmental adaptation and group management, and to assist with determining which students should be referred for evaluation. By educating and supporting teachers, therapists can have a positive influence on the school experiences of hundreds of children.

The School to Work Opportunities Act (1994) and IDEA (1997) both reflect the high priority placed on preparing students for gainful employment. Middle and high school students who have emotional and behavioral problems are considered by many to be among the most difficult to transition successfully into independent living and satisfying, economically adequate work (Carson, Sitlington, & Frank, 1995; Maag & Katsiyannis, 1998; Wagner, 1995). Although no universally successful means have been identified, research to date indicates that the most promising interventions include individualized planning that involves the student and parents. The intervention should also include social skills training and support, classroom education regarding work values and life skills, and actual work experience in positions that involve a good fit between students and jobs (Maag & Katsiyannis, 1998). Age- and situational-appropriate occupations should be emphasized over performance components training, and environments should be structured to facilitate students' success (Brollier, Shepherd, & Markley, 1994). Occupational therapists are able to provide any and all of these services, and they can serve educational teams, as well as transitional planning specialists.

The idea of school-based occupational therapists providing psychosocially oriented intervention is innovative. Based on a review of the special education literature, Schultz (1992) believed that teachers would welcome the kind of assistance that occupational therapists can provide in improving students' social skills. School administrators who appreciate the shortage of therapists to meet even the traditional referrals may initially be less encouraging. School-based therapists who are committed to providing holistic services need to educate and persuade colleagues regarding the potential effectiveness of occupational therapy approaches to help students meet central academic goals by developing essential psychosocial skills. This may be approached directly through inservices and program development, and indirectly by incorporating psychosocial goals into students' individual education programs. Trends in inclusionary and transitional education have created an atmosphere in which occupational therapy leadership in comprehensive holistic intervention approaches are needed and will be welcomed.

Case Study 2: Darnell
Part A

Darnell was an 8-year-old second grader who was referred for an occupational therapy evaluation because his handwriting was slow and illegible. The teacher completed a Preassessment Checklist (Figure 30-1), indicating that Darnell often exhibited problems with incomplete and careless work, disorganized work habits, and peer relations characterized by teasing and rejection, as well as the handwriting difficulty that precipitated the referral.

1. What assessment tools and methods would you choose to use with Darnell? What information would you want to obtain from these?
2. What other educational team members would you include in your evaluation? How and why?
3. Does your assessment battery provide information about the student as a person, his environment, and his occupational performance?

Part B

During the evaluation session Darnell was polite and compliant. His affect was generally sad, and he made frequent self-disparaging comments, such as, "I'm not good at this." When motor testing was completed, the occupational therapist asked about Darnell's feelings about school this year and whether he had anyone in his class with whom he played on a regular basis. He reported feeling "okay" about school in general, but said, "I don't have any friends at school. They all say I'm fat and dumb." Darnell's fine motor skills were significantly below average.

4. What are this student's key strengths and limitations?
5. What kinds of long- and short-term treatment goals would you formulate? How can these goals be written to relate directly to Darnell's academic performance?
6. What intervention approach do you recommend?

NAME:_____ AGE:_____ DOB:_____ GRADE:_____

SCHOOL:_____ TEACHER:_____

Thank you for your referral to OT services. Your completion of the following will help us to effectively plan evaluation and intervention.

Difficulties Observed in Pupil Behavior	never	seldom	occasionally	often	always
Has trouble following directions					
Cries easily					
Has difficulty with balancing (climbing steps)					
Fatigues easily					
Has difficulty with matching shapes (3-5 yr.)					
Has difficulty identifying letters & numbers (5 + yr.)					
Has reading problems (6 + yr.)					
Has poor awareness of self in space; bumps into children, desks, and walls					
Seems "nervous" or anxious					
Easily frustrated, gives up quickly					
Confuses directional concepts (up and down, in and out, before and behind)					
Has poor understanding of spatial concepts					
Over-reacts to unexpected touch and/or sound					
Dislikes removing outer garments or standing close to classmates					
Unable to control distractibility					
Unable to control over-activity					
Has difficulty in independent work habits					
Disorganized in manner of working, inexact, careless					
Does not participate in classroom and playground activities; "withdrawn"					
Does not automatically hold paper while writing					
Ignores or cannot use one side of body in gross motor activities					
Aggressive behavior					
Disregards the feelings of others					
Makes decisions impulsively					
Is teased or rejected by peers					
Is socially immature					

figure 30-1   Preassessment checklist for occupational therapy services in public schools.

7. From what other school services would Darnell benefit?

Part C

Darnell was enrolled in 30 minutes per week of occupational therapy with two other second graders. The group worked on developing writing and cutting skills by making group collages with themes, such as, "I can be a friend by. . ." and "The five best things about me are. . . ," by drawing pictures of what they would like to be doing 20 years in the future, and by writing and illustrating collective stories. Group members discussed their ideas and, with guidance and encouragement from the therapist, began to listen to one another, express their ideas, and give and accept positive feedback. The boys shared ideas about how to make friends and cope with teasing and rejection. Darnell and another boy developed a friendship that continued outside of the sessions. The group members voted to name themselves "The Tuesday Club," adding to their sense of belonging. Additionally, the therapist worked with Darnell's teacher on adaptations that would facilitate improved organization, handwriting performance, and social interactions. Together they designed a chart to reward desirable behaviors. Finally, the occupational therapist advised the parents regarding recreational opportunities, such as YMCA day camp and Boy Scouts, which would further enhance Darnell's social and motor skills.

8. In designing a behavioral charting program for Darnell, what would be three target behaviors to reinforce? (These should relate to problems with academic performance.)

9. What adaptive techniques might help with organization, handwriting, and social interaction?

After one semester of occupational therapy, Darnell's grades improved significantly. His mother reported that he no longer resisted attending school on most days, and Darnell reported satisfaction with his school performance and social life. The teacher was pleased both with Darnell's progress and with her success in using a behavior charting system. At that point the occupational therapist reduced intervention to biweekly monitoring and occasional consultation with the teacher.

The therapist in this example met the concerns of the referring teacher, who could not read the student's writing, and the concerns of the student, who felt isolated and anxious at school. Both problems significantly impaired the student's academic progress and were effectively and efficiently addressed through a combination of direct service and consultation.

▪ OUTPATIENT MENTAL HEALTH SERVICES

Children and adolescents who seek *outpatient mental health services* usually have significant behavioral disturbances. Typically, the young person's problems have caused moderate to severe levels of disturbance for family, school, or community members by the time mental health care commences. The primary goals of outpatient mental health services are the diagnosis and management of mental health problems to improve functioning within the community and the prevention of crises necessitating hospitalization.

The child's initial contact with an outpatient mental health facility usually consists of an intake interview exploring the nature and severity of the child's and the family's problems. Responses to the interview form the basis for decisions regarding appropriate evaluation and intervention. In many cases, the intake interviewer is a social worker or a paraprofessional who is trained in mental health screening. Possible dispositions include outpatient evaluation at a later date or crisis evaluation with immediate short-term intervention.

Outpatient mental health services may be provided through freestanding clinics, hospital-based programs, community mental health centers, health maintenance organizations, and private practice offices. Funding sources may include the clients' families, private insurance, Medicaid, federal grants, and state monies (Manderscheid & Sonnenschein, 1992). The agency's sources of funding influence the types of clientele served and the types of services provided. For example, private for-profit services are generally affordable only by upper-income families with generous insurance plans. These programs may offer special services such as yoga or academic tutoring, in addition to the traditional interventions. Middle- and lower-income families usually seek services that are partially publicly funded and therefore more basic (Tuma, 1989).

The Diagnostic and Statistical Manual of Mental Disorders, Fourth Edition (DSM-IV) (APA, 1994) is used to classify clinical problems into diagnostic categories. Children and adolescents seek services from community and outpatient mental health services for help with problems ranging from attention deficit disorder to schizophrenia. Service provision often begins with screening and crisis intervention. Comprehensive evaluation of the child and family may consist of interviews, play sessions, and standardized psychologic or developmental testing. Therapy may be provided for the individual child or parent, couples, groups, and families. Parent education groups, pharmacotherapy, and case management may also be available. Some mental health centers offer primary prevention services such as public education, wellness programs, and consultation to public schools. Other services include vocational training, respite care, and day care services (Homonoff & Maltz, 1991).

Frames of reference used in outpatient programs vary with the philosophies of the specific facilities, but they commonly draw from cognitive, behavioral, family systems, neurobiologic, and psychodynamic theories (see Table 30-1). Treatment approaches are most commonly goal-focused, time limited, and involve the family and school. Clients generally attend one or two 1-hour sessions per week for a specified period. In publicly funded mental health centers, payment for services is based on the individual's income. Third-party payers have varied levels of coverage for mental health care. Therapeutic modalities commonly include play therapy (for young children), talking, expressive art, therapeutic board games, group discussions, and family discussions. Staffing patterns may take the form of multidisciplinary, interdisciplinary, or transdisciplinary models and typically include psychologists, social workers, and psychiatrists, with some combination of psychiatric nurses, licensed counselors, and trained paraprofessionals (Manderscheid & Sonnenschein, 1992).

The number of occupational therapists who currently

work with children and adolescents in community-based mental health practice is relatively small. In 1990, approximately 9.2% of all practicing occupational therapists specialized in mental health, and only 14.8% of these worked with clients younger than 19 years of age (AOTA Member Survey, 1990). Work with children and adolescents who have significant emotional and behavioral problems is extremely challenging. A well-developed understanding of developmental and biopsychosocial theories and their occupational therapy applications, as well as excellent communication and behavioral management skills, are required. Personal maturity and comfort with role sharing are needed. Empathy and the ability to relate to troubled children and their families must coexist with the knowledge that often the clients' values and behaviors run counter to those of the therapist. Many communities lacking in social resources such as work training and social activities may not be able to provide comprehensive programs for these children and families.

With the challenges inherent in community-based mental health practice come some compelling rewards. Children and adolescents bring a sense of spontaneity and energy to treatment that is found less often in adult clients. The crafts, games, and daily living activities that are so much a part of occupational therapy are extremely motivating and developmentally appropriate for most young people. The therapeutic relationships formed with many young clients can be powerful in their capacity to facilitate positive change, giving therapists a tremendous sense of accomplishment. Working with clients within the context of their families, schools, and communities affords the greatest opportunities for generalizing therapeutic effects into everyday living. Additionally, occupational therapists have a unique combination of skills, for example, expertise in developmental evaluation, sensory integration evaluation and therapy, and activities-based therapy, that is highly valued by intervention teams (Case-Smith, 1994). Client and public education regarding issues such as parenting, stress reduction, and child development are needed services that occupational therapists can provide. Teaching childcare workers, educators, and vocational trainers ways of promoting effective social and work-related behavior is a valuable consultation service. Service coordination and interfacing with other service agencies are also important roles well suited to occupational therapists (Adams, 1990). Program planning and administration are areas of mental health practice in which occupational therapists can excel (Nielson, 1993). Such services may be provided in clinical or community settings, including the public schools or clients' homes.

In 1992, congress authorized the Comprehensive Community Mental Health Services for Children and their Families Program. This program provides federal funding through demonstration grants to states and communities and is designed to promote effective ways to organize, coordinate, and deliver mental health services and supports for individual children and their families. Cultural competence is a critical goal of the program, and each grant must document that the policies and practices of each agency address the impact of and show respect for the race, culture, and ethnicity of the children and families they serve. The agencies that have been receiving funding provide a broad array of services, including occupational therapy and are designed to meet the multiple and changing needs of children and adolescents with serious emotional disturbances and their families. The projects place emphasis on family involvement and support and linkage between home and school. Many of these projects involve day treatment services for culturally diverse children and adolescents (U.S. Department of Health and Human Services, 1997).

Day treatment programs are offered in a variety of settings, including psychiatric hospitals, community mental health facilities, and schools for students with special needs (Pruitt & Kiser, 1991). Such programs provide a middle step between outpatient intervention and hospitalization and are becoming popular for clinical and economic reasons (Erker, Searight, Amant, & White, 1993). Clients attend programming from 4 to 6 hours per day, 5 days per week, and are at home during evenings and weekends (Block & Lefkovitz, 1992).

Day treatment may facilitate a child's transition from the hospital back to the home and community, provide crisis stabilization, allow comprehensive evaluation, or serve as an intensive therapeutic alternative to outpatient or inpatient treatment (Pruitt & Kiser, 1991). Programming often follows a psychoeducational model and may include vocational evaluation and training for adolescents (Nelson & Condrin, 1987). A psychiatrist or psychologist who specializes in child and adolescent mental health typically leads intervention teams. Other team members are listed in Table 30-1 and often include occupational therapists.

Occupational therapy activities are selected to motivate and facilitate self-awareness and communication skills, develop grooming and etiquette habits, and teach life skills such as cooking and community mobility. Crafts, role-playing exercises, cooperative action games, and therapeutic board games are popular modalities in such occupational therapy programs. Working with the client's parents, childcare providers, teachers, job coach, or school-based occupational therapist can facilitate the transition from intensive day treatment programs to the community and public school and enhance the carryover of interventions and goals. The family may also benefit from assistance with locating and securing social and leisure resources. Case Study 3 describes how a consultative model of intervention may be used to assist with the transition of a client from day treatment back to full community involvement. The focus in this example is on educating and problem solving with personnel from another agency.

Case Study 3: Mario
Part A

Mario was 17 years of age and had diagnoses of mild mental retardation, anxiety disorder, and impulse control disorder. He had a lifelong history of poor socialization with nonfamily members, separation anxiety, and occasional temper tantrums. Mario was admitted to day treatment after a series of explosive episodes during which he broke furniture and a window.

1. To what kinds of services would you expect Mario to have access in a day treatment program?
2. What are the current needs for assessment? What team members would address these needs and how?

Part B

Mario, his family, and the treatment team decided that Mario would begin a job-training program following discharge from day treatment. It was determined that the occupational therapist would serve as the liaison between the treatment and the job-training program. The administrators at the job-training site expressed both interest and a little trepidation at the notion of working with a client who had a history of psychiatric disturbance with aggressive behavior.

3. What job-training programs are available in your area? Who administers them? How are they funded?
4. What are three ways that occupational therapists can help to dispel negative stereotypes regarding persons with mental illnesses?
5. How might a therapist meet the client's and work programs' needs in this case?

Part C

To facilitate his transition, the occupational therapist accompanied Mario and his mother to Mario's first appointment at the job-training program. As the job trainer and Mario discussed the program's operations, the therapist made suggestions to increase Mario's chances of success. One suggestion was for Mario to write the program schedule into his pocket calendar and to negotiate with the job trainer any times needed for psychiatric or medical appointments. Another suggestion was for the job trainer to provide Mario with a written list of basic expectations for participation in the program, such as arriving on time, wearing appropriate clothing, and bringing a sack lunch. Mario's mental health problems were discussed, and the therapist was able to clarify the nature of the disorder and the behavioral cues that had been effective in therapy, as well as information about Mario's medications.

6. What are the legal and therapeutic issues involved in discussing a client's medical or psychiatric issues with a community member? What is your opinion of this therapist's actions?
7. In what other ways could Mario's transition be facilitated into this new environment?

Part D

Once Mario began the job-training program, the occupational therapist remained available on an as-needed basis. Things progressed smoothly until Mario graduated from the sheltered training site into competitive employment with a job coach. At this point Mario began to display anxiety, and he occasionally became verbally threatening to his supervisor and co-workers. The job coach called the occupational therapist who helped to analyze the process. It was learned that Mario was acting out when he was given what he perceived as conflicting directives from different supervisors. It was also observed that Mario did not interact with co-workers, even if they greeted him.

8. How could these problems be addressed?

Part E

The therapist met with Mario, the coach, and the supervisors to negotiate a plan. It was decided to (1) assign Mario routine tasks that needed to be performed the same way each time, as much as possible; (2) limit Mario's supervision to one person at a time; and (3) encourage Mario to verbalize his feelings of confusion, anxiety, and frustration to his supervisor before he felt overwhelmed. The therapist assisted Mario and his supervisor in writing and signing a behavioral contract that outlined consequences for behavioral outbursts: a 30-minute break after the first outburst and suspension without pay for the remainder of the day if there was a second outburst. Finally, the therapist spent some time in the company lunchroom helping Mario meet and find some commonalities with his co-workers. Once Mario was integrated with his colleagues and supervisor, he was able to demonstrate his full potential as a reliable and capable worker.

▪ RESIDENTIAL TREATMENT CENTERS

Residential Treatment Centers present an environment that is more restrictive and intensive than a day treatment program, but less restrictive than an acute care hospital setting. The number of residents living in care centers for emotionally disturbed children and adolescents has approximately doubled between 1970 and 1990 when it reached 27,785 (Manderscheid & Sonnenshein, 1994). Lengths of stay in residential treatment centers vary considerably and are influenced by funding constraints, the facility's philosophy, and the needs of the client and family (Spreat & Jampol, 1997). Placement may last from weeks to years (Durrant, 1993). Approximately 15% of residential treatment centers serve children with severe chronic disabilities such as severe mental retardation and autism (Tuma, 1989). Other facilities serve children who are unable to function in home and community settings due to behavioral problems that have grown out of chronic neglect and abuse (Spreat & Jampol, 1997). Program philosophies range from highly structured and intensively therapeutic to more naturalistic and home-like environments. Facilities vary in size from a few to hundreds of residents. Children and adolescents who require residential treatment are usually troubled by combinations of psychologic, social, behavioral, and family problems that are severe and chronic enough to warrant extended periods of care and respite.

The primary goals of residential treatment facilities are to provide safe and nurturing living environments while preparing children and adolescents for a successful return to the community and their families, foster homes, or independent living arrangements. The staffing reflects the facility's philosophies and target populations. Most programs are largely staffed by trained paraprofessionals (sometimes called "houseparents") who provide round-the-clock care. Psychotherapists and administrators, who may be social workers, psychologists, or psychiatrists, provide supervision. Educational services for the children may be provided on-site or through the local public school system.

Traditionally, occupational therapists are not full-time staff members. Some residential treatment facilities may contract for services that include consultation to the house staff regarding the residents' developmental needs and limitations, ways to organize and guide household responsibilities to include the residents, and ways to teach self-care and community living skills. Other occupational therapists provide services within their school programs, addressing goals related to academic and social performance.

Children who live in even the most deluxe institutional settings do not have access to many occupational experiences that are a part of the daily cultures of others. Direct intervention with the children and adolescents could include many of the goals and approaches outlined in the discussion of occupational therapy in day treatment programs. Often the therapists intervene to facilitate the resident's participation in community activities such as shopping, playing sports, participating in activity clubs, and attending church. Opportunities for as much family interaction as possible during such activities increase the benefits of such experiences (Spreat & Jampol, 1997).

A small but growing area of occupational therapy psychosocial practice is the *juvenile justice system*. Juve-

nile justice and mental health service systems have always worked closely together to evaluate and rehabilitate young offenders (Mulvey, 1984). Children and adolescents who steal, vandalize property, or assault others may enter either the mental health or the correctional system, depending on whether the behavior is interpreted as a symptom of a conduct disorder or a violation of the law (Tuma, 1989). Occupational therapists are increasingly involved in the comprehensive psychiatric evaluations of children and adolescents who are either under consideration for psychiatric commitment or who are to be tried as adults. Youth offenders who are enrolled in diversional programs or who are being treated in state or other psychiatric facilities may also receive occupational therapy.

■ INPATIENT PSYCHIATRIC HOSPITALS

Inpatient psychiatric hospitals provide the most restrictive, intensive, and costly therapeutic intervention. It is generally reserved for children and adolescents who pose a serious safety risk to themselves or others, who have complicating medical conditions, or who are considered to have poor prognoses if treated as outpatients (Mabe, Riley, & Sunde, 1989). Inpatient psychiatric units may be found in general hospitals, state psychiatric hospitals, and private psychiatric hospitals. There was a burgeoning of inpatient facilities from the middle 1970s through the 1980s, when reimbursement for such care was abundant. This trend ended and reversed with the advent of managed mental health care and increased controls by third-party payers on admissions and lengths of stay (Dalton & Forman, 1992). Despite such shifts in service availability, there will always be a need for the rapid diagnosis and stabilization that such specialized facilities provide.

Child and adolescent inpatient psychiatric units are usually locked facilities that are staffed by nurses and paraprofessionals who are trained in the care and management of severely impaired patients (Dalton & Forman, 1992). Very often patients are hospitalized when in crisis, such as after a suicide attempt, an assault, or a psychotic episode. Sometimes patients are admitted for comprehensive psychological and medical evaluation of complex chronic problems. In most cases the length of stay is limited to days or weeks, with the goal being rapid discharge to less costly and restrictive treatment alternatives.

The treatment team is interdisciplinary and may include psychiatrists, nurses, paraprofessional direct care staff, social workers, recreational therapists, psychologists, special educators, and music therapists, as well as occupational therapists (see Table 30-1). Trainees representing these professions may also circulate through the team. Frames of reference reflect a variety of psychosocial theories, with behavioral and neurobiologic approaches among the most commonly used (Dalton & Forman, 1992).

Occupational therapists who work with children and adolescents who are experiencing acute psychiatric problems have an important role in diagnosis, stabilization, and discharge planning. Activities within a locked hospital unit are typically quite structured, limiting opportunities for individual choices and participation in many occupational roles. Often the occupational therapist's evaluation of hospitalized children includes observation of the patient performing activities that are motivating and require the cognitive, social, and adaptive skills needed at home and school. Additionally, occupational therapists evaluate the child's performance levels as they compare with developmental norms. This information allows the team to predict more reasonably how the youth performs when coping with the demands of community settings.

It is essential for members of any interdisciplinary team to combine their unique perspectives on each patient's needs into a cohesive and coherent plan that is mutually agreeable. This cohesion is especially important when working with patients who are challenging and often volatile. The following case study illustrates how an occupational therapist recognized a programmatic need and worked with an administrator and interdisciplinary team to implement changes.

Case Study 4
Part A

One common goal of psychiatric treatment with adolescents is to facilitate a youth's identification with the peer group. This developmentally appropriate goal may be met counterproductively, such as when the patients group together to perform antisocial activities like smuggling alcohol into the unit or assisting a peer in running away from the hospital. This type of dynamic occurred in the adolescent psychiatric unit of a large teaching hospital about twice per year, usually soon after a large influx of new patients entered the unit. The traditional manner of response to such group behavior was unit restriction, during which time the regular schedule of therapies, school, and passes was suspended. During unit restriction the patients, nurses, and therapists gathered several times daily to try to facilitate the adolescents' understanding of the group process and their individual roles in contributing to the negative behaviors. Often this was a lengthy and painful process because of the adolescents' limited comfort and skills in communicating their feelings and concerns. Meetings were characterized by periods of silence and blaming, and they often ended in frustration on all sides.

1. What are the benefits and costs of the current approach to group dysfunction?
2. How does the described approach fit with the value of client-centered care?

Part B

The occupational therapist hypothesized that the group meetings would be more productive if the patients had basic communication skills and a better sense of their own values and feelings. The therapist met with the program director and proposed incorporating daily self-awareness and assertiveness groups into the unit restriction protocol in an effort to catalyze the unit restriction process. The director approved the idea and suggested presenting it to the rest of the team for feedback. Other team members were less enthusiastic because they viewed occupational therapy as fun and rewarding to the patients. They thought that this would undermine the punitive aspects of unit restriction.

3. How would you respond to the other team members' concerns? Do you think that other professionals and clients may often view occupational therapy as mainly entertaining? Why?
4. How could you gain the team's support for trying a new approach?
5. What kinds of activities would you want to do with the clients? How could these be structured to maintain discipline and the spirit of "restriction?"

Part C

The occupational therapist explained that the highly structured activities would develop skills that are foundational to the verbal processing that was needed. Inappropriate behavior would lead to suspension from the session. The team agreed to a trial of occupational therapy during unit restriction with the provision that if the misbehavior increased, the sessions would discontinue. Unit nurses and staff were invited to observe or join the sessions, at their discretion.

The adolescents, many of whom felt bored, isolated, and confused by the unit restriction, immediately welcomed the occupational therapy sessions. Initial sessions facilitated learning and applying words to express feelings about being hospitalized, being a part of the patient group, and the causes and effects of unit restriction. Subsequent sessions were devoted to teaching concepts and skills related to assertive communication.

The incidence of group behavior was significantly decreased, and as a result the unit, staff members had to cope with fewer disciplinary problems. Most importantly, the patients discussed pertinent issues during process meetings. They were able to explore and understand the group's responsibility to the progress of each member and each individual's responsibility to the betterment of the group. The ensuing maturation led to the development of a positive peer group culture in which the majority discouraged individual antisocial behaviors.

Staff members were pleasantly surprised to observe that the occupational therapy sessions were clearly related to the goals of the unit restriction, and they expressed their support by direct feedback and by helping to prepare the room and gather the patients for sessions. Additionally, the occupational therapist believed that her treatment philosophy and skills were better understood by the rest of the team, the result being, greater job satisfaction.

■ SUMMARY

Children and adolescents with emotional, cognitive, and behavioral problems are unable to participate satisfactorily in home, school, and community life. Social problems such as poverty, family sociopathic conditions, and cultural violence have been linked with an increased incidence of psychosocial dysfunction in young people (Constantino, 1993; Prothro-Stith, 1991; Wolfner & Gelles, 1993). Such social problems are steadily increasing in our country, while mental health services for young people continue to be inadequate in quantity and quality. Occupational therapists who work with young people have the knowledge and skills to help improve their clients' occupational functioning by addressing key psychosocial needs. This may be accomplished through individual and group therapy, program development, and consultation. Pediatric occupational therapists in all settings need to become psychosocial practitioners to meet effectively the urgent and growing needs of young people and their families.

References

Adams, R. (1990). The role of occupational therapists in community mental health. *Mental Health Special Interest Newsletter, 13* (1), 1-2.

Agrin, A. (1987). Occupational therapy with emotionally disturbed children in a public school. *American Journal of Occupational Therapy, 7,* 105-114.

American Occupational Therapy Association. (1990). *Member Data Survey.* Rockville, MD: American Occupational Therapy Association.

American Psychiatric Association. (1994). *Diagnostic and statistical manual of mental disorders* (4th ed.). Washington, D.C: American Psychiatric Association.

Blackorby, J., & Wagner, M. (1996). Longitudinal post school outcomes of youth with disabilities: Findings from the National Longitudinal Transition Study. *Exceptional Children, 62,* 399-413.

Block, B., & Lefkovitz, P. (1992). *Standards and guidelines for partial hospitalization.* Alexandria, VA: American Association for Partial Hospitalization.

Broillier, C., Shepherd, J., & Markley, K. (1994). Transition from school to community living. *American Journal of Occupational Therapy, 48,* 346-353.

Carson, R., Sitlington, P., & Frank, A. (1995). Young adulthood for individuals with behavioral disorders: What does it hold? *Behavioral Disorders, 20,* 127-135.

Case-Smith, J. (1994). Defining the specialization of pediatric occupational therapy. *American Journal of Occupational Therapy, 48,* 791-802.

Cohen, J., Brennan, C., & Sexton, B. (1984). *A social cognitive approach to the prevention of adolescent substance abuse. Intervention I: Sixth grade. (A manual).* New Haven, CT: Yale University School of Medicine, The Consultation Center.

Constantino, J. (1993). Parents, mental illness, and primary health care of infants and young children. *Zero to Three, 13* (5), 1-10.

Coulton, C., Korbin, J., Su, M., & Chow, J. (1995) Community level factors and child maltreatment rates, *Child Development, 66,* 1262-1276.

Dalton, R., & Forman, M. (1992). *Psychiatric hospitalization of school-age children.* Washington, D.C: American Psychiatric Press.

Davidson, D. (1995). Physical abuse of preschoolers: Identification and intervention through occupational therapy. *American Journal of Occupational Therapy, 49,* 235-243.

Davidson, D., & LaVessar, P. (1998). Facilitating adaptive behaviors in school-aged children with psychosocial problems. In J. Case-Smith (Ed.) *AOTA self-study series: Occupational therapy: Making a difference in school based practice.* Bethesda, MD: American Occupational Therapy Association.

Durrant, M. (1993). *Residential treatment: A cooperative, competency-based approach to therapy and program design.* New York: W.W. Norton.

Erker, G., Searight, H.R., Amant, E., & White, P. (1993). Residential versus day treatment for children: A long-term follow-up study. *Child Psychiatry and Human Development, 24,* 31-39.

Florey, L. (1989). Nationally speaking: Treating the whole child: Rhetoric or reality? *American Journal of Occupational Therapy, 43,* 365-368.

Gresham, F., & Elliot, S. (1993). Social skills intervention guide: Systematic approaches to social skills training. *Special Services in the Schools, 8,* 137-158.

Homonoff, E., & Maltz, P. (1991). Developing and maintaining a coordinated system of community-based services to children. *Community Mental Health Journal, 27,* 347-358.

Humphry, R. (1995). Families who live in chronic poverty: Meeting the challenge of family-centered services. *American Journal of Occupational Therapy, 49,* 687-693.

Hunter, J., & Powell, G. (1990). Failure to thrive. In C. Semmler & J. Hunter (Eds.). *Early occupational therapy intervention.* Gaithersburg, MD: Aspen Publications.

Individuals with Disabilities Education Act of 1997 (Public Law 117-05), 20 U.S.C. 1401.

Individuals with Disabilities Education Act of 1990 (Public Law 101-476), 20 U.S.C. 1401(a)(17).

Knitzer, J. (1982). *Unclaimed children.* Washington, D.C: Children's Defense Fund.

Maag, J., & Katsiyannis, A. (1996). Counseling as a related service for students with emotional or behavioral disorders: Issues and recommendations. *Behavioral Disorders, 21,* 293-305.

Maag, J., & Katsiyannis, A. (1998). Challenges facing successful transition for youths with E/BD. *Behavioral Disorders, 23,* 209-221.

Mabe, P., Riley, W., & Sunde, E. (1989). Survey of admission policies for child and adolescent inpatient services: A national sample. *Child Psychiatry and Human Development, 20,* 99-111.

Manderscheid, R., & Sonnenschein, M. (Eds.). (1992). *Mental health, United States, 1992.* Rockville, MD: U.S. Department of Health and Human Services.

Martin, K., Lloyd, J., Kauffman, J., & Coyne, M. (1995). Teachers' perceptions of educational placement decisions for pupils with emotional and behavioral disorders. *Behavioral Disorders, 20,* 106-117.

Mulvey, E. (1984). Judging amenability to treatment in juvenile offenders: Theory and practice. In R. Price & J. Monahan, (Eds.). *Children, mental health, and the law.* Beverly Hills, CA: Sage Publications.

National Advisory Mental Health Council. (1990). *National plan for research on child and adolescent mental disorders.* Washington, D.C: National Institute of Mental Health.

Nelson, R., & Condrin, J. (1987). A vocational readiness and independent living skills program for psychiatrically impaired adolescents. *Occupational Therapy in Mental Health, 7,* 105-113.

Nielson, C. (1993). Occupational therapy and community mental health: A new and unprecedented turn. *Mental Health Special Interest Newsletter, 16* (3), 1-2.

Offard, D., & Fleming, J. (1991). Epidemiology. In M. Lewis (Ed.). *Child and adolescent psychiatry: A comprehensive textbook.* Baltimore: Williams & Wilkins.

Peloquin, S. (1993). The patient-therapist relationship: Beliefs that shape care. *American Journal of Occupational Therapy, 47,* 935-942.

Pickens, J., & Field, T. (1993). Facial expressivity in infants of depressed mothers. *Developmental Psychology, 29,* 986-988.

Prothro-Stith, D. (1991). *Deadly consequences: How violence is destroying our teenage population and a plan to begin solving the problem.* New York: Harper Collins.

Pruitt, D., & Kiser, L. (1991). Day treatment: Past, present, and future. In M. Lewis (Ed.). *Child and adolescent psychiatry: A comprehensive textbook.* Baltimore: Williams & Wilkins.

School-to-Work Opportunities Act of 1994, 20 U.S.C.A. § 6101 et seq. (West 1996).

Schultz, S. (1992). School-based occupational therapy for students with behavioral disorders. *Occupational Therapy in Health Care, 8,* 173-196.

Shure, M., & Spivack, G. (1982). Interpersonal problem-solving in young children: A cognitive approach to prevention. *American Journal of Community Psychology, 10,* 341-356.

Solomon, P., & Evans, D. (1992). Service needs of youths released from a state psychiatric facility as perceived by service providers and families. *Community Mental Health Journal, 28,* 305-315.

Spreat, S., & Jampol, R. (1997). Residential services for children and adolescents. In R.T. Ammerman & M. Hersen (Eds.). *Intervention in the real world context: Handbook of prevention and treatment with children and adolescents* (pp. 106-133). New York: John Wiley & Sons, Inc.

Tuma, J. (1989). Mental health services for children: The state of the art. *American Psychologist, 44,* 188-199.

United States Department of Education. (1993). *Fifteenth annual report to Congress on the implementation of the individuals with disabilities education act.* Washington, D.C: United States Government Printing Office.

United States Department of Health and Human Services. (1997). *Caring for every child's mental health: Communities together campaign: Fact sheet.* Rockville, MD: United States Department of Health and Human Services, Substance Abuse and Mental Health Services Administration, Center for Mental Health Services.

Vondra, J. (1990). Sociological and ecological factors. In R.T. Ammerman & M. Hersen (Eds.). *Children at risk: An evaluation of factors contributing to child abuse and neglect* (pp. 149-165). New York: Plenum Press.

Wagner, M. (1995). Outcomes for youths with serious emotional disturbance in secondary school and early adulthood. *Future of Children, 5* (2), 90-112.

Walker, R., & Bunsen, T. (1995). After high school: The status of youth with emotional and behavioral disorders. *Career Development for Exceptional Individuals, 18,* 97-107.

Weissberg, R. (1985). Developing effective social problem-solving programs for the classroom. In B. Schneider, K.H. Rubin, & J. Ledingham (Eds.). *Peer relationships and social skills in childhood* (Vol. 2). New York: Springer-Verlag.

Weissberg, R., Caplan, M., & Bennetto, L. (1988). *The Yale New Haven problem solving (SPS) program for young adolescents.* New Haven, CT: Yale University.

Williamson, G. (1993). Enhancing the social competence of children with learning disabilities. *Sensory Integration Special Interest Section Newsletter, 16,* 1-2.

Wolfner, G., & Gelles, R. (1993). A profile of violence toward children: A national study. *Child Abuse and Neglect, 17,* 197-212.

chapter 31

Transition Services: From School to Adult Life

Karen C. Spencer

key terms

Legal mandates
Transition services
Collaborative teaming
Ecologic approaches
Community-referenced assessment
Interagency linkages
Models of service delivery

■ CHAPTER OBJECTIVES

1. Define transition services for youth and young adults with disabilities.
2. Describe the mandate for transition services based on federal legislation.
3. Describe collaborative teamwork as it applies to the school-to-adult life transition process.
4. Describe an ecologic service model as it relates to transition-age students.
5. Describe the interagency linkages needed for effective transition services.
6. Identify the role of occupational therapy in the transition process, including assessment, program planning, and service delivery.
7. Compare alternative models of service delivery, including direct service, consultation, monitoring, and service coordination.

Individuals with disabilities may spend from 12 to 18 years receiving some form of education. Education is viewed as a way to develop the knowledge, skills, and experiences that are needed to assume productive adult roles. These adult roles can include pursuing post-secondary education, maintaining paid employment, vol-unteering, living in the community, and maintaining meaningful relationships.

Occupational therapists have valuable contributions to make to the transition process as youth with disabilities move from school to a variety of adult roles, activities, and environments. With a focus on promoting human performance of essential occupations in a variety of natural contexts, occupational therapy personnel can help design and implement effective transition services. These services may be characterized as a collaborative venture involving the student, his or her family, members of the educational team, including occupational therapists, and as needed, representatives from adult service agencies which provide vocational, residential, or recreational services.

This chapter discusses federal legislation related to mandated transition services, describes "best practice" models for the delivery of transition-related services, and presents specific roles for occupational therapy personnel in the transition process for youth with disabilities.

■ LEGISLATIVE BACKGROUND

Since the passage of Public Law 94-142, The Education for All Handicapped Children Act of 1975 (EHA), special education and related services have been made available through the public education system to the nation's children and youth who have disabilities. Occupational therapy was described in the EHA as a "related service." Related services were intended to complement and extend the efforts of teachers by helping children and youth with disabilities to participate more fully in and to obtain maximum benefit from their educational program.

The EHA and its subsequent amendments (Individuals with Disabilities Education Act, [IDEA], 1990, 1997) guarantee a free and appropriate education for all children with disabilities. An appropriate education is one in which children with disabilities acquire, to the maximum extent possible, the skills, knowledge, and behaviors that will ultimately help them function successfully as adults. After initial passage of the EHA, several major benefits were realized:

1. Formal mechanisms were established to identify and bring children with disabilities into the public education process.

2. Parents and guardians were identified as essential members of the educational team and were provided with legal rights related to their child's education.

3. All identified children were provided with Individualized Education Programs (IEPs) developed by an educational team that included the student's parents or guardians.

As with many public law and policies, the full intent of the EHA has never been fully realized. Negative post-school outcomes have been reported for many youths with disabilities and, in large part, demonstrate the shortcomings. For these individuals the benefits of a free public education have not consistently translated into community living, gainful employment, income, social connections, or quality of life. A national, longitudinal study of young adults who completed special education programs revealed that a large percentage of research participants entered adult lives characterized by isolation, dependency, and nonproductivity (Blackorby & Wagner, 1996). The poor transition outcomes experienced by the nation's youth with disabilities (Wagner, 1989, 1995) as well as the associated human and economic costs helped spur the passage of the EHA amendments in 1990. For the first time, these amendments directly mandated school-to-adult life transition planning and services for youths with disabilities. Additionally the 1990 amendments renamed the EHA, the Individuals with Disabilities Education Act (IDEA) (Public Law 101-476). This name change reflects the commitment of the federal government to use respectful, nonstigmatizing language when referring to people with disabilities.

The new focus on school-to-adult life transition processes and the 1990 federal mandate for transition services represented a significant change for the special education system nationwide. Schools were given the responsibility to provide comprehensive, individualized transition services for all special education students. Transition services were defined in the law as . . .

> . . . a coordinated set of activities for a student, designed with an outcome-oriented process, which promotes movement from school to post-school activities, including post-secondary education, vocational training, integrated employment (including supported employment), continuing and adult education, adult services, independent living, or community participation. The coordinated set of activities shall be based on the individual student's needs, taking into account the student's preferences and interests, and shall include instruction, community experiences, the development of employment, and other post-school adult living objectives, and, when appropriate, acquisition of daily living skills and functional vocational evaluation (P.L. 101-476, pp. 1103-1104).

Transition services, mandated by IDEA, reflect the major performance areas that are typically addressed by occupational therapy: work or education, independent living (including activities of daily living), and community participation, which may include community mobility and transportation, access to community services and activities, recreation and leisure, and socialization and relationships. Among the other highlights of the 1990 amendments was the requirement for interagency involvement during transition planning and the delivery of services. The IEP was identified in the law as the forum for discussing and documenting interagency involvement. For example, if a student required supported employment or independent living services that were provided by a community-based, non-school agency, a service commitment would be formally documented on the IEP.

As the central feature of special education for students, the IEP also provides a structure for individualized transition planning. During the IEP process for a transition-aged student, a team meets to discuss the student's needs and abilities. Discussion is followed by goal setting and the development of a written, individualized program of education and related services. The IEP is a legal document that is intended to provide assurances and accountability for the delivery of appropriate services.

The IEP team for a transition-aged student is composed of the student, school personnel (administrators, teachers, related services, and others as needed), and the student's parents or guardians. The student's presence at the IEP meeting requires that all other team members pay close attention to their own communication and create a comfortable environment that respects the student and allows him or her to participate and lead the process to the maximum possible extent. Student presence at the IEP meeting requires professionals to abandon jargon and negative labeling and to focus on the student's strengths and abilities.

In 1997, IDEA was amended and re-authorized (P.L. 105-17). Perhaps the most far-reaching change is the requirement for all educators and related service personnel to consider each student in terms of his or her progress and involvement in the *general education curriculum.* This requirement is in contrast to local educational policies that did not expect children with disabilities to use the general education curriculum and to be evaluated as part of general education outcomes. The 1997 amendments clearly intend that children with disabilities gain greater access to general education and in doing so, improve the knowledge and skills required to function as literate, productive citizens.

These IDEA provisions emphasized that, once a child has been identified as being eligible for special education, the connection between special education and related services and the child's opportunity to experience and benefit from the general education curriculum should be strengthened (IDEA, 1997, §300.347, p. 55091).

For many special educators and related service personnel, this new focus on helping students achieve within the general curriculum creates exciting opportunities and some difficult challenges. Under the 1997 amendments, services provided to students with disabilities outside the general education environment must be justified in the IEP. In many cases, transition services will be provided to students in community settings and not solely in the classroom. Statements justifying community experiences give therapists the opportunity to explain the importance of evaluation, problem solving, and to practice in a natural context to prepare youth for successful transition to community living and work (Giangreco, 1996; Rainforth & York-Barr, 1997).

With the new focus on enabling students with disabilities to participate to the maximum possible extent in the general education curriculum, the 1997 amendments added related services to the list of transition services that may be provided to a student. Furthermore, the 1997 amendments specify the attendance of related service professionals (including contracted therapists) at IEP meetings when it is appropriate.

In addition, the IEP team must consider the student's transition-related needs by age 14 and a formal statement of transition services and any interagency responsibilities must be stated in the IEP by age 16. The 1990 amendments had specified age 16 as the starting point for transition planning and services. This change recognizes that for some students the transition from school to adult life will be a complex process requiring adequate time for long-range planning. If the transition process begins at 14 years of age, students are more likely to have the necessary services and supports in place when they complete high school.

From an occupational therapy perspective, the 1997 amendments change the way services are designed and justified. First, the IEP requirement to specify how a child's disability affects his or her participation in the general education curriculum requires occupational therapists to understand the general curriculum. Most school districts publish general education "standards." These standards are an essential resource for occupational therapists who must become informed about general education expectations for different age groups.

Second, student assessment by the occupational therapist must now address discrepancies between the child's performance and the expectations established by the general curriculum. Educationally relevant assessment focuses on how the child actually performs in the educational environment and what supports, services, or adaptations are needed to maximize that performance. An occupational therapist must complete functional observations and determine present levels of performance within the general education curriculum. Evaluation must be directly relevant to planning each student's IEP and transition goals.

Third, the 1997 amendments strengthen the role of assistive technology in educating students with disabilities, including those who are transition-aged. Individual technology needs must be addressed during the IEP process for all special education students. This does not mean that all students will need or receive assistive technologies. It does mean, however, that technology of potential benefit to the student must be consistently addressed by education teams during the IEP process to ensure that each student has an opportunity to receive technology services. In many school districts, occupational therapists are instrumental in the provision of assistive technology assessments and services and are therefore in an excellent position to help implement the assistive technology portion of IDEA.

Adding further emphasis to nationwide transition efforts that began in 1990, the federal School-to-Work Opportunities Act of 1994 (P.L. 103-239) was enacted by Congress. Unlike IDEA, this law does not differentiate between students with and without disabilities, nor does it target only the public education system for action. All students may participate in school-to-work initiatives, and multiple agencies and programs share responsibility for developing and implementing a comprehensive system of school-to-work activities. According to the National School-to-Work Learning and Information Center (1996), the act . . .

. . . provides seed money to States and local partnerships of business, labor, government, education, and community organizations to develop school-to-work systems. This law doesn't create a new program. It allows States and their partners to bring together efforts at education reform, worker preparation, and economic development to create *"A system to prepare youth for the high-wage, high-skill careers of today's and tomorrow's global economy"* (p. 1).

With federal seed money, states are allowed to design school-to-work systems that meet local needs that can be implemented with local partners. With positive employment outcomes in mind, school-to-work systems in every state are expected to provide learners with a highly relevant education, marketable skills, and valued credentials that are recognized by employers. To achieve these outcomes, each state's system must include three main elements (National School-to-Work Learning and Information Center, 1996):

1. *School-based learning* in the classroom based on occupational skill standards that are defined by businesses and the schools.

2. *Work-based learning* that provides students with active hands-on learning opportunities in the workplace. At community work-sites, students may participate in direct work experience, training, mentoring, or career exploration.

3. *Connecting activities* that link classroom-based and on-the-job learning activities, match students with community employers, train community mentors, and generally build bridges for students between school and the workplace.

For over a decade, the national, state, and local focus on the transition of students from school to productive, adult roles has required teachers and related service personnel to become well informed about any and all resources and programs that could benefit their students. For students who have disabilities, IDEA and the School-to-Work initiatives can be coordinated, therefore expanding student learning opportunities. Occupational therapists are well qualified to design and deliver transition services as defined in IDEA and School-to-Work initiatives, thereby contributing to positive post-school outcomes for youth with disabilities.

It is now understood that for most students, optimal learning takes place through highly relevant activities and across a variety of environments where skills can be generalized and practiced. The School-to-Work initiatives affirm the value of experiential learning related to employment for all students. While promoting the inclusion of students with disabilities in the general curriculum, IDEA also recognizes that a student's successful transition from school to adult life requires opportunities to learn and to practice skills in a variety of relevant school and nonschool learning environments. These environments may include the classroom, school lunchroom, home, public transit bus, work site, community recreation facility, and a variety of other relevant settings. Occupational therapy practitioners are well prepared to provide identified students with needed services by (1) using environmentally referenced, situational assessments that examine discrepancies between the environmental demands (e.g., general curriculum, community job expectations) and the student's performance, (2) directly teaching needed skills in relevant contexts and providing students with opportu-

nities to practice, (3) changing or adapting environments to facilitate optimal student performance given his or her current skills, and (4) adapting or changing tasks within an environment to support student performance (Dunn, Brown, & McGuigan, 1994). Occupational therapy, therefore, can assist students with disabilities to perform essential roles and activities in school and in a wide range of real-life settings and situations.

■ "BEST PRACTICE" FOR TRANSITION

Transition services clearly emphasize outcomes. This means that IEPs are specifically developed with the student's eventual school-to-adult life transition in mind. The student's educational program, therefore, must prepare him or her to perform the desired and necessary adult roles in a variety of current and anticipated community environments. Effective transition services are evaluated based on the extent to which graduated students and young adults actually achieve meaningful work roles, live in the community, engage in chosen recreation activities, and have ongoing positive social relationships. Accountability for these types of outcomes has significant implications for how teachers and related service personnel provide transition-related services. A description of the "best practices" related to the design and delivery of transition services follows. For the purposes of this introductory chapter, the best practices related to the school-to-adult life transition process include three major features:

1. The use of *collaborative teaming* among professionals, agencies, the student, and family members (NICHCY, 1993; Rainforth & York-Barr, 1997; Wehman, 1992)

2. The use of an *ecologic curriculum* that focuses on the interactions between the student and his or her environments (Brown et. al., 1979; Rainforth & York-Barr, 1997; Sample, Spencer, & Bean, 1990)

3. The establishment and use of *interagency linkages* to facilitate the smooth transfer of support and training from the school to adult and community agencies when the student exits public schools (Everson & McNulty, 1992; Halloran, 1992; NICHCY, 1993)

Collaborative Teaming

Rainforth and York-Barr (1997) describe collaboration within an educational context as "an interactive process in which individuals with varied life perspectives and experiences can join together in a spirit of willingness to share resources, responsibility, and rewards in creating inclusive and effective educational programs and environments for students with unique learning capacities and needs" (p. 18). For transition-aged students, collaboration is viewed as an effective way for a team to help the student achieve his or her goals as related to future adult living. The primary team member is the student. Other team members may include the student's family, friends and classmates, teachers, related service professionals, representatives of adult service agencies, and others. The collaborators on the team must have a shared sense of purpose that is driven not only by the student, but also by the student's unique interests, abilities, and needs. Central to effective collaborative teamwork is each team member's ability to share the responsibility for student outcomes and not to work solely from their discipline's perspective. For example, the occupational therapist, teacher, and paraprofessional may all work with a student who has significant motor limitations toward the goal of completing written classroom assignments. This would be an appropriate transition goal because it is grounded in the general education curriculum, and it is based on the student's anticipated need for literacy as an adult and on the aspirations for post-secondary education. The occupational therapist may oversee and coordinate an assessment of the student's technology-related needs and abilities, followed by the selection of specific hardware and software for adapted computing. With the technology in place, then the occupational therapist may spend time working with the student, teacher, and paraprofessional who will be involved in the day-to-day use of the technology in the classroom. Therefore a collaborative working relationship is established, with the team sharing responsibility for meeting the *student's* goal of completing written work. There is no need for separate goals to guide each member of the team.

Collaboration requires a commitment on the part of the different team members to teach each other and to learn from each other across traditional disciplines or professional boundaries (Lyon & Lyon, 1980; Giangreco, 1996). Collaboration also requires services to be delivered in functional, real-life situations (Rainforth & York-Barr, 1997). In the previous example, the occupational therapist would be working with the student in the classroom where other students are also engaged in written work. Occupational therapy services would not be provided in a separate location that is isolated from the real-life demands of the student's classroom.

In addition to the need for collaboration among the team members at the student's school, there is a need for collaboration between the school and other community agencies related to transition (NICHCY, 1993). As students with disabilities approach the end of their school career, many will need ongoing supports or services. These services may help the young adult obtain and maintain community employment, live in the community, and participate in social and recreational activities. To achieve a smooth transition from the supports and services of the schools to the supports and services of other external community agencies requires extensive communication and collaboration. It is therefore considered the best practice to include community agencies in the transition planning process. These agencies are also potential providers of some transition services, although

the student is still enrolled in school (Everson & McNulty, 1992). A word of caution, however, is in order: members of collaborative, interagency transition teams must create or identify services or supports based on the individual student's needs. They must refrain from simply matching students with available "slots" in existing programs or agencies (Mount, 1987). This strategy requires time and effort on the part of all members of the team to maintain clear communication and to conduct planning and services that are truly in the best interests of any student who is making the difficult transition from familiar education environments to an array of separate community services and settings.

Collaborative teamwork can clearly benefit transition-aged students when the diverse perspectives, backgrounds, and skills of team members can be brought together to create effective services and to solve challenging problems. Team members themselves can also benefit because collaboration promotes the establishment of cooperative and caring relationships among team members characterized by communication, shared responsibility, and mutual support (Rainforth & York-Barr, 1997). Members of collaborative teams have a sense of belonging and do not have a strong need to compete with other team members for status or authority.

Ecologic Curriculum

For the purposes of this chapter, curricula are viewed as carefully selected, sequenced activities and learning materials used primarily by teachers to guide classroom teaching. General education curricula reflect the "standards" that have been adopted by a school district or a state and may be commercially developed and purchased by a school, or they may be locally designed and developed by the education professionals who use them. Regardless of the source, curricula are widely viewed as structured guides for teaching groups of children. For students enrolled in special education, the general curriculum serves as an overarching framework within which individualized educational services and supports are provided (IDEA, P.L. 105-17, 1997). Furthermore, IDEA requires students who receive special education services be evaluated based on the general education standards that apply to all students. Naturally, there will be students who, because of their disability, cannot meaningfully participate in traditional evaluation procedures *or* who cannot perform at a level commensurate with their peers. In these situations, alternative measurable assessments must be used on a regular basis to demonstrate levels of learning and progress.

The individualization of the general education curriculum for students with disabilities is accomplished through the IEP process. The IEP, conceived in federal law, is viewed as a blueprint guiding the day-to-day implementation of each student's educational program. Theoretically, no two students enrolled in special education should have the same IEP. Each student's individual interests, needs, abilities, goals, and anticipated performance environments must be used to guide IEP development.

Brown and others (1979) first described a broad curricular model for students with significant disabilities that addressed student performance in essential life domains: domestic (home), vocational, community, and leisure. These domains were later expanded to include school (York & Vandercook, 1991), where children and youth spend a great deal of time. This domain-based curriculum is highly relevant for transition-aged students because it focuses the efforts of teachers and related service personnel on enhancing student performance in areas that are essential for productive and meaningful adult life (Spencer & Sample, 1993; York & Vandercook, 1991). It considers each student as a unique individual who must function in a variety of contexts both while in school and as an adult.

A domain-based curriculum for transition-aged youth specifies to some extent *how* and *where* transition services should be delivered. The *how* aspect of service delivery relates to collaborative teaming among members of the education team and the use of highly relevant learning materials and activities. The *where* aspect of service delivery relates to the team's use of highly relevant teaching and learning environments to include the school, home, and assorted community environments. Taken together, the *how* and *where* aspects of a transition curriculum may be termed *ecologic*, focusing on the interaction between the student and the environments in which he or she participates (Rainforth & York-Barr, 1997). The use of ecologic models is considered "best practice" for students with significant disabilities (Rainforth & York-Barr, 1997; Williams, Fox, Thousand, & Fox, 1990), including those students who are approaching the transition from school to adult life.

An effective ecologic curriculum is based on some core principles that must be embraced by all members of a student's educational team, including the occupational therapist. These principles include the following:

1. Age-appropriate placement of the student with same age peers with and without disabilities.

2. Integration of education and related services.

3. Use of community-referenced, ecologic assessment.

4. Active involvement of the student in planning and decision making.

5. Instruction in a variety of relevant, school and community environments.

6. Evaluation of the extent to which students are achieving targeted transition outcomes.

Age-appropriate placement of students with disabilities in educational activities alongside their chronologic age peers, with and without disabilities, has been deemed the best practice (Giangreco, Cloninger, & Iverson, 1998; Williams et. al., 1990). The inclusion of students who have disabilities in typical educational activities and environments is believed to promote student performance, offer rich opportunities for learning, provide age-appropriate role modeling, increase awareness among all students of diverse learning styles and abilities, and provide opportunities for relationship building that is so important during adolescent development. Age-appropriate placement does not mean that students with disabilities are simply placed in a typical class or at a community job site. Appropriate support services and resources that facilitate the student's full inclusion and maximum participation in the environment must accompany these placements.

Total responsibility for meeting the needs of students with disabilities cannot fall solely on the teacher. It must be shared among different members of the student's education team. The occupational therapist may be identified as an essential support person for a given student. The occupational therapist may work in the classroom or on a job site directly with a student, consult with the teacher or employer on how to best adapt activities to accommodate student abilities, or train a teacher or paraprofessional to implement specific occupational therapy recommendations throughout the course of the student's day.

Integrating education and related services brings members of the team together to address a student's goals. An integrated approach is best explained using the following example:

> Amelia is an 18-year-old student who wants to live in the community after she completes high school. At her IEP meeting a transition goal to use neighborhood services was developed. Amelia has significant cognitive, communication, and mobility limitations that currently interfere with her ability to access and use services and businesses in her neighborhood. To meet her transition goal, the team identified the need for Amelia to begin to participate in purchasing needed food and personal items at her neighborhood grocery store. An integrated approach was developed involving the teacher, speech-language pathologist, and occupational therapist. Amelia's special education teacher developed strategies with Amelia that allowed her to shop from a pictured list of items. Amelia's speech-language pathologist worked with Amelia at the grocery store, teaching her to initiate a transaction and functionally communicate with grocery store employees. The occupational therapist, addressing the same goal, worked with Amelia to devise a way for her to carry grocery items and move safely around the store. In addition to their own specific responsibilities, each professional worked with Amelia in the grocery store environment and communicated what occurred to the other team members so that efforts were overlapping, complementary, and reinforcing.

Community-referenced assessment (ecologic assessment) is considered an essential feature of the best transition-related practice with youth and young adults (Rainforth & York-Barr, 1997; Spencer, Murphy, Bean, & Schelly,

1991; Spencer & Sample, 1993; Woolcock, Stodden, & Bisconer, 1992). The purpose of a community-referenced or ecologic approach is to identify student performance needs and abilities in the environments that he or she is expected to use as an adult. For example, if the team seeks to identify the student's interests, needs, and abilities as they relate to future employment, the assessment must take place, to a large extent, in actual employment settings. Systematic and careful observation of the student's performance during actual work tasks is completed to identify discrepancies between the demands of the job and the student's current performance level. Services are subsequently designed to reduce these discrepancies as the student acquires context-specific work skills. Because of the highly individual nature of transition planning, services, and environments for any given student, traditional discipline-specific assessments are not recommended (Giangreco, Cloninger, & Iverson, 1998; Rainforth & York-Barr, 1997). Collaboration among team members during an ecologic assessment process will yield the most valid and useful information that can then be used to design or adjust services and supports.

The *active involvement of the student in planning and decision making* is considered one of the most important aspects of effective transition services (Halloran, 1992; Sands & Wehmeyer, 1996; Ward, 1992; Wehmeyer & Sands, 1998). The ultimate goal of education according to Ward (1992) is for students to actively participate in and fully manage their own lives.

> Professionals can facilitate the development of self-determination skills by involving youth with disabilities in the transition planning process. . . . The goal is for students to assume control (with appropriate levels of support) over their transition program, and identify and manage its various components (p. 389).

Active involvement of the student in planning and decision making related to his or her transition requires the thoughtful attention of the professional members of the educational team. The format of the IEP meeting may need to be adjusted to facilitate student involvement. For example, the student (with or without support) may prepare the agenda, introduce team members, or chair the meeting. To assume these functions, it is likely that the student would need help preparing for the meeting. This preparation should include some discussion of possible transition goals, activities, and timetables. During the IEP meeting, the attending professionals must follow the student's lead and keep discussions constructive by focusing primarily on the student's strengths and abilities.

Effective transition services require the delivery of *instruction in a variety of relevant, school and community environments* (Brown et. al., 1979; Giangreco et. al., 1998; Rainforth & York-Barr, 1997; Udvari-Solner, Jorgenson, & Courchane, 1992). In many cases, students

with disabilities, particularly those with severe disabilities, have difficulty learning needed skills. This problem, combined with the associated challenge of identifying optimal learning styles and teaching approaches, requires the attention of both education and related service professionals. In addition to difficulty with learning, students with significant disabilities may be unable to readily transfer or generalize learning to new environments or situations. For these reasons, it is best to provide education and related services in the actual environments that the student will be using, which allows for explicit teaching to the real-life demands of a particular environment and eliminates the need for the student to transfer skills. For example, if a student is learning to prepare simple meals to eat at his or her home, it is best to provide meal preparation training in that home environment. Meal preparation in a different kitchen environment may not promote acquisition of skills that transfer to the home.

Implementation of an ecologic curriculum requires periodic *evaluation of the extent to which students are achieving targeted transition outcomes* (Hasazi, Hock, & Cravedi-Cheng, 1992). Given the focus of an ecologic curriculum on preparing students to function in five major life domains (domestic, school, community, leisure, and vocational), best practice would require ongoing evaluations of the extent and quality of performance in each domain. Without periodic evaluation of the overall effectiveness of transition services, decisions regarding local educational practices and policies will not be well informed. Accountability for the expenditure of public resources on transition services also requires such an evaluation.

Transition outcomes that may be tracked by school districts include the extent to which students are (1) employed in the community, (2) living in the community, (3) satisfied with their lives, (4) using community services, (5) socially connected, and (6) participating in chosen leisure activities. These outcome data can be helpful to the members of the educational team who are responsible for designing and implementing individualized transition services. Occupational therapists, as members of educational transition teams, can specifically benefit from feedback regarding the efficacy of occupational therapy services.

Interagency Linkages

Although transition services, as mandated in IDEA to be initiated by the school on behalf of students with disabilities, Congress did not intend for schools to have total responsibility for the entire transition process. The need for *interagency linkages* became a part of the law in 1990, indicating the need for shared responsibility between local education agencies and adult or community service agencies, such as state vocational rehabilitation agencies (NICHCY, 1993). The interagency linkages envisioned by Congress included shared financial responsibility for the cost of needed transition services, including the sharing of personnel resources and expertise.

Implementing the vision from Congress of interagency linkages and shared resources is, without a doubt, challenging. This task is viewed as an administrative responsibility that should not fall solely on already overextended teachers and related-service personnel (NICHCY, 1993). Education and related-service personnel responsible for the implementation of transition services must know, however, who the other transition "players" and agencies are and must be prepared to invite them to participate fully in the transition process. The potential benefits of clear interagency linkages, however difficult to implement, are many.

> Establishing such interagency linkages can be of enormous benefit to students planning for transition. This is because, as students with disabilities leave the public education system, their entitlement to educational, vocational, and other services ends. In the place of one relatively organized service provider (the school system), there may now be a confusing array of many service providers (e.g., the local vocational rehabilitation agency, school-to-work systems, the state department of mental health, developmental disability councils, community service boards, the federal social security system). Individuals with disabilities who have left school become responsible for identifying where to obtain the services they need and for demonstrating their eligibility to receive the services. Therefore, for many students with disabilities, identifying relevant adult service providers, establishing eligibility to receive adult services, and having interagency responsibilities and linkages stated in the IEP, all while in school, will be necessary to ensure a smooth transition from school to adult life (NICHCY, 1993).

Linking the resources of different agencies can, to a great extent, facilitate the smooth transition of students with disabilities from school to an array of other services. Failure to initiate and formalize these connections while the student is still in school can result in the student being left out of services, sitting for extended periods on waiting lists, or losing skills because of the lost opportunity to participate in active learning. The importance of strong interagency linkages cannot be overstated.

■ OCCUPATIONAL THERAPY'S ROLE IN TRANSITION

The focus of transition services is on helping students with disabilities acquire essential skills that are needed for meaningful and productive adult life. This is consistent with occupational therapy's focus on promoting individual performance of essential life occupations, including participation in activities of daily living, work, school,

and leisure. In addition, an understanding of context and environment in the design and delivery of transition services is essential and represents one of occupational therapy's unique contributions to the transition process for students with disabilities. Context includes temporal and environmental aspects. Temporal aspects may relate to an individual's age, level of maturation, life stage, status along a continuum of ability and disability, and the time it takes to accomplish a given task. Environmental aspects of context include both the non-human and human (social) characteristics of context. Objects, tools, and buildings are examples of non-human contextual variables. Human or social characteristics of a given context may include friends and family members, social roles and expectations, and cultural features such as values, beliefs, and customs.

> Occupational therapy is most effective when it is imbedded in real life. If occupational therapists evaluate individual performance without considering the context of the performance, there is a great risk of interpreting the behavior inappropriately (Dunn et. al., 1994).

Three main areas for occupational therapy involvement in transition are presented and include: (1) evaluation, (2) service planning, and (3) the delivery of transition-related services.

Evaluation

Evaluation using an ecologic curriculum requires that the student, family, occupational therapist, and other members of the educational team, envision a desirable future for the student (Mount, 1987; Mount & Zwernik, 1988; Rainforth & York-Barr, 1997). This requires considering the student in the five major performance domains: domestic, school, vocational, community, and leisure. In general, the student and the team envision a future that includes a home in the community, use of assorted community services and amenities, some sort of job or productive activity, ongoing relationships, and participation in chosen recreational or leisure activities. These aspects of life are those that most people, with or without disabilities, envision for themselves.

In addition to clarifying a positive vision for the future, the team must also discuss the student's long-term needs for resources and supports that will allow the vision to become reality. For example, a young adult with significant disabilities may require long-term job support in the form of a job coach who provides on-the-job training and other supports needed to maintain employment. Another individual may require short- or long-term, in-home support with personal hygiene, dressing, and meal preparation to live in the community.

Evaluation follows the establishment of a vision of a high-quality life in the community *and* the team's identification of areas in which the student is likely to need support (Giangreco, 1996). The occupational therapist and other members of the collaborative team must assess the extent to which the student can currently achieve this vision based on existing skills and experience. The team also identifies discrepancies between the level that the student needs to be functioning for a successful transition and his or her current level of performance. Evaluation, therefore, must include observation of the student's performance in the actual situations and environments he or she is likely to encounter as a young adult. To conduct an ecologic transition evaluation, the team must do the following:

1. Specify the environments in which the student will participate (domestic, school, vocational, community, and in leisure.)

2. Prioritize the performance environments considered to be most essential in the short term and those that will become more important over time.

3. Identify the activities that occur naturally in the selected, prioritized environments. The student's actual performance of relevant activities in relevant environments provides essential information from which the team can plan and make decisions.

4. Divide the responsibility for conducting different parts of the assessment among members of the educational team. Family members as well as professionals may share responsibilities during the assessment process.

5. Conduct the assessment by actually observing student performance during activities in the selected environments. Based on careful observation, discrepancies between the environment and activity demands and the student's ability to perform should be noted. This type of *discrepancy analysis* forms the heart of the assessment and guides planning and decision making.

6. Record the evaluation findings for the purposes of communicating with all members of the educational team, including the student and his or her parents. It is recommended that a consistent recording format be used, such as the one presented in Figure 31-1.

7. Present the findings to the team during the IEP meeting. With all the needed information before them, the team can proceed with planning transition services using an ecologic model.

The following is an example of a transition-related assessment completed by an occupational therapist:

> Ron is 16 years of age and is enrolled in his neighborhood high school. He is about to attend his IEP meeting, and his team has already discussed what a desirable future for Ron would look like. Ron's desired future includes living in the community with other people that he chooses, shopping at his neighborhood grocery store, and having a few ongoing and close friendships. Ron is very sociable, enjoys music, communicates with a combination of sign language and words, and walks slowly with a walker. Ron has cerebral palsy and severe mental retardation.

In preparation for the IEP, members of the team have been assigned to gather information about Ron's current performance in domestic, vocational, school, community, and recreational domains. An ecologic assessment format was chosen with different members of the team coordinating assessment activities in each domain. The occupational therapist, with specific skills in assessing activities of daily living in the home environment, coordinated an assessment of Ron's performance in the domestic domain. This involved a trip to Ron's home, an interview with Ron and his mother, and direct observation of Ron during dressing, meal preparation, and eating activities. Evaluation findings are presented, in part, in Figure 31-2.

The occupational therapist also collaborated with the teacher to evaluate Ron's use of public transportation. While the teacher evaluated Ron's ability to follow a bus schedule, identify correct stops, pay, and communicate with the bus driver, the occupational therapist focused on the physical barriers that interfered with Ron's ability to ride the bus. This type of shared responsibility for an aspect of the assessment reflects collaborative teamwork.

Transition Service Planning

The mechanism for planning transition services is the IEP. Members of the team come together with assessments to discuss the student's identified abilities, interests, and needs. A useful way to approach the development of an IEP for transition has been clearly developed by Sample and others (1990). Specifically, an IEP meeting is held and the student and team members who know the student well and who have information to contribute to the planning effort are in attendance. One member of the team facilitates the meeting and guides discussion around five questions:

1. What are the dreams for the student when he or she leaves school? The team records these dreams as *Transition Goals*.

2. What is the student able to do now? The team records current student abilities as *Current Levels of Function*.

3. What does the student need? Needs relate to the discrepancies between what the student is able to do now in all five performance domains (domestic, school, vocational, community, and leisure) and the level of performance needed for an effective transition. *Student Needs* also encompass the types of services and supports needed to maximize performance in the different transition domains.

4. What is the student going to do this year? The team records this year's plan as *Annual Goals*.

5. Who, what, when, where, and how? Responsibility for implementation of the transition plan is assigned to members of the team and recorded as *Characteristics of Services*. In addition to the delegation of responsibility, the nature of services is determined and must be consistent with an ecologic curriculum approach.

Student: _____

Date and time of assessment: _____

Persons involved and roles: _____
_____

Domain: ___ Domestic
         ___ School
         ___ Vocational
         ___ Community
         ___ Recreation

Environment observed (describe general environment along with physical, social, and cultural attributes):

Activities observed in this environment:
1.
2.
3.

STUDENT PERFORMANCE

Strengths/interests	Supports needed/barriers
Activity:	
add pages as needed	

Summary:

figure**31-1**   Ecologic assessment. *(Modified from Spencer, K., Murphy, M., Bean, G., & Schelly, C. [1991]. Vocational needs assessment: A functional, community-referenced approach. In K. Spencer [Ed.]. From school to adult life: The role of occupational therapy in the transition process [pp. 185-213]. Fort Collins, CO: Office of Transition Services Department of Occupational Therapy, Colorado State University.)*

A useful way to organize and summarize transition planning during the IEP meeting is to write main points on a blackboard or flip chart for all team members to see. The five questions previously listed serve as headings (Figure 31-3). This type of recording allows all members of the team to follow the process and to actively participate in decisions.

The role of the occupational therapist during transition service planning is to contribute information (based on evaluation results) and to share ideas for service delivery (goals, learning activities, and learning environments) that will help the student ultimately achieve his or her transition goals. The occupational therapist may contribute information about the student in all domains or

Student: Ron Hunt

Date and time of assessment: October 3, 1994, 7:30AM-9:00AM

Persons involved and roles: Ron Hunt, student; Marie Hunt, mother; Sara Clark, occupational therapist

Domain: X   Domestic
           ___ School
           ___ Vocational
           ___ Community
           ___ Recreation

Environment observed (describe general environment along with physical, social, and cultural attributes):

The assessment took place at Ron's home, which is located in a quiet, older residential neighborhood with large trees and off-street sidewalks. The single-level, three bedroom house has five steps up to the entrance. Ron lives with his mother and a younger sister who is 13 years old. Assessment activities took place in the well-equipped kitchen and in Ron's bedroom and bathroom.

Activities observed in this environment:
1. Clothing selection, dressing, grooming
2. Breakfast preparation and eating
3. Lunch preparation/packing

STUDENT PERFORMANCE

Strengths/interests	Supports needed/barriers
Activity: Clothing selection, dressing, grooming.	
Ron selected a matching shirt and pants from his closet that were appropriate for the cool season.	Ron's mother, Marie, does Ron's clothes shopping and buys clothes in basic colors and styles that can be mixed and matched.
	Clothes are washed and hung in the closet by Marie.
Ron located socks and shoes, which he put on independently while sitting down.	Ron's shoes have velcro closures.
Ron combed his hair while looking in the mirror in the bathroom.	Marie verbally directed Ron to comb his hair. She also "touched up" his hair combing job.
	Marie schedules Ron's haircuts with the local barber.
Ron located his toothbrush and opened and squeezed a small amount of toothpaste onto his toothbrush. He brushed his teeth while receiving verbal guidance from his mother.	Marie verbally reminded Ron to brush his teeth. During the activity she verbally cued him to "brush the back teeth, top teeth," etc.
Ron independently located his wallet and pocket comb and put these in his rear pants pocket.	
Ron and Marie "talked" about plans for the day as Ron got ready. Ron used gestures, basic sign language, and "yes" and "no" to communicate. Ron initiated communication by saying "Mom!" loudly.	Marie communicates primarily by asking Ron "yes" and "no" questions, or she asks Ron to "show me."

figure 31-2   Example of ecologic assessment.

Question #1	Question #2	Question #3		Question #4	Question #5
Transition goals	Current levels of function	Student learning needs	Support/ training needs	Annual goals	Characteristics of services

figure31-3   Form to record a transition plan.

on one or two domains, depending on the areas evaluated and on how the team has divided the responsibilities. It is important to remember that transition and annual goals belong to the student and not to the members of the educational team. Effective transition planning requires that the team work in a collaborative manner, respecting the input of the student, family members, teachers, and related service personnel.

Implementation

The delivery of occupational therapy services in the schools requires close collaboration between the occupational therapists and the entire team. An ecologic approach is also required for transition-related occupational therapy services to be considered best practice. The specific focus of occupational therapy intervention for transition-aged students is to maximize student performance of essential roles and activities in real-life situations and environments.

The student's IEP for transition, specifically the student's long-term transition goals, determines the involvement of occupational therapy services in the student's program. These services may be delivered in a number of ways based on the needs of the student and the resources of the team:

1. *Direct service* provided by the occupational therapist to the student.

2. *Consultations with the student's core educational team,* including the student, family members, and other school personnel.

3. *Consultations with community agencies* that share responsibility for the implementation of transition-related services.

4. *Monitoring* of services designed by the occupational therapist but delivered primarily by other team members.

5. *Service coordination* or management of a particular student's overall transition program.

To illustrate direct service approaches for transition-aged students, some examples are useful. Consider a student with limited movement caused by severe and persistent spasticity. Direct occupational therapy services for this student may include evaluating, designing, and testing a wheelchair positioning device that allows him or her to maintain an upright seating position needed to complete school assignments and to work in the community. Direct occupational therapy services could also include teaching the student how to use an environmental control unit system that increases the ability to independently manage and control the home environment. For example, the occupational therapist may directly teach the student to use wheelchair-mounted switches to operate telephones, unlock and open doors, turn lights on and off, and turn a television or radio on and off.

Direct occupational therapy services may occur in a variety of environments. If the student's needs relate to home management and community living, it is best for direct services to take place in the student's home (e.g., teaching adapted techniques for dressing and grooming). If the needs are vocational, services are most appropriately delivered in the relevant community or job settings (e.g., teaching the student how to safely enter and exit a public bus when balance problems exist). For many students, transition-related needs are present in the area of school performance. In this situation, the occupational therapist may deliver direct services to the student in his or her classroom (e.g., modifying assignments and writing methods), during lunch period (e.g., eating with the use of adaptive equipment), or during extracurricular school activities (e.g., learning how to function effectively in a locker room). However, the occupational therapist must be *sensitive* to the stigma that any type of "special" or "different" services can have on a teenager or young adult. If the direct services involve unusual equipment, activities, or additional adults nearby, the student may strongly resist participating. If this is the case, direct service may result in resistance, and other less invasive intervention strategies should be considered, such as limited direct services paired with consultation.

Consultation with the student's core educational team is a frequently used service model for transition-aged youth. It requires that the occupational therapist have excellent listening, observing, and communication skills. Consultation fits well within a collaborative team framework where information is readily shared with team members and where no one team member is viewed as having ultimate "authority" or decision-making responsibility (Dettmer, Dyck, & Thurston, 1996; Hanft & Place, 1996; Pugach & Johnson, 1995). Although all team members have unique knowledge, experience, and perspectives, these attributes are blended within a collaborative team. The consulting occupational therapist is invited to the team because he or she is viewed as having knowledge or experience that complements the experience and knowledge of other team members. Occupational therapy input may be conveyed through discussion and joint problem-solving sessions with the student and other members of the team, or through demonstrations for and training of team members.

Unlike direct services, consultation requires ongoing communication and problem solving with many other players. It is incumbent on the consulting occupational therapist to listen and communicate in an effective way that helps other team members evaluate alternatives and make decisions. The consultant and the other members of the team share accountability for these decisions. Occasionally, the team may choose not to accept the consulting occupational therapist's suggestions. This may happen for a variety of reasons, two of which are mentioned here. Ineffective consulting may be attributed to the occupational therapist's failure to effectively listen and interpret the team's needs. In this situation the occupational therapist may carry his or her own agenda into the consulting situation, rendering him or her unable to listen to or hear what other team members are requesting. The result is an occupational therapist advocating and making recommendations that do not match what the team perceives as needs or priorities. A second reason that consultation may not be well received is the team's perception that they lack the expertise, time, or resources to carry out the occupational therapist's recommendations. The recommendations may be sound, but team members perceive that they do not have the resources and time to implement them, resulting in limited follow-through. The consultation effort, therefore, remains incomplete unless the occupational therapist stays

involved and helps the team identify implementation alternatives.

To increase the likelihood of effective occupational therapy consultation with the team, it is strongly recommended that the occupational therapist maintain involvement with the student and his or her team over time. This continuing contact makes it possible for the occupational therapist to evaluate the extent to which information has been received, understood, and acted on by team members. It also allows for new information to be gathered and for further clarification or modification of recommendations. Effective consultation, therefore, is more than a one-time event. Ideally, it is an ongoing "conversation" with the consultant, the student, and other team members.

From the school district's perspective, occupational therapy consultation with the student's core educational team is often viewed as a way for the occupational therapist to have a greater influence on the educational environment than direct service can achieve. A strong relationship between the occupational therapist and a core educational team can clearly benefit individual students and families, as well as an interdisciplinary group of professionals. The benefits to the team include identifying solutions that may help more than one student, learning to solve problems interactively, and gaining a better awareness of the expertise and roles of different team members. The ultimate goal of consultation is to enable the person or persons seeking the consultation to solve current and future problems in a more skillful way (Dunn, 1988; Hanft & Place, 1996).

Consider a 16-year-old student who was working on community job skills as a part of his transition program.

> The student had a work-study position in the laundry area of the local hospital. The teacher, paraprofessional, job coach, and speech pathologist had all recognized that the student could not perform some of the required job tasks despite his strong motivation to work. To address the student's difficulties on the job, the team requested consultation from the school's occupational therapist. After an assessment of the student's current job performance and interviews with the employer, the student, and the job coach, the occupational therapist met with the other team members for discussion and joint problem solving. It was determined that the student lacked the coordination and strength to safely push the heavily loaded laundry carts and was unable to manipulate and load up to six bedsheets simultaneously into the large presser. Additionally, the student lost track of the number of towels he had folded and frequently overstocked the clean laundry carts, causing clean linens to fall on the floor. On the positive side, the student was skillful at folding towels and small linens, locating supplies, asking for help, and interacting with coworkers in a friendly way. During one consultation session, the occupational therapist and the team identified the need to revise the stu-

dent's job description to include more towel folding and linen cart stocking, which would replace pushing the large carts and pressing sheets. As this idea was being negotiated with the employer, the occupational therapist continued to seek ways to facilitate accurate counting of towels and other items that get stocked onto the clean linen carts. The therapist finally devised a jig that was built by the paraprofessional to eliminate the student's need for counting. The jig was a workstation adaptation resembling a box that was carefully constructed to hold exactly eight folded towels. When the jig was full, the student moved the stack of towels to the cart, making each stack on the cart exactly the right size. The next consultation session occurred at the job site between the occupational therapist, student, job coach, and employer. During this time, the jig was tested, modified, and determined to be effective. The jig idea was then extended to other items that go on the clean laundry carts. A final consultation session was held approximately 2 weeks after the student had begun using the jigs at work. The purpose of this session was to evaluate the student's progress on the job and the effectiveness of the recent job modifications. When it was determined that the student was performing well, the occupational therapy consultation ended.

Consultation with community agencies represents another type of consultation that can benefit transition-aged students with disabilities. Although similar to the consultation that occurs between the occupational therapist and other members of the student's core educational team, consultation with community agencies tends to be short-term and specific. Because a student's entitlement to public education services ends when he or she exits high school (typically between the ages of 18 and 21), it is important for members of the educational team to work with the community agencies and employers who are likely to become involved with the student after high school. For this reason, the occupational therapist may need to consult with prospective community employers, community job placement agencies, local residential service providers, and others to create and maintain opportunities for the student to participate in meaningful adult roles and activities after exiting the public school system.

An example of occupational therapist involvement with a community employer may illustrate the nature of consultation with community agencies.

Renee is a 19-year-old student who sustained a brain injury when she was a sophomore in high school. She is now working part-time at a local sporting goods store and hopes to continue working there after she completes high school. The employer has reported that Renee has difficulty following through with assigned tasks, though she seems to understand the task. The occupational therapist, who is familiar with the student and the job tasks, offers to consult with the employer. The purpose of the consultation is to identify strategies that will help Renee perform her job more effectively. The consulting occupational therapist visited the job site while Renee was working and spent time observing her job performance, characteristics of the job environment, and the student's interactions with her job coach and the employer. Based on these observations, the occupational therapist recommended the following:

1. The employer *shows* the student what to do rather than *telling* her what to do.
2. The student's job coach develops a small, inconspicuous notebook that lists routine job tasks and materials. The student is then asked to carry the notebook and use it as a guide when she is unsure about certain procedures.
3. The employer provides the student with daily, positive feedback in the quiet of the office at the end of each day.
4. The materials used on the job are modified to accommodate the student's need to use one hand for most tasks. This includes locating a wheeled cart that the student can use to transport cleaning supplies and merchandise for restocking more conveniently.

These recommendations were shared with Renee, her employer, and her job coach at an informal meeting at the job site. After some discussion, the recommendations were modified slightly and resources were identified to obtain and adapt a wheeled cart for Renee. The occupational therapist then followed up within a week to check on Renee's progress and the employer's satisfaction. A few additional adjustments were made to Renee's cart during this visit. To be certain that Renee was maintaining adequate job performance, the occupational therapist made a second follow-up visit 2 weeks later. When it was determined that Renee and her employer were both pleased, the consultation ended. The occupational therapist, however, made it clear that if new needs should arise, she would be available to re-enter the job site to help solve problems.

Monitoring of services that are designed by the occupational therapist but delivered primarily by other members of the team represents a fourth model for occupational therapy service provision. Monitoring requires the occupational therapist to be involved in assessing the student's performance and needs, intervening for a short period, and then turning over responsibility for ongoing intervention to other members of the team. When responsibility for actual service delivery is turned over to other team members, the occupational therapist begins a monitoring role. Although similar to consultation, monitoring differs in the sense that the occupational therapist continues to maintain primary responsibility for student outcomes and must continue regular contact (at least twice a month) with the student for the duration of the intervention (AOTA, 1987). The occupational therapist's responsibility continues, despite delegating the day-to-day implementation of the program to another person. This person may be a teacher, paraprofessional, or anyone who has regular, daily contact with the student.

Before monitoring is selected as the approach, it must be determined that the persons identified to implement the services are sufficiently skilled and available to carry out the program. The occupational therapist must provide training and supervision to ensure that the services being delivered are those that are needed (AOTA, 1994).

Monitoring can be an effective approach to service delivery for a student who is learning to use an adapted computer to communicate and complete school assignments. After a thorough assessment of the student's assistive technology needs and the acquisition of an adapted computer, the occupational therapist may design services to teach the student to become independent in the use of the computer. These services may involve the student's use of alternative computer access methods such as a head-mounted switch with specific software. The occupational therapist teaches the student, teacher, and paraprofessional how to set up and use the equipment. Once the teacher and paraprofessional demonstrate proficiency with the assistive technology, the occupational therapist then reduces involvement to occasional but regular visits to assess the student's progress and make adjustments when necessary. Should the student fail to make expected progress toward independent computer use, the occupational therapist would evaluate and redesign the intervention. The following case study provides an example of monitoring.

Amy was in the 8th grade, and she attended regular education classes with the support of special education and related services. Diagnosed with severe athetoid cerebral palsy, her motor skills were quite low, requiring that she use a powered wheelchair and a number of adaptive devices. At the age of 14, she continued to progress well in the regular curriculum. However, Amy's ability to write and manipulate materials was limited by ballistic arm movements and poor control of shoulder movements; however, she demonstrated some isolated control of finger movements once her arm was stabilized on a surface. She began using a virtual, on-screen keyboard at age 12, when she was in the 5th grade. The occupational therapist helped to set up a system for her at the time. The occupational therapist set up an arm board to stabilize her left arm and hand where her control was greatest. Then Amy was able to use a large track ball with the virtual keyboard. A row and column scanning system was used. Her word processing with the on-screen keyboard was slow but more accurate than it was with direct selection using the keyboard and the keyguard.

Amy made steady progress in speed and accuracy with the track ball and the on-screen keyboard, and the occupational therapist continued to monitor her progress. However, by the time Amy entered the 7th grade, the curriculum required extensive report writing and she was unable to maintain the pace of her classmates. Her progress was not satisfactory, although the number of written assignments was reduced.

At this time, the occupational therapist recommended that she use the software program, *Co-Writer*. This software helps to reduce keystrokes by predicting the intended word based on one or two initial letters. The therapist also wrote several "macros" to help reduce the number of keystrokes Amy had to make in written assignments. When these keyboarding aides appeared successful, the occupational therapist provided consultation to Amy's teacher regarding use of *Co-Writer* software and provided a written list of macros to assist Amy. The occupational therapist continued to monitor her progress that semester to help her become an accurate, efficient user of *Co-Writer*. Given Amy's overall academic progress, keyboard skills are likely to be important assets when future employment opportunities are considered.

Monitoring can be an effective way to deliver transition-related services. It requires an intensive, up-front investment of time followed by decreased involvement from the occupational therapist. When monitoring is effective, the people who work most frequently with the student acquire the skills needed to implement occupational therapy recommendations throughout the student's day. This infusion of occupational therapy into the student's overall education program can significantly increase the efficacy of occupational therapy (Giangreco, 1986).

Service coordination refers to the efforts of one member of a student's transition team to assist the student and his or her family with coordination and management of the many details associated with transition-related services.

As students approach the school-to-adult life transition they experience changes in their day-to-day activities and the accompanying support services and resources. Students who need ongoing, transition-related support beyond high school may need assistance with identifying the resources to assist with community employment, living, recreation, or post-secondary education. These supports and services do not come from the schools but rather from an array of adult and community service agencies. To assure the student's smooth transition from the familiar surroundings of the school to new and unfamiliar adult roles, service coordination may be essential if needed supports and services are to be in place *before* the student exits the public school system. Proactive coordination of transition-related services can prevent gaps in service and unnecessary "down-time" for the student.

The role of the transition service coordinator requires skill in working directly with the family and the student so that their choices and interests are reflected in all planning activities. The service coordinator also needs to know, understand, and communicate effectively with other team members including the student, teachers, related service personnel, and adult service agencies. Maintaining a broad view of the student's current performance and performance needs across all domains (domestic, school, vocational, community, and leisure) constitutes a third skill of a transition service coordinator.

The occupational therapist has an understanding of human performance needs in different environments as well as training and skill in communication, group dynamics, individualized assessment, and service delivery. The occupational therapist is, therefore, well suited to work as a transition service coordinator. This role requires keeping the interests, preferences, and abilities of the student foremost in mind while working with available resources to identify or create needed services. The service coordinator then facilitates the transition process by supporting (and gently prodding) other team members to complete their assessment or service responsibilities, managing a transition time line, linking resources and services, and most importantly, helping the student participate to the maximum extent in all decisions related to his or her transition services.

■ SUMMARY

What happens to people with disabilities after they complete 12 to 18 years of public education? This question has received a great deal of attention from legislators, researchers, teachers, and related service personnel (including occupational therapists) over the years. Public education is often viewed as an "investment" in the future of society and specifically in youth. As with all investments, there is a desire to obtain a positive and profitable return on the investment. The return on the education investment for children and youth with disabilities relates to their eventual and successful transition from school to a productive and meaningful adult life.

Responsibility for the delivery of transition services clearly rests with all members of the IEP team, including occupational therapy personnel (Brollier et. al., 1994; Dunn, 1991; Spencer & Sample, 1993). The ability of occupational therapists and certified occupational therapy assistants to focus on the needs of youth in the context of their approaching adult roles and performance environments adds strength to an educational team charged with designing and implementing transition services. Occupational therapy assessment and intervention related to a student's performance of school roles, activities of daily living, work, and recreation are consistent with the transition services mandated in federal law and are essential components of effective transition planning and service delivery. Occupational therapy personnel may assume roles in consulting, providing direct service, monitoring occupational therapy programs, or coordinating transition service. Each role requires an understanding of the overall public educational context, the transition processes for students with disabilities, and each student's unique abilities, interests, and needs.

STUDY QUESTIONS

1. Consider the school-to-adult life transition process for a student with significant disabilities. How would this be similar or different from your own transition from high school to new and different adult roles?

2. What does an occupational therapist bring to the transition process for students with disabilities? How would you describe the occupational therapist role to a high school teacher? A transition-aged student? A transition-aged student's parent?

3. Explain how the role of occupational therapy may be affected by the requirement to work within the framework of the general education curriculum.

4. What skills do you have that will help you work as a collaborative team member? What skills do you think you will need to develop?

5. What would an ecologic assessment have looked like for you during your initial transition from high school to the adult world?

References

American Occupational Therapy Association. (1987). *Guidelines for occupational therapy services in school systems.* Rockville, MD: American Occupational Therapy Association.

Blackorby, J., & Wagner, M. (1996). Longitudinal postschool outcomes of youth with disabilities: Findings from the national longitudinal transition study. *Exceptional Children, 62* (5), 399-413.

Brollier, C., Shepherd, J., & Markley, K. (1994). Transition from school to community living. *American Journal of Occupational Therapy, 48,* 346-353.

Brown, L., Branston-McLean, M.B., Baumgart, D., Vincent, L., Falvey, M., & Schroeder, J. (1979). Using the characteristics of current and future least restrictive environments in the development of curricular content for severely handicapped students. *American Association for Education of the Severe and Profound Handicapped Review, 4* (4), 407-424.

Dettmer, P.A., Dyck, N.J., & Thurston, L.P. (1996). *Consultation, collaboration, and teamwork for students with special needs.* Boston: Allyn and Bacon.

Dunn, W. (1988). Models of occupational therapy service provision in the school system. *The American Journal of Occupational Therapy, 42* (11), 718-722.

Dunn, W. (Ed.). (1991). *Pediatric occupational therapy: Facilitation of effective service provision.* Thorofare, NJ: Slack.

Dunn, W., Brown, C., & McGuigan, A. (1994). The ecology of human performance: A framework for considering the effect of context. *The American Journal of Occupational Therapy, 48* (7), 595-607.

Education of All Handicapped Children Act of 1995 (Public Law 94-142). 20 U.S.C., 1400, et seq.

Everson, J., & McNulty, K. (1992). Interagency teams: Building local transition programs through parental and professional partnerships. In F. Rusch, L. Destefano, J. Chadsey-Rusch, L.A. Phelps, & E. Szymanski (Eds.), *Transition from school to adult life: Models, linkages, and policy* (pp. 342-351). Pacific Grove, CA: Brooks/Cole.

Giangreco, M. (1986). Effects of integrated therapy: A pilot study. *Journal of the Association for Persons with Severe Handicaps, 11* (3), 205-208.

Giangreco, M. (1996). *Vermont interdependent services team approach: A guide to coordinating educational support services (VISTA)*. Baltimore: Brookes.

Giangreco, M.F., Cloninger, C.J., & Iverson, V.S. (1998). *Choosing outcomes and accommodations for children: A guide to educational planning for students with disabilities* (2nd Ed.). Baltimore: Brookes.

Halloran, W. (1992). *Transition services requirement: Issues, implications, challenge.* Washington, D.C: United States Department of Education.

Hanft, B.E., & Place, P.A. (1996). *The consulting therapist.* San Antonio: Therapy Skill Builders.

Hasazi, S., Hock, M., & Cravedi-Cheng, L. (1992). Vermont's post-school indicators: Using satisfaction and post-school outcome data for program improvement. In F. Rusch, L. Destefano, J. Chadsey-Rusch, L.A. Phelps, & E. Szymanski (Eds.), *Transition from school to adult life: Models, linkages, and policy* (pp. 485-506). Pacific Grove, CA: Brooks/Cole.

Individuals with Disabilities Education Act Amendments of 1990 (Public Law 101-476). 20 U.S.C., 1400 et seq.

Individuals with Disabilities Education Act Amendments of 1997 (Public Law 105-517). 20 U.S.C., 1400 et seq.

Lyon, S., & Lyon, G. (1980). Team functioning and staff development: A role release approach to providing integrated educational services for severely handicapped students. *Journal of The Association for the Severely Handicapped, 5* (3), 250-263.

Mount, B. (1987). *Personal futures planning: Finding directions for change. Unpublished doctoral dissertation.* Athens, GA: University of Georgia.

Mount, B., & Zwernik, K. (1988). *It's never too early, it's never too late: A booklet about personal futures planning.* St. Paul, MN: Metropolitan Council.

The National School-to-Work Learning and Information Center. (1996). *School-to-Work.* Washington D.C: The National School-to-Work Learning and Information Center, 400 Virginia Ave, Room 150. Available: www.stw.ed.gov/general/whatis.htm

NICHCY: National Information Center for Children and Youth with Disabilities. (1993). Transition summary. *NICHCY, 3* (1), 1-19.

Pugach, M.C., & Johnson, L.J. (1995). *Collaborative practitioners collaborative schools.* Denver: Love Publishing.

Rainforth, B., & York- Barr, J. (1997). *Collaborative teams for students with severe disabilities: Integrating therapy with educational services* (2nd ed.). Baltimore: Brookes.

Reauthorization of the Individuals with Disabilities Education Act of 1990. (1997). (Public Law 105-17). Proposed regulations for assistance to states for education of children with disabilities, 62 Fed. Reg. 55068.

Sample, P., Spencer, K., & Bean, G. (1990). *Transition planning: Creating a positive future for students with disabilities.* Fort Collins, CO: Office of Transition Services, Department of Occupational Therapy, Colorado State University.

Sands, D.J., & Wehmeyer, M.L. (1996). *Self-determination across the life span.* Baltimore: Brookes.

School-to-Work Opportunities Act of 1994 (Public Law 103-239). 108 Stat 568.

Spencer, K., Murphy, M., Bean, G., & Schelly, C. (1991). Vocational needs assessment: A functional, community-referenced approach. In K. Spencer (Ed.), *From school to adult life: The role of occupational therapy in the transition process* (pp. 185-213). Fort Collins, CO: Office of Transition Services Department of Occupational Therapy, Colorado State University.

Spencer, K., & Sample, P. (1993). Transition planning and services. In C. Royeen (Ed.), *Classroom applications for school-based practice* (pp. 6-48). Rockville, MD: American Occupational Therapy Association.

Udvari-Solner, A., Jorgenson, J., & Courchane, G. (1992). Longitudinal vocational curriculum: The foundation for effective transition. In F. Rusch, L. Destefano, J. Chadsey-Rusch, L.A. Phelps, & E. Szymanski (Eds.), *Transition from school to adult life: Models, linkages, and policy* (pp 285-320). Pacific Grove, CA: Brooks/Cole.

Wagner, M. (1989). *The transition experiences of youth with disabilities: A report from the national longitudinal transition study.* Menlo Park, CA: SRI International.

Wagner, M. (1995). Outcomes for youths with serious emotional disturbance in secondary school and early adulthood. *Future of Children, 5* (2), 90-112.

Ward, M. (1992). Introduction to secondary special education and transition issues. In F. Rusch, L. Destefano, J. Chadsey-Rusch, L.A. Phelps, & E. Szymanski (Eds.), *Transition from school to adult life: Models, linkages, and policy* (pp. 387-389). Pacific Grove, CA: Brooks/Cole.

Wehman, P. (1992). *Life beyond the classroom: Transition strategies for young people with disabilities.* Baltimore: Brookes.

Wehmeyer, M.L., & Sands, D.J. (1998). *Making it happen: Student involvement in education planning, decision making, and instruction.* Baltimore: Brookes.

Williams, W., Fox, T.J., Thousand, J., & Fox, W. (1990). Level of acceptance and implementation of best practices in the education of students with severe handicaps in Vermont. *Education and Training in Mental Retardation, 25* (2), 120-131.

Woolcock, W., Stodden, R., & Bisconer, S. (1992). Process- and outcome-focused decision making. In F. Rusch, L. Destefano, J. Chadsey-Rusch, L.A. Phelps, & E. Szymanski (Eds.), *Transition from school to adult life: Models, linkages, and policy* (pp. 219-244). Pacific Grove, CA: Brooks/Cole.

York, J., & Vandercook, T. (1991). Designing an integrated education for learners with severe disabilities through the IEP process. *Teaching Exceptional Children, 23* (2), 22-28.